HEALTH PROMOTION
Throughout the Lifespan

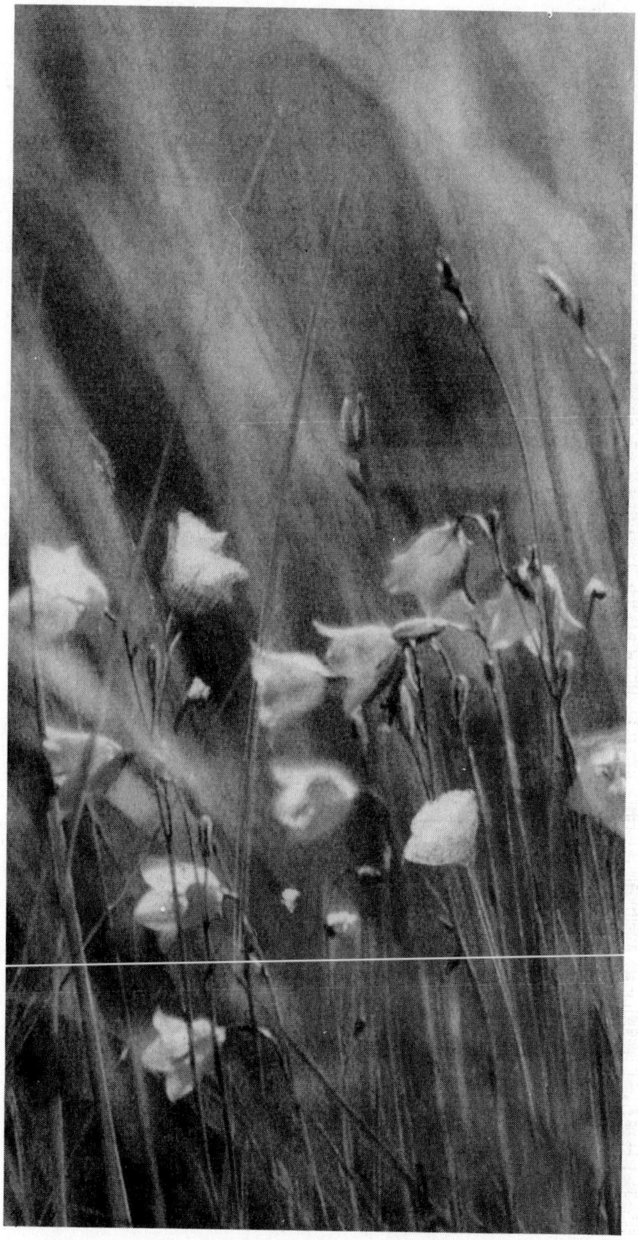

THIRD EDITION

HEALTH PROMOTION
Throughout the Lifespan

CAROLE LIUM EDELMAN, RN, MS, CS
Director of Nursing
The Osborn Retirement Community
Rye, New York;
Associate Faculty Member
Columbia University
School of Nursing
New York, New York;
Fellow
Brookdale Center on Aging
Hunter College
New York, New York

CAROL LYNN MANDLE, PhD, RN
Associate Professor
Boston College
Graduate School of Nursing
Chestnut Hill, Massachusetts;
Associate for Research
and Consultation
Beth Israel Hospital
Boston, Massachusetts;
Clinical Nurse Specialist
and Scientist
Mind-Body Medical Institute
and New England Deaconess Hospital
Boston, Massachusetts

illustrated

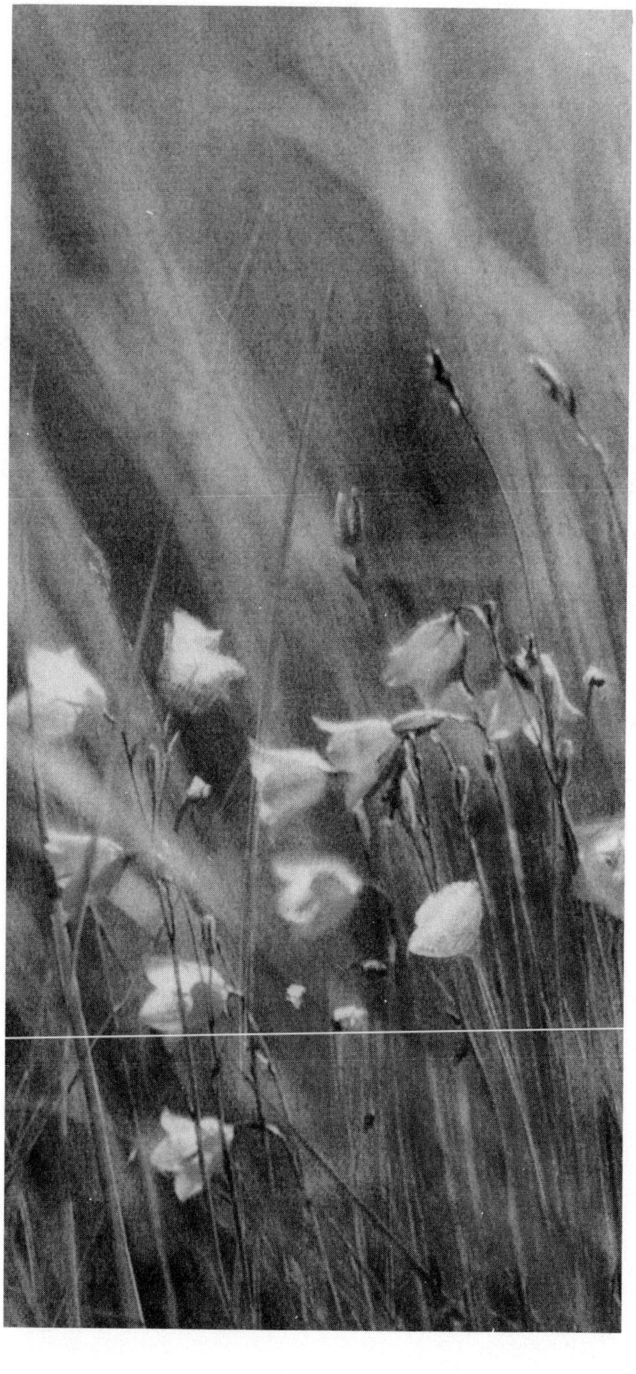

Mosby
St. Louis Baltimore Boston Chicago London Madrid
Philadelphia Sydney Toronto

Mosby
Dedicated to Publishing Excellence

Executive Editor: N. Darlene Como
Senior Developmental Editor: Laurie Sparks
Project Manager: Barbara Bowes Merritt
Editing and Production: The Bookmakers, Incorporated
Designer: John Beck
Manufacturing Supervisor: Kathy Grone
Cover Art: The Bookmakers, Incorporated

THIRD EDITION

Printed in the United States of America

Mosby-Year Book, Inc.
11830 Westline Industrial Drive
St. Louis, Missouri 63146

Library of Congress Cataloging in Publication Data

Health promotion throughout the lifespan / [edited by] Carole Lium Edelman, Carol Lynn Mandle. – 3rd ed.
p. cm.
Includes bibliographical references and index.
ISBN 0-8016-7786-6
1. Health promotion. 2. Nursing. 3. Medicine, Preventive.
I. Edelman, Carole. II. Mandle, Carol Lynn.
[DNLM: 1. Nursing. 2. Health Promotion. WY 100 H4343 1994]
RT90.3.H435 1994
613 – dc20
DNLM/DLC
for Library of Congress

94-1467
CIP

95 96 97 / 9 8 7 6 5 4 3 2

Contributors

Mary E. Abrums, RN, MN
Doctoral Student, Anthropology
University of Washington
Seattle, Washington

Donna Behler, MSN
Clinical Specialist
King Faisal Hospital
Saudi Arabia

Barbara Woods Bodnar, RN, MS
Medical Surgical Clinical Specialist
Westchester County Medical Center
Valhalla, New York

Philip Boyle, PhD
Associate for Medical Ethics
The Hastings Center
Briarcliff Manor, New York

Joni Cohen, RN, MN
Mental Health Therapist
Los Angeles, California

Rebecca Cohen, RN, EdD
Northern Illinois University
School of Nursing
DeKalb, Illinois

Katherine Smith Detherage, PhD, RN, CNAA
Chief of Nursing
Anthony L. Jordon Health Center
Rochester, New York

Carole Lium Edelman, RN, MS, CS
Director of Nursing
The Osborn Retirement Community
Rye, New York
Associate Faculty Member
Columbia University
School of Nursing
New York, New York
Fellow
Brookdale Center on Aging
Hunter College
New York, New York

Lea Edwards, BSN, MEd
Lea Edwards Associates
Management Consultant
Fairfax, Virginia

James A. Fain, RN, PhD
Associate Dean/Associate Professor
School of Nursing
Yale University
New Haven, Connecticut

Gail Park Fast, MN
Coordinator, Childbirth Education Program
Yakima Valley Memorial Hospital
Yakima, Washington

Ellen Flaherty, RN, MS, GNP
Gerontological Nurse Practitioner
The Osborn Retirement Community
Rye, New York

Marilyn Frank-Stromborg, EdD, NP
Professor, School of Nursing
Northern Illinois University
DeKalb, Illinois

Terry T. Fulmer, PhD, RNC, FAAN
Anna C. Maxwell Chair of Nursing Research
Professor
Columbia University School of Nursing
New York, New York

Carol Scheel Gavan, MS
Assistant Professor
State University of New York
Health Science Center
Division of Nursing
Syracuse, New York
Doctoral Candidate
Columbia University

Geraldine V. Go, PhD, RN, CS
Professor
College of New Rochelle
New Rochelle, New York

Rosemary Gruber-Wood, MS
Staff Educator
New England Medical Center
Boston, Massachusetts

Krishan Gupta, MD
Associate Professor of Medicine
New York Medical College
Hawthorne, New York

Lois A. Hancock, MSN, ARNP
Lecturer
University of Washington
School of Nursing
Seattle, Washington

June Andrews Horowitz, PhD, RN, CS
Associate Professor and Chairperson
Psychiatric-Mental Health Nursing Department
Boston College
School of Nursing
Chestnut Hill, Massachusetts

Dennis T. Jaffe, PhD
Professor
Department of Psychology
Saybrook Institute
San Francisco, California

Sally Stark Johnson, RN, MSN
Lecturer
Boston College
School of Nursing
Chestnut Hill, Massachusetts

Nancy T. Koge, RN, MS
Associate Director of Nursing
The Ruth Taylor Geriatric and Rehabilitative Institute
Westchester County Medical Center
Hawthorne, New York

Elizabeth C. Kudzma, DNSc, MPH
Chairperson and Professor
Curry College
Division of Nursing Studies
Milton, Massachusetts

Jeanette Lancaster, RN, PhD, FAAN
Dean, University of Virginia
School of Nursing
Charlottesville, Virginia

Carol Lynn Mandle, PhD, RN
Associate Professor
Boston College
Graduate School of Nursing
Chestnut Hill, Massachusetts
Associate for Research and Consultation
Beth Israel Hospital
Boston, Massachusetts
Clinical Nurse Specialist and Scientist
Mind-Body Medical Institute and New England Deaconess Hospital
Boston, Massachusetts

William Martimucci, MD
Medical Director
The Osborn Retirement Community
Rye, New York

Ann Marie McCarthy, RN, PNP, PhD
Post-Doctoral Fellow
College of Education
University of Iowa
Iowa City, Iowa

Nancy Curro McCarthy, RN, EdD
Associate Dean of Graduate Programs
Boston College
Graduate School of Nursing
Chestnut Hill, Massachusetts

Nancy Milio, PhD
Professor of Nursing and Health Administration
School of Nursing
School of Public Health
University of North Carolina
Chapel Hill, North Carolina

Katherine E. Murphy, MN, FNP
Family Nurse Practitioner
Teen Health Center
Seattle King County Health Department
Seattle, Washington

James A. O'Donohoe, JCD
Associate Professor of Theological Ethics
Boston College
Chestnut Hill, Massachusetts

Ellen F. Olshansky, DNSc, RN, C
Associate Professor
Department of Parent and Child Nursing
University of Washington
Seattle, Washington

Sharon L. Pederson, MS
Clinical Specialist
Westchester County Medical Center
Valhalla, New York

Anne Griswold Peirce
Assistant Professor
Director of Doctoral Studies
Columbia University
New York, New York

Susan Pennacchia, RN, MSN
Nursing Program Director
Lake Sumter Community College
Leesburg, Florida

Johanne Quinn, PhD, RN
Education Consultant
North Carolina Board of Nursing
Raleigh, North Carolina

Jan Schurman, MN, FNP
School Nurse Practitioner
Seattle Public Schools
Seattle, Washington

Susan Simmons, PhD
Senior Policy Analyst
Office on Women's Health
Office of the Assistant Secretary for Health
Department of Health and Human Services
Washington, D.C.

Arlene Spark, RD, FACN
Assistant Professor of Nutrition
Graduate School of Health Sciences
Department of Medicine
Department of Pediatrics
New York Medical College
Valhalla, New York

Terry Tippet, RNC, MSN
Vanderbilt University
School of Nursing
Nashville, Tennessee

Carol L. Wells-Federman
Clinical Nurse Specialist
Division of Behavioral Medicine
New England Deaconess Hospital
Boston, Massachusetts

**To our wonderful families, friends, students, and colleagues –
that they promote health in themselves and others.**

Preface

The case for promoting and protecting health and preventing disease and injury has been established by many accomplishments. Americans are taking better care of themselves now. Public concern about physical fitness, good nutrition, and avoidance of health hazards such as smoking has gone beyond a fad and has become ingrained in the American lifestyle.

Encouraging positive health changes has been a major effort of individuals, the government, health professionals, and society in general. In the United States, public and private attempts to improve the health status of individuals and groups traditionally have focused on reducing communicable diseases and health hazards. Now a growing concern exists to reduce costs of health services, increase life expectancy, and improve the overall quality of life.

Personal lifestyles are known to influence health status, and nurses can use specific strategies to help their clients maintain and adopt positive lifestyle behaviors. Indirect health information and informed decision or direct health education and resulting health promotion, health protection, and disease and injury prevention practices all can lead to the adoption of healthy lifestyles.

Health promotion advances require a better understanding of risk and behavior, as well as intervention measures. Ten categories may be identified as important determinants of health status:

1. Smoking
2. Nutrition
3. Alcohol use
4. Habituating drug use
5. Driving
6. Exercise
7. Sexuality and contraceptive use
8. Family relationships
9. Risk management
10. Coping and adaptation

Nursing measures designed to assist individual efforts to change and improve behavior in these areas can lead to a decrease in morbidity and mortality.

Nurses who undertake health promotion strategies also need to understand the basics of health protection and disease and injury prevention. Health *protection* is directed at population groups of all ages and involves adherence to standards, infectious disease control, and governmental regulation and enforcement. The focus of these activities is reducing exposure to various sources of hazards, including those related to air, water, foods, drugs, motor vehicles, and other physical agents.

Disease and injury *prevention* services are provided to the individual by health care providers and include immunizations and screenings, as well as health education and counseling. To implement prevention strategies effectively, it is essential to develop cross-cutting activities targeted to and tailored for all age groups in various settings, including schools, industries, the home, the health care delivery system, and the community.

Throughout the history of the United States, the public health community has assessed the health of Americans. In 1789 the Reverend Edward Wigglesworth developed the first American mortality tables through his study in New England. "The Report of a General Plan for the Promotion of Public and Personal Health" was completed by Dr. Lemuel Shattuck in 1880. *Healthy People,* the Surgeon General's report on health promotion and disease prevention, was first published in 1979. These databases have provided an assessment of health status and risk for evaluation and future planning not only to health policy makers and care providers but to individuals, families, and communities as well.

The current U.S. government report, *Healthy People 2000: National Health Promotion and Disease Prevention Objectives,* lists three goals to be achieved by the year 2000:

1. Increase the span of healthy life for Americans.
2. Reduce health disparities among Americans.
3. Achieve access to preventive services for all Americans.

This report presents many opportunities in the form of measurable targets, or objectives, which are organized into 22 priority areas within four broad categories: health promotion, health protection, preventive services, and surveillance and data systems.

The information in this book is based on these goals and the possibility of their achievement. Specific objectives relevant to the content of each chapter are included in boxes and are linked to common health problems and appropriate nursing interventions and outcomes. Our intent is to develop and present the related theory and skills that the nurse must understand and practice when providing care.

The focus of the book is on *primary prevention inter-*

vention, based on the Leavell and Clark model; its three main components are health promotion, specific health protection, and prevention of specific diseases. Health promotion is the intervention designed to improve health, such as providing adequate nutrition, a healthy environment, and ongoing health education. Specific protection and prevention are the interventions used to protect against illness, such as massive immunizations, periodic examinations, and safety features in the workplace.

In addition to primary prevention, this book discusses *secondary prevention intervention,* focusing specifically on screening. Such programs include blood pressure, glaucoma, and diabetes screening and referral. We address only this aspect of secondary prevention, not the acute component.

This text is presented in five parts, each forming the basis for the next: Foundations for Health Promotion, Assessment for Health Promotion, Interventions for Health Promotion, Application of Health Promotion, and Trends.

Unit One describes the foundational concepts of promoting and protecting health and preventing diseases and injuries, including diagnostic, therapeutic, and ethical decision making. Unit Two focuses on individuals, families, and communities as clients and the factors affecting their health. The functional health pattern assessments developed by Dr. Marjory Gordon serve as the organizing framework for assessing the health of individuals, families, and communities. Unit Three discusses theories, methodologies, and case studies of nursing interventions, including screening, health education counseling, stress management, and crisis intervention. Unit Four also uses Dr. Gordon's functional health patterns, emphasizing developmental, cultural, ethnic, and environmental variables in assessing the developing person through the eight developmental phases of the lifespan. The final chapter, in Unit Five, discusses changing population groups and their health needs and related implications for research and practice in the next century. Throughout the text, research abstracts have been added to highlight state-of-the-art and the science of nursing practice and to demonstrate to the reader the relationship between research, practice, and outcomes.

Throughout these units, the evolving profession of nursing and the changing health care systems, including future challenges and initiatives for health promotion, are described. Emphasis is placed upon the current concerns of reducing health care costs while increasing life expectancy and improving the quality of life for all Americans.

The current trend to emphasize the developing health of people mandates that the nurse understand the many issues that surround individuals in social, work, and family settings, including the biologic, inherited, cognitive, psychologic, environmental, and sociocultural factors that can put their health at risk. Most important, nurses can intervene to promote health by understanding the diverse roles these factors play in the person's beliefs and health practices, particularly in the areas of disease and injury prevention and protection and of health promotion. Achieving such effectiveness requires nurses to collaborate with other health care providers and integrate practice and policy while developing interventions, considering the ethical issues within individual, family, and community responsibilities for health.

Acknowledgments

We had the good fortune of receiving much assistance and support from many friends, relatives, and associates. Our colleagues read chapters, gave valuable advice and criticism, helped to clarify concepts, and provided case examples.

We also acknowledge the contributions of all the authors. In developing this text, they gave the project their total commitment and support. Their professional competence aided greatly in the development of the final draft of the manuscript. We acknowledge the contributions of Jeanette Lancaster, Marilyn Frank-Stromborg, Rebecca Cohen, and Jim Fain, whose material on mental health, cancer, and research has been integrated throughout the unit on application of health promotion. Special mention must be given to the secretarial and administrative contributions of Megan O'Brien. Her consistent consideration for deadlines, assistance in drawing, and meticulous work kept order when time was of the essence.

The editors worked and learned from each other during the planning and development of this book; throughout the entire process close contact prevailed. They seemed to become the book, and in turn the book now reflects them.

Both family and friends helped in the work and tolerated the many demands placed on them.

Fredric Edelman gave immeasurable strength, joy, and happiness during the second and third editions. Lenora Pennacchia provided much encouragement and support throughout. My children, Megan, Heather, and Deirdre, brought joy to me as a weary author and editor. Their patience was persistent and truly appreciated. (C.E.)

In the continued development of health, I acknowledge the dimensions of the faith in God and strength of my mother, sister, and aunt; the love of marriage and family with Robert, Jonathan, David, and Elizabeth; the commitments of nurses to social justice in the care of all people; and the knowledge we are just beginning. (C.L.M.)

Contents

HEALTH PROMOTION
Throughout the Lifespan

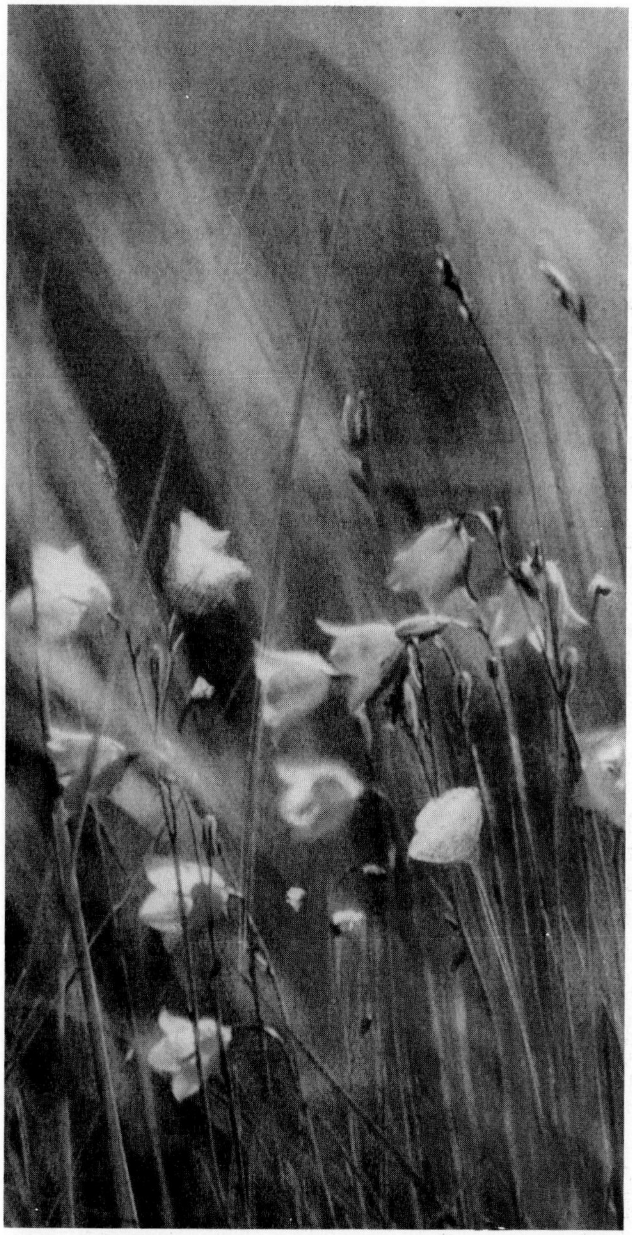

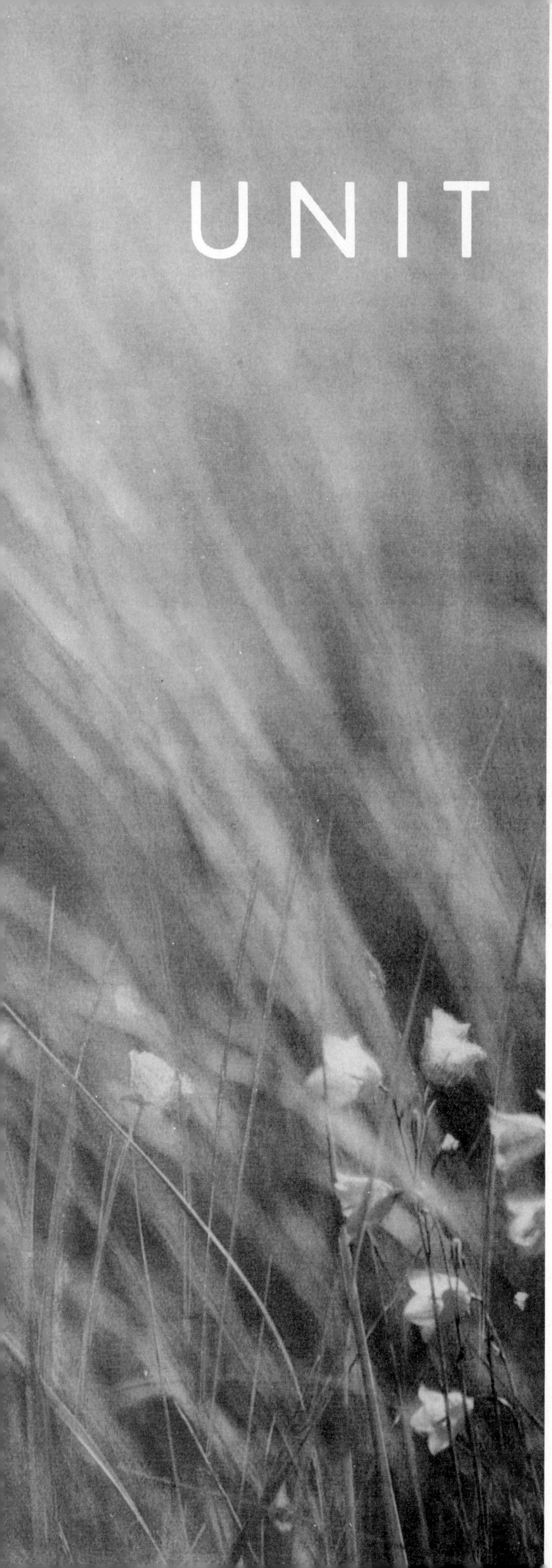

UNIT ONE

Foundations for Health Promotion

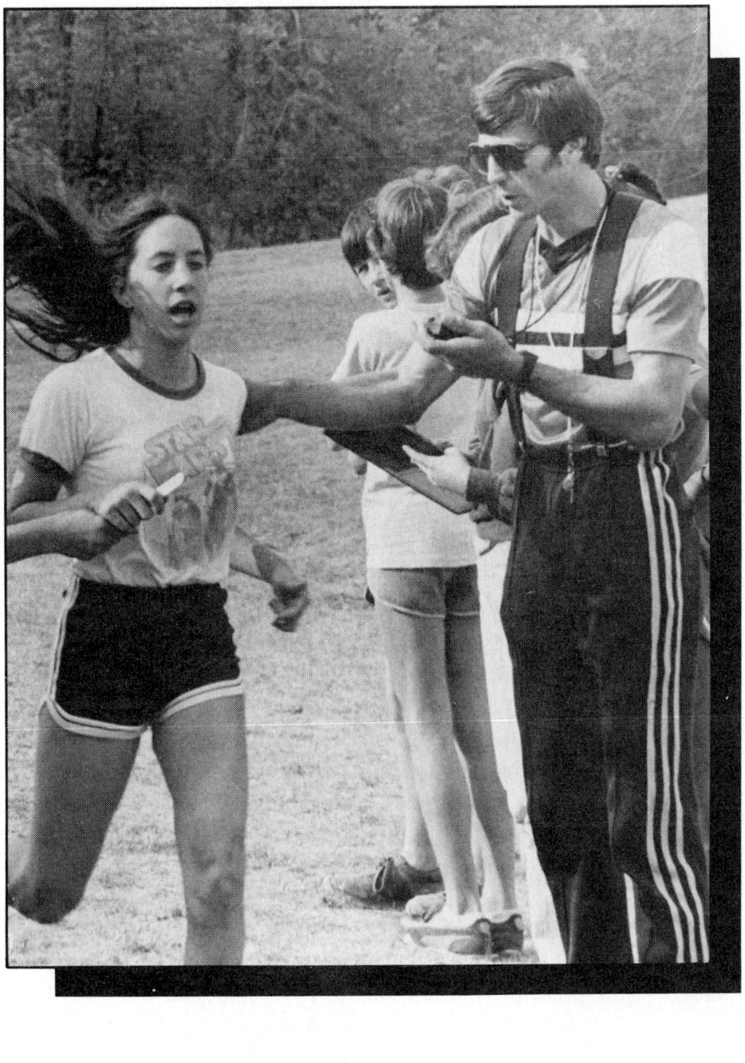

CHAPTER 1

Health Defined: Objectives for Promotion and Prevention

Carole Lium Edelman

Nancy Milio

Objectives

After completing this chapter, the nurse will be able to

- *List four of the U.S. Surgeon General's goals for health for the year 2000.*
- *Define the term* health *as used in this textbook.*
- *Examine the historical evolution of health.*
- *Analyze a typical case history (Frank Thompson).*
- *Discuss three views of Frank Thompson's health problem.*
- *Differentiate between health promotion and specific protection.*
- *Explain the three levels of prevention: primary, secondary, and tertiary.*
- *Discuss nursing activities in primary prevention and intervention.*
- *Describe the role of the nurse in health promotion and protection.*

In 1979, health agencies became aware of and began using the published report, *Healthy People: The Surgeon General's Report on Health Promotion and Disease Prevention*. This report presented to the American people some formidable challenges. Among these challenges were the prevention and reduction of major illnesses such as heart disease, cancer, and stroke.[39]

Though many of the 1979 Healthy People Objectives were achieved, many were not; yet the coordination among health professionals was considered so positive, the focused effort nationally toward better health so valuable, and the commitment so impressive that objectives were developed for the year 2000. It was not until the issuance of *Healthy People 2000* that a subtle, but compeling, shift was noted in the primary emphasis upon health promotion and individual responsibility.[32] Health was considered to be a positive concept, and individuals were viewed as able to influence their own health and the health of the nation. Although the 1990 report used the same triad of strategies for health as the 1979 report, the order in which these tactics were pursued changed. The emphasis was on health promotion first then health protection, and finally preventive services (see Table 1-1).

Healthy People 2000 is a broad-based initiative led by the U.S. Public Health Service (PHS) to improve the health of all Americans through an emphasis on prevention, not just the treatment, of health problems over the next decade. The Year 2000 National Health Objectives begin with three broad goals (see box on p. 5). National health objectives to reduce preventable death, disease, and disability form the cornerstone of this effort. Released at a conference in Washington, D.C., on September 6-7, 1990, the National Health Promotion and Disease Prevention Objectives set out a prevention agenda for the 1990s with quantifiable targets for improving health status, reducing risk factors for disease and disability, and improving services. Priorities are grouped in Table 1-1 in three major categories: health promotion, health protection,

Table 1-1. Priority groups of *Healthy People 2000*

Health promotion	Health protection	Preventive services
Physical activity and fitness	Unintentional injury	Maternal and infant health
Nutrition	Occupational safety and health	Heart disease and stroke
Tobacco	Environmental health	Cancer
Alcohol and other drugs	Food and drug safety	Other chronic conditions
Family planning	Oral health	HIV infection
Mental health		Sexually transmitted diseases
Violent behavior		Immunization and infectious disease
Educational and community-based programs		Clinical preventive services

Adapted from American Hospital Association Fact Sheet: *Healthy people 2000*, Chicago, 1990, The Association.

❑ ❑ NATION'S YEAR 2000 GOALS

1. *Increase the span of healthy life for Americans.* Data indicate that Americans had a life expectancy of 73.7 years in 1980 (it was actually 75 in 1987). However, on average, only 62 of those years were spent in a healthy state; 11.7 years included dysfunctions such as acute and chronic illnesses, impairments, and handicaps. One goal of the Year 2000 National Health Objectives is to decrease the number of dysfunctional years.
2. *Reduce health disparities among Americans.* Even as average life expectancy lifespan for African Americans has actually declined since 1986. The average life expectancy for Whites in 1988 was 75.6. For Blacks it was 69.4. Furthermore, Whites experience fewer years of dysfunction than do Blacks or American Indians, although more years of dysfunction than experienced by Hispanics. One goal of the Year 2000 National Health Objectives is to reduce this disparity.
3. *Achieve access to preventive health services for all Americans.* One of the reasons for the disparity between ethnicity and life expectancy is the inequitable use of preventive health services. For example, whereas 79% of white pregnant women received first-trimester prenatal care, only 61% of black pregnant women did. The result is that the infant mortality rate for black infants is 17.9 deaths per 1000 live births, but the rate for Whites is only 8.6. Another result of the inequitable use of preventive health services can be found in the death rate statistics for people age 74 and younger. In 1987, the death rate for Whites was 367 per 100,000 population, whereas for Blacks it was 628 per 100,000 population. One goal of the Year 2000 National Health Objectives is to assure access to preventive services for all Americans so as to improve health and ensure years of healthy life.[33]

and preventive services. In addition, the specific health problems of different age groups and income groups are highlighted (see box on p. 6) for *Healthy People 2000* priorities. Throughout this text, the *Healthy People 2000* objectives will be discussed. Each of the chapters relates the specific content of the chapter to this national health-promotion framework.

MEANING OF HEALTH

The meaning of health is viewed in many contexts: historic and cultural, social and personal, scientific and philosophic. These meanings, sometimes contradictory and often overlapping, will always exist in the varied contexts of human experience. Health relates to all aspects of our lives: from physical well-being to our social interactions, our mental and emotional capacities, and even our spiritual lives. Defining our state of health at any one time involves assessing the very complex interaction of all these facets of our health, as well as ordering them in terms of their value to us. It is meaningless, then, if not outright impossible, to assess someone else's health without involving that person in the assessment.[14] It is important, however, for health professionals, policymakers, and the public to share a common understanding of health so they can work together to find more effective ways to promote health.

In exploring the various meanings of health in this chapter, we first outline the hypothetical life of a man we call "Frank Thompson" to present some of the major related factors that promote and damage health in many persons. We then continue with the views of health to help the nurse focus on the definition of health used in this text as well as see its historic evolution. Next, we briefly consider the three levels of prevention for effective health promotion and specific protection, examining the nurse's role in these areas, as applied to Frank Thompson's health history.

HEALTHY PEOPLE 2000 PRIORITIES

HEALTH PROMOTION

Physical activity and fitness
Nutrition
Tobacco
Alcohol and other drugs
Family planning
Mental health and mental disorders
Violent and abusive behavior
Educational and community-based programs

HEALTH PROTECTION

Unintentional injuries
Occupational safety and health
Environmental health
Food and drug safety
Oral health

PREVENTIVE SERVICES

Maternal and infant health
Heart disease and stroke
Cancer
Diabetes and chronic disabling conditions
HIV infection
Sexually transmitted diseases
Immunization and infectious diseases
Clinical preventive services

SURVEILLANCE AND DATA SYSTEMS

AGE-RELATED

Children
Adolescents and young adults
Adults
Older Adults

From *Healthy people 2000: national health promotion and disease prevention objectives*, Washington, DC, 1990, Superintendent of Documents, US Government Printing Office.

FRANK THOMPSON: BACKGROUND OF THE MAN

Frank Thompson's large brick home sits off a sparsely traveled country road. Not many yards away stands the uninhabited shack of hand-hewn slabs of timber where Frank was born during World War II.

Frank grew up knowing the odds he faced as a poor tenant farmer. He helped his father Ben with their small tobacco and corn crops, neither of them aware of the hazardous chemicals in the pesticides they used to raise sallable crops – chemicals that would later affect Ben's life. As his father often reminded him, Frank had to do better than others in school so that he would not be doomed to the tenant farmer's life. Frank's school attendance was erratic, however, interrupted by the frequent demand of tending field crops. Thin and often tired, he had recurrent streptococcal infections. The school nurse helped the Thompsons get the necessary medication for Frank's initial infection, but they were never able to afford the penicillin needed for preventing recurrent ones.

Intent on helping at home and building something better for his future and inspired by the early work of Martin Luther King, Jr., Frank managed to more than make up for his lost time at school. He not only passed college entrance examinations but was awarded one of the new equal opportunity grants, which offered a choice of attending any of the Ivy League schools in the Northeast. Instead, he chose a prestigious southern university and eventually earned a master of business administration (MBA) degree. He married Sada, his long-time girlfriend, and the two planned their future.

Armed with his new MBA and a good job in a large local sales firm, Frank built their new house. He was determined to rise in the company, which he did. First as a salesperson and then as division head, he traveled to regional meetings, sometimes accompanied by Sada and their three children. Frank's dream was to share the pleasures of his success with his family. He wanted to use part of his earnings to help his brothers and sisters with their college educations.

The new way of life meant, of course, little time for relaxation and frequent attendance at business luncheons and career-promoting social occasions. He kept late hours and long weekends. Good food, drinks, and cigarettes helped him relax before and after important business and social encounters; these softened the edges of hard bargaining and were symbols of status as well.

Not surprisingly, Frank was gaining weight. He had long had a persistent cough, probably a result of his smoking habit, developed during the early years of his career. Frank's physician, whom Frank visited regularly at the corporation's health maintenance organization (HMO), said Frank's blood pressure and serum lipids were both higher than normal and that he now had chronic bronchitis. The physician urged Frank to do what Frank as a well-read man knew: cut down on smoking, drinking, and eating saturated fats and calories; get more exercise;

and above all, relax. The nurse tried to help him set up a plan to follow this advice. Frank had no time for exercise. Rather than relax, Frank had to try harder, but he also had to appear relaxed, a characteristic deemed essential for a prospective vice president. To meet these goals, he tended to drink and smoke more. Then Sada pointed out that his chance for promotion might actually improve if he lost some weight. He registered for a physical fitness program designed for executives, one he could attend on Sunday mornings and before work on weekdays. At his first workout, the classic sharp pain gripped his chest, and Frank had a massive heart attack.

Weeks later, Frank was convalescing at home after being well cared for at the university's renowned coronary care facilities. Most of the services were covered by his medical insurance plan. The company's disability pension protected 80% of his earnings; in this he was more fortunate than most employed people, who get only about half that amount.

Frank's dreams of promotion were shattered, however; at best he could go to the office only two or three times a week for many months to deal with routine matters. He would do no traveling, business-related or otherwise, for a long time.

The Problem

What was Frank Thompson's problem? The answer depends on whom you ask; each point of view focuses on different aspects of Frank's life. His physician would say that Frank had a coronary heart disease with an acute myocardial infarction, hypertension, hyperlipidemia, chronic bronchitis, and obesity. His nurse might add that he overate, overdrank, smoked, was too sedentary, and lived a stress-provoking life. Frank's employer saw a man too disabled to take on new responsibilities and perhaps unable to continue doing his previous work. To Frank's children the problem meant he could no longer take them on jaunts or play with them as he had. His wife Sada knew their plans for educating their children might suffer and that Frank and she could never move into a new dream house. The office personnel managing Frank's health insurance and pension programs would say that he had an expensive disease, and the state health planner would point out that Frank's problem was one more of a growing number of disabling illnesses resulting from preventable causes.

To Frank the health problem meant fear of dying, pain, and dependence and frustration – he might never be able to realize his dreams for himself and his family. Although potentially in his prime, Frank suddenly saw himself as far older than his years, both in body and in social achievement. He believed he had met his limits, since he would never again have the freedom to choose his future.

The Cause

The cause of Frank's health problem again depends on who defines the problem, as well as the purpose and time perspective used in defining the cause.

Frank's physician and nurse, to save his life and prevent complications, focus on his immediate situation and its most apparent cause, a myocardial infarction resulting from coronary atherosclerosis and repaired with the tools of coronary intensive care. Earlier they had taken a broader time perspective when they advised Frank to cut down on smoking, which was contributing to both his bronchitis and hypertension, and to change his high-saturated-fat diet and sedentary habits, which contributed to his weight problem and aggravated his high blood pressure. Their purpose was to prevent these conditions leading to what the statistical risks predicted: coronary heart disease and heart attack.

Frank's employer, also taking a narrow time perspective, saw the cause of the problem as heart disease. The company, however, was interested in the immediate cause, not to determine treatment but to foresee the consequences for Frank's job.

Frank and his family used a broader perspective than the medical personnel or the corporation. They knew that to achieve the family's economic and educational goals and still spend time together, they could not have lived much differently than they had. As is true of Americans, they had been willing to live with Frank's job pressures and lifestyle. The family members were aware of their impoverished roots and had no wish to go back. Frank's friends took an even broader view of the problem's cause, seeing the family's past rural-poor economic status as inevitably resulting in illness and other disadvantages, such as the pressures of having to strive harder.

Health planners used the longest time frame and broadest perspective in viewing Frank as illustrative of a pattern of preventable disabling illness that stifles persons in their prime. The planners looked to public and private community patterns and policies that can make healthful habits and living conditions easier but often make them harder to achieve. Such patterns and policies – often beyond the awareness of individuals – span a wide spectrum: work schedules, work load, and stress and safety in work environments; affirmative action programs for jobs and wages; availability of nonautomobile transport systems and recreational facilities and economically accessible sound housing for safety and exercise; farm price subsidies for food and tobacco crops that affect buying patterns; and excise taxes and regulation of health-damaging drugs such as alcohol and nicotine.[23]

What was the actual cause of Frank's problem?

In the real world it is not possible to separate one cause from another – causes are not single factors. In Frank's case, the sources of illness are found in the many interrelationships that make up his life. To try to treat or change each factor as though it were a separate entity can have only a limited effect in improving overall health.

Frank has several health problems. His hyperlipidemia – a biologic, adaptive response to the pressures in his life as well as to his diet, weight gain, lack of exercise, and smoking – could not sustain him indefinitely and eventually clogged his coronary vessels and became maladaptive. His hypertension, the result of his diet and time-constrained lifestyle, was also a biologic effort to adjust to his life situation that contributed to the imbalance between his total resources as a person and the demands of his family and the economic world. Frank's smoking was a psychosocial means to help him relieve some of the emotional pressures; it may have served this short-term purpose but only at a silently rising cost to his health. Cigarette use by persons who have hypertension or high serum cholesterol multiplies their risk of coronary heart disease.[21,22,28]

DEFINITIONS OF HEALTH

Health can be better understood if each person is seen as a part of a complex, interconnected biologic and social system. This ecologic view is useful to those who promote health.

Persons involved in health promotion should consider the meaning of health, since a focused definition clarifies their work and enhances the quality of the health care system. Health is used to describe a number of entities: a *philosophy* of care (health promotion, health maintenance), a *system* (the health care delivery system), *practices* (good health practices), *behaviors* (health behaviors), *costs* (health care costs), *insurance,* and so on. We therefore can see why confusion continues regarding use of the term *health.*

Until recently, literature dealing with health care focused almost exclusively on sickness, illness, and disease. Educational curricula taught treatment for identified symptomatology. Health coverages paid only for treatment of illness, with little or no provision for health promotion or health maintenance activities. Recent scientific and economic developments, such as improved methods for prevention and early detection of illness, mandate reexamination of the more medically oriented definition of health.[40]

For this text, health is equated with a state we define as *wellness.* Wellness activities are synonymous with the activities identified under primary prevention in the Leavell and Clark Model (see Table 1-4 later in this chapter) that promote health. The following section briefly reviews the historic development of the concept of health in order to provide the background for examining more recent definitions.

Historical and Contemporary Views

HISTORICAL

The ancient Greek physicians believed health was a condition of perfect body equilibrium. When the forces, or humors, that constituted the core of the human body were perfectly balanced, a person was healthy. Disturbed balance resulted in disease. The ancient Greeks viewed health as one of the greatest goods. In fact, the cult of Hygenia claimed that health was the foremost good and "the most desirable thing."[36] However, other cults cautioned against the glorification of health. The stoic philosophers did not view health as an absolute value, but they did emphasize the idea that health was necessary for the practice of virtue.[4]

Health was perceived by the New World Indians as the relationship among human beings, nature, and the supernatural.[9] Being healthy was considered natural or in harmony with nature, whereas being unhealthy was unnatural or contrary to nature. The ancient Chinese believed that human activity and health were nothing more than the reflection of a vital body force derived from cosmic energy.[15]

In some sources tracing the origins of modern English, the heading "health" is followed by a reference to "whole."[29] "Whole" is derived from "hole" in middle English and from "hol" in old English, meaning being safe or sound and whole of body. Such definitions fit into the dimensions of health commonly quoted today – physical, psychologic, and environmental.

CONTEMPORARY

Beginning early in the 20th century, Western science attempted to understand how things work by analyzing their components rather than focusing on the interconnection of the parts or their relation to the surroundings. Health was thus defined in more restrictive terms appropriate to the tools used in medical science. The body often was equated to a machine, with emphasis placed on both diagnostic tools and repair mechanisms. For example, an advertisement in the New York City subway system pronounced the human body a wonderful machine that should be taken to a physician once a year for an overhaul. Although put in more sophisticated terms, the prevalent medical view of health problems today still reflects such a restricted view.

This current medical outlook usually uses nonvoluntary and organic expressions.[36,40] Various phases are given such distinct labels as "diagnosis," "symptoms," or most recently, "risk factors," which are thought to predispose a person to disease. With the "medicalization" of many problems, the medical model or framework recently has been expanded to include problem drinking, child abuse, learning disabilities, delinquency, and crime.[10] This definition of health focuses on the individual with a problem, with care directed at the diseased organ, symptom, or risk factor. Health and illness are viewed as the extremes on a continuum: either one's absence indicates the other's presence. Using such a medical model, a person is deemed healthy and medical care no longer needed when the focus of treatment disappears. Thus, it is assumed that a disease-free population is a healthy population.[31]

The health literature of the 1950s through the 1970s focused on preventative health, as did the national objectives of *Healthy People*.[42] During this period, multiple studies were conducted to investigate behavior and the relationship to health promotion. A majority of the studies were designed to explain why people fail to use preventive health services (see Table 1-2). These studies dealt primarily with a single preventive action. In the late 1970s, a few studies attempted to determine why people act as they do regarding a range of health promotion, health protection, and illness prevention behaviors. The studies of the 1980s indicate a lack of clarity regarding relationships among variables in complex explanatory behavior, contributed to the weak association of social and psychologic variables and health behavior. Therefore, Kulbok recommended further explorations of the fundamental natures of the concepts of health and health behavior as being essential to nursing research on health promotion.[19]

Margaret Newman,[26] a nurse theorist, made further progress in developing a definition of health in the late 1970s, stating that health is a synthesis of disease and nondisease. Her concepts are listed in the box on p. 10. Newman uses the concepts of time, space, movement, and consciousness as a framework for viewing "health as the totality of life processes, with disease included as a process. Everyone has a certain kind of health, including those in excellent, good, fair, or poor condition. Health is measured on a graded scale, just as is disease or disability."[26] It may be affected by disease vectors, inherent and acquired characteristics, and environmental variables.

Although an emphasis upon health promotion over preventive health was beginning to be evident in the health literature in the 1980s, inconsistency of definitions and

***Table 1-2.* Preventive health behavior: a summary of research: 1958-1980**

Author and year	Sample N/design	Operationalization of concept
Hochbaum (1958)	Random N = 1201 survey	Chest radiograph in past 7 years
Kegeles (1963)	Random N = 277 survey	One dental checkup in past 3 years
Haefner and Kirscht (1970)	Nonrandom N = 166 experiment	Physician visit in absence of symptoms Radiograph in absence of symptoms
Belloc and Breslow (1972)	Random N = 6928 survey	7 hours of sleep Eat breakfast almost every day Eat between meals rarely or occasionally Weight/height ratio relative to desirable mean: 5% below to 5% above Physical activity: active sports, swim, exercise often Cigarette smoking history: never Amount drink: none, 1-2 at a time
Bullough (1972)	Nonrandom N = 806 survey	Checkup for a new baby, immunization for older children, checkup for older children, dental care for older children, mother's dental care, prenatal care first trimester, postpartum checkup, percentage of pregnancies planned, last pregnancy planned
Cummings et al. (1979)	Random N = 286 survey	Received swine flu shot
Harris and Guten (1979)	Random N = 842 survey	Five clusters of health-protective behaviors: personal health practices, safety practices, preventive health care, environmental hazard avoidance, harmful substance avoidance
Mechanic and Cleary (1980)	Nonrandom N = 302 survey	Takes few risks Prepared for health emergencies Drinks (heavily) Smokes Wears seat belt: most recent time Preventive medical care Physically active Exercise

Adapted with permission from Chinn PL, editor: *Advances in nursing theory development,* Rockville, Md, 1983, Aspen.

❑ ❑ NEWMAN'S CONCEPTS OF HEALTH

1. Health includes conditions described as illness or pathology.
2. Pathologic conditions can be considered a manifestation of the total pattern of the individual.
3. The pattern of the individual that eventually manifests itself as pathology is primary and exists before structural or functional changes.
4. Removal of the pathology only will not change the pattern of the individual.
5. If becoming ill is the only way an individual's pattern can manifest itself, then this illness represents a form of health for that person.
6. Health is an expansion of consciousness.

the variety of terms used posed problems for nursing.[3] Research abstracts were reviewed to select nursing research on health promotion or preventive health behavior. The list included 30 nursing research reports (Table 1-3).

The most quoted and criticized definition of health is unquestionably that of the World Health Organization (WHO),[44] which reflects a philosophic ideal, encompassing optimal mental, physical, and emotional well-being and not merely the absence of disease. Criticism points to this definition's abstractness, simplicity, vagueness, and unsuitability for scientific interpretation. Within the WHO definition, however, three characteristics essential to a more positive conceptualization of health can be found: (1) a concern for the individual as a total system rather than the sum of various parts, (2) a view of health that identifies both internal and external environments, and (3) a fulfillment of an individual's role in life.[45]

***Table 1-3.* Nursing studies of health promotion behavior (1980-1990)**

Author and year	Sample/N characteristics	Design	Behavior
Hautman and Harrison (1982)	Nonrandom N = 100 18-88 years 71% female	Survey Closed- and open-ended interview	General: diet, exercise, vitamins, rest, activity, meditation, health food, herbs
O'Brien (1982)	Nonrandom N = 125 Adult Mexican-American migrant workers	Qualitative Observation and interview observed	No preventive behaviors Maintain low level of wellness
Brown, Muhlenkamp, Fox, and Osborn (1983)	Nonrandom N = 67 18-90 years 75% female White predominantly	Survey Cross-sectional Questionnaire	General: safety, nutrition, prevention, substance use, relaxation, exercise (24 items)
Cox, Sullivan, and Roughman (1984)	Nonrandom N = 203 adults over 34 years females	Survey Questionnaire and secondary analysis	Specific (risk reduction): counseling, amniocentesis (prenatal, genetic, diagnostic)
Alexy (1985)	Nonrandom N = 152 27-66 years 68% male	Experimental	Specific (at-risk): weight, alcohol, exercise, seat belt, self-breast exam
Kulbok (1985)	Probability N = 3025 20-64 years 60% female	Survey Cross-sectional Telephone interview Secondary analysis	General: fitness, dental checkup, health protection, harmful consumption (16 items)
Laffrey (1985)	Random (household) N = 95 18-69 years 61% female, white	Survey Cross-sectional Questionnaire	General: dental care, nutrition, relaxation, exercise, sleep/rest (15 items)

From Kulbok P, Baldwin P: From preventive health behaviors to health promotion: advancing a positive construct of health, *Adv Nurs Sci* 14(4):50-64, 1992.

Table 1-3. **Nursing studies of health promotion behavior (1980-1990) – cont'd**

Author and year	Sample/N characteristics	Design	Behavior
Muhlenkamp, Brown, and Sands (1985)	Nonrandom N = 175 17-84 years 81% female	Survey Cross-sectional Questionnaire	General: same as Brown et al. (1983)
Walsh (1985)	Random N = 140 adults	Survey Cross-sectional Questionnaire	General: nutrition, exercise, substance use, stress management, safety practices, medical awareness, and self-care
Duffy (1986)	Nonrandom N = 59 18-51 years Female	Qualitative Interview Diary	General: exercise, nutrition, substance use decline, health care, personal health (physical/emotional), safety, health knowledge, work on community programs (53 card sort items)
Laffrey (1986)	Random (household) N = 59 19-66 years 34 females	Survey Cross-sectional Questionnaire	General: same as Laffrey (1985)
Murdaugh and Hinshaw (1966)	Nonrandom N = 66 22-83 years 67% female	Survey Cross-sectional Questionnaire	Specific: smoking, exercise
Pender and Pender (1986)	Nonrandom N = 377 18-66 years 60% female White predominantly	Survey Cross-sectional Questionnaire	Specific: exercise regularly, maintain weight, avoid stress (15 items)
Murdaugh and Verran (1987)	Random N = 41 22-83 years 61% female	Survey Cross-sectional Questionnaire	Specific: smoking, exercise
Sennot-Miller and Miller (1987)			
Study A	Random N = 60 26-70 years 50% female	Survey Cross-sectional Questionnaire	Specific: (C-V risk-reduction): maintain normal BP, diet low in cholesterol, ideal weight, alcohol a/drink/day or less, low stress, eat limited refined sugar, no salt at table, exercise daily, 1-mile walk, strenuous exercise 4 times/week, do not smoke (10 items)
Study B and C	Nonrandom N = 55 & 68 mean of 20 90% females	Survey Cross-sectional	
Study D	Nonrandom N = 83 61% female	Survey Cross-sectional Questionnaire	
Walker, Sechrist, and Pender (1987)	Nonrandom N = 952 18-88 years 46% female	Survey Cross-sectional Questionnaire	General: self-actualization, health responsibility, exercise, nutrition, interpersonal support, stress management (48 items)
Denyes (1988)	Nonrandom N = 369 mean of 16.4 12-20 years	Survey Cross-sectional Questionnaire	General: self-care actions, specific: action that meets universal self-care requisites (22 items)
Duffy (1988)	Nonrandom N = 262 35-65 years Female	Survey Cross-sectional Questionnaire	General: same as Walker et al. (1987)

Continued.

Table 1-3. **Nursing studies of health promotion behavior (1980-1990) – cont'd**

Author and year	Sample/N characteristics	Design	Behavior
Kulbok, Earis, and Montgomery (1988)	Nonrandom N = 1856 14-19 years 76% female 84% black	Survey Cross-sectional Questionnaire	General: problem (health negating) group/individual activities, conventional (health promoting) (26 items)
Muhlenkamp and Broerman (1988)	Nonrandom N = 172 17-84 years 81% female White predominantly	Survey Cross-sectional Questionnaire	General: same as Brown et al. (1983)
Walker, Volkan, Sechrist, and Pender (1988)	Nonrandom N = 452 18-88 years 66% female	Survey Cross-sectional Questionnaire	General: same as Walker et al. (1987)
Woods et al. (1988)	Nonrandom systematic N = 528 18-45 years Female White predominantly	Qualitative Interview	General: practicing health lifestyle
Aaronson (1989)	Nonrandom N = 529 18-41 years Female	Survey Questionnaire Telephone interview	Specific (risk factors) caffeine, alcohol, smoking
Riffle, Yoho, and Sams (1989)	Nonrandom N = 113 56-94 years 78% female 93% white	Survey Cross-sectional Questionnaire	General: same as Walker et al. (1987)
Walker (1989)	Random N = 173 17-40 years	Survey Cross-sectional Questionnaire	General: same as Walker et al. (1987)
Yarcheski and Mahon (1989)	Nonrandom N = 165 15-21 years 50% female 77% white	Survey Questionnaire Cross-sectional	General: same as Brown et al. (1983)
Laffrey (1990)	Nonrandom N = 85 22-88 years 80% female	Semi-structured Interview and Questionnaire	General: nutrition, exercise, well-being, relaxation, sleep/rest, health professional, work-school, substance avoidance, moral behaviors, hygiene, and general environment

Recognizing a need for a major shift in focus from illness to health, WHO formulated a campaign for health for all by the year 2000.[16] It implies a collective responsibility to provide access to health care to everyone worldwide, starting with our own national areas of need.[43] During a series of three WHO health conferences in 1991, experts attending the conference stated that health promotion in America was misdirected. In addition, the gap widened between health promotion as practiced in the United States and the "world view" of health promotion pursued in other countries. The differences are particularly strong in three areas: equity, power, and scope. (See box on p. 13 for explanations of these terms, and see Appendix 1-1 for an example of a Canadian health promotion model.)

Lay Concepts of Health

During the mid-1980s, research in health promotion showed that professionals and consumers of health services do not share the same ideas concerning health.[8] This difference in perception may be the main reason for

❑ ❑ HEALTH PROMOTION: UNITED STATES VERSUS WHO VIEW

Equity. In the world view of health promotion, the goal of equal access to health carries more importance than optimizing each person's individual health. The WHO emphasizes providing basic health services to all people before moving on to the more sophisticated needs of subgroups.

Power. In other countries, power and control are central issues in health promotion. "Health Promotion in Developing Countries: A Call to Action," a 1990 WHO strategy document, declares: "Focus of health promotion is social action for health." The goal is to give people a voice in changing unhealthy environments. Showing people how to adapt to or make the most of their situations through behavioral changes has less value. "Knowledge alone, without adequate supportive systems and facilities, is not enough to lead people to action." In the United States, most health promotion efforts steer clear of political involvement for social action.

Scope. In the world of community, the scope of health promotion includes broad social aspects of quality of life. Good housing, safe transportation, basic education, good food supplies, and strong social relationships are within the domain of health promotion. American health promotion rarely addresses these broader determinants of health.

Adapted from World Health Organization: Health promotion in developing countries: a call for action, *Am J Health Promotion* 6(3):174, 1992.

consumers' low adherence to professional advice or health messages.

In the late 1980s, the lay adult populations continued to cite three themes that define health. These are the absence of illness, a functional capacity, or a positive condition. In all studies reviewed by Colantonio,[8] health as "the absence of illness" surfaces to some degree. The idea of health as a functional capacity was held by a notable proportion of subjects in these studies and was defined as being able to do what one has to do. A good mental state, described as feeling good, was included in the definition of health by 66% of the sample consisting of middle- and working-class people in Quebec.[8] The most recent and extensive study on French Canadian lay concepts of health performed revealed 41 themes of health, grouped under 10 subheadings.[8] In congruence with other contemporary health promotion studies, thematic groupings, such as physical aptitude, absence of sickness, a positive condition expressed as vital psychologic well-being, and reference to the body were found in D'Houtand's results.

Overall Concept

The health status of any individual or any population is a sustainable balance involving complex responses between a person's internal (physiologic and psychologic) and external (environmental) factors. Thus, health initially is conceived as a biologic state, with genetic endowment the starting point of the definition.

The case of Frank Thompson previously outlined can clarify this definition of health. Frank's biologic status intertwined with social forces and other life-long behavior patterns in an attempt to meet the demands on him. He created some stresses, whereas others were imposed. Although his lifestyle was supported by his family, Frank could not maintain the difficult balance between all the demands. His myocardial infarction was a way of saying, "It's too much."

The interconnections between biophysical, psychologic, and environmental causes and consequences did not end with Frank's heart problem. That attack was only the most dramatic sign of health-damaging responses outweighing health-promoting ones. The "tip of the iceberg" analogy is frequently used to illustrate the importance of identifying individuals with subclinical symptoms. High blood lipids, high blood pressure, obesity, smoking, and persistent worrying, less obvious earlier, were no less important than the infarction in shaping the status of Frank's health.

The infarction and resulting disability also permanently shaped Frank's environment. His limited ability to work cut his income and thus his children's education, his family's leisure activities and chances of moving, and his dying father's medical care. The concern and uncertainty surrounding these and daily living patterns also would affect interfamilial relationships. Frank's entire life, internal and external, was changed.

Frank's problem illustrates how causes and effects in life and health tend to merge into constant, inseparable interconnections between persons and their worlds. A person's health status is not a state but, rather, a web of relationships. Health is not an achievement or a prize but a high-quality interaction between a person's inner and outer worlds that provides a continuing capacity to respond to the demands of the biologic, psychologic, and environmental systems of these worlds.

The people of the United States only recently have begun to see the imbalance between their natural habitat and the basis for production of their goods and services: reliance on nonrenewable resources and relentless use of croplands. Environmental pollution, acute poisoning, cancer, and cardiovascular disease are signs of the United States population's unstable relationship with the external world – an imbalance that cannot be sustained humanely in long-term projections. The critical concept is the *sustainable* or *stable* (but not static) relationship that should be present in this interconnected network that fosters health and life.

Health and Illness as Part of a Continuum

It is easy to think of health or wellness as the lack of disease and of illness and disease as interchangeable terms. Health and disease, however, are not simply antonyms, and disease and illness are not synonyms. Disease literally means "without ease." Disease may be defined as a failure of an organism's adaptive mechanisms to counteract adequately the stimuli and stresses to it, resulting in functional or structural disturbances. This definition is an ecologic concept of disease using a multifactorial perspective rather than limiting factors to search for a single cause. This approach is closer to reality and also increases the chances of discovering those factors that may be susceptible to intervention.

Health and disease must be inseparable – if disease did not exist, there would be no need to discuss health. The difficulty is to determine at what point health and disease meet and whether they are mutually exclusive. If the set of responses is not sustainable – as in Frank Thompson's life – illness results. Illness stems from *human responses,* whether by individuals or society, that place persons in an imbalanced, unsustainable relation with their worlds and therefore decrease their ability to survive and to create higher standards for the quality of life. Illness is a disenabling response, a mismatch between needs and resources available to meet those needs, and a signal to individuals and populations that the present balance is not working. Illness diminishes the ongoing capacity to respond and thus future capabilities. When persons can no longer respond and maintain the essential sustaining balance of relationships between inner and outer worlds, they die.[24]

Disease is a biomedical term, whereas illness is a state of being. Illness has social and psychologic as well as biomedical components; a person can have a disease without feeling ill, as occurs in asymptomatic hypertension. The theory that health and illness are dynamic patterns changing with time and social circumstance leads to the conclusion that judgments of healthiness must be made often during the life cycle. This urges the nurse to reiterate that most health evaluations are relative, based on a series of perceptions and observations rather than on a limiting standard of measurement. Health arises from a finely graded continuum of functional ability and disability, not from mutually exclusive categories.

Neither health, illness, nor disease is static or stationary. Behind every condition is the phenomenon of almost constant alteration. These conditions are continuing processes – a battle by human beings to maintain a positive balance agaionst biologic, physical, mental, and social forces tending to disturb their health equilibrium.

High-Level Wellness

The term *wellness* has been looked upon as a reaction to a preconceived preoccupation with illness. Use of this term suggests a health continuum in which illness lies on one end, wellness lies on the other end, and health spans the whole (Fig. 1-1). In this model, health is a state of being that can be characterized by any degree of illness or wellness.[5]

Wellness in the sense used in this text signifies something quite different from good health. Good health exists as a relatively passive state of freedom from illness in which the individual is at peace with his or her environment – a condition of relative homeostasis.[25] Wellness is conceptualized as dynamic, a condition of change in which the individual moves forward, climbing toward a higher potential of functioning. High-level wellness for the individual is an integrated method of functioning that is oriented toward maximizing the individual's potential within the environment in which she or he is functioning.[25]

This definition does not imply that there is an optimum level of wellness but rather that wellness is a progression toward a satisfactory level of functioning. High-level wellness, therefore, involves (1) the progression forward and upward toward a higher potential of functioning, (2) an

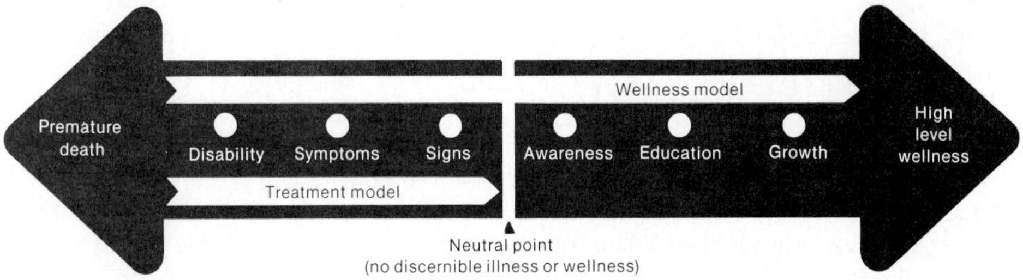

Fig. 1-1. Wellness-illness continuum. Moving from center to left shows progressively worsening state of health. Moving to right of center indicates increasing levels of health and well-being. Treatment model can bring client to neutral point, where symptoms of disease have been alleviated. Wellness model, which can be used at any point, directs client beyond neutral and encourages him or her to move as far to right as possible. It is not meant to replace treatment model on left side of continuum but to work in harmony with it. If client is ill, treatment is important, but he or she should not stop there. (Redrawn from Ryan RS, Travis JW: *Wellness workbook,* Berkeley, Calif, 1981, Ten Speed Press.)

open-ended and ever-expanding tomorrow with its challenge of fuller potential, and (3) the integration of the whole being.[25]

The challenge posed by the concept of high-level wellness is how it can be achieved within everyday living and for humankind as a whole. The challenge must be met by both individuals and groups, and within the context of various ideologies, races, religions, and cultural patterns.[25]

LEVELS OF PREVENTION

Prevention in a narrow sense means averting the development of disease. In a broad sense it consists of all measures, including definitive therapy, that limit the progression of disease at any point of its course. Leavell and Clark[20] define three levels of prevention: primary, secondary, and tertiary. Each level of prevention occurs at a distinct point in the development of the disease process and requires specific nursing interventions:[6]

Primary – includes generalized health promotion as well as specific protection against disease

Secondary – emphasizes early diagnosis and prompt treatment to halt the pathologic process, thereby shortening its duration and severity and enabling the individual to return to a former state of health at the earliest time possible

Tertiary – not only stops a disease process but prevents complete disability. The objective is to return the affected individual to a useful place in society within the constraints of the disability

Although these levels of prevention are disease-oriented, they provide guidelines for nurses to follow in making effective, positive changes in the health status of their clients. Within the three levels of a prevention program there are five steps, as shown in the Leavell and Clark model (Table 1-4). These include health promotion and specific protection (primary prevention); early diagnosis, prompt treatment, and disability limitation (secondary prevention); and restoration and rehabilitation (tertiary prevention).

Since some confusion exists in the interpretation of these concepts, a consistent understanding of primary, secondary, and tertiary prevention is essential. The levels of prevention operate on a continuum and may overlap in practice. The nurse must clearly understand the goals of each level to effectively intervene in keeping persons healthy.

Primary Prevention

Primary prevention is true prevention; it precedes disease or dysfunction. Primary prevention is not therapeutic, does not use therapeutic treatments, and does not involve symptom identification. Primary prevention intervention includes health promotion as well as specific protection, and its purpose is to decrease the vulnerability of the individual or population to illness or dysfunction. This intervention also encourages individuals and groups to become more aware of the primary health level, the optimal health level possible, and the means of improving

***Table 1-4.* Three levels of prevention**

Primary prevention		Secondary prevention		Tertiary prevention
Health promotion	Specific protection	Early diagnosis and prompt treatment	Disability limitations	Restoration and rehabilitation
Health education Good standard of nutrition adjusted to developmental phases of life Attention to personality development Provision of adequate housing and recreation and agreeable working conditions Marriage counseling and sex education Genetic screening Periodic selective examinations	Use of specific immunizations Attention to personal hygiene Use of environmental sanitation Protection against occupational hazards Protection from accidents Use of specific nutrients Protection from carcinogens Avoidance of allergens	Case-finding measures: individual and mass Screening surveys Selective examinations to Cure and prevent disease process to Prevent spread of communicable disease Prevent complications and sequelae Shorten period of disability	Adequate treatment to arrest disease process and prevent further complications and sequelae Provision of facilities to limit disability and to prevent death	Provision of hospital and community facilities for retraining and education to maximize use of remaining capacities Education of public and industry to use rehabilitated persons to fullest possible extent Selective placement Work therapy in hospitals Use of sheltered colony

Modified from Leavell H, Clark AE: *Preventive medicine for doctors in the community,* New York, 1965, McGraw-Hill.

health; they are also taught to use appropriate primary preventive measures.

HEALTH PROMOTION

Since health promotion is a new and emerging field, definitions of it vary. O'Donnell[27] has defined health promotion as "the science and art of helping people change their lifestyle to move toward a state of optimal health. A more complex definition was proposed by Kreuter and Dwore[18] in a paper commissioned by the Public Health Service. Their definition stated that health promotion is "the process of advocating health in order to enhance the probability that personal (individual, family, and community), private (professional and business), and public (federal, state, and local government) support of positive health practices will become a societal norm."[27]

Health promotion is, therefore, not just exercise and nutrition information but is proactive decision making at all levels of care. A few of the strategies identified within this decision-making process are screening, self-care of minor illness, readiness for emergencies, successful management of chronic disease, environmental changes to enhance good nutrition, and no-smoking policies within an organizational setting.[12] Based on the significance of the health promotion activities within the health care system, efforts must be made to identify the multiple determinants of health, identify relevant health promotion strategies, and delineate issues relevant to economic constraints.

Health promotion efforts, unlike those directed at specific protection against certain diseases, focus on maintaining or improving the general health of individuals, families, and communities. These activities are carried on at both the public level, such as government programs promoting adequate housing, and the personal level. Nursing interventions are directed toward developing the resources of persons to maintain or enhance their well-being.[35]

Two strategies of health promotion involve the individual and are either passive or active. *Passive* strategies involve the client as a passive participant or recipient. Examples of passive strategies are (1) to maintain clean water and sanitary sewage systems to decrease infectious diseases and improve health and (2) to introduce vitamin D in all milk so that children will not be at high risk for rickets when little sunlight is available. Many health professionals believe in these passive strategies, since compliance with individual therapeutic regimens tends to be low.

Active strategies depend on the individual becoming personally involved to adopt a proposed program of health promotion (see Unit Two). Examples that involve changes in lifestyle are (1) daily exercise as part of a physical fitness plan and (2) a stress management program as part of daily living. A combination of both active and passive strategies is best for making an individual healthier. However, such strategies depend on mass application for their economic benefits; controversy surrounds the optimal balance between these two strategies.

This text is almost entirely concerned with active strategies and the nurse's role in these strategies. Some passive strategies are presented, but with the implicit belief that full health primarily results from activities generated within the individual. This does not deny that passive strategies also have a valuable role; however, they must be used within a context in which individual clients are encouraged and taught more and more to assume responsibility for their own health.

Although health promotion would seem a practical and effective mode of health care, the major portion of health care delivery is geared to respond to acute and chronic disease. Preventing some chronic disease and adding new dimensions to the quality of life are not as simple; these actions are more closely associated with everyday living and the lifestyles adopted by individuals, families, communities, and nations. Such habits as eating, resting, exercising, and handling anxieties appear to be transmitted from parent to child and from social group to social group, as part of cultural, not genetic, heritage. These activities may be taught in subtle ways, but they may influence behavior as much as genetic inheritance. Although the causal relationship between behavior and health may be appreciated only dimly by the public, it sould be apparent to health professionals.

Health promotional strategies have the potential of enhancing the quality of life from birth to death. Good nutrition, for example, is adjusted to various developmental phases of life, accounting for the rapid growth and development in infancy and early childhood, the physiologic changes associated with adolescence, the extra demands during pregnancy, and the many changes occurring in the elderly. Other individual activities are adapted to the person's needs for optimal personality development at all ages. As seen in Unit Four, much can be done on a personal or group basis through counseling and properly directed parent education to provide the environmental requirements for the child's proper personality development. Community participation is also an important factor in promoting individual and group health (see Chapters 7 and 8).

Personal health promotion most commonly is provided by health education. An important function of nurses, physicians, parents, and allied health professionals, health education involves more than providing health information, since it is concerned principally with effecting useful changes in human behavior. The goal is the inculcation of a sense of responsibility for one's own health and a shared sense of responsibility for avoiding injury to the health of others. For children this implies encouragement of those child-rearing practices that foster normal growth and development – personal and social as well as physical. Health education nurtures health-promoting habits, values, and attitudes that must be learned through practice. These in turn must be reinforced through systematic instruction in hygiene, bodily function, physical fitness, and use of leisure time. Another goal is understanding appropriate use of health services; for example, the semiannual visit to a dentist may teach the child to become a regular dental client, even though this is not the primary purpose of the visit.

Health promotion interventions must continually demonstrate that they are effective and cost saving to a degree, rarely or never expected of any acute care intervention.[42] Available research clearly shows an increase in longevity, decrease in mortality and morbidity, and improvement in quality of life for individuals who have been involved in health promotion activities. Although empiric data linking risk factors, health promotion activities, and outcomes are inconclusive,[41] evidence from research does not support the idea that health promotion programs actually save money. In fact, significant reductions in cost may not appear for several years after program implementation.[13]

SPECIFIC PROTECTION

This aspect of primary prevention focuses on protecting persons from disease by providing immunization and reducing exposure to occupational hazards, carcinogens, and other environmental health risks (see Table 1-4). Primary prevention intervention is considered health protection because it emphasizes shielding or defending the body from injury. Nursing intervention to prevent a specific health problem is easier than promoting well-being among individuals, groups, or communities, since the variables are delineated more clearly in prevention than in promotion, and the potential influences are less diverse.

Secondary Prevention

Although primary prevention measures have decreased the hazards of infectious diseases, chronic disease and other conditions that preclude a healthy life are still prevalent.

Secondary prevention ranges from providing screening techniques and treating early stages of disease to limiting disability by averting or delaying the consequences of advanced disease. Screening, which also involves health teaching, primarily establishes case findings in an early stage of disease, when treatment is more effective. This has become an important aspect in the control of chronic disease and cancer, as well as in providing early diagnosis and treatment of nutritional, mental, and other problems.

Delayed recognition because of incomplete knowledge of some disease process in early secondary prevention results in the need to limit future disability in the late stage of secondary prevention. Certain economic environmental changes may aid in preventing sequelae, but the preventive measures primarily are therapeutic to arrest the disease and prevent further complications.

Tertiary Prevention

Tertiary prevention occurs when a defect or disability is permanent and irreversible. It involves minimizing the effects of disease and disability by surveillance and maintenance aimed at preventing complications and deterioration. Tertiary prevention focuses on rehabilitation to help persons attain and retain an optimal level of functioning regardless of their disabling condition. Its objective is to return the affected individual to a useful place in society and make maximal use of remaining capacities. The responsibility of the nurse is to see that disabled persons are rehabilitated in such a manner that they can live and work according to the resources still available to them. When persons have a stroke, rehabilitating these individuals to their highest level of functioning is an example of tertiary prevention.

THE NURSE'S ROLE

Evolving demands are placed on the nurse and the nursing profession as a result of changes in society, especially changes in modern technology, social consciousness, and the quality and types of health care. Emphasis has shifted from acute, hospital-based care to preventive, community-based care.[17] All these changes that affect the health care delivery system affect nursing. Nursing role changes must parallel delivery system changes, and more importantly, as the largest group of health care workers, nurses must anticipate societal changes if they are to continue to develop with public and professional accountability.[9] Nurses need to be on the forefront of change.[1]

The health objectives for the year 2000 are, in general, health promotion. This section discusses the many nursing roles in health promotion, with a view toward future horizons and the nurse's roles with the client and the broader role in society.

Role Defined

The term *role* is defined by social scientists as the functioning of individuals in a group and the learning of a social role as an aspect of personality that is acquired with other habits.[33] A role assigned by society is different than a role achieved by the individual. The nurse today has many roles, and societal changes have placed new demands on the nursing profession.

Within these roles, nurses are assuming more active involvement in the prevention of disease and promotion of health. They are more independent in their practice, place greater emphasis on promoting and maximizing health, and more than ever are accountable morally and legally for their professional behavior.

Nursing Roles in Health Promotion and Protection

Although nurses often work with clients on a one-to-one basis, they seldom work in isolation in their practice. Within today's health care system, nurses work with other nurses, physicians, social workers, nutritionists, psychologists, therapists, and clients. In the role of *caregiver,* the nurse is a member of a team and needs to communicate extensively with other team members as a *collaborator.* As an *advocate,* the nurse is speaking and acting on behalf of a person or group; the nurse explains and interprets the client's or family's feelings and position to others. The nurse may be a *facilitator* and *coordinator* of services for the client to prevent duplication of services and to ensure that needs are met. In addition, the nurse may serve as a *consultant* to other health care providers, to clients, or to agencies within the community that provide health services. The nurse may also be a *deliverer of services,* an *educator,* and a *researcher.*

ADVOCATE

The nurse can be an advocate by (1) assisting clients to obtain what they are entitled to from the system and (2) trying to make the system more responsive to their needs. One example of client advocacy involves speaking to the local social service department before referral to pave the way for the family members who need to receive health benefits.

FACILITATOR AND COORDINATOR

The nurse acts as coordinator to prevent duplication of services. When several team members visit a client, the nurse usually facilitates and coordinates the total plan. An example of coordination is ensuring annual health examinations by having all family members checked and arranging any care plan with the other team members. Nurses are evolving into the role of Care Manager.

CONSULTANT

Because of their knowledge in health promotion and disease prevention, nurses often mediate the interaction of clients and others. Consultative exchanges can occur with school teachers, legislators, or other persons who maintain a working relationship with the client. Some nurses have very specialized areas of expertise, such as gerontology, pediatrics, or obstetrics, and are equipped and prepared to provide information as consultants in these areas of specialization. For example, a gerontologic nurse specialist might be on a community planning board and offer advice about what type of health promotional activities should be considered in planning a new senior citizens' housing development.

DELIVERER OF SERVICES

The nurse also delivers services, such as health education and counseling in health promotion. Visible, direct nursing care often gives credibility to these semidirect and indirect services.

EDUCATOR

Health practices are derived from scientific theory in the United States to put such health components as good nutrition, industrial and highway safety, immunization, and specific drug therapy within the grasp of the total population. Even with these rich resources, society falls far short of attaining the goal of maximal health for all. Since the problem is not lack of knowledge but lack of application, it is incumbent on nurses to add teaching to their roles. To teach effectively, the nurse must know some essential things about the learner and the teaching-learning process (see Chapter 11).

In addition to their storehouse of scientific knowledge, nurses committed to their teaching role know that individuals are unique in their response to efforts designed to change their behavior. To expand options in teaching method, nurses should explore the literature to find various ways to present health information; records of personal experiences also can be used to improve teaching. Teaching may range from a chance remark by the nurse based on a perception of desirable patient behavior to structurally planned teaching according to patient needs. Selection of methods most likely to succeed involves the establishment of teacher-learner goals. Health promotion and protection rely heavily on the individual's ability to use appropriate knowledge. Teaching is one of the major primary preventions available to avoid the major causes of disability and death today.

RESEARCHER

Nursing research is a creative, disciplined endeavor that seeks answers to inquiries about variables that affect a client's health and illness. Although many nurses do not have to do nursing research, all active and practicing nurses have a responsibility to read about and critically analyze research studies and incorporate the findings into daily practice. (See Chapter 4 on the nursing process and

❑ ❑ GOALS OF PEW HEALTH PROFESSIONS COMMISSION FOR PRACTITIONERS OF 2005

Care for the community's health
Expand access
Emphasize primary care
Participate in coordinated care
Provide clinical care
Ensure cost-effectiveness
Practice preventive and supportive care
Involve patients as partners
Change patient behavior
Apply technology appropriately
Accommodate expanded accountability
Manage information
Provide ethical counseling
Function in a racially and culturally diverse society
Continue to learn

From Pew Health Professions Commission: Healthy America practitioners for 2005, an agenda for action for U.S. health professional schools, Durham, NC, June 1991.

development. See Chapters 16 through 24 for specific health promotion research studies.)

The goal of the Pew Health Professions Commission is to assist the nation's health professional schools in producing practitioners for the year 2005 (see the box above). The Pew Commission believes that the United States must have practitioners with expanded abilities and new attitudes to meet society's evolving health care needs.[30]

Despite its many facets, the role of the nurse, to be successful, must be based on a balance between the population's health needs and the nursing profession's effective contributions. (See Chapter 3 for Nursing Agenda for Health Care Reform.)

IMPROVING PROSPECTS FOR HEALTH

Population Effects

In 1989, life expectancy at birth reached a record high of 75.3 years. The difference in life expectancy for males and females has narrowed since the late 1970s; however, women are still exptected to outlive men by an average of 6.8 years. Life expectancy increased for the white population, but it remained unchanged from the previous year for the black population. This resulted in a widening gap in life expectancy between the black and white populations. Although the difference in life expectancy between the white and black populations narrowed from 7.6 years in 1970 to 5.6 years in 1984, it increased to 6.4 years in 1988 and 6.8 years in 1989. Life expectancy for black males again declined between 1988 and 1989, as it has every year since 1984, with the exception of 1987, when it remained unchanged. Life expectancy for black females has fluctuated since 1982, showing no clear trend.[33]

Cultural and social economic changes within our population unequivocally impact lay concepts of health promotion. The myth that all Americans are alike – white and middle class – has been prominent in the delivery of health care for many years.[37] However, predications are that by the year 2000, one third of all Americans will be ethnic minorities.[11] By the year 2050, it is predicted that the majority of Americans will not be of white European descent but a mixture of all the ethnic and racial mixes of the world. Taken together as a potent for future health promotion strategies, these facts about the population proclaim that health promotion as it is now viewed by lay people may not be meeting the coming needs of the future American population.

More important than population size is the projected age distribution. Considerable growth is expected in the proportion of the population 25 years of age and older. For example, the post-World War II baby boom will increase the number of persons in the 65 and older age group between the years 2010 and 2030. The drop in births after 1960 will decrease the number entering the 65 and older age group and result in a more stable population pattern by 2050.[38] Analysis of these population trends and projections helps health professionals determine future and changing needs. In addition, analysis of the social environment is necessary for social policy related to health.

Shifting Problems

The provision of personal health services must be combined with nonpersonal or environmental services. Environmental pollution is a complex and increasingly hazardous problem. Diseases related to industry and technology, including accidents and trauma, have become an important threat to health.

The physical and psychic stresses of a rapidly changing and fast-paced society present daily problems, such as economic pressures and poor health habits. Obesity, especially from lack of exercise, is at least partly a product of modern technology. The ingestion of potentially toxic, nonnutritive, high-fat foods is another contributing factor to poor health (see Chapter 12).

The use of cigarettes, drugs, and alcohol is a further example of factors that negatively affect health. Environmental conditions produce both physical and socioeconomic limitations. Emphasis on the application of complex technologic advancements *after* the manifestation of disease is not only costly but has minimal effect on improving health. An orientation toward illness clearly focuses on effects rather than on causes of disease.

There has been a substantial change in wellness patterns: infectious and acute diseases were the major causes of death in the early part of this century, whereas chronic conditions, heart disease, cerebrovascular accident (stroke), and cancer are the major causes today. The diagnosis and treatment of disease, which were so successful in the past, are not the total answer for today's needs, which are closely related to and affected by biochemical makeup and environment, especially lifestyle.

In the health belief model, belief in the efficacy of an action implies belief that an action will be beneficial in reducing the perceived health threat. For a health behavior to occur, potential barriers such as cost and level of complexity of the behavior must not outweigh the benefits as the individual perceives them. The difference between the individual's perception of the barriers to action and belief in the efficacy of the action influence the state of readiness to take action and thereby influences the likelihood of action.[34] In addition to perceived susceptibility, severity, efficacy, barriers, and modifying factors, internal (somatic) or external (social or cultural) cues must be present and strong enough to trigger an individual to act.[34]

Toward Solutions

Solutions are not simple or easy but can be directed in two major directions: individual involvement and government involvement. The first concentrates on actions of the individual, especially those related to lifestyle, beginning early in life with the young child. The learning and inherent changes involved require an attitudinal change, which is perhaps the most difficult to effect. About one fifth of the population is faced with problems in getting the basic necessities of food and shelter. The other four fifths, whose basic necessities have been met, must overcome problems that result from affluence.

Motivational factors play a large role in influencing attitudinal change. As discussed in Chapter 11, programs for health promotion and health education are only part of the answer. Financial incentives for prevention may be another motivating factor, and health advocacy by professionals in the health field is critical. In addition, private and public action at all levels is needed to protect against possible environmental hazards. Since toxic agents in the environment can present health hazards that may not be detected for years, it is necessary for individuals to monitor industrial and agricultural production processes to reduce exposure to potentially toxic agents. The government's involvement in health may signal an increasing trend. Health care expenditures have escalated rapidly; illness care is not the answer.

Legislation as well as financing that relates to primary prevention is discussed in Chapter 3. Government activity, in the form of legislation, is currently increasing in this area. For example, bicycle safety, seat belts, and a graduated tax on cigarettes are specific areas of concern. The area of health planning presents one of the most important future areas of government. The redirection of the existing health care delivery system to put more emphasis on primary prevention is probably the most difficult and the most far-reaching goal; however, an emphasis on a wellness system is necessary to improve the health of the U.S. population.

SUMMARY

The way we define health and health problems is important, since our definitions influence how we attempt to improve health and care for health problems. Frank Thompson's health was affected by such obvious immediate, personal factors as his diet and employment pressures. Yet his problems had their roots in the social and economic conditions of his parents; in his own early history of illness, education, and work; and in his and his family's hopes and aspirations. Those, such as his physician, who defined Frank's problem in immediate biomedical terms, used the tools of personal services to help repair the short-term effects of his heart attack. Those, such as public health planners, who saw Frank's problem on a longer-term population basis, sought policy solutions to the problem of preventing cardiovascular disease.

The view taken in this text is that a broad and longer-term perspective of health can guide us more effectively toward promoting health, even as we deal with individual problems on a day-to-day basis.

Health is a sustainable balance within internal forces (ourselves) and between these forces and the environment (external forces). It allows us to move through life free from the constraints of illness, limited only by the winding down of our biologic clock's genetically programmed capacity. In this sense, health means keeping in time with our biologic clocks as persons and populations.

Illness is the speeding up of an individual's biologic clock as a result of the imbalanced relations that human choices – intertwined social and political, professional and personal choices – create. As individuals, we cannot turn back our life's clock. As a society, we may yet have time to slow the onslaught of chronic disability and shift the direction, slow the pace, and humanize the scope of economic and social life.

To shift directions in today's health care patterns may be possible only if nurses and other health professionals do what is expected of them as leaders in the care of health: to work with others through open processes; to give leadership in finding the vision and the path; and to inform, educate, and reeducate themselves, their colleagues, the media, and the general public.

The responsibility of nurses as health professionals today calls for seeing the health problem in new ways and helping others to do the same. It means developing new roles and looking at the problem through others' eyes as well, including those of the client, the public, other professionals, and other nations. It also means evaluating the social as well as individual consequences, the long-term as well as short-term effects, and the public as well as private interests that are involved when deciding on the set of tools to use in the care of health.

References

1. Afifi LA, Swanson E: *Health promotion in times of economic constraint: issues in decision making, vol 4,* Des Moines, 1992, University of Iowa.
2. American Hospital Association fact sheet: *healthy people 2000,* Chicago, 1990, The Association.
3. Balog JE: The concept of health and techniques of conceptual analysis, *Health Education,* pp 10-12, 1988.
4. Baumann B: Diversities in conceptions of health and physical fitness, *J Health Hum Behav* 2(1):40, 1961.
5. Brubaker BH: Health promotion: a linguistic analysis, *Adv Nurs Sci,* p 2-14, 1988.
6. Burns CR: The nonnaturals: a paradox in the western concept of health, *J Med Phil* 1(3):202, 1976.
7. Chinn PL, editor: *Advances in nursing theory development,* Rockville, Md, 1983, Aspen.
8. Colantonio A: Lay concepts of health, *Health Values* 12(5):36, 1988.
9. Dolan JA: *Nursing in society – a historical perspective,* ed 14, Philadelphia, 1978, WB Saunders.
10. Dubos R: Human ecology, *WHO Chronicle* 23:499, 1969.
11. Farrell J: The changing pool of candidates for nursing, *J Prof Nurs* 4(3):185-230, 1988.
12. Folding J: The proof of the health promotion pudding, *J Occup Med* 30(2):113-115, 1988 (editorial).
13. Foote A, Erfut J: The benefit to cost ratio of work-site blood pressure control programs, *JAMA* 265(10):1283-1286, 1991.
14. Greenberg J, Dintiman G: *Exploring health, expanding the boundaries of wellness,* Englewood Cliffs, NJ, 1992, Prentice Hall.
15. Huard P, Wong M: *Chinese medicine,* New York, 1964, McGraw-Hill (Translated by B Fielding).
16. Is health promotion in America misdirected?: An international conference report, *Am J Health Promotion* 6(3): 23-25, 1992.
17. Keller MJ: *Health needs and nursing care of the labor force.* In Fromer MJ, editor: *Community health care and the nursing process,* ed 2, St Louis, 1983, Mosby.
18. Kreuter M, Devore R: Update: reinforcing the case for health promotion, *Fam Comm Health* 10:106, 1980.
19. Kulbok P, Baldwin P: From preventive health behaviors to health promotion: advancing a positive construct of health, *Adv Nurs Sci* 14(4):50-64, 1992.
20. Leavell H, Clark AE: *Preventive medicine for doctors in the community,* New York, 1965, McGraw-Hill.
21. Logan R, et al: Risk factors of ischemic heart disease in normal men aged 40, *Lancet* 1(8031):949, 1978.
22. Maglacas A: Health for all: nursing's role, *Nursing Outlook* 36(2):66-71, 1988.
23. Milio N: A framework for prevention: changing health-damaging to health-generating life patterns, *Am J Public Health* 66(5):435, 1976.
24. Milio N: *Promoting health through public policy,* Philadelphia, 1981, FA Davis.
25. Neilson E: Health values achieving high level wellness 12(3):5, 1988 (editorial).
26. Newman MA: *Theory development in nursing,* Philadelphia, 1979, FA Davis.
27. O'Donnell M: Definition of health promotion, *J Health Promotion* 1(1):4, 1987.
28. Papenfuss RI: Health promotion: issues for AAHE in the 1980s, *Health Educ,* 1988.
29. Partridge E: *Origins – a short etymological dictionary of modern English,* New York, 1966, Macmillan.
30. Pew Health Professions Commission: Healthy America practitioners for 2005, an Agenda for action for U.S. health professional schools, Durham, NC, June 1991.
31. Powles J: On the limitations of modern medicine, *Sci Med Man* 1:1, 1973.
32. Public Health Service: *Healthy people: the surgeon general's report on health promotion and disease prevention,* Health and Human Services, PHS Pub No 7955071, Washington, DC, 1990, US Government Printing Office.
33. Public Health Service: US Health and Human Services, Washington, DC, 1992, vol 40, no 8, suppl 2, US Government Printing Office.
34. Redeker N: Health beliefs and adherence in chronic illness, *Image J Nursing Scholarship* 20(1):18-22, 1988.
35. Shetland ML: *An approach to role expansion – the elaborate network.* In Spradley BW, editor: *Contemporary community nursing,* Boston, 1975, Little, Brown.
36. Temkin A: *The double faces of Jarus: and other essays in the history of medicine,* Baltimore, 1977, Johns Hopkins University Press.
37. Tripp-Reimer T, Afifi LA: Cross-cultural perspectives on patient teaching, *Nurs Clin North Am* 24(3):613-619, 1989.
38. Uhlenberg P: Changing structure of the older population of the USA during the twentieth century, *Gerontologist* 17:197, 1977.
39. US Department of Health and Human Services, Public Health Service: *Healthy people 2000: new objectives to promote health, prevent disease,* Prevention Report, Office of Disease Prevention and Health Promotion, Washington, DC, 1990.
40. Veatch R: The medical model: its nature and problems, *Hastings Center Studies* 1(3):59, 1973.
41. Warner K: Wellness at the worksite, *Health Affairs (Millwood),* 9(2):63-79, 1990.
42. Warner K, Wickizer TM, Wolfe RA, et al: Economic implications of workplace health promotion programs: review of the literature, *J Occup Med* 30(2):106-112, 1988.
43. Wilson RJ: *The sociology of health: an introduction,* New York, 1970, Random House.
44. World Health Organization: *Constitution,* Geneva, 1947, World Health Organization.
45. World Health Organization: *Health promotion for working populations,* Tech Rep Series 765, Geneva, 1988, World Health Organization.
46. World Health Organization: Health promotion in developing countries: a call for action, *Am J Health Promotion* 6(3):174, 1992.

APPENDIX 1-1: OTTAWA CHARTER FOR HEALTH PROMOTION

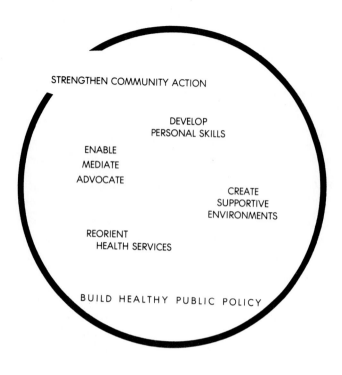

The first International Conference on Health Promotion, meeting in Ottawa this 21st day of November 1986, hereby presents this charter for action to achieve Health for All by the year 2000 and beyond.

This conference was primarily a response to growing expectations for a new public health movement around the world. Discussions focused on the needs in industrialized countries but took into account similar concerns in all other regions. It built on the progress made through the Declaration on Primary Health Care at Alma Ata, the World Health Organization's Targets for Health for All document, and the recent debate at the World Health Assembly on intersectoral action for health.

Health Promotion

Health promotion is the process of enabling people to increase control over, and to improve, their health. To reach a state of complete physical, mental, and social well-being, an individual or group must be able to identify and realize aspirations, to satisfy needs, and to change or cope with the environment. Health is, therefore, seen as a resource for everyday life, not the objective of living. Health is a positive concept emphasizing social and personal resources as well as physical capacities. Therefore, health promotion is not just the responsibility of the health sector but goes beyond healthy lifestyles to well-being.

PREREQUISITES FOR HEALTH

The fundamental conditions and resources for health are peace, shelter, education, food, income, a stable ecosystem, sustainable resources, social justice and equity. Improvement in health requires a secure foundation in these basic prerequisites.

ADVOCATE

Good health is a major resource for social, economic, and personal development and an important dimension of quality of life. Political, economic, social, cultural, environmental, behavioral, and biologic factors can all favor health or be harmful to it. Health promotion action aims at making these conditions favorable through *advocacy* for health.

ENABLE

Health promotion focuses on achieving equity in health. Health promotion action aims at reducing differences in current health status and ensuring equal opportunities and resources to *enable* all people to achieve their fullest health potential. This includes a secure foundation in a supportive environment, access to information, life skills, and opportunities for making healthy choices. People cannot achieve their fullest health potential unless they are able to take control of those things which determine their health. This must apply equally to women and men.

MEDIATE

The prerequisites and prospects for health cannot be ensured by the health sector alone. More importantly, health promotion demands coordinated action by all concerned: by governments, by health and other social and economic sectors, by nongovernmental and voluntary organizations, by local authorities, by industry, and by the media. People in all walks of life are involved as individuals, families, and communities. Professional and social groups and health personnel have a major responsibility to *mediate* between differing interests in society for the pursuit of health.

Health promotion strategies and programs should be adapted to the local needs and possibilities of individual countries and regions to take into account differing social, cultural, and economic systems.

What Health Promotion Action Means

BUILD HEALTHY PUBLIC POLICY

Health promotion goes beyond health care. It puts health on the agenda of policy makers in all sectors and at all levels, directing them to be aware of the health consequences of their decisions and to accept their responsibilities for health.

Health promotion policy combines diverse but complementary approaches, including legislation, fiscal measures, taxation, and organizational change. It is coordinated action that leads to health, income, and social policies that foster greater equity. Joint action contributes to ensuring safer and healthier goods and services; healthier public services; and cleaner, more enjoyable environments.

Health promotion policy requires the identification of obstacles to the adoption of healthy public policies in nonhealth sectors and ways of removing them. The aim must be to make the healthier choice the easier choice for policy makers as well.

CREATE SUPPORTIVE ENVIRONMENTS

Our societies are complex and interrelated. Health cannot be separated from other goals. The inextricable links between people and their environment constitute the basis for a socioecologic approach to health. The overall guiding principle for the world, nations, regions, and communities alike is the need to encourage reciprocal maintenance – to take care of each other, our communities, and our natural environment. The conservation of natural resources throughout the world should be emphasized as a global responsibility.

Changing patterns of life, work, and leisure have a significant impact on health. Work and leisure should be a source of health for people. The way society organizes work should help create a healthy society. Health promotion generates living and working conditions that are safe, stimulating, satisfying, and enjoyable.

Systematic assessment of the health impact of a rapidly changing environment, particularly in areas of technology, work, energy production, and urbanization, is essential and must be followed by action to ensure positive benefit to the health of the public. The protection of the natural and built environments and the conservation of natural resources must be addressed in any health promotion strategy.

STRENGTHEN COMMUNITY ACTION

Health promotion works through concrete and effective community action in setting priorities, making decisions, planning strategies, and implementing them to achieve better health. At the heart of this process is the empowerment of communities, their ownership, and control of their own endeavors and destinies.

Community development draws on existing human and material resources in the community to enhance self-help and social support and to develop flexible systems for strengthening public participation and direction of health matters. This requires full and continuous access to information, learning opportunities for health, as well as funding support.

DEVELOP PERSONAL SKILLS

Health promotion supports personal and social development through providing information, education for health, and enhancing life skills. By so doing, it increases the options available to people to exercise more control over their own health and over their environments and to make choices conducive to health.

Enabling people to learn throughout life, to prepare themselves for all of its stages, and to cope with chronic illness and injuries is essential. This has to be facilitated in school, home, work, and community settings. Action is required through educational, professional, commercial, and voluntary bodies and within the institutions themselves.

REORIENT HEALTH SERVICES

The responsibility for health promotion in health services is shared among individuals, community groups, health professionals, health service institutions, and governments. They must work together toward a health care system which contributes to the pursuit of health.

The role of the health sector must move increasingly in a health promotion direction, beyond its responsibility for providing clinical and curative services. Health services need to embrace an expanded mandate which is sensitive and respects cultural needs. This mandate should support the needs of individuals and communities for a healthier life and open channels between the health sector and broader social, political, economic, and physical environmental components.

Reorienting health services also requires stronger attention to health research as well as changes in professional education and training. This must lead to a change of attitude and organization of health services, which refocuses on the total needs of the individual as a whole person.

Moving into the Future

Health is created and lived by people within the settings of their everyday life; where they learn, work, play, and love. Health is created by caring for oneself and others, by being able to make decisions and have control over one's life circumstances, and by ensuring that the society in which one lives creates conditions that allow the attainment of health by all its members.

Caring, holism, and ecology are essential issues in developing strategies for health promotion. Therefore, those involved should take as a guiding principle that, in each phase of planning, implementation, and evaluation of health promotion activities, women and men should become equal partners.

COMMITMENT TO HEALTH PROMOTION

The participants in this conference pledge

- to move into the arena of healthy public policy and to advocate a clear political commitment to health and equity in all sectors
- to counteract the pressures toward harmful products, resource depletion, unhealthy living conditions and environments, and bad nutrition and to focus attention on public health issues such as pollution, occupational hazards, housing, and settlements
- to respond to the health gap within and between societies and to tackle the inequities in health produced by the rules and practices of these societies
- to acknowledge people as the main health resource; to support and enable them to keep themselves, their families, and friends healthy through financial and other means; and to accept the community as the essential voice in matters of its health, living conditions, and well-being
- to reorient health services and their resources toward the promotion of health and to share power with other sectors, other disciplines, and most importantly, with people themselves
- to recognize health and its maintenance as a major social investment and challenge and to address the overall ecologic issue of our ways of living

The Conference urges all concerned to join them in their commitment to a strong public health alliance.

CALL FOR INTERNATIONAL ACTION

The Conference calls on the World Health Organization and other international organizations to advocate the promotion of health in all appropriate forums and to support countries in setting up strategies and programs for health promotion.

The Conference is firmly convinced that if people in all walks of life, nongovernmental and voluntary organizations, governments, the World Health Organization, and all other bodies concerned join forces in introducing strategies for health promotion – in line with the moral and social values that form the basis of this charter – Health for All by the Year 2000 will become a reality.

❑ ❑ ❑

This charter for action was developed and adopted by an international conference, jointly organized by the World Health Organization, Health and Welfare Canada, and the Canadian Public Health Association. Two hundred and twelve participants from 38 countries met from November 17-21, 1986, in Ottawa, Canada to exchange experiences and share knowledge of health promotion.

The Conference stimulated an open dialogue among lay, health, and other professional workers; among representatives of governmental, voluntary, and community organizations; and among politicians, administrators, academics, and practitioners. Participants coordinated their efforts and came to a clearer definition of the major challenges ahead. They strengthened their individual and collective commitment to the common goal of Health for All by the Year 2000.

This charter for action reflects the spirit of earlier public charters through which the needs of people were recognized and acted upon. The charter presents fundamental strategies and approaches for health promotion, which the participants considered vital for major progress. The Conference report develops the issues raised, gives concrete examples and practical suggestions regarding how real advances can be achieved, and outlines the action required of countries and relevant groups.

The move toward a new public health is now evident worldwide. This was reaffirmed not only by the experiences but by the pledges of Conference participants who were invited as individuals on the basis of their expertise. The following countries were represented: Antigua, Australia, Austria, Belgium, Bulgaria, Canada, Czechoslovakia, Denmark, England, Finland, France, German Democratic Republic, Federal Republic of Germany, Ghana, Hungary, Iceland, Ireland, Israel, Italy, Japan, Malta, the Netherlands, New Zealand, Northern Ireland, Norway, Poland, Portugal, Romania, St. Kitts-Nevis, Scotland, Spain, Sudan, Sweden, Switzerland, Union of Soviet Socialist Republics, United States, Wales, and Yugoslavia.

CHAPTER

2

Changing Populations and Health

Geraldine V. Go

Objectives

After completing this chapter, the nurse will be able to

- *Provide a brief history of immigration patterns to the United States.*
- *Define ethnicity, the process of ethnicization, ethnic group and minority group, race, and culture.*
- *Explain the functions of ethnicity, values, and value orientations.*
- *Contrast the folk health care system from the Western view.*
- *Identify health problems of Asian-Pacific Islanders and Hispanics, Blacks, and Native Americans.*
- *Describe health-related aspects of the culture of Asian-Pacific Islanders, Hispanics, Blacks, and Native Americans.*
- *Describe the impact of homelessness on the individual, family, and community.*
- *Discuss the health problems of homeless individuals and families and individuals afflicted with AIDS.*
- *Identify short- and long-term measures in alleviating homelessness.*
- *Explain how preventive care for HIV/AIDS can be culturally sensitive.*
- *Identify major movements and their goals in meeting the challenge of the health care of changing populations.*

Successful emergence of the 21st century will require a critical look at both the past and the present. Populations will be required to look at their nations, communities, and families relative to the impact of rapid social, political, and economic events which have shaped their present and continue to have a bearing on their futures.

> The year 2000 appears ahead on the calendar of the Nation's history like a turning point. It may well be like any other year in the ongoing lives of people who inhabit this country and the world. But, from the perspective of history, the year 2000 will bring to its conclusion, a tumultuous century, characterized by astounding scientific achievements, devastating world wars, and explosive population growth.[116]

The growth and, more important, the diversity in the population requires special attention.

The increase in population diversity presents major challenges for nations such as the United States. These challenges are clearly evident as one examines the economic, social, and political impact of the emergence of ethnic groups; increases in minority group members; and increases in elderly population, homeless persons, and individuals afflicted with the human immunodeficiency virus (HIV)/acquired immunodeficiency syndrome (AIDS).

Who will meet the challenges presented by these changing populations? What are the priorities that warrant attention? How can life be better for these Americans in the next century? The answers to these questions could come from the collaborative efforts of both public and private sectors of society. Improved health of Americans is the key to a quality life, not only for every individual, but also for families and the nation. "The health of a people is measured by more than death rates. Good health comes from reducing unnecessary suffering, illness, and disabilities. It comes from an improved quality of life. Health is thus best measured by citizens' sense of well-being. The health of a nation is measured by the extent to which the gains are accomplished for all the people."[116] Since the health of changing populations is a major concern for the coming century, an understanding of these populations and their current status is a preliminary step in preparing to meet the challenges for the 21st century.

CHANGING POPULATIONS IN THE UNITED STATES

Changes in the numbers and diversity of the population can be attributed to large-scale immigrations which were largely voluntary.[40] Voluntary immigrations are generally motivated by the individual's or group's quest for one or more of the following ends: (1) educational opportunities, (2) economic benefits, (3) social improvements, and (4) political and religious freedom.[97] A brief look at the patterns of immigration to the United States provides information on the population diversity accomplished over a certain period of time.

Immigration to the United States

The number of early immigrants is difficult to estimate because "their arrival was not officially documented by the government until 1820."[50] Kitano and Daniels,[66] in their study of immigration trends and their effects, identified the first two periods of immigration prior to 1820. They called the first period Colonial, during which neither "Great Britain nor the American colonies had effective control of immigration and when the overwhelming number of all immigrants came from the British Isles and were Protestant."[66] The second period was dated 1775-1820 and was called the era of American Revolution. Gonzalez[50] provides a clear outline of immigration periods from 1820 to the present. Table 2-1 shows the different periods, the people, and their numbers.

Table 2-1. **Immigration periods: 1820-1980**

First Period: Old Immigrants, 1820-1880		
	Germany	3,052,126
	Ireland	2,829,206
	England	962,651
	Canada	654,660
Second Period: New Immigrants, 1881-1920		
	Italy	4,114,603
	Austria-Hungary	3,925,034
	Germany	2,443,565
	Ireland	1,529,144
	England	1,499,367
Third Period: Depression and War Years, 1921-1950		
	Canada	1,204,760
	Germany	752,838
	Italy	581,004
	England	291,428
	Ireland	260,725
	Poland	252,331
Fourth Period: Immigration Reform, 1951-1970		
	Canada	791,262
	Mexico	753,748
	Germany	668,561
	Caribbean	593,304
	China	577,877
	Italy	399,602
	England	330,623
Fifth Period: Third World Immigration, 1971-1980		
	Mexico	640,300
	Philippines	355,000
	Korea	267,600
	Cuba	264,900
	Vietnam	172,800
	India	164,100
	England	137,400
	Italy	129,400
	China	124,300

From Gonzalez JL: *Racial and ethnic groups in America,* Dubuque, Iowa, 1990, Kendall/Hunt.

Immigrants who came to the United States between 1820 and 1881 were called "old immigrants."[50,60,66] These immigrants came from northern and western Europe. "They quickly blended into and reinforced the British, Protestant majority who had become the predominant element of America's population during the colonial period."[60] One group were the Catholic Irish who came from the south of Ireland. A small number were fleeing religious and political persecution under British rule. The great immigration of the Irish occurred when a series of potato crop failures brought famine and hardships, which forced families to seek economic survival elsewhere.[60]

In the period between 1881 and 1920, many people from Europe arrived on American shores. Of these, the Italians, who numbered close to 4 million, were the largest group, and they comprised the "new immigrants."[50]

The third period of immigration was identified with the Great Depression and World War II, two major events responsible for the drastic reduction in the number of immigrants.[66] At the close of the war, immigration policies were enacted to accommodate refugees, American citizens, and legal aliens separated from spouses during the war.[11] This period also encompassed the years when the

National Origins Quota System (NOQS) reduced the volume of immigration from other countries such as the Orient. Most of the immigrants during this period were from the countries of the old immigrants.[66]

The last period, Third World Immigration, was facilitated by the abolition of the NOQS. In 1965, President Lyndon Johnson signed the Immigration and Nationality Act. The goals of this act were to (1) provide for the unification of families; (2) increase the pool of skilled and educated aliens; (3) ease population problems caused by environmental and social upheavals; (4) facilitate international exchange programs; and (5) prevent entry of poor aliens, those with health problems, or those with criminal records.[50]

It is important to note that only with the ending of the quota system did any shift come about in the pattern of arrivals. "By and large, the shift has been in favor of those whom the old quota system was designed to exclude – southern and eastern Europeans and Orientals. The new law's preference system gave most immigrant visas to relatives of American citizens which favored the eastern Europeans and Orientals."[83]

***Table 2-2.* Comparison of the 1980 and 1990 census of Asian and Hispanic populations**

	Number in thousands	
	1980*	1990†
Asian and Pacific Islander	3,501	7,273
Chinese	806	1,645
Filipino	775	1,406
Japanese	701	847
Asian Indian	362	815
Korean	355	798
Vietnamese	262	614
Other	NA	821
Hispanics	14,608	22,354
Mexicans	8,740	13,495
Puerto Ricans	2,014	2,727
Cubans	803	1,043

*Yetman NR: *Statistical appendix 1: racial and hispanic population in the United States, 1970-1980.* In *Majority and minority: the dynamics of race and ethnicity in American life,* Boston, 1985, Allyn & Bacon.
†US Department of Commerce, New York City Bureau of the Census: *Telephone report of the 1990 census.*
NA, not available.

Refugee Movement

Another type of immigration which changed and increased the U.S. population was the immigration of refugees. Prior to 1965, there was an increase in the number of immigrants seeking political asylum. In the 1960s and 1970s, political refugees from Cuba, Vietnam, and Indochina were admitted by the thousands. The Immigration and Naturalization Act of 1976 created the Select Commission on Immigration and Refugee Policy. In addition, the passing of the Refugee Act of 1980 broadened the definition of refugee. This new definition allowed the entry of more Cubans. In 1986, the Immigration Reform and Control Act made an important provision – the legalization of undocumented aliens.[50]

In this century then, the abolition of the National Origins Quota System and the series of refugee acts increased the numbers of two ethnic groups, namely, the Hispanics and Asians or Orientals. Table 2-2 shows a comparison between 1980 and 1990 census data on these two groups.

As immigrants begin to settle in a new land, they are exposed to the host culture. Do they lose their identity? What becomes of their culture, customs, traditions, and values?

Immigrants to Ethnics

Decades of studies and deliberations among social anthropologists, sociologists, and other scientists have produced two major opposing perspectives. "The analysis of ethnicity in American sociology has been dominated by an argument between the assimilationist and the pluralistic perspectives."[125]

The assimilationist position maintains that cultural differences between groups disappear as generations pass. The earliest proponent of this position was Zangwill[127] who saw all the races of Europe coming to the United States, the melting pot. "The melting pot theory was the first attempt to analyze what was happening to immigrants in the United States."[29]

The pluralistic view strongly maintains the need for continued persistence of the immigrants' culture. The position of cultural pluralism developed as a response to the question, regarding the relationship of immigrant populations to the host culture.[29] This perspective appears to have stronger support in the literature on ethnicity. How immigrants maintain their identity can be explained further by an understanding of the concept of ethnicity.

The Concept of Ethnicity

The word ethnicity was derived from the Greek word *ethos*, which meant tribe, race, nation, or people. More recently, it has come to be associated with customs, socialization, and cultural patterns rather than biologic origins.[71] Individuals with a sense of their ethnicity tended to have a "sense of belonging or fellow-feeling"[94] shared with other members of the same ethnic group. This shared sense might be manifested in "kinship patterns, physical contiguity (as in localism or sectionalism), religious affiliation, language or dialect forms, tribal affiliations, nationality, phenotypical features, or a combination of these."[97]

Isajiw[62] suggested that "ethnicity refers to an involuntary group of people who identify themselves and/or are identified by others as belonging to the same involuntary group." Though this definition referred more to an ethnic group, it contained an important element identified in Staiano's[104] definition. This author defined ethnicity as a process, "an on-going response, a reaction to the categorical ascription of others as well as a reaction to the creation and incorporation of symbols into the collective identity." Both definitions incorporated the process of identifying ethnic group members by other individuals. This identification could be clearly understood as the process of ethnicization.

The Process of Ethnicization

DeSantis and Benkin[33] stated that individuals are perceived as ethnics by virtue of their being in a foreign land. Natives are, therefore, not ethnics in their own countries. The process of becoming an ethnic is initiated by the social processes resulting from large-scale immigration when natives leave their countries with regional identities as opposed to a national one.[25]

Sarna[96] proposed a model of ethnicization based on ascription and adversity. He proposed that immigrants, upon entry into a new land, are identified based on a classification scheme such as the Immigration Commission's Dictionary of Races. The use of race as a classification criterion is subscribed to and reinforced by the government, schools, churches, the political machine, the media, and the public at large. As immigrants begin to de-emphasize their regional identities and view themselves according to a classification scheme intelligible to others, then they have become ethnics. Through this process of ascription, the immigrants' self-definitions and others' definition of them merge into one. This ascribed classification is accepted by the immigrants as "part of defense against prejudice and hostility." Barth[6] proposed that the emergence of a printing press and mutual and benevolent societies are considered ethnic symbols and serve to unite ethnics. Ethnic symbols are "routine items internal to the culture and/or race" and are emphasized by ethnics to differentiate themselves. Further, ethnics create new symbols in an effort to stimulate solidarity and self-consciousness.[96] For example, the author's friends and church members organized an ethnic organization to facilitate the maintenance of cultural traditions which foster the ethnic identities of their American-born children.

Racial, Ethnic, and Minority Groups

Race, considered a biologic term, refers to a grouping of individuals who share distinct physical characteristics such as skin color, hair texture, or facial features.[7,39,48] (See Fig. 2-1.) A *racial group* may be defined as "a group of people of the same race who interact with one another and who develop some common cultural characteristics."[39] On the other hand, an *ethnic group* is a "collectivity within a larger society"[41] with its markedly contrasting values, rituals, and maintenance of separate institutions thus, differentiating it from the larger society.[93] Both racial and ethnic groups share commonalities which strengthen the individual's sense of identity and belonging.

Often an ethnic group is identified as a minority group, but each may be distinct from a sociologic perspective. A *minority group* is "any group that has less than its proportionate share of wealth, power, and/or social status."[39] The identity of the minority group is made in relation to the dominant group defined as "a collectivity within a society which has a preeminent authority to function as guardians and sustainers of the controlling value system and as prime allocators of rewards in society."[97] A minority may consist of a particular racial, religious, or occupational group.[7] A group may be identified as either a minority group or an ethnic group or both.

The process of becoming an ethnic and identification with an ethnic group serve many functions. Ethnicity plays an important role in the life process of an individual by conveying the orientations, values, role expectations, norms, and social responsibility, patterns of involvement, commitment, loyalty, and solidarity.[71] The person's values and perceptions about health and illness evolve from the socialization process within one's ethnic group. A sense of ethnicity also inspires the person to form a network of individual and group relationships "crystallized by frequent associations and identifications with common origins."[125] The importance and emphasis placed by individuals on their families and relatives as sources of formal and informal support during illness and crises are significant aspects of ethnic culture. Ethnicity provides the guidelines for the organization of individual and group life through established and integrated life patterns.[71] Specific roles and expectations regarding different life situations facilitate optimal functioning of individuals. For example, in certain ethnic groups, male and female members assume different culturally designated roles related to coping with the illness of a parent. Last, ethnicity provides a "cultural screen"[5] through which value systems of other groups are evaluated. This function is operational when ethnics select which health care system would best serve them, that is, their own folk system or the Western system. This will be discussed more fully under "Health as a Value."

Culture, Values, Value Orientations

Ethnicity is evidenced in customs which reflect the socialization and cultural patterns of the group. Culture, as an element in ethnicity, consists of shared patterns of values and behaviors that are characteristics of a particular

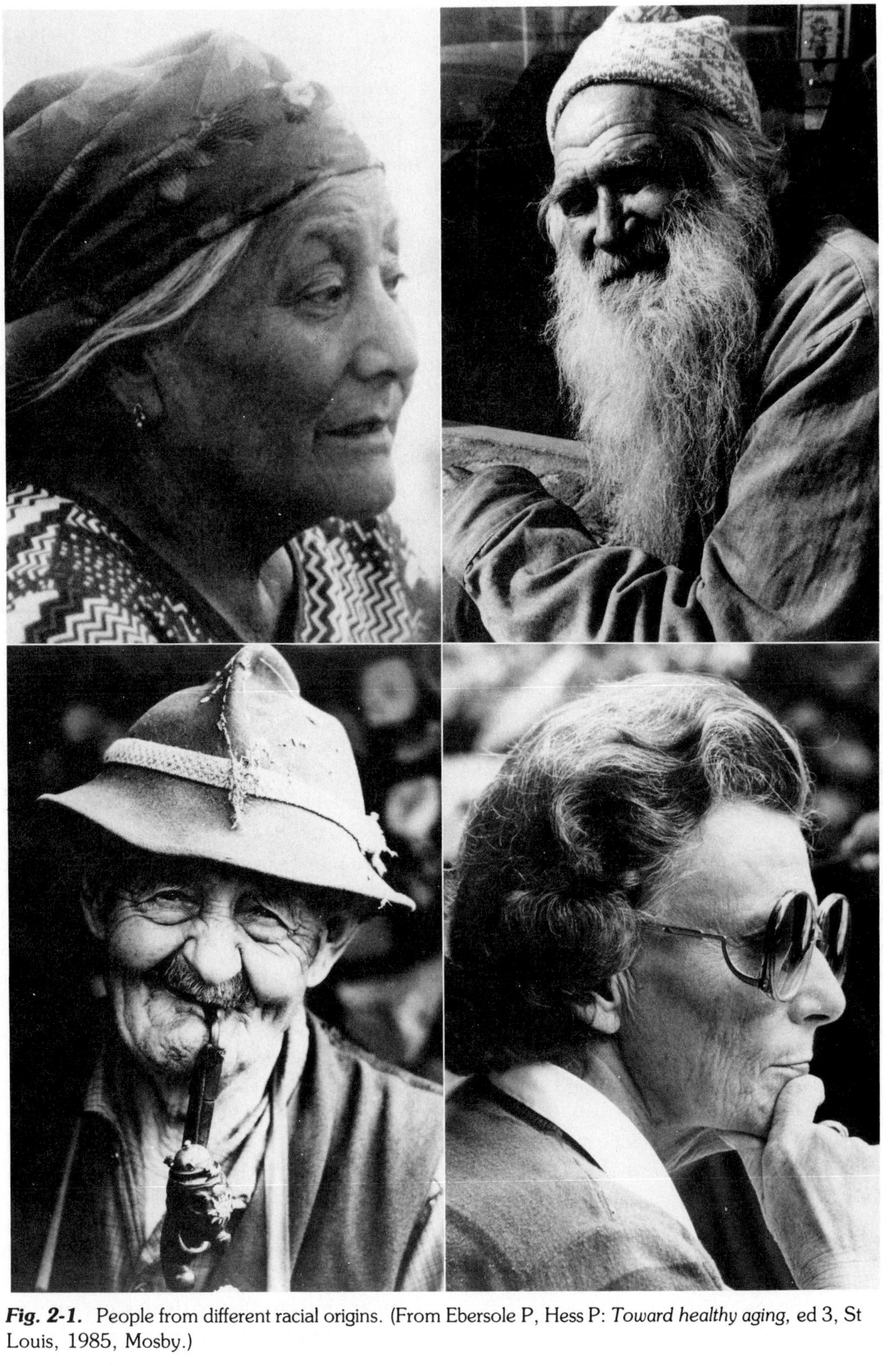

Fig. 2-1. People from different racial origins. (From Ebersole P, Hess P: *Toward healthy aging,* ed 3, St Louis, 1985, Mosby.)

***Table 2-3.* Cultural value orientations**

Theme	Solution types A	Solution types B	Solution types C
What is man's innate human nature?	*Evil:* Either unalterable or perfectible only with discipline and effort	*Mixed:* A combination of good and evil: lapses in behavior are unavoidable, but self-control is possible	*Good:* Unalterable or corruptible
What is man's relationship to nature?	*Destiny:* Man is subjugated to nature: fatalism, inevitability	*Harmony:* Man and nature exist together as a single entity	*Mastery:* Natural forces are to be overcome and put to man's use
What is man's significant time dimension?	*Past:* Focus is on ancestors and traditions	*Present:* The time is "now"; little attention is paid to the past; future is considered vague or unpredictable	*Future:* Orientation is toward progress and change; not content with present; past considered "old-fashioned"
What is the purpose of man's being?	*Being* (Dionysian): Spontaneous expression of impulses and desires; nondevelopmental in focus	*Being-in-becoming* (Apollonian): Self-contained and inner controlled; detachment that brings enlightenment; development and self-realization paramount	*Doing* (Promethean): Active striving and accomplishment; competition against externally applied standards of achievement
What is man's relationship with his fellow men?	*Lineal:* Continuity through time; heredity and kinship ties; ordered succession	*Collateral:* Group goals primary focus; family orientation	*Individual:* Personal autonomy and independence; authority not absolute; group goals submerged; individual goals dominate

From Kluckhohn FR: *Dominant and variant value orientations.* In Kluckhohn C, Murray HA, editors: *Personality in nature, society, and culture*, ed 2, New York, 1953, Knopf. Reprinted by permission of The Estate of F.R. Kluckhohn.

group.[78] *Culture* "consists of symbols, values, and beliefs regarding the self, and others, the external social world, events of nature, and events of history."[30] These values and behaviors which relate to basic areas of life are incorporated into cultural patterns, and they survive through the teaching-learning process,* though one may see innovations from time to time.

Cultural values determine what behaviors are desirable and how particular behaviors are interpreted and judged. *Values*, as shared elements of a symbolic system, serve as criteria of the desirable.[69] "They influence the selection from available modes, means, and ends of action."[28]

Value orientations, learned and shared through the socialization process, reflect the personality type of a particular society. Those that are shared by the majority of the group are the dominant value orientations. Kluckhohn's[69] model on value orientations incorporates themes regarding basic human nature, the relationships of human beings to nature, human beings' time orientation, valued personality type, and dominant modality of relationship between and among human beings. Table 2-3 on cultural value orientation provides the solutions to the themes proposed by Kluckhohn.[69]

HEALTH AS A VALUE

Leininger, the pioneer and founder of Transcultural Nursing, stated that a "cultural value of particular interest to health personnel is the heightened emphasis on optimum health for all American citizens."[75] Further, health care is believed by many individuals to be a fundamental right for all citizens.[1] However, this value and belief meet complex implementation issues because many barriers exist. For instance, health care for poor Americans is less than optimum because of their inability to pay for services. Therefore, accessibility has a limited definition for these individuals. In addition there are many barriers

*References 49, 54, 57, 67, 72, and 81.

which prevent individuals from seeking preventive care, including (1) difficulties getting to the facilities; (2) long waiting periods in clinics; and (3) unattractive, impersonal surroundings of health care facilities. Fragmentation of care and ethnocentric, impersonal attitudes of some health care providers place individuals in uncomfortable situations when intimate and personal information are sought from them. Health care insurance is not affordable by many poor Americans whose priorities are their basic needs of food, clothing, and shelter rather than health care. For ethnic groups, health as a value may have different definitions, and their behaviors may reflect this. A discussion of the health beliefs and practices of selected ethnic groups in subsequent pages will clarify this statement.

Incongruent beliefs and attitudes about health and the use of health care services of ethnic groups and the rest of the population, particularly health care providers, are major barriers in introducing improvements in health status of ethnic group members. Leininger[76] stated that

> in general professional nurses and other health care personnel tend to support the cultural value of optimum health, for it is viewed as their primary interest and their professional raison d'être. Their desire to promote this professional health value among cultural and subcultural groups whose health values differ significantly from theirs may well get in the way of being a helpful professional person.

Therefore, it is imperative that a closer scrutiny of folk health care systems and the Western view be considered. This may give health care professionals an understanding of how these can coexist and provide optimum benefits to individuals.

FOLK AND WESTERN HEALTH CARE

"Health policies and practices in the United States have been formulated within the context of Western scientific and cultural values."[1] Therefore, differences in perceptions, orientations, and values of ethnic groups regarding health and illness could create potential difficulties in health care situations.

"The practice of Western medicine is viewed as professional care."[16] In professional care, there is an emphasis on curative approaches based on "scientifically proven methods and research data to the exclusion of treatments which may not have a basis in research."[1] Care is provided by a professional group who claims a kind of authority which "involves not only skill in performing a service, but also the capacity to judge the experience and needs of others."[106] Folk systems, on the other hand, embody the beliefs, values, and treatment approaches of a particular cultural group. These values are a product of cultural development, and they are not based on "the conceptual framework of medicine."[16] Folk health practices are seen in a variety of settings, including community groups, kinship groups, private homes, and healers' shrines. "Folk healers range from priests and shamans to fortune tellers, astrologers, and geomancers. Unlicensed practitioners such as lay midwives, bone setters, some dentists, and herbalists are part of the folk sector, as are religious practitioners such as spiritualists, Christian Science healers, and users of scientology."[16]

Other areas of differences between folk and Western health care systems are summarized in Table 2-4.

***Table 2-4.* A comparison between folk and Western health care systems**

Criteria	Western	Folk
Philosophy of care	Curative	Curative
Approach to care	Fragmented specialization Often impersonal	Personalized
Setting for services	Institutions	Homes, community, and other social places
Treatments	Technology Approved pharmacologic agents	Herbs, charms, amulets, massage, meditation
Providers	Licensed professionals	Healers, shamans spiritualists, priests, other lay unlicensed therapists
Support for care	Other ancillary personnel and agencies	Family, relatives, friends
Payment for services	Third-party insurers Personal funds	Negotiable
Philosophy of health	Influenced by the professional's definition and dealt with in terms of illness and treatment	Reflected as a quest for harmony with nature
Definition of disease	The result of cause–effect phenomena and the cure is achieved by scientifically proven methods	Illness is an imbalance between the person, the physical, social, and spiritual worlds

The Ethnic Group's Choice

The choice of health care system varies among different ethnic groups and among individuals within the same group. Often, there is a combined use, in different degrees and at different times, of the services and resources from each system. Situational factors – including access, perceived degree of severity of the illness and its symptoms, previous experiences with each system, ability to pay for the services and treatments – may singly or in combination influence which system to approach.

Scott[99] conducted a study of health and healing among five ethnic groups, including Bahamians, Cubans, Haitians, Puerto Ricans, and southern U.S. Blacks. The study indicated that each ethnic group practiced different healing practices. It also showed that reliance on the ethnic group's folk healing system continued because "the scientific health care system is not sufficiently relevant to multiethnic populations in urban U.S. areas."

Ethnic individuals' preference for their own folk healing systems is motivated by their familiarity and even close acquaintance with the folk healer who usually speaks the same language and is knowledgeable of the folk beliefs, customs, and traditions of the ethnic group. Easy access and the individual's perceived ability to pay for the healer's services are real advantages when compared to difficulties getting appointments, long waits, and unfamiliar institutional settings in the Western system.

When folk healing practices are not effective, the individual may turn to Western health care. Health care professionals such as nurses should, in their assessments, "determine what folk treatments clients have used and what benefits were obtained without demeaning the clients or their health beliefs."[13] Through a culturally sensitive assessment process, nurses can determine the specific folk remedies clients are using and whether their continued use would interfere with the prescribed therapeutic regimen. Tripp-Reimer, Brink, and Saunders[110] have developed a tool for cultural assessment which can be extremely useful for nurses in working with ethnically diverse clients. In addition, Geissler[47] suggested a taxonomy of nursing diagnoses for culturally diverse clients.

Health care professionals must avoid an ethnocentric perspective when working with ethnic groups. An ethnocentric perspective which sees that "all other ways are inferior, unnatural, or perhaps barbaric"[44] is a major obstacle in establishing and maintaining good working relationships with consumers of health care services.

Ethnic groups will continue to use folk remedies and healing. Therefore, health care professionals need to take a look at the many positive aspects of folk systems. The holistic approach, incorporation of family and support systems, consideration of the individual's viewpoint, and the caring approach are just a few of the more positive aspects of folk systems that Western health care systems are recognizing. It is believed that the blend of both would optimize health care for ethnic Americans.

ASIAN-PACIFIC ISLANDERS

Asian-Pacific Islanders comprise the second largest ethnic group in the total U.S. population. According to the Bureau of Census, there were just slightly over 7 million Asians in 1990 compared to the 3.5 million in 1980.[8] Table 2-2 on p. 27 shows the comparison of the groups in 1980 and 1990. A complete discussion of the immigration history of each Asian group is beyond the scope of this chapter. Kitano and Daniels[66] classify Filipinos as Asians, whereas Samoans, Guamanians, and Hawaiians are identified as Pacific Islanders. Asian-Pacific Islanders are naturalized citizens or legal residents of the United States whose parents or ancestors have their origins from one or a combination of Asian countries, namely China, Japan, Korea, Southeast Asia, and Vietnam.

A look at the status of Asian-Pacific Islanders reveals that they are doing relatively well in their new home (see box below). "Like all Americans, education has been the primary key to Asian American success. By investing time, energy, and resources in higher education, Asian Americans have been able to move up steadily in the hierarchy of occupations."[58] The importance of education from the Asian-Pacific Islanders' perspective is evident in both secondary and higher education. For instance, the 8% dropout rate of Asian-Pacific Islanders from 10th grade was the lowest.[114] A greater number of Asian-Pacific Islanders earned bachelor's, master's, and doctor's

❑ ❑ ASIAN-PACIFIC ISLANDERS

1990 U.S. Population: 7,273,662, or 3%
Median Age: 30.4 years
High School Education: 82% among 25 years and older
Four or More Years College: 39% among 25 years and older
Marital Status: 80% married couples
Labor Force Participation: Male: 72%
Female: 56%
Median Earnings: Male: $26,760
Female: $21,320
Family: $42,250*
Poverty Level: 11%

From Bennett CE: *The Asian and Pacific Islander in the United States: March 1991 and 1990*, US Bureau of the Census, *Current population reports, P 20-459*, Washington, DC, 1992, US Government Printing Office.

*There were 3 or more earners in 19% of the families.

***Table 2-5.* Comparison among Whites and ethnic groups by higher education degrees conferred**

	White	Black	Hispanic	Asian-Pacific Islander	American Indian Alaskan Natives
Total number in 1990 U.S. population	199,686,070	29,986,060	22,354,059	7,273,662	1,959,234
High school class 1980 attending 4-yr college					
Full-time	8.3	5.6	6.2	18.3	6.6
Part-time	4.2	3.3	4.3	8.3	1.0
Associate degrees conferred: 1989-1990	368,529	52,278	22,062	13,426	3,525
Bachelor's degrees conferred: 1989-1990	882,996	61,074	32,686	39,059	4,338
Master's degrees conferred: 1989-1990	251,518	15,331	7,905	10,646	1,108
Doctor's degrees conferred: 1989-1990	25,793	1,145	783	1,282	102

From US Department of Education, National Center for Education Statistics, Office of Educational Research and Improvement: *Digest of Education Statistics 1992*, Washington, DC, 1992, US Government Printing Office.

degrees in 1989-1990 compared to Hispanics and Native Americans. (See Table 2-5.)

Health Problems of Asian-Pacific Islanders

Variations in the health status of Asian-Pacific Islanders are due primarily to sub-cultures within the larger group. As a group, Asian-Pacific Islanders suffer from cardiovascular disease and cancer, their leading causes of death. Also, many show a high incidence of tuberculosis and hepatitis B, which is linked to high incidence of liver cancer, cirrhosis, and other chronic liver problems. The incidence of tuberculosis in Southeast Asians is 40 times higher than the rest of the total U.S. population.[116] Compared to the general population, Chinese have a higher prevalence of eye pathologies, malnutrition, dental caries, and mental disorders.[13] Issues related to mental disorders are probably related to the combination of stress of adjustment, lack of adequate family support, and conflicting cultural values.[26]

Health-Related Cultural Aspects

Asian-Pacific Islanders share many commonalities in their traditional values. Chang[24] summarized these important values:

1. The family is an extended one with grandparents, uncles, aunts, and cousins considered as part of the household.
2. Within the family, there is differential treatment based on age and gender. The elderly male is usually the considered head.
3. The family's interests and honor supersede that of the individual; therefore, every member strives to avoid those situations which may bring shame to the family.
4. Older individuals are respected, and their authority is unquestioned. In addition, filial piety assures loyalty and devotion from children.
5. The maintenance of harmony is a priority, so Asians have a strong emphasis on the avoidance of conflict and direct confrontations.
6. Strong emotions or feelings are suppressed and discouraged. Self-control and bravery are upheld even in pain, hardships, and strong emotional conflicts.
7. There is a strong emphasis on the recognition of people with authority, so disagreement with them is avoided.

Asian Americans try to inculcate these values in their children. Many find the task difficult because some of these values conflict with the dominant cultural values (i.e., passivity) to avoid conflict versus assertiveness. Exposure of Asian American children to different cultures in schools and their neighborhoods facilitates their adoption of other cultural beliefs and attitudes in their socialization. In addition, employment of immigrant women outside the home have exposed children to other caretakers. In addition, the likelihood of absent grandparents who are important transmitters of culture has contributed to the identification of children with the dominant host culture.[119]

Asian folk medicine and philosophies have a strong Chinese influence as the result of early Chinese migration all over Asia. Therefore, the folk medicines of Filipinos, Japanese, Koreans, and Southeast Asians are imbued with Chinese influence.

The Taoist religion was the philosophic and theoretic foundation and basis of Chinese medicine. According to the Tao doctrines, humans are microcosms within the universe. Achieving harmony between the two is essential because the energies of both intertwine. Two forces, Yin and Yang, keep innate energy (called Chi) and sexual energy (called Jing) in balance. Yin is feminine, negative dark, and cold; whereas Yang is masculine, positive, and warm. An imbalance in energy can be caused, for instance, by yielding to strong emotions or eating an improper diet. Both humans and the universe, in their interactions, are susceptible to the forces of the earth, fire, water, metal, and wood.[55]

Asian folk medicine uses a wide variety of herbs, roots, leaves, seeds, tree bark, and parts of flowers for healing purposes. In Chinatown, New York City, there are several drug stores which sell these varieties of folk remedies.

Some aspects of Asian folk medicine have gained popularity within the Western system of health care. Of these, the one best known is acupuncture. The acceptance of this treatment, as an adjunct rather than a replacement for Western treatment, may pave the way for the use of other folk remedies. Other alternate treatment modalities which are slowly gaining wide acceptance are meditation, therapeutic touch, massage, imagery, relaxation, and bipolarity. (See Chapters 13 and 14 for further discussions.)

HISPANIC AMERICANS

The Hispanic population in the United States numbered 19.4 million, or 8.1% of the total 1980 U.S. population.[111] Their increasing numbers are seen in the 1990 census, which documented 23 million, or 8.9% of the total population.[46] According to the author's descriptions between ethnic and minority designations, Hispanic Americans comprise the largest ethnic group in the United States (see box on this page for current information).

Hispanic Americans immigrate from many countries. In March 1991, the Hispanic population consisted of 62.6% Mexicans, 13.6% Central and South Americans, 11.1% Puerto Ricans, 4.9% Cubans, and 7.6% other Hispanics.[46]

California, Texas, Arizona, Colorado, and New Mexico have the largest Hispanic population. California and Texas have 55.2% of the total Hispanic population; New York has 10.9%; Florida has 7.6%; Illinois has 4.1%; and New Jersey has 3.3%.[45]

Hispanics are making educational strides. For example, from the total Hispanic population, there was a rise from 32% in 1970 to 51% in 1988 in the number of Hispanics, 25 years and older, completing 4 or more years of high school. College-level education also increased from 5% in 1970 to 10% in 1988. Although these strides in education are promising, Hispanics in the 10th grade had the second highest dropout rates in 1989.[114]

❑ ❑ HISPANIC AMERICANS

1990 U.S. Population: 22,354,059, or 8.6%
Median Age: 26.2 years
High School Education: 51%
Four or More Years College: 9.7%
Marital Status: 56.7% married couples
Labor Force Participation: Male: 78%
Female: 51%
Median Earnings: Male: $14,000
Female: $10,000
Family: $23,400
Poverty Level: 25%

From Garcia JM, Montgomery PA: *The Hispanic population in the United States: March 1991*, US Bureau of the Census, Current Population Reports, Series P 20-455, Washington, DC, 1991, US Government Printing Office.

Language often acts as a barrier as demonstrated by the fact that 50% of school dropouts are not fluent in English. This lack of language skill also comprises their inability to find suitable employment.

Health Problems of Hispanic Americans

Although cardiovascular disease and cancer are the first and second causes of morbidity and mortality among Hispanics, incidence of these diseases is lower among Hispanics than among the general population. However, Hispanics have higher rates of diabetes, alcohol-related problems, mortality from homicides, and AIDS.[121] Hispanics receive less preventive health care. For instance, in 1987 only 39% of Hispanic women received prenatal care during their first trimester of pregnancy.[116]

The difficulties experienced by Hispanics in receiving appropriate health care services are identical to the poor. In addition, many Hispanic Americans may not readily seek care because of their continued reliance on their folk system of healing and their difficulties negotiating the health care system because of a language barrier.

Health-Related Cultural Aspects

Each sub-group of the Hispanic population has distinct cultural beliefs and customs. However, a common heritage determines similar values and beliefs. For instance, among all Hispanics, the emphasis on family and religion are the two most important aspects of their culture.

The family is the most important source of support.[85] The needs of the family as a whole supersede that of the individual. In times of illness and crisis, the family is there for the individual.[13] Older family members and relatives are accorded courtesy and respect and are often consulted on important matters.[77,86]

Hispanics' dependence on their spiritual strength to aid them in their illness and dying is seen in their praying.[82] Hispanics put their trust in God and believe that harmony with God is essential in maintaining health. Furthermore, an offense to God warrants punishment.[13]

Hispanics attribute the origins of disease and illness to (1) spiritual or natural punishments, (2) hot and cold imbalances, (3) magic, (4) dislocation of internal organs, (5) natural diseases, and (6) emotional and mental origins.[27]

The hot and cold concept of disease was derived from the Hippocratic theory of pathology. Illness occurs when there is an imbalance.[87,121] This concept of hot and cold guides Hispanics when they categorize illnesses and select appropriate treatments. For example, rheumatic fever is considered a cold illness. Therefore, through the process of neutralization, a hot treatment would correct the imbalance. In this instance, penicillin, considered a hot substance, would be an acceptable treatment.

Hispanics still resort to many home remedies and consult a folk healer, the "curandero."[82] Curanderos use a variety of folk remedies, including prayers, rituals, herbs, and the laying on of hands.[34]

Among Hispanics there is a continued use of folk remedies to augment Western approaches as long as these do not harm the individual. The individual's belief in the folk remedy can have positive effects on the person's well-being. Therefore, Western health care professionals need to find the ways which will blend the two systems to the optimum benefit of Hispanic individuals and families.

BLACK AMERICANS

Currently, there are 29 million Black Americans, or 12.1% of the total population.[9] Black Americans constitute the largest minority group, a designation consistent with the definitions set forth in the previous pages. The identification of Black Americans as a minority group in spite of the ethnic diversity was summed up in this statement: "The case of Black Americans is unique in its history of slavery, of extreme segregation, exclusion, and discrimination."[91]

Black Immigration to the United States

The immigration history of Blacks to the United States is significantly different from that of Europeans, Asians, and Hispanics. The beginning of Black America is recorded as the time when Blacks were crew members in a pirate ship that docked in America in 1619.[10] In their study of black migration, Johnson and Campbell[64] wrote that although Blacks had participated in many types of migration, they noted that the predominant type in Blacks had been the forced or impeled type imposed by explorers of the New World, Spain, and Portugal. In the New World, many thriving industries had high demands for labor which the Native Americans could not fill. Africans were captured and sold as slaves. In the history of black slavery, an estimated 6 million Africans were brought to America and enslaved.[10] Thus, the saga of centuries of injustices began. This chapter touched only a very small part of history but one that had a lasting impact to the current status of Black Americans (see box below).

An extensive study of Black Americans conducted collaboratively by the Committee on the Status of Black Americans, Commission on Behavioral and Social Sciences and Education, and the National Research Council revealed gains in areas such as education and employment. However, these gains are far from being adequate to meet the social, economic, and health care needs of Black Americans.

Educationally, Blacks have made substantial gains, but they continue to experience less-than-optimum standards in schools and educators. Blacks' achievement outcomes are far below those of Whites. For instance, in 1988, black eighth graders' performance in mathematics showed that 27.6% were below basic knowledge, compared to 15.5% in the White population. Furthermore, black 10th graders had a dropout rate of 22%, compared to the 15% for Whites.[114] In 1988, the college enrollment of black males and females 18 to 24 years of age was 25.0% and 30.5%, respectively, compared to 39.4% for white males and 36.9% for white females.[115] Further,

❑ ❑ BLACK AMERICANS

1990 U.S. Population: 29,986,000, or 11.7%
Median Age: 27.9 years
High School Education: Male: 71.9%
Female: 77.9%
Four or More Years College: Male: 16.7%, 35 to 44 years old
Female: 14.5%, 35 to 44 years old
Marital Status: 50.2% married couples
Labor Force Participation: Male: 70.1%
Female: 57.8%
Median Earnings: Male: $20,430
Female: $17,390
Family: $20,210
Poverty Level: 30.7%

From Bennett CE: *The Black population in the United States: March 1990 and 1989,* US Bureau of the Census, Current population reports Series P 20-448, Washington, DC, 1991, US Government Printing Office.

in all levels of higher education, Blacks lag behind Whites as seen in Table 2-5.

Based on 1989 data, Blacks experienced a 30.7% poverty level, compared to the 10.0% experienced by Whites. The median earnings of black males were about 69% of White males' median earnings. In contrast, black females' median incomes were about 98% of white females' earnings. This could be attributed to black female workers' longer work hours and job tenure compared to white female workers.[9]

The information presented paints a bleak socioeconomic profile that increases Blacks' risk for many health problems.

Health Problems of Black Americans

A complex set of social, economic, and environmental factors could be identified as contributors to the current health status of Black Americans. However, poverty may be the most profound and pervasive determinant of the health status of Black Americans.[91] In the United States, health care is a commodity which can be purchased according to an individual's ability to pay.[39] Furthermore, health care is expensive. Needless to say, individuals and families below the poverty level or those who lack adequate resources are the most affected.

Poor people do not have the resources to purchase health care insurance. This limits their access to health care services such as prenatal and maternal care, childhood immunizations, dental checkups, well-child care, and a wide range of preventive services. Decreased resources for preventive care may necessitate the more expensive services such as emergency room care and intensive care in times of severe illness.

Two indexes of the effects of poverty can be seen in the high rates of infant and maternal mortality. Despite the changes in living conditions, advances in infection control, and improved standards in neonatal care, Blacks still experience high infant mortality rates. The black infant mortality rate for 1989 was 18.6% compared to 8.1% for the white population.[90]

Black American children, living below the poverty level, suffer numerous health problems, including malnutrition, anemia, and lead poisoning. These and the lack of immunizations combine to inhibit normal growth and development and, in turn, affect school performance.

Poverty-stricken families and their children usually live in depressed socioeconomic areas where housing conditions are unsafe and unhygienic. Unsafe buildings and other environmental structures cause injuries and accidents to young children. Toddlers and young children have fallen to their deaths from windows that were unprotected by metal railings. Older people suffer falls and other injuries from poorly lit stairways and hallways. Other hazards include uncollected garbage and abandoned buildings often used as dump sites and meeting places for a variety of illegal activities.

High hospital admission rates and stays for all Blacks are attributed largely to adolescent pregnancies and reproductive-related conditions. Homicide, motor vehicle accidents, and suicides are also high in adolescent Blacks. For black males 15 to 34 years of age, homicide is the leading cause of death. AIDS among Blacks, which is triple in occurrence compared to Whites, is the current major health problem.[92]

The black population suffers approximately the same death rates from cardiovascular disease and cancer as the general population. However, black men have a 25% higher risk for all cancers and a 45% higher incidence of lung cancer. A higher rate of death in Blacks occurs after diagnosis of cancer. Diabetes is 33% more prevalent. Severe high blood pressure is more common in both males and females.[116]

Health-Related Cultural Aspects

Differences in cultural beliefs, attitudes, and practices exist between rural and urban Black Americans; however, they share common basic cultural beliefs. Black culture is centered on the family and religion.[109] Billingsley,[12] a leading black sociologist, recognizes the family as the strongest institution for Blacks. There are strong kinship bonds extended to grandparents, aunts, uncles, and cousins. The family is considered the strongest source of support, especially in times of crisis and illness. Within the family there is usually a key member who is consulted on important decisions.[13]

"For some Black Americans, religion has functioned principally as an escape mechanism for the harsh realities of daily life. The Black church has created self-respect out of poverty and it functions in promoting a high level of self-esteem."[14] In church services, Blacks have a feeling of oneness as they respond to the minister and pray and sing in the style characteristic of their African heritage.[105] Comer[31] sees the Black church as a place to release emotions, including frustrations and helplessness, toward the daily injustices they have to face.

Black Americans see life as a process rather than just a physical state.[103] In this process, they believe that in order to remain well, harmony with nature must be maintained. Therefore, illness is considered a state of disharmony.[63]

Black Americans continue to use their own traditional health system, particularly if they lack access to the Western health care system. Traditionally, roots, herbs, potions, oils, powders, tokens, rituals, and ceremonies are still used in many Southern communities. There is also use of healers, including (1) the elder who is knowledgeable on herbs, (2) the spiritualist who focuses more on psychologic problems, and (3) the voodoo priest who is considered to be powerful and can cause desired events.[65]

As indicated in the previous discussions regarding the folk health practices of both Asian and Hispanic Americans, Black Americans' folk healing beliefs and practices can augment the Western system. Black Americans often find comfort and solace in the support that their religious leader or traditional healer can give them. Health care providers must find an appropriate place for these nontraditional modalities in caring for Black Americans.

NATIVE AMERICANS

Native Americans, referred to as "bronze-skinned men and women from northern Asia,"[88] populated America thousands of years before Columbus's discovery. Chroniclers of Native American history believe that these people came to Alaska via land bridges now known as the Bering Strait.[36,37,108] Native Americans came to be known as Indians, a label given by Columbus when he encountered the natives in the West Indies which he mistook for the East Indies. This label extended to all native peoples of North and South America, from the Arctic to Tierra del Fuego.[36]

Prior to 1492, there were 5 million Native Americans. Columbus's discovery brought colonization and settlement by various European groups who numbered 75 million by 1890. The ancestral lands of the Native Americans were usurped, and the Native Americans were forced by the settlers to labor on farms and mines. Thousands died from disease, the hard labor, and attempts to escape slavery.[37] Other events such as the removal of the Southeastern tribes in 1830, the Navajos' Long March to Fort Sumner in 1864, and the tragedy of Wounded Knee in 1890 caused the Native American population to dwindle to 250,000 by 1890.[108] The 1890 Census, the first to obtain a complete census of American Indians, reported a growth of 237,000 in 1900 to 357,000 in 1950. The period from 1950-1980 was a time of rapid growth, as the American Indian population grew to nearly 1.4 million.[113]

Native Americans are currently concentrated in Oklahoma, California, Arizona, New Mexico, Alaska, Washington, North Carolina, Texas, New York, and Michigan. Of the total Native American population of almost 2 million, 62.3% live on reservations and 37.7% live on Indian lands.[118] There are 542 tribes, most of which have less than 1000 members. Cherokees and Navajos comprise 25% of the total Native American population.[74] For other information, refer to the box on this page.

Native Americans, the smallest of the ethnic groups discussed in this chapter, also experience the minority group status. In important aspects of life such as educational attainment and income levels, Native Americans lag behind Whites and major ethnic groups. For example, the percentage of Native Americans in the eight grade who performed below basic knowledge and skill in mathematics was the highest, and the percentage of the same group able to do advanced mathematics was the lowest compared to Whites, Asians, Blacks, and Hispanics. In 1989, the dropout rates for 10th graders was 36%, the highest compared to Whites, Asians, Blacks, and Hispanics.[114] Native Americans' percentages for higher-education degrees are low in proportion to their total numbers. For example, in 1989-1990 there were only 102 Native Americans who earned doctoral degrees. Of these, 54 were doctors of medicine.[115] Table 2-5 (p. 33) provides more information on other higher-education degrees.

Income levels for Native Americans in 1990 were low, with a median household income of $20,025, compared with $30,056 nationally. Poverty levels for families was 23.7%, compared with 10.2% nationally.[118]

Low educational attainment and income levels combined with higher rates of poverty are socioeconomic issues which affect the health and quality of life. Native Americans experience the many negative situations which confront poor people, not only in their own reservations but in the larger society as well.

❑ ❑ NATIVE AMERICANS

1990 U.S. Population: 1.9 million
Median Age: 23.5 years
High School Education: 56% (based on 1980 census)*
Four or More Years College: 8% (based on 1980 census)*
Median Earnings: Males: NA
Females: NA
Family: $20,025
Poverty Level: 23.7%

From U.S. Indian Statistics, *Denver Post*, August 18, 1992.
*U.S. Department of Commerce, Bureau of the Census: *We, the first Americans*, Washington, DC, 1989, US Government Printing Office.

Health Problems of Native Americans

Many of the health problems of Native Americans could be linked directly to social and economic conditions.[123] These conditions predispose these people to illnesses and health problems that afflict the poor. Some of these have been discussed under the section on Black Americans.

Most of the excess deaths of Native Americans can be attributed to unintentional injuries, cirrhosis, homicide, suicide, pneumonia, and complications of diabetes. Among Native American males younger than 44 years, unintentional injuries account for one fifth of all deaths each year. Of these, 75% are related to alcohol use.[116]

Among the Sioux and other tribes of the Northern Plains, cancers of the lung are the most common. Adults in these tribes show a 50% to 60% rate of smoking.[107]

The highest known prevalence of diabetes and its associated condition, obesity, is found among Pimas whose eating patterns show a preference for high-carbohydrate, high-fat, low-protein foods.[123] The relationship of unhealthy lifestyles to heart disease and cancer is being addressed by a study because of the high morbidity and mortality rates from these diseases.[107]

Cirrhosis is another chronic problem that afflicts Native Americans more frequently than other groups. Alcohol use affects nearly 95% of all Native American families.[116]

The health problems of Native Americans are complicated by difficult access to health care. Those living on reservations and are served by the Indian Health Service may find that this federally funded agency may not provide the services they need. Those who live in rural areas are underserved by inadequate facilities and qualified personnel. Among first professional-degree graduates in 1989-1990, only 52 Native Americans earned the Doctor of Medicine degree, compared to 12,127 Whites, 887 Blacks, 554 Hispanics, and 1351 Asian-Pacific Islanders.[115]

Health-Related Cultural Aspects

Native Americans are, in general, present oriented; therefore, they emphasize events that are now occurring, rather than those that will be happening. They value cooperation, rather than competition. Sharing of resources is an important component of this cultural value.[55]

Native Americans place great importance on their families and relatives. Three or more generations may form an extended kinship system, enlarged by membership of nonrelatives included through various religious ceremonies.[55]

Though there is great diversity among Native American groups with regards to their beliefs and practices concerning health, illness, and healing, they share a common philosophic base. They believe that a state of health exists when a person is in total harmony with nature. The earth is treated as a living thing and should be treated with respect. Failure to do so harms the body and vice versa.[13,53]

Illness is viewed not as an alteration in the person's physiologic state but, rather, as an imbalance between the ill person and natural or supernatural forces.[68,120]

A renowned Native American healer, Medicine Grizzlybear Lake[73] wrote, "A patient's sickness can be directly traced to committing a violation against natural and spiritual laws, or they may have inherited the violation. This causes the individual to get out of balance, and disharmony causes illness: mentally, physically, emotionally, and spiritually."[74]

Various rituals and healing ceremonies, believed to restore balance when illness occurs, may be carried out by the medicine man or woman believed to have hypnotic powers, the gift of mind reading, and expertise in concocting drugs, medicine, and poisons.[120] The medicine man or woman, called the *shaman*, is called to effect a cure.[32] The shaman is usually a powerful individual in the tribe. Although the power and reverence given to the shamans may vary in different tribes, shamans are nevertheless important because they serve as "keepers of the faith and religion and try to promote spirituality, good health, and good living for the people."[74]

THE CHANGING URBAN POPULATION: HOMELESS PERSONS

Homelessness is a complex social and economic problem which affects the individual, family, and society. The Stewart B. McKinley Homeless Assistance Act (Public Law 100-77) defined the homeless person as one who does not have a fixed, regular, and adequate nighttime residence. Further, the person's nighttime residence may be (1) a supervised or publicly operated shelter designed for temporary living quarters, (2) an institution serving as temporary residence for those requiring institutionalization, or (3) any public or private place not intended for regular sleeping accommodations.[61]

Ropers[95] provided a brief historical view of homeless people in the United States from the end of the Civil War to the emergence of places known as "skid rows." (Skid rows were geographic concentrations of homeless persons, at least since the period after the Civil War.) "Some views of skid row claim that side rows emerged and persisted because they were depositories of deviants, drunks, addicts, and social misfits." Persons who frequented skid rows were labeled as skid row bums and were "generally older, white, uneducated, alcohol dependent men."[15] "Contrary to the traditional stereotypes of homeless people, the homeless of the 1980's are not all single, middle-aged male alcoholics. Neither are they all mentally-ill people made homeless as a by product of the policy of deinstitutionalization of mental health care."[89] The homeless of the 1980s present different characteristics with regards to age, gender, marital status, educational levels, and other important variables.

Burt[18] and colleagues, through the Urban Institute, conducted a comprehensive survey of urban homeless persons. The investigator and associates stratified 178 cities with a population of 100,000 or more (1984 data) by city and size. The investigators felt that "the vast majority of the homeless would be found in cities [where shelter and other services are located]."[18] New York, Los Angeles, Philadelphia, Chicago, Detroit, and Houston, with over 1 million people, were automatically included. An additional 14 cities were randomly selected from the remaining strata. A random sample of 1074 homeless persons drawn from users of soup kitchens and shelters provided the data for this study.

This study of homeless persons showed that single men accounted for 73% of the total sample. Single women and women with children were also represented but in smaller percentages. Both Blacks and non-Hispanics showed significant representation in all categories of both males and females. This sample of homeless persons had mean ages between 30 and 39 years for all categories. This finding indicated that society's concept of homeless persons as older individuals is a stereotype.

Single status (i.e., never married or divorced/separated) appeared to be a major factor related to homelessness. The only exception was widowed status in both genders. Single status also appeared to be strongly related to the length of homelessness. Single men had a mean of 41 months, and single women had a mean of 33 months.

With regards to educational status, a large percentage of the sample either completed 11th grade or graduated from high school. The percentage of homeless persons with college education was very low. The relationship between educational status and employment was not shown. The homeless persons' employment history might help explain their situation. Single men who never worked a steady job had a mean of 50 jobless months, while this was 41 months and 46 months for single women and women with children, respectively.

The diversity of the homeless population and strong indicators leading to homelessness can be clearly seen in this study. Lack of a college education and inability to obtain and/or maintain a steady job characterized this sample. Interesting data from this study point to homelessness as a women's issue as well as a public health problem.[18]

Factors Leading to Homelessness

The major factors leading to homelessness are (1) lack of housing for low-income individuals and families, (2) tightening of eligibility criteria to receive public assistance, and (3) deinstitutionalization policies without adequate community support for the mentally ill.[89]

Inadequate housing in the 1980s for low-income individuals and groups resulted from skyrocketing increases in rents and mortgages.[19,95] In a 1987 statement to the U.S. House, Honorable George Miller, Chairman of the Select Committee on Children, Youth, and Families, declared

> Limited affordable housing and insufficient AFDC [Aid to Families with Dependent Children] grants contribute to family homelessness. . . . Families are a large percentage of the two and a half million people who are displaced from their homes every year as a result of eviction, revitalization projects, economic development plans, and spiraling rent inflation. One half low rent dwellings continue to be lost each year as a result of condominium conversions, abandonment, arson, and demolition.[117]

The ability of families to afford even low-income housing was related to deindustrialization, which began in the 1970s, and subsequent unemployment. Between 1945 to 1975, the average national unemployment rate was 4.6%. By early 1984, it had more than doubled.[95]

The deinstitutionalization of mental patients in the 1960s and the lack of well-planned and organized community resources, such as psychiatric services, housing, and outpatient services to the discharged, increased the numbers of homeless individuals. Some of the housing facilities were "often poorly-regulated, or unregulated, with little or no attention to the health of resident."[70]

The most visible of the homeless, the mentally ill, numbered 433,722 between 1955 and 1983.[95] In Burt's study,[18] slightly more than half of the homeless adult sample had been in one type of institution, including mental hospitals, inpatient settings for chemical dependency, or prison.

Loss of or changes in public assistance programs may have had a major contribution to the homeless situation. Individuals and families receiving general assistance, Social Security income supplemental payments, food stamps, and AFDC found that their benefits had lost purchasing power because of double-digit inflation. In addition, substantial cuts in federal programs, such as the AFDC, affected at least 500,000 low-income families.[95] Furthermore, the tightening of eligibility criteria for federal assistance programs occurred in the face of increased poverty levels.[89]

A state of homelessness is a complex problem involving personal, social, economic, and political ramifications. Although only three major factors have been identified as causing or leading to homelessness, it is not "known how much of the problem can be attributed to family issues, psychiatric disorders, substance abuse, criminality, or a combination of these individual and social system forces."[19]

Health Problems of Homeless Persons

Compared to the general population, homeless individuals experience illness and injuries to a much greater extent.[89] Homeless individuals lack appropriate health care because they do not have health insurance. Facilities which provide some services may be difficult to reach when transportation expenses are involved. The long waits and the unpleasant surroundings of clinics can deter the individual from seeking care. Homeless persons suffer malnutrition and related problems such as anemia and growth problems in children. Use of alcohol and drugs are common.[122] Drapkin[35] identified trauma as one of the major causes of morbidity and death. Even following trauma treatment in an emergency room, the injured homeless person is highly susceptible to a wide range of infections. Lack of hygienic facilities; inadequate resources to carry out the therapeutic regimen; lack of proper nutrition; and lack of a safe, comfortable place to convalesce optimize conditions for complications to occur. Other common health problems of the homeless are tuberculosis, peripheral vascular problems, pediculosis, skin problems, uncontrolled diabetes and hypertension, and in the winter months, hypothermia.[35]

Current and Future Strategies to Alleviate Homelessness

Since homelessness is a multifaceted problem, current strategies have only begun to reveal the tip of the problem. Current short-term measures have limited potential in meeting the basic needs of the homeless, and long-term solutions have begun to drain resources. Therefore, strategies, both short and long term, must be holistic in philosophy, planning, implementation, and evaluation. In addition, "Health and social programs are more likely to be effective if they are planned in areas frequented by the homeless, rather than traditional settings, which may be inconvenient and less responsive to this group."[100]

Ropers[95] suggested that the first step in alleviating the homeless problem is to correct the public's perception of the nature of the population affected. Priority attention should be given to those who provide services to homeless persons. Left uncorrected, these health care workers' stereotypical notions could interfere in health care situations.

Strategies to alleviate homelessness have been primarily short term in nature. Both public and private sectors have been involved in collaborative efforts to meet the emergent needs of the homeless. Current short-term strategies have included the provision of shelters which are both publicly funded and supported by religious or nonprofit organizations. Affordable housing, subsidized by the government, has helped to get individuals and families off the streets. In New York City, housing projects aimed at rehabilitating vacant buildings have provided a very limited number of residences. Long-term projects must be envisioned to accommodate low-income individuals and their children. The Stewart B. McKinley Homeless Assistance Act, passed on July 27, 1987, was an effort to address the long-term solutions to the homeless situation. This Act appropriated funds for the Emergency Shelter Grant Program, Transitional Housing, Permanent Housing for the Handicapped, federal loans for the rehabilitation of single-room occupancy dwellings, and supplemental assistance for facilities to assist homeless persons.[20] Health care, alcohol and drug abuse rehabilitation services, mental health services, and emergency community programs were also funded.

Private funding sources have been available for housing programs. For example, the Robert Wood Johnson Foundation with the Department of Housing and Urban Development and the Department of Health and Human Services, supported community projects which focused on mental health, social services, and housing needs of the chronically mentally homeless.[20] More of these sources must be obtained by community grants proposals. However, as in many cities with large numbers of homeless individuals, such as New York City, problems cannot be solved by housing alone. Homeless people need gainful employment opportunities as long-term strategies.[56]

Increasing employment opportunities for homeless persons can be both short- and long-term goals. Homeless people who are temporarily housed in shelters may be encouraged to contribute toward their daily keep by using their abilities and willingness to assume responsibilities for those tasks essential to the maintenance of the shelter.[20] Furthermore, they can be given temporary work assignments by the government or private agencies which contribute to the operation of the shelter. An example of a long-term strategy in New York City was the creation of the Work Experience Program which gave homeless people training. The skills and attitudes they gained from the experience allowed them to compete for jobs in the economic sector. There is a need for both the government, at all levels, and the private sector to support such short- and long-term strategies.

A variety of short-term measures which provide essential services to meet the basic needs of homeless individuals have been successful in many communities. Programs managed by self-help groups include "drop-in social clubs, financial benefits and other advocacy programs, temporary and transitional housing placements, street outreach programs, and multiservice centers."[20]

Large philanthropic organizations such as the Robert Wood Johnson Foundation and the Pew Memorial Trust, in collaboration with the U.S. Conference of Mayors, have sponsored health programs for the homeless.[112] Continued collaboration among these groups is essential in meeting the basic health care needs such as preventive care through screening of communicable diseases such as tuberculosis.

The efforts of both the public and private sectors deserve recognition. However, many more short- and long-term strategies need to be implemented in order that homelessness does not become a permanent characteristic of the U.S. population. Current programs for the homeless should undergo evaluations to determine cost-effectiveness and success in alleviating the problems of homeless people. Furthermore, there needs to be a critical analysis of the many governmental programs which provide assistance to low-income individuals and families who have a higher risk for homelessness. The reform process needed to revitalize federal, state, and city programs is a monumental task for policy makers. What should guide them in their work when there are so many priorities? In considering the viability of each program, legislators and policy-making bodies need to consider the basic strategy of prevention as opposed to crisis management. Multiple problems which drain available resources and lead to more serious long-term difficulties should be the priority areas for action.

Worth mentioning are some efforts of nurses who are providing solutions to the health care problems of homeless persons and families. Models of care delivery which view the homeless situation as a multifaceted phenomena include the approach used by nurses in the City Coalition for Health Care for the Homeless in a southwestern city. Funded by the Robert Wood Johnson Foundation and the Pew Memorial Trust, this agency uses the Tool for Referral Assessment of Continuity to coordinate referrals and service provision.[100] Another project, the Nursing Center for the Homeless in Buffalo, New York, is directed by Dr. Juanita Hunter, a nurse. Funded by the U.S. Public Health Service, the Center collaborates with other agencies in providing primary care. Nurses see the discharge of homeless persons as the biggest challenge, given the many actual and potential physical and social problems of these individuals.[59] The Center's process of follow-up care is analogous to the process of rebuilding connections with home, families, adequate source of income, and adequate health care services as proposed by Francis.[43]

Homelessness is everyone's problem, and people can ultimately affect the establishment of priorities and reform the agenda that will facilitate improved quality of life. Increasing awareness and knowledge of the current status of homeless people would facilitate understanding of the problem and its ramifications. This understanding would serve as an excellent guide in providing input, taking necessary action, and making the final decision as to what would make a healthy nation.

PERSONS WITH HUMAN IMMUNODEFICIENCY VIRUS (HIV) AND ACQUIRED IMMUNODEFICIENCY SYNDROME (AIDS)

In an official publication dated June 5, 1981, the Centers for Disease Control (CDC) described the deaths of five individuals who succumbed to severe cases of pneumonia.[52] These were the first cases of AIDS. Since then, more than 115,000 cases had been reported by the end of 1989.[21] Projections indicate that by the end of 1993, there will be 390,000 to 480,000 cases in the United States.[23] Since the recognition of the human immunodeficiency virus in 1984, the World Health Organization (WHO) has estimated that the number of HIV-infected adults may be as many as 20 million in the year 2000.[102] In the United States, there are roughly 1 million people infected with HIV. Over one third of cases reported among adult and adolescent women were attributed to heterosexual contact.[17] By the end of 1990, there were 15,894 cases of AIDS in women.[22]

"Despite uncertainty about the incidence of HIV infection and the ultimate magnitude of the problem, HIV and AIDS are a growing threat to the health of a nation and will continue to make major demands on health and social systems for many decades."[116] The projected costs of AIDS in 1992 is $8 billion to $16 billion in health care costs for 175,000 cases.[98]

HIV/AIDS in Ethnic and Minority Groups

Many misconceptions about the transmission of the disease, its incidence, and prevalence still exist. "Despite the disproportionate number of diagnosed AIDS cases among ethnic minorities, the misconception that AIDS is only a 'gay, white male disease' continues to exist."[38] This misconception evolved because "the earliest cases of AIDS that aroused physicians' concern involved white gay men who had unexpected opportunistic infections."[80] With increased and improved methods of monitoring, the United States is seeing different statistics. The disproportionately high incidence of AIDS in ethnic/minority populations can be seen in the 1988 data which showed 26% cases in Blacks and 14% in Hispanics, whereas these groups composed only 12% and 7% of the total U.S. population, respectively.[42] Selik and colleagues[101] did a study through the AIDS Program, Center for Infectious Disease, CDC, between 1981 and 1988. They measured the relative risk (RR) of ethnic/minority groups. The RR in a given group was the ratio of the cumulative incidence of AIDS in that group to the cumulative incidence of AIDS in a reference group. Cumulative index (CI) was equated to the number of AIDS cases reported from June 1, 1981 to January 18, 1988 per million population of the same race/ethnicity. The reference group used was the white population. The highest RRs were seen in central cities' black and Hispanic heterosexual adults who were intravenous drug users. Compared to Whites' RR of 1.0 with a CI of 50.5, Blacks' RR was 6.2 with a CI of 315.6, and Hispanics' RR was 8.8 with a CI of 446.4

Current treatment of AIDS remains disappointing. The battle against the spread of AIDS can be won through zealous preventive measures including serologic testing and modification of sexual practices.[52] However, there are many issues involved in instituting these preventive strategies with ethnic and minority groups.

HIV/AIDS PREVENTION IN ETHNIC AND MINORITY GROUPS

The perception that AIDS is an epidemic has generated a great deal of anxiety on the part of the public but more importantly has challenged the health care system. AIDS presents a unique set of attributes which make it a formidable challenge from all dimensions. It has "the potential for rapid spread through sexual intercourse and needle-sharing; the profound multisystem dysfunction caused by the virus; and the public's lack of empathy, sometimes even hostility toward infected persons."[51]

At the present time, the most significant attribute of AIDS is its uncontrollability. Although progress has been made in several treatment modalities, an effective cure or vaccine is elusive in the future. Therefore, "the only effective avenue for dealing with the problem, for the foreseeable future is prevention at all levels: primary, secondary, and tertiary."[102]

Primary prevention is a necessity at this stage of the AIDS epidemic. There are many desirable effects from primary prevention even though many may disagree with its effectiveness. Benefits from primary preventive strategies may include possible reductions in other sexually-transmitted diseases, the birth of fewer AIDS afflicted babies, lessened use of intravenous illicit drugs, and lower rates of teenage pregnancy.[102]

Preventive efforts directed at ethnic minorities must take into consideration the group's culture and its perceptions of this disease. "Prevention efforts and risk-reduction activities occur within a framework that incorporates norms, tastes, preferences, shared language, and the like within segments of that community."[80]

Blacks' and Hispanics' misperception that AIDS is a gay man's disease must be first corrected before any preventive teaching can take place. Health care workers must impress the fact that heterosexual contact is a vehicle for transmission of HIV.[92]

The importance of the family in Hispanic and Black cultures can be a positive aspect for preventive teaching. Hispanic and Black American families can serve as effective channels for communicating preventive measures. For example, preventive teaching can be done with small groups of individuals who are closely related to each other. Older members' awareness of the disease and its transmission may help in giving appropriate advice to younger members. Key family members could motivate behavior changes in younger members.

Communicating information regarding AIDS and its transmission should be done in ways that will not embarrass the individual. If openness and candidness are not one of the cultural norms of a particular group, a teaching or information session in an outpatient setting may not be appropriate. People may be more receptive in a more familiar setting such as the church or a community social hall.

The language of the health care recipient must be taken into consideration. For example, Hispanics will be more receptive to materials and information in Spanish even though they may speak and understand English. They may also be more comfortable with a health care professional from the same ethnic group.

Individuals from ethnic/minority groups may share their traditional health beliefs with a health care professional in the course of an assessment interview in a variety of possible health care interactions. The professional's attitude should be one of openness and receptivity rather than ridicule or amusement. For example, for the Puerto Rican woman, the prophylactic use of condoms may not be well received because her culture has socialized her to cater to the male who considers condom use as unromantic.[124]

Finally, health care professionals need to consider whether their teachings conflict with the individual's religious beliefs. For instance, the use of condoms may be prevented by religious tenets.[84] Perhaps consulting the religious leader may give the health care professional information as to why individuals would be resistant to certain preventive measures. The religious leader may also be asked to participate in preventive teaching. The respect he or she commands from the congregation may serve as a strong motivation for people to change their attitudes and behaviors. Knowledge of the individual's religious ties may provide valuable information on support networks and potential avenues for organizing preventive activities.[81] Sensitivity to cultural beliefs and practices of ethnic and minority groups is a positive aspect of preventive care. Health care professionals must always be receptive of cultural information which facilitate their working with these groups. Care that is culturally-sensitive not only promotes a positive working relationship but also optimizes health and improves the quality of life.

THE NATION'S RESPONSE TO CULTURAL DIVERSITY

Healthy People 2000

The nation has mobilized its energies to promote the health and quality of life for all Americans by the next century. The challenge is acknowledged in *Healthy People 2000.* "It is a product of a national effort involving professionals and citizens, private organizations and public agencies from every part of the country."[116] This statement declares the need for both the individual and governmental efforts in achieving the goals stated in the document. The following are the broad goals proposed:

1. Increase the lifespan of healthy life for Americans.
2. Reduce health disparities among Americans.
3. Achieve access to preventive services for all Americans.

Within these broad goals are specific objectives for different age groups and special populations such as the elderly, ethnic/minority groups, people with low income, and people with disabilities. Included are objectives for health promotion, health protection, and preventive services. Specific strategies to meet the objectives incorporate input from everyone involved, including the target individual and/or group.

Nursing's Agenda for Health Care Reform (NAHCR)

Another major national move, spearheaded by the American Nurses' Association (ANA) and the National League for Nursing (NLN), is endorsed by over 40 national nursing organizations. The present U.S. health care system is in crisis because quality of care, access to services, and costs are becoming insurmountable barriers for many Americans. NAHCR calls for a basic core of essential health care services to be available to everyone with a restructured health care system that will focus on consumers and their health. The focus will shift from an illness and cure model to one of orientation toward wellness and care. Care delivery settings would include familiar and convenient sites, such as school, workplaces, and homes.[3]

The proposals set forth by NAHCR are congruent with the goals of *Healthy People 2000*. Furthermore, NAHCR explicitly addresses active consumer participation and responsibility for "personal health, self-care, and informed decision-making in selecting health care services."[3] This particular statement of goals emphasizes the contribution of ethnic individuals whose traditional health care practices will be carefully considered in their plan to maintain optimum health.

THE NURSING PROFESSION'S RESPONSE TO CULTURAL DIVERSITY

Nursing's *Code of Ethics* explicitly states the commitment to people in that "the nurse provides services with respect for human dignity and the uniqueness of the client unrestricted by considerations of social or economic status, personal attributes, or the nature of health problems."[2] In addition, The ANA has an active Council on Cultural Diversity which works to help nurses develop culturally sensitive care.

Ethnicity and culture are attributes of individuals which nurses must consider in their interactions with consumers of their services. Cultural sensitivity is an important dimension, particularly in this era "when members of some minority groups are demanding culturally-relevant health care that incorporates their specific beliefs and practices."[4]

Nurses have been making many positive moves toward understanding culturally diverse populations. One major move has been the formal establishment of the field of transcultural nursing pioneered by Leininger, a nurse scholar with a strong interest in anthropology. "The field of transcultural nursing has opened the doors to discover fresh perspectives about human care and different ways to serve humanity."[76] Her early visions have come to reality with the establishment of the Transcultural Society in 1974. This organization is the major group which supports the work of transcultural nurses. Another major achievement was the establishment of the *Journal of Transcultural Nursing* to encourage worldwide sharing of transcultural ideas.[76]

Major organizations such as the ANA and the NLN publish culturally relevant materials to guide students, clinicians, and educators. There are also a cadre of nurses whose research on the relationship of cultural practices and beliefs of individuals and families give professionals a sound base for improving practice and designing cost-effective and humanistic health care strategies.

SUMMARY

The health of a nation is a concern of all. Individuals and groups need to collaborate in optimizing conditions which improve the quality of life. Good health, as a major determinant of the quality of life, should be a right for all regardless of socioeconomic or cultural backgrounds.

The challenge posed by ethnic and minority group individuals is particularly important as the U.S. population is becoming more diverse. The important role of cultural beliefs and practices must be emphasized in health care situations for effective and humanistic care.

The nation, but especially the nursing profession, have given their visions, creativity, energy, and commitment to assure a more healthy people by 2000.

References

1. Adams LM, Knox ME: *Traditional health practices: significance for modern health care*. In Van Horne M, editor: *Ethnicity and health: vol 7, Ethnicity and public policy series*, Milwaukee, 1988, University of Wisconsin System Institute on Race and Ethnicity.
2. American Nurses' Association: *Code of ethics*, Kansas City, Mo, 1985, The Association.
3. American Nurses' Association: *Executive summary: nursing's agenda for health care reform*, Kansas City, Mo, 1991, The Association.
4. Andrews MM: Cultural perspectives on nursing in the 21st century, *J Prof Nurs* 8(1):7-15, 1992.
5. Banks JA, Gay G: Ethnicity in contemporary American society: toward the development of a typology, *Ethnicity* 5:238-251, 1969.
6. Barth F: *Introduction*. In Barth F, editor: *Ethnic groups and boundaries: the social organization of cultural differences*, Boston, 1969, Little, Brown.
7. Bauwens E, Anderson S: *Social and cultural influences on health care*. In Stanhope F, Lancaster J, editors: *Community health nursing*, ed 3, St Louis, 1992, Mosby.
8. Bennett CE: *The Asian and Pacific Islander in the United States: March 1991 and 1990*, US Bureau of the Census, Current population reports, Series

P 20-459, Washington, DC, 1992, US Government Printing Office.
9. Bennett CE: *The Black population in the United States: March 1990 and 1989,* US Bureau of the Census, Current population reports, Series P 20-448, Washington, DC, 1991, US Government Printing Office.
10. Bennett L: *Before the Mayflower: a history of Black America,* ed 6, Chicago, 1992, Johnson Publishing.
11. Bennett MT: *American immigration policies: a history,* Washington, DC, 1963, Public Affairs Press.
12. Billingsley A: *Black families and the struggle for survival,* New York, 1974, Friendship Press.
13. Blais KK: *Ethnic and cultural values.* In Kozier B, Erb G, Olivieri R, editors: *Fundamentals of nursing: concepts, process and practice,* ed 4, Redwood City, Calif, 1991, Addison-Wesley Nursing.
14. Bloch B: *Nursing care of Black patients.* In Orque MS, Bloch B, Monrroy LS, editors: *Ethnic nursing care: a multicultural approach,* St Louis, 1983, Mosby.
15. Bowdler J: Health problems of the homeless in America, *Nurs Prac* 14(44): 47, 50, 51, 1989.
16. Boyle JS, Andrews MM: *Transcultural concepts in nursing care,* Glenview, Ill, 1989, Scott, Foresman/Little, Brown.
17. Brookmeyer J: Reconstruction and future trends of the AIDS epidemic in the United States, *Science* 253:37-41, 1991.
18. Burt MR: *Over the edge,* New York, 1992, Russell Sage Foundation.
19. Caton CL: *Homelessness in historical perspective.* In Caton CL, editor: *Homeless in America,* New York, 1990, Oxford University Press.
20. Caton CL: *Solutions to the homeless problem.* In Caton CL, editor: *Homeless in America,* New York, 1990, Oxford University Press.
21. Centers for Disease Control: *AIDS weekly surveillance report: United States, January 2, 1989,* Atlanta, 1989, US Department of Health and Human Services.
22. Centers for Disease Control: *HIV/AIDS surveillance,* Atlanta, 1991, Centers for Disease Control.
23. Centers for Disease Control: *MMWR* 39(7):110-119, 1990.
24. Chang B: *Asian-American patient care.* In Henderson G, Primeaux M, editors: *Transcultural health care,* Menlo Park, Calif, 1981, Addison-Wesley.
25. Charsley SR: *The formation of ethnic groups.* In Cohen A, editor: *Urban ethnicity,* London, 1974, Tavistock Publications.
26. Chen-Louie T: *Nursing care of Chinese American patients.* In Orque MS, Bloch B, Monrroy LS, editors: *Ethnic nursing care: a multicultural approach,* St Louis, 1983, Mosby.
27. Clark M: *Health in the Mexican American culture,* Berkeley, 1970, University of California Press.
28. Clark M, Anderson BG: *Culture and aging: an anthropological study of older Americans,* Springfield, Ill, 1967, Charles C Thomas.
29. Clark M, Kaufman, Pierce RC: Exploration of acculturation: toward a model of ethnic identity, *Human Org* 35(3): 231-238, 1976.
30. Cohler BJ, Grunebaum H: *Mothers, grandmothers, and daughters: personality and child care in three generation families,* New York, 1981, John Wiley & Sons.
31. Comer JR: *Beyond black and white,* New York, 1972, New York Times Book.
32. Daugherty RD: *People of the salmon.* In Josephy M, editor: *America in 1492: the world of the Indian people before the arrival of Columbus,* New York, 1992, Alfred A Knopf.
33. De Santis G, Benkin R: Ethnicity without community, *Ethnicity* 7:137-143, 1980.
34. Dorsey PR, Jackson HQ: *Cultural health traditions: the Latino/Chicano perspective.* In Branch MF, Paxton PP, editors: *Providing safe nursing care for ethnic people of color,* New York, 1976, Appleton-Century-Crofts.
35. Drapkin A: *Medical problems of the homeless.* In Caton CL, editor: *Homeless in America,* New York, 1990, Oxford University Press.
36. Driver HI, editor: *The Americas in the eve of discovery,* Englewood Cliffs, NJ, 1964, Prentice Hall.
37. Embree ER: *Indians of the Americas,* New York, 1973, Collier Books.
38. Evans PE: Minorities and AIDS, *Health Educ Res* 3(1):113-115, 1988.
39. Farley JE: *Majority-minority relations,* ed 2, Englewood Cliffs, NJ, 1988, Prentice Hall.
40. Feagin JR: *Racial and ethnic origins,* Englewood Cliffs, NJ, 1978, Prentice Hall.
41. Feinstein O, editor: *Ethnic groups in the city,* Lexington, Mass, 1971, Heath Lexington Books.
42. Fleming AF, et al, editors: *The global impact of AIDS,* New York, 1988, Alan R Liss.
43. Francis MB: Homeless families: rebuilding connections, *Public Health Nurs* 8(2):90-99, 1991.
44. Galanti GA: *Caring for patients from different cultures,* Philadelphia, 1991, University of Pennsylvania Press.
45. Garcia A: *The changing demographic face of Hispanics in the United States.* In Sotomayor M, editor: *Empowering Hispanic families: a critical issue for the 1990's,* Milwaukee, 1991, Family Service America.
46. Garcia JM, Montgomery PA: *The Hispanic population in the United States: March 1991,* Current population reports Series P 20-455, Washington, DC, 1991, US Government Printing Office.
47. Geissler EM: Nursing diagnosis of culturally diverse patients, *Inter Nurs Rev* 38(5):150-152, 1991.
48. Giger JN, Davidhizar RE: *Transcultural nursing,* St Louis, 1991, Mosby.
49. Goldschmidt W: *Introduction.* In Goldschmidt W, editor: *Exploring the ways of mankind,* New York, 1971, Holt, Rinehart, & Winston.
50. Gonzalez JL: *Racial and ethnic groups in America,* Dubuque, Iowa, 1990, Kendall/Hunt.
51. Gostin LO: *Hospitals, health care professionals, and persons with AIDS.* In Gostin LO, editor: *AIDS and the health care system,* New Haven, Conn, 1990, Yale University Press.
52. Grinek MD: *History of AIDS,* Princeton, NJ, 1990, Princeton University Press.
53. Hanley CE: *Navajo Indians.* In Giger JN, Davidhizar RE, editors: *Transcultural nursing,* St Louis, 1991, Mosby.
54. Havilland WA: *Cultural anthropology,* New York, 1975, Holt, Rinehart, & Winston.
55. Henderson G, Primeaux M: *The importance of folk medicine.* In Henderson G, Primeaux M, editors: *Transcultural health care,* Menlo Park, Calif, 1981, Addison-Wesley.
56. Hirschl T, Momeni JA: *Homelessness in New York: a demographic and socioeconomic analysis.* In Momeni JA, editor: *Homelessness in the United States (vol. 1 state surveys),* New York, 1989, Greenwood Press.
57. Holmes LD: *Other cultures, elder years: an introduction to cultural anthropology,* Minneapolis, 1983, Burgess Publishing.
58. Hsia J: *Asian Americans in higher education and at work,* Hillsdale, NJ, 1988, Lawrence, Erlbaum Associates Publishers.
59. Hunter JK: Making a difference for homeless patients, *RN* 55(12):48-53, 1992.
60. Hutnacher JJ: *A nation of newcomers: ethnic minority groups in American history,* New York, 1967, Dellwood Press.
61. Institute of Medicine: *Homelessness, health, and human needs,* Washington, DC, 1988, National Academy Press.
62. Isajiw W: Definitions of ethnicity, *Ethnicity* 1:111-124, 1974.
63. Jacques G: *Cultural health traditions: a Black perspective.* In Branch MF, Paxton PP, editors: *Providing safe nursing care for ethnic people of color,* New York, 1976, Appleton-Century-Crofts.
64. Johnson DM, Campbell RR: *Black mi-*

gration in America, Durham, NC, 1981, Duke University Press.
65. Jordan WC: The roots and practice of voodoo medicine in America, *Urban Health* 8:38-41, 1979.
66. Kitano HL, Daniels R: *Asian Americans: emerging minorities,* Englewood Cliffs, NJ, 1988, Prentice Hall.
67. Kluckhohn C: *Culture and behavior,* New York, 1962, Free Press.
68. Kluckhohn C, Leighton D: *The Navaho,* New York, 1962, Doubleday.
69. Kluckhohn F: *Dominant and variant value orientations.* In Kluckhohn C, Murray HA, Schneider DA, editors: *Personality in nature, society, and culture,* ed 2, New York, 1953, Knopf.
70. Knight K, et al: A comparison of the health status of residents in sheltered care facilities in Monmouth County, New Jersey, *Public Health Nurs* 8(3): 182-189, 1991.
71. Kolm R: *Ethnicity in society and community.* In Feinstein O, editor: *Ethnic groups in the city,* Lexington, Mass, 1971, Heath Lexington Books.
72. Kroeber AL: *Anthropology,* New York, 1948, Harcourt, Brace, & World.
73. Lake MG: *Native healer,* Wheaton, Ill, 1991, Quest Books.
74. *Lakota Times:* Census figures misleading, 12(23):A1.
75. Leininger MM: *Nursing and anthropology: two worlds to blend,* New York, 1970, John Wiley & Sons.
76. Leininger MM: Transcultural nursing: quo vadis (where goeth the field?), *J Trans Nurs* 1(2):33-45, 1990.
77. Marin BV: *Hispanic culture: implications for AIDS prevention.* In Boswell J, Hexter R, Reimisch J, editors: *Sexuality and disease: metaphors, perceptions, and behavior in the AIDS era,* New York, 1989, Oxford Press.
78. Marshall PA: Cultural influences on perceived quality of life, *Sem Oncol Nurs,* 6(4):278-284, 1990.
79. Mason JO: *Letter to the Honorable Louis W. Sullivan.* In U.S. Department of Health and Human Services: *Healthy People 2000,* PHS 91-50212, Washington, DC, 1990, US Government Printing Office.
80. Mays VM: *AIDS prevention in Black populations: methods of a safer kind.* In Mays VM, Albee G, Schenider SF, editors: *Primary prevention of AIDS,* Newbury Park, Calif, 1989, Sage Publications.
81. Mead M: *Sex and temperament in three primitive societies,* New York, 1963, Morrow-Quill Paperback.
82. Monrroy LS: *Nursing care of Raza/Latina patients.* In Orque MS, Bloch B, Monrroy LS, editors: *Ethnic nursing care: a multicultural approach,* St Louis, 1983, Mosby.
83. Moquin W, editor: *Makers of America: emergent minorities 1955-1970, vol 10,* Encyclopaedia Britannica Educational Corporation, Chicago, 1971, William Benton Publishers.
84. Muir MA: *The environmental context of AIDS,* New York, 1991, Praeger.
85. Murillo N: *The Mexican American family.* In Wagner NN, Haug MJ, editors: *Chicanos: social and psychological perspectives,* St Louis, 1971, Mosby.
86. Murillo N: *The Mexican American family.* In Martinez RA, editor: *Hispanic culture and health care,* St Louis, 1978, Mosby.
87. Murillo-Rohde I: *Hispanic American patient care.* In Henderson G, Primeaux M, editors: *Transcultural health care,* Menlo Park, Calif, 1981, Addison-Wesley.
88. Nabokov P, editor: *Native American testimony,* New York, 1991, Penguin Group.
89. National Academy of Science Report: *Homelessness, health and human needs: summary and recommendations.* In McKenzie N, editor: *The crisis in health care: the ethical issues,* New York, 1990, Penguin Group.
90. National Center for Health Statistics: *Monthly vital statistics report,* 40(8), Jan 7, 1992.
91. National Research Council: *A common destiny: Blacks and American Society,* Washington, DC, 1989, National Academy Press.
92. Perales CA: *Social services for people with AIDS: the state perspective.* In David RE, Ginzberg E, editors: *The AIDS patient: an action agenda,* Boulder, 1988, Westview Press.
93. Pettigrew TF: *Ethnicity in American life: a social-psychological perspective.* In Feinstein O, editor: *Ethnic groups in the city,* Lexington, Mass, 1971, Heath Lexington Books.
94. Place LF: *The ethnic factor.* In Berghorn FJ, Schafer D, editors: *Dynamics of aging,* Boulder, 1981, Westview Press.
95. Ropers RA: *The invisible homeless,* New York, 1988, Human Science Press.
96. Sarna J: From immigrants to ethnics: toward a new theory of ethnicization, *Ethnicity* 5:370-378, 1978.
97. Schermerhorn R: *Comparative ethnic relations: a framework for theory and research,* Chicago, 1970, University of Chicago Press.
98. Scitovsky AA, Rice DP: AIDS: the cost in dollars, *Internist* 28:9-15, 1987.
99. Scott CS: *Health and healing practices among five ethnic groups in Miami, Florida.* In Bauwens EE, editor: *The anthropology of health,* St Louis, 1978, Mosby.
100. Sebastian JG: *Vulnerable populations in the community.* In Stanhope M, Lancaster J, editors: *Community health nursing,* ed 3, St Louis, 1992, Mosby.
101. Selik RM, Castro KG, Pappaioanou M: Racial and ethnic differences in the risk of AIDS in the United States. *Am J Public Health,* 78(12):1539-1545, 1988.
102. Shannon GW, Pyle GE, Bashshur RL: *The geography of AIDS: origins and course of an epidemic,* New York, 1990, Guilford Press.
103. Spector RE: *Cultural diversity in health and illness,* ed 2, New York, 1985, Appleton-Century-Crofts.
104. Staiano K: Ethnicity as a process: the creation of an Afro-American identity, *Ethnicity* 7:27-33, 1980.
105. Staples R: *Introduction to Black sociology,* New York, 1976, McGraw-Hill.
106. Starr P: *Social transformation of American medicine,* New York, 1990, Basic Books.
107. Strong Heart Study Newsletter, 4(2), Public Health Service Indian Hospital, Rapid City, SD.
108. Taylor CF, editor: *The Native Americans,* New York, 1991, Smithmark Publishers.
109. Thomas DN: *Black American patient care.* In Henderson G, Primeaux M, editors: *Transcultural health care,* Menlo Park, Calif, 1981, Addison-Wesley.
110. Tripp-Reimer T, Brink PJ, Saunders JM: Cultural assessment: content and process, *Nurs Outlook* 32:78-82, 1984.
111. U.S. Bureau of the Census: *Summary population and housing characteristics CPH-1-1,* Washington, DC, 1990, US Government Printing Office.
112. U.S. Conference of Mayors: *The growth of hunger, homelessness, and poverty in America's cities in 1985: a 25 city survey,* Washington, DC, 1986, Conference of Mayors.
113. U.S. Department of Commerce, Bureau of the Census: *We, the first Americans,* Washington, DC, 1989, US Government Printing Office.
114. U.S. Department of Education: *Indian nations at risk: an educational strategy for action,* Washington, DC, 1991, Indian Nations Risk Task Force.
115. U.S. Department of Education, National Center for Education Statistics, Office of Educational Research and Improvement: *Digest of education statistics 1992,* Washington DC, 1992, US Government Printing Office.
116. U.S. Department of Health and Human Services: *Healthy people 2000,* PHS 91-50212, Washington, DC, 1990, US Government Printing Office.
117. U.S. House Select Committee on Children, Youth and Families: *The crisis in homelessness: effects on children and families hearings,* Serial No 72-23, Washington, DC, 1987, US Government Printing Office.
118. U.S. Indian Statistics: *Denver Post,* August 17, 1992.

119. Valencia-Go GN: *Integrative aging in widowed immigrant Filipinas: a grounded theory study, Order Number 8923910,* Ann Arbor, Mich, 1989, University Microfilms International.
120. Verrill AH: *The American Indian: North, South, and Central America,* New York, 1927, New Home Library.
121. Westburg J: Patient education for Hispanic Americans, *Patient Educ Counsel* 13:143-160, 1989.
122. Wiecha JL, Dwyer JT, Dunn-Strobecker M: Nutrition and health services needs among the homeless, *Public Health Report* 106(4):364-374, 1990.
123. Wilson UM: *Nursing care of American Indian patients.* In Orque MS, Bloch B, Monrroy LS, editors: *Ethnic nursing care: a multicultural approach,* St Louis, 1983, Mosby.
124. Worth D: *Minority women and AIDS: culture, race, and gender.* In Feldman DA, editor: *Culture and AIDS,* New York, 1990, Praeger.
125. Yancey WL, Ericksen EP, Juliani RN: Emergent ethnicity: a review and reformulation, *Am Soc Rev* 41(3):391-402, 1976.
126. Yetman NK, editor: *Statistical appendix table 1: racial and Hispanic populations in the United States: 1970-1980.* In *Majority and minority: the dynamics of race and ethnicity in American life,* Boston, 1985, Allyn & Bacon.
126. Zangwill I: *The melting pot: drama in four acts,* New York, 1921, Macmillan.

CHAPTER

3

Health Policy and the Delivery System

Carole Lium Edelman

Carol Scheel Gavan

Objectives

After completing this chapter, the nurse will be able to

- *Discuss key developments in the history of health care that (1) influenced the philosophic basis of American health care and (2) separated preventive from curative measures.*
- *Differentiate between private and public sectors in the delivery of health care.*
- *Describe the mechanisms by which health care in the United States is financed in both private and public sectors.*
- *Identify the role of government agencies responsible for new legislative acts.*
- *Discuss the nurse's role in influencing health policy.*
- *Differentiate between the Medicare and Medicaid program.*

In 1977, the World Health Assembly of the World Health Organization (WHO) decided that the "new social target of governments and of WHO should be the attainment by all people of the world by the year 2000, a level of health that permits them to live socially and economically productive lives."[12] This was the birth of the "health for all by the year 2000" movement.[12] To date, every country, every member state of WHO has done something toward the attainment of "health for all."[12] However, the level of achievement tends to be very unbalanced with some countries having more difficulty moving toward this goal because of shrinking health care budgets.

The health care delivery system in the United States is currently experiencing significant changes. Although health care is often equated with medical care, which focuses on the treatment of illness, this chapter presents the evolution and ongoing development of a broader concept of health based on the definition of health described in Chapter 1.

The complexities of the health care system necessitate an understanding of the system as a whole before focusing on the intermingled causative factors that have created a huge, fragmented enterprise. Many of today's problems have their roots in the decisions and directions of the past. It is not possible to identify and analyze current problems or to devise solutions without first exploring how the system developed to its present state.[7]

The relevance of the split between preventive and curative measures is apparent when the organization and financing of the delivery system is examined. The United States has established a system that uses two basic divisions of society to provide service: the private sector and the public sector. The merger of public health and welfare policies in the public sector is rooted in the Puritan ethic inherent in the historical development of the United States. An understanding of the history and development of the health care delivery system enables the nurse to apply principles to daily care. With the focus shifting to community health care, the nurse must be aware especially of the issues surrounding the developing health care system.[22]

The historical development of health planning is explored briefly to better understand the current status of health planning, its relationship to national health insurance planning, and its impact on the system. This discussion points out the essential link between health planning and health care financing to deal with the scarcity and rising costs of basic resources.

HISTORY AS HEALTH CARE

The beginnings of new epochs always go unnoticed. Regardless if the new era is one of light or darkness, it is only after dawn has brightened the sky or deep twilight has fallen that humanity fully comprehends the change that has occurred. Only then can people see in retrospect the point where they turned into a path of no return.[7]

Early Influences

Historical records of early civilizations (Egyptian, Indian, Chinese, Aztec, Greek) show that ancient peoples were concerned with disease and practiced various methods of treatment. The earliest views of health can be viewed as holistic, in the sense of having a world view. Primitive peoples understood illness in mystical terms; sickness and cure theories were tied to the cosmic view of life, with natural and supernatural forces often inseparable.

Most of the primitive peoples of the world practice cleanliness and personal hygiene as part of their religious world view. For thousands of years, epidemics were viewed as divine judgments on human wickedness, with a gradual awareness that pestilence is caused by natural causes, such as climate and physical environment.

In the Middle Ages, infectious diseases in epidemic proportions (i.e., leprosy, bubonic plague, smallpox, tuberculosis) were the leading causes of death. A breakthrough in understanding the disease process did not occur until the development of bacteriology in the 19th century. In fact, it was not until the 20th century that infectious diseases were mastered and were no longer the leading causes of death. Details of these influences are presented in the remainder of this section. Clearly, health was viewed in terms of survival and absence of disease until the dread infectious diseases were conquered.

Industrial Influences

The population of the Western world increased beginning in the 1600s when America was first being explored. The New World had many things to offer the explorers. An adequate food supply made it possible for the population to live longer, and advances in transportation made distribution of food supplies and other goods and services possible. Then an influence of manufacturing in the 18th century through the invention of the flush toilet and cast iron pipe, made sanitary engineering possible and saved many lives by preventing diseases such as typhoid, paratyphoid, and gastroenteritis.

Socioeconomic Influences

Although the Elizabethan Poor Laws (1601) in England provided a system of relief for the poor, including infants, sick and elderly persons, and those in the workhouses, a new Poor Law was enacted in 1834 based on the harsher philosophy that regarded pauperism among able-bodied workers as a moral failing. If the worker did not earn a subsistence level income, the attitude toward that worker was punitive and suspicious.

These Poor Laws are the legal implementation of the Protestant ethic that our Puritan forebearers brought to the United States. Persons are held directly accountable for their state in life, and health maintenance is the responsibility of the individual. The far-reaching implications of this ethic can be seen today in the organization, financing, and delivery of health services.

Public Health Influences

Edwin Chadwick (1800-1890) is known as the father of British and American public health. He established an English Board of Health, which emphasized environmental sanitation but which excluded physicians except in times of crisis. In addition, he was secretary of the Poor Law Commission, which strove to improve the health of the masses for economic reasons. Chadwick's rationale was that disease among the poor was a major factor in their inability to support themselves. Thus, governmental health and welfare policies have been joined in England since the 19th century.

In the United States, Lemuel Shattuck began the public health movement, using the British system as the model, with public health services and welfare combined despite the contradictory emphasis. Public health has focused on improving health of the poor, whereas welfare has dictated subsistence at the minimal level. Thus, the influence of the Puritan ethic on the American health care system is apparent in the emphasis on the value of work and the attitude toward the poor. Today, health and welfare departments continue their contradictory approach to the poor. The Medicaid Law of 1965 is a good example of this ambivalence. Medicaid is charged with the provision of health services to the medically indigent; but when state budgets are cut, income eligibility levels are decreased to remove people from the roles, or specific services such as dental services or medications are denied. Medicaid plans vary from state to state.

Scientific Influences

Until the 20th century, epidemics of infectious disease (e.g., plague, cholera, typhoid, smallpox, influenza) were the most critical health problems and major causes of death and disability for Americans. Scientific advances in the 19th century by Pasteur (germ theory), Koch (origin of bacterial infection), Lister (antisepsis), and Ehrlich (chemotherapy) expanded public health from its earlier concentration on sanitation to control of communicable disease using a broad biologic base. Public health became a major force in decreasing death rates and increasing life expectancy through the application of bacteriology. Environmental conditions were improved by developing systems that safeguard water, milk, and food supplies; promote sanitary sewage disposal; and monitor the quality of urban housing.

The discovery and use of sulfonamides and antibiotics to treat bacterial infections between 1936 and 1954 reduced the death rate to its lowest point in history, with deaths caused by primary infections reduced to 4% as compared with 33% just 50 years earlier. The death rate did not change significantly between 1954 and the middle of the 1960s, when another decline in the death rate began. This decline has continued into the 1990s.

Special Population Influences

Today, poor and homeless represent special populations that both are large enough and include enough of America's most vulnerable citizens to warrant particular concern in the Year 2000 Health Objectives. For these disadvantaged, issues of preventing disease and promoting good health often are secondary to the problems associated with everyday survival.

The acquired immunodeficiency syndrome epidemic of the 1980s will still be a worldwide endemic problem at the end of the 21st century, since no effective vaccine has been developed and successfully implemented worldwide. New, unimagined, and even unimaginable diseases will arise; and their effects, by definition, will be completely unpredictable.

Political and Economic Influences

Political and economic considerations are basic to the health care system. Politics determines who the decision makers are, and economics defines what and how resources are distributed.

The effect of economics and politics on the delivery of health care is illustrated by the situation in the United States after the Great Depression. The emergence of Roosevelt's New Deal had an impact on health care, specifically in the passage in 1935 of the Social Security Act, which authorized grants-in-aid to the individual states to improve state and local public health programs. Funds were available for "categorical assistance" programs, wtih cash grants first given to needy blind and aged individuals and later to disabled persons as well. Medical care was an allowable budget item, but payments often went for food, shelter, or other needs. In addition, the Social Security Act served as the basis for other assistance programs, such as Medicaid and Medicare, through subsequent amendments.

Split between Preventive and Curative Measures

An orientation toward prevention has not been part of the traditional medical educational system because of the exclusion of physicians from early public health policies and the nature of medical education. Voluntary hospitals (those organizations which are not for profit) had a monopoly on clinical medical education dating back to the 18th century.[7] These hospitals were concerned with the treatment of overt disease, with a focus on activity and observable effects; persons attracted to clinical medicine then, as with those now, were "activists."

The division between clinical medicine and public health is reinforced further by the custom of payment for a measurable act – in this case, treatment of visible illness. Monetary value cannot be placed on such "intangibles" as preventive services. In addition, the Hippocratic Oath, the basic philosophy of Western medicine, designates the physician's primary responsibility to the client as an individual. This may prevent or prohibit the physician from seeing the broader needs of society, even if these needs coincide with those of the client.

The advances that conquered infectious disease involved a combination of social, educational, and medical efforts that integrated preventive and curative health care. On the other hand, the shape of our current health care system stems from the 1850s, when separation of administration and staff for curative services (acute, chronic, and psychiatric illnesses) became the norm.[7]

The link between environmental health and personal medical care developed when sanitarians realized that their efforts alone were not sufficient to prevent and cure the diseases of the population as a whole; improvement of personal health also was necessary. The early preventive services directed at individuals originated in medical practice rather than public health but were associated either with welfare medicine or with salaried medical practice in factories. Community health centers that developed in the United States before World War I limited their scope to prevention and health education and, with the exception of some prenatal clinics, generally were located in poor neighborhoods. Thus, the delivery of preventive services developed separately from clinical medicine and became associated with public health. Physicians, educated in hospitals, were interested in individuals in whom prevention had failed and whose illnesses brought them to the hospital ward.

Despite the separation of preventive and treatment services, the benefits of prevention eventually were incorporated into clinical medicine for individuals. Preventive and early detective measures became a part of pediatrics and obstetrics in the early part of the 20th century when vaccines and vaginal cytology became available and accepted. Later in the 20th century, internal medicine incorporated early detection of diseases such as diabetes, glaucoma, obesity, and hypertension. A shift to preventive medicine for the individual thus occurred, but the separate educational programs for public health and medicine still divided these areas. It was not until the 1960s that the emphasis began to turn from individual to societal values.[7] The U.S. focus on individual change toward better fitness, stress management, nutrition, and medical self-care must follow other countries' focus on health promotion efforts that call for changing the environment to support health.

This new emphasis toward societal values parallels another evolution in the role of health in society. Increasingly, health care is regarded as a right rather than a privilege, with an increased governmental involvement in and concern for the protection of that right. The future holds many more changes in the ongoing development of the role of health.[5]

Access to health care is influenced by individual health needs, financial resources, and the health care delivery system. Each of these factors may be affected by the prevailing public policy established by federal, state, and local government. Technologic developments, chronic illness, and the aging population each have an independent as well as interrelated impact on access to health care and the delivery of health services. Some claim that using "big ticket" technology rather than alternatives is unjust or unfair. Applying the principle of justices in the health care system has implications for both access and resource allocation. Daniels suggests that "justice will require us to make decisions about which technologies and services it is more important to disseminate under conditions of moderate scarcity."[4]

An example of prioritizing health care services is the Oregon plan which was developed in 1989. At the time, a coalition of Oregon legislators, policy makers, and health care professionals created a new plan that attempts to ensure equitable and universal access to health care by prioritizing types of care. Critics call it unrealistic and a dangerous rationing scheme. Proponents argue it is better than the current system that denies thousands of citizens access to basic care.[2]

ORGANIZATION OF THE DELIVERY SYSTEM

The health care delivery system in the United States is a complex interrelationship involving providers, consumers, and settings, with both private and public sectors providing services (Table 3-1). The public sector includes voluntary and nonprofit agencies as well as official or governmental agencies. Delivery of services is organized on three levels in both sectors: local, state, and national. Each of the three levels consists of private providers along with official or voluntary public agencies. Since the nurse is often the professional who assists the health consumer through the complex delivery system, a basic understanding of the system's organization is essential.

Private Sector

INDEPENDENT PRACTICE

Traditionally, a person enters the health care system by contracting directly with a physician for individual care on the basis of fee-for-service. Free choice of provider has been the hallmark. Private practice is basically disease ori-

***Table 3-1.* Organization of U.S. health care delivery**

	Private sector (independent practices)	Public sector (public health agencies)	
	Proprietary	Official	Voluntary
Source of money	Fee-for-service or salary	Taxes	Voluntary contributions or fee-for-service
Accountability	Individual client	Citizens	Source of funds
Purpose, duties	Independent contractor operating within professional ethics	Prescribed or mandated by law	Free to experiment and support research

ented, with some areas of specific protection – such as routine physical examinations, immunizations, and screening – according to the type of practice.

Most physicians are in private practice. Since specialists tend to focus on their area of expertise, it is easy for them to lose sight of the whole person. The nurse encourages the client to employ the specialist intelligently and maintain collaboration between specialists when more than one is involved.

Private care may be delivered in an inpatient (hospital) or an outpatient (ambulatory) setting; the latter is defined as any setting where the individual is not a bed patient. The setting most frequently used in private practice is the physician's office or the outpatient clinic. Over the past few years, same-day surgery centers have become another setting for surgical procedures.

Physicians in primary care can have a positive effect on health behaviors in very cost-effective ways. For example, the simple offering by a general practitioner of advice to stop smoking to clients who come to the doctor for some reason other than smoking results in a 5% quit rate at the end of 1 year.[4]

PREFERRED PROVIDER ORGANIZATIONS

Preferred provider organizations (PPOs) are another delivery method in the private sector developed in the 1980s. PPOs are networks of doctors and hospitals that have agreed to give the sponsoring organization discounts from their usual charges. These doctors and hospitals may be the same ones the sponsors use for their health maintenance organizations (HMOs), or they may be different.

PPOs usually do not exercise tight management over medical care. They may require doctors to obtain the plan's approval before sending clients to the hospital, but members are not required to choose a primary care physician. Members of a basic PPO can go to any doctor in the network. A criticism of PPOs is the inability to control costs. As long as network doctors are used, the organization may pay 80% or 90% of medical bills and, in some plans, 100%. Outside the network, the organization may pay only 60% to 70%.

GATEKEEPER PPOs

Gatekeeper PPOs also have networks of hospitals and doctors who have agreed to give discounts. But in these arrangements, the sponsoring organization may pay more attention to the quality of the doctors. It may also more tightly control the use of medical services, much the way an HMO does.

EXCLUSIVE PROVIDER ORGANIZATIONS

A number of managed-care companies have taken their gatekeeper PPOs one step further. They have created plans that pay no benefits if members go outside the network. These plans, called exclusive provider organizations (EPOs), resemble HMOs but are usually regulated under state insurance laws, not the statutes governing HMOs. As a result, they may lack some consumer safeguards, such as quality formal grievance programs.

HEALTH MAINTENANCE ORGANIZATIONS

Health maintenance organizations deliver comprehensive health maintenance and treatment services for a group of enrolled persons who pay a prenegotiated and fixed payment. The HMO accepts responsibility for the organization, financing, and delivery of health care services for those who are members. Two models of delivery link HMOs and providers (physicians and other professionals).[21]

The traditional and most predominant HMO structure offers primary care in a multispeciality group practice setting with salaried providers – as at Kaiser-Permanente – often linked to the HMO's own hospital in the case of large HMOs or involved in contract agreements with community hospitals in the case of smaller HMOs. Alternatively, providers are paid a capitation rate – a fixed sum per patient per unit of time regardless of the volume of service, such as in the Puget Sound Group Health Cooperative.[23]

Another newer delivery model of a type of HMO that is increasing in popularity is an individual or independent practice association (IPA) that combines a prepayment mechanism with individual practice for providers who see their prepaid clients as well as their fee-for-service clients in their own offices. Providers are paid a prenegotiated fee-for-service by the intermediary IPA that contracts with employers to supply a benefit package in exchange for a fee-per-person contract.[23] IPAs have low start-up costs and are easy to organize but may not be as cost-effective as traditional group model HMOs.[23]

Opt-out or point-of-service HMOs, the latest fashion in managed care (see box on p. 52 for glossary of managed care terms), are regular HMOs with one critical difference. As we explain in the accompanying report, in a regular HMO, all care is delivered by plan physicians, and in return,the client pays either nominal copayments or nothing at all. Medical care outside the HMO may require the client to cover the entire cost. In an opt-out arrangement, the employer's plan will pay some of the cost, usually 60% or 70% for care outside the HMO. The HMO's usual grievance procedures and quality assurance programs will apply as long as the client stays within the network. Outside the network, the client loses the HMO's oversight of the care received.

Public Sector

The public sector contains official and voluntary public health agencies operating at the local, state, federal, and

❑ ❑ A GLOSSARY OF MANAGED CARE

Capitation. A preset payment based on membership, not services delivered. Usually expressed in units of per member per month (PMPM).

Case rate. A set amount of reimbursement based on the diagnosis, regardless of resources consumed. Similar to the DRG method of reimbursement.

EPO. Exclusive provider organization. Limits enrollees to providers belonging to one organization. They may or may not be able to use outside providers at an additional out-of-pocket cost.

HMO. Health maintenance organization; the prototypical managed care model. Provides health care in return for a preset, prepaid amount of money on a per member per month basis. The enrollee is limited to certain providers and historically could not go outside the plan for services; this has now changed in some HMO models.

Managed care. A system that seeks to control costs by monitoring the delivery of care and by limiting access to specialists and costly procedures.

Managed competition. A system designed to control costs through competition, not price controls. Organized groups of physicians and other practitioners, hospitals, insurers, and HMOs compete for customers by offering standardized benefit packages.

Per diem. Reimbursement based on a set rate per day rather than on charges.

PPO. Preferred provider organization. Contracts with independent providers for services at a discount. Limits enrollee choice to a list of "preferred" hospitals, physicians, and providers; the enrolled pays more out of pocket for using a provider who is not on the list.

Stop loss. A form of protection for hospitals that limits their financial losses in extreme cases when medical expense exceeds a certain limit.

Utilization review. A system used to monitor diagnosis, treatment, and billing practices. The purpose of the system is to lower costs by discouraging unnecessary treatment.

From *The New York Times*, Sept 23, 1993.

international level. Health promotion and protection and disease prevention receive greater emphasis in this sector than in the private sector.

SOURCE OF POWER

The U.S. Constitution is based on the sharing of sovereign power between federal and state governments. The powers of the federal government in relation to health are not delineated specifically in the Constitution; they are derived from the financial authority to tax and to spend for the general welfare and from powers delegated to the government by the states, which reserve police power. *Police power,* the basis of the states' role in health, means the states have the obligation and duty to protect the health and welfare of their citizens.[17] Police power generally is delegated by the state governor or legislature to a specific health agency, usually the public health department. The public health officer thus can arrest an individual who has a communicable disease, such as tuberculosis, and refuses treatment to protect citizens from the potential risk of contracting the disease. The police power also permits states to require licenses of professions dealing in the public sector, such as nurses, physicians, and beauticians, that affect the public health.

State health authority also is based on the Tenth Amendment, which reserves to the states or to the people those powers not delegated to the federal government by the Constitution. The states in turn use their powers to create local government, delegating authority in health to local governments.

INFLUENCE OF POLITICAL PHILOSOPHY

The prevailing political philosophy toward societal health needs affects the relationship among federal, state, and local governments, such as the 1930 New Deal philosophy discussed previously. This trend toward increased federal government involvement continued during the Kennedy-Johnson era, when the government focused on societal needs and health care to an unprecedented degree. During the Nixon-Ford era, a "New Federalism" movement called for less federal encroachment into states' responsibilities and greater state and local responsibility related to the introduction of revenue sharing.

The Reagan era version of "New Federalism" included procompetition and deregulation policies as a means of dealing with limited finances (see the financing discussion later in this chapter). Clearly, the federal government's role swings back and forth according to political philosophy.

During George Bush's term as president, little change occurred in moving new legislature ahead toward health care reform. During his 4 years in the Oval Office, President Bush worked toward two principal efforts – the "Health Summit" convened in 1991 and the report issued by the Social Security Advisory Commission. These provided no concrete solutions about how to solve the deep-set problems endemic to our health care system.

PRESIDENT CLINTON'S HEALTH CARE PROPOSAL

In September, 1993, President Clinton proposed a health benefits package for all Americans. Americans would receive a health care security card that will guarantee a comprehensive package of benefits over the course of an entire lifetime. With this card, an individual is covered if they lose their job or switch jobs. In addition, individuals are covered for hospital care, doctor visits, emergency and lab services, diagnostic services, and substance abuse and mental health care. Equally important and for the first time, this program would provide a broad range of preventive services, including regular checkups and well-baby visits.

This "standard package," which under Clinton's health care reform plan would become the mandatory minimum coverage that all health plans would be required to provide, includes a significant expansion in mental health benefits and drug and alcohol abuse treatment coverage over what most Americans now have. In the areas of mental health and long-term care, Clinton opted for an approach that emphasizes primary and preventive care. Long-term care coverage extends to 100 days per year. Dental coverage is limited to nonemergency dental care for children and emergency dental care for adults, although the plan envisions that adult dental coverage would be phased in by the year 2000. Children would be covered for eyeglasses and routine eye care exams; adults would not.

The benefit package is a key element in Clinton's overall health reform plan. Under the terms of the program, the standard package would determine not only the minimum level of care but how much consumers would have to pay out of pocket – or with the help of their employers – to add benefits. (See the box below for the vocabulary of Clinton's health care reform proposal; see Table 3-2 for Clinton's plan and the alternatives to his plan.)

MANAGED COMPETITION

According to the administration proposal, competing health care plans could include extra benefits as a way to attract customers. Prices could vary between competing plans in a given region; but plans would not be allowed to charge different people different prices for the same standard benefits, except for some permitted variation in charges for the elderly who use more medical services.

Managed competition, the basis for the Clinton proposal, incorporates the coordinated delivery system of managed care, but also encompasses large purchasing

❑ ❑ VOCABULARY OF CLINTON'S HEALTH CARE PLAN

Employer Mandate. The Clinton plan's requirement that employers pay at least 80% of the cost of health coverage for their workers.

Guaranteed National Benefit Package. The standard comprehensive coverage that all Americans would receive under the President's proposal.

Health Alliances. Purchasing groups that, under the Clinton plan, would each buy health care services for thousands of consumers. The alliances would be of two types: regional health alliances, whose creation would be the states' responsibility, and corporate health alliances. A corporate alliance could be established by any large employer (in general, one with more than 5000 workers). These employers would have the option of joining a regional alliance instead.

Health Plans. The networks of doctors, hospitals and insurers that would provide coverage through contracts negotiated with regional or corporate alliances.

Managed Competition. A policy, partly embraced by the President, that combines free-market forces with government regulation. Large groups of consumers buy health care from networks of providers. The aim is to create business competition, thereby restraining prices and encouraging quality of care.

Medicaid. The existing federal-state program of health coverage for the poor. Under the Clinton plan, Medicaid beneficiaries would be folded into the health alliance system.

Medicare. The existing federal program of health coverage for the elderly and the disabled. Under the Clinton plan, a state could apply to the government for permission to include Medicare beneficiaries in the alliance system, and a person who was already included in an alliance upon turning 65 could remain.

National Health Board. A seven-member federal panel that would be appointed by the President to oversee the states' creation of regional health alliances, interpret the guaranteed benefits package, enforce a national health care budget, monitor the quality of care and investigate pharmaceutical companies' prices for new drugs if evidence suggested prices were unreasonably high.

National Health Security Card. An identification card that would serve as proof of a person's eligibility for the government-guaranteed package of benefits. All citizens and legal aliens would be eligible.

Single-Payer Option. A provision of the Clinton plan that a state would be allowed to enact as an alternative to the system of regional health alliances. Under the alternative, the state would make direct payments to health care providers, with no intermediaries.

From *The New York Times*, Sept 23, 1993.

Table 3-2. **Health care: Clinton's plan and the alternatives**

	McDermott (single-payer)	Clinton	Chafee	Cooper	Gramm	Michel
Coverage	All legal residents would have access to a standard medical benefits package, administered by the states, with the government paying the bills. Would cover all medically necessary procedures, excluding cost of private hospital rooms and cosmetic surgery.	All legal residents would be required to be insured, choosing from at least three plans providing standard benefits: a health maintenance organization, fee-for-service, or a combination plan. Plans would be administered by large corporate employers or by regional purchasing alliances.	Individuals would be required to obtain insurance for a standard benefits package. Employers would be required to offer it. Individuals could also buy insurance through purchasing alliances. Vouchers to subsidize the poor would become available as the system produced savings.	Purchasing cooperatives would reduce cost of insurance and make it more affordable. The Federal Government would pay insurance premiums for individuals below the poverty level and subsidize them for people with incomes up to twice the poverty level.	Employers would be required to offer workers at least three choices, including their existing health insurance arrangements, membership in an HMO or other provider, and a tax-free savings account to cover medical expenses that exceed $3000 in a year.	Employers would be required to offer workers at least one insurance plan and a tax-free medical savings account. Insurance companies that sell to small employers would be required to offer both kinds. Expansion of community and migrant health care centers would expand access to care.
Benefits	Complete payment for doctors' and hospital bills, prescription drugs, mental health care, substance abuse, and other medically necessary treatment.	Complete coverage of hospital, doctors' and prescription drug bills. Some coverage for mental health and substance abuse. Prescription drug and limited long-term care added to Medicare benefits.	Complete coverage of doctors' and hospital bills, prescription drugs, substance abuse, limited mental health coverage. Customers could choose a catastrophic plan instead.	Would be set by a national health board.	Unspecified.	To be established by National Association of Insurance Commissioners.

Payments	Substantial payroll taxes would be imposed on employers, replacing insurance most employers now pay. Individuals would pay nothing.	Employers would pay 80% of cost of average insurance, but no more than 7.9% of payroll. Subsidies for small, low-wage employers. Individuals would pay up to 20% of premiums. Subsidies for the poor. Copayments, deductibles and $3000 family limit in fee-for-service plans. None for preventive care. Would bar penalties for pre-existing conditions.	No employer payments required. No controls on premium payments. Benefits commission could set standards for copayments and deductibles, subject to Congressional approval. Would limit higher insurance rates for those with pre-existing conditions.	No employer payments required. No control of premium payments, copayments, or deductibles, except no deductibles or copayments allowed for preventive care. Would prohibit cancellations and higher payments for pre-existing conditions.	No employer payments required. No control of premium payments, copayments or deductibles. Would limit and subsidize higher rates for those with pre-existing conditions, except those caused by individual behavior like smoking.	No employer payments required. No control of premium payments, copayments and deductibles. Would limit higher insurance rates for those with pre-existing conditions.
Major additional financing provisions	Being developed.	New taxes of $105 billion on tobacco and on large corporate employers that stay out of regional purchasing alliances. Reductions of $238 billion in anticipated growth of Medicare and Medicaid from 1995 to 2000.	Would cut $213 billion in growth of Medicare and Medicaid from 1995 to 2000. Would limit tax deductibility of employer-paid insurance plans. Self-employed could deduct full cost of standard health insurance.	Would raise $16 billion by preventing employers from deducting costs of insurance beyond the cost of basic plans and $6.5 billion by slowing Medicare increases. Would allow self-employed to deduct full cost of standard insurance.	Would slow Medicaid growth by $113 billion and Medicare growth by $62 billion from 1994 to 1998; would gain $16 billion in additional taxes from lower business expenses. Self-employed could deduct health insurance up to average cost for all employees.	Would save $17 billion by reducing Medicare subsidies, and altering Federal retirement rules.
Additional cost containment (All plans would save by standardizing medical claim forms.)	Would establish annual national health budgets. National health board would set standards for pricing of covered services.	National health board would establish national and regional budgets. Insurance premium increases would be limited by the board.	Expects competition to produce savings.	Expects competition to produce savings.	Expects competition to produce savings.	Expects competition and preexemption of state rules on basic coverage to produce savings.

From *The New York Times*, Oct 17, 1993.

Continued.

***Table 3-2.* Health care: Clinton's plan and the alternatives – cont'd**

	McDermott (single-payer)	Clinton	Chafee	Cooper	Gramm	Michel
Malpractice reform	None.	Plans would have to establish mediation or arbitration as alternatives to court. Unhappy claimants would need a certificate from independent doctors that the claim has merit before going to court. Would hold lawyer's fees to one third of award, the current practice.	Would require mediation, then alternative dispute resolution. If case was appealed to the courts, loser would pay winner's costs and lawyer's fees. Pain and suffering damages would be limited to $250,000. Would limit lawyer's fees to 20% of award.	Would require alternative dispute resolution initially. If decision was appealed, loser would pay winner's court costs and lawyer's fees. Pain and suffering damages limited to $250,000. Lawyer's fees held to 25% of first $150,000, and 10% of rest of award.	Would require loser in court to pay the winner's costs and attorney's fees. Pain and suffering damages limited to $250,000. Lawyer's fees limited to 25% of awards.	Would require mediation, then alternative dispute resolution. If case was appealed to the courts, loser would pay winner's costs and lawyer's fees. Pain and suffering damages would be limited to $250,000. Would limit lawyer's fees to 20% of award.
Administration	Benefits would be established by a health security board, which would also set pricing standards. The states would provide and structure their individual plans for health services.	A national health board could revise benefits. It would set budgets and approve operations of regional and corporate insurance purchasing alliances. The alliances would contract with health plans, distribute information to consumers and collect premiums. Corporate alliances allowed for employers of 5000 or more.	A national commission would set benefits. States would have to establish health insurance purchasing cooperatives for small businesses and individuals. There could be more than one in a geographic area, and they could operate across state lines. Multistate employer plans would be regulated by the Department of Health and Human Services.	A national health board would establish benefits. States would create health plan purchasing cooperatives that exclude large employers (size to be determined) to make insurance available at reduced cost to small business.	None.	States could establish voluntary insurance purchasing cooperatives.

From *The New York Times*, Oct 17, 1993.

groups (health insurance purchasing cooperatives) made up of businesses, government employees, or individuals. These groups negotiate with the provider networks' payer sources – most commonly an insurer of health maintenance organizations – for service. All the accountable health plans, as the integrated network of provider and payer sources are referred to, would offer a uniform set of health services. This would enable the purchasing cooperatives to shop around for their best deal and force the accountable health plans to compete for their business. Fig. 3-1 shows survey results of the American consumer's choice for managed competition versus increased government regulation of health care.

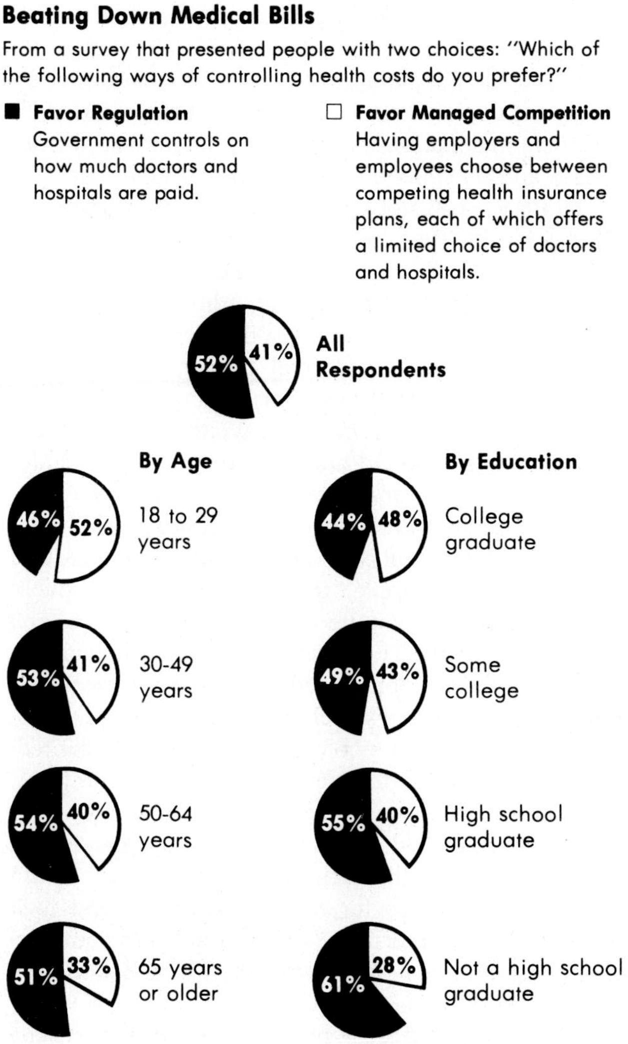

From a nationwide survey of 1,149 adults conducted Nov. 3, 1992 (election night) by Louis Harris & Associates for the Henry J. Kaiser Family Foundation and the Harvard School of Public Health. Those with no answer are not shown.

Fig. 3-1. Results of a survey asking consumers for their preferences between government regulation of health care costs and managed competition. (From *The New York Times*, March 14, 1993.)

The health care market, not the government, is the driving force behind these networks which are currently being formed in major metropolitan areas. However, doctors, hospitals, executives, and insurers say they are also trying to position themselves for success under any legislation Congress might pass in 1994. The competition to establish these networks is being intensified by the belief that whoever moves first will be able to profit by controlling the shape of the new health system.

NURSING'S ROLE IN THE SEARCH FOR HEALTH CARE REFORM

Nursing organizations are also banking on the growing pressure from government and private health insurers to reduce medical bills. The agenda from the nursing community, "Nursing's Agenda for Health Care Reform" (see the box below), would steer Americans away from an emphasis on high technology care favored by physicians toward a preventive health care approach favored by nurses.[1]

Since nurses in primary care do focus on health promotion and disease prevention, they are in a unique position to open the door to universal, affordable health care. The first major point in nursing's agenda is to provide primary care in familiar, community settings such as schools, community clinics, factories, and home.[22] Recognizing the importance of nursing's input on key issues, President Clinton invited the American Nurses' Association (ANA) to join his team to help assess the health care systems and assist his administration's search for adapting new health care delivery system changes.

OFFICIAL AGENCIES

Official agencies are tax supported and, therefore, are accountable to the citizens and the government through

NURSING'S NATIONAL AGENDA FOR HEALTH CARE REFORM

- Universal access to health care
- Empowerment of consumers
- Wellness and health as priorities
- Integration of public and private resources
- Managed care and primary health care as delivery models of care
- Objection to increased health care
- Direct consumer access to a variety of professional care providers including nurses

From American Nurses' Association: *Nursing's agenda for health care reform*, Washington, DC, 1990, The Association.

elected or appointed officials or boards. The purpose and duties of official agencies are prescribed or mandated by law. This discussion is from the perspective of the individual gaining knowledge of or access to the health care system.

Local Level. The *health department* of a town, city, county, township, or district is the local health unit and usually the first line of access and health responsibility for the population it serves. The chief administrator, the *health officer,* is appointed by the mayor, board of health, or some other executive governing body.

The local health department's role and functions usually center on providing direct services to the public and depend on the state mandate and community resources. The usual range of functions includes six basic categories of service that are detailed in Table 3-3.

Local governments, but usually not health departments, have the responsibility for providing general health care services for the poor (see the Medicaid section later in this chapter).

State Level. Public health services are organized by each state, with wide variation from one state to another. The chief administrator usually is a state health officer or commissioner appointed by the governor. One agency, typically the state health department, carries out the primary responsibilities in policy, planning, and coordination of programs and services for local units under its jurisdiction.

Federal Level. The U.S. Department of Health and Human Services (DHHS) is the main federal body concerned with the health of the nation. Established as a separate body in 1979, DHHS was formerly part of the Department of Health, Education, and Welfare (HEW). The U.S. Public Health Service (PHS) is the major component of DHHS concerned with health matters.

The major functions of the PHS are (1) assisting state and local communities with the development of health resources and education for the health professions; (2) assisting with the delivery of health services to all Americans; (3) supporting and conducting research in health-related sciences to disseminate scientific information; (4) protecting the people against impure and unsafe foods, drugs, and cosmetics and other potential hazards; and (5) providing national leadership for communicable disease control and prevention plus other health functions.

The PHS consists of eight agencies. The first seven are (1) the Health Resources and Services Administration (HRSA); (2) the Centers for Disease Control and Prevention (CDC); (3) the Food and Drug Administration (FDA); (4) the National Institutes of Health (NIH); (5) the Alcohol, Drug Abuse, and Mental Health Administration (ADAMHA); (6) the Agency for Toxic Substances and Disease Registry (ATSDR); and (7) the Indian Health Service. The eighth and newest agency, the Agency for Health Care Policy and Research, was created by Congress in December 1989. These subsidiaries provide leadership, protect the public, conduct research, and provide treatment. For example, the FDA protects the public against unsafe and impure drugs, food, cosmetics, and other hazards; the 11 institutes of the NIH provide for research and education related to many health problems, ranging from dental research to cancer treatment.

Other departments involved in health care at the federal level include (1) the Veteran's Administration (VA), an independent agency directly under the president, which provides health care services for four categories of veterans; and (2) the Department of Defense, which sponsors health care for military personnel and their dependents, covered under an insurance program purchasing health care in the private sector from Blue Cross/Blue Shield.

Departments engaged in health-related activities include (1) the Department of Agriculture, providing inspection and research related to crops and animals as well as providing food stamps; (2) the Department of Housing and Urban Development (HUD), involved in constructing such facilities as rural hospitals and neighborhood clinics; and (3) the Department of Labor, providing preventive services in the workplace through the Occupational Safety

***Table 3-3.* Local health department: role and functions**

Category of service	Basic functions
1. Vital statistics	Record births, deaths, marriages
2. Laboratory facilities	Testing: bacteriology, virology, and immunology Detect: chronic and metabolic disease
3. Communicable disease control	Investigate outbreaks; maintain free clinics for immunization and early diagnosis and treatment of tuberculosis and venereal disease
4. Environmental health and safety	Supervise food, water, and milk supplies, sanitary conditions in public eating places, and sanitary waste disposal; control water and air pollution; inspect health facilities
5. Personal health services	Provide preventive maternal and child health (MCH) services (well-baby clinics, prenatal clinics) and adult health services (health inventories and surveys)
6. Public health education and information	Maintain public health nursing services and health education system, including preventive and rehabilitative services in chronic disease control

and Health Administration (OSHA).

Over the last few years, government agencies have demonstrated an awareness that infection control procedures in the hospital can help protect hospital employees from acquiring blood-borne diseases. In 1987, following the first documented reports of occupationally acquired human immunodeficiency virus (HIV) in health care employees, the ANA and some labor unions petitioned the OSHA to issue an emergency infection control standard. OSHA responded by enforcing a series of guidelines developed by the CDC 4 years earlier. In these guidelines, hepatitis B is cited as a major health risk to health care personnel – a more significant risk than HIV. A recent study revealed that after a 2-year training evaluation period, physician compliance with infection control procedures increased from 20% to 80% and nurse compliance from 50% to 86%.[14] The OSHA laws mentioned above were implemented in 1992.

Despite their need for health promotion and disease prevention, people with disabilities face numerous problems gaining access to health promotion programs and preventive services. The barriers are financial, social, physical, and logistical.

Starting in 1992, health care providers, both as employers and providers of public services, were required to comply with requirements of the Americans with Disabilities Act (ADA) of 1990. The ADA is considered the most sweeping civil rights legislation since the Civil Rights Act of 1964. The two parts of the ADA that apply most directly to health care providers are the prohibitions on employment discrimination and the requirements for provision of services to persons with disabilities. An example of health care provider accommodation is to install wheelchair lifts in the shuttle bus systems they operate.

On November 5, 1990, President Bush signed the Patient Self-Determination Act which took effect in December 1991. This law was designed to increase client involvement in decisions regarding life-sustaining treatment by ensuring that advanced directives for health care are available to physicians at the time medical decisions are being made and that clients who have not prepared such documents are aware of their legal right to do so. As a condition of Medicare and Medicaid payment, the Patient Self-Determination Act requires health care facilities to have the following:

1. Policies and procedures in advanced directives
2. Client choice in the medical record
3. Client facility policy and procedures
4. Facility staff and community education about advanced directives

The federal agency that has major accountability for control of the environment is the Environmental Protection Agency (EPA). Established in 1970 as an independent (nondepartmental) government agency, its responsibilities include quality and pollution control of air and water; control of solid waste disposal, radiation hazards, and toxic substances; and pesticide regulation. Functions of the EPA include (1) conducting research on pollution control and the effects of pollution on humans, (2) developing criteria and promulgating national standards for pollutants, and (3) enforcing compliance with these standards.

International Level. The World Health Organization (WHO), established as a specialized agency of the United Nations in 1948, directs and coordinates international health. It assists governments in strengthening health services and furnishing technical assistance as well as encouraging and coordinating international scientific research.

Voluntary Sector

VOLUNTARY AGENCIES

The voluntary (or not-for-profit) health movement, which began in 1882, stems from the good will and humanitarian concerns that are part of the nongovernment, free-enterprise heritage of the people of the United States. Powerful forces in the health field, voluntary agencies, foundations, and professional associations are nonprofit entities that maintain a tax-free status (see Table 3-4).

Voluntary agencies are influential in promoting health affairs at the national policy level and often have significant impact on health legislation. Their prominent role in public influence was demonstrated by the American Cancer Society's early mass media announcements concerning the health hazards of smoking. In addition, voluntary agencies have stimulated research advances, as in the development of the polio vaccine by Jonas Salk in 1954 for the prevention of paralytic poliomyelitis.

Philanthropic foundations provide valuable stimulation to the health field and operate under fewer constraints than other sources in supporting research or training projects. Historically, foundations tend to be less formal in their review and grant procedures and provide support for untried research projects.

Nurses interested in research or advanced clinical study that relates to the special interests of voluntary agencies or foundations will find grant monies available to support their work. Most libraries contain references detailing specific grant interests and monies available.

Professional associations, organized at the national level with state and local branches, are powerful political forces. The American Medical Association's role in opposing legislation for comprehensive health insurance (endorsed by the ANA) is a good example. Nurses may support their professional organizations, the ANA and the National League for Nursing (NLN), to influence the direction of health policy. Membership and active participation are the first steps (see Table 3-3).

***Table 3-4.* Voluntary agencies, foundations, and professional associations**

	Voluntary agencies	Foundations	Professional associations
Types/examples	Focus on specific populations, e.g., American Red Cross, National Society for Prevention of Blindness, National Association for Mental Health	Rockefeller Foundation Ford Foundation	American Nurses' Association (ANA) American Medical Association (AMA) American Hospital Association (AHA)
Purpose	Provide public and professional educational programs to improve services and quality of facilities and personnel	Provide support for research	Provide political influence, information, forum on current issues Support research and innovation
Financing	Contributions from individual citizens, business, and industry	Private philanthropy	Dues from individual members

FINANCING HEALTH CARE

Costs

The health care industry is one of the largest industries in the United States today and accounts for an ever-increasing share of national resources.

During the 1960s and 1970s, when a rapid growth in federal expenditures occurred, federal funds were an important source of new monies for health care. The Medicare and Medicaid programs accounted for most of the increase in public spending, as well as the bulk of federal health expenditures.

The 1980s experienced reduced growth both in overall federal expenditures and in federal health spending. In fact, 1984 showed the beginning of a trend toward decreased growth of federal health expenditures that continues to date.[18] Health care analysts credit federal cost containment measures with this trend.[10,18] (See discussion of the prospective payment system later in this chapter.)

Increasingly in the 1980s, with less money available for health care, the nation's employers, who are generally the payers of health care costs, are experimenting with different payment mechanisms, such as employee cost sharing, self-insurance, and alternative delivery systems.[8] The effects of this influx of business into health care and the subsequent emphasis on competition to resolve the financial problems have not been fully realized.

Changes in hospital care – more outpatient services, shorter inpatient stays, and more care of chronic than acute illness – mean that hospitals have less opportunity to offer prevention or health promotion education to clients. Also, work force shortages, especially in nursing, and inadequate resources or reimbursement may prevent health care professionals from offering the range of educational efforts called for in the 1990 Objectives, such as counseling in safety belt use, nutrition education, physical fitness regimens, and stress-coping skills. Given the lack of progress toward some key objectives such as infant mortality among minorities and the lack of access to private health insurance, "It is perhaps time to elevate financing for preventive services to the status of an objective if risk reduction and health status objectives are to be achieved for all populations" by the year 2000.[27]

Health care costs are approaching 12% of the Gross National Product (GNP). Health care is expected to cost over $756 billion in 1991.[27] If nothing is done to control expenditures, health care spending is expected to reach $1.2 to $1.3 trillion by 1995 – an increase of some $500 billion in less than 5 years. At this rate, if the system remains unchanged, spending will reach between $2.1 and $2.7 trillion by the year 2000.[19] (See Table 3-5 for cost of treatment for selected preventable conditions.)

An increasing portion of the health care pie is being used by the elderly through private sources (out-of-pocket, insurance, and/or Medicare premiums) and the shrinking amount paid through public funds. Unlike those under age 65 who rely on employee-paid insurance as the major source of health care payments, public funds are a major source for those over 65.[24]

In the past, one of the principal ways that providers (mainly hospitals and physicians) have offset the decrease in revenues generated by public sector clients is to increase the costs for their private clients. This cost shifting will become increasingly more difficult with the growing emphasis on cost control by the major purchaser of health care.[28] The problem of how to finance health care coverage will remain a major concern for this country in the 1990s and beyond.

Sources

Government monies in the public sector generally travel from federal to state to local level. This system of allocation has been predominant since World War II. However,

***Table 3-5.* Costs of treatment for selected preventable conditions**

Condition	Overall magnitude	Avoidable intervention*	Cost per patient†
Heart disease	7 million with coronary artery disease 500,000 deaths/yr 284,000 bypass procedures/yr	Coronary bypass surgery	$ 30,000
Cancer	1 million new cases/yr 510,000 deaths/yr	Lung cancer treatment Cervical cancer treatment	$ 29,000 $ 28,000
Stroke	600,000 strokes/yr 150,000 deaths/yr	Hemiplegia treatment and rehabilitation	$ 22,000
Injuries	2.3 million hospitalizations/yr 142,500 deaths/yr 177,000 persons with spinal cord injuries in the United States	Quadriplegia treatment and rehabilitation Hip fracture treatment and rehabilitation Severe head injury treatment and rehabilitation	$570,000 (lifetime) $ 40,000 $310,000
HIV infection	1-1.5 million infected 118,000 AIDS cases (as of Jan 1990)	AIDS treatment	$ 75,000 (lifetime)
Alcoholism	18.5 million abuse alcohol 105,000 alcohol-related deaths/yr	Liver transplant	$250,000
Drug abuse	Regular users: 1-3 million, cocaine 900,000, IV drugs 500,000, heroin Drug-exposed babies: 375,000	Treatment of drug-affected baby	$ 63,000 (lifetime)
Low birth weight baby (LBWB)	260,000 LBWB born/yr 23,000 deaths/yr	Neonatal intensive care for LBWB	$ 10,000
Inadequate immunization	Lacking basic immunization series: 20% to 30%, age 2 and younger 3%, age 6 and older	Congenital rubella syndrome treatment	$354,000 (lifetime)

Data compiled from various sources by the Office of Disease Prevention and Health Promotion, 1991.
*Examples (other interventions may apply).
†Representative first-year costs, except as noted. Not indicated are nonmedical costs, such as lost productivity to society.

in the early 1970s, a decentralization of federal decision-making bodies occurred with a conversion to 10 regional areas and a consultant consolidation of grant programs to develop "general revenue sharing" in 1973. This general revenue sharing transferred money from the federal government directly to the local governments based on population and relative economic status.

In 1982 a major change in the federal financing system occurred with the implementation of the Omnibus Budget Reconciliation Act (P.L. 97-35), which combined 20 programs into four block grants (six programs remained categorical).[22] These block grants were given to the states to administer; and the states' total funding was reduced by 21%, which combined with inflation amounted to 30%.[20] In 1983 congressional consensus changed, and funding was not further reduced.

What are the effects of block grants? With long initiation times, carry-over funds, and different administrations in each state, it is hard to tell. Some groups are claiming, however, that because states may spend these funds in various ways, many communities have had reductions in lead poisoning programs, rodent control, drug abuse programs, prenatal and delivery services, and other areas.

Local programs can create problems with inequities because of an unequal distribution of resources; the stigma of being poor and racial prejudice compound the inequities. In addition, state-funded benefits with varying eligibility requirements and exclusions have created different programs and unequal distribution. Welfare is one example; requirements and benefits vary widely from state to state. Welfare and Medicaid are both state administered; and the unequal distribution of funds has led to proposals to federalize them, similar to the Supplemental Security Income (SSI) program that provides public assistance to the aged, blind, and disabled.

Mechanisms

Although some physicians and other professionals in the private sector are paid on a fee-for-service basis by clients or third-party private or public-supported insurance, most health workers, including nurses in institutional or community agencies and in the military, receive wages or salaries. Since most nurses are salaried, the separation of nursing costs from all other health-related costs is very difficult. Without documentation of specific nursing costs, it is also difficult to validate the need for skilled nursing services.

In recent years, nurses – especially nurse practitioners – have begun to enter independent practice to provide direct client services. This may be viewed as a logical outgrowth of seeking higher levels of professionalism. The Nurse Practice Acts of some states encourage nurses to use their knowledge more comprehensively than many agencies sanction. In independent practice, the nurse is directly accountable to clients and is paid either directly or by third parties (see Table 3-6). The philosophic and realistic issues of private nursing practice range from questions about the equity of fee-for-service to the practical problems of setting up such a practice.

Controversy surrounds the fee-for-service system. Advocates say that the one-to-one relationship cements the bond between client and provider. Opponents say that it sets up two systems – one for clients who can pay and one for those who cannot. Opponents also claim that fee-for-service costs go up more rapidly than in other systems. Independent practice becoming commonplace in nursing's future depends on decisions about reimbursement by third parties in both private and public sectors.[27]

Alternate forms of payment are salary and capitation. The *salary* system involves a straight amount for services provided in a time frame. This system provides the employer with a fixed nursing income that is protected from changes in supply and demand, includes fringe benefits, and obviates fee collection problems. The salary system's flexibility makes it easier to fill unpopular jobs or jobs in underserved areas than with other payment mechanisms.[10] Disadvantages of this system include a limit on income and constraints on schedules, vacations, and peer review. The nurse may have to meet goals other than personal ones.

In the *capitation* system, such as in an HMO, each physician providing care receives a flat annual fee for each client regardless of how often services are used. Individuals who enroll in an HMO pay a fixed amount on a monthly basis whether they use the services; prepayment provides an incentive to provide efficient care. The objective is to keep persons healthy to prevent costly services. Cost consciousness dictates that illness be treated as early as possible and in the most cost-effective setting. Capitation is simple to administer: no third-party insurance payments are present, and the HMO bears the risk of illness. In other words, preventive primary care that deters the need for costly hospitalizations keeps costs down and the savings revert to the organization. On the negative side, however, clients may make unnecessary visits, and the increased number of clients necessary to provide more monies may decrease comprehensive care. At present no conclusive data exist on the outcomes of this system compared to other programs. (See further discussion of HMOs in the following Insurance section.)

Two major points are evident from this discussion of financing health care: (1) the cost of health care is rising at an increasingly rapid rate, and (2) government influence and involvement in health care are increasing, with Medi-

***Table 3-6.* Federal reimbursement for nurses in advanced practice: current status—current direct federal reimbursement for nursing services**

	Nurse providers			
Federal programs	**Nurse practitioner**	**Certified nurse midwife**	**Certified reg'd. nurse anesthetist**	**Clinical nurse specialist**
Medicare				
Part A	No	No	No	No
Part B	Yes*	Yes	Yes	Yes†
Medicaid	Yes‡	Yes	State discretion	State discretion
Champus‖	Yes	Yes	Yes	Yes§
FEHB¶	Yes	Yes	Yes	Yes

Prepared by Pamela Mittelstadt, RN, MPH, American Nurses' Association, Washington, DC, 1992.
*Limited to nursing facilities and rural areas
†Limited to rural areas
‡Limited to Pediatric NPs and Family NPs
§Limited to certified psychiatric nurse specialists
‖Civilian Health and Medical Program of Uniformed Services
¶Federal Employee Health Benefit Program

care and Medicaid consuming two thirds of public funds for health.[27] Rising health care expenditures, with a growing portion in the government's domain, signal increased federal interest to control costs.

The government's interest in hospital treatment cost containment is exemplified by the passage of P.L. 98-21, the Social Security Amendments of 1983, which mandate the establishment by the Health Care Financing Administration of a prospective payment system (PPS) for Medicare. This means providers are paid at preset rates based on 467 diagnosis-related group (DRG) categories that are used to classify the illness of each Medicare client. Rates for each diagnosis are established according to regional and national amounts based on each hospital's urban and rural cost experience.

This revolutionary PPS cost-containment mechanism was the first in a series of changes for the health care industry. Predictions are that prospective payment for services and facilities excluded from the present system, including psychiatric services, long-term care, rehabilitation, and home health care, will be followed by prospective payment for physicians.[11,13]

The impact of prospective payment on nurses revolves around a fundamental issue: documentation of nursing service costs and the contribution of nursing to provider revenues. Since nursing service is an undocumented part of hospital costs, nursing care for clients has been affected by prospective payment.

Cost-containment measures in the early 1980s forced hospitals to economize, often holding back salary increases for nurses and laying off other health care workers, thereby increasing nurses' tasks and responsibilities. Trends in the late 1980s, during a full-blown nursing shortage (an estimated 200,000 to 300,000 nursing vacancies nationwide in July 1988),[10] were toward increasing nurses' salaries and instituting other incentives to recruit and retain nurses. Creative measures to attract nurses include paying tuition for nursing education in exchange for a pledge to work in the hospital after graduation (as at Crouse-Irving Memorial Hospital School of Nursing, Syracuse, New York) or paying tuition for a nurse, spouse, and children to attend a sponsoring university if the nurse agrees to work at the hospital for a designated time (as at Loyola University Medical Center, Chicago).[10]

Clearly, a means of documenting nursing services is needed, such as the separate item specified on accounting forms for hospital nurses' services that New Jersey and Maine have instituted. New Jersey has a plan for calculating the amount of nursing time needed for different DRGs in terms of "relative intensity measures" (RIMs). Maine has a law requiring that its hospitals determine nursing costs for different DRG classifications and report the resulting data to the state's rate-setting commission annually. Only by documenting the value of nursing services can nurses prevent budget cuts that affect nursing care delivery; such services are now an indistinguishable part of the hospital budget.

Studies monitoring and evaluating the use of Medicare services show changes in practice patterns under prospective payment. Included are a decline in hospital services: fewer hospital admissions with shorter stays and some decline in services provided, contrasted with an increase in use of posthospital services; a substantial increase in outpatient services; and a slight increase in Medicare-supported home care and nursing home use.[9] These practice pattern changes slowed the rate of increase in Medicare costs between 1983 and 1986.[9]

Quality of care concerns are more difficult to evaluate, but early results of evaluation studies on utilization and mortality statistics do not suggest problems of access to inpatient care or increases in mortality related to the implementation of prospective payment.[6] The evaluation process is ongoing.

Insurance

There are some very positive elements of the health care system in America, one of which is highest quality acute care facilities in the world. In addition, the health care system covers approximately 67% of Americans through health insurance.[14]

That is not to say that there are not also problems ailing the system. Over 30 million Americans have no health insurance. These people receive health care, but they do so through the back door of the health care system – the emergency room door. This is the most inefficient and most costly way of providing care.[16]

Insurance refers to individual payment to a fund to provide protection for each contributor against financial losses resulting from an unlikely but possible occurrence. Medical insurance began in this tradition in 1847, with payments made to offset income lost as a result of an accident. Sickness benefits began as an extra and again emphasized loss of income. Blue Cross and Blue Shield originated reimbursing general health care costs in the 1930s.

The term *insurance* is really a misnomer, since health care is often required and is not a rare occurrence. *Assurance* is the term used in England to mean coverage for expected happenings (life assurance), whereas insurance covers unexpected happenings such as fire and theft.

PRIVATE HEALTH INSURANCE

Private health insurance, together with the individual expenditures in fee-for-service discussed earlier, accounts for more than half of all national health expenditures. Private health insurance covers more than two thirds of all persons in the United States who have health care coverage. In addition, a majority of the elderly, most of whom have Medicare coverage, purchase private insurance to supplement Medicare.[11] Coverage under private health insurance varies widely in terms of specific provisions, reimbursement amount for covered services, and limitations or restrictions. *Basic insurance* plans provide specified protection for the most costly services: inpatient and outpatient hospital services, including laboratory procedures and inpatient physician fees. *Major medical insurance* extends coverage to include such services as office visits to physicians or other providers, prescribed medicines, ambulance services, and durable medical equipment. The beneficiary pays a deductible and coinsurance, and the insurer pays a specified share of covered expenses up to a maximum limit. *Comprehensive insurance* combines features of both basic and major medical insurance.

In the private sector there are four types of organizations that provide health care insurance: (1) the traditional insurance companies, including the earliest insurer, Blue Cross/Blue Shield, a nonprofit charitable organization, and for-profit commercial insurance companies; (2) PPOs acting as "brokers" between insurers and health care providers; (3) HMOs, independent prepayment plans; and (4) self-insurance plans, in which employers take on the role of insurer.

Organized at the state and local level, Blue Cross and Blue Shield generally complement each other, with Blue Cross reimbursing hospitals and Blue Shield covering physicians and other providers. Today, Blue Cross sponsors 63 organizations, Blue Shield administers 65 plans, and 50 of these plans are administered jointly.[11]

Once the principal source of health care reimbursement, in 1987 Blue Cross/Blue Shield plans received less than 25% of the group insurance market share.[8]

After World War II insurance companies began to provide health insurance plans in competition with Blue Cross and Blue Shield. Today, more than 1000 commercial, profit-making insurance companies, such as Metropolitan Life and Aetna, offer individual, family, and group health policies that cover (1) hospitalization and in-hospital physician and office-based care coverage, (2) major medical expenses directed primarily at catastrophic illness, or (3) cash payments as a flat sum of money per day of hospitalization. Other types of private insurance plans designed to supplement Medicare, called Medigap plans, reimburse only deductibles and coinsurance payments associated with Medicare.

PPOs (discussed earlier in the Organization section) act as "brokers" between private insurers and health care providers.[8]

HMOs (discussed earlier in the Organization section) attempt to lower health care costs by emphasizing preventive rather than curative care, thus possibly decreasing the severity of some illnesses. Outpatient care is the focus, with lower hospitalization rates than in the fee-for-service area, almost entirely as a result of lower admission rates. HMOs tend to utilize fewer services, with emphasis on the least costly means of providing a needed service.

Employers in the 1980s, faced with increasing costs for health care insurance for their employees, are using their influence as payers to experiment with employee cost sharing, self-insurance, and alternative delivery systems, such as PPOs and HMOs, to moderate their outlays for health care coverage.[8]

Self-insurance means an employer (or union) assumes the claims risk of its insured employees, often self-funding or paying insurance claims from an established fund, such as a bank or trust account. Self-insurance gives employers a financial advantage, including an exemption from state taxes on health insurance premiums and interest earnings on reserves prior to claims payment.[8]

A 1987 Health Insurance Association of America (HIAA) study of group health insurance trends estimates that over 60% of Americans with employer-provided health care coverage are enrolled in a plan with some kind of self-insurance.[8] In 1987, half of the commercial insurance plans and one fourth of the Blue Cross/Blue Shield plans were self-insured[8] (see Table 3-7).

Medicare

Medicare is a federal insurance program that provides funds for medical costs to persons 65 years of age and older plus certain persons under age 65 who are disabled. Federal Medicare legislation, Title XVIII of the amendments to the Social Security Act, went into effect in 1966 after decades of debate. The intent was to protect the elderly against the catastrophic financial debts often incurred in treating chronic illness. This was the first time that federal legislation was enacted to remove financial barriers to medical care for the elderly.[9]

Since 1973, two groups of disabled persons under age 65 also have been able to receive Medicare benefits: (1) those totally and permanently disabled who qualify for Social Security can receive disability benefits for 2 years and (2) those who require hemodialysis of kidney transplantation.[9]

Medicare, Part A, basic hospital insurance, is financed by payroll taxes under the Social Security system. (See Table 3-8 for an explanation of benefits of Medicare, Part A.) Medicare, Part B, is supplementary voluntary medical insurance supported by general tax revenues and by the subscriber or person buying the insurance. (See Table 3-9 for an explanation of benefits of Medicare, Part B.)

Psychiatric benefits have not changed for inpatient care; they are still a lifetime limit of 190 days. However, the Omnibus Reconciliation Act of 1987 increased outpatient psychiatric coverage from $250 to $450 per year and in 1989 and thereafter to $1100 per year. Thus, Medicare has made provisions for financially catastrophic acute illness but not for catastrophic chronic illness, except for end-stage renal disease. In addition, continual health needs are not provided through Medicare, such as

***Table 3-7.* Conventional Blue Cross/Blue Shield (BC/BS) versus group health maintenance organization (HMO)**

Area of comparison	BC/BS/master medical	HMO
Persons covered	Individual Family Group	Individual Family Group
Ages covered	Prenatal to age 65; supplementary options to extend Medicare after age 65	All ages; an option for Medicare after age 65
Geographic area covered	No restrictions in United States	Specific geographic service area; if outside area, emergency coverage *only*
Payment mechanism	Annual premium; hospitals and physicians bill BC/BS directly Extended benefits: insured pays provider and bills BC/BS, which pays 80% of *reasonable* charges for *covered* services	Capitation fee (flat annual fee regardless of services used); client pays minimal fee at time of service
Insurance rating	Experience rating*	Community rating†
Preventive and health maintenance services	None	Physical examinations for infant and child; immunizations; preventive dentistry; eye examinations
Illness	Inpatient and outpatient hospital care; physician care; emergency services; diagnostic laboratory tests; diagnostic and therapeutic radiologic services	Inpatient and outpatient hospital care; physician care; emergency services; diagnostic laboratory tests; diagnostic and therapeutic radiologic services
Availability of services	Variable; hospital emergency rooms—24 hours a day, 7 days a week	24 hours a day, 7 days a week

*Based on use of services, with variations in premium rate.
†Determined by average of high-cost and low-cost individuals and groups, with same fee for all members regardless of age, sex, and health condition.

***Table 3-8.* Medicare (Part A): hospital insurance-covered services for 1992**

Services	Benefit	Medicare pays	You pay
Hospitalization			
Semiprivate room and board, general nursing, and miscellaneous hospital services and supplies.	First 60 days 61st to 90th day 91st to 150th day* Beyond 150 days	All but $652 All but $163 a day All but $326 a day Nothing	$652 $163 a day $326 a day All costs
Skilled nursing facility care			
You must have been in a hospital for at least 3 days and enter a Medicare-approved facility generally within 30 days after hospital discharge.†	First 20 days Additional 80 days Beyond 100 days	100% of approved amount All but $81.50 a day Nothing	Nothing $81.50 a day All costs
Home health care			
Medically necessary skilled care.	Part-time or intermittent care for as long as you meet Medicare conditions	100% of approved amount; 80% of approved amount for durable medical equipment	Nothing for services; 20% of approved amount for durable medical equipment
Hospice care			
Pain relief, symptom management, and support services for the terminally ill.	If you elect the hospice option and as long as doctor certifies need	All but limited costs for outpatient drugs and inpatient respite care	Limited cost sharing for outpatient drugs and inpatient respite care
Blood	Unlimited if medically necessary	All but first 3 pints per calendar year	For first 3 pints‡

1992 Part A monthly premium: None for most beneficiaries.
$192 if you must buy Part A (premium may be higher if you enroll late).

From US Department of Health and Human Services: *Medicare benefits booklet, Social Security Administration,* Washington, DC, 1993, US Government Printing Office.
*This 60-reserve-days benefit may be used only once in a lifetime.
†Neither Medicare nor private Medigap insurance will pay for most nursing home care.
‡To the extent the blood deductible is met under one part of Medicare during the calendar year, it does not have to be met under the other part.

***Table 3-9.* Medicare (Part B): medical insurance-covered services for 1992**

Services	Benefit	Medicare pays	You pay
Medical expenses			
Doctors' services, inpatient and outpatient medical and surgical services and supplies, physical and speech therapy, ambulance, diagnostic tests, and more.	Medicare pays for medical services in or out of the hospital	80% of approved amount (after $100 deductible)	$100 deductible* plus 20% of approved amount and limited charges above approved amount†
Clinical laboratory services			
Blood tests, biopsies, urinalyses, and more.	Unlimited if medically necessary	100% of approved amount	Nothing for services
Home health care			
Medically necessary skilled care.	Part-time or intermittent skilled care for as long as you meet conditions for benefits	100% of approved amount; 80% of approved amount for durable medical equipment	Nothing for services; 20% of approved amount for durable medical equipment
Outpatient hospital treatment			
Services for the diagnosis or treatment of illness or injury.	Unlimited if medically necessary	80% of approved amount (after $100 deductible)	$100 deductible plus 20% of billed charges
Blood	Unlimited if medically necessary	80% of approved amount (after $100 deductible and starting with 4th pint)	First 3 pints plus 20% of approved amount for additional pints (after $100 deductible)‡

1992 Part B monthly premium: $31.80 (premium may be higher if you enroll late).

From US Department of Health and Human Services: *Medicare benefits booklet, Social Security Administration,* Washington, DC, 1993, US Government Printing Office.

*Once you have had $100 of expenses for covered services in 1992, the Part B deductible does not apply to any further covered services you receive for the rest of the year.

†If your doctor does not accept assignment.

‡To the extent the blood deductible is met under one part of Medicare during the calendar year, it does not have to be met under the other part.

routine physical exams, vision care (including eyeglasses), medication, dental care, and private duty nursing care. Furthermore, custodial care, whether at home or in a nursing home, is not covered. This is the most costly and financially catastrophic service.

The limits in Medicare coverage mean that the elderly pay a substantial portion of their own health care costs beyond the expected 20%, especially if they have a chronic illness. The main population at risk, the elderly, may not have financial access to preventive health services, such as periodic examinations or screening for early detection of such diseases as high blood pressure, glaucoma, and diabetes.

More states are placing tighter limits on the amount doctors can charge their Medicare patients. A Pennsylvania law, effective November 1992, bars physicians from charging beneficiaries more than the amount approved by Medicare. Medicare pays for 80% of "approved charges." Approved charges are determined by Medicare to be "reasonable" for the care rendered. The client is then liable for the remaining 20% of the approved charges. Clients also may be liable for amounts that doctors charge that exceed the sum approved by Medicare. However, beginning in 1993, this amount will decrease as caps are established for physician fees.

Medicaid

Medicaid is an assistance program managed jointly by the federal and state governments to provide partial or full payment of medical costs for categories of individuals and families of any age who are too poor to pay for the care. Medicaid legislation, Title XIX of the amendments to the Social Security Act, went into effect in 1967 and was amended again in 1972. The federal government provides funds to states on a cost-sharing basis, according to the per capita income of each state, to guarantee medical services to eligible Medicaid recipients. Table 3-10 compares Medicare and Medicaid.

Persons eligible for Medicaid are those groups who receive cash payments from welfare programs established under Social Security – Aid to Families with Dependent Children (AFDC) and Supplemental Security Income (SSI). The "categorically needy" are children of AFDC families and those covered by SSI, namely, the aged, the blind, and the totally and permanently disabled. Also, the Deficit Reduction Act of 1984 (P.L. 98-369) added three other eligible groups: (1) poor children up to age 5, (2) poor pregnant women who would qualify for AFDC if their children were born, and (3) pregnant women in two-parent families with an unemployed principal wage earner.[13] In addition, states may provide Medicaid for the "medically needy" or persons whose income and assets fall within a needy standard set by each state.

States administer Medicaid under broad federal requirements and guidelines. Basic health services mandated are (1) inpatient and outpatient care, (2) laboratory and radiologic services, (3) physicians' services, and skilled nursing facility services for persons over age 21. Other services, such as dental care, eyeglasses, or intermediate care facility services, may be added at the state's option.

By 1973 the federal government required states to provide Medicaid programs for early and periodic screening, diagnosis, and treatment (EPSDT) of persons under age 21. The EPSDT provision signified the federal government's recognition of the need for primary prevention and health promotion. The emphasis on prevention rather than treatment – the focus of this text – was a positive approach toward health and required the development and implementation of new methods of health care delivery. The EPSDT program has five phases: (1) outreach and case findings, (2) screening, (3) testing, (4) compiling and reporting results, and (5) follow-through and treatment.

When Ronald Reagan took office in 1981, his administration quickly succeeded in decreasing Medicaid funding by nearly $1 billion and nearly succeeded in capping the amount of Medicaid funding granted to each state.[3] By 1983, interest groups began to mobilize and gather data on the poor state of children's health and the inadequacies of Medicaid policies. In June 1992, a joint House and Senate budget resolution appropriated an additional $200 million for Medicaid for fiscal year 1984. The Con-

***Table 3-10.* Comparison of Medicare and Medicaid**

	Medicare (Title XVIII)	Medicaid (Title XIX)
Type of program	Insurance	Assistance
Source of money	Part A—social security tax Part B—tax revenues and voluntary premiums	General tax revenues
Level of administration	Federal (same in all states)	Federal and state (varies from state to state)
Eligible persons	1. Persons over age 65 2. Those qualifying for disability under social security 3. Persons of any age with kidney disease requiring dialysis and transplant	Required: Categorically needy persons receiving the following: Welfare AFDC (Aid to Families with Dependent Children) SSI (Supplemental Security Income) OAA (Old Age Assistance) AB (Aid to the Blind) ATPD (Aid to Totally and Permanently Disabled) Optional: Medically indigent persons unable to pay for medical care
Services	Part A 1. Hospital insurance (compulsory) 2. Posthospital care—ECF (extended care facility) 3. Home health services Part B—voluntary (optional) medical insurance 1. Physicians' services 2. Outpatient hospital services 3. Home health services 4. Other medical services	1. Inpatient and outpatient hospital care 2. Laboratory and radiologic tests 3. Physicians' services 4. Skilled nursing facility services for persons age 21 and over 5. Home health services 6. Family planning services 7. Rural health clinic services 8. EPSDT (early and periodic screening, diagnosis, and treatment) for persons under age 21 9. Optional services according to state's choice

solidated Omnibus Budget Reconciliation Act (COBRA, 1985) continued the trend begun in 1984 in that it expanded the scope of those eligible for Medicaid coverage. When the Gramm-Redman-Hollings deficit reduction bill was signed into law in 1985, Congress exempted Medicaid from across-the-board cuts.

A law (P299-504) known as the Omnibus Reconciliation Act was passed and signed by President Reagan in 1987. This law gave the states the option of extending automatic Medicaid coverage to pregnant women and to children younger than 5 years of age in families with incomes below the federal poverty level but over the states' AFDC eligibility level. Building on the momentum of the late 1980s, Congress enacted legislation in 1989 that mandated Medicaid coverage for pregnant women and children up to age 6 with family incomes less than 133% of the federal poverty level.[3]

As the expansion of Medicaid eligibility places serious financial burdens on state governments, state policy makers are examining ways of improving access to health care while simultaneously holding down costs. (See Table 3-11 for percentage increases in Medicaid budgets.)

President Clinton's 1993 budget package brought with it new mandates for Medicaid eligibility. In addition to having the 30-month spenddown increased to 36 months, individuals can no longer look to the living trust as a method of protecting assets.

There are several states which are participating in the Robert Wood Johnson model program of purchasing long-term care insurance to protect a specific amount of money. Once the insurance monies are paid out up to that amount, the insured individual qualifies for Medicaid. This program is considered an attempt to cut Medicaid costs for long-term care of those individuals over the age of 65.

States determine Medicaid eligibility as well as covered benefits and provider payment mechanisms; thus, Medicaid programs vary widely from one state to another and may be inadequate to meet the health care needs of covered individuals. In addition, since eligibility is tied to the receipt of cash assistance and each state can set the income level for cash assistance wherever it deems appropriate, many poor persons who cannot afford to pay for health insurance are not covered.

***Table 3-11.* Percentage increases in Medicaid budgets (1975-1990)**

Year	Total	Federal	State
1975	23.5	21.0	26.9
1976	15.9	17.7	13.5
1977	16.8	16.9	16.7
1978	10.8	10.0	11.9
1979	14.8	14.9	14.8
1980	18.5	18.6	18.4
1981	17.8	17.3	18.4
1982	6.8	2.6	12.2
1983	7.7	8.4	7.0
1984	7.7	5.8	9.8
1985	8.7	12.7	4.1
1986	9.6	10.3	8.7
1987	10.0	9.8	10.3
1988	9.7	11.0	8.0
1989	13.2	13.6	12.7
1990*	15.8	16.3	15.2

Source: US House of Representatives, Committee on Ways and Means: *Background material and data on programs within the jurisdiction of the Committee on Ways and Means*, Washington, DC, 1990, US Government Printing Office.

*Current law estimate.

The Uninsured

The number of Americans without health care insurance of any kind has increased since the late 1970s. Without health insurance, low-income families must rely on a frequently fragmented and difficult-to-use public system of health care. Regular preventive care, including prenatal care, immunization, and well-child care, is sometimes difficult to get; and its availability may not be well understood. Only when families do not have to make a choice between food on the table and a visit to the doctor or clinic will adequate care for those most at risk be provided.

Today, more than 60 million Americans are either uninsured or underinsured. This fact alone cries out for health care reform. Now the system's inability to contain costs is placing more and more Americans with "adequate" insurance coverage at risk of hardship when major illnesses do occur. Employers and employees alike are desperately seeking solutions to the dual problems of using health care costs and increased premium rates that threaten basic coverage for most American workers and their dependents.

THE CANADIAN HEALTH CARE SYSTEM

Contrary to what some in the U.S. health care industry would suggest, Canada does not have "socialized medicine." Medicare, as Canada's health care system is called, is simply a social insurance plan much like Social Security and Medicare for older people in the United States. Canada's doctors do not work on salary for the government.

Canadians pay for health care through a variety of federal and provincial taxes, just as Americans pay for Social Security and Medicare through payroll taxes. (See Fig. 3-2 for a comparison of health care spending between Canada and the United States.) The government of each province pays the medical bills for its citizens. Because the government is the primary payer of medical bills, Canada's health care system is referred to as a "single-payer arrangement." Benefits vary somewhat among the

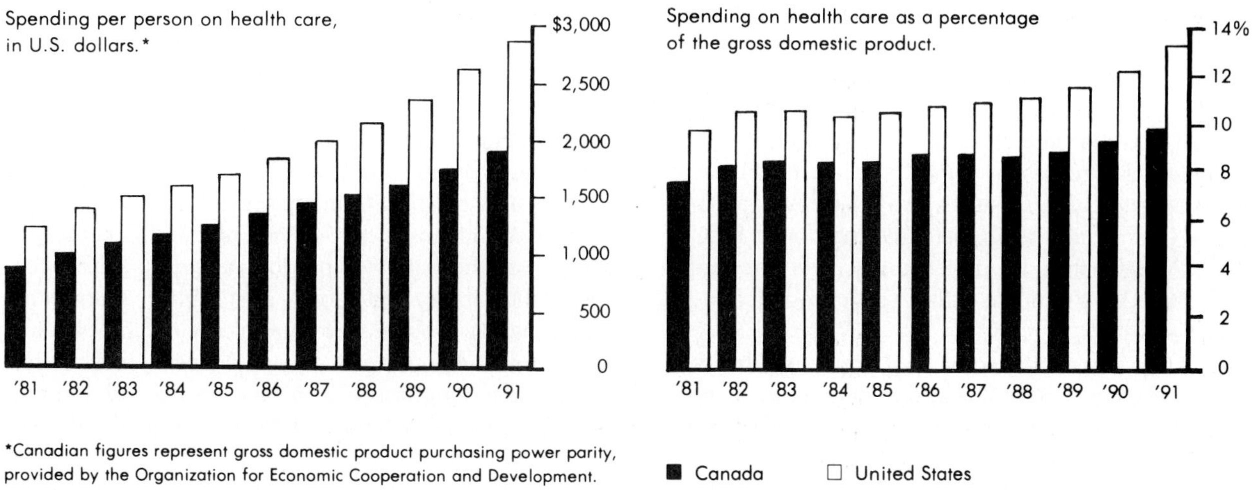

Fig. 3-2. Spending on health care. (From *The New York Times,* March 14, 1993.)

provinces, but most cover – in addition to hospital, medical care, long-term care, and mental health services – all prescription drugs for people over age 65. Private insurance exists only for those services the provincial plans do not cover.

Although each province runs its own insurance program as it sees fit, all are guided by the five principles of the Canada Health Act, as shown in the box to the right. A single-payer system such as described above is the best system for the growing number of consumers shut out of the private insurance market and the even larger number who have reasons to fear their coverage might disappear at any time.

FIVE PRINCIPLES OF THE CANADA HEALTH ACT

1. **Universality.** Everyone in the nation is covered.
2. **Portability.** People can move from province to province and from job to job or onto the unemployment roles and still retain their health coverage.
3. **Accessibility.** Everyone has access to the system's health care providers.
4. **Comprehensiveness.** Provincial plans cover all medically necessary treatment.
5. **Public administration.** The system is publicly run and publicly accountable.

INFLUENCING HEALTH POLICY

The primary responsibility of the nurse is to the client served, whether the client is an individual, family, group, or community.

Since health cannot be separated from its environment, it is essential that nurses become involved in all aspects of planning for health to maximize the health potential of all Americans. This involvement needs to include attention to policy decisions and political action. Policy affects the broader aspects of environment, the biophysical and socioeconomic conditions of homes, schools, workplaces, and communities as well as the health care delivery environment. By virtue of numbers, nurses, the largest group of health care providers in the United States, have tremendous potential power to influence decision making.

Participating in policy decision making requires the nurse to take a proactive stance to determine needs before a problem arises. Policy development and change take place on many levels: from within the nurse's agency or work group to the community, state, and national levels. At the institutional level clinical decisions influence policy just as management issues do. The nurse should examine the rationale behind an existing or planned policy and determine whether it is relevant now. Nurses are empowered by their education and experience to use their people skills and to apply change theory to influence policy development and change.

Much health-related decision making is the result of legislation at the local, state, or national level. *Laws,* rules enforced by a ruling authority by which society is governed, and *regulations,* agency or department rules developed for the implementation of laws, define what services are being offered to whom and who will pay how much.

Politics, or the use of power to promote a needed change, is an arena for nursing's participation that is part of this nation's democratic heritage. The nurse can be politically involved in many ways. Bumper stickers proclaim that 1 of every 44 registered voters is a nurse. Voting, after becoming well informed on current issues and candidates, is a major way for nurses to be actively involved. The nurse should get to know the politically influential people in the community and disseminate information learned from them to others.

The nurse can run for political office (many nurses now represent their local constituencies, and there is increasing visibility at the state and national levels) and support colleagues who represent nursing's interests. Financial contributions to N-PAC (Nurses for Political Action Coalition), ANA's political arm, increases the power base of nurses. Membership in professional and community groups provides the nurse with a collective voice to influence legislators.

Legislators are influenced by the information that they receive and the source of that information. (Vested interest groups were discussed previously.) The process of trying to persuade legislators to vote for or against measures important to the interest group represented is *lobbying*. A *lobbyist* is a registered representative of a special interest group. The ANA has relocated to Washington, D.C., and employees nurse lobbyists. The lobbyists need to receive input from nurses individually and as a group.

A legislator can be approached personally or via telephone, telegram, of mail. Legislators have staffs of experts in the applicable areas of their involvement, and each legislator is assigned to certain committees. To understand the legislative process, the individual nurse needs to follow the progress of a bill. It is essential that nurses become politically aware and active to enable the collective voice of nursing to reach its full potential.

It is the responsibility of nurses to become well informed. As well-informed, empowered professionals, nurses play a significant role in supporting appropriate legislative initiatives that promote and protect the health of the public.

SUMMARY

Historical perspective and description of the present health care delivery system in the United States provide a framework for the analysis of trends, values, and needs related to health. The current U.S. system, or nonsystem as it has been frequently called, concentrates on the delivery and financing of illness care. Not only is the real purpose of health care – the promotion of health – the lacking in policy, delivery, and financing, but the care that does exist focuses on short-term, episodic disease patterns that were predominant in the first half of the 20th century instead of on those that will predominate during the second half of the century and into the 21st century. Current and future health problems are chronic in nature, requiring long-term continuous delivery and financing mechanisms. A change in emphasis and direction is needed and must be reflected in federal health policy and goals for the year 2000 and beyond.

The U.S. government provides the legal underpinnings for protecting and controlling the environment for health and delivery of health care services through the enactment of laws and the regulation of financing for the system. Social policy as a reflection of society's values has changed from a laissez-faire approach in the 1850s to one, since the 1970s, in which the central federal government has a prominent role in organizing and financing health care.

In 1993, President Clinton's initiation of the Health Security Program caused Congress to take note. In promoting health security for all U.S. citizens, the current system would provide universal coverage, equal access, and managed care through competition. If President Clinton is successful in gaining congressional and consumer support for this program, the United States will offer its citizens the most sweeping national program since Social Security in 1935. As part of this national program and equally important for both health care and economic reason, this program, for the first time, would provide a broad range of preventive services including regular check-ups and well-baby visits.

References

1. American Nurses' Association: Nursing's agenda for health care reform, Washington, DC, 1992, The Association.
2. Capuzzi C, Garland M: The Oregon plan: increasing access to health care, *Nurs Outlook* 38(5):200, 1990.
3. Cohen S: The politics of medicaid 1980-1989, *Nurs Outlook* 38(5): 229, 1990.
4. Daniels N: *Justice and the dissemination of big ticket technologies.* In Arras H, Rhoden N: *Ethical issues in modern medicine,* ed 3, Mountain View, Calif, 1989, Mayfield.
5. Editorial, *Am J Health Promotion* 6(3): 174, 1992.
6. Eggers P: Prospective payment system and quality: early results and research strategy, *Health Care Financing Rev* (ann suppl):29, 1987.
7. Freyman JG: *The American health care system: its genesis and trajectory,* Huntington, NY, 1980, Kriefer Publishing.
8. Gabel J, et al: The changing world of group health insurance, *Health Affairs* 7(3):48, 1988.
9. Guterman S, et al: The first three years of Medicare prospective payment: an overview, *Health Care Financing Rev* 9(3): 67, 1988.
10. Hevesi D: Shortage of nurses forces a rise in salaries, *The New York Times,* July 31, 1988.
11. Koch AL: *Financing health services.* In William S, Torrens P, editors: *Introduction to health services,* ed 3, New York, 1988, John Wiley & Sons.
12. Little C: Health for all by the year 2000, *Nurs Health Care* 13:4, 1992.
13. McCarthy C, Thorpe KE: *Financing for health care.* In Jonas S, editor: *Health care delivery in the U.S.,* ed 3, New York, 1986, Springer Publishing.
14. Miramontes H: Progress in establishing safety protocols based on CDC and OSHA recommendations, Infection Control Hospital, *Epidemiology* 11:561-562, 1991.
15. Mittelstadt P: *Federal reimbursement for nurses in advanced practice: current status,* Washington, DC, 1992, American Nurses' Association.
16. Moley K: Insurance gaps create inefficiency, *McKnight's Long Term Care News,* p 10, 1992.
17. Northrup C: *Governmental, political and legal influences on the practice of com-*

munity health nursing. In Standhope M, Lancaster J, editors: *Community health nursing: process and practice for promoting health,* ed 2, St Louis, 1988, Times Mirror/Mosby College Publishing.
18. Pearson C: National health expenditures 1986-2000, *Health Care Financing Rev* 8(4):1, 1987.
19. Sharp N: The issue of reimbursement, *Nurs Management* 23(6):17, 1992.
20. Shonick W: *Public health services: background and present status.* In William S, Torrens P, editors: *Introduction to health services,* ed 3, New York, 1988, John Wiley & Sons.
21. Sorkin AL: *Health care and the changing economic environment,* Lexington, Mass, 1986, Lexington Books.
22. Stanhope M, Lancaster J, editors: *Community health nursing: process and practice for promoting health,* ed 2, St Louis, 1988, Times Mirror/Mosby College Publishing.
23. Thorpe KE, Thorpe J, Barhydt-Wezenaar N: *Health maintenance organizations.* In Jonas S, editor: *Health care delivery in the U.S.,* ed 3, New York, 1986, Springer Publishing.
24. US Department of Health and Human Services: *Medicare benefits booklet, Social Security Administration,* Washington, DC, 1993, US Government Printing Office.
25. US Department of Health and Human Services, Public Health Service: *Healthy people 2000,* Washington, DC, 1990, US Government Printing Office.
26. US House of Representatives, Committee on Ways and Means: *Background material and data on programs within the jurisdiction of the Committee on Ways and Means,* Washington, DC, 1990, US Government Printing Office.
27. Waldo DR, Levit KR, Lazenby H: National health expenditures, 1985, *Health Care Financing Rev* 8:1, 1986.
28. Wilensky G: Filling the gaps in health insurance: impact on competition, *Health Affairs* 7(3):133, 1988.

CHAPTER

4

Nursing Process

Carole Lium Edelman

Ellen Flaherty

Nancy T. Koge

Barbara Woods Bodnar

Sharon L. Pederson

Objectives

After completing this chapter, the nurse will be able to

- *Describe the historical development of the nursing process.*
- *Identify nursing scholars and theorists who contributed to the nursing process.*
- *Discuss the importance of utilizing the nursing process to advance the science of nursing and maintain standards of care.*
- *Identify the relationship between the five phases of the nursing process and the standards to guide nursing practice developed by the American Nurses' Association.*
- *List the overall categories of knowledge and skills required for using the nursing process.*
- *Identify assessment tools that assist in data gathering to reflect the whole person.*
- *Discuss the limitations of the currently accepted classification of nursing diagnoses when applied toward health promotion.*
- *Discuss the client's role as a decision maker responsible for self-initiated changes to improve their current health status as well as the nurse's role in enhancing the client's self-care.*

OVERVIEW OF THE NURSING PROCESS

Delivery of nursing care via a systematic, problem-solving approach is not a new concept when considering that nursing has existed in some form throughout history. In the 20th century, public attitudes about nursing as a profession have changed, as have nurses' approaches to their own practices. The recent trend toward health promotion and prevention has stimulated nursing to validate its significant contribution to health care. Use of the nursing process, as discussed here, provides nurses with a *systematic* and *standardized* way to organize the care they provide. This care delivery enables nurses to fulfill their responsibility to society in a scientific manner and to continue providing a meaningful service to humanity.

Historical Overview

In the past, nursing might have been defined as nurturant care of ill or infirmed persons. In addition to carrying out the medical regimen of physicians in hospitals, nurses functioned intuitively to promote health restoration in sick persons. Until the 19th century, educational preparation was not required of most nurses, nor was any rationale offered for nursing activities.

Changes in societal views of women, as well as advances in medical science during the 1700s and 1800s, precipitated change in nursing status. Educational programs were developed, and physicians wrote textbooks on nursing technique and sick care to upgrade skills so that the nurse could better carry out the health care provider's regimen.[6]

Florence Nightingale recognized that nurses could do more to promote well-being than merely carry out physicians' orders. In her book *Notes on Nursing,* published in 1859, she describes areas that affect human health, such as nutritional adequacy, hygiene, and sensory stimulation. She also addresses environmental aspects of care, including ambient temperature, noise, ventilation, cleanliness, and light. In a chapter devoted to observing the sick, she defines the purpose of observation: "It is not for the sake of piling up miscellaneous information or curious facts, but for the sake of saving life and increasing health and comfort."[25]

In 1955, Lydia Hall became the first person to describe nursing as a process in a presentation on the quality of nursing care.[9] In her philosophy, she describes three interrelated spheres of nursing. The "care" represents the nurturing component; the nurse provides client comfort by attending to basic activities of daily living. Theory for this part of nursing is based on the biologic and natural sciences. The "core" represents nursing activities to help patients become aware of feelings about their level of health. This is accomplished through the nurse's use of reflection as a therapeutic communication technique. Clients' awareness of their feelings ultimately leads them to conscious decision making regarding the existing state of health. The "cure" aspect of nursing involves those activities done in collaboration with other health team members such as the physician. The nurse carries out prescribed treatment measures while acting as a client advocate[9] (Fig. 4-1).

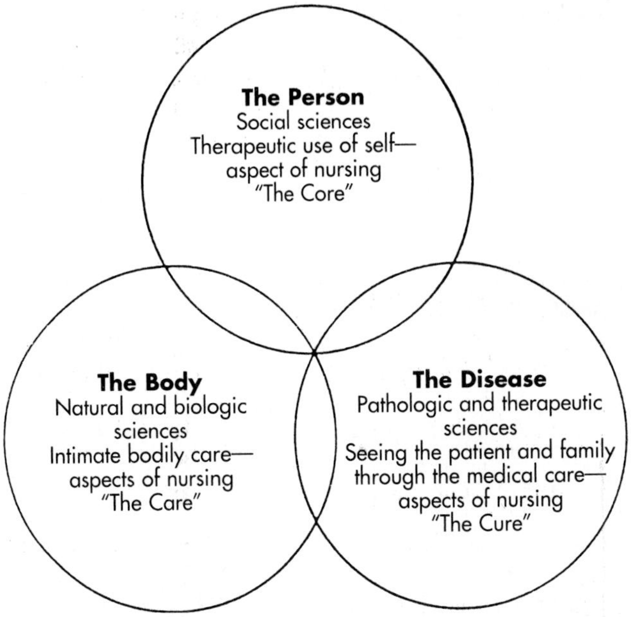

Fig. 4-1. Hall's core, care, and cure diagram. (From Hall L: Nursing – what is it?, *Can Nurse* 60[2]:151, 1964. Reproduced with permission.)

Orlando[28] was the first nursing theorist to use the term *nursing process.* She identified the three components of the process that occurred during a nurse-client interaction as (1) client's behavior, (2) nurse's reaction, and (3) nurse's action. The process begins with the presentation of a particular client behavior, either verbal or nonverbal. The nurse reacts by exploring the behavior and validating this perception with the client's own view. An analogy may be drawn from Orlando's client's behavior/nurse's reaction to the assessment phase of the nursing process described later in this chapter. The nurse extracts information about the client behavior for later use in analyzing the problem and developing subsequent nursing actions.

Another model of nursing activities analogous to the nursing process is the five D's described by Knowles[15] in 1967: (1) discover, (2) delve, (3) decide, (4) do, and (5) discriminate. *Discovery* is the nurse's acquisition of new knowledge that will contribute to nursing care. *Delving* may be defined as acquiring information about a client (data collection). *Deciding* includes consideration of the client's problems and designing nursing approaches to resolve these problems. In *doing,* the nurse actually carries out these approaches. *Discrimination* distinguishes differences in client problems and needs. The following list aligns Knowles's five D's to the nursing process described in this chapter:

- Discover – knowledge base of the nurse
- Delve – assessment
- Decide – diagnosis and planning
- Do – implementation
- Discriminate – evaluation

During the 1960s, although the present nursing process had not been acknowledged as an accepted model of nursing practice, nursing authors wrote about selected components of the process and outlined ways to organize nursing practice.

McCain[22] described a tool nurses could use to assess their clients' functional abilities (Table 4-1). Assessment

***Table 4-1.* Development of the nursing process: historical overview, 1859-1968**

Theorist	Year	Contribution
F Nightingale	1859	Described areas affecting human health (e.g., nutritional adequacy, hygiene, and sensory stimulation) Addressed environmental aspects of care (e.g., ambient noise, ventilation, cleanliness, and light) Defined purpose of observation: "It is . . . for the sake of saving life and increasing health and comfort."[25]
L Hall	1955	First person to describe nursing as a process. Described three interrelated spheres of nursing: 1. "Care" or nurturing component; theory based on biologic and natural sciences 2. "Core" or nursing activities to help patients become aware of feelings about their level of health; accomplished through use of reflection as a therapeutic communication technique 3. "Cure" or those activities done in collaboration with other health team members; carrying out of prescribed treatment measures while acting as a client advocate[9]
JJ Orlando	1961	First theorist to use term "nursing process" Identified the three components of the process that occurs during the nurse-client interaction as (1) client's behavior, (2) nurse's reaction, and (3) nurse's action[28]
RF McCain	1965	Described a tool nurses could use to assess patients' functional abilities. Suggested use of data acquired to formulate nursing diagnoses and to proceed with a plan of care[22]
L Knowles	1967	Described a model analogous to the nursing process: • Discover—knowledge base of the nurse • Delve—assessment • Decide—diagnosis and planning • Do—implementation • Discriminate—evaluation[15]
Western Interstate Commission on Higher Education	1967	Published manuscript defining clinical content for graduate nursing programs Defined steps in the nursing process as "perception, communication, interpretation, intervention, and evaluation"[5]
H Yura and M Walsh	1967	Outlined the four-step nursing process: assessment, planning, implementation, and evaluation[41]
L Lewis	1968	Described the same four-step process as Yura and Walsh Provided the nurse with a tool that ensures that care is designed to meet the needs of the whole individual[18]
LM McPhetridge	1968	Wrote about personalizing the nursing process through use of a nursing history Emphasized need to consider the client's perception of his or her existing state[24]

factors included mental status, emotional status, sensory perception, and motor ability. She suggested that nurses use the data acquired to formulate nursing diagnoses and proceed with a plan of nursing care.

McPhetridge[24] wrote about personalizing nursing care through use of a nursing history. The format emphasizes the need to consider the client's perception of his existing state, as opposed to relying on mere objective assessment in identifying problems. For example, under the nutrition section the client is asked if he considers himself to be overweight, underweight, or close to proper weight.

In 1967 the Western Interstate Commission on Higher Education published a manuscript defining clinical content for graduate nursing programs. The nursing process was defined as ". . . that which goes on between a client and nurse in a given setting; it incorporates the behaviors of client and nurse and the resulting interaction. The steps in the process are: perception, communication, interpretation, intervention, and evaluation."[5] Also at this time, the Catholic University of America Press published the first edition of *The Nursing Process,* edited by Yura and Walsh,[41] who outlined the four-step nursing process: assessment, planning, implementation, and evaluation.

In 1968, Lewis described the same four-step nursing

process as Yura and Walsh. According to Lewis, this model provides the nurse with a tool that ensures that care rendered is designed to meet the needs of the whole individual. The nurse systematically identifies problems or needs through a thorough assessment of the person's physical, emotional, spiritual, and social milieu. Goals are formulated to restore or maintain wholeness in one or more of these assessment areas; then a specific plan of action is developed and implemented. The nurse then determines the success of the plan by measuring whether goals were achieved. Lewis comments on this highly individualized care: "The nurse who functions on this level should find increasing satisfaction in her caring role as she acts as a thinking, responsible, goal-directed member of the health team, contributing to the comfort, development and happiness of those she serves."[18]

Acceptance of nursing in its own right offering a valuable service and having a unique responsibility within the health care system also was reflected in public policy. In 1972, under the sponsorship of the New York State Nurses's Association, the following amendments to the New York State Education Law in relation to the practice of nursing were enacted into law:[26]

DEFINITIONS

1. *Diagnosing in the context of nursing practice means identification of and discrimination between physical and psychosocial signs and symptoms essential to effective execution and management of the nursing regimen. Such diagnostic privilege is distinct from a medical diagnosis.*
2. *Treating* means selection and performance of those therapeutic measures essential to the effective execution and management of the nursing regimen and execution of any prescribed medical regimen.
3. *Human responses* are those signs, symptoms, and processes that denote the individual's interaction with an actual or potential health problem.

Nursing Process Redefined

The nursing process is a combination of two words, nursing and process. Throughout the literature various definitions of nursing can be found, with many interpretations reflecting the authors' different philosophies. The one used as a reference point for this chapter was adopted by the American Nurses' Association (ANA) in 1980, when it issued a social policy statement presenting a current view about the nature and scope of nursing practice. This definition of nursing captures the evolution of nursing from Nightingale to the present: "Nursing is the diagnoses and treatment of human response to actual or potential health problems."[1]

The word *process* has fewer interpretations, and for purposes of this discussion Webster's definition suffices: "The action of passing through continuing development from a beginning to a contemplated end; the actions of continuously going along through each of a succession of acts, events, or developmental stages."[40]

With nursing and process thus defined, what then is the nursing process? Lewis claims it is "the key which opens the door to the patients' problems and to the ways of solving them."[18] Marriner states that it is the "application of scientific problem solving to nursing care."[20] The nursing process is aptly described by Yura and Walsh as "an orderly, systematic manner of determining the client's problems, making plans to solve them, initiating the plan or assigning others to implement it, and evaluating the extent to which the plan was effective in resolving the problems identified."[41]

Notice how many times the word *problem* appears in these definitions. Do these definitions seem applicable for use with healthy clients? Must nurses always assume that problems exist? Is it possible that no problems exist? What about potential problems?

In fairness to the authors cited, although the word *potential* is not offered in their definition, they do include the possibility of potential problems in their work. If the nursing process is intended to determine the client's actual problems as well as his or her potential problems, this concept can apply to healthy clients if it is agreed that everyone has the potential for problems. A problem, however, whether actual or potential, connotes a negative image that is incongruent with wellness; it does not seem helpful when conceptualizing the well person approaching the self-actualizing end of the health continuum.

A more positive and acceptable idea is to view every individual as having the capacity for improving his or her level of health. An individual without any identified actual or potential problems could be assisted to improve health practices to achieve an even higher level of wellness. Consider the following hypothetical client: A 32-year-old male of normal weight is free of hereditary risk factors for disease. He pursues a wellness lifestyle that includes good nutrition, daily exercise, and adequate recreation. He avoids smoking and drinking, enjoys his work, relates well to people, and has periodic health examinations. Physical examination results are within normal limits. This individual decides to join a wellness resource program because he would like to know how to increase his self-awareness.

This scanty profile is intended to demonstrate that this person may be assessed to have no actual or potential problems. Perhaps the nursing process needs to be redefined to apply it to this individual. It seems easier to use the nursing process when actual or potential problems exist than when no problems exist. However, after assessing the client to be healthy and judging him to have no existing problems, the nurse can plan for a periodic reassessment of wellness. The client is responsible for keeping such appointments and seeking reassessment sooner if he suspects a problem.[41] The nurse's behavior might help the client to maintain his level of wellness, but it does not indicate that he will be assisted to improve on his health practices.

It is difficult to estimate how many individuals are at or near the self-actualizing level of the health continuum, since no way exists to measure this. The hypothetical client just presented may be a rarity; nurses encounter both healthy clients with potential problems and those with actual problems. A proper definition should encompass individuals at all levels of illness and wellness:

The nursing process is a systematic progression through a series of purposeful steps to assess and diagnose the client's actual or potential problems, to assess behaviors indicative of health promotion, and to plan with the client actions that will assist recovery, maximize potential until death if recovery is not possible, prevent disruption in health, and maintain and improve the present level of wellness.[29]

Phases of Nursing Process

The phases of the nursing process are[19]

1. Assessment
2. Diagnosis
3. Planning
4. Implementation
5. Evaluation

The steps in the process follow a logical progression, but two or more may be operating at once (Fig. 4-2).[41] For example, while teaching a client breast self-examination, the nurse observes an ulcerated nevus beneath the left breast. Further inquiries into this assessment may lead to additional nursing diagnoses.[23]

The nursing process is continuous and cyclic; it does not end with the final phase of evaluation. Feedback on the client's progress or lack of progress toward goal achievement directs reassessment, reordering of priorities, new goal setting, and revision of the care plan.[1] For example,

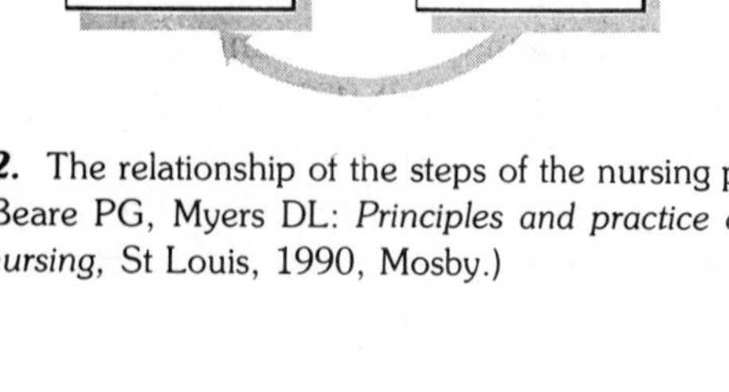

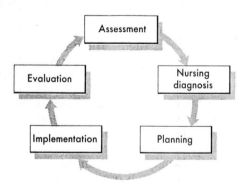

Fig. 4-2. The relationship of the steps of the nursing process. (From Beare PG, Myers DL: *Principles and practice of adult health nursing,* St Louis, 1990, Mosby.)

a healthy male client sets two goals for himself in an effort to modify his lifestyle: increase physical activity and change his eating habits. He is making progress with these goals when suddenly his democratic and benevolent boss is terminated and replaced by an authoritarian figure. The client fails to progress further toward his stated goals and identifies his work environment as highly stressful. This feedback concerning lack of progress toward stated goals (dietary habits and exercise), combined with new data (job stress), may lead to a reordering of priorities. Ineffective stress management becomes the number one priority. Revision of the nursing plan of care and new goal setting (stress reduction) can then occur.

Each of the phases in the nursing process is discussed in detail later in this chapter.

Scope of Nurses' Knowledge

The nurse should consider the following questions: (1) What broad overall categories of knowledge and skills are required by the nurse using the nursing process with clients at all levels of the wellness-illness continuum?, (2) Are there any specific categories of knowledge and skills needed during the different phases of the nursing process?, and (3) Does a nurse collaborating with healthy clients require any additional areas of knowledge and skill?

Yura and Walsh[41] state that the nurse must have intellectual, interpersonal, and technical skills to use the nursing process. *Intellectual* skills require the nurse to be able to solve problems and make judgments; *interpersonal* skills require the nurse to be able to communicate, listen, and demonstrate compassion; and *technical* skills require the nurse to be able to use equipment and carry out procedures.

In response to the second question, Yura and Walsh[41] describe a four-phase nursing process, with nursing diagnosis included in the assessment phase. Since this chapter presents a five-step process, that of Gordon[8] is used to discern the knowledge base necessary for the diagnostic phase. Table 4-2 depicts the widely divergent areas of knowledge and skills that a nurse must integrate to proceed through each phase of the nursing process, with decision making a part of every step.[41]

In answering the third question, a review of the table of contents in the current literature advocating health promotion suggests that a nurse must possess not only the knowledge areas cited in Table 4-2 but also a knowledge of health-promoting and illness-preventing strategies.[4,31] The following areas are important: risk-factor identification, risk-appraisal tools, stress-management techniques, lifestyle modification strategies, teaching/learning strategies, leadership and change theory, self-responsibility ethics, exercise and physical fitness, and self-development practices.

Table 4-2. **Knowledge base in nursing process**

Phases	Knowledge and Skills
Assessment	Emphasis on intellectual and interpersonal skills Knowledge areas: basic human needs, anatomy and physiology, human behavior, major causes of morbidity and mortality, human growth and development, basic pathophysiology and psychopathology, cultural beliefs, major religions, family and social organizations, economic patterns, chemistry, physics, microbiology, psychology, sociology, mathematics, literature, art, philosophy, and theology
Nursing diagnosis*	Emphasis on range of norm for 11 functional health patterns (age norms) and their natural development during lifespan; on variations in patterns related to cultures, environment, disease, and other influences; and on common dysfunctional patterns (nursing diagnoses) and indicators of these patterns
Planning	Emphasis on intellectual and interpersonal skills Knowledge of biologic, physical, and behavioral sciences as well as nursing knowledge, clinical experience, and knowledge resources—persons, books, and ability to seek out consultation
Implementation	Emphasis on intellectual and interpersonal as well as technical skills
Evaluation	Highly intellectual activity

Adapted from Yura H, Walsh M: *The nursing process*, ed 2, New York, 1978, Appleton-Century-Crofts.

*Data from Gordon M: *Nursing diagnosis: process and application*, New York, 1982, McGraw-Hill.

A nurse caring for a client in any environment and at any level of the health-illness continuum should be familiar with all these areas. The question is one of usage: How often will the nurse caring for seriously ill hospital clients use the strategies of exercise and physical fitness? It is understood that life-threatening situations are assigned the highest priority. The nurturative aspect of nursing practice is highly visible in the acute care setting. On the other hand, a nurse in a group practice setting working with clients seeking health-promoting behavior may use these strategies daily.

Holistic Approach

The holistic perspective reminds the nurse to view a person as a whole consisting of integrated parts: "Each individual is unique and represents a complex interaction of body, mind, and spirit."[30] A disruption in the functioning of one health pattern can adversely affect the whole. Likewise, maximizing the functioning of one health pattern can contribute to the emergence of a more integrated whole. Nursing has distinguished itself from other health disciplines by focusing on the basic human needs that affect the total person rather than on one aspect or problem or limited need fulfillment.[41]

For the nursing process to be holistically applied to healthy clients, the components of the process should include the biopsychosocial components of the whole person moving through a constantly changing environment from one developmental stage to the next (Fig. 4-3).

During the *assessment* phase, the nurse should use a standardized assessment format to assist in the gathering of data reflective of the whole person. Gordon's typology of 11 functional health patterns[8] is well suited for this purpose. According to Gordon, "Each pattern area is a biopsychosocial expression of the whole person . . . Human development occurs in these patterns; thus they also provide for developmental assessment of client-environment interaction.[8] A change in one pattern area is reflected in other areas because the patterns are interdependent. For example, parents having difficulty handling the behavior of their brain-damaged child (coping and stress tolerance pattern) may become irritable and hostile toward each other as a result of suppressed guilt feelings and then experience sexual problems (sexuality and reproductive pattern).

The pattern areas provide nurses with a useful way of organizing complex data. Once the data are collected and analyzed, findings may emerge that indicate actual, potential, or no problems. The findings should be reviewed within the context of the client's whole situation to ensure that a nursing diagnosis is not made in isolation.

For example, a 44-year-old overweight man, at the insistence of his physician, has been on a weight-loss plan for 3 weeks and has gained 4 pounds. The client is asked to describe a sample menu for a 1-day, 1200-calorie diet and has difficulty listing the correct foods. The nurse diagnoses the problem as noncompliance with the weight-reducing plan related to knowledge deficit. Since no positive change in the problem status occurred as predicted (no demonstrated weight loss), the nurse should now consider whether the etiologic factor was incorrect or other factors were operating. The client did not know the appropriate foods for a 1200-calorie diet. However, the client's wife was present when the instructions were presented. She was interested, wrote everything down, and has been selecting and preparing foods according to the plan. The client did not pay much attention to the nutri-

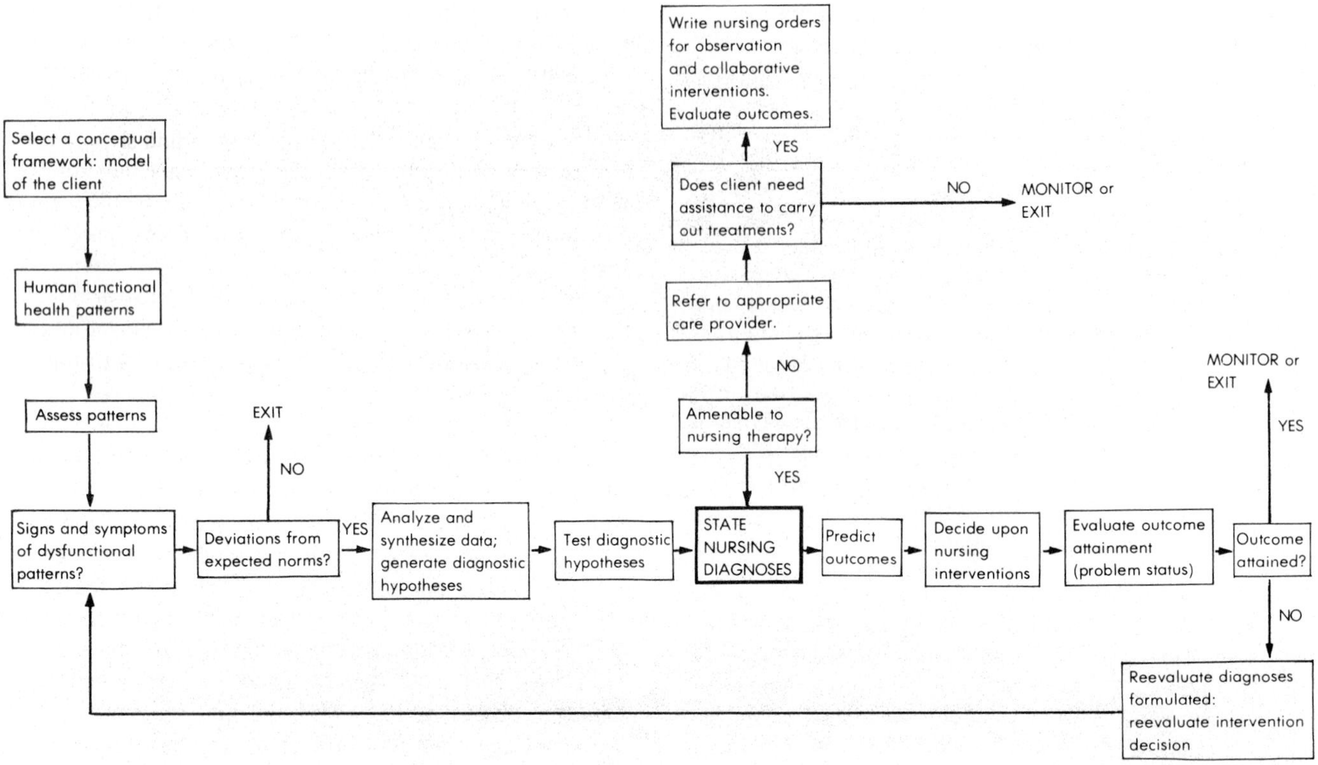

Fig. 4-3. Components of the nursing process. (From Gordon M: *Manual of nursing diagnosis 1993-1994,* St Louis, 1993, Mosby.)

tional information regarding the diet because he knew his wife would handle this. The nurse then learns that the man is the headwaiter at a famous restaurant and has been "sneaking" food from the chef. With more information about the client's total situation, should the nurse still conclude that the noncompliance was caused by a knowledge deficit? Or was the nursing diagnosis made in isolation? Are there other alternatives to explore, such as past failure to achieve weight loss, motivation to change, and the employment situation? Failure to consider the person holistically can result in erroneous diagnoses.

During the *planning* phase the nurse assists the client to prioritize his problems or, if no problems exist, determine areas for improvement that lead toward high-level wellness. The nurse and client together explore health problems and concerns and establish mutually agreeable goals. Before offering solutions for the client to choose, the nurse considers age, sex, lifestyle, education, and socioeconomic and cultural background, as well as coping ability and his physiologic and emotional status as they affect suggested solutions.

A client with an actual or potential problem selects a behavior from the proposed alternatives. A client with no problem but with identified areas for improvement chooses behaviors that will enhance further growth. It is important for the client, not the nurse, to select strategies the client believes will be most feasible to implement. If the nurse is to assist the client toward health promotion, the nurse must try to view the world from the client's eyes. Each client carries out health-protecting and health-promoting behaviors in ways that fit his or her lifestyle.[4] For example, in one popular progressive relaxation technique, the individual (with closed eyes) focuses on relaxing various muscle groups and then passively concentrates on pleasant scenes or experiences from the past.[33,34] Usually the client is asked to imagine drifting weightlessly through space or sitting on the warm sands of a beach with gentle breezes blowing and palm trees swaying. This stress-reduction approach, used routinely with clients trying to manage the stress in their lives, would not be appropriate to the client who can eliminate tension only by running. Imagery of quiet tranquil places may not meet the individualized needs of those clients who become more stressed when asked to assume a passive posture. The imagery could be modified so that the client imagines running in a favorite place. Realistic goals set the stage for sound health planning and effective implementation.

To meet the changing needs of the client, the plan should remain flexible. Periodic review of progress toward goals should occur, with plans for revision to create a more viable and positive growth experience for the client.[10] The plan developed with the client during the nursing process provides him or her with the opportunity to express behaviors he or she will use to maintain health, such as continuing to refrain from smoking, and behaviors that will be initiated to promote self-actualization, such as joining a community arts council and developing an interest in sculpting.

ASSESSMENT

Assessment, the first phase of the nursing process, involves collecting data about the client to identify actual or potential problems as well as strengths and areas in need of improvement. The assessment must be comprehensive to develop a holistic plan that will meet the needs of each client.

Maibusch points out "that a reasonable explanation must be given for any conclusion or nursing diagnosis arrived at, and that there must be a connection between the indicators and the nursing diagnosis. Unless assessment data are included, the accuracy of a diagnosis cannot be evaluated at a later date."[19]

Data Collection

The type of data includes a health history, physical examination, functional health pattern assessment, and risk factors. Since this nursing process is wellness oriented rather than problem oriented, and since the health assessment focuses on healthy clients, the nurse can assume that such clients will be available for ongoing visits to the clinic or center. The nurse then can plan to collect the data over several visits to avoid a time-consuming and overwhelming comprehensive assessment.

A nursing data base for assessment of healthy clients is given in the box on pp. 80-86. It includes sections on health history, physical examination, and functional health patterns.

HEALTH HISTORY

The history format is designed to elicit information on the following factors:

1. Demographic data
2. Current and past medical problems
3. Family medical history
4. Surgical and (if appropriate) obstetric history
5. Childhood illnesses
6. Allergies
7. Current medications
8. Psychologic status
9. Social history
10. Environmental background
11. Review of systems

This part of the nursing data base, excluding the review of systems, can be completed by the client; the nurse should check with the client for completeness. When reviewing the data base, the nurse may need to offer assistance in completing the tool if the client appears not to have understood terms or to have low reading skills. The nurse notes any data that signal a potential or actual problem area and clarifies with the client any information that seems ambiguous. If a client admits having allergies, the nurse attempts to find out what actions the client took and the consequences. If the client is presently taking medications, the nurse inquires about the dosage, action, and side effects. With any admission to present illness, the nurse determines the onset, setting in which it occurred, symptoms, treatments, and response to treatments, as well as what the meaning of illness is to the client.

The psychologic screening provides some indication of the client's present feelings. An admission to feelings of sadness and depression usually signals the need for further exploration. The social history, which includes the environmental category, is not extensive in scope but provides guidelines to obtaining information about the client's living space and social networks as well as indicating developmental progress through school and adult life (marriage, work, financial status). In the review of systems, the nurse asks questions in the different systems to obtain subjective data apparent only to the client, such as joint pain and itching. (For a detailed list of suggested guideline questions to be reviewed in each system, see Bates.[2])

PHYSICAL ASSESSMENT

A complete physical examination should follow the health history, since it provides the nurse with an opportunity to gather objective data. For example, the nurse observes swelling of the knees and a diffuse macular rash of the upper torso in the client who complained of joint pain and itching. These objective data are found to complement the health history's subjective data. The physical examination can verify the client's subjective data, although in some instances this is not sufficient and the client must be referred for further tests. For example, the client complains of frequent abdominal cramping and bouts of diarrhea following the ingestion of certain foods. A gastrointestinal series and/or allergy testing ordered by the physician may be necessary to objectify the subjective complaints. No attempt is made here to provide guidelines for the technique of conducting a physical assessment (for more information, see Bates[2]).

As for technique and environmental factors conducive to effective interviewing during the entire nursing data-collection process, many excellent sources are available.[2,7,24] An important consideration for nurses interviewing well or ill clients is the ability to remain sensitive to the clients' behavior and to view them as unique individuals. Nurses must avoid stereotyping, which is inconsistent with the

❑ ❑ NURSING ASSESSMENT DATABASE

Name ______________________ Age ________ Sex ________
Address ______________________ Race ______________________
City, state ______________________ Religion ______________________
Phone number ______________________ Occupation ______________________
Marital status ______________________ Place of employment ______________________
Private physician ______________________ Education ______________________

Health History

Check the problems that you presently have or have had that were diagnosed and treated by a physician.

Yes	No	Problem
____	____	Alcoholism
____	____	Anemia
____	____	Bleeding trait
____	____	Bronchitis
		Cancer
____	____	Breast
____	____	Cervix
____	____	Lung
____	____	Uterus
____	____	Other
____	____	Cirrhosis
____	____	Colitis
____	____	Depression
____	____	Diabetes
____	____	Emphysema
____	____	Fibrocystic breasts (lumps in breast)
		Heart problems
____	____	Heart attack
____	____	Coronary disease
____	____	Rheumatic heart
____	____	Heart valve problem
____	____	Heart murmur
____	____	Enlarged heart
____	____	Heart rhythm problem
____	____	Other

Yes	No	Problem
____	____	High blood pressure
____	____	High blood fats
____	____	Cholesterol
____	____	Triglycerides
____	____	Obesity (more than 20 pounds overweight)
____	____	Pneumonia
____	____	Polyps in colon (overgrowths in colon)
____	____	Rheumatic fever
____	____	Stroke
____	____	Suicide
____	____	Tuberculosis
____	____	AIDS/HIV
____	____	STDs
____	____	Hepatitis

In the past year have you had

Yes	No	
____	____	Chest pain on exertion relieved by rest?
____	____	Shortness of breath lying down, relieved by sitting up?
____	____	Unexplained weight loss of more than 10 pounds?
____	____	Unexplained rectal bleeding?
____	____	Unexplained vaginal bleeding?

Family Medical History

Check items that apply to your blood relatives (parents, grandparents, siblings, children).

Yes	No	Illness
____	____	Anemia
____	____	Bleeding trait
____	____	Cancer
____	____	Diabetes
____	____	Heart disease

Yes	No	Illness
____	____	High blood pressure
____	____	Mental illness
____	____	Stroke
____	____	Suicide
____	____	Tuberculosis

Check the items that apply.

Yes	No	
____	____	Father died of heart attack before age 60
____	____	Mother died of heart attack before age 60

Yes	No	
____	____	Mother or sister had breast cancer

Surgical History

List any operations and dates ______________________________

Females: describe obstetric history (if appropriate) ______________________________

List childhood illnesses ______________________________

Immunizations	**Yes**	**No**		**Yes**	**No**
Tetanus	____	____	Rubella (German measles)	____	____
Pertussis	____	____	Mumps	____	____
Diphtheria	____	____	Flu	____	____
Polio	____	____			
Measles	____	____			

List any allergies (food, drugs, other) ______________________________

List current medications (if appropriate) ______________________________

Psychologic History

Mark the frequency with which you have the feelings listed by placing a check mark in the appropriate column (*M*—Most of the time; *S*—some of the time; *R*—rarely or none).

M	**S**	**R**	
____	____	____	Feel sad, depressed?
____	____	____	Wish to end it all?
____	____	____	Feel tense and anxious?
____	____	____	Worry about things generally?
____	____	____	More aggressive and hard driving than friends?
____	____	____	Have an intense desire to achieve?
____	____	____	Feel optimistic about the future?

Social History

Family members (parents, siblings, spouse, children, grandparents)
List family members, their ages, and health status or cause of death ______________________________

Educational history (schools attended, diplomas or degrees earned) ______________________________

Marital history (how many years; any past or present difficulties) ______________________________

Work history (types and places of employment) ______________________________

Leisure time activities ______________________________

Financial status (plans for retirement, insurance, medical coverage) ______________________________

Continued.

NURSING ASSESSMENT DATABASE—cont'd

Environmental Background

Place of residence: apartment ________ home ________ Do you own? Yes ________ No ________
Travel time to work or school ________
Means of transportation ________
Environmental pollutants in area of residence ________
Place of residence in past and travel history ________

Describe present neighborhood (noisy or quiet; location to shopping, social, cultural, and religious centers) ________

Review of Systems

Head and neck ________
Skin ________
Respiratory ________
Cardiovascular ________
Gastrointestinal ________
Genitourinary ________
Reproductive ________
Musculoskeletal ________
Central nervous ________
Endocrine ________
Circulatory ________

Physical Examination

Height ________ Weight ________
Blood pressure ________ Pulse ________ Respirations ________ Temperature ________

Functional Health Pattern Assessment

The nurse should use these questions as a basis to explore the health patterns listed.

1. Health perception and health management pattern
   How has your general health been?
   Describe the most important things you do to stay healthy.
   Which statement is more like you?
   "If it's meant to be, I will stay healthy."
   or
   "If I take care of myself, I will stay healthy."
   Regularly use dental floss?
   Has had dental examination in past 2 years?
   Has had eyes checked in past 2 years?
   Seeks professional advice for unusual physical or mental changes?
   Has smoke detector in house?
   Has emergency phone numbers posted?
   Wears seat belt?
   (If responsible for children) Keeps medicines and cleaning products in locked cabinet?
   Women
   Has had Pap test within a year? Conducts monthly breast self-examinations?
   Men
   Conducts monthly testicular examinations?

   Any concerns about current health practices?
   Behaviors you think you should change? Would like to change?

Functional Health Pattern Assessment—cont'd

Strengths and areas for improvement ______________________________

Weaknesses and problem areas ______________________________

2. Nutritional and metabolic pattern
   Describe typical daily food and fluid intake.
   Any supplements? Appetite? Discomfort? Diet restrictions?
   Heals well or poorly?
   Skin problems?
   Dental problems?
   Drinks less than three alcoholic beverages (including beer) per week?
   Drinks less than five soft drinks per week?
   Drinks less than three cups of coffee or tea per day?
   Any foods avoided? Why?
   Snacks between meals? What kind?
   Limits intake of refined sugars (junk foods, desserts)?
   Adds salt to food? Cooking? At the table?
   Checks ingredients in prepackaged food?
   Describe cooking facilities.
   Limits intake of high-cholesterol foods?
   Uses foods containing polyunsaturated fats?
   Adds bran to diet to provide roughage?
   Eats at least one uncooked fruit or vegetable a day?
   Knows ideal weight? Current weight? Recent changes?
   Considers self overweight? Underweight? Ideal weight?
   Any concerns in this area?
   Behaviors you think you should change? Would like to change?

Strengths and areas for improvement ______________________________

Weaknesses and problem areas ______________________________

3. Elimination pattern
   Describe bowel elimination pattern.
   Frequency? Character? Discomfort? Laxatives?
   Describe urinary elimination pattern.
   Frequency? Problems with control?
   Excess perspiration?
   Odor problem?
   Do you have to get up during the night to go to the bathroom? If so, how often?
   Any concerns?
   Behaviors you think you should change? Would like to change?

Strengths and areas for improvement ______________________________

Weaknesses and problem areas ______________________________

Continued.

NURSING ASSESSMENT DATABASE—cont'd

Functional Health Pattern Assessment—cont'd

4. Activity and exercise pattern
   Describe daily pattern of activity
   Has sufficient energy for desired and required activities?
   Exercise? Type? How often?
   Spare time activities?
   Climbs stairs rather than rides elevator?
   Participates in any strenuous exercise or sports?
   Engages in warm-up exercises?
   Participates in sports for competition or enjoyment?
   Any concerns?
   Behaviors you think you should change? Would like to change?

Strengths and areas for improvement ______________________

____

____

Weaknesses and problem areas ______________________

____

____

5. Sleep and rest pattern
   Describe sleep pattern.
   Generally rested and ready for daily activities after sleeping?
   Any onset problem? Aids? Dreams? Nightmares? Early awakening?
   Takes time to relax each day? How?
   Enjoys spending time without planned activities?
   Any concerns?
   Behaviors you think you should change? Would like to change?

Strengths and areas for improvement ______________________

____

____

Weaknesses and problem areas ______________________

____

____

6. Cognitive and perception pattern
   Has hearing difficulties? Aids?
   Has difficulties with vision? Wears glasses or contact lenses? Any pain? Discomfort?
   Changes in memory? Describe.
   New interest areas?
   Easiest way to learn things?
   Any difficulty learning?
   Estimate of reading ability
   Likes to read?
   Any concerns?
   Behaviors you think you should change? Would like to change?

Strengths and areas for improvement ______________________

____

____

Weaknesses and problem areas ______________________

____

____

7. Self-perception and self-concept pattern
   How would you describe yourself?
   Most of the time, do you feel good or not so good about yourself?
   Perceives self as being well accepted by others?
   Any recent body changes? Changes in the things you do? Is this a problem for you?

Functional Health Pattern Assessment—cont'd

Any changes in the way you feel about your body? Yourself?
Has an enthusiastic and optimistic outlook?
Enjoys expressing self through arts, hobbies, or sports?
Continues to grow and change? Describe.
Enjoys work or school?
Member of community group? How active?
Proud of self?
Respects own accomplishments?
Finds it easy to express concern, love, and warmth to others?
Enjoys meeting and getting to know new people?
Can accept constructive criticism easily and not react defensively?
Looks forward to the future?
Any concerns?
Behaviors you think you should change? Would like to change?

Strengths and areas for improvement ______________________________

Weaknesses and problem areas ______________________________

8. Role and relationship pattern
   Any family problems? Difficulty handling? Describe.
   (If appropriate) Problems with children? Difficulty handling? Describe.
   Finds it easy or difficult to communicate with others?
   If difficult, with whom? Actions taken to resolve?
   Belongs to social groups?
   Enjoys family? Friends?
   Has at least three close friends?
   Things generally go well for you at work or school?
   Enjoys touching other people? Being touched by others?
   Finds it easy or difficult to express love, warmth, and concern to those you care about?
   Any concerns?
   Behaviors you think you should change? Would like to change?

Strengths and areas for improvement ______________________________

Weaknesses and problem areas ______________________________

9. Sexuality and reproductive pattern
   Any problems or changes in sexual relations? Describe.
   (If appropriate) Use of contraceptives? Any problems?
   Any concerns?
   Behaviors you think you should change? Would like to change?
   Number of sexual partners?
   Use of safe practices? Describe.
   Number of pregnancies? Of living children?
   Menstrual cycles? Describe (regular, experience discomfort, bloating).
   Practice BSE? Regularly? When?

Strengths and areas for improvement ______________________________

Continued.

NURSING ASSESSMENT DATABASE—cont'd

Functional Health Pattern Assessment—cont'd

Weaknesses and problem areas ______________________

10. Coping and stress tolerance pattern
    Tense much of the time? Causes? What helps?
    Who's most helpful when you're distressed? Available now?
    Any big change in your life recently?
    Practices any methods of relaxation? Meditation? Yoga?
    Considers it acceptable to cry, feel sad, angry, or afraid? Can laugh at self?
    Able to say no without feeling guilty?
    Any concerns?
    Behaviors you think you should change? Would like to change?

Strengths and areas for improvement ______________________

Weaknesses and problem areas ______________________

11. Value and belief pattern
    How important is "health" to you?
    Generally get things out of life that you want?
    Is religion important? Is it a help when difficulties arise?
    Are you satisfied with how you spend a typical work day? School day? Leisure day?
    Any concerns?
    Behaviors you think you should change? Would like to change?

Strengths and areas for improvement ______________________

Weaknesses and problem areas ______________________

Developed by Bodnar B, Pederson S in Edelman C, Mandle C: *Health promotion throughout the lifespan*, St Louis, 1986, Mosby.

concept of wholeness.[21] If nurses are insensitive to the individuality of the client, they are liable to become selectively blind and deaf, which can result in suppression of significant data about the person being interviewed.

FUNCTIONAL HEALTH PATTERNS

Gordon[8] has suggested that the nursing profession take action to delineate the basic areas of assessment applicable to all clients and has proposed 11 structural areas as a step in unifying nurses' approach to assessing clients. In addition, Gordon argues that the assessment conducted in the 11 functional areas prepares the nurse more easily to formulate a nursing diagnosis using the National Classification of Accepted Diagnoses.[14] For clarification, refer to Gordon.[8] Gordon's typology of functional health patterns are shown in the box on pp. 87-88.

While assessing the client during the data collection process, nurses begin to construct a pattern from the client's description and their own and their own observations.

Pattern recognition, according to Gordon, "prevents superficial data collection that can lead to errors in diagnoses.[8] This assessment approach encourages the nurse to assist the client in reviewing the patterns in his or her life and their impact on his or her health. The questions selected in the health perception and health management section address the client's ability to engage in self-care practices that maintain and promote health. Two questions are superficially aimed at discerning the client's *locus of control* in this section: whether the client believes that his or her health status is under his or her own control or governed by chance. Individuals who believe that their health is largely self-determined would be classified as internals.[37] Locus of control, a measurable concept in

NURSING DIAGNOSTIC CATEGORIES BY FUNCTIONAL HEALTH PATTERNS*

HEALTH PERCEPTION-HEALTH MANAGEMENT PATTERN

Altered health maintenance
Ineffective management of therapeutic regimen
Total health management deficit
Health management deficit (specify)
Noncompliance (specify)
High risk for noncompliance (specify)
Health-seeking behaviors (specify)
High risk for infection
High risk for injury (trauma)
High risk for poisoning
High risk for suffocation
Altered protection

NUTRITIONAL-METABOLIC PATTERN

Altered nutrition: high risk for more than body requirements *or* high risk for obesity
Altered nutrition: More than body requirements *or* exogenous obesity
Altered nutrition: less than body requirements *or* nutritional deficit (specify)
Ineffective breastfeeding
Effective breastfeeding
Interrupted breastfeeding
Ineffective infant feeding pattern
High risk for aspiration
Impaired swallowing *or* uncompensated swallowing impairment
Altered oral mucous membrane
High risk for fluid volume deficit
Fluid volume deficit
Fluid volume excess
High risk for impaired skin integrity *or* high risk for skin breakdown
Impaired skin integrity
Pressure ulcer (specify stage)
Impaired tissue integrity (specify type)
High risk for altered body temperature
Ineffective thermoregulation
Hyperthermia
Hypothermia

ELIMINATION PATTERN

Constipation *or* intermittent constipation pattern
Colonic constipation
Perceived constipation
Diarrhea
Bowel incontinence
Altered urinary elimination pattern
functional incontinence
Reflex incontinence
Stress incontinence
Urge incontinence
Total incontinence
Urinary retention

ACTIVITY-EXERCISE PATTERN

High risk for activity intolerance
Activity intolerance (specify level)
Fatigue
Impaired physical mobility (specify level)
High risk for disuse syndrome
High risk for joint contracture
Total self-care deficit (specify level)
Self-bathing–hygiene deficit (specify level)
Self-dressing–grooming deficit (specify level)
Self-feeding deficit (specify level)
Self-toileting deficit (specify level)
Altered growth and development: self-care skills (specify level)
Diversional activity deficit
Impaired home maintenance management
Dysfunctional ventilatory weaning response (DVWR)
Inability to sustain spontaneous ventilation
Ineffective airway clearance
Ineffective breathing pattern
Impaired gas exchange
Decreased cardiac output
Altered tissue perfusion (specify)
Dysreflexia
High risk for peripheral neurovascular dysfunction
Altered growth and development

SLEEP-REST PATTERN

Sleep-pattern disturbance

COGNITIVE-PERCEPTUAL PATTERN

Pain
Chronic pain
Pain self-management deficit (acute, chronic)
Uncompensated sensory deficit (specify)
Sensory-perceptual alterations: input deficit *or* sensory deprivation
Sensory-perceptual alteration: input excess or sensory overload
Unilateral neglect
Knowledge deficit (specify)
Impaired thought processes
Uncompensated short-term memory deficit
High risk for cognitive impairment
Decisional conflict (specify)

SELF-PERCEPTION–SELF-CONCEPT PATTERN

Fear (specify focus)
Anxiety
Mild anxiety
Moderate anxiety
Severe anxiety (panic)
Anticipatory anxiety (mild, moderate, severe)
Reactive depression (situational)
Hopelessness

Continued.

NURSING DIAGNOSTIC CATEGORIES BY FUNCTIONAL HEALTH PATTERNS—cont'd

SELF-PERCEPTION—SELF-CONCEPT PATTERN—cont'd

Powerlessness (severe, low, moderate)
Self-esteem disturbance
Chronic low self-esteem
Body image disturbance
High risk for self-mutilation
Personal identity disturbance

ROLE-RELATIONSHIP PATTERN

Anticipatory grieving
Dysfunctional grieving
Disturbance in role performance
Unresolved independence-dependence conflict
Social isolation
Social isolation *or* social rejection
Impaired social interaction
Altered growth and development: social skills (specify)
Relocation stress syndrome *or* relocation syndrome
Altered family processes
High risk for altered parenting
Altered parenting
Parental role conflict
Parent-infant separation
Weak mother-infant attachment *or* parent-infant attachment
Caregiver role strain
High risk for caregiver role strain

ROLE-RELATIONSHIP PATTERN—cont'd

Impaired verbal communication
Altered growth and development: communication skills (specify)
High risk for violence

SEXUALITY-REPRODUCTIVE PATTERN

Sexual dysfunction
Altered sexuality patterns
Rape-trauma syndrome
Rape-trauma syndrome: compound reaction
Rape-trauma syndrome: silent reaction

COPING AND STRESS-TOLERANCE PATTERN

Ineffective coping (individual)
Avoidance coping
Defensive coping
Ineffective denial *or* denial
Impaired adjustment
Post trauma response
Family coping: potential for growth
Ineffective family coping: compromised
Ineffective family coping: disabling

VALUE-BELIEF PATTERN

Spiritual distress (distress of human spirit)

From Gordon M: *Manual of nursing diagnoses: 1993-1994,* St Louis, 1993, Mosby.
*Diagnoses accepted by the North American Nursing Diagnosis Association appear in boldface type.
NOTE: If the main treatment for a diagnosis (e.g., drugs or surgery) is outside the scope of nursing practice, the problem is placed under a closely related functional pattern. For example, impaired gas exchange mainly influences the activity-exercise pattern. Syndromes are placed under the pattern corresponding to the causative factor (e.g., disuse or relocation).

psychology, can be useful in predicting which types of individuals will and will not be more effective in changing behavior patterns to promote health.[3] It may be necessary first to assist externally controlled individuals to a more internal orientation if behavior changes are to be successful.

For nurses interested in clarifying the beliefs of clients concerning their health management, instruments for measurement are available.[39] In addition, for the nurse interested in a more extensive assessment of nutritional practices, activity patterns, and level of physical fitness, as well as indicators of stress, a wide variety of measurement scales also are available. Some of these tools include the Nutrition Health, and Activity Profile,[27] the Adult Physical Fitness Profile,[8] and the Life-Change Index to Measure Stress.[12,15]

Functions of self-actualization, although not specifically referred to in Gordon's typology, are subsumed in the category, self-perception and self-concept. Behaviors that indicate the actualizing pattern include being able (1) to demonstrate creative expression appropriate to one's developmental level, (2) to express love humanistically, (3) to express needs freely to another person, (4) to build and maintain meaningful relationships, and (5) to demonstrate a zeal for living.[4]

The section on functional health patterns is designed for the nurse to ask specific questions, circle or mark significant findings, and ascertain whether the client has any additional concerns. Toward the end of the section, the nurse asks if the client thinks he or she should change certain behaviors or if he or she would like to change others. The client may think he or she *should* stop smoking, as this is detrimental to his or her health, but *would like* to join a community group, learn how to deal with stressors at work, and lose 15 pounds. The "shoulds" and the "likes" may provide some clues as to the priority to change the client is considering. Finding out what behavioral changes are most important to the client will lead to more successful goal setting and implementation. In questioning what the client thinks he or she should change, the nurse should inquire about barriers that might exist for preventing this change. Finally, the section contains space for the nurse to list the strengths and weaknesses of the pattern area as well as areas for improvement and potential or actual problems. This will prove useful later in trying to determine the nursing diagnoses and plans for intervention.

RISK FACTORS

To ensure the comprehensiveness of the nursing assessment, health hazards must also be reviewed so that the client can identify risks for illness or injury. Aware of the risks and contributing factors, the client can then decide if he or she wants to maintain or improve his or her health status by taking risk reduction actions. Risk factors are not included in the nursing data base, since an excellent tool has already been developed by Pender (Fig. 4-4).[31] Pender's risk appraisal tool is comprehensive but lengthy; it does not have to be conducted with the nursing data base in one visit.

Pender[31] has classified risk factors into five categories: (1) risk for cardiovascular disease, (2) risk for malignant disease, (3) risk for auto accidents, (4) risk for suicide, and (5) risk for diabetes. Contributing factors, such as habits, family and personal medical history, sex, age, the environment, and lifestyle patterns are included. Information gained from analysis of relevant risk factors can alert the nurse and client about actual or possible risks to health. In addition, awareness of risk factors can serve as a motivator to initiate behavior that will prevent illness and optimize health.

Since recent blood cholesterol levels for all adults over age 20, regardless of age and sex, are part of the risk factor review, Fig. 4-5 has been included to augment Pender's appraisal form.

After the data have been collected from the health history, physical examination, functional health pattern typology, and risk appraisal form, the nurse reviews, summarizes, and analyzes it. From this the nurse is able to formulate a nursing diagnosis, the second step of the nursing process.

NURSING DIAGNOSIS

Nursing diagnosis, with its Greek origin meaning "to distinguish," conveys the idea of skilled clinical judgment, as the nurse sifts through assessment data and defines the client's response patterns.[17] Titler points out that critical thinking, concept development, and problem-solving activities are important components of learning diagnostic reasoning.[37]

Nursing diagnoses are derived from health status data. The data base; the information base the nurse has gathered and stored; and the logical use of inductive, deductive, and intuitive processes lead to these diagnostic conclusions.[4]

Marriner defines the nursing diagnosis as a "combination of signs and symptoms that indicate an actual or potential problem."[20] Gordon expands on this and says that nursing diagnoses "describe actual or potential health problems that nurses by virtue of their education and experience are capable and licensed to treat.[8] Unlike the theme of this chapter, which is focused on health orientation, both definitions reflect an attitude of problem orientation. What then can be done with the nursing diagnosis in relation to the nursing process applied toward healthy clients? Moreover, what can be done with the classification of nursing diagnoses, in which the vast majority are problem focused?

One answer is for the nursing process to end once a decision is reached that no actual or potential problems exist; this negates the need for nursing diagnoses.[38] The definition of nursing diagnosis also could be expanded to include not only a statement about actual or potential problems but also one that considers clients with no problems who have a curiosity, interest, or desire to further enhance their knowledge and health practices to maximize their health potential.

Lee and Frenn[17] elucidate a real need for diagnostic statements that reflect a generally healthy population seeking nursing care when the primary objective is promotion of health and personal well-being.

Healthy clients who function effectively will seek the consultative services of the nurse to assist them to develop their potential, if such clients perceive that the nurse recognizes their need for further development.

Thus, in order for positive nursing diagnoses to be useful, they must be congruent with clients' perceptions of their well-being as expressed in their responses. Development of positive nursing diagnoses that reflect health-promotion and health-protection models would enable the needs of healthy populations served by nurses to be named and further examined.[17]

Data Analysis

Assuming that interested nurses will continue to submit health-oriented categories and that many healthy clients will have potential problems, we now review the components of the nursing diagnosis. The components accepted by the North American Nursing Diagnosis Association (NANDA) include (1) a brief statement of the problem (P), (2) its etiology (E), and (3) the signs and symptoms that constitute its defining characteristics (S).[14] An example follows: individual coping pattern, maladapative (P);

Risk Factor		→ Increasing Risk →					
Risk for cardiovascular disease							
Sex and age		Female under 40	Female 40-50	Male 25-40	Female after menopause	Male 40-60	Male 61 or over
Family history (parents, siblings)	High blood pressure	No relatives with condition		One relative	Two relatives		Three relatives
	Heart attack	No relatives with condition	One relative with condition after 60	Two relatives with condition after 60	One relative with condition before 60		Two relatives with condition before 60
	Diabetes	No relatives with condition		One or more relatives with maturity onset		One or more relatives with preadolescent or adolescent onset	
Blood pressure*	Systolic	120 or below	121-140	141-160	161-180	181-200	Above 200
	Diastolic	70 or below	71-80	81-90	91-100	101-110	Above 110
Diabetes		No diagnosis	Maturity onset, controlled	Maturity onset, uncontrolled	Adolescent onset, controlled		Adolescent onset, uncontrolled
Weight*		At or slightly below recommended weight	10% overweight	20% overweight	30% overweight	40% overweight	50% overweight
Serum triglycerides* (mg/dl) fasting		150 or below		151-400	401-1000		Above 1000
Percentage of fat in diet*		20%-30%		31%-40%	41%-50%		Above 50%
Frequency of exercise*	Recreational	Intensive recreational exertion (35-45 minutes at least 4 times a week)		Moderate recreational exertion	Minimal recretional exertion		No recreational exertion
	Occupational	Intensive occupational exertion		Moderate occupational exertion	Minimal occupational exertion		Sedentary occupation
Sleep patterns* (hours per night)		7-8		More than 8			4-6
Cigarette smoking*	No. per day	Nonsmoker	1-10	11-20	21-30	31-40	Over 40
	No. years smoked	Nonsmoker	Less than 10	11-15	16-20	21-30	31 or more
Stress*	Domestic	Minimal		Moderate	High		Very high
	Occupational	Minimal		Moderate	High		Very high
Behavior pattern* (particularly males)		*Type B* Relaxed, appropriately assertive, not time dependent, moderate to slow speech			*Type A* Excessively competitive, aggressive, striving, hyperalert, time dependent, loud and explosive speech		
Air pollution*		Low		Moderate			High
Use of oral contraceptives* (females)		Do not use oral contraceptives		Under age 40 and use oral contraceptives	Over age 35 and use oral contraceptives		Over age 40 and use oral contraceptives

*Indicates risk factors that can be fully or partially controlled.

†Serum lipid analysis is also recommended to determine low-density (beta) and high-density (alpha) lipoprotein levels. Evidence suggests that high-density lipoprotein (HDL) carries cholesterol from tissues for metabolism and excretion. An inverse correlation appears to exist between HDL and coronary artery disease.

‡Chemicals such as asbestos, nickel, chromates, arsenic, chlormethyl ethers, radioactive dust, petroleum or coal products, and iron oxide.

Fig. 4-4. Risk appraisal form. In each row, circle item that best describes current life situation or behavior. (From Pender NJ: *Health promotion in nursing practice*, ed 2, Norwalk, Conn, 1987, Appleton & Lange.)

Risk Factor		→ Increasing Risk →					
Risk for malignant diseases							
Breast cancer (women)	Age	20-29	30-39		40-49		50 or over
	Race	Oriental			Black		White
	Family history (grandmother, mother, sister)	None	Mother, sister, or grandmother	Mother and grandmother			Mother and sister
	Onset of menstruation	Over age 12					Under age 12
Pregnancy*	Time	First pregnancy before age 25		First pregnancy after age 25			No pregnancies
	No.	Three or more			One or two		None
	Weight*	0% to 40% overweight					More than 40% overweight
	Personal history	No evidence of dysplasia or previous breast cancer		Breast dysplasia			Previous breast cancer
Lung cancer Cigarette smoking*	No. per day	Nonsmoker	1-10	11-20	21-30	31-40	Over 40
	No. years smoked	Nonsmoker	Less than 10	11-15	16-20	21-30	31 or more
Occupational exposure to toxic chemicals‡	Years of exposure	Less than 1	1-5	6-10		11-15	Over 15
	Frequency and intensity of exposure	Low frequency and low intensity	Low frequency, moderate intensity (or vice versa)	Moderate frequency, moderate intensity		Moderate frequency, high intensity (or vice versa)	High frequency, high intensity
Cervical cancer	Onset of sexual activity*	Before age 16	Age 16-21		Age 22-27		After age 28
	Number of sexual partners*	Two		Three			Four or more
	Marital status*	Single					Married
	Sexual partner*	Circumcised					Uncircumcised
Colorectal cancer	Age	Under 45					Over 45
	Personal history	No history of ulcerative colitis	Ulcerative colitis less than 10 years			Ulcerative colitis more than 10 years	
	Fiber content of diet*	High		Moderate			Low
	Weight* (men)	Less than 40% overweight					More than 40% overweight
	Rectal bleeding or black bowel movement	Never		Occasionally			Frequently

Continued.

Risk Factor		→ Increasing Risk →				
Risk for malignant diseases—cont'd						
Uterine and ovarian cancer	Age	Under 45				Over 45
	Weight*	Less than 40% overweight				More than 40% overweight
	Vaginal bleeding other than during menstrual period	Never		Occasionally		Frequently
Skin cancer	Complexion	Dark		Medium		Fair
	Sun exposure (without protection)	Never or seldom		Occasionally		Frequently
Risk for auto accidents						
Alcohol consumption*		Nondrinker	Occasionally small to moderate consumption	Frequently small to moderate consumption	Occasionally heavy consumption	Frequently heavy consumption
Miles driven per year*		Under 5000	5001-10,000		10,001-20,000	Over 20,000
Use of seat belt*		Always	Usually		Occasionally	Never
Use of shoulder harness*		Always	Usually		Occasionally	Never
Use of drugs or medication that decrease alertness*		No use	Occasional use		Moderate use	Frequent use
Risk of suicide						
Family history		No history		One family member		Two or more family members
Personal history*		Seldom experience depression	Periodically experience mild depression	Frequently experience mild depression	Periodically experience deep depression	Frequently experience deep depression
Access to hypnotic medication*		No access		Access to small or limited dosages		Unlimited access to large dosages
Risk for diabetes						
Weight*		Desired weight	15% overweight	30% overweight	45% overweight	More than 45% overweight
Family history (parent or sibling)		None		Either parent or sibling		Both parent and sibling

Fig. 4-4, cont'd. Risk appraisal form.

related to divorce (E); as evidenced by inability to make decisions (S). Gordon's premise that data collection in the 11 functional health pattern areas can assist nurses in the formulation of a nursing diagnosis is illustrated by the following example:

Mrs. B. J., a 40-year-old full-time secretary for an insurance company. Height – 5 feet, 3 inches; weight – 156 pounds, medium frame.

Nutritional and metabolic pattern: rarely eats breakfast, has a Danish pastry and coffee at work; snacks at night watching television, mostly on junk foods such as ice cream, potato chips, pretzels, and soda.

Activity and exercise pattern: no regular exercise; sits most of the day at work typing. Activity includes housework and some gardening; recreation consists of watching television, dining out with other couples.

Coping and stress pattern: tension occurs occasionally with husband over disciplinary actions toward sons, ages 11, 12, and 13. Responds to stressful situations by eating.

Analyzing the data may require the nurse to refer to the *Manual of Nursing Diagnosis: 1993-1994*[8] or to a similar

Criterion	Action
If total blood cholesterol <200	Repeat total blood cholesterol in 5 years or at physical examination Recommend general diet
If total blood cholesterol 200-239 and • No CHD and <2 risk factors (see below)	Repeat total blood cholesterol annually; Step 1 diet
• CHD present or ≥2 risk factors If total blood cholesterol ≥240	Determine LDL
If LDL <130	Repeat total blood cholesterol in 5 years; Recommend general diet
If LDL 130-159 and • No CHD and <2 risk factors	Repeat total blood cholesterol annually; Step 1 diet
• CHD present or ≥2 risk factors If LDL ≥160	Clinical evaluation; Step 1 or 2 diet Diet goals: LDL <160 or LDL <130 if CHD present or ≥2 risk factors

Continue dietary treatment for 6 months. If goals not met, consider drugs.

Risk factors for coronary heart disease (CHD)

- Male sex
- Family history
- Cigarette smoking
- Hypertension
- HDL <35 mg/dl
- Diabetes mellitus
- Cerebrovascular disease or occlusive PVD
- Severe obesity

Dietary treatment

	Step 1 diet	**Step 2 diet**
Saturated fat	<10% of calories	<7% of calories
Dietary cholesterol	<300 mg/day	<200 mg/day

Drugs

First-line drugs*	**Daily dosage range**	**Major side effects**	**Precautions**
Cholestyramine	2-6 packets 8-24 grams	GI upset, constipation	Can decrease absorption of other drugs administered simultaneously; sudden cessation may cause toxicity from other drugs.
Colestipol	2-6 packets 10-30 grams	GI upset, constipation	Can decrease absorption of other drugs administered simultaneously; sudden cessation may cause toxicity from other drugs.
Nicotinic acid	1.5-6.0 grams	Flushing	

*Probucol, gemfibrozil, clofibrate, and lovastatin may be considered for use when bile acid sequestrants or nicotinic acid produce an insufficient reduction in cholesterol. They also may be used in combination with sequestrants.

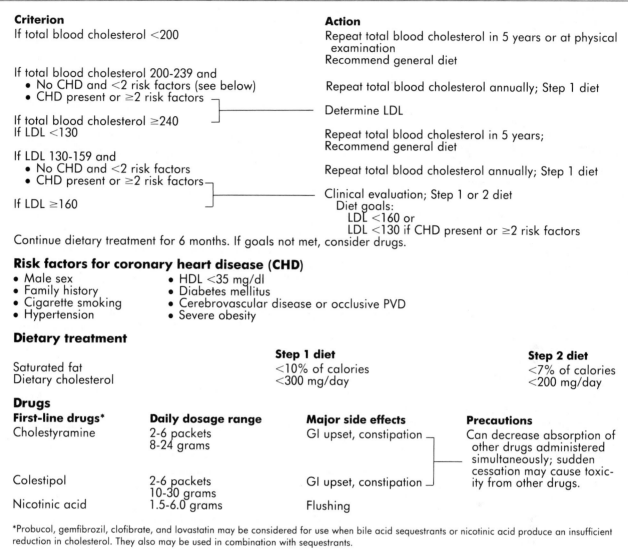

Fig. 4-5. Adult treatment guidelines, National Cholesterol Education program. Guidelines apply to all adults over the age of 19 years. (From the National Institutes of Health.)

reference. The nurse may find scanning the list of accepted nursing diagnostic categories (see box on pp. 87-88) to be particularly helpful. In the above example, three possible diagnostic judgments emerge:

1. Alteration in nutrition – more than body requirements
2. Impaired physical mobility
3. Ineffective individual coping

Which diagnosis is appropriate for Mrs. B. J.? Considering the etiology and characteristics for each of the diagnostic categories chosen, the nurse should notice that the second diagnostic category can be eliminated. (At present, no category deals with alteration in mobility – less than body requirements.) That leaves the first and third choices, which are now broken down according to the classification of Kim and Moritz.[14]

Alteration in nutrition – more than body requirements (P) has its etiology (E) in an excessive intake in relation to metabolic need, and the signs and symptoms of the defining characteristics (S) involve

1. Weight 10% over ideal for height and frame
2. Weight 20% over ideal for height and frame*
3. Triceps skin fold greater than 15 mm in men and 25 mm in women*
4. Sedentary activity level
5. Reported or observed dysfunctional eating patterns
6. Pairing food with other activities
7. Concentrating food intake at end of day
8. Eating in response to external cues, such as time of day and social situation

*Critical defining characteristic.

9. Eating in response to internal cues other than hunger, such as anxiety

The other choice is classified as ineffective individual coping (P), with an etiology (E) based on (1) situational crisis and (2) maturational crisis – both with a defining characteristic identified as a verbalization of inability to cope or inability to ask for help* – and (3) personal vulnerability, with these defining characteristics:

1. Inability to meet role expectations
2. Inability to meet basic needs
3. Inability to problem solve*
4. Alteration in societal participation
5. Destructive behavior toward self or others
6. Inappropriate use of defense mechanism
7. Change in usual communication pattern
8. Verbal manipulation
9. High illness rate
10. High rate of accidents

Mrs. B. J. has not verbalized any inability to cope or problem solve or to meet basic needs and role expectations. If she had, these characteristics would lead to a nursing diagnosis of ineffective individual coping. On the other hand, Mrs. B. J. is 20% over her ideal weight for height and frame (based on weight table for adult women). Her activity pattern is mainly sedentary. She concentrates high-calorie snacks at the end of the day and eats in response to anxiety. These defining characteristics lead to an appropriate diagnosis of alteration in nutrition – more than body requirements.

Once the health problem is clearly recognized and labeled as a nursing diagnosis, the nurse and client can work together to identify personal health goals and possible behavior change, which comprise the plan of nursing care. The plan includes priorities and approaches to achieve the goals derived from the nursing diagnoses. For Mrs. B. J., the reduction of food intake with changes in eating behvavior is the primary intervention, but attempts should be made to increase her activity level and generate alternative solutions to coping with stress in her home situation. As mentioned, all the functional health patterns are interrelated; thus, a change in one pattern area is reflected in the other areas. When a problem is diagnosed in one area, the etiologic factors usually are found in one or more of the other pattern areas.[8] Mrs. B. J.'s overweight condition is the result of overeating and poor dietary habits, combined with a sedentary lifestyle and an unhealthful response to situational stress.

PLANNING

Once nursing diagnoses have been derived, planning care may proceed. Diagnoses based on a comprehensive health assessment provide a foundation from which a highly individualized plan of care may emanate, a plan that is clearly within the realm of nursing accountability and professional authority.

Prioritizing nursing diagnoses, the first step in planning, helps the nurse and client carry out planning in an organized fashion. The nurse, working with the client and family, may set goals of care suited specifically to each identified diagnosis. Formulating goals serves to facilitate prescription of appropriate interventions. Goal setting provides the means for reaching a mutual agreement with the client on the expected achievements and also for measuring the success of suggested interventions.

Planning care is a rational activity that draws on the nurse's intellectual skills. A knowledge of biologic and behavioral sciences, as well as an ability to synthesize client information gained through assessment, govern the nurse's ability to help the client develop an effective plan or care. Interpersonal skills assist the nurse in working with the client and family to maintain a relationship of mutual trust and respect. The client's faith in the nurse's judgment lead to greater satisfaction with the plan developed for self-improvement, which should increase the client's will to carry it out.

Priority Setting

Established diagnoses must be ranked according to priority; the nurse cannot focus attention on a number of areas at once. The client's perception of priorities is crucial in establishing a mutually acceptable plan. Smitherman states, "If the patient, family, and the nurse are focusing their efforts in the same direction, a successful resolution of the problem is more likely than if they are going in opposite directions."[36] If the nurse and the client are unable to reach agreement on the ordering of priority in certain areas, compromise should be sought. A nurse's unwillingness to recognize and accept the client's view may contribute to the deterioration of a therapeutic relationship.

A frequently cited framework for prioritizing is Maslow's hierarchy, consisting of five areas of basic human need: physiologic, safety, love and belonging, esteem of self and others, and self-actualization.[21] The lowest level on the hierarchy encompasses basic physiologic needs such as food, water, and oxygen. As a person proceeds upward in need satisfaction, higher-level needs emerge. The individual may progress from meeting physiologic needs to meeting the need for safety from physical or psychologic harm, the social need for loving and fulfilling relationships, the need for self-esteem, and the need to be valued by others. The highest level of fulfillment is self-actualization. At this level, energy is directed to attainment of the individual's maximum potential as a human being. This person appreciates the aesthetic value of life, since other need areas are basically fulfilled. The individual is content to pursue the beauty of life, to consummate interpersonal relationships, and to achieve peace and satisfaction with the world at large. This person may be thought of as healthy in the purest sense, operating at a level where a sustainable balance within the self and between self and the environment is reality.

In planning care for the healthy person, it may be assumed that lowest level needs have already been satisfied. Attention to basic physiologic needs is not the focus of the client or the nurse; the client may be viewed as independent and competent in self-care. Thus, the nurse serves to direct the client in areas of self-improvement and to facilitate the ability to carry out activities to reach a higher level of functioning.

Examining levels of need, the nurse may find that fulfillment does not proceed in a clearly hierarchic order. For example:

Ms. D., 35 years old, nulliparous, with a generally healthy appearance physically, psychologically, and socially, comes to the health center. A history of breast cancer in her family has prompted her visit, since she has a knowledge of the risk of breast cancer associated with familial history and nulliparity. Ms. D. has already learned breast self-examination (BSE) from a self-enhancement group for women to which she belongs. Assessment reveals that her technique for BSE is correct; however, she does not practice it on a regular monthly basis. Further investigation reveals that practicing BSE is a possible threat to her self-esteem; she was raised in an environment where it was not proper for a woman to touch her breasts. This stigma prevents Ms. D. from practicing regular BSE. The nursing diagnosis might be noncompliance with health preventive practice – namely, BSE – related to disturbance in self-concept.

Prioritizing in this situation, using Maslow's hierarchy, may first lead the nurse to identify the diagnosis at the level of safety needs. BSE is ultimately practiced to validate the absence of a physical problem or to promote early detection. However, on further analysis, the nurse may deduce that the problem is at the self-esteem level. Ms. D. has a knowledge of the need for BSE and understands how it can help protect her; the threat to her self-image prevents her from practicing the technique. Therefore, planning should be directed at changing the notion she has about what persons think about women who touch their breasts.

Prioritizing in planning care for the healthy individual must be done with the participation of the client, the family, or both. Unlike illness care, in which the client is dependent on the nurse's clinical judgment in setting priorities of physical care, the healthy client is at a more independent level of biopsychosocial functioning and can be responsible for carrying out the plan of care. The client's agreement with the nurse on the sequential focus of the plan may dictate how much motivation there is to carry out the prescribed actions. The client's participation ultimately will dictate the plan's effectiveness.

Goal Setting

A goal may be defined as a condition or state to be brought about through a course of action. In nursing care, planning the goal is a statement of the plan's aim so the nurse and client know the expected result. What specifically is the client going to achieve as a result of cooperating in the nursing process?

Different authors use various terminology to define goals. Objectives, outcome criteria, or expected outcomes are all used in the literature and seem to have the same functional meaning: each describes the end result of care plan implementation.[20,41] For consistency and clarity, the term *goal* is used here to describe the expectations associated with the care plan. The word *outcome* is used in reference to weighing the consequences of possible nursing interventions. Maibusch has defined nursing outcomes as "the status at discharge of all nursing diagnoses identified during an episode or encounter of care."[19]

In setting goals, as in prioritizing, it is imperative that the client and/or the family be included. Expectations of interventions developed by the nurse and client reflect the knowledge and experience of the nurse as well as the client's and family's self-awareness. The goal derived in this manner should be better suited to the client's unique life situation than one based on only the nurse's perceptions. In viewing the client's particular life situation, as previously stated, the nurse must consider age, developmental level, sociocultural milieu, sex, and spirituality. An analysis of the client's strengths and weaknesses in these areas guides the nurse in structuring a plan that will capitalize on strengths and result in more effective goal attainment. In the previous example of Ms. D., who needs to practice regular BSE, an obvious strength is her belonging to a self-enhancement group for women. The nurse may suggest a goal that encorporates the client's involvement with this group: *Client will verbalize feelings elicited by BSE with group leader.* Formulation of such a goal would be preceded by the nurse's validating that the self-enhancement group leader is an appropriate resource in this situation.

SHORT-TERM AND LONG-TERM GOALS

Goals of care may be long term or short term. Establishing long-term goals first assists in organizing and generating an individualized plan of care. Long-term goals usually are stated in more general terms than short-term ones. For example, in setting goals for Ms. D., dietary patterns may be considered. Based on the nurse's knowledge that a high-fat diet increases the risk for breast cancer, the nurse might propose a long-term goal for Ms. D.: *Client will reduce intake of dietary fat.* Short-term goals that define specific behaviors leading to attainment of the long-term goal might include (1) *Client will identify foods in her diet that are high in fat;* and (2) *Client will develop a diet plan that is nutritionally sound and reflects a reduction in fat intake.*

Setting precise goals provides the nurse and client with an agreeable direction for care. Short-term goals are useful in evaluation; after implementation of the plan of care, referring to stated short-term goals tells the client and nurse whether the plan has been effective in reaching the long-term goal. For this reason, short-term goals must be stated in measurable behavioral terms. Using action verbs, such as "the client will *identify, demonstrate, list,* or *state,*" ensures that attainment of the stated goal can be evaluated objectively. It is wise to avoid terms such as "the client will *understand, appreciate,* or *know,*" since these imply a subjective behavior and cannot be measured effectively.[20]

In addition to being stated in specific behavioral terms, the short-term goal should be given a time frame for attainment. Progress in short-term goal achievement will reflect movement toward the long-term goal. Some short-term goals may take only a few days to accomplish, whereas others may take weeks. Dating each one will ensure that evaluation occurs within a realistic period. For example: *Client will develop a diet plan that is nutritionally sound and reflects a reduction in fat intake by next meeting, Nov. 20.* If the client reports to the nurse on the said date with the appropriate diet plan, that particular short-term goal has been achieved.

Reassessment must take place in areas of unmet goals. Redefining the goals themselves, setting a new date for attainment, or implementing a different strategy for care may be warranted.

Intervention

Succinctly stated goals facilitate the prescription of interventions designed for goal achievement. Each short-term goal should be analyzed and possible actions to meet the goal enumerated. In selecting appropriate interventions, all facets of the client's situation must be considered. According to Yura and Walsh, "Nursing actions must be clear, purposeful, moral, capable of being accomplished, and adapted to the particular life situation, beliefs, and expectations of the client."[41] Systems of codification for the interventions practiced by nursing have been proposed. Maibusch[19] describes a seven-element taxonomy, which has the following categories: (1) surveillance/observation, (2) supportive measures, (3) assistive measures, (4) treatments/procedures, (5) emotional support, (6) teaching, and (7) coordination of care.

The nurse and client together generate possible interventions. The breadth and number of alternatives depend on the nurse's experience, knowledge, and ability to utilize appropriate resources, as well as on the client's experience and self-awareness in terms of strengths and limitations. The possible outcomes of each alternative intervention should be considered. Checking the pros and cons of each outcome help the nurse and client decide which interventions are best suited to assist the client toward goal achievement. Ultimately the decision regarding which interventions will be included on the plan of care is left to the client. The nurse, however, as the client's counselor, is responsible for providing guidance and using interpersonal and communication skills to help the client examine alternatives and their possible consequences. Kilpack and Dobson-Brassard[13] state that there is a definite and direct relationship between effective communication and the quality of nursing care.

Until the plan is put into action, the nurse cannot be sure that selected interventions will effect appropriate changes to meet stated goals. The nurse, therefore, should keep a record of all alternative actions for future reference. If evaluation and reassessment reveal a lack of movement toward goal achievement, a previously identified intervention may be the appropriate second or third option in a plan for action.

The nursing care plan should be recorded and filed with other client information. It must be available for easy reference by all health care providers working with the particular client.[38] The client should be given a copy to serve as an implicit contract between nurse and client. The care plan delineates areas for self-improvment, potential problems, identified problems (nursing diagnoses), the goals of care for each diagnosis, and actions the client and nurse are responsible for carrying out to achieve goals. The box on p. 97 shows an example format for the written nursing care plan.

A plan should be written for each nursing diagnosis identified. The number next to the diagnosis reflects the priority assigned to it during the initial stages of planning. The completed nursing care plan reflects specific attention to each nursing diagnosis. Once planning is over, goals have been stated, initial interventions chosen, and all information recorded on the care plan format, implementation may occur.

IMPLEMENTATION

The nursing care plan instructs the nurse and client on how to proceed through the implementation phase. Given the groundwork laid down during assessment and planning, the nursing care plan can be put into effect. Nursing activity during implementation may involve teaching or counseling,[32,35] and certain activities may be delegated to other health team members. The client and family are responsible for carrying out designated activities. What action takes place, in what order, and by whom is predetermined by the care plan. The success of implementation depends heavily on the extent to which assessment and planning were comprehensive, accurate, and indi-

❏ ❏ NURSING CARE PLAN

Client: Jane Doe No.: 1 Date: 3-14-94	Diagnosis: Noncompliance with health preventive practice, namely, low-fat diet, related to lack of knowledge
Long-term goal:	Client will reduce intake of dietary fat.
Short-term goals	**Interventions**
1. Client will identify foods in her diet that are high in fat.	a. Refer to dietician for counseling regarding high- vs. low-fat diet b. Have patient list foods in present diet that are high in fat c. Assist patient to select optional foods that are lower in fat
2. Client will develop a diet plan that is nutritionally sound and reflects a reduction in fat intake.	a. Have patient keep a diary of intake for 1 week b. Review diet diary with patient on next visit

vidualized. Implementation should continue until goals are met or additional data suggest that the care plan needs revision.[36]

Collaboration and Referral

Given the holistic nature of nursing, it is inconceivable that the nurse can meet all the client's health care expectations. In carrying out the comprehensive health assessment as previously prescribed, the nurse readily may identify personal strengths and limitations with regard to selected areas of client health. The nurse must have a usable system for delegating activities and referring clients to appropriate resources in order to implement a plan of care that addresses the client as a total physical, psychologic, social, and spiritual being.

In certain instances, the nurse is the one who will implement care for the client; expertise in given areas will determine if the nurse can accommodate the client or must delegate activity. For instance, the nurse and client have determined the potential for growth in the area of family dynamics. The given agency has a nurse whose areas of expertise include family interactional patterns; the client's nurse delegates that part of the care to the family care expert. Collaboration between the two nurses is essential to provide continuity of care delivery. When certain parts of care implementation are delegated, comprehensive data must be provided for the delegated nurse to allow an informed delivery of care. The nursing care plan must remain flexible so that revision is based on team members' communication of additional assessment data and the client's nurse's own constant reassessment. Validation of assessment data with the client and/or the family should also be ongoing to ensure the client is following the current care plan.[39] In providing for client input, the nurse implies her respect for him as an individual. The client who has a high "reflexive self-concept" (what he thinks the person with whom he is interacting thinks of him) is more apt to be satisfied with care delivery.[1] This, in turn, may affect his level of motivation to achieve stated health goals.

For areas of care that require the expertise of other health professionals, the nurse must have a system to identify appropriate client resources, as well as a knowledge of the qualifications and reputations of resource persons within the community. The ability to refer to appropriate health care providers reflects the nurse's professional competence. A client's dissatisfaction with the care rendered by a referred person may influence the nurse's credibility with the client and those around him or her.

As the coordinator of the client's health care, the nurse must reassess continuously the client's status and movement toward goals of care.[11] The nurse's ability to mobilize resources, to recognize progress, and to initiate appropriate change when necessary are critical in the successful implementation of a care plan.

EVALUATION

Evaluation, the fifth component of the nursing process follows the implementation of actions by both client and nurse as prescribed in the nursing plan of care. Its purpose is to measure the client's progress or lack of progress toward goal achievement, as determined through a collaborative effort between nurse and client. "The client's progress or lack of progress toward goal achievement directs reassessment, reordering of priorities, new goal setting, and revision of the plan of nursing care."[1] Thus, the nursing process is a continuing cycle. Evaluation is a purposeful, goal-directed activity that occurs during attainment of short-term goals and after attainment of long-term goals.

Measurement of Progress

Progress or lack of progress toward goal achievement is measured through evaluation of the outcome criteria specified by short-term goals. During the planning phase, the nurse and client formulate goals depicting desired client behavior or clinical status. These goals specify what behavior or clinical status is needed for the correction of the problem and include a deadline for evaluation.[31] The box below shows an example of such a care plan.

By the dates specified, the client is able to first correctly plan a daily menu for a 1500-calorie diet and then show a weight loss of 2 pounds. It could be concluded that the client has exhibited the desired behaviors necessary toward resolving the problem of being overweight. Can it also be concluded that the client actually met with the nutritionist, decreased between-meal snacking, and counted the calories of foods eaten? No, not unless he was observed doing all of these things. The client could have gone to the library to research the contents of a 1500-calorie diet and starved himself for 2 days before his visit with the nurse. If the client cheated, he or she will probably not continue to lose weight steadily, but it will appear that he or she has reached the established short-term goals.

Thus, the nurse largely must depend on the subjective reports of the client when dealing with healthy clients. In the situation described, the nurse asked the client to write down a menu plan for a 1500-calorie diet and also weighed the client. The nurse then was able to evaluate progress via objective data. Other objective data can be obtained through laboratory measurements. A client trying to reduce cholesterol intake could have a serum cholesterol test, and the nurse looking at the results would have objective evidence of the client's progress toward adhering to a low-cholesterol diet. It is more likely, however, that nurses working in wellness-oriented centers will have to depend on indirect observation or the client's verbalized participation to evaluate progress.[16] However, the focus for application of the nursing process in assisting clients toward health promotion implies that action resides with the self-directed, self-responsible client. The nurse should be primarily available as a valuable resource for instruction, motivation, and evaluation to enhance the potential success of the client in learning.[31]

❑ ❑ NURSING CARE PLAN FORM

Nursing diagnosis	Intervention	Short-term goal
Alteration in nutrition—more than body requirements (Date 8/1/94)	Client confers with nutritionist about the content of a 1500-calorie diet; decreases number of between-meal snacks; and counts calories of foods to be eaten.	By 8/8/94 client can plan on paper a daily menu for a 1500-calorie diet. By 8/15/94 client will show a weight loss of 2 pounds.

DOCUMENTATION

An ongoing documentation of the nurse's involvement in assisting the client toward health promotion is essential, especially since the nurse is accountable to the individual and larger community. Documentation is essential for legal accountability and assurance of provision of appropriate standards of care (see box below). According to standards established by the ANA, the licensed professional nurse is responsible for directly and indirectly measuring and observing signs which signify the client's response to care. Standards of care include guidelines for collecting data, the utilization of nursing diagnoses, and planning and evaluating the efficacy of care.[5] The documentation of the nursing process ensures the standards of care have been met.[3]

An evolving method of documenting the nursing process in the 1990s will be through computerization of the client's record. There are many reasons for implementing computerized documentation systems (see box below).

THE RELATIONSHIP OF THE NURSING PROCESS TO THE RESEARCH PROCESS

As previously discussed, the nursing process is a systemic progression through a series of purposeful steps to assess and diagnose the client's actual or potential need or problems and to plan with the client interventions to reach a goal. Through evaluation, the nurse and client review the outcome and reassess the need to continue with the intervention or plan for new ones.

The research process is a systemic inquiry that utilizes scientific methods to answer questions and solve problems. Data collected provide evidence to support findings which answer clearly defined questions or problems. Like the nursing process, research is a process that consists of

❑ ❑ REASONS FOR COMPUTERIZING MEDICAL RECORDS

Reduces the burden of documentation
Facilitates the nursing process
Enables the nurse to transmit information more quickly
Provides constant quality reports
Encourages research through the establishment of a database

a purpose, set of actions, goal setting, and evaluation. The purpose provides direction to the process, with methodologies arranged to achieve identifiable goals and evaluate outcome measures. The process is continuous and can be amended or redesigned.[3] Comparison of both processes are shown in Table 4-3.

Table 4-3. **Comparison of nursing process to research process**

Nursing Process	Research Process
Assessment	Knowledge to identify nursing
	Phenomena
	Review of literature
Nursing diagnoses	Identification of problem
Planning	Research methodology
	Formulate hypotheses
	Research design
	Select sample
Implementation	Data collection
	Data analyses
Evaluation	Outcome measures
	Interpret results

SUMMARY

The nursing process is an important tool in assisting healthy individuals to maintain and promote their level of health. Modifying the definition of the nursing process and enlarging the scope of the diagnostic categories is necessary to follow the evolution of the nursing process, which parallels society's transition from a disease-oriented to a health-oriented system of care. Nursing must move from its largely nurturant activities to a more preventive and generative practice.

The health assessment approach delineates the types of data to be collected; use of a standardized assessment format incorporating Gordon's typology of 11 functional health patterns can unify nurses' approach to assessing healthy clients. The nursing process must be used in a holistic manner, with the client as active participant responsible for the outcomes of health care.

The nursing process is not new, nor is it unique, but its application toward healthy individuals demands creative nursing strategies. Nurses are involved deeply in today's evolving health care system and will continue to be a major voice in the future.

References

1. American Nurses' Association: *Nursing: a social policy statement,* Kansas City, Mo, 1980, The Association.
2. Bates B: *A guide to physical examination,* ed 5, New York, 1990, JB Lippincott.
3. Beare P, Myers DL: *Principles and practice of adult health nursing,* St Louis, 1990, Mosby.
4. Blattner B: *Holistic nursing,* Englewood Cliffs, NJ, 1981, Prentice Hall.
5. *Defining clinical content, graduate nursing programs, medical and surgical nursing,* Boulder, 1967, Western Interstate Commission on Higher Education.
6. Dietz LD, Lehohky AR: *History and modern nursing,* Philadelphia, 1967, FA Davis.
7. Getchell B: *Physical fitness: a way of life,* ed 4, New York, 1992, John Wiley & Sons.
8. Gordon M: *Manual of nursing diagnosis: 1993-1994,* St Louis, 1993, Mosby.
9. Hall L: *Nursing: what is it?,* Richmond, 1959, Virginia State Nurses' Association.
10. Hames CC, Joseph DH: *Basic concepts of helping: a holistic approach,* New York, 1980, Appleton-Century-Crofts.
11. Hegyvary ST, Hausmann RKD: *The relationship of nursing process and patient outcomes,* NLN Pub No 21-2194, New York, 1987, National League for Nursing.
12. Holmes T, Rahe R: The social readjustment rating scale, *J Psychosom Res* 11: 213, 1967.
13. Kilpack V, Dobson-Brassard S: Intershift report: oral communication using the nursing process, *J Neurosci Nurs* 19:5, 1987.
14. Kim M, Moritz D, editors: *Classification of nursing diagnoses,* ed 5, New York, 1982, McGraw-Hill.
15. Knowles L: *Decision making – a necessity for doing,* New York, 1967, Appleton-Century-Crofts.
16. Kulbok PA, Baldwin JH: From preventive health behavior to health promotion: advancing a positive construct of health, *Adv Nurs Sci* 14(4):50, 1992.
17. Lee HA, Frenn MD: Nursing diagnoses for health promotion in community practice, *Nurs Clin North Am* 22:4, 1987.
18. Lewis L: *This I believe . . . about the nursing process – key to care.* In Browning MH, Minehan PL, editors: *The nursing process in practice,* New York, 1974, American Journal of Nursing.
19. Maibusch RM: *The nursing minimum data set: benefits and implications for clinical nurses,* NLN Pub No 41-2199, New York, 1987, National League for Nursing.
20. Marriner A: *The nursing process: a scientific approach to nursing care,* ed 3, St Louis, 1983, Mosby.
21. Maslow AAH: *Motivation and personality,* New York, 1954, Harper & Row.
22. McCain, RF: Nursing by assessment – not intuition, *Am J Nurs* 65:82, 1965.
23. McCourt A: *Models, activities, and issues.* In Kim M, Moritz D, editors: *Classification of nursing diagnoses,* ed 5, New York, 1992, McGraw-Hill.
24. McPhetridge LM: Nursing history: one means to personalize care, *Am J Nurs* 68:68, 1968.
25. Nightingale F: *Notes on nursing,* London, 1859, Harrison & Sons. Reprint: Philadelphia, 1946, Edward Stern.
26. Nurse Practice Act, New York State, 1973, Sections 6901 and 6902.
27. *Nutrition, Health, Activity Profile,* Pacific Research Systems, PO Box 64218, Los Angeles, CA 90064.
28. Orlando JJ: *The dynamic nurse patient relationship: function, process and principles,* New York, 1961, GP Putnam & Sons.
29. Pearson A, Vaughan B: The nursing process: a literature review, *Midwifery* 3:3, 1987.
30. Pelletier K: *Mind as healer, mind as slayer,* New York, 1977, Dell Publishing.
31. Pender N: *Health promotion in nursing practice,* ed 2, Norwalk, Conn, 1987, Appleton & Lange.
32. Redman BK: *The process of patient education,* ed 6, St Louis, 1988, Mosby.
33. Rushton CA: Attitudes to the nursing process, *New Zealand Nursing Forum* 16(2): 11, 1988.
34. Samuels M, Bennet H: *The well body book,* New York, 1973, Random House.

35. Sheehan J: Conceptions of the nursing process amongst nurse teachers and clinical nurses, *J Adv Nurs* 16(3):333-342, 1991.
36. Smitherman C: *Nursing actions for health promotion*, Philadelphia, 1981, FA Davis.
37. Titler MS: Implementation of nursing diagnoses in nursing education, *Nurs Clin North Am* 22:4, 1987.
38. Turner SJ: Nursing process, nursing diagnoses, and care plans in a clinical setting, *J Nurs Staff Development* 7(5):239-243, 1991.
39. Walton I: The nursing process in perspective: a literature review. In Henderson V: The nursing process in perspective, *Adv Nurs* 12:6, 1987 (editorial).
40. *Webster's new international dictionary*, Springfield, Mass, 1992, C & C Merriam.
41. Yura H, Walsh M: *The nursing process: assessing, planning, implementing, evaluating*, ed 4, Norwalk, Conn, 1983 Appleton-Century-Crofts.

CHAPTER

5

Nurse-Client Relationship

June Andrews Horowitz

Objectives

After completing this chapter, the nurse will be able to

- *Describe the process of values clarification.*
- *Examine the elements and process of communication.*
- *Analyze differences between functional and dysfunctional communication.*
- *Apply knowledge of values clarification and communication to development of the helping relationship.*
- *Understand the significance of the nurse-client relationship in all aspects of clinical practice.*

The interpersonal context of the nurse-client relationship is the milieu in which nursing care occurs. Practice is shaped by a one-way interest of the nurse in the client, which Peplau[37] describes as "professional closeness": the nurse's ability to focus on the interests, concerns, and needs of the client. This one-way focus enables nurses to detach their own self-interest and needs from the client situation so that they are free to promote positive changes in the client.

When the goal is health promotion, the nurse-client relationship is the primary vehicle for assisting persons to engage in positive health practices. Active health promotion strategies require personal involvement. Individuals, families, and communities must make choices that are likely to optimize their health potential if health promotion is to be successful. Nurses and other care providers cannot force the outcome of their health promotion efforts, but they can use the nurse-client relationship as the arena for health promotion activities. Without a nurse-client relationship, nurses' health promotion efforts are severely limited and may be reduced to the status of friendly advice. Therefore, the interpersonal context is the essence of health promotion. Kasch suggests, "Nursing action might be conceptualized as a process of social interaction."[22] Essential to this process are values clarification, communication, and the helping relationship.

VALUES CLARIFICATION

Definition

Values are qualities, principles, attitudes, or beliefs about the inherent worth of an object, behavior, or idea.[33,55] Values guide action by sanctioning certain behaviors and negating others. There are two types of values: cognitive and active. *Cognitive* values are those stated as being ascribed to intellectually. *Active* values, in contrast, are those physically acted out.[35] It is important to judge the power of a given value by its ability to influence action. For example, a nurse may claim to value the worth of all persons equally but treat clients of various races differently and provide the most time and concern for those similar to the nurse's own self. This cognitive value has little power to shape the nurse's behavior. If the nurse treated clients of all races with equal respect, the value would also be active and have great power to motivate behavior.

Many forces shape values. They are passed down from

one generation to another and color the individual's identity, goals, and sense of personal meaning. Values are imbedded in the culture and taught within a family and social context, thus giving meaning to the life events and happenings outside the family's boundaries. From consciously and unconsciously held values, a repertoire of behavioral responses to events is developed over time.[14,19]

Once established, however, values are not static. Life events and social processes can spark a reappraisal of personal values. Values clarification is a method whereby a person purposely seeks to discover what his or her values are and what importance these values have.[41,53] Values clarification does not tell a person how to act but rather assists the person in recognizing what values are held to evaluate how they influence action.

The client's and nurse's values both will color their interaction – values influence expectations, norms for interactions, interpretations of messages exchanged, and goals. Sensitivity to possible discrepancies in values and respect for the client's values are essential if the nurse hopes to engage the client in a therapeutic relationship.

The box below outlines seven steps in the valuing process.[41] The first three steps of choosing involve a cognitive process; the next two steps involve the affective or emotional domain; and the final steps involve behavior.[50]

The nurse uses values clarification for two purposes: (1) to examine personal values and their potential influence on nursing care and (2) to assist clients to identify their values and to reflect on their connection to health-related behaviors. The box to the right lists suggestions for putting values clarification into action.

Values clarification becomes a clinical aim when clients' values lead to behaviors that conflict with the nurse's value of promoting health. For example, a nurse tells a childbirth education class of pregnant women and their coaches that use of cocaine is dangerous: it poses serious risks to the fetus and to the newborn. After the class, one woman comments, "Do you really think that using coke just once in a while is bad for the baby? I'm sick of being told that I can't do things because of the baby." In this example, a conflict in values is clear. Intervention would need to be aimed at examination of how the client's wish for gratification clashes with her desire to have a healthy child. The nurse also must weigh his or her own values related to health promotion for the client and the fetus against respecting a client's right to decide about her own health behaviors. When values conflict, an ethical dilemma results. Resolution of this conflict and success of subsequent interventions rest on the ability of the nurse and client to examine the conflicting values and their outcomes, and to acknowledge responsibility for the decisions made.

Values and Therapeutic Use of Self

The self, the most precious and unique of all human endowments, is a personal concept of one's individuality as distinct from other persons and objects in the world. The terms *self-concept* and *self-esteem* also are used to refer to individuals' judgments and attitudes concerning themselves. The critical importance of having an overall high self-concept has been demonstrated by clinicians and researchers in studies of children's behavior. Children

❑ ❑ THE VALUING PROCESS

Choosing

1. Choosing freely.
2. Choosing from possible alternates.
3. Choosing after careful consideration of potential outcomes of each alternative.

Prizing

4. Cherishing and being happy with personal beliefs and actions.
5. Affirming the choice in public, when appropriate.

Acting

6. Acting out the choice.
7. Repeatedly acting in some type of pattern.

❑ ❑ TECHNIQUES FOR ASSISTING CLIENTS TO CLARIFY VALUES

Identify the client's values

- "What is important to you?"
- "Which of the following statements sounds most like the way you think?"
- "What do you value most in life?"

Use reflection to restate the value and make it explicit

- "In what you've just told me, I hear that it is very important to you that . . ."
- "I understand that you value . . ."

Identify value conflicts or conflicts between values and actions

- "What connection does this value have to your current health or illness and to the healthy behaviors, interventions, or treatments needed to maintain or restore your health?"
- "How does this particular value affect your behavior and health?"
- "What are some ways you could put your values into action?"
- "Are your actions consistent with your values? If not, what might you change?"

with positive self-concepts approach tasks and new experiences with confidence; they expect to succeed and be accepted by others. In contrast, children whose self-concepts are weak or negative tend to shy away from challenges and attention. According to Patterson, "They are likely to live in the shadows of social groups, listening rather than participating, and preferring the solitude of withdrawal above the interchange of participation."[34]

Self-concept evolves throughout life. From birth, family experiences and parental identification mold the child's sense of identity. Studies have demonstrated positive relationships between the self-reliance, self-esteem, and self-confidence of parents and children.[10,46] To cultivate children's self-esteem so that they have a realistic perception of strengths and weaknesses, parents should avoid (1) focusing excessively on negatives, (2) failing to give feedback concerning abilities and limitations, and (3) leaving the child without a sense of belonging.[18-20]

Sullivan,[51] founder of the Interpersonal School of Psychiatry, which has influenced the evolution of psychiatric nursing theory and practice, stressed the importance of early parent-child experiences in molding the child's self-concept. Positive, rewarding, anxiety-free interactions contribute to security, esteem, and positive self-view. Negative experiences colored by a moderate degree of anxiety contribute to the child's sense of "bad me," that is, a sense of incompetence, insecurity, and negative self-concept. The "bad me" serves a purpose by reflecting a realistic view of those areas of self that are not positive. In contrast, the "not me" portion of the self emerges from highly anxiety-laden experiences and represents the dissociation of part of the self. A healthy self-concept would include a large "good me"; a small "bad me"; and little or no "not me" portions. Multiple positive but realistic appraisals from significant others, most important the parents, assist the young child to develop such a healthy self-view.[18]

Joel has aptly summarized the importance of the parents' role in shaping the child's self-concept: "The purpose of nurturing a child's self-concept is to provide him or her with an internal sense of self that realistically reflects his or her abilities and limits the consensus of reflected appraisals from the world. An adequate self-concept, then, includes a relatively nondistorted view of self balanced by a sense of one's inherent value, importance, and potential."[20]

The self is not only developed in response to reflected appraisals of others. Genetic endowment, experiential opportunities, and the individual's own action shape self-concept. Persons can accept or reject the appraisals of others and modify their behavior. The ability to control actions and evaluate outcomes of interactions allows individuals to modify and alter their views of self. As such, the self is dynamic, changing through interaction with the outside world and in response to the various maturational and situational crises of life.

The ability to examine, reflect on, and evaluate the self is a uniquely human talent. Campbell defines this quality of self-awareness as "the dynamic, conscious and active gaining of knowledge about the psychological, physical, environmental and philosophical components of the inner self."[4] Self-awareness also involves interactions between the self and the external world and the symbolic connections created by the person. The self includes an unconscious component that is only partially accessible and a force that influences behavior.

Self-awareness is influenced by the degree to which a person has an accurate conception of all dimensions of the self.[16] The Johari window provides a schema for understanding the various components of the self (Fig. 5-1). There are four recognized components of the self: (1) the public self, which is shown to others; (2) the semipublic self, which is seen by others but may be outside the individual's awareness; (3) the private self, which is known to the individual but not revealed to others; and (4) the inner self, which is the unconscious portion not known even to the individual because its content is too anxiety provoking.[3,16]

Altogether, these windowpanes represent the total self. Three principles guide understanding of how the self functions in this representation: (1) change in one portion influences all other portions; (2) the smaller the first portion, the poorer communication will be; and (3) interpersonal learning enlarges the first portion and decreases the size of one or more other portions.[28] Thus the goal of self-awareness is to increase the size of the first windowpane while reducing the size of the other three areas (Fig. 5-2).[52]

Consider the differences between windows A and B of Fig. 5-2. Window A represents a person with little self-awareness. Note that windowpane number 4 is large, suggesting that a good deal of the person's experiences, thoughts, and feelings are repressed or suppressed, probably a result of associated anxiety. It also suggests a large "not me" portion of the self. In contrast, window B repre-

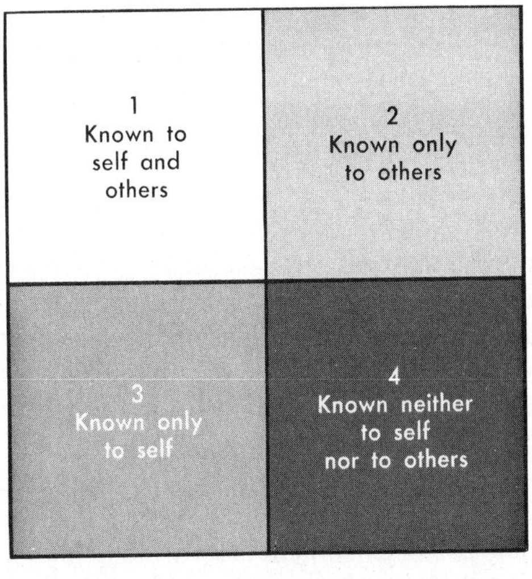

Fig. 5-1. Johari window. (Redrawn from Luft J: *Group processes: an introduction to group dynamics,* Palo Alto, Calif, 1970, National Press Books.)

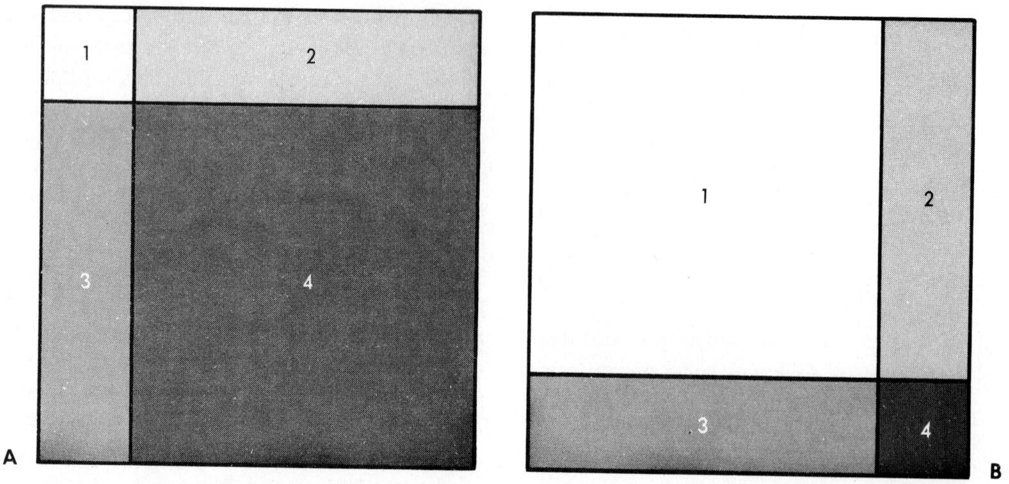

Fig. 5-2. Johari windows illustrating varying degrees of self-awareness. **A,** Person has little self-awareness. **B,** Person has great amount of self-awareness. *1,* Public; *2,* semipublic; *3,* private; and *4,* inner self. (From Sundeen SJ, et al: *Nurse-client interaction: implementing the nursing process,* ed 4, St Louis, 1989, Mosby.)

sents a person who is open to the world and is comfortable with his or her self-concept.

The goal of high self-awareness, as illustrated in window B of Fig. 5-2, is reached through three steps.[4,50] The first step is *listening to oneself* and paying attention to emotions, thoughts, memories, reactions, and impulses. Often persons tune out their feelings and thoughts because they are anxious or because they are in a hurry to accomplish some other task. Without self-reflection, individuals act automatically and lose some of the meaning of living. To improve the ability to listen to oneself, ask questions such as the following:

What am I feeling now? What emotions have I experienced today and in the past day or so? What were my thoughts?

What events led up to these thoughts and feelings?

What actions did I take? Did my behavior fit with my thoughts and feelings, or was there a lack of harmony?

Was I aware of my reactions at the time they took place?

(For the nurse) How have I responded in clinical situations lately? In response to a particularly happy, sad, or difficult situation, how did I react? In what way might I alter my actions now?

The second step is *listening to and learning from others.* Feedback from others can cause anxiety when it conflicts with self-image – even when that image is distorted. In response, the feedback is ignored or translated incorrectly to preserve self-image and reduce anxiety. However, this pattern of responding limits knowledge of the self; it inhibits the ability to examine the appraisals of others and to grow as a result. It is helpful to ask, "What feedback have I received today?" and "What is the other person trying to tell me now?" A person can also ask others directly for feedback. For example, a student nurse might ask another student how he or she comes across to a client. The feedback could be used to alter aspects of behavior that are ineffective or problematic before asking the faculty member for evaluative feedback.

The third step is *self-disclosure;* sharing aspects of the self enriches interpersonal life. Through self-disclosure, persons come to know themselves better because they have held thoughts, actions, and feelings up to the light for examination with others. Self-disclosure has been called a symptom of a healthy personality and the means to achieving it.[21,50]

Why is it important for the nurse to clarify personal values and to increase self-awareness? The things we value and our ability to understand ourselves influence our behavior. The nurse uses behavior in interactions with clients. The self is the nurse's greatest tool; to use it effectively, the nurse must be fully aware of how it functions. When unexamined values and aspects of the self, or "unconscious material," motivate a great deal of the nurse's behavior, therapeutic use of self becomes impossible. The nurse's needs must be kept in check so that the client's needs can be met.[39] Self-awareness and acceptance of personal beliefs free the nurse to direct energy toward meeting the client's needs. Openness to self generates openness to others and acceptance of differences among people – qualities essential to a therapeutic use of self. In addition, the nurse's and client's definitions of a situation are derived from active construction and interpretation of experience. These definitions generate actions to follow.[22] The nurse's and client's systems of beliefs and values will serve as lenses through which to focus their interactions.

COMMUNICATION PROCESS

Communication is far more than simply talking with others or imparting information. Communication is the arena of all thought and relationships shared between people.[31] As such, it is crucial to human life and growth. In conjunction with use of scientific and technologic advances, communication is an essential tool of the nurse.

Communication has been defined as "a process by which information is exchanged between individuals through a common system of symbols, signs, or behavior."[43] This exchange involves all the modes of behavior that an individual uses, consciously or unconsciously, to affect another person. It includes the spoken and written word as well as nonverbal communication – gestures, facial expressions, movement, bodily messages or signals, and artistic symbols.[11,43]

Communication is important to clients. In a national telephone survey of 6455 adults recently discharged from medical and surgical services of 62 hospitals across the United States, Cleary and colleagues[7] found that the most common complaint (45% of reported complaints) was that patients were not told about the daily routine of the hospital. Other top problems identified by the respondents also relate to inadequate or poor communication with the clinicians. Frequently cited complaints included not being told whom to ask for help; the physician or nurse in charge not being available to answer questions; the physician or nurse not explaining, before a test, how much discomfort or pain to expect; not getting understandable answers from nurses or physicians in response to important questions; not being given adequate privacy while receiving important information about one's condition; and physicians and nurses sometimes talking in front of the patient as if he or she weren't there. Clearly, the results of this study show that clients perceived multiple problems in communication that adversely affected the quality of care received.

The implications for clinical practice and outcome evaluation are clear. "Regardless of what a patient was told, if he or she does not remember being given certain information, communication has failed. Thus, we do not interpret negative responses as necessarily indicating failure to offer information, education, or opportunities to ask questions. Rather, they may reflect a need to improve communication."[7] Nurses and other health care professionals must understand the critical importance of effective communication – without it, care fails to help the clients.

Function and Process

The functions of communication have been delineated by Ruesch and Bateson:[43]

1. To obtain and send messages and to retain information.
2. To use the information to arrive at new conclusions and to reconstruct past and look forward to future events.
3. To begin and to modify physiologic processes.
4. To influence others and outside events.

Communication transports information, both interpersonally and intrapersonally, and provides the basis for action.

The process of communication consists of input, flow and transformation, output, and feedback. Nurses must be able to diagnose communication difficulties in any of these components. *Input* involves taking in information from outside the individual or group. Once taken in, input must be transformed in some manner to be used. For example, food must be broken down for use as energy, and symbols must be translated into ideas. The flow of processed input refers to the way information is analyzed and stored within the individual or the way it is transmitted from person to person within a human system (group, family) before communication with the external environment occurs. The outcome of information processing, *output,* involves further exchange with the environment or other person. A new information exchange is triggered at this point in the cycle by the response called *feedback,* a monitoring system through which the person or group controls the internal and external responses to behavior (output) and accommodates appropriately. The idea of a feedback loop shows the dynamic nature of communication: each piece of communication is both a stimulus, designed to elicit a response, and a response to a different stimulus (Fig. 5-3).[3,54]

In analyzing interpersonal communication, two types of feedback can be identified: positive (encouraging change) and negative (encouraging homeostasis or no change). The following mother's commands to her toddler illustrate these types: (1) *positive* – "Try that again, walk to Mommy"; and (2) *negative* – "Don't walk there, it's not a safe place." The first statement shows the mother's attempt to encourage the child to continue new behavior; the second illustrates her effort to curtail undesired behavior. Rather than meaning "good" or "bad," the labels positive and negative feedback refer to system change and homeostasis. Both types are needed, depending on the situation.

The notion of the situational context of communication is important. The context of communication is the setting in both a physical and psychosocial sense. Thus the context includes the relationship between sender and receiver; their previous experiences, feelings, values, cultural norms, and age and developmental stage; and the physical location.[18,22,50,52,56]

Types

All human communication occurs in three forms: verbal, nonverbal, and metacommunication. Each affects the meaning and influences the interpretation of the message.

VERBAL

Verbal communication is the transmission of messages through the use of spoken or written words. Words, as symbols for ideas, impart meaning defined by a specific language. The ability to communicate through the use of

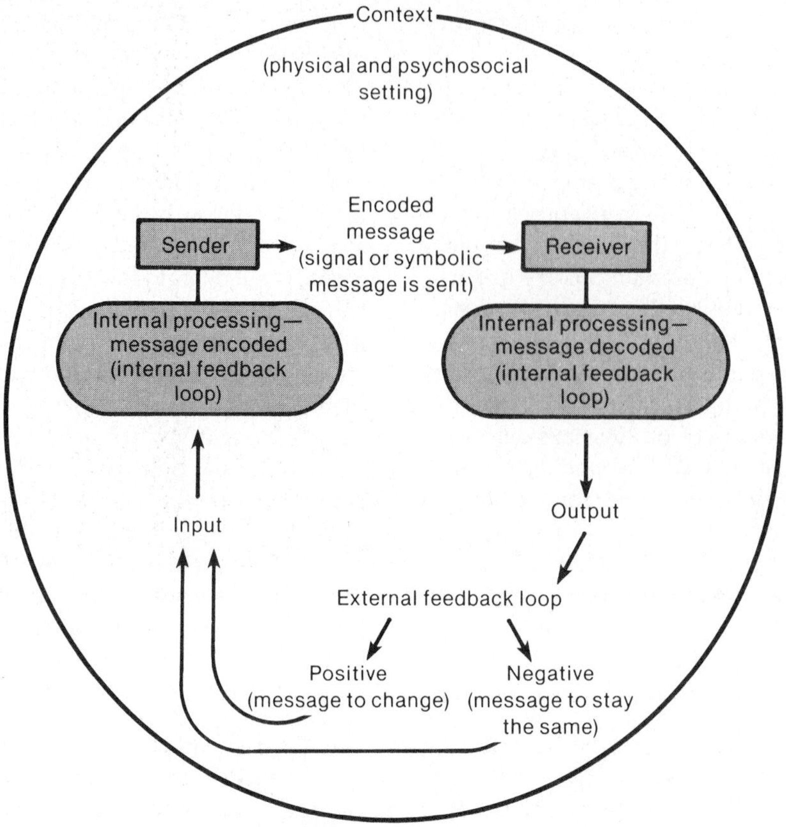

Fig. 5-3. Communication system.

language is a uniquely human attribute and a most critical ability.

The complexity of learning to use language is demonstrated by the skills that are needed before a child can begin to associate any particular sound to a particular class of objects. These skills include (1) the concept of object, (2) some degree of object constancy, (3) knowledge that characteristics vary in importance, and (4) space-object coordination.[25] In addition to development of these cognitive skills, according to Chomsky,[6] a built-in "language acquisition device" (LAD) is required for the child to process language heard (linguistic input), to generate rules, and to comprehend and construct grammatical speech.[32] Although some data appear consistent with this theory, other evidence is less supportive. However, it is clear that linguistic development primarily rests on maturation and changes in the brain, particularly increasing specialization in neural structure and functioning, including the emergence of cerebral dominance or laterality of brain function. Once begun, the process of language acquisition progresses in geometric fashion. By adolescence, mastery of sophisticated language skills should be evident.[18,29]

The importance of language development is apparent in its three functions: (1) informing the person of others' thoughts and feelings, (2) stimulating the receiver of a message by triggering a response, and (3) serving a descriptive function by imparting information and sharing observations, ideas, inferences, and memories.[54] The ability of verbal communication to fulfill these functions is influenced by the communicator's social class, culture, age, and milieu.

NONVERBAL

Nonverbal communication or language encompasses all messages sent that are not spoken or written. Movement, facial and eye expressions, gestures, appearance, and vocalization or paralanguage all constitute nonverbal modes of communication (Fig. 5-4).[2,9]

Although all communication has the potential for being misunderstood, Blondis and Jackson[2] point out that nonverbal communication is particularly subject to misunderstanding because it does not always reflect the sender's conscious intent. Nonverbal messages also tend to be nebulous, without specific beginnings and endings. As such, nonverbal communication "is constant, flowing, and dynamic – a two-way mime performed on the stage of the subconscious."[2]

The channels of nonverbal communication are the five senses. The ability to see, hear, smell, touch, and taste assists in the perception of messages. The senses can be

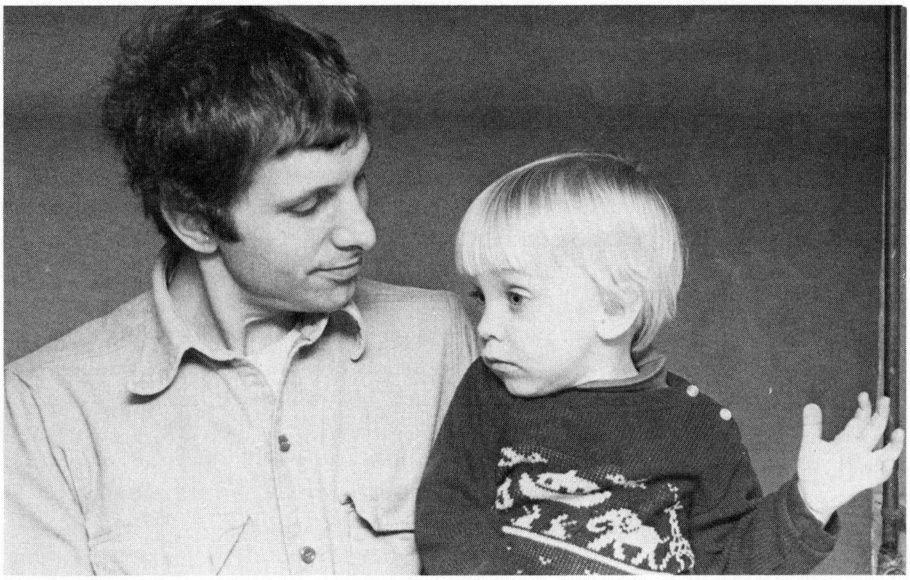

Fig. 5-4. Nonverbal cues are important components of communication. (Photograph by Douglas Bloomquist.)

tuned to differing aspects of communication; for example, the receiver might hear the sender laugh but see a sad facial expression. Both messages are crucial to interpretation of the communication.

Body Motion or Kinetic Behavior. Body motion or kinetic behavior includes facial expression (or facies), eye movements, movements of the body, gestures, and posture.[2]

When observing facial expression, the nurse should notice the affect or emotion that is communicated. Does the person appear happy or sad; alert, distracted, or sleepy; or contented, agitated, or anxious? The degree of emotion expressed should also be noted. Does the person's face express what is generally considered an excessive degree of feeling for the situation, or too little or none at all?

Eye movements are closely related to facial expression. Eyes, in conjunction with movement of other facial muscles, move in ways that convey affect. Eye contact conveys messages of interest or trust; lack of eye contact can imply lack of interest or anxiety; constant eye contact can send a message of hostility.

It is important to note that all these messages are bound culturally and situationally. Interpretations of nonverbal behavior, particularly facial and eye expressions, are rooted in the context of the communication. For example, avoidance of direct eye contact between some persons can be a sign of respect in certain circumstances and cultures.

Appearance. Appearance is an overall notion of how persons present themselves. The nurse must consider whether the person's appearance seems appropriate to the context.

Paralanguage. Paralanguage is vocalization, other than expression of words, and includes many aspects of sound, such as tone, pitch, and tempo of speech. Sounds of crying, groaning, gasping, and grunting are all examples of paralanguage.[2] Infants begin their vocal communication with paralanguage. Although some authors classify paralanguage as verbal communication,[51] it seems more appropriate to view it as nonverbal communication because words, the hallmark of verbal communication, are not used.

Importance. The importance of nonverbal communication must not be overlooked by health care providers. Because this communication has great power to transmit information about another's thoughts and feelings, the nurse must observe carefully; even a silent client can reveal much. The significance of nonverbal communication is best captured by the axiom, "What people do is often more important than what they say."[23]

METACOMMUNICATION

Besides verbal and nonverbal, a type of communication called metacommunication refers to a message about the message. Watzlawick and others discuss it in relation to the impossibility of not communicating, in other words, "one cannot not communicate."[54] Even in silence, the person is transmitting a message about what is being communicated.

Metacommunication is the relationship aspect of communication. In a sense it involves reading between the lines or going past the surface content of the message to glean nuances of meaning. When the content and the relationship – or metacommunication aspects – of a message are incongruent, it may be difficult to interpret the communication accurately, leaving the receiver uncomfortable and confused.

The importance of metacommunication is particularly clear in relation to communication between adults and children. If nonverbal or verbal messages are conflicting, the young child becomes confused. Trust is diminished and the child's emergent self-concept can be compromised. The child will not learn to trust personal reactions and interpretations and may find communicating a risky enterprise (Fig. 5-5).

GROUP PROCESS

In group settings a special type of metacommunication is called *process*. A basic principle of group theory states that all communication has a content and a process aspect. Content is what is said; process is the relationship aspect of what is communicated. For example, consider two clients in a therapy group who always support each other by agreeing with each other and offering additional comments or criticism to any group member who disagrees. Although this pairing between the two clients offers them some protection from anxiety that may result from self-examination and feedback, it isolates them and curtails feedback from others. Examination of this group process is an essential task. The nurse leader and clients could transform this problematic situation into a learning opportunity by doing the following: (1) identifying the pattern, that is, pointing out the behavior after it has occurred frequently enough; (2) helping the paired clients and other group members to consider what needs are being met through this pattern; (3) looking at each person's role in fostering this process (Why have other group members failed to confront the paired clients?); and (4) discussing potential outcomes of changing the behavior. The principles embedded in these steps for examining group process can be applied in clinical situations when greater self-understanding is a goal.

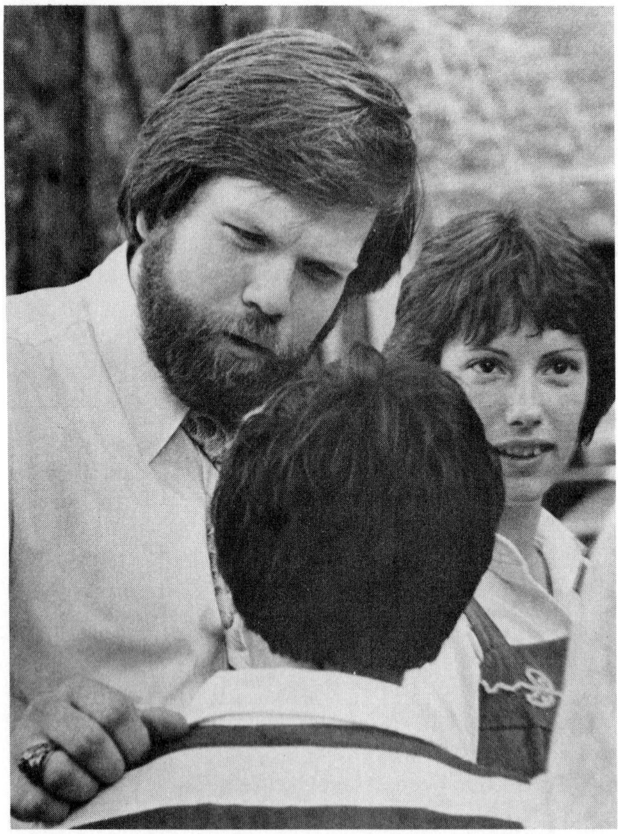

Fig. 5-5. Children typically are open and direct about what they think and feel. It is important for adults to respect their expression of thoughts, emotion, and judgments. (Photograph by David S. Strickler.)

Functional Communication

Understanding what makes communication functional will improve the nurse's ability to assess clients' needs and to intervene effectively. See the box below for steps to functional communication.

To state the case firmly, the sender needs to make the content and the metacommunication congruent; if they conflict, the message is confusing. For example, a married man is working with a new woman in the office. The man verbally denies that he is sexually attracted to the woman; but his dress, facial expression, and posture, and the topics he introduces are all provocative. Clearly the man's levels of communication are not congruent. His verbal statements about his intent are disconfirmed by his nonverbal communication; his metacommunication, or message about the message, tells others to disregard what he says and to "listen" to his nonverbal cues. To make his communication functional, he needs to reflect on his feelings; bring any anxiety, fears, or wishes into awareness; and adjust his metacommunication to his professional role.

To clarify and qualify the message, the sender must give a complete message. Important features of the message should be emphasized, and specifics of any request must be stated, not assumed. The message's importance also must be indicated. To illustrate, a wife mentions to her husband that it is nearly June. The husband responds that he had noticed how warm the weather was becoming. On the surface this communication may seem functional, until the intent of the wife's message is considered.

STEPS TO FUNCTIONAL COMMUNICATION

1. Firmly state the case.
2. Clarify and qualify the message.
3. Seek feedback.
4. Be receptive to feedback when it is received.

The wife meant to imply that June is the month of their anniversary. She hoped that her husband would somehow know that she wanted him to comment on their anniversary plans. To make this communication functional, she needed to expand the message ("Our anniversary is coming up") and clarify her wish for a response ("What shall we do to celebrate?"). In addition, she needed to show how important the message was ("I'd really like to do something special this year").

One technique for clarifying and qualifying messages is called the "I statement," in which the sender states what he or she wants, feels, thinks, or plans (including likes and dislikes). For example, "I felt hurt when you forgot our anniversary last year."

Questions can clarify and qualify depending on the type asked. Open-ended questions tend to elicit a descriptive response, not a one-word answer. For example, "Tell me about what you did at school today" is likely to yield a fuller description from the child than the question, "Did everything go OK at school today?" However, direct questions that seek a one-word answer are useful when a specific piece of information is sought. "Did you pass your math test today?" may be a better approach than, "What was the math test like?" when the issue of passing the test is important to discuss. Also, for clients experiencing difficulty in expressing more than the most simple thoughts, it can be helpful to ask direct questions that call for brief replies, such as, "Did you eat breakfast?" This approach is particularly useful with clients who are depressed, regressed, cognitively impaired, or unable to handle complex information or communication at a particular time.

Seeking feedback is another element of functional communication. Consensual validation, confirming that both sender and receiver understand the same information, calls for the use of the clarification skills just described. In family communication the parent, as sender, should model this behavior for children by asking the child, as receiver, to explain his or her sense of the message and how to ask the sender for further explanation. For example, "I want you to clean your room" (message from parent) can be followed by, "Tell me how you think you will do that?" (validating that child and parent agree about what the task entails). This style of seeking validation can be adapted to nurse-nurse and nurse-client interactions.

It is also crucial for the sender to be open to feedback. A "no questions" attitude blocks functional communication, whether in the home, classroom, or clinical setting. Children, students, clients, and even other nurses may be afraid to question anyone in authority or may assume that the person should magically know what is intended or expected. For example, a client may avoid confronting a nurse who fails to explain the treatment plan and then communicates that the client should know what and how to follow through. Statements by the sender such as, "Tell me what you think" and "what is your understanding of what I said" are helpful.

The art of receiving messages involves many of the same processes as sending. Evaluation of the intent of the message, both the content and the metacommunication, is the first step. Because this task is difficult, particularly if the content and metamessage are not congruent, the receiver frequently must ask for clarification and validate the understanding of the message.

LISTENING

Effective listening, an important part of communication, is more than passively taking in information; it is actively focusing attention on the message. Asking questions to explore what is meant helps the receiver in reaching an accurate assessment of the message's intent.[57]

Effective listening is essential if the nurse is to assist the client and to understand him or her as a person. The nurse's failure to listen to the client may be caused by anxiety; lack of experience, which leads to excessive talking by the nurse; preoccupation with personal thoughts; or lack of practice.[50]

RESPECT

Holding the client in esteem and giving special attention to concerns connote respect. Effective listening is the most appropriate way to convey respect to the client, followed by focusing on the client's needs and providing feedback.

EMPATHY

In empathy nurses experience the client's feelings by drawing on emotions and experiences and placing themselves in the client's situation. According to Ehmann, "We gain something from empathy. We achieve a close communication with another person, and a deeper, fuller appreciation and understanding of him as an individual. In another sense, when a person empathizes with us, we experience the reassuring feeling that we are being understood and accepted."[12] With empathic understanding the nurse acknowledges the affective domain of personal experiences and uses this knowledge to appreciate the client's reactions. Empathy enables the listener to share human experiences as the basis for providing care.

FLEXIBILITY

In flexibility a balance exists between control and permissiveness.[11] In overcontrol every message is monitored; in exaggerated permissiveness anything can be communicated in any way. For communication to be functional, rules should be laid down about what is appropriate, without rigid prescriptions that inhibit any meaningful interchange. For example, the rule that nurses will not answer questions concerning intimate details of their lives sets an appropriate limit; however, that does not mean that nurses should refuse to answer any question from a client.

SILENCE

Silence between persons is often uncomfortable for the nurse, who is somewhat insecure about what should occur during a "therapeutic" encounter. However, silence can be very useful when used carefully. When a patient is seeking a verbal response, silence can be perceived as a lack of interest.[50] At other times, silence allows clients to reflect on what is being discussed or experienced, lets them know that the nurse is willing to wait until they are ready to say more, or simply provides them with comfort and support. Each situation needs individual evaluation by the nurse, with sensitivity to the client's needs. Rather than asking a flurry of questions to break the silence, the nurse should allow the client to decide when to comment or should make brief comments that do not demand answers, such as, "It can be helpful to take time to think about what we've been discussing." Also, comments such as, "Try putting your thoughts (or feelings) into words," can assist the client to share these thoughts or feelings when silence is blocking rather than improving the communication.[26]

HUMOR

Humor is part of being human. It relieves tension, reduces aggression, and creates a climate of sharing. It can block communication when it is used to avoid subjects that might be uncomfortable or when it excludes other persons. Humor can also inflict emotional pain and communicate negative views or stereotypes about particular persons or groups through jokes concerning race, ethnicity, culture, country of origin, occupation, age, or gender and sexual activity. A direct response to the latent content or message in such humor is an effective way to curtail its use and minimize its effect. For example, "That kind of joke makes me very uncomfortable. I don't find it funny to describe (insert the specific group in question) that way, and I would like you to stop."[45] In order to be helpful, the meaning of the humor must be understood and its purpose supportive to the client. Clarification of the meaning should be used when there is doubt or concern.

TOUCH

Touch is an interesting means of nonverbal communication for nurses, who often touch clients during administration of care. The nurse's concern can be expressed by a gentle or soothing application of touch. Yet in some instances touch is not appropriate. In interactions with acutely disturbed psychiatric clients, for example, touch might be misinterpreted; a psychotic client might think the nurse is attacking, and a very anxious client might be startled if touched. It is important for the nurse to evaluate the context and meaning of touch to the client on the basis of knowledge about the client and interpretation of feedback. Appropriate use of touch is illustrated in Fig. 5-6.

SPACE

Space between communicators varies according to the type of communication, the setting, and the culture. Hall[17] has researched *proxemics*, or use of space between communicators, and has identified four common zones of space used in interaction in North America:

1. Intimate space – up to 18 inches (45.5 cm); used for high interpersonal sensory stimulation (Fig. 5-7).
2. Personal space – 18 inches to 4 feet (45.5 to 120 cm); appropriate for close relationships in which touching may be involved and good visualization is desired (Fig. 5-8).
3. Social-consultative space – 9 to 12 feet (270 to 360 cm); less intimate and personal, requiring louder verbal communication (Fig. 5-9).
4. Public space – 12 feet and over (360 cm and over); appropriately used for formal gatherings, such as speech giving (Fig. 5-10).

Understanding the appropriate distance for a given type of interaction assists the nurse to make the nonverbal and verbal communication congruent. Awareness of

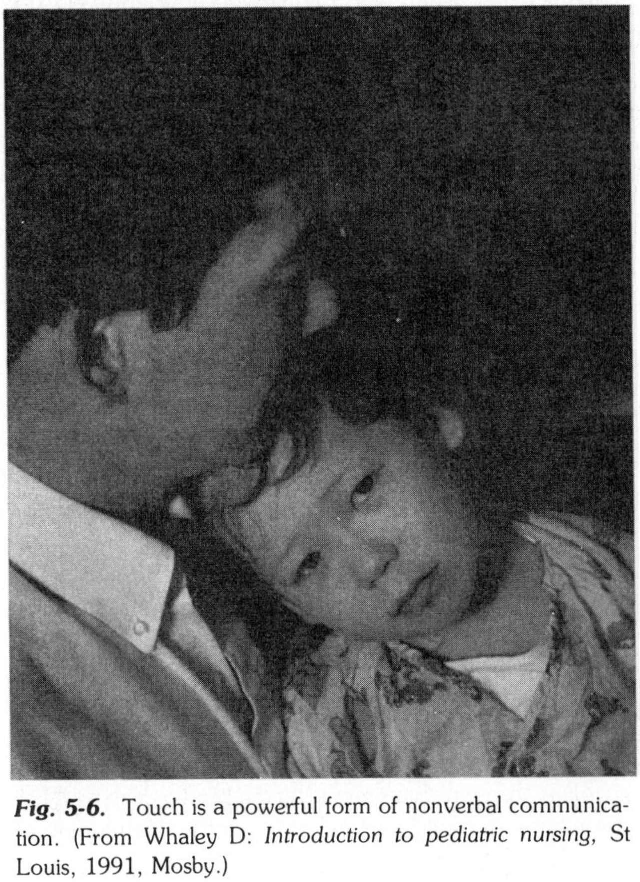

Fig. 5-6. Touch is a powerful form of nonverbal communication. (From Whaley D: *Introduction to pediatric nursing,* St Louis, 1991, Mosby.)

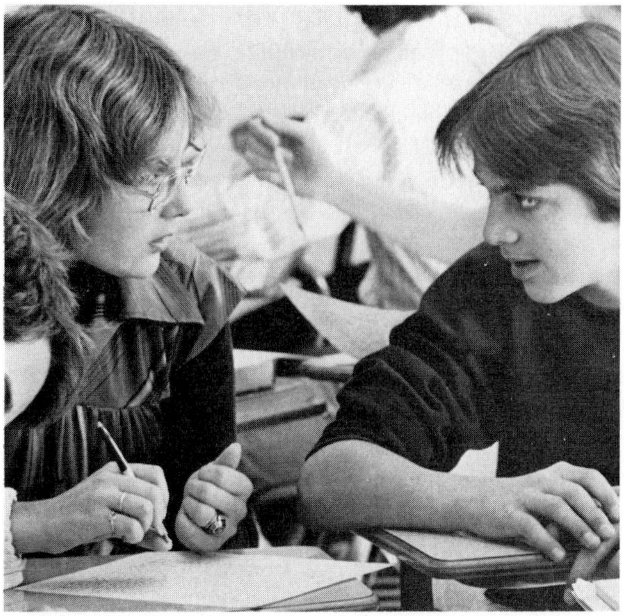

Fig. 5-7. Intimate distance communication. (Photograph by Douglas Bloomquist.)

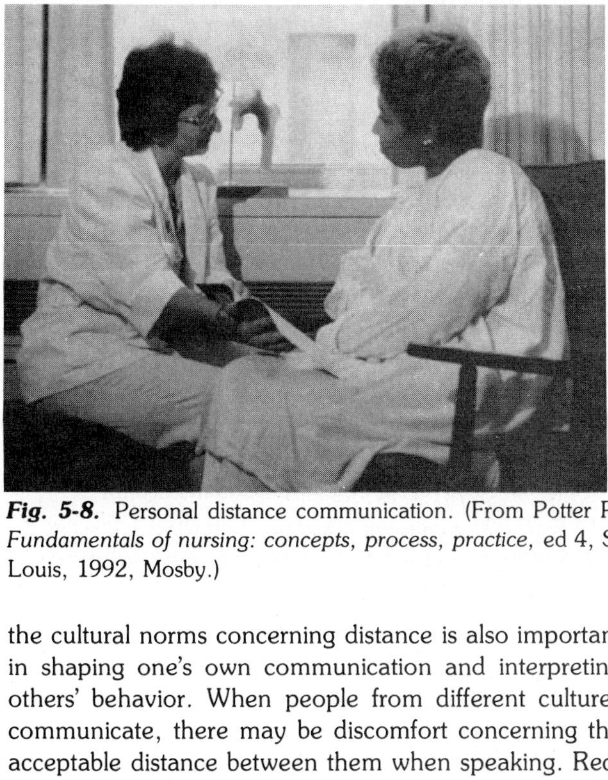

Fig. 5-8. Personal distance communication. (From Potter P: *Fundamentals of nursing: concepts, process, practice*, ed 4, St Louis, 1992, Mosby.)

the cultural norms concerning distance is also important in shaping one's own communication and interpreting others' behavior. When people from different cultures communicate, there may be discomfort concerning the acceptable distance between them when speaking. Recognition of differences assists the nurse to adjust the distance and interpret the meaning of this nonverbal communication.

ASSESSMENT AND DIAGNOSIS

Examination of clients' communication is an essential part of any nursing assessment. McFarland and Naschinski[30] conducted a validation study concerning etiologic factors

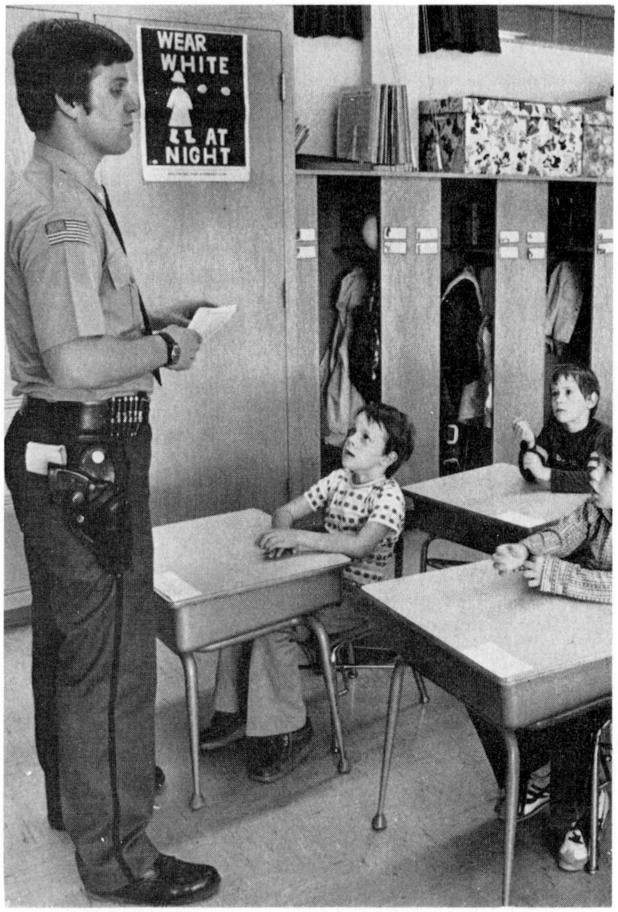

Fig. 5-9. Social-consultative distance communication. (Photograph by David S. Strickler.)

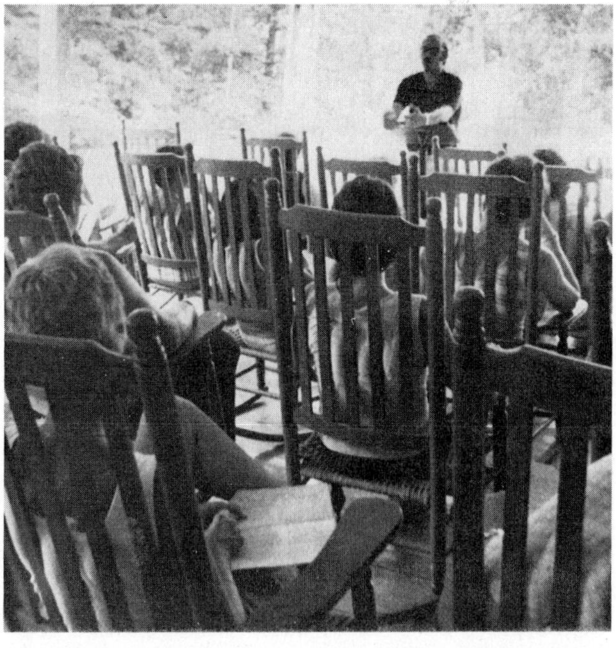

Fig. 5-10. Public distance communication. (Photograph by David S. Strickler.)

and defining characteristics of the nursing diagnosis of impaired communication. The related factors, defining characteristics, and outcome criteria related to the diagnosis are given in the boxes on this page and at the top of p. 113. The nursing diagnosis of impaired verbal communication can be defined as "the state in which an individual experiences a decreased or absent ability to use or understand language in human interaction."[27] Although further research is needed to validate the diagnostic label of impaired communication, this material can assist nurses in their efforts to identify disordered communication to the degree of specificity needed to understand and diagnose the difficulty with the goal of promoting functional communication.[29,30]

❑ ❑ ❑

Functional communication is characterized by the many traits and components discussed in this chapter. However, communication is more subtle and intricate – it cannot be reduced to a set of parts and principles; its roles and nuances are far more complex and variable. It is a special human ability to communicate by language and symbols. When communication is healthy, it enables persons to bridge the gap between themselves, to move from being alone to being together – clearly one of the crucial tasks of living.

HELPING RELATIONSHIP

A helping relationship is a process in which one person promotes the development of another by fostering that person's maturation, adaptation, integration, openness, and ability to find meaning in the present situation.[31,39] The nurse-client relationship emerges from purposeful encounters; this helping relationship is created through the nurse's application of scientific knowledge, understanding of human behavior and communication, and commitment to the client. The nurse-client relationship is the foundation of clinical nursing practice – the essential element of care in every setting with every client in every situation. Techniques, technology, interventions, and contexts vary; but the relational aspect of nurses' practice is the glue that produces a cohesive whole allowing nurses to see clients holistically as unique persons.

The power of the nurse-client relationship and its implications for health promotion are illustrated in a long-term follow-up program for persons with ischemic heart disease.[13] Frasure-Smith and Prince reported the outcomes of a life stress monitoring program involving monthly telephone assessment of discharged patients' experiences of cognitive and behavioral symptoms of stress. When the

❑ ❑ FACTORS RELATED TO IMPAIRED VERBAL COMMUNICATION

Developmental or age-related stages(s)
Mechanical impairment(s)
Physical condition(s)
Severe physical or psychosocial stress(es)
Extreme anger
Severe anxiety or panic
Moderate to severe depression
Significant impairment of perception
Unrealistic or inadequate self-concept
Cultural differences
Faulty communication skills

From Thompson JM, et al, editors: *Mosby's manual of clinical nursing*, ed 2, St Louis, 1989, Mosby.

❑ ❑ OUTCOME CRITERIA FOR CLIENT GOAL OF SUCCESSFUL COMMUNICATION

Attendance to appropriate input

1. Oriented to person, place, and time.
2. Selects and responds to relevant stimuli.
3. Perception is accurate.
4. Absence or control of physical symptoms.

Clear, concise understandable messages

1. Absence of speech impediments.
2. Selects and organizes words appropriate to the receiver and context.
3. Speaks dominant language.
4. Uses effective communication techniques.
5. Uses appropriate amount of verbiage.
6. Expresses feelings appropriately.

Congruent nonverbal and verbal communication

1. Expresses congruent nonverbal behaviors.
2. Expresses congruent verbal and nonverbal behavior.
3. Balances use of verbal and nonverbal behavior.

Sends and receives feedback

1. Listens actively.
2. Examines effects of behavior on others.
3. Asks for and receives feedback.
4. Sends feedback to others.

Experiences gratification from communication

1. Reports satisfaction from communication.
2. Reports a sense of high self-esteem.
3. Reports or shows a willingness to assume responsibility for communication.
4. Sends and receives confirmation when communicating.

From Thompson JM, et al, editors: *Mosby's manual of clinical nursing*, ed 2, St Louis, 1989, Mosby.

❑ ❑ DEFINING CHARACTERISTICS OF IMPAIRED VERBAL COMMUNICATION

Disorientation
Too little or too much attention to stimuli
Speech impediments
Physical conditions
Inability to speak dominant language
Inability or reluctance to speak
Disregard for speaker
Reliance on nonverbal communication
Inability to organize words
Inappropriate selection of words
Use of unfamiliar words
Inconsistent verbal and nonverbal messages
Message inappropriate to context
Excessive or insufficient verbiage
Ill-timed message
Inadequate listening skills
Disparity of punctuation
Absent or inappropriate feedback
Discordant information
Disconfirmation
Absence of gratification
Inability or reluctance to express feelings
Withdrawal from interaction
Unrestrained or inappropriate emotional expression
Imaginary or false perceptions
Incongruent communication styles
Lack of assertive skills

From Thompson JM, et al, editors: *Mosby's manual of clinical nursing,* ed 2, St Louis, 1989, Mosby.

monitoring indicated that the patient was experiencing 5 or more out of 20 symptoms (or was readmitted to the hospital without having a high stress score), the patient received home-based nursing interventions designed to reduce stress. Individually tailored interventions combined teaching, support, and counseling or referral strategies. The outcome was dramatic. Over the program year, treatment-group participation decreased risk by a factor of about 50%. The researchers suggested that, "beta-blockade and program participation had parallel effects on sympathetic arousal. . . . While the medication may have reduced sympathetic effects at cardiac receptor sites, the program may have lowered general background levels of fear and anger, thereby lowering sympathetic tone."[13] This apparent synergistic impact may also have resulted from increased patient compliance with prescribed medications associated with program participation. In either case, the effect of the nurse-client relationship in stress reduction and reduction in morbidity and mortality must be recognized.

No perfect profile or personality of a helping person exists. Certain traits, however, enable the nurse to be an agent of therapeutic care. Such characteristics of a helping person, which can be nurtured without thwarting the nurse's own unique personality, include[5,31,40,50,56]

1. Self-awareness and self-reflection
2. Openness
3. Self-confidence and strength
4. Genuineness
5. Concern for the client
6. Respect for the client
7. Knowledge
8. The ability to empathize
9. Sensitivity
10. Acceptance
11. Creativity
12. Ability to focus and confront

The process of values clarification, as described earlier, can assist the nurse to nurture these personal characteristics. Counseling clients can serve many purposes and is useful in a variety of settings (see box below).

Characteristics

No recipe is available for a successful nurse-client relationship. Techniques and concepts serve only as tools. As a nurse develops and evaluates a helping relationship, several guides may be useful.

PURPOSEFUL COMMUNICATION

Purposeful communication means that the nurse focuses communication for a particular aim. Social chit-chat – communication without a goal – should not make up the bulk of nurse-client interaction. This does not mean the

❑ ❑ PURPOSES OF HELPING RELATIONSHIP

To identify and reduce or resolve problematic feelings, anxiety, and stress.
To clarify conflicts, needs, and goals.
To make decisions after considering alternatives, variables, and differing perspectives; to set short- and long-term goals.
To clarify and strengthen values; to consider the consequences of values and related behavior.
To cope with situational or maturational crises.
To problem solve effectively.
To gain insight and self-understanding.
To reduce psychopathology and mental health problems.

Adapted from Litwick L, Litwick J, Ballou M: *Health counseling,* New York, 1980, Appleton-Century-Crofts.

nurse should never discuss a social topic; nevertheless, there should be some purpose: discussing the weather with a somewhat disoriented elderly client serves the purpose of orienting that client to the environment. Client goals guide the nurse in focusing communication.

RAPPORT

Rapport is a harmony and affinity between people in a relationship.[42] It is the nurse's responsibility to establish an atmosphere in which rapport can develop, using many of the traits listed for a helping person. It is important to be genuine, open, and concerned to let the client know that his or her concerns interest the nurse and that working together may alleviate some of his or her difficulties and encourage growth.

TRUST

Trust is the reliance on the ability, character, and behavior of a person; it involves a sense of certainty that the other will carry out responsibilities and promises, and an expectation that the outcome of interaction need not be feared.[52] The nurse can encourage the client to be trustful by (1) modeling trust for the client by trusting the client to do as promised; (2) clearly defining the relationship parameters and expectations, particularly the purpose and specifics of time, place, and anticipated behavior; (3) being consistent; and (4) willingly examining nurse and client behaviors that interfere with trust.

EMPATHY

Empathy is feeling with another person and also understanding the dynamic meaning of behavior.[52,55] Nurses do not empathize by switching the focus of the interaction to themselves or by sympathizing ("I know exactly how you feel; that happened to me once."); they use personal experience to appreciate the client's own feelings and experiences.

"Empathy is a pervasive phenomenon in the life experience of all people. It allows people to feel the feelings of another and respond to and understand that person's experience on his or her terms."[24] Using this understanding while maintaining personal boundaries is the essence of empathy in the helping relationship.

GOAL DIRECTION

A helping relationship is special in its goal-directed nature; unlike most human relationships that focus on mutual benefit, it exists solely to meet some need or promote the growth of the client. Although a side benefit is often gratification, learning, or growth for the nurse, the relationship is client centered.

As previously stated, goals are formulated as desired client behaviors. Short-term goals are changes likely to be achieved within 10 days to 2 weeks; long-term goals are all others. All goals should be stated in measurable terms and focus on a positive change or in a decrease of a problematic behavior.

Ideally the client works with the nurse to establish goals. However, some clients – such as those who are seriously depressed, psychotic, or organically impaired – are unable to do this. When the client is unable to negotiate appropriate goals, the nurse establishes realistic goals and shares them with the client. The client is free to participate or to reject efforts to reach the goals.

ETHICAL DECISION MAKING

Ethical decision making is closely linked with the goal-directed nature of helping relationships. The nurse often may wish to set goals that the client does not wish to reach; the nurse must remember that the problem belongs to the client, as does the choice of care alternatives. The nurse assists the client in decision making, with the decision based on the client's value system. However, the nurse should not take a laissez-faire approach and avoid assisting the client. The nurse's responsibility is to help the client examine values, identify conflicts, and prioritize. Action follows from understanding values and the best available information.[44]

This approach to decision making requires the nurse and other health care professionals to find a balance "between the goals of cure and the goals of care."[1] Both the client and the nurse must bring interpreted facts and their own clarified values to the interaction to establish goals. Recognizing this interplay, the nurse must clarify personal values, subsequently respect the client's rights, and act to support and protect the client's and family's integrity.

Six steps in ethical decision making have been identified by Stuart and Sundeen:[50]

1. Gather background information – consider what information is known and whether a dilemma exists and its context.
2. Identify the ethical components – consider underlying issues and who is affected.
3. Clarify roles – consider the rights and obligations of all involved parties.
4. Explore options – consider the alternatives, including aims and potential outcomes.
5. Apply ethical principles – consider relevant criteria, ethical theories, scientific facts, and personal philosophy.
6. Resolve the dilemma – consider the legal and social constraints and ramifications, the goal and method of implementation, and evaluation.

Purposeful application of these steps enables the nurse to respect the client's rights and integrity while assisting in making difficult decisions.

Therapeutic Techniques

Sometimes individuals new to the concept of the helping relationship assume either that they are bound to "say the wrong thing" and cause terrible damage to the client or that they will learn some magical phrases and questions to create instant rapport. No nurse or other professional is so powerful that a "wrong word" could destroy the client's self-concept or self-esteem. Even clients with physical and emotional problems are resilient and have coped, at least to some degree, with a lifetime of stresses. Alternately, there is no magical saying that the nurse can always plug into an interaction and then communicate successfully. Although some techniques are often useful, they must be applied with purpose, skill, and attention to the context and individuality of the client. The following approaches, therefore, should be viewed as guidelines for effectively shaping the nurse-client relationship.

KEEP CLIENT IN FOCUS

Nurses must first master the ability to focus on the client's needs by orienting the client to who they are and the purpose of the interaction; nurses should avoid delving into their own personal lives.[33] It can be difficult to avoid nurse-directed conversation; a useful rule of thumb is for nurses to answer or respond to obvious questions and to switch the focus back to the client when other questions are asked. For example:

Client: (looks at nurse's wedding ring): "Are you married?"
Nurse: "Yes, I am."
Client: "What does your husband do?"
Nurse: "Rather than get off to a discussion about me, let's get back to planning how you will manage at work."

This focus also involves acknowledging the client's intent by stating that portion of the client's message that is clear, seeking validation, and helping the client to clarify the rest of the message. Davis[11] calls the acknowledgment the principal tool by which the helping professional promotes communication and encourages the client to seek further improvement.

APPLY CONCEPT OF LEARNING

Peplau's operational definition of learning[38] serves as a guide for collecting data about the client and assisting the client to acquire new knowledge and develop skills to explain events, to change, and to solve problems. The steps in the definition and verbal strategies that the nurse can use to promote each step are listed in Table 5-1.

CLARIFY CONTENT AND MEANING

Table 5-1 presents many suggestions for helping the client to observe, describe, analyze, formulate, and validate. Because clarification by the nurse is so important, however, it merits emphasis as a distinct technique. The use of *who, what,* and *where* questions and statements beginning with phrases such as, "tell me," "go on," "describe to me," "explain it to me," and "give me an example," assist the client to expand on and clarify the content and meaning of what is communicated. By seeking feedback (see Table 5-1, step 5), the nurse further assists the client to explain the meaning.

In clarifying, the nurse should avoid threatening, detective-like questions. Questions that begin with "why" often increase the client's anxiety because they demand reasons, conclusions, analysis, or causes.[36] Generally it is more helpful to reformulate questions to obtain data first and to help the client analyze and formulate.

USE REFLECTION

Reflection is the restatement of what the client has said in the same or different words. This technique can involve paraphrasing or summarizing the main point made by the client to indicate interest and to focus the discussion. Effective use of this approach does not include frequent, parrotlike repetition of the client's statements.

EMPLOY CONSTRUCTIVE CONFRONTATION

Confronting a client means that the nurse points out a specific behavior and then assists the client to examine its meaning or consequences. For example:

Nurse: "You are 20 minutes late for our meeting."
Client: "Oh, I didn't notice the time."
Nurse: "What were you doing that interfered with your being on time today?" *or* "What do you think is going on with you that you didn't notice the time when you are usually very aware of it?"

This type of confrontation is not an angry exchange but a purposeful way of helping the client to examine personal actions and their meaning.

USE PRONOUNS CORRECTLY

Some clients have difficulty in separating themselves from others or in specifying the object or subject in their language. Such clients misuse pronouns by referring to "we," "us," "they," "him," "her," and so forth without clearly identifying the referent. The client will make statements such as, "They don't like me. They told me I was useless." The nurse can clarify by asking, "Who are they?" or "To whom are you referring?" In addition, the nurse must be careful to use separate pronouns when speaking of herself or himself and the client. For example, when communicating with clients with disordered thinking, the nurse should say "you and I" rather than "let's" or "we" to assist such clients in maintaining personal boundaries.[38]

***Table 5-1.* Peplau's concept of learning**

Steps of learning	Nursing strategies
1. Observation: ability to attend to events and people	Encourage use of the senses and memory: "Tell me about what happened." "Describe it to me."
2. Description: ability to remember and share details of an experience	Encourage fuller use of memory and verbal skills: "Tell me exactly what happened next." "What did you think or feel at the time?" "Give me an example." (Other who, what, where, and when questions that elicit a sequential account)
3. Analysis: ability to examine parts of an experience and see relationships	Encourage comparison of components and their classification (for example, fact vs. fantasy or speculation): "What meaning does this have for you?" "What's the connection?" "Tell me what your part was."
4. Formulation: ability to state outcome of step 3 in systematic expression	Encourage restatement of data in verbal or written format: "Sum up what happened." "What pattern is there?" "Tell me the essence of it."
5. Validation: ability to compare perceptions and conclusions resulting from the previous steps	Encourage verbal comparison: "Do you mean . . .?" "What might you do to find out how the other person sees it?" "Let me tell you what I understand you to be saying."
6. Testing: ability to try out results from previous steps (particularly 4) in new situations	Encourage consideration of use in other present and future situations: "What would you do the next time?" "What difference does understanding this make?"
7. Integration: ability to add new to past knowledge for future use	Encourage development of new picture or idea with appropriate adjustment or former one: "Tell me how you see it now." "In what way has your view changed?"
8. Utilization: ability to apply outcome of previous steps with anticipation and insight	Encourage application in new situations by role playing and/or practice in appropriate settings: begin process again (steps 1 to 8) in examining outcome of step 8.

Adapted from Peplau HE: *Process and concept of learning.* In Burd S, Marshall M, editors: *Some clinical approaches to psychiatric nursing,* New York, 1963, Macmillan; and O'Toole A, Welt SR: *Interpersonal theory in nursing practice,* New York, 1989, Springer.

USE SILENCE

Allowing a thoughtful silence at intervals helps the client to talk at his or her own pace without pressure to perform for the nurse. It also permits time for reflection. Silence can be particularly helpful to the depressed or physically ill person in reducing pressure and conserving energy. After several moments the nurse can help the client by asking him or her to try sharing thoughts. For example: "Try putting your thoughts into words," "What are you thinking (or feeling) now?" or "I'll be here when you feel ready to talk."

ACCEPT COMMUNICATION

Allowing the client to communicate verbally and nonverbally in his or her own fashion makes the client feel safe and respected. This does not mean that the nurse always agrees with the client or tolerates inappropriate behavior, such as verbal or physical abuse; but within the established limits of the setting, acceptance of the client's mode of communication is an important ingredient in a helping relationship.

Barriers to Effective Communication

Barriers to effective communication, which can originate with the nurse, the client, or both, include the following.

INEFFECTIVE TECHNIQUES

The most obvious block is the nurse's failure to use the types of therapeutic techniques just described. Lack of knowledge or experience can limit the nurse's ability to assess the client's needs and repertoire of skills. Supervision and study can help the nurse apply the steps of the nursing process, using effective intervention approaches.

Communication is also ineffective when some part of the communication-feedback loop breaks down. Failure to send a clear message, receive and interpret the message correctly, or provide useful feedback can interfere with communication. It is the nurse's responsibility to diagnose the source of the communication breakdown and take steps to correct it by using knowledge of the communication process and appropriate therapeutic techniques.

ANXIETY

When the nurse or client is highly anxious during an interaction, perception is altered; and the ability to communicate effectively is curtailed sharply. The use of defense mechanisms, such as denial, projection, or displacement, reduces anxiety at the expense of understanding the true meaning of an interaction. Anxiety and use of defenses distort reality and lead to disordered communication. The nurse should identify the anxiety and its source and use anxiety-reducing interventions to enhance the interpersonal communication.*

ATTITUDES

Biases and stereotypic notions can limit both the nurse's and the client's ability to relate. When the problem is the client's, the nurse can assist in examining those views that interfere with the client's relationships. When the problem is the nurse's, openness to examination of personal behavior in the supervisory relationship is crucial. If the nurse fails to examine attitudes toward the client, negativity may be communicated, and the interaction may be distorted.

GAPS BETWEEN NURSE AND CLIENT

Related to attitudinal barriers is the idea that gaps in age, sociocultural background, race, ethnicity, or language can block functional communication between the nurse and client. These factors can cause differences in perception and block mutual understanding. The nurse can assist the client to recognize how perceptions may be different and to clarify meanings. (For additional discussion, see Chapter 2).

RESISTANCE

Resistance comprises all phenomena that inhibit the flow of thoughts, feelings, and memories in an interpersonal encounter,[8] as well as behaviors that interfere with therapeutic goals. Resistance arises from anxiety when the person feels threatened. To reduce this anxiety, the person implements resistant behavior, most often in the form of avoidance behavior, such as being late, changing the subject, forgetting, blocking, or becoming angry.

The nurse should first identify the behavior, whether nurse's or client's, and then attempt to interpret it in the context of the interaction. Exploration of possible threats in the relationship, goals, or a particular topic can lead to understanding the source of the resistance and finding the ability to handle such difficulties. Anxiety reduction is often a necessary step in dealing with resistant behavior.

TRANSFERENCE AND COUNTERTRANSFERENCE

Transference is reacting to another person in an exchange as if that person were someone from the past.[48] It may involve a host of feelings generally classified as positive (love, affection, regard) or negative (anger, dislike, frustration). The usual transference reaction involves an important figure from the past, such as a mother or father; however, at times it may be more general and include all authority figures. Something about the other person's characteristics, behavior, or position triggers this response. Clients in a therapeutic relationship often develop strong transference feelings toward the helping professional because of the interaction's intensity and the care provider's authoritative or nurturing role.

Countertransference is the same phenomenon but is experienced by the health care professional. The nurse experiences many feelings toward the client; these are not problems unless they remain unanalyzed and become potential blocks to the nurse's ability to work effectively with the client. For example, if a nurse has deep feelings for the client and thinks the client cannot possibly function after discharge without the nurse's aid, the nurse is likely to distort the client's abilities, encouraging a childlike dependency and interfering with the person's progress. This nurse needs to examine personal feelings to understand their source. Once understood, countertransference reactions generally cease to interfere with the relationship.

In working with the client's transference reactions, the nurse helps the client examine his or her feelings and thoughts about the nurse. The client can compare and contrast the nurse with persons from his or her past to better comprehend the present reality.

SENSORY BARRIERS

When the client has any sensory limitations, the nurse may need to use great skill in communicating. Use of the other senses to send or receive messages should be tried. Special help often is available from trained therapists and teachers; for example, many agencies have access to interpreters for deaf clients. Nurses must be as creative as possible, learn from the client and others who are skilled

*For those who wish to explore interventions for reducing anxiety, refer to a psychiatric nursing text, such as Stuart GW, Sundeen SJ: *Principles and practice of psychiatric nursing,* ed 4, St Louis, 1991, Mosby; or Haber J, et al: *Comprehensive psychiatric nursing,* ed 4, St Louis, 1992, Mosby.

in alternate forms of communication, and make needed referrals.

FAILURE TO ADDRESS CONCERNS OR NEEDS

The failure to meet the client's needs or to recognize concerns is the most serious barrier to effective interaction. It can arise from (1) an inadequate assessment, (2) lack of knowledge, (3) inability to separate the nurse's needs from the client's, and (4) confusion between friendship and a helping relationship, including unrecognized or unresolved sexual issues. To correct such a problem, the nurse first should recognize that a barrier to relating with the client exists. Using the supervisory process to determine the problem's source, the nurse then takes corrective action, such as obtaining more information or knowledge or performing a self-assessment with values clarification and examination of reactions, biases, and expectations.

Setting

The setting of nurse-client interaction can affect the goals and the nature of the communication. Sometimes the nurse has only minimal control over the setting, as in a busy clinic, health center, inpatient unit, or the client's home. Although far from the ideal of a quiet, pleasant, well-lit private office, such typical nursing settings can be used effectively by creating a sense of private space. Curtains can be drawn, doors shut, and two chairs pulled to a corner to shape an environment for interaction. When possible, nurses should seek offices or rooms to see clients privately. In research conducted by Cleary and colleagues, former hospital patients stressed the importance of establishing privacy during significant communication or imparting of health information by nurses and physicians[7] (Fig. 5-11).

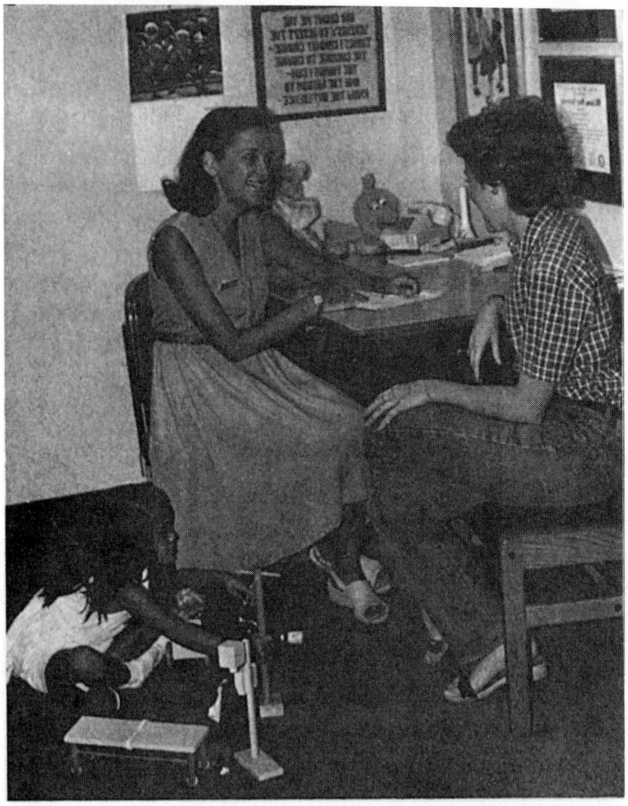

Fig. 5-11. The interpersonal context of the nurse-client relationship is the optimal milieu for health promotion. (From Wong D: *Essentials of pediatric nursing,* ed 4, St Louis, 1993, Mosby.)

The most important aspect of any setting is that the nurse and client are able to attend to each other. The nurse's attention to the client helps create such an atmosphere. Second, the nurse can assess the possible influence of such factors as lighting, noise, temperature, comfort, physical distance, and privacy; potentially disturbing factors can be altered or controlled within the limits of the setting. The nurse also can acknowledge verbally that some aspect, such as an interruption or noise, is bothersome. This technique shows the client that the nurse recognizes possible concentration difficulties and is sharing the environment with the client.

Stages

Nurse-client relationships follow sequential phases, which may overlap, vary in length, or involve issues that appear over time rather than in a set sequence. The orientation or introductory, working, and termination phases have been identified.[52]

ORIENTATION OR INTRODUCTORY PHASE

This stage begins when the nurse and client meet. This meeting typically involves some feeling of anxiety; neither knows what to expect. It is the nurse's job to help structure the interaction by discussing several topics during the initial and sometimes first few meetings:

1. What to call each other
2. Purpose of meeting
3. Where, when, and how long meetings will be
4. Termination date or time for review of progress
5. Confidentiality–with whom clinical data will be shared
6. Any other limits related to the particular setting

Discussion of these issues establishes the contract or pact and involves a mutual understanding of the parameters of the relationship and an agreement to work together.

During the orientation phase, many nursing students inexperienced in setting up a nurse-client contract pass through several stages themselves.[49] First, they feel moderate to severe anxiety. Second, they use defense mechanisms such as denial, and social conversation with clients predominates. Third, they question their ability and may project hostility to the staff. Finally, students adjust to and are interested in what the clients say; anxiety is lowered, and the working stage is beginning.

WORKING PHASE

It is during this phase that the major tasks of the relationship are met. Goals are set, and the nurse and client mutually work toward their accomplishment. Problem solving, coping with stressors, and efforts to gain insight are all part of the working phase. The nurse and client see each other as unique individuals.

Resistant behaviors commonly are seen during this phase.[50] As the nurse and client become closer and work on possibly anxiety-producing problems, the client may pull away through use of defense mechanisms. Overcoming the resistance becomes an important nursing task.

TERMINATION PHASE

Termination marks the end of the relationship established in the nurse-client contract or negotiated in accordance with the limits of the contract. Ending a relationship can cause anxiety in both the client and the nurse.[47] Because termination represents a loss, it can trigger feelings of sadness, frustration, and anger. It is the loss of a relationship and the loss of future involvement, with attendant realistic expectations or fantasies. Termination also reawakens feelings of past unresolved losses, such as a death or divorce.

It is important that the client work through any feelings related to the termination. The client requires the nurse's assistance to experience the feelings of loss and to connect present reactions to past real or symbolic losses. Other important interventions follow:

1. Let the client know why the relationship is to be terminated.
2. Remind the client of the date and how many meetings are left during the latter period of the relationship.
3. Collaborate with other staff so that they are aware of how the client is reacting and any special needs the client may have at this time.
4. Assist the client to identify other people with whom it is possible to have a relationship.
5. Review the gains and the goals that remain.
6. Discuss the pros and cons experienced during the relationship to help the client develop a realistic appraisal.
7. Make any referrals for follow-up care.

Both nurse and client can learn much during termination. The process directs both to examine problems and progress in the relationship, as well as feelings and reactions. Termination experience also helps the nurse and client gain practice in ending relationships and in exploring reactions, which can be most helpful when future losses occur.

SUMMARY

Working with clients offers many challenges and rewards to the nurse. Although some aspects of this work are predictable, each client is unique and provides a chance for the nurse to learn, grow, and help in new ways. This chapter provides guidelines for developing therapeutic relationships but does not guarantee success or an easy job. It is the desire and skill of the individual nurse that bring this information to life. The blend of the nurse's artistry, humanity, knowledge, skill, and ethics sparks concern and the ability to help another human being to communicate effectively.

The nurse-client relationship is the primary arena for health promotion. Values clarification, communication, and the helping relationship are its core components. It is useful to consider how nurses can apply this knowledge to their role beyond the confines of individual nurse-client encounters. To promote real change in health and health care, nurses can focus on their value of caring, communicate their worth and the importance of their work to others, and nurture their professional nurse-nurse relationships. Suzanne Gordon, a journalist who has observed the world of nursing, provides the following analysis and challenge:

> Today, nurses continue to deliver essential care and are helping to transform the entire health-care system. And yet, their work goes largely unacknowledged. In a world transformed by women's liberation, nurses' innovations in care and their experiments in understanding the nature of cooperation and collaboration are some of the best kept secrets of the gender revolution. . . . To create this new health-care system, nurses need to be far less humble and far more assertive in promoting their profession and its achievements. For this to succeed, however, they need advocates and allies – among patients, families, politicians, business people, and journalists – who understand that quality health care is dependent not only on heroic intervention and the promise of cure, but also on the efforts of hundreds of thousands of women and men who provide the care without which the cure would be impossible.[15]

References

1. Benoliel JQ: Ethics in nursing practice and education, *Nurs Outlook* 31(4):210, 1983.
2. Blondis MN, Jackson BE: *Nonverbal communication with patients: back to the human touch,* ed 2, New York, 1982, John Wiley & Sons.
3. Burd S, Marshall M: *Some clinical approaches to psychiatric nursing,* New York, 1963, Macmillan.
4. Campbell J: The relationship of nursing and self-awareness, *Adv Nurs Sci* 2(4):15, 1980.
5. Carter FM: *Psychosocial nursing: theory and practice in hospital and community,* New York, 1976, Macmillan.
6. Chomsky N: *Syntactic structures,* The Hague, 1957, Mouton.
7. Cleary PD, et al: Patients evaluate their hospital care: a national survey, *Health Affairs,* Winter:264, 1991.
8. Clement J: The helping relationship: choices and dilemmas, *Iss Ment Health Nurs* 1(4):17, 1978.
9. Cooper J: Actions really do speak louder than words, *Nursing* 9(4):113, 1979.
10. Coopersmith S: *The antecedents of self-esteem,* San Francisco, 1967, WH Freeman.
11. Davis AJ: The skills of communication, *Am J Nurs* 63:66, 1963.
12. Ehmann VE: Empathy: its origin, characteristics, and process, *Perspect Psychiatr Care* 9(2):72, 1972.
13. Frasure-Smith N, Prince R: Long-term follow-up of the ischemic heart disease life stress monitoring program, *Psychosomatic Med* 51:508, 1989.
14. Friedman MM: *Family nursing: theory and practice,* Norwalk, Conn, 1992, Appleton-Lange.
15. Gordon S: What nurses know, *Mother Jones* 17(5):46, 1992.
16. Haber J, et al: *Comprehensive psychiatric nursing,* ed 4, St Louis, 1992, Mosby.
17. Hall E: *The silent language,* Garden City, NY, 1973, Doubleday/Anchor Press.
18. Horowitz JA: *Human growth and development across the life span.* In Wilson HS, Kneisl CR, editors: *Psychiatric nursing,* ed 3, Menlo Park, Calif, 1988, Addison-Wesley.
19. Horowitz JA, Hughes CB, Perdue BJ: *Parenting reassessed: a nursing perspective,* Englewood Cliffs, NJ, 1982, Prentice Hall.
20. Joel LA: *A psychosocial perspective on parenting.* In Horowitz JA, Hughes CB, Perdue BJ: *Parenting reassessed: a nursing perspective,* Englewood Cliffs, NJ, 1982, Prentice Hall.
21. Jourard S: *The transparent self,* rev ed, New York, 1971, Van Nostrand Reinhold.
22. Kasch CR: Toward a theory of nursing action: skills and competency in nurse-patient interactions, *Nurs Res* 35:226, 1986.
23. King M, Novik L, Citrenbaum C: *Irresistible communication: creative skills for the health professional,* Philadelphia, 1983, WB Saunders.
24. Kneisl CR, Wilson HS: *The psychiatric nurse and the interdisciplinary mental health team: personal integration and professional role.* In Wilson HS, Kneisl CR, editors: *Psychiatric nursing,* ed 4, Redwood City, Calif, 1992, Addison-Wesley.
25. Lindsay PH, Norman DA: *Human information processing: an introduction to psychology,* ed 2, New York, 1977, Academic Press.
26. Litwick L, Litwick J, Ballou M: *Health counseling,* New York, 1980, Appleton-Century-Crofts.
27. Luft J: *Group processes: an introduction to group dynamics,* ed 3, Palo Alto, Calif, 1984, Mayfield.
28. Luft J: *Of human interaction,* Palo Alto, Calif, 1969, National Press Books.
29. McFarland GF, Naschinski CE: *Impaired verbal communication.* In Thompson JM, et al, editors: *Mosby's manual of clinical nursing,* ed 2, St Louis, 1989, Mosby.
30. McFarland GK, Naschinski CE: Impaired communication: a descriptive study, *Nurs Clin North Am* 20:775-785, 1985.
31. Murray RB, Huelskoetter MM: *Psychiatric/mental health nursing: giving emotional care,* ed 3, Norwalk, Conn, 1991, Appleton-Lange.
32. Murray RB, Zentner JP: *Nursing assessment and health promotion: strategies through the life span,* ed 5, Norwalk, Conn, 1993, Appleton-Lange.
33. Parad H, Caplan G: *A framework for studying families in crisis.* In Parad H, editor: *Crisis intervention: selected readings,* New York, 1965, Family Service Association of America.
34. Patterson GR: *The aggressive child: victim and architect of a coercive system.* In Mash EI, Handy LC, Hamerlynck A, editors: *Behavior modification and families. 1. Theory and research,* New York, 1976, Brunner/Mazel.
35. Pendagast E, Sherman C: A guide to the genogram family systems training, *Family* 5(1):3, 1977.
36. Peplau HE: *Basic principles of patient counseling,* ed 2, Philadelphia, 1964, Smith Kline and French Laboratories.
37. Peplau HE: *Interpersonal relations in nursing,* New York, 1991, Springer.
38. Peplau HE: *Process and concept of learning.* In Burd S, Marshall M, editors: *Some clinical approaches to psychiatric nursing,* New York, 1963, Macmillan.
39. Peplau HE: Professional closeness: as a special kind of involvement with a patient, client, or family group, *Nurs Forum* 8:342, 1969.
40. Peplau HE: Talking with patients, *Am J Nurs* 60(7):964, 1960.
41. Raths L, Harmin M, Simon S: *Values and teaching,* Columbus, Ohio, 1978, Charles E Merrill Publishing.
42. Rogers C: *Client-centered therapy,* Boston, 1965, Houghton Mifflin.
43. Ruesch J, Bateson G: *Communication: the social matrix of psychiatry,* New York, 1987, WW Norton.
44. Ryden MB: An approach to ethical decision-making, *Nurs Outlook* 26:705, 1978.
45. Satir V: *Conjoint family therapy,* ed 3, Palo Alto, Calif, 1983, Science and Behavior Books.
46. Sears RR: Relation of early socialization experience to self-concepts and gender role in middle childhood, *Child Dev* 41:267, 1970.
47. Sene BS: "Termination" in the student-patient relationship, *Perspect Psychiatr Care* 7(1):39, 1969.
48. Singer E: *Key concepts in psychotherapy,* ed 2, New York, 1970, Basic Books.
49. Stacklum M: New student in psychology, *Am J Nurs* 81:762, 1981.
50. Stuart GW, Sundeen SJ: *Principles and practice of psychiatric nursing,* ed 4, St Louis, 1991, Mosby.
51. Sullivan HS: *The interpersonal theory of psychiatry,* New York, 1953, WW Norton.
52. Sundeen SJ, et al: *Nurse-client interaction: implementing the nursing process,* ed 4, St Louis, 1989, Mosby.
53. Uustal D: Values clarification in nursing: application to practice, *Am J Nurs* 78:2058, 1978.
54. Watzlawick P, Beavin JH, Jackson DD: *Pragmatics of human communication: a study of interactional patterns, pathologies and paradoxes,* New York, 1967, WW Norton.
55. *Webster's ninth new collegiate dictionary,* Springfield, Mass, 1983, Merriam-Webster.
56. Wilson HS, Kneisl CR: *Psychiatric nursing,* ed 4, Redwood City, Calif, 1992, Addison-Wesley.
57. Young D, Friedman M: *Family communication patterns.* In Friedman M: *Family nursing: theory and assessment,* New York, 1986, Appleton-Century-Crofts.

CHAPTER

6

Ethical Issues Relevant to Health Promotion

Carol Lynn Mandle

Philip Boyle

James A. O'Donohoe

Objectives

After completing this chapter, the nurse will be able to

- *Describe ethics as "humanizing," that is, pertaining to the development of the whole person.*
- *Contrast philosophic to theologic ethics.*
- *Describe the relationship of norm to value.*
- *Describe three traditional theoretic approaches in philosophic ethics: egoism, Kantianism, and utilitarianism.*
- *Describe three traditional theoretic approaches in theologic ethics: Jewish, Catholic, and Protestant.*
- *Describe three contemporary theoretic approaches in philosophic ethics: Frankena's theory of obligation, Firth's ideal observer theology, and Rawls's justice as fairness.*
- *Define the nature of the discipline of health care ethics today.*
- *Describe the role and limitations of professional codes of ethics in nursing today.*
- *Identify the principles of ethics stressed in professional codes of ethics for nursing today.*
- *Contrast the influences of ethics versus laws in the nursing profession and health promotion today.*
- *Discuss factors to consider in moral decision making.*
- *Describe key components in the ethical positions confronting the following ethical dilemmas within health promotion: research, stewardship over one's own health, contraception, abortion, genetic therapy, and reproductive technology.*
- *Delineate a method for analyzing ethical dilemmas in health promotion.*
- *Discuss paradigmatic cases of ethical dilemmas in health promotion.*

The previous chapters have examined the biologic, psychosocial, economic, philosophic, and theologic dimensions of keeping healthy. In this chapter the ethical dimensions of these important issues are discussed. Since there are many misunderstandings about the discipline of ethics, before some major ethical issues of interest to healthy people are examined, it is necessary to describe basic ethical notions, before presenting a discussion on the specific questions of health care ethics. In addition, fundamental notions on the nature and techniques of ethical decision making must be set forth. Then specific ethical issues of interest to healthy people can be considered.

TOWARD AN UNDERSTANDING OF ETHICS

The Nature of Ethics

As indicated, many persons do not properly understand the discipline of ethics. They tend to think of it as something repressive and suppressive, if not destructive, of the growth and development of the person. This was well expressed recently by a contemporary student who advised a friend about to enter college: "Keep away from the study of ethics; it declares that everything you would like to do is illegal, immoral, or bad for your health."

Nothing could be further from the truth; ethics is concerned with the humanization process. It proclaims its share of "oughts" and "ought nots"; but this is done so that men and women can become what they are destined to be: fully developed and mature human beings.

Throughout the centuries many definitions of ethics have been proposed. For some persons ethics is an attempt to discover the behavioral implications of being human. For others it is a study of the origins and nature of those "oughts" and "ought nots" that constitute the pursuit of what the classic authors called the *verum humanum,* "that which embodies total humanization." Above all, ethics is a search for what shapes the human being, for what contributes to the growth and development of the person. It is an attempt to discover all those elements that are required to make and keep life human so that a person may achieve the goals of the humanization process and thus live as properly and well as possible.[47,67]

The word *ethics* is derived from the Greek *ethos,* "the customary way of acting," or the manner of action that contributes to the growth of the human person. It is interesting to observe that in its very primitive sense the Greek word referred to a stall in which animals were kept. By means of this stall and the protection it guaranteed, the animal placed in it would be in a position to become as perfectly as possible what it was destined to be, despite, or possibly as a result of the stall's confinement.

Often the word *morality* is used as a substitute for ethics. Morality is merely a synonym for ethics. It is derived from the Latin *mosmoris,* which also signifies "the customary way of acting," in the sense of that which "customarily" brings about true humanization. The term *moral ethics* is thus redundant and should not be used. A person engaged in the study of how human beings should act is involved in the study of "ethics," if one employs the Greek root, or in the study of "morality," if one uses the Latin root.

Relationship between the "Is" and the "Ought"

The study of ethics is concerned with the discovery of humanizing "oughts" and the discouragement of dehumanizing "ought nots." Where are these to be found? Most traditional forms of thinking have always located the "ought" in the "is"; what the person ought to do is always rooted in what the person actually is. An automobile, precisely because of what it *is, ought* to be able to transport its owner; a power mower *ought* to be able to cut grass. One cannot expect the car to cut the lawn or the power mower to be a means of transportation. What these machines *ought* to do is very much related to what each *is.*

Ethics is not concerned with any type of oughts; it is concerned solely with *humanizing oughts.* To do this effectively, ethics must begin with a consideration of what constitutes the human being, what the person *is.* In other words, every system of ethics articulates its oughts in the light of and as a consequence of the manner in which it conceives the essence of the human person. Every ethical system proceeds from and is rooted in a basic *anthropology,* an understanding of what constitutes the human being. A system's anthropology constitutes the point of departure for the formulation of its ethics.

In a pluralist society like our's, we meet a considerable number of ethical systems, many of which differ radically from the others. One group favors abortion as a practical and humanizing solution for an unwanted pregnancy, and another classifies such an action as the direct taking of an innocent life. One group favors euthanasia for those with terminal illnesses; another denounces such an action as the unjust taking of human life. One group suggests artificial insemination from a donor as a humanizing solution to the problem of sterility; another sees it as totally dehumanizing because it is contrary to the meaning of coitus, an act of love between husband and wife. Differing solutions to human problems are rooted in differing understandings of what constitutes the human person. Every ethical system that articulates humanizing oughts and dehumanizing ought nots finds the source of its teaching in a specific understanding of what shapes that elusive entity known as *human nature.*

Types of Ethics

As stated, all systems of ethics are rooted in a specific anthropology. The "oughts" and "ought nots" that they set forth find their origin in a specific understanding of human nature. Thus the source of such understandings must now be sought by seeking the answer to a specific question: "Where can human beings discover the elements that constitute their nature?" To answer that question, the distinction between philosophic and theologic ethics must be made.

Philosophic ethics grounds its comprehension of human nature in human reason. It tries to formulate an understanding of human nature by means of a rational and comprehensive examination of these elements that distinguish members of the human race from animals and other forms of subhuman existence. It proceeds from the premise that all things fundamentally reasonable contribute to the humanizing process. Stating that the use of reason distinguishes human beings from all other creatures, this form of ethics teaches that, if properly applied, human reason can determine those elements essential to the growth and development of the person. To accomplish this task in a competent manner, philosophic ethics employs a variety of auxiliary science, such as psychology and sociology.

Theologic ethics also bases its comprehension of human nature in the use of reason. However, it does so by using human reason as enlightened by means of a religious faith, or affirmative acceptance of a divine revelation, which in turn is a sort of divine "breakthrough." By means of this revelation, God communicates some knowledge of the divine nature and that of the human beings God has created. For those unfamiliar with theology, it is important to point out that the knowledge about God or God's people God communicates is in no way contrary to human reason but rather supplements it. Theologic ethics therefore attempts to articulate the ethical implications of being a believer: one who accepts and takes to heart the revelatory communications made by a gracious God. Such systems include Muslim ethics, Jewish ethics, and Christian ethics, which has been subdivided into Catholic and Reformed (Protestant) ethics at least since the 15th century.

Even though one can distinguish in theory between philosophic and theologic ethics, it is important to remember that theology cannot be separated from philosophy. Theologic ethics is not merely a system of pious platitudes devoid of rational foundation, but a science that attempts an accurate articulation of a religious faith by using other sciences, such as philosophy, psychology, sociology, cultural anthropology, reproductive physiology, and history.

Elements of Ethics

According to Dyck, "Ethics as a discipline . . . is a systematic analysis of what things are right or wrong, good or bad, virtuous or evil (normative ethics); of what is meant or conveyed by these moral terms to see whether or to what extent judgments involving them can or cannot be rationally justified (metaethics); and of specific moral decisions and policies, and what ethics can contribute to such decisions and policies (moral policy)."[27]

Ethics is thus a normative science. Unlike sociology, it is not merely content to observe what human beings are doing; it is especially concerned with what human beings ought or ought not to be doing. In other words, ethics lays down certain *norms* that are to be followed if the humanization process is to be accomplished; it is concerned with precepts, rules and regulations, principles, and guidelines. Ethics tries to answer the question, "What ought I do and what should I avoid if I am to become a mature human being?" As a normative discipline, ethics tries to point out what human beings ought to do or refrain from doing if they are to achieve the *verum humanum*.

Ethics is also concerned with *metaethics*. It is not merely content to lay down the "what" in regard to human activity; it also attempts to articulate the "why" behind the what. Ethics tries to show why we need norms, how they should be formulated, and the type of language that should be employed in their formulation. It also endeavors to point up the specific value that underlies the norm. Any humanizing good is called a value; the norm's function is to indicate how to achieve the particular good. Norms are rooted in and depend on values. As insights into values change, norms must be modified accordingly. As a metaethical discipline, ethics does not merely articulate norms to achieve humanization; it also explores why. As Ladd writes, "Metaethics encompasses three broad categories of questions. The first . . . concerns the connection between morality and conduct; . . . the second . . . concerns the connection between beliefs about right and wrong and facts about the real world; . . . the third . . . concerns the logical relationship between the ethical propositions of various degrees of generality, for example, all embracing super principles . . ., moral rules and practices, and individual, here-and-now moral decisions."[47]

As a discipline ethics does not stop at setting forth "whats" and "whys"; it also attempts to respond to "how." How should the person act if he or she is to respond to the proposed norms and the justification for them? It is the function of ethics to attempt an answer to the following question: "How can I, as the person I am and existing in these specific circumstances, best achieve the purpose for which the norm was set forth?" Besides knowing the norm or appreciating the reasons governing its formulation, the ethical person must also be able to choose the method to use in each existential situation.

In the past many believed the work of ethics was done whenever norms were set forth. Today persons are becoming more and more conscious of the added need to be conscious of values and able to formulate an ethical strategy or policy. Just as the metaethical and strategy questions of ethics were neglected in the past, the renewed emphasis on them today may lead to a neglect of the normative question. It is very difficult to keep these three questions in proper focus, but it must never be forgotten that ethics is not merely about norms, metaethics, and strategy taken singly. All three elements are correlated and therefore must be seen as essential elements in the study of ethics as a discipline.

Ethical Theory

Ethical theory refers to a workable system that provides a proper framework within which a person can determine and distinguish morally appropriate actions. How can a person discover how to act in the light of the existential situation? Should one look merely to the rule, or should one also look to the consequences that can result from keeping or even breaking the rule?

Most ethical textbooks distinguish two types of ethical theory: deontology and teleology. Two things should be noted: (1) the deontology-teleology dichotomy was formally introduced into the study of ethics only 50 or 60 years ago; and (2) the terms are often used in different senses by different authors. Some ethicists employ them as mutually exclusive, while others see them as overlapping in many instances if not at least complementary in most instances.

Deontology, or formalism, as it is often called, is more concerned with what the act to be performed *is* rather than what it *does*. Its basic premise is that the moral act does not depend entirely on the consequences of the act; there are duties or obligations affecting actions that have ethical validity independent of the consequences. Some deontologists admit that the rightness or wrongness of some actions under certain conditions can be determined by some consideration of their consequence, but they are adamant in maintaining that there are certain actions that are "intrinsically evil" – actions always wrong no matter what the consequences or circumstances.[7]

At present most authors would distinguish four principal paradigms in deontology: (1) the Judeo-Christian, (2) the Kantian, (3) the Oxford Intuitionist, and (4) the contemporary version of the contract theory, as formulated by John Rawls.

In the *Judeo-Christian* model the moral life is seen as consisting in total obedience to the plan of God, as made manifest through revelation or through the positive legislation enacted by the faith community. As a consequence, it holds that certain absolute prohibitions exist that the moral person will never contravene no matter what the consequences. This position is evidenced in the writings of the so-called classic Roman Catholic moral theologians, who taught that actions such as direct abortion, direct contraception, direct killing, and active euthanasia could never be permitted despite the consequences. In the case of actions forbidden but not "intrinsically evil," these same authors teach that some exceptions are permitted through a careful application of the *principle of the double effect*. This asserts that we may never purposefully do evil, even for a good reason, but may for a proportionate reason; it permits unintended evil consequences that might flow from a good action. It is based on many actions having two effects – one good and the other evil – and on a significant difference existing between doing evil and permitting it as a side effect of a good action. Traditionally, the principle is described as follows: it is licit to posit an action which has two foreseen effects, one good and the other bad, if four conditions are verified all at the same time: (1) if the action taken in itself is good or at least morally indifferent, (2) if the good effect is not produced by means of the bad effect, (3) if only the good effect is directly intended, and (4) if there is a proportionate reason for placing the action and permitting the bad effect. Thus a hysterectomy on a pregnant woman who has developed cancer of the cervix would be considered an indirect abortion and hence licit (the expulsion of the nonviable fetus is a side effect of the life-saving procedure), whereas the taking of a nonviable fetus from a woman who has developed renal toxemia would be considered a direct abortion and hence illicit (the saving of the woman's life would be a side effect of the direct taking of the nonviable fetus).

In the *Kantian* system,[27] the morally upright person is always prepared to do whatever moral duty requires. It teaches that all persons are subject to a "categorical imperative," which is based solely on the formal nature of the law and which unconditionally requires every rational being to act only on maxims regarded as universal laws of nature. It requires that these maxims be followed no matter what the consequences of the act. In other words this system sees all moral imperatives as unconditional and admits to no exceptions.

The *Oxford Intuitionists*[27] seem to hold on to the intrinsicalism of the deontologists but shy away from their absolutism. They hold that the determination of the moral rightness or wrongness of a specific act depends on its intrinsic nature. However, they believe that the consequences of the act are always, but not totally, relevant to its rightness. An act is morally correct if its right-making properties outweigh its wrong-making ones.

Rawls would retain the intrinsicalism common to the Intuitionists, but he stresses the values that arise from a satisfaction of the proper conditions of human association, such as freedom, autonomy, human rights, dignity, self-respect, and the just distribution of jointly produced primary goods.[66]

Before considering teleology, it should be mentioned that a fairly sizeable group of contemporary Roman Catholic moral theologians are introducing some modifications of the system proposed by the classic moral theologians. The theory they propose has been given different names by different authors, but it is commonly referred to as "mixed consequentialism," "an ethic of proportionality," or "an ethic of relationality and proportionality." These theories center around the denial that any action can be intrinsically evil apart from any consideration of consequences and circumstances.[41] In determining the morality of any action, consequences must be given due consideration without giving them the entire and sole consideration. These moral theologians evaluate consequences in terms of needs and purposes to be established, not by the subjective preference of the moral agent (subjectivism) or merely abstract laws (legalism), but by the nature of the human person considered within the dimensions and implications of individual and communal attributes.

Teleology, or consequentialism as it is sometimes called, is an ethical theory that is more concerned with what the act *does* than with what the act *is*. It maintains that no action as such can be termed intrinsically evil; the principal determinant of the morality of any act is its *consequences*. The morally good action is one that produces the best consequences, either for the moral agent or for human society.

Teleology manifests itself today in various forms, such as ethical *hedonism* (only the moral agent's good is to be considered), ethical *elitism* (only the good of those most gifted in society is to be considered), ethical *parochialism* (only the good of the moral agent's appropriate in-group should be taken into consideration), and ethical *universalism* (the good of all humankind is to be taken into consideration).

The most common and most widely championed teleologic theory is *utilitarianism,* which holds that established rules are "useful rules of thumb" but not unbreakable and exceptionless prescriptions. Its foundation is the *principle of utility,* which teaches that in all circumstances the greatest possible balance of value over disvalue for all persons affected must be sought. It is based on an evaluative calculus, that would enable one to conduct one's moral life in a rational manner comparable to that of the efficient businessperson. Just as this person maximizes profits, so the moral person maximizes the net balance of good over bad, pleasure over pain, and happiness over unhappiness. The single, exceptionless principle for the utilitarian is that the right action is the one that, by means of empirical calculation, produces the greatest amount of good for the greatest number.

A perusal of contemporary ethical literature shows that utilitarians make a distinction between *rule* utilitarianism and *act* utilitarianism. In the act form, the rightness of an act is determined by its conformity with all the compulsory social rules that pass the test of utility. In the rule type, the only right-making property is "optimificity": the act has consequences at least as good as those of any other alternate acts open to the agent. Rule is less radical than act utilitarianism and most likely originated to defend utilitarianism against the objection that it pays no attention to moral principles and rules. For that reason it maintains that the correct act is prescribed by a set of rules whose general acceptance in society will produce more utility than the acceptance of any other set of rules.

Closely allied to utilitarianism is the so-called situation ethics. This system is motivated by concern for human well-being, decisionally flexible in its method, and guided in its judgments by the greatest good realizable rather than by adherence to prefabricated norms or moral rules. It weighs each case on its own merits, clinically and consequentially. For many who profess this method of moral discourse, there is only one serious ethical question: "What is the best thing to do in this case, for this particular person, and for this particular ethical dilemma?"

TOWARD AN UNDERSTANDING OF HEALTH CARE ETHICS

The Nature of the Discipline

As in other areas of life, the principles and theories of ethics just mentioned are applied to the human relationships of health care to provide ways by which persons can systematically reason through ethical issues and dilemmas. Davis and Aroskar[20] state, "Health care ethics, sometimes also called medical ethics, biomedical ethics, and bioethics, is normative ethics specific to the health science in that it raises the questions of what is right or what ought to be done in a health science situation that calls for a moral decision." They believe health care ethics addresses four interrelated areas: clinical, allocation of scarce resources, human experimentations, and health policy.

The recent increases in knowledge and their applications in technologies have increased the complexities of the ethical issues and dilemmas within each of these areas. Consequently, individuals, both clinicians and clients, potentially have great power over the quantity and quality of human life. "Health care ethics does not promote a particular moral lifestyle, nor does it campaign for particular life values. Its role has been defined as functioning to sensitize or raise the consciousness of health professionals (and the lay public) concerning ethical issues found in health care settings and policies; and to structure the issues so that ethically relevant trends of complex situations can be drawn out."[11,20]

Based on the holistic perspective of the person, nursing requires its members to consider the wholeness of each patient, as well as themselves, in ascribing to particular theories of ethics. To be a nurse requires the willing assumption of ethical responsibility in every dimension of practice. A nurse cannot act morally unless he or she has developed a strong moral self and constructed a moral system that supports each act.[32,59,80]

In making each decision, one is deciding, determining, what type of person one is and wants to become. All nursing judgments are therefore also ethical judgments; no dichotomy exists between nursing or clinical judgments and decisions and ethical decisions. Every nursing decision is either an ethical nursing decision or an unethical one. The nurse, or anyone, first needs a sensitivity to and an ability to recognize the presence of ethical issues.[49]

In addition to personal values and beliefs, the nurse's development of a moral self is influenced by the ethics of the profession. What is a good nurse? How should a good nurse interact? What supports a nurse to do what ought to be done? Perhaps the single greatest cause for confusion, stress, and misunderstanding in nursing today is an inadequate definition of the nursing role, particularly the meaning of professionalism in nursing. What are the roles, rights, and responsibilities of patients? Of nurses? Of other health care providers and agency administrators? The patient, the nurse, the physician, and the administrator are all human beings with relatively unique roles and concurrent, often undefined, but frequently overlapping rights and responsibilities that demand mutual knowledge and respect. Informal and formal professional ethics provide some assistance in addressing these questions.[43,50,56]

Professional Oaths and Codes of Ethics

Informal professional ethics are not readily reduced to writing. They are acquired by the nurse through socialization. The content of *ad hoc,* clinical advice from superiors, as well as from peers, contains these covert messages of what is right and what is wrong to do in particular situations.

The other classification is *formal* professional ethics, as represented in writings, usually by health care organizations and frequently in the format of codes. The purpose of ethical codes is to provide a framework for each nurse to generate personal ethical decisions, but within the guidelines of the profession. Professional codes indicate a profession's acceptance of the responsibility and trust invested to it by society. On entering a profession, each person inherits this responsibility and trust. The ethical codes of a profession therefore provide a primary means for the exercise of self-regulation by the profession and each professional in it.

Increasingly, the primary relationship of the nurse is defined to be to his or her client.[3] Historically this responsibility has not been clear and frequently has been quite different. The nurse has been responsible to the church, the administration of the health care agency, other health care providers (especially physicians), and the socially selected member(s) of the client's family. This multiplication of responsibilities has presented ethical dilemmas to the nurse because of the conflicting demands of who should be the decision makers.[21,48]

These multiple perspectives of responsibilities are particularly evident in the *Florence Nightingale Pledge.* This oath was constructed in 1863 by a committee appointed by the Farr Training School of Harper Hospital in Detroit (see the box to the right).

Before the industrialization of the 19th century, nursing was primarily practiced within religious communities. In this context, the ethics of the particular denomination guided the ministrations of the nurses. With the social changes of industrialization in England, nurses came from more varied backgrounds and manifested a wider range of beliefs and abilities; many were even of marginal social development and character. Nightingale organized and developed nurses during the Crimean War. Her ideals are reflected in this pledge, which has been taken by nurses throughout the world.

The *Code for Nurses* (see box on p. 127), adopted by the American Nurses' Association in 1950, has been revised many times, most recently in 1985. This revision, less prescriptive than previous revisions, relies more on the individual nurse's accountability to the client, whose right of self-determination is affirmed.[1]

In addition, in 1953 the International Council of Nurses' (ICN) *Code – Ethical Concepts Applied to Nursing* – (see box on p. 128) was developed and accepted. It was revised in 1965 and 1973. Its extraordinary challenge has been to provide guidelines that can be applied to all cultures and to the various developmental stages of nursing in countries throughout the world.

Both codes are accompanied by interpretive statements that further explain and illustrate their intent. The welfare of the recipient of nursing care is emphasized in both, demonstrating that they are codes of ethics rather than the codes of professional etiquette that exist for some other professions.

In addition, other ethical guidelines address more specific nursing concerns, such as research, particular populations, and health care agencies. The American Nurses' Association's *Human Rights Guidelines for Nurses in Clinical and Other Research*[2] exemplifies the profession's concerns about those who participate in scientific investigations or whose care is impinged on by such research.

❑ ❑ FLORENCE NIGHTINGALE PLEDGE FOR NURSES

I solemnly pledge myself before God and in the presence of this assembly to pass my life in purity and to practice my profession faithfully.

I will abstain from whatever is deleterious and mischievous, and will not take or knowingly administer any harmful drug.

I will do all in my power to elevate the standard of my profession, and will hold in confidence all personal matters committed to my keeping, and all family affairs coming to my knowledge in the practice of my calling.

With loyalty will I endeavor to aid the physician in his work, and devote myself to the welfare of those committed to my care.

❑ ❑ AMERICAN NURSES' ASSOCIATION CODE FOR NURSES

1. The nurse provides services with respect for human dignity and the uniqueness of the client unrestricted by considerations of social or economic status, personal attributes, or the nature of health problems.
2. The nurse safeguards the client's right to privacy by judiciously protecting information of a confidential nature.
3. The nurse acts to safeguard the client and the public when health care and safety are affected by the incompetent, unethical, or illegal practices of any person.
4. The nurse assumes responsibility and accountability for individual nursing judgments and actions.
5. The nurse maintains competence in nursing.
6. The nurse exercises informed judgment and uses individual competence and qualifications as criteria in seeking consultation, accepting responsibilities, and delegating nursing activities to others.
7. The nurse participates in activities that contribute to the ongoing development of the professional's body of knowledge.
8. The nurse participates in the profession's efforts to implement and improve standards of nursing.
9. The nurse participates in the profession's efforts to establish and maintain conditions of employment conducive to high quality nursing care.
10. The nurse participates in the profession's efforts to protect the public from misinformation and misrepresentation and to maintain the integrity of nursing.
11. The nurse collaborates with members of the health professions and other citizens in promoting community and national efforts to meet the health needs of the public.

American Nurses' Association: ANA Publication Code No G-56 42M 11/86R, Kansas City, Mo, 1985.

Ethical Principles Currently Stressed

Beaucamp and Childress[10] believe that moral principles govern laws of conduct, as codes of conduct by which one directs one's life or actions or as generalizations that provide a basis for reasoning. Moral principles are statements that convey a directive or prescriptive force, an internal suggestion that the person uses in guiding behavior.

Rawls[67] has developed five criteria for moral principles: generality, universality, publicity, imposition of an order, and finality. *General* (versus particular) descriptions of the properties and relations of principles are preferred. *Universality* refers to the application of principles to all people. *Publicity* of principles is needed to ensure their public acknowledgment and acceptance by a society. The principle, according to Rawls, also should impose an *order* on conflicting claims between persons. *Finality* holds that the reasoning processes from such principles is conclusive in moral decision making.

Meeting these criteria, Davis and Aroskar[20] suggest principles that nurses can effectively apply to identified ethical issues and dilemmas in direct client care and health policy-making levels: principles of respect for persons, of beneficence, and of justice. The principle of respect for persons includes not only autonomy and self-determination of the individual, but recognition that the individual is a member of the human community. This adds the dimensions of duties and obligations to others, as well as to one's self in making moral judgments.[57] Dworkin[27] defines self-determination as an individual's exercise of the capacity to form, revise, and pursue personal plans for life.

Bok[12] identifies two ways to interfere with legitimate, autonomous choices by patients. These are overt coercion and deception. She defines deception as manipulating the information reaching patients so that they accept what they would not have chosen had they been correctly informed.

The two principles of doing good and of not doing harm – beneficence and nonmaleficence – are particularly relevant in caring for healthy people. These are best developed by Frankena,[36] who has defined four components: (1) one ought not to inflict evil or harm; (2) one ought to prevent evil or harm; (3) one ought to remove evil; and (4) one ought to do or promote good to or for anyone. The duty not to inflict evil or harm takes priority over the other components.

Role of Justice and Rights

Many different perspectives on justice are found in our society in general and especially in nursing care today. One particularly strong current concern is delivering care in a just manner. At present, health care is distributed according to the client's and third-party's ability to pay. Rawls's principle of justice as fairness provides assistance in developing a more just allocation of resources. Fairness is based on the perspective of the needs of the least advantaged in society: "Each person participating in a practice or affected by it, has an equal right to the most extensive liberty compatible with like liberty for all."[66]

The concepts of rights are used in many different ways in our society. Currently the word "rights" is so overused that it is misused. Rights are most effectively understood as rationally demonstrable claims enabling a person to have access to all those things necessary to achieve development as a person. Rights are rooted in needs: biologic (needs for bodily existence and sustenance), psychosocial (needs for love, affection, respect), ethical (needs for insights into right and wrong), and spiritual (needs flowing from the soul).

The papal encyclic *Pacem in terris*[37] – a document issued by the Roman Catholic church – describes four kinds of

INTERNATIONAL COUNCIL OF NURSES' CODE—ETHICAL CONCEPTS APPLIED TO NURSING

The fundamental responsibility of the nurse is fourfold: to promote health, to prevent illness, to restore health, and to alleviate suffering.

The need for nursing is universal. Inherent in nursing is respect of life, dignity, and rights of man. It is unrestricted by considerations of nationality, race, creed, color, age, sex, politics, or social status.

Nurses render health services to the individual, the family, and the community and coordinate their services with those of related groups.

Nurses and People

The nurse's primary responsibility is to those people who require nursing care.

The nurse, in providing care, promotes an environment in which the values, customs, and spiritual beliefs of the individual are respected.

The nurse holds in confidence personal information and uses judgment in sharing this information.

Nurses and Practice

The nurse carries personal responsibility for nursing responsibility for nursing practice and for maintaining competence by continual learning.

The nurse maintains the highest standards of nursing care possible within the reality of a specific situation.

The nurse uses judgment in relation to individual competence when accepting and delegating responsibilities.

Nurses and Practice—cont'd

The nurse when acting in a professional capacity should at all times maintain standards of personal conduct which reflect credit upon the profession.

Nurses and Society

The nurse shares with other citizens the responsibility for initiating and supporting action to meet the health and social needs of the public.

Nurses and Co-Workers

The nurse sustains a cooperative relationship with co-workers in nursing and other fields.

The nurse takes appropriate action to safeguard the individual when his care is endangered by a co-worker or any other person.

Nurses and the Profession

The nurse plays the major role in determining and implementing desirable standards of nursing practice and nursing education.

The nurse is active in developing a core of professional knowledge.

The nurse, acting through the professional organization, participates in establishing and maintaining equitable social and economic working conditions in nursing.

Adopted by the ICN Council of National Representatives, Mexico City, May 1973.

rights: moral (natural), legal (positive), human, and socioeconomic. *Moral* rights are natural rights that exist before and independent of social conventions or legal rules. A person has a moral right when he or she is guided by moral principles or the principles of an enlightened conscience.[36]

All human beings have the right to be shown respect for their persons and for their good reputation. They also have the right to be free in searching for truth, in expressing opinions, and in pursuing art. Moral rights also give the push the right to share in the benefits of culture, including education and truthful information about public events, and the right to privately and publicly worship God.

In contrast, *legal* or positive rights are either recognized, conferred, or protected by law or by some other social or political enactment. For example, the right to private property, even of productive goods, is an effective safeguard of the dignity of the human person.

Human rights are moral rights of fundamental importance, for example, to food, water, health care, and liberty. They are held equally by all human beings and are unconditional and unalterable. *Socioeconomic* rights are claims to have those processes, which are generally basic to the pursuit of human rights. They can include the right to free initiative in the economic field, the right to work, and the right to a proper wage.

Moral rights therefore are the source and basis of all rights: the right to life and to all the means necessary and suitable for its proper development. Some rights are basic because they are necessary for the development of the person. All rights, however, are inseparably connected in the person who is their subject, with respective duties or responsibilities. The right of every person to life, for example, is correlated with the duty to preserve it.

Clearly a person's right necessitates duties, responsibilities, and obligations of others to acknowledge and respect the right. Because of the social implications of right, societies frequently exercise control over them. It is one thing to have a right and another to be able to exercise it, since in certain situations conflicts in rights can arise (e.g., whenever the rights of one person clash with similar rights in another, especially when both have a legitimate claim on the same object). Such conflicts frequently occur in health care decisions. A person's right to freedom versus society's right to have someone immunized for the safety of others is an example of an ethical dilemma.

In our society, however, there is no legally recognized claim or right to health care. An individual may request care, but one has no legal right to health care, with the exception that certain states impose legal duties on physicians and hospitals to treat people in life-threatening emergencies. Affirmations to rights to health care are addressing moral rights and generally have no legal obligations or duties of others.

Relationship to Civil Law

Fenner[30] describes the evolution of contemporary law from two sources: legislation and judicial decision. Law enacted by legislative bodies (federal, state, local) is termed statutory. Law created by judicial decision is termed case or common law.

The purpose and function of statutory law is to maintain or promote the rights of the state to uphold the social order and to protect the rights of the individual. Law that deals with the protection of the rights of the individual is civil law. Violations of civil law are termed torts and include acts that harm the individual or the individual's property.

As citizens, nurses are subject to all of the laws of society. Nurses are also governed by laws specific to them. Nurse practice acts and the related rules and regulations, for examples, are the basis for providing nursing care.

There are statutes governing the practice of nursing within each state. These laws usually delineate minimal educational preparation to apply for registered nurse licensure and the scope and limitations of nursing practice standards and minimal continuing education. Increasingly, the various levels of nursing education and practice are differentiated.

Other laws also govern the practice of nursing. For example, in 1979 the legislature of the Commonwealth of Massachusetts enacted a patient's bill of rights, Chapter 214, into law. This legislation was supplemented into its current (1987) provisions (see box on pp. 130-131). In contrast to other codes of rights, this bill has the power of the law enforcing it.

Fenner[30] discusses four principles of law, that provide a base on which many of the processes of the legal system function. The fundamental principle on which all law is based is a concern for justice and fairness. It seeks to protect the rights of one party from infringement by the actions of another party. The characteristic of change is the second principle of law. As change occurs in society, change in the legal system is also necessary. The recent changes in laws created by the accumulation of health care knowledge and technology are effective examples. The third principle of law is that an action is judged on the basis of what a similarly trained and experienced, reasonable, and prudent person would do under similar circumstances. This has become an increasingly challenging principle for the nursing profession because of the evolving, multiple levels of nursing education and specialization of practice. The last principle of law is that each individual has rights and responsibilities. As discussed, the powers or privileges that each person possesses have attendant responsibilities.

Smith and Davis[75] describe four relationships between ethics and law. An individual's actions can be (1) ethical and legal, (2) unethical and illegal, (3) ethical and illegal, and (4) unethical and legal. The last two relationships present particularly perplexing situations for nurses.

The requirements of the professional codes of nursing often exceed, but are never less than, the requirements of the law. Punishments for violations of laws and codes, however, are quite different. Violations of the law can become civil or criminal liabilities and accordingly be punished. In contrast, professional associations may reprimand, censure, suspend, or expel a professional from membership. For both types of violations, the nurse loses the respect of the community, especially colleagues who share the obligation as peers adhering to legal and professional requirements. Familiarity with appropriate processes to fulfill ethical and legal requirements can enable the nurse to practice more effectively.

The dichotomy between codes and laws is becoming clouded in some states. In addition, conflicts and contradictions are developing between what the law states and what is regarded as good ethics. In Oregon, for example, the American Nurses' Association Code of Ethics has become incorporated into the State Nurse Practice Act, that is, law. In such situations the nurse who violates an article of the code can also lose the license to practice nursing, or worse. This becomes a difficult and controversial dilemma. When for example, in section 1.5 it is illegal for a nurse to refuse to advise a patient where a legally sanctioned but (in the nurse's opinion) unethical treatment, such as abortion, is available.

The nurse has an ethical and legal right, even in military service, of conscientious objection from participating in any procedure she considers morally objectionable. With this right, as with all rights, there are concomitant responsibilities. For example, during the hiring process the nurse has the responsibility to inform the potential employer of his or her conscientious moral objections to any moral issues, such as abortion. If, however, the nurse is unexpectedly confronted with the moral issue in any emergency situation, the nurse's responsibility is the patient's safety until he or she can withdraw from the care when alternate staff become available.

❑ ❑ MASSACHUSETTS PATIENTS' AND RESIDENTS' RIGHTS STATUTE MASSACHUSETTS GENERAL LAW, EXCERPTS FROM CHAPTER III

111:70E. Patients' and Residents' Rights.

Section 70E. As used in this section, "facility" shall mean any hospital, institution for the care of unwed mothers, clinic, infirmary maintained in a town, convalescent or nursing home, rest home, or charitable home for the aged, licensed or subject to licensing by the department; any state hospital operated by the department; any "facility" as defined in section three of chapter one hundred and eleven B; any private, county or municipal facility, department or ward which is licensed or subject to licensing by the department of mental health pursuant to section nineteen of chapter nineteen; or by the department of mental retardation pursuant to section fifteen of chapter nineteen B; any "facility" as defined in section one of chapter one hundred and twenty-three; the Soldiers Home in Holyoke, the Soldiers' Home in Massachusetts; and any facility set forth in section one of chapter nineteen or section one of chapter nineteen B.

The rights established under this section shall apply to every patient or resident in said facility. Every patient or resident shall receive written notice of the rights established herein upon admittance into such facility, except that if the patient is a member of a health maintenance organization and the facility is owned by or controlled by such organization, such notice shall be provided at the time of enrollment in such organization, and also upon admittance to said facility. In addition, such rights shall be conspicuously posted in said facility.

Every such patient or resident of said facility shall have, in addition to any other rights provided by law, the right to freedom of choice in his selection of a facility, or a physician or health service mode, except in the case of emergency medical treatment or as otherwise provided for by contract, or except in the case of a patient or resident of a facility named in section fourteen A of chapter nineteen; provided, however, that the physician, facility, or health service mode is able to accommodate the patient exercising such right of choice.

Every such patient or resident of said facility in which billing for service is applicable to such patient or resident, upon reasonable request, shall receive from a person designated by the facility an itemized bill reflecting laboratory charges, pharmaceutical charges, and third party credits and shall be allowed to examine an explanation of said bill regardless of the source of payment. This information shall also be made available to the patient's attending physician.

Every patient or resident of a facility shall have the right:

(a) upon request, to obtain from the facility in charge of his care the name and specialty, if any, of the physician or other person responsible for his care or the coordination of his care;

(b) to confidentiality of all records and communications to the extent provided by law;

(c) to have all reasonable requests responded to promptly and adequately within the capacity of the facility;

(d) upon request, to obtain an explanation as to the relationship, if any, of the facility to any other health care facility or educational institution insofar as said relationship relates to his care or treatment;

(e) to obtain from a person designated by the facility a copy of any rules or regulations of the facility which apply to his conduct as a patient or resident;

(f) upon request, to receive from a person designated by the facility any information which the facility has available relative to financial assistance and free health care;

(g) upon request, to inspect his medical records and to receive a copy thereof in accordance with section seventy, and the fee for said copy shall be determined by the rate of copying expenses;

(h) to refuse to be examined, observed, or treated by students or any other facility staff without jeopardizing access to psychiatric, psychological, or other medical care and attention;

(i) to refuse to serve as a research subject and to refuse any care or examination when the primary purpose is educational or informational rather than therapeutic;

(j) to privacy during medical treatment or other rendering of care within the capacity of the facility;

(k) to prompt life saving treatment in an emergency without discrimination on account of economic status or source of payment and without delaying treatment for purpose of prior discussion of the source of payment unless such delay can be imposed without material risk to his health, and this right shall also extend to those persons not already patients or residents of a facility if said facility has a certified emergency care unit;

(l) to informed consent to the extent provided by law;

(m) upon request to receive a copy of an itemized bill or other statement of charges submitted to any third party by the facility for care of the patient or resident and to have a copy of said itemized bill or statement sent to the attending physician of the patient or resident; and

(n) if refused treatment because of economic status or the lack of a source of payment, to prompt and safe transfer to a facility which agrees to receive and treat such patient. Said facility refusing to treat such patient shall be responsible for: ascertaining that the patient may be safely transferred; contacting a facility willing to treat such patient; arranging the transportation; accompanying the patient with necessary and appropriate professional staff to assist in the safety and comfort of the transfer, assure that the receiving facility assume the necessary care promptly, and provide pertinent medical information about the patient's condition; and maintaining records of the foregoing.

Every patient or resident of a facility shall be provided by the physician in the facility the right:

(a) to informed consent to the extent provided by law;

(b) to privacy during medical treatment or other rendering of care within the capacity of the facility;

(c) to refuse to be examined, observed, or treated by students or any other facility staff without jeopardizing access to psychiatric, psychological or other medical care and attention;

(d) to refuse to serve as a research subject, and to refuse any care or examination when the primary purpose is educational or informational rather than therapeutic;

(e) to prompt life saving treatment in an emergency without discrimination on account of economic status or source of payment and without delaying treatment for purposes of prior discussion of source of payment unless such delay can be imposed without material risk to his health.

(f) upon request, to obtain an explanation as to the relationship, if any, of the physician to any other health care facility or educational institutions insofar as said relationship relates to his care or treatment, and such explanation shall include said physician's ownership or financial interest, if any, in the facility or other health care facilities insofar as said ownership relates to the care or treatment of said patient or resident.

(g) upon request to receive an itemized bill including third party reimbursements paid toward said bill, regardless of the sources of payment;

(h) in the case of a patient suffering from any form of breast cancer, to complete information on all alternative treatments which are medically viable; and

Every maternity patient, at the time of preadmission, shall receive complete information from an admitting hospital: on its annual rate of primary caesarian sections; annual rate of repeat caesarian sections; the annual percentage of women who have had a caesarian section who have had a subsequent successful vaginal birth; the annual percentage of deliveries in birthing rooms and labor-delivery-recovery rooms; the annual percentage which were externally monitored only; the annual percentage which were internally monitored only; the annual percentage which were both internally and externally monitored; the annual percentage utilizing inductions, epidurals and general anesthesia; and the annual percentage of women breast-feeding upon discharge from said hospital.

Any person whose rights under this section are violated may bring, in addition to any other action allowed by law or regulation, a civil action under sections sixty B to sixty E, inclusive, of chapter two hundred and thirty-one.

No provision of this section relating to confidentiality of records shall be construed to prevent any third party reimburser from inspecting and copying, in the ordinary course of determining eligibility for or entitlement to benefits, any and all records relating to diagnosis, treatment, or other services provided to any person, including a minor or incompetent, for which coverage, benefit or reimbursement is claimed, so long as the policy or certificate under which the claim is made provides that such access to such records is permitted. No provision of this section relating to confidentiality of records shall be construed to prevent access to any such records in connection with any peer review or utilization review procedures applied and implemented in good faith.

No provision herein shall apply to any institution operated or listed and certified by The First Church of Christ, Scientist, in Boston, or patients whose religious beliefs limit the forms and qualities of treatment to which they may submit.

No provision herein shall be construed as limiting any other right or remedies previously existing at law.

111:70F. HLTV-III Test; Confidentiality; Informed Consent

Section 70F. No health care facility, as defined in section seventy E, and no physician or health care provider shall (1) test any person for the presence of the HTLV-III antibody or antigen without first obtaining his written informed consent; (2) disclose the results of such test to any person other than the subject thereof without first obtaining the subject's written informed consent; or (3) identify the subject of such tests to any person without first obtaining the subject's written informed consent.

No employer shall require HTLV-III antibody or antigen tests as a condition for employment.

Whoever violates the provisions of this section shall be deemed to have violated section two of chapter ninety-three A.

For the purpose of this section "written informed consent" shall mean a written consent form for each requested release of the results of an individual's HTLV-III antibody or antigen test, or for the release of medical records containing such information. Such written consent form shall state the purpose for which the information is being requested and shall be distinguished from written consent for the release of any other medical information, and for the purpose of this section "HTLV-III test" shall mean a licensed screening antibody test for the human T-cell lymphotrophic virus type III.

DECISION MAKING: NATURE AND TECHNIQUES

Contemporary ethical literature puts heavy emphasis on the decision-making process being vitally important for the moral agent. This primarily has resulted both from the present focus on the dignity and freedom of the human person, and from the personal responsibility demanded of those who possess such dignity and freedom. One can speak of "morality" only when the action under discussion is performed by a human being possessing knowledge and freedom and capable of using them in a responsible fashion.

As a consequence of this contemporary development, there is less emphasis in ethical writing on moral "fiat" issued by persons in authority to be obeyed almost blindly and without questioning by their human subjects. The moral agent has become a decision maker rather than a passive recipient for a neatly packaged moral judgment handed down from above. That is as it should be, but it can be counterproductive when decision making is expected of those who were never allowed or taught to make decisions.

Whenever one is faced with making a moral decision, one also is faced with making a practical judgment about the rightness or wrongness of a projected action. Considerable effort must be made to decide where one's moral obligation is located. In other words, decision making is a process by which an individual – in the throes of a moral dilemma and often in the presence of a series of conflicting opinions about the binding force of a specific ethical rule – attempts to discover where his or her true obligation lies.

Decision making is a difficult and demanding task. How one goes about making moral decisions will influence greatly the type of person one will become.[44]

The following guidelines contribute to making a good moral judgment:

1. Assemble all the relevant data (facts, norms, principles, rules, interpreations of the rules).
2. Realize that all personal judgments contain a good deal of subjectivity; as a result of personal prejudices and previous history, no one can claim to be totally objective.
3. Understand that all personal judgments have communal dimensions: human existence is coexistence; consultation of the many voices in the community is essential; and reflection on the possible consequences of your decision on the community is imperative.
4. Realize that every human judgment is fallible; these are judgments of people who can err and who can both deceive themselves and be deceived in their comprehension of the situation.
5. Understand that personal judgments do not create the truth of themselves but are practical judgments of what appears to be the proper method of procedure here and now.
6. Know the distinction between superego and conscience; the superego makes decisions out of a desire to gain approval, whereas conscience makes decisions out of a desire to do what is just and loving.

This is a most important distinction. Glaser[38] makes the following observations:

1. The basis for action in the superego is the fear of low withdrawal, whereas for conscience it is a call to commit oneself in abiding love.
2. Superego is static (cannot function creatively in a new situation), whereas conscience is dynamic (sensitive to values and grows in each new situation).
3. Superego is authority oriented (it responds to command rather than to value), whereas conscience is value oriented (it responds to values as perceived in the here and now).

Superego is atomized (individual acts are seen in isolation), whereas conscience is global (individual acts are seen as part of a larger pattern).

Superego guilt depends on the weight of the authority figure rather than on the density of the value in question, whereas conscience guilt depends on the density of the value in question and not on the weight of the authority figure.

Whenever one studies the history of ethical thought, one always comes across some serious advice on the nature of decision making. None is more clear and to the point than that offered by Thomas Aquinas in his *Summa Theologiae*. He lists eight qualities as essential for what he calls "the prudent decision":

1. *Memoria:* the ability to recall to mind universal principles and commandments as well as the accumulated wisdom of the past
2. *Intellectus:* the ability to penetrate to the central values at stake and the ability to grasp the unique situation in its true meaning
3. *Ratio:* the ability to reason from insights and experience new insights
4. *Docilitas:* the ability to be open to new learning and to profit by the experience of others
5. *Solertia:* the ability to come to a decision without undue delay
6. *Providentia:* the ability to exercise foresight, which gauges the effects or consequences of the decision
7. *Circumspectio:* the ability to take into consideration and weight all possible circumstances
8. *Precautio:* the ability to anticipate obstacles and prepare to surmount them

These guidelines provide profound insights into human psychology. Decision making can be greatly enriched if one heeds their practical advice.

From an ethical perspective there are many issues in addressing one's care of self. Most prominent is the dilemma of self-determination or autonomy versus the common good. This argument is between the rights and responsibilities of the individual and those of society and is related to the quality versus the sanctity of life discussions.

A second area of ethical concern is the application of the principles of informed consent, particularly an individual's right to truth. What does an individual need to know to make informed decisions about personal health? A third issue is that of nonmaleficence and beneficence, which reminds one not to inflict harm or evil, to prevent harm, to remove evil, and to promote good. This principle applies to the care of self as well as to the care of others.

That last area of ethical dilemma for healthy people is the allocation of care resources. Who should receive the money, time, and space allocations for health care in our society? Is it just to give resources to the well for increased health when the ill are suffering?

Each human being has the capability of learning about self. This increased consciousness of self is essential for good stewardship of one's life and health. An individual learns self-care thorugh the care received from others. In the beginning of life these significant others are primarily from the family. Gradually they include broader and broader circles of the community, including health care providers. In the context of this organized community a person grows and develops as an individual. In receiving truthful information from others within this context of a just community, an individual can make well-informed decisions about life. There is always, however, an attempt to negotiate the rights and responsibilities of the individual with those of the community: balancing autonomy and self-determination with the common good presented with varying degrees of truthfulness and justice. What then are a person's rights and responsibilities for health, and what are the community's rights and responsibilities for the health of an individual and that of the whole community? Because of the very intimate nature of health, it is difficult to disagree that the primary responsibility for an individual's health rests with that individual, not the community. It seems especially difficult for the nurse or anyone else to acknowledge that his or her first responsibility is to self, that is, to practice effective health promotion and prevention and not get sick.

This has not been clear, however, in Western health care. Health has become so technologized that an individual may be more likely to depend on others, such as professional specialists, than the self. Perceiving one's body, mind, and spirit is a subjective experience, which is difficult to describe to oneself, let alone to others.

As discussed in Chapter 9, communities, cultures, and religious groups have developed specific guidelines for the promotion of health and prevention of illness. Leininger[50] and Spector[76] identify many of these prescribed health practices. Varying cultures and religions emphasize contrasting recommendations for rest, activity, nutritional intake, and so on.

Some groups absolutely prohibit ingesting certain food or drink, such as pork or alcohol. Others advise individuals to wear protective metals and jewelry. Although these are differences between the health prescriptions of specific cultures and religions, the theme of wholeness is generally included. Clearly, groups throughout the world and history recognize the influence of the body, mind, and spirit on one another and on the promotion of health for the individual.

Nurses can use these culturally and religiously prescribed guidelines to health to anticipate concerns and desired activities of clients. With the many religious beliefs and practices in our society, however, the nurse is advised to explore these issues individually with each client. Many religious people, for example, believe that disease and trauma are the direct punishments for moral evil and sin instead of the result of physical evils.[15]

In making decisions about personal health, an individual is affirming a commitment to health or illness, to life or death. The person who makes a commitment to life strives for wholeness in every dimension of being. Perhaps many decide not to choose, which is a decision for illness and death.

The Jewish religion, however, presents very strong affirmations. The Old Testament presents the Jewish view as profoundly life affirming. Ashley and O'Rourke state, "It constantly emphasizes the idea that God gives his friends health, security, children and long life and God has created men and women for life and wishes to prolong it for them . . . thus disease, aging and death are not willed by God, but only permitted by Him as . . . the inevitable consequence of human commitments to death rather than to life."[5]

This tradition continues with Christianity. Braaten and Braaten believe the role of the body is addressed to Christianity: "Energy, courage, zest for life and willingness to undertake arduous endeavors are all bound up with bodily health. Attempting a harmonious balance of exercise, diet, rest and positive mental attitude is, therefore, a duty of the human body-person, as it certainly is of the Christian who recognizes the material world and the body as precious gifts from the Creator."[14]

Personal responsibility for health means manifesting a health-affirming lifestyle, which is a rarity today. Stress; insufficient time for rest, exercise, and nutrition; and chemical abuse (cigarettes, alcohol, drugs) do not provide the individual with the substance for health. It is typical that many individuals "live without clear commitments or goals, suffering from the emptiness, meaninglessness, and absurdity of life, in a loneliness that never seeks deep level communication with others." To be healthy, other choices need to be made. Unhealthy behaviors have been rejected for a quality life to be developed.

Stewardship of one's health involves one's own spirit, mind, and body, as well as the community and environment. Ashley and O'Rourke[5] have formulated the *principles of stewardship and creativity:*

1. We are ethically obliged to use our natural environment and our multidimensional human nature as precious gifts, with profound respect for their intrinsic teleology.
2. We are also obliged to use our creativity as an equally precious gift to improve our environment and our nature, with a caution set by the limits of our actual knowledge and by the risk of destroying that same creativity.

A clear example of the ethical dilemma of self-determination versus the common good surrounds the 1967 federal standard for highway safety, which declared that the states require motorcycle riders to wear helmets. (A threatened reduction in highway and safety funds encouraged compliance.) Although few data were available to document the costs and benefits, it seemed to be a logical step to prevent injuries and save lives. Many individuals believed this legislation was an infringement on their liberties. The ethical controversies are well discussed by Watson[81] and others. Perkins[60] attempts to summarize the issues by asking, "What variables are most significant in the cause of motorcycle accidents?" Different answers may be found, such as motorcyclists involved in accidents having inadequate driver training and therefore not being able to take appropriately evasive actions.

The quest for greater autonomy in caring for the self is also well demonstrated in the currently popular self-help health literature. Many of these publications clearly have the position that the health problems of the individual are interwoven into the health problems of the society. Any interventions that do not consider this relationship are thus inadequate.[53]

Health care providers are concerned that many of these publications do not meet Frankena's principles of nonmaleficence, of not doing harm.[35] Several weight-reducing diet manuals, for example, have prescribed deficient nutritional patterns. Consumers of these recommended diets subsequently have experienced severe complications.

There are many examples of a person's responsibilities for health. A theme throughout these choices is the individual's use of time. Ruthmann[70] discusses that our society's present attitudes toward work and leisure are more utilitarian than the Puritan philosophy, which values industry, punctuality, and thrift, from which it grew. As Lauer and Mlecko state, "Utilitarians live consciously or unconsciously by the principle that only useful activity is valuable, meaningful and moral."[49] In a more psychosocial perspective Ruthmann discusses that the tendency to assume that the more one does, the more one is alive, is really a subtle way of running away from one's self. For an individual to develop a more balanced life, Ruthmann[70] believes that one has to experience acceptance of self as a good person and not what one can produce. This is the same process as Erikson's fifth stage of identity development in adolescence.

Many different criteria are posed to define the quality of life. As discussed, ancient Greek ethical theories proposed two types of standards for evaluating the value of a human life: perfectionist and utilitarian standards. The perfectionist standard specifies a given number of qualities, such as the ability to reason, as being necessary for a valuable life. Today's self-actualization theories are derived from this perspective. Utilitarian standards are based on the net utility (utility minus net utility) of a life. Varieties include the consideration of pleasure minus pain and fulfillment of desire minus nonfulfillment of desires.

Another perspective of the quality of life is developed in Judaism and Christianity. Judeo-Christian sanctity-of-life ethic appears to be rooted in deontologic theory. It gives equal value to each human life regardless of the condition or abilities of the person on the basis of inherent values. McCormick[53] describes the Judeo-Christian tradition as being midway between the extremes of medical vitalism, which says life is an absolute to be preserved at all costs, and medical pessimism, which is based on the idea that only the fittest have a right to life and health care.

The danger in current arguments, however, is the polarization of these positions, precluding one from the other. The mixed consequentialism apprpoch seems to take this into consideration. This position seems to develop the argument combining both perspectives for a more balanced approach to the value of a human life.

The Code for Nurses states that nursing encompasses the promotion and restoration of health, the prevention of illness, and the alleviation of suffering. This is partly accomplished by arriving at the best decisions declared by the circumstances, the client's rights and wishes, and the highest standards of care. The measures used to provide assistance should enable the client to live with as much comfort, dignity, and freedom from anxiety and pain as possible. The varying definitions of quality of life vary with the context, and a client's self-determination to define quality of life to make the corresponding decisions for his own life are clearly affirmed.[55]

The same answer is given in the 1982 study of ethical problems by the president's commission,[62] which posed the question: "What are the values that ought to guide decision making in the provider-patient relationship or by which the success of a particular interaction can be judged?" Their answer was "Promotion of a patient's well-being and respect for a patient's self determination." As discussed throughout this text, well-being is difficult to define consistently because of minimal objective criteria and the legitimate subjective perspectives of clients.

In conclusion, optimal health is a challenge for each person to become more fully human, using acceptable means to obtain meaningful ends. Health is a means of living the kind of life and fulfilling the kind of goals an individual has chosen based on the meaning one finds in life. The nurse has an opportunity in each phase of the nursing process to help a client develop a meaningful appraisal of his own condition in life.[23,24]

SELECTED ETHICAL ISSUES

Research

Confronting the ethical dilemmas of research in health care is not new. What is new is the rapid development of knowledge and technology in our society. As previously discussed, this knowledge gives health care providers great potential control over the quantity and quality of human life, which is where the complexities of ethical issues and dilemmas accelerate. From an ethical perspective the fundamental dilemma in research with human beings involves "individual rights versus societal rights, the right balance between present lives and future lives, individual morality and statistical morality, immediate benefits versus future benefits and science versus therapy."[46]

Experimentation can mean either the use of interventions not adequately accepted or the use of interventions designed to accept or reject a newly posed hypothesis. The first generally allows for greater accuracy in the prediction of the outcomes, including desirable and undesirable effects.

Investigational treatments may also be distinguished according to their therapeutic benefits. In therapeutic research a client usually receives direct benefits from a research project, such as increased knowledge about his own health and ways to prevent problems for which he is at risk. On the other hand, in nontherapeutic research the subject generally receives no direct benefits and may actually experience a loss, such as blood for samples; it is hoped the data results obtained will benefit future clients.[46]

A second fundamental ethical issue in human experimentation is the informed consent of the subject. Informed consent is a generally accepted component within health care, especially with procedures that are invasive or have less predictable outcomes. Virtually all codes of ethics affirm the principle of informed consent, which Ramsey[65] defines as the cardinal canon of loyalty that joins persons together in health care practice and investigation. The problem, however, is actually obtaining it. What does fully informing the subject consist of? How can the experimenter explain the outcomes when he or she cannot accurately predict? Can a person really give truly free and voluntary consent?[2,30,61]

How can a researcher adequately inform a client about the complexities of current DNA research, including unknown, irreversible genetic and immunologic processes? How does one describe the potential risks of psychosocial research? Can one reasonably predict the benefits and risks to the individual versus society? How does one differentiate altered interventions from experimental interventions? Such questions confront today's nurse, whose knowledge base and scope of responsibilities change on an almost daily basis.

Two rights are specified within this document. First is the right to freedom from intrinsic risk of injury, which demands that the individual be informed of the extent of potential risks. Sometimes it is difficult for investigators to explain adequately potential risks because of inadequate knowledge and the anticipated benefits for the individual and humanity.

The second is the right of privacy and dignity. It is equally difficult for the investigator to estimate what is invasion of privacy and a threat to the dignity of an individual, especially in today's pluralistic society. Presumptions of the other person's perspectives are inappropriate. All aspects of the investigation (instruments, protocols, techniques) should be reviewed with the subject. When anonymity or confidentiality may be sacrificed, additional consent must be obtained.

Individuals who are particularly vulnerable to exploitation through research are specifically addressed. The use of captive audiences, including prisoners, military personnel, students, children, and fetuses, in research requires special justification by investigators.

The other commitment of the nurse, however, is to society as a whole. Balancing the rights of the individual with the rights and benefits of society has been difficult to weigh, especially in preventive interventions, such as immunization and fluoridation. For the nurse these responsibilities most commonly include ensuring that clients are informed that they are on experimental protocols and seeing that informed consent documents are truly free and informed.

The mechanisms for these protection of rights are identified as being ensured by informed consent, agency review committees, and professional organizations. To fulfill these professional obligations, "each nurse must develop an awareness of the issues and a framework for dealing effectively with emerging human rights problems."[2]

These concerns about individual rights and duty and autonomy become even more intensified when one considers particularly vulnerable clients: the fetus, children, mentally compromised patients, and prisoners. Some ethicists argue that no experiments should be performed on these groups; it would be better to limit health care research than to limit the rights and autonomy of such individuals. In practice, however, any new intervention, even revised assessment, teaching, or counseling protocols, is an investigation.

Gray[40] lists five basic principles that are generally accepted in research with human beings:

1. A research subject is a person who volunteered to participate in the research on the basis of having all the necessary information so that his or her decision

will be a truly informed one.

2. The research subject should be allowed to withdraw from the study at any point if and when he or she wishes to do so.
3. All necessary risks should be eliminated in the research design, and, if appropriate, the reserach design should have been tried out with prior animal studies (which are separately addressed).
4. The benefits of the study, either to society or to the individual or preferably both, should outweigh the risks to the subject involved.
5. The experimentation should be conducted only by individuals qualified to do so.

All professional health care agency and political codes of ethics generally contain these principles.

World War II marked society's formal concern with matters related to human experimentation. The atrocities of the war, particularly those committed by Nazi physicians, necessitated a worldwide response. The results included the Nuremberg and Helsinki declarations, landmark documentations in human experimentation specifying the relationship between experimenter and subject. The ethical values of human freedom and the inviolability of the human person are the foundation of these codes.[56]

They were followed by many other more specific codes. These were also developed because of the rapid explosion of knowledge and technology during and after World War II. People needed guidelines to make decisions about the application of massive amounts of data in political, health care, and work environments. Included among these codes are the *Code for Nurses* (American Nurses' Association, 1950), the *Principles of Research and Experimentation* (World Medical Association, 1954), *Principles of Medical Ethics* (American Medical Association, 1971), and the *Department of Health, Education and Welfare Guidelines* (1974), which were revised in the 1981 *Basic Health and Human Services Policy for Protection of Human Research Subjects.*[1]

The American Nurses' Association *Code for Nurses* provides general guidelines for nurses participating in research. The value of research and protection of human rights are emphasized. Inherent is "respect for each individual to exercise self-determination, to choose to participate, to have full information, and to terminate participation without penalty."

The *Code for Nurses* emphasizes the self-determination of clients:

> Whenever possible, clients should be fully involved in the planning and implementation of their own health care. Each client has the moral right to determine what will be done with his/her person; to be given information necessary for making informed judgments; to be told the possible effects of care; and to accept, refuse or terminate care. These same rights apply to minors and others not legally qualified and must be respected to the fullest degree permissible under the law. . . . The nurse must also recognize those situations in which individual rights to self-determination in health care may temporarily be altered for the common good.[1]

The near impossibility of full and informed consent seems to be reflected in the Department of Health and Human Services' regulations, which emphasize "reasonably" informed consent in the following guidelines:[9]

1. A fair explanation of the procedures to be followed and their purposes including identification of any procedures that are experimental
2. A description of the attendant discomforts and risks reasonably to be expected
3. A description of the benefits reasonably to be expected
4. A disclosure of appropriate alternative procedures that might be advantageous for the subject
5. An offer to answer any inquiries concerning the procedures
6. An instruction that the person is free to withdraw his/her consent and to discontinue participation in the project or activity at any time without prejudice to the subjects

In 1975, the American Nurses' Association established a Commission on Nursing Research that developed *Human Rights Guidelines for Nurses in Clinical and Other Research.*[2] This document publicly affirms the nursing profession's obligation to develop scientific knowledge toward improving nursing practice and patient care. Thus two sets of human rights are addressed with commitments. First is the commitment to support qualified nurses to conduct research and have access to related resources. The second commitment is to the human rights of all people who participate in research, especially subjects who are directly or indirectly involved with nursing care. The right of self-determination of each subject is a critical issue; each nurse has an obligation to support this moral and legal right of the individual.

Within these guidelines the need is emphasized for special protection of the human rights of the individual when "the focus of care is not specifically directed toward meeting the needs of the client or subject . . . especially when the probable outcomes are unknown or doubtful."[2] Individual health care agencies are encouraged to develop written statements and guidelines.

The inescapable moral responsibility therefore rests with the nurse who is conducting, participating in, or has knowledge of the clinical investigation. This individual's level of sensitivity and ability to implement basic ethical principles determine the proper approach to the ethics of the research processes.[36,54]

Stewardship over One's Own Health

The title of a recent movie and play asks the question, "Whose life is it anyway?" This seems to be the core question in approaching the stewardship of one's own health.

In addition to who decides, What is health? This question is addressed from multiple perspectives in Chapter 1.

Contraception

From the beginnings of recorded history, men and women have been interested in the possibility of controlling births while not limiting the pleasure of human coitus. A variety of methods have been devised, many of which gave rise to some serious ethical problems. As might be suspected, these ranged from the possibility of physical harm to the morality of government intervention in curbing population growth.

In contemporary society, which is marked by a great deal of sexual freedom as well as a failure to examine and appreciate the real meaning of human coitus, contraception has become, for many, matter-of-fact and unfortunately, something utterly devoid of any ethical dimensions. Since birth limitation is something usually practiced by healthy persons, it deserves consideration in this text.

Contraception can be understood as the employment of any mechanical, chemical, pharmaceutical, or surgical means of preventing sexual intercourse from resulting in the generation of offspring. As such, it is distinguished from so-called periodic continence (rhythm) and natural family planning systems, which entail the use of no mechanical, artificial, or unnatural means.

Throughout history there has been much discussion about the ethical implications of contraception, but it is only within the past hundred years, with the technologic development of better and safer methods of contraception and with serious discussions about the world population problem, that the matter has become a highly controversial issue. The heart of the discussion may be found in the varying understandings of the meaning of human coitus. Traditionally it has been seen as an expression of love, which is open to the possibility of the generation of human life. Whether it is permissible to separate these two values for the sake of other values has been the dominant theme in contemporary ethical discussion. Is it moral to use human coitus as a means of expressing love while eliminating the possibility of its resulting in the conception of a new human being through the use of some artificial means? The proper answer to that question depends on one's comprehension of the meaning of human coitus.

Most secular humanists see no problem in the employment of mechanical, chemical, pharmaceutical, or surgical means to separate the production of human life from the act of lovemaking. They tend, however, to question the morality of contraception done out of purely self-centered motives, performed in a manner that would infringe on the rights of either or both marriage partners, or entailing the use of a contraceptive device that might be harmful to physical or mental health.

The Jewish tradition has a long history of rabbinic teaching on the morality of contraception. There is no law as such in the Hebrew scriptures that constitutes an outright condemnation of contraception. However, Judaism's strong emphasis on fertility generally led many of its researchers to look with disfavor on the practice. From the 16th century there were some indications of the existence of a singular rabbinic interpretation that seemed to permit the use of contraceptives by women for a good reason. Nevertheless this position was strongly opposed by official rabbinic teaching until the 20th century.[45] However, at present many rabbinic authorities permit the use of the diaphragm and the annovulant pills. In practice, on the other hand, it seems that most cultural but nonpracticing Jews follow the ethical stance set by the secular humanists.

From the very beginnings of the Protestant Reformation many of those responsible for the movement were strongly opposed to contraception, since they saw it as an unlawful interference with nature as well as an illicit separation of love and life. However, in the period from 1880 to 1930, as medical opinion shifted its disapproval and as various groups were formed to encourage the practice of "family planning," many Protestant denominations modified this opposition. In 1930 the bishops of the Anglican Church, by a vote of 193 to 67, approved a cautious acceptance of methods other than those of sexual abstinence to avoid parenthood. From that time the major Protestant churches all publicly abandoned their absolute (deontologic) prohibition of contraception by married couples. Nevertheless most of them still require good reasons for doing so, whether medical, economic, social, or eugenic.

The Roman Catholic position on the morality of artificial contraception is well known by health care professionals. It goes back as far as the so-called Alexandrian Rule (circa A.D. 150), which held that sexual intercourse was lawful only within the context of marriage and only for the purpose of procreation, an opinion that became the official teaching of the church for more than a millennium. After a short period of tentative reconsideration in the 1960s, the traditional teaching was reaffirmed in 1968, when Pope Paul VI, in the encyclic letter *Humanae Vitae,* declared that every act of marital intercourse had to be kept open to procreation:

> The Church calling men back to the observance of the norms of natural law, as interpreted by constant doctrine, teaches that each and every marriage act must remain open to the transmission of life. That teaching, often set forth by the official church, is founded upon the inseparable connection, willed by God and unable to be broken by man on his own initiative, between the two meanings of the conjugal act: the unitive meaning and the procreative meaning.

Anyone familiar with the current writing by Roman Catholic theologians on this issue knows that the teaching of the encyclic occasioned a good deal of disagreement within the confines of the Roman communion. Everyone concerned agreed with the values announced by the intrinsic connection between "love and life," but there was strong dissent from the rule which the Pope formulated as a result of these values. He taught that every contraceptive act contradicts the basic unity that should exist between marital love and fertility. The theologian dissenters continued to insist that this need not always be the case. They believed that whenever there is a conflict, that is, whenever it is imprudent to continue to procreate and equally imprudent to abstain from coitus, contraception is not wrong provided that the marriage itself is open to procreation.

As a result of this controversy there are two current opinions within the Roman Catholic community on the morality of contraception: that of the traditional deontologists and that of the so-called proportionalists or mixed consequentialists. The first hold that any act of contraception is "objectively wrong" because it breaks the intimate connection between love and life, but they maintain that if any couple should practice it in good conscience, if they are unable to appreciate the values involved because of their particular circumstances, their action could be considered "subjectively defensible." The proportionalists hold that the contraceptive act is a "premoral evil," that is, it introduces disorder between the values of love and life; but it does not become a "moral evil," that is, a sin if the value to be achieved by the practice of contraception is proportionate to the disvalues it can cause.

Many episcopal conferences, or geographic groupings of Roman Catholic bishops, issued pastoral guidelines for their congregations in the light of the teaching set forth by *Humanae Vitae*. Of practical interest for those nurses who may be asked about this issue by Roman Catholic clients are the statements of the Indonesian and South African bishops. According to the Indonesians,

> There are parents who are troubled because from the one side they feel the obligation to regulate births, but from the other they are not able to fulfill their obligation by temporary or absolute sexual abstinence. In these circumstances, they decide responsibly and do not need to feel that they have sinned if they employ other means provided that the means employed do not go against human life . . . and provided that medical responsibility is upheld.*

According to the South African bishops,

> In this conflict of duties (another pregnancy is unacceptable for serious reasons and a regime of continence would threaten family peace, marital fidelity or the future of the marriage . . .) their (i.e. the parents) responsible decision, though falling short of the ideal will be subjectively defensible since the aim is not the selfish exclusion of pregnancy but the promotion of the common good of the family. They will, however, remain open to a revision of their practice, to a deeper grasp of the teaching of the church, and where possible, to the removal of those circumstances that prevent the realization of the ideals of marriage. Those who fail to respond to the high standard proposed will not readily reproach themselves with serious fault, unless their motives are wholly selfish, materialistic or pleasure seeking, contradicting the fundamental duties of responsible parenthood.†

The practice of contraception presents a serious dilemma for many healthy people. A decision to practice it must not be taken lightly, since the attitude chosen has direct consequences on the couple's appreciation of the meaning and purpose of human coitus. For that reason no couple should undertake the practice of contraception without competent spiritual counseling and medical advice. The first will help them to avoid a decision that might be harmful to a proper evaluation of the role of human sexuality within the context of marriage, and the second will help them to avoid decisions that might prove injurious to physical and mental health. This is especially true whenever there is danger that a couple is operating out of selfish and hedonistic reasons, as well as whenever consideration is being given to the possibility of permanent sterilization (tubal ligation in the female and vasectomy in the male). At present these procedures are practically irreversible and exclude the possibility of future children if there should be a subsequent marriage, as with widows or widowers, or if a sudden turn of events, such as the death of an only child, would make a future pregnancy desirable.

Abortion

At present more than 1.5 million legal abortions are reported each year in the United States, and government statistics show that one out of every nine women of reproductive age has had one. These facts shed some light on the magnitude of the ethical issue faced by health care personnel. The basis of the difficulty can be stated as follows: How can we reconcile, relate, and balance the rights of the mother with the rights of nascent life in such a way that it can be translated into public policy? Those who take a "pro-life" stance on this issue continue to debate with those who take the "pro-choice" stance, and yet nothing seems to result.

There is obviously no easy solution to this problem; it is one of the most complex ethical issues facing contemporary society. This was well stated by Glaser, one of the most outstanding Roman Catholic moralists in the United States today, when he wrote:

> Abortion is a matter that is morally problematic, pastorally delicate, legislatively thorny, constitutionally insecure, ecumenically devisive, medically normless, humanly anguishing, racially provocative, journalistically abused, personally biased and widely performed. It demands a most extraordinary discipline of moral thought, one that is penetrating without being impenetrable,

*Origins 3:42, 1974.

†Ibid.

humanly compassionate without being morally compromising, legally realistic without being legally positivistic, instructed by cognate disciplines without being determined by those informed by tradition without being enslaved by it.[38]

It must also be remembered that in our society the "abortion debate" occurs within the context of religious and philosophic pluralism. It deeply concerns all people of good will, since as it goes to the core of our vision of what the human being is and of what constitutes the human being's right to life. Yet in a technologically sophisticated society such as ours there is often very little patience with philosophizing and theologizing; a "practical and efficient" solution is preferred.

A variety of reasons has been proposed to justify abortion: to protect the life of the mother, to safeguard the physical and mental health of the mother, to act as a remedy against injustices caused by rape or incest, to prevent the birth of defective children, to vindicate the right of the woman to determine her own reproductive capacities and have control over her body, to protect the reputation of a violated woman, and to alleviate economic, sociologic, or demographic problems.

The ethical issue centers around the difficult question of the beginning of human life. The ultimate judgment on this question remains within the realm of philosophy or theology; biologic, genetic, or scientific data alone will not suffice. When human life begins is essentially a human judgment to be made by philosophy or theology but always taking into consideration the data supplied by the biologic and empiric sciences.

Many theories discuss the beginnings of human life, and each employs differing criteria for arriving at such a determination. In general, these criteria can be reduced to two: (1) the individual-biologic criterion, which seems to place the beginning of human life at conception or at very early stages of development; and (2) the relational and conferral-of-rights criteria, which usually accept a rather late point in development for the beginning of a life that can be regarded as truly human.

In contemporary society there seem to be four basic stances on the ethics of abortion, offered by those in the tradition of secular humanism and by the three major religious groupings – Jewish, Protestant, and Roman Catholic. However, within each of these systems one can find a number of nuances that give rise to a variety of opinions when it comes to practical cases. This discussion focuses on the principal position of each group.

The United States Supreme Court decisions handed down in 1973 seem to reflect the basic tenet of the so-called secular humanist group: the individual woman's right to privacy encompasses the decision to terminate a pregnancy; and this right to abort is fundamental enough to override any interest the state might have in protecting fetal life. Many of those ethicists who follow utilitarianism or situationism would make this position their own.

Traditional Judaism is very cautious about the morality of abortion. Its position can be identified with that of the late Chief Rabbi of Israel, Issar Unterman, who saw any abortion as "akin to homicide" and therefore allowable only in cases of corresponding gravity, such as saving the life of the mother. Against today's background of more causal abortion, most rabbis seem to adhere to this opinion and allow abortions only for serious reasons.[29]

In American Protestantism the perspectives on abortion range along a continuum from antiabortion to abortion-on-demand, including perhaps the group affirming the justifiable-but-tragic abortion in certain situations when there is a serious conflict of values. Ramsey,[65] a deontologist, represents the antiabortion position; Gustafson,[42] a mixed consequentalist, seems to hold the "justifiable-but-tragic position"; Fletcher,[33] taking a utilitarian or situationist approach, seems to favor the abortion-on-demand position.

Among Roman Catholic ethicists the official opinion on abortion is deontologic. It is stated in the *Declaration on Abortion* issued by the Vatican in 1974:

The right to life is no less to be respected in the small infant just born than in the mature person. In reality, respect for human life is called for from the time that the process of generation begins. From the time that the ovum is fertilized, a life is begun which is neither that of the father nor of the mother; it is rather the life of a new human being with his or her own growth. . . . One can never approve of abortion; but it is above all necessary to combat its causes.

This position is totally in conformity with the statement issued in 1965 by the Second Vatican Council: "Life from its conception is to be guarded with the greatest care. Abortion and infanticide are horrible crimes."

However, it should be noted that a growing number of contemporary Roman Catholic theologians are tentatively arguing that there might be some legitimate exceptions to the general rule prohibiting abortions. Arguing from a position of proportionalism or mixed consequentialism, some of those theologians seem to permit what traditional moralists would call "directly forbidden actions" whenever certain disvalues can be minimized. Thus some hold that abortion to save the life of the mother might be permitted, but only in that specific case, since no other possible cause could be proportionate to the direct taking of the life of an unborn child.

This section on the question of the morality of abortion is necessarily brief and incomplete. As mentioned, the abortion issue is extremely complex and problematic. However, it must never be forgotten that it is a question intimately connected with the meaning and value of human existence. As stated by a prominent Protestant ethicist:

The "cure" of the abortion epidemic can be no less profound than its causes. If, as right-wing critics affirm, its source is in the heart of man, its remedy must penetrate to similar depths. Neither cool debate nor heated polemics can move men at such levels. Only the example of sincere regard for others can rekindle the conviction that all life is sacred and bound together in mystery so that the death of the least diminishes each. When a fetus is aborted no one asks for whom the bell tolls. No bell is tolled. But do not feel indifferent and secure. The fetus symbolizes you and me and our tenuous hold upon a future here at the mercy of our maker.[60]

Genetic Therapy

Within the past several decades, advances in molecular biology have enabled scientists to acquire extraordinary insights into genetics and human genetic development. Even at this moment there is a definite possibility that geneticists can eliminate deleterious genes from the human gene pool and add desirable genes that will improve human individuals and the human species. Advances in this area have already begun to affect the manner in which parents, together with their physicians and genetic counselors, make decisions about parenthood and childbearing. Such extraordinary developments will have considerable impact on the human race in the future, thus they are observed with great interest by ethicists, who very frequently pose the question: "If we can do it, should we?" The possibility of genetic therapy can bring with it great blessings for the human race, but one would be naive if one did not admit that it can also cause considerable damage. As a consequence, the ethicist must evaluate constantly the so-called advances that genetic therapy can accomplish. In trying to perform this duty, the ethicist must ask two questions: (1) To what extent do human beings have the right to interfere in the genetic processes? and (2) What effect will such interferences have on basic social structures, such as marriage and the family?

Some ideas on the various methods proposed for genetic control should be mentioned. First, there is the phenomenon known as *eugenics,* which might be described as "planned breeding"; it has been used successfully in the development of hybrid breeds of cattle and certain food products. This involves the selection and recombination of genes already existing in the human gene pool. Two types of eugenics are envisioned: (1) positive eugenics, or preferential breeding of so-called superior individuals to improve the genetic stock of the human race; and (2) negative eugenics, or discouragement or legal prohibition of reproduction to individuals who carry defective genes. The first type urges the development of sperm banks for the purpose of storing frozen sperm taken from outstanding people, as well as the development of the process known as cloning or transplantation of nuclei from one cell to another to make an exact copy of a certain perfect specimen of humanity. The second type urges genetic counseling or the provision for abortion or sterilization, on either a voluntary or an enforced basis.

A second method proposed for genetic control is *genetic engineering,* the alteration of the individual's genetic complement. This entails the changing of a particular molecule in the complex structure of the gene, either to eliminate a certain deleterious trait or to improve the genotype. This process, for example, might be employed to control such genetic diseases as sickle cell anemia or Tay-Sachs disease.

A final method proposed by geneticists is called *euthenics* or *euphenics.* These terms describe techniques for correcting defects in individuals after they have been born. Thus if a person is born with defective liver cells and lacks some needed enzyme, it might be possible to extract one or two liver cells, modify their DNA (deoxyribonucleic acid), and reimplant them.[33,73]

Genetic therapy has great possibilities, but it is not without its problems. First, there is immense disagreement on what an ideal genetic inheritance might be. Care must be taken that the concept of genetic illness be not broadened to include genetic liabilities. Second, many modes of genetic therapy involve some of the most radical contemporary scientific experiments and projections and therefore involve serious human risks. Third, by treating successfully some age-old illnesses of genetic origin, modern medicine enables persons to survive and reproduce in situations when they could not have done so in the past. This can interfere with the processes of natural selection, which operate in a cruel manner toward many individuals but at the same time strengthen the human species. Fourth, genetic therapy can very often entail manipulation of persons. Geneticists need to be careful that they do not attempt to "play God," and they must also be careful not to harm the evolutionary process and ecology. Finally, because genetic therapy represents such a major enhancement of human powers, it has within its grasp the makings of unprecedented totalitarianism. Techniques for genetic therapy can become techniques for more ambitious programs of reconstituting the human genetic heritage, producing a superrace or even the breeding of a new race of human chimeras or imaginary monsters who can do menial tasks.

Ramsey,[64,65] a deontologist, submits that those who would project a program for genetic engineering should seriously consider the implications of two basic ethical principles: (1) the separation of the spheres of procreation and marital love as something forbidden by the nature of human parenthood, and (2) the difference between therapy and experimentation and their relationship to informed consent. For those reasons Ramsey is opposed to techniques that would require artificial insemination from donors and the whole procedure of cloning.

Fletcher,[34] a consequentialist-utilitarian, would permit any form of genetic engineering that could offer an optimal or maximal degree of desirable consequences. For him, to be human is to be a maker, a selector, and a designer;

coital reproduction is less human than laboratory reproduction, which is more rationally contrived and hence more human.

Gustafson,[42] a consequentialist-deontologist, believes that societal benefits should count in genetic decisions but not at all costs, just as individual rights should be respected, but not at all costs. He thinks that in the processes employed by genetic engineering scientists should try to hold in balance two intransigent elements of moral discourse: (1) the utter complexity of human reality, and (2) the abiding need to attempt to bring our decisions under objective rational scrutiny so that any resultant moral policies might be kept truly human.

Curran,[18] an advocate of an ethics of relationality and proportionality, insists on a proper understanding of "human stewardship," that is, the ability we have to control our own destiny with the context of constitutive principles. He disagrees with Ramsey's approach, which he believes restricts human stewardship unnecessarily, but he also disagrees with Fletcher, who seems to attribute too much power to human stewardship. Curran suggests that we should all be very critical of utopian schemes in the field of genetics, since this science will never completely overcome our inherent human limitations. He warns against any technologic practice that seems to now ignore the dignity of the human person in the concern for pragmatic adaptability.

Many ethicists are critical observers of the genetic engineering scene. They believe we are just witnessing the beginning of genetic therapy and thus should be very cautious to steer a middle course between native enthusiasm and rigid opposition. They also hold that it is the role of the ethicist to exercise a critical function in regard to the programs suggested by those competent in the field of genetic therapy. The ethicist must be ready to pose hard questions, always keeping in mind not only what the therapy can accomplish but also what the therapy entails in relation to the demands of human nature, as properly understood. Ethicists must check on the experimentation that genetic therapy may require. They must demand that any experimentation employed respect human dignity, receive previous informed consent, and not totally subordinate the good of the individual to the goals of scientific advancement. Finally, all persons involved in the field of genetic therapy should keep in mind two basic ethical principles: (1) the principle of human stewardship over human existence, and (2) the principle governing the meaning of human coitus as something involving love and life.

Genetic therapy has great possibilities for the advancement of the human race, but it also has great possibilities for harm. At present its potential is largely unknown. Thus it is important to resist the technologic enthusiasm insisting that everything possible should be tried or is at least desirable.

Reproductive Technology

Many married couples today are plagued with problems of infertility. They are very anxious to have children of their own, but for various reasons one is found to be infertile. In the past little could be done to help these people; however, today reproductive technology can come to the rescue by means of artificial insemination and in vitro fertilization. Both procedures can help infertile couples, but the techniques are not without their difficulties from a moral point of view.

Artificial insemination is of two kinds: it may be done by means of sperm taken from the husband (AIH) or by means of sperm obtained from a donor (AID). The discussions about the morality of these procedures center around the origins of the sperm. Most ethicists would have no difficulty with AIH, but many of them have real difficulty with AID.[69]

In regard to the morality of homologus artificial insemination, all secular humanists, most Protestant and Jewish ethicists, and some contemporary Roman Catholic moralists agree that it is a morally legitimate intervention to overcome chronic infertility. The strongest opposition to it in the past came from the majority of Roman Catholic moralists who, following the teaching of Pope Pius XII in 1951, held that AIH is immoral because a child born in that manner is the product of a laboratory intervention and not the fruit of an act expressive of the spouses' personal love. As indicated, this argument is not accepted today by a number of responsible Roman Catholic theologians, who would agree with the majority of their Roman Catholic colleagues if procreation occurred routinely in this manner. However, when it is done by way of exception to help a concerned couple to achieve the fruit of their love, it is not contrary to the nature and purpose of the marital act. These theologians base their opinion on the conviction that parenthood is not principally a matter of biologic begetting, but a broader human function: a man and a wife accepting responsibility to care for and rear a child.[79]

Ethicists from almost every theologic and philosophic persuasion voice strong opposition to donor artificial insemination (AID). With few exceptions, Roman Catholic and Jewish ethicists take exception to this as a legitimate means for overcoming marital infertility. Roman Catholic moralists list the following reasons for their objections: (1) AID violates the marriage contract, in which exclusive, nontransferable, and inalienable rights to each other's bodies for procreative acts are exchanged; (2) it can lead to or at least foster the acceptability of adultery; and (3) it creates a "stud farm" approach to marriage. Jewish ethicists employ similar arguments: "By reducing human generation to stud-farming methods, AID severs the link between the procreation of children and marriage, indispensable to the maintenance of the family as the most basic and sacred unit of human society. It would enable women to satisfy their craving for children without the necessity to have homes and husbands.[45]

Protestant ethicists offer a more diversified point of view. Fletcher,[33] speaking from the situationist-utilitarian point of view, holds that AID does not violate the marriage bond because the mutual agreement of the spouses to permit the use of sperm taken from a third party in no way constitutes a break in conjugal fidelity. Ramsey,[65] however, writing from a deontologist viewpoint, voices strong opposition to such a position. He believes AID illicitly separates that which God joined together: the spheres of personal love and procreation.

The discussion about the morality of AID and AIH will continue, with the key issue being to what extent such practices can disturb or destroy the connection between the unitive and procreative dimensions of marital sexuality. However, it seems proper to conclude that the pro and con arguments in regard to AID have a substantial validity and can be safely followed in practice.

Closely allied to the problem of artificial insemination is the problem of in vitro fertilization. Whereas insemination can be a remedy for male sterility, fertilization can often be offered as a remedy for female infertility. To date there have been several successful attempts at fertilization in this manner, but it is legitimate to suppose that there have also been an even greater amount of failures. Even though the procedure is fairly new, there is abundant ethical literature on the subject. One of the best is a *Commonweal* editorial.

The authors of the editorial identified three possible approaches to the problem. First, they cited the "anathema" approach. This evaluates in vitro fertilization as something morally unthinkable, a gross and depersonalizing interference in the natural reproductive process, and a procedure that places a severe risk on an unborn person, demands a consent that obviously can never be given, and inevitably involves the foreseeable rejection of fertilized ova or even the calculated abortion of defective fetuses. Second, they cited the "assimilation" approach; neither the end nor the means involved in this procedure are drastic departures from what people have already been doing. The end and purpose is an ancient one – to help childless couples to have offspring – and the means employed are merely an extension of the intervention human beings already accept whenever nature proves to be harsh or recalcitrant. Third, they cited the "apprehension" approach; in vitro fertilization will loosen human procreation just that much more from the knot of personal determincy, sexual intimacy, and marital relations. It has great possibilities for moral and social misuse, and it moves human reproduction one more step toward becoming another form of manufacturing.

Having proposed these three approaches to the issue, the editors of *Commonweal* offer a critique of each of them. They found the first approach (anathema) to be too naive about "nature" and too negative toward human control. In addition, they thought it was too unrealistic about risks, too certain about possible abortions, and too dogmatic in its tone. The second approach (assimilation) was labeled as "deluding." The authors believed that its attempt to justify today's developments because they are not much different from yesterday's is to pile ambiguity on ambiguity and to construct a morality based on sand. The third approach (apprehension) seemed to be the most reasonable, and they listed some of the chief sources of their own concern: (1) the loss of zygotes or mini-abortions (one researcher failed in attempts to transfer 200 fertilized ova); (2) the problem of fetal damage and deformity once that transfer has been accomplished, a risk to which the fetus could give no consent; (3) the drift toward donor in vitro fertilization and surrogate wombs; (4) the possibility of viewing the zygote as a "product" and the child as a "consumer item"; (5) the restriction of the issue to purely individual benefits – with limited resources we should not be pouring money into life-creating technologies when other more basic health needs are going unmet; and (6) the publicity given to such cases can lead people to false hopes and thus delay the decision to adopt.

The morality of reproductive technology is far from totally determined, and the weight of contemporary literature on the subject suggests caution. In these matters, as in so many others that influence the pursuit of the *verum humanum,* it is the role of the ethicist to keep asking pertinent and substantial questions. If this is not done seriously, publicly, and continually, there is a real danger that we will end up identifying the humanly and morally good with what is possible technologically.

HIV Screening

The ethical dilemmas between individual liberty and privacy and public health and safety occur in all matters related to HIV infection. For the individual, measures to control the spread of HIV may involve the invasion of privacy; constraints on drug use, sexual conduct, and procreation; and limitations on liberty.[6] Because of the stigmatization of those at risk for AIDS[25] (that is, homosexuals, bisexuals, or drug abusers), confidentiality of screening and counseling is a particular concern.

Cases of HIV infection, as defined by the Centers for Disease Control, are reportable to public health authorities throughout the United States (see Chapter 10). Reporting requirements also vary from state to state.[39,74] In Missouri, for example, all positive test results must be reported to the State Health Department, along with the name, address, and telephone number of the person who has tested positive. Individual clinicians and staff have a duty to keep all aspects of the screening confidential.

Many organizations such as insurance companies, branches of the military, and prisons have mandatory

HIV testing. Some people contend that society has the right to know who is infected and who is at risk. They contend this would increase the knowledge of the development and spread of HIV and eventually improve the efficacy of prevention strategies.

Others contend that routine testing and screening are not in the individual's or public's interest, and the potential consequences (especially discrimination and cost) outweigh the potential benefits from testing asymptomatic persons who lack at risk patterns of behavior.

The informed consent process should include pre- and post-test teaching and counseling so the individual understands the implications and consequences of the testing process. Crisis intervention needs to be provided for individuals who have adverse reactions after being informed of the test results.[74,82] Also, health care providers are subjected to the specific legal requirements. (See Massachusetts General Law 111:70F on p. 131 of this chapter as an example.)

All the questions about HIV testing revolve around one central moral issue: to what extent should the identification of possible carriers and the undertaking of preventive health measures be a matter of private choice and to what extent one of public health responsibility? Ethically, these distinctions should reflect society's concerns for individuals, as well as for the common good.[51,72,82]

CASE STUDIES: A METHOD FOR ETHICAL ANALYSIS

Moral issues, which often seem complex and irresolvable, sometimes leave the nurse overwhelmed, if not paralyzed. Take for example the case of providing teenagers with information about contraception. The issue presents so many competing, almost unreconcilable, interests that some nurses might simply avoid addressing this teenage health issue. The nurse is committed to health promotion and has a long-range vision of the health and socioeconomic effects of teenage pregnancy on both mother and child. Simultaneously, the nurse sees that some parents have other interests that mightily resist anyone outside the family providing information to their children that they find morally objectionable. In these debates, pitting parents, teenagers, and the government against one another, does any means exist for a nurse to sort out the conflict?

Ethical analysis occurs on several levels – those of facts, of values, and of reflection on method[4] (Fig. 6-1). To set the stage for analysis of these three levels, a nurse would first need to ask the question: "What issues must be decided?" For example, in the act of providing teenagers with information on contraception, more than one moral issue needs to be decided. Each subissue will, alone or together, help clarify whether a nurse can offer education about contraception. Who should ultimately decide what information an adolescent receives – the parents, the nurse, the government, or the teenager him or herself? What criteria should be used to balance the health prerogative of the adolescent with the interests of the parents to raise a teenager as they see fit? To what extent, if ever, should the common good of society prevail over the rights of the parents?

1. GATHER AND ASSESS FACTS
   - A. What facts do you see as important?
   - B. What facts are needed?
2. IDENTIFY AND CHARACTERIZE THE VALUES IN CONFLICT
   - A. What values are in conflict? (Autonomy vs. Beneficence)
   - B. How can each of the values be characterized?
   - C. What are the general rules associated with these values? (i.e., the patient is the primary decider in health care)
   - D. Is there any stronger justification for one or another value?
3. NAME AND EVALUATE THE METHOD
   - A. What method of ethics do you use to resolve your problem? (Emotivism, divine commands, legalism, etc.)
   - B. Do different theories arrive at similar or dissimilar answers?

Fig. 6-1. Ethics work-up.

Gather and Assess Facts

A careful examination of questions at various levels of ethical consideration might expiditiously resolve any moral conflicts. For example, it would be important to examine whether all facts have been gathered and assessed. For initiating a teenage education program on contraceptives, for example, although the list is not exhaustive, the following questions might be relevant:

- Does the nurse see positively what part of the content is creating the conflict?
- Are there any alternatives to providing teenagers with sensitive information?
- Are any alternatives conflict free?
- If not, which education options are most effective in reducing teenage pregnancy?
- What are the risks of not offering the education program?
- What programs have other health promoters in similar circumstances elected to employ?
- What are the views of parents in a given region of the country about providing teens with this information?
- What are the parents' cultural and religious perspectives?
- Other than the parents and the adolescents, who else will be affected by employing a health promotion strategy?

In some cases, facts alone might resolve the conflict. For example, under the assumption that a nurse would be required to utilize her or his time only on programs proven to show some benefit, it would be important for the nurse to establish which information program is likely to work. If, for example, only one is proven effective, this fact will surely indicate which moral course of action to follow. More frequently, the relevant facts – such as the effectiveness of an education program – will be unclear. Nurses may be compelled to act by circumstances beyond their control, but it is preferable that they attempt to identify the facts to the extent possible in order to claim they have done a morally adequate analysis.

Identify and Characterize Values

At the values level, a nurse must identify and characterize the ethical values in conflict. Sometimes the conflict may be a communication problem or an administrative or legal uncertainty rather than a genuine clash of values. In the case of providing contraceptive information to teenagers, values will pull in opposing directions. The value of protecting the health of the adolescent who could become pregnant, the so-called value of "beneficence," pulls in favor of providing education. The value of autonomy or self-determination also has a bearing on this case as one honors a teenager's ability to consent to a health promotion strategy. There is also the value society might have in wanting to avoid an unwanted pregnancy that can carry with it social and economic costs. Pulling in the opposite direction are the value of allowing parents to direct and control a child's education and the value of resisting promiscuity. None of these values is likely to be a sufficient justification for a given course of action. Even so, the moral analysis at the values level includes clarifying the meaning of specific value concepts. The term *beneficent,* for example, is ambiguous. There is little shared understanding about whose perspective should be used to judge beneficence – that of the nurse who is committed to avoiding teenage pregnancy or that of the parents who want to direct the moral education of their offspring? Also beneficence – "doing good for others" – can mean, from one perspective, considerate, respectful, and compassionate care. Therefore, part of the analysis will entail characterizing a concept and estimating whether there is any consensus in society on the concept. A good place to start is by looking to national consensus statements on ethics, such as those of the President's Commission for the Study of Medicine and Biomedical and Behavioral Research[61] and the American Nurses' Association codes of ethics.[1]

Name and Evaluate Method

Once the values in conflict have been identified and characterized, it is sometimes obvious which value or competing interest prevails. Ethical and legal consensus, as found in the president's commission, for example, might prefer one value to another; and this is a solid indicator that good reasons favor acting in accord with the regarded value. At times, however, no clear value preference exists, and a nurse must identify alternative courses of action. Each strategy would be evaluated to determine its consistency with moral values. In particular, strategies must be judged to determine which most minimizes damage to cherished values.

Even when reasonable people reasonably disagree over alternative courses of action, ethical analysis continues. Clarity can be gained by moving to a final level of ethical analysis – the level of ethical method. This level of analysis focuses on the method nurses use to select the values in conflict. For example, did the nurse use his or her emotions, intuitions, a divine command, prevailing social opinion, a code, or the course of action that produced the greatest good for the greatest number in society? These methods are theories our conscience employs; and while there is no agreed-upon method employed by all, nonetheless some methods are more acceptable than others because they are open to rational argumentation.

THE ETHICS OF HEALTH PROMOTION: CASES

The approach included here is not an attempt to offer an exhaustive set of cases that a health promotion nurse will confront. Rather, cases are selected from representative situations that provide insight into the common features a nurse confronts in daily practice.

Case 1: The Limits of Health Promotion

Marsha works for an HMO in the far Northwest, and her nursing responsibilities include monitoring and addressing preventive health needs of patients identified as at risk by an institutional assessment scale. As individual HMO patients are identified as being at higher risk for preventable disease, she must, on those patients' next several visits, take time to persuade them to make lifestyle changes. Recently, a patient, Ms. Jones, told her HMO primary care physician that she resented being required to spend the first 15 minutes of her visit with that "preachy nurse, Marsha." Ms. Jones told Marsha that she did not welcome her moralism. She stated she had struggled all her life with moderate obesity and noted that in light of the tension of her recent divorce and fights with her children she was not going to give up the few joys left in her life – chocolate, scotch, and an occasional cigarette.

Marsha is perplexed about how to handle the situation because Ms. Jones seems to come in a pound or two heavier at each visit. Marsha thinks that if she is not relentless she will be negligent and that her nonaction will harm Ms. Jones. But if Marsha persists it will subject Ms.

Jones – already unhappy and stressed – to even more pressure. Marsha ponders the alternatives. Should she simply hand Ms. Jones her institutional profile on the next visit? Or should she exaggerate the future problems of morbidity and morality associated with Ms. Jones's habits in order to gain compliance? Or, if Ms. Jones remains noncompliant, should Marsha use a bluff by threatening to recommend that Ms. Jones be dropped from HMO coverage? If noncompliance endures, should Marsha actually recommend that Ms. Jones be dropped from the HMO because she is too great a health risk for the organization?

PERSONAL RESPONSIBILITY FOR HEALTH

Like most ethical controversies, the case of Marsha poses several separate ethical issues. The fundamental issue here, as in all health promotion cases, is establishing who is responsible for personal health. It might seem obvious to most people that a person is individually responsible for his or her health. Yet actions that involve coercion or behavior modification by a health promoter to entice a client could be viewed to imply that the responsibility for health resides with the health promoter. So who is primarily responsible for promoting personal health? Based on the noncontroversial Golden Rule – "Do unto others as you would have them do unto you" – it could be argued that each person is obligated to care for personal health needs within his or her capability so as not to place undue burdens on others. On this account, Ms. Jones is primarily rseponsible for her health.

AUTONOMY

Marsha's concern about whether she can manipulate the facts or coerce Ms. Jones into a healthy lifestyle raises a second issue, closely tied to issues of autonomy and informed consent. Even if Ms. Jones is personally responsible for her health, should a health provider use every means possible to gain compliance, including bending the truth or applying pressure? A long tradition in Western bioethics and Anglo-American law holds that each competent individual is autonomous, with the capability for self-determination. Practically speaking, this means that competent persons can, without interference, do with their bodies as they please, so long as the interests of others are not harmed.[6] Even outside the health care environment, an individual's choice to act autonomously is respected, and not restrained, because the foundations of a free society demand that each member refrain from trammeling other members' autonomy. If reasons are found to restrict others' self-determination, these same reasons would restrict anyone's self-determination. The obligation to respect others' autonomy is stringent in health care because "the outcome that will best promote the persons' well-being rests on the subjective judgment about the individual."[7] This judgment is best made by the individual and further strengthens obligations to respect an individual's autonomy.

TRUTH-TELLING

In the case of Ms. Jones, autonomy considerations mean that she is free to do what she wants with her health; and to accomplish this, she needs accurate information about the risks and benefits of living different lifestyles. Ms. Jones might be willing to trade long-term health prospects for short-term enjoyment; but to make such a choice she needs a realistic appraisal, not one where the facts have been manipulated by Marsha. More important, Ms. Jones – not Marsha – is the final decision maker as to how she will live. Coercion by Marsha that interferes with Ms. Jones's ability to freely determine which lifestyle to adopt runs at odds with cherished notions of autonomy and informed consent.

ACCESS TO HEALTH CARE

The thorniest moral issue Marsha considers is whether Ms. Jones forfeits her access to HMO care because of noncompliance. Since each person is responsible for his or her health, why should an HMO be responsible for an individual who adopts a risky lifestyle? Part of the answer fits squarely into the long-standing debate over the right to health care in the United States. Specifically, if there is a right to health care, does a patient forfeit that right if she brings illness upon herself? This question is critical for those involved with promoting healthy lifestyles because they will constantly face clients who adopt risky lifestyles, such as driving motorcycles without wearing helmets or cars without fastening seat belts, or practicing unsafe sex in the age of AIDS.

Although public opinion polls indicate that a majority of Americans believe a right to health care exists,[19] philosophers and policy makers have found it difficult to establish such a right. One argument, based on the Golden Rule, suggests that when a patient has exhausted the ability for self-care, society responds by supplying the needed help on the basis that any member of society could find him or herself in like circumstances. Society is not absolved from ensuring this right merely because patients seemingly bring their illness upon themselves, according to the president's commission.[63] Society retains an obligation to ensure access to health care on the basis that it is difficult to prove the patient actually caused her illness; and if forfeiting access to health were institutionalized, then injustice would be created for the ill who never abused their bodies. Nonetheless, the president's commission states that those who consciously adopt unhealthy and risky behavior should avoid unfairly placing the burdens on others in society. Ms. Jones is effectively asking other HMO members to subsidize her risk, yet risk takers should assume a greater burden for the cost of such behavior.

FORFEITING HEALTH CARE?

Marsha finds herself in a moral quandary as to whether to inform the HMO of Ms. Jones's unhealthy lifestyle. Ms. Jones is likely to be dropped, and she will find enrollment in another plan difficult and costly. The ethical analysis hinges on whether private organizations have the responsibility to assume Ms. Jones's risks. Those who would object to the HMO's action assume, in part, that insurers and the HMO have a social responsibility to ensure access to health care. However, the existence of a free market economy in health care makes it difficult to require that private organizations, like HMOs, assume risks greater than those they maintain they can afford.

Case 2: Behavior Modification

Jean works part time as head of an antismoking campaign for a county health department. Her county has endorsed a ban on smoking in public spaces, such as county buildings, train stations, malls, and theaters, to name a few. As part of the campaign, county police have recently cracked down on convenience stores that sell tobacco products to teenagers. Jean is pleased with her public health efforts in the community.

Jean also wears another hat; she substitutes at a visiting nurse association, especially when they are understaffed or overwhelmed with the number of home care clients. One client Jean has been visiting for the past 2 months is Regis, a 62-year-old man. Regis has been a chain smoker all his life. His wife can barely tolerate going into his smoke-filled room, let alone watch her husband smoke. Jean has persuaded her to cut the number of his cigarettes by telling him that only one or two remain. Even in his cognitively impaired state, Regis realizes cigarettes are being withheld, and he protests. Jean believes that they have the perfect opportunity to slowly reduce Regis's daily consumption of cigarettes and that this can further be reenforced with appropriate health education. Since the cost of reduction to Regis is merely emotional irritation, Jean believes she is justified because on balance a stronger public health message about healthy habits is sent to his family and friends who visit.

For some who support the growing surge of antismoking endeavors, Jean's actions pose little ethical conflict. Upon closer inspection, this case's subtleties, especially Jean's humane manipulation, are significant. Behavior modification strategies, central to health promotion, are usually so benign as to rarely be perceived as offensive. The case of Jean focuses the ethical issue on whether there are any limits to such everyday humane manipulation – the coaxing, cajoling, coercing – needed to promote healthy lifestyles. Complicating ethical matters is Regis's cognitive ability.

DETERMINING COMPETENCY

As was established in the case of Marsha, there is an agreed-upon rule of autonomy that competent people can do as they please with their bodies so long as the interests of others are not harmed. Regis's competency complicates the ethical issue. Factually it must be determined to what degree he is competent. Even if Regis is shown to be noncompetent, the problem is more difficult because there is a sizable ethical and legal agreement that caretakers are obligated to follow what the competent patient's wishes would have been.[77]

Is Regis competent? Most clients, in particular the elderly, are presumed to be noncompetent simply because of sensory, functional, or cognitive impairment, with no factual determination of the case. Yet, strong presumption exists in law and ethics that a person is competent until proven otherwise. Even working with this presumption, the more vulnerable the patient becomes, the more likely it is that quick (and probably incomplete) estimation of competence will be made and that the patient will have little strength to object. Surely Jean should not base her estimation of Regis's competency on his agreement with her that nonsmoking is a healthy habit. Many other means of determining noncompetency exist, exceeding the possibility for evaluation here.[71] Nurses can be more certain that they are acting appropriately, though, if they presume patients to be competent and admit only rigorous evaluations of noncompetency before overriding a patient's autonomy.

PROXY DECISION MAKING

Had Regis been shown to be incapacitated, which is not the case, his health care proxy, either someone he appointed or someone who knows him and has his best interests in mind, would be required to make a choice whether to comfort him by assisting his smoking. As preposterous a dilemma as this seems, the issue is driven by ethical obligations of health care agents. When they make decisions for the incapacitated, health care agents are held to one of two decision-making standards: if possible, the decision should accord with the known wishes of the patient, or, where the patient's wishes cannot be known, they should be in harmony with the patient's best interests. Even if preference is given to Regis's wishes, however, no one is ever obligated to participate in actions that he or she finds morally objectionable.

LIMITS TO COERCION

The case of Regis and Jean presents a more pressing ethical issue in health promotion, namely, the limits of behavior modification. The subtle denial, almost negation, of free will by humane manipulation is the locus of ethical concern. A common feature of professional and private life is getting others to do what we want by teasing or taunting, prodding or punishing. Given this very natural and ordinary feature of human life, is it possible to allege truly that some kinds of behavioral modification are morally indefensible? One way to tease apart the issue is to consider free will as separate from the ability to act on it. It is safe to say that all people who cherish freedom would find coercive behavior objectionable. Likewise it is fair to say that in spite of other persons' cajoling, coaxing, and pressuring, individuals are able to choose freely. In Regis's case however, he might retain his free will but be unable to smoke without assistance.

OBLIGATIONS TO THE PROFESSION

Should Regis's wife, or anyone else for that matter, assist him to smoke, given that he is physically unable to do it for himself? Restraining his smoking deprives him of one of his few joys in life, yet smoking creates an unhealthy condition for him and for those who assist him. With growing medical evidence of smoking's ill effects and with a general understanding that there is little more justification for placing our bodies in harm's way for no good reason, then some reason exists to resist smoking or helping others to smoke. As in all ethical questions, reasonable alternatives must be investigated. Should Regis's wife tell him that she and others would not assist because of the secondary smoke, as opposed to manipulating him by telling him she was low on cigarettes? Equally important, if Jean was going to join in the bluffing, perhaps lying, she must be concerned that others will perceive that health promoters are the types of nurses who will bluff, perhaps lie, to accomplish their goals. If the client-nurse relationship is based, in part, on trust that the nurse will tell the truth, then to adopt patterns of deception could undermine this particular relationship and give the impression that health promotion nurses, as a class, are willing to break their trust to meet a goal.

Case 3: Maternal-Fetal Conflicts

Eli, a public health nurse, works in a women's health center in the state of South Carolina, where she cares for Ms. Smith, 26 years old, who is 8 months pregnant with her second child. Ms. Smith has a history of cocaine and alcohol abuse. Roger, her 6-year-old first child, has been found to have fetal alcohol syndrome and is expressing learning disabilities in school. Without success, Eli has tried every strategy possible to dissuade Ms. Smith from abusing drugs during this second pregnancy. Eli wonders whether she should pursue legal means, including having Roger placed in foster care and, for the sake of the fetus, having Ms. Smith charged with child abuse when the child was born for supplying the infant with drugs in utero.

Eli is aware that Jennifer Johnson of Florida was convicted for becoming pregnant while addicted to drugs and carrying the pregnancy to term.[58] Prosecutors argued that Ms. Johnson delivered drugs through the umbilical cord during the 60 to 90 seconds between birth and the time the cord was cut. In the lower court, Ms. Johnson was convicted of two counts of drug delivery but acquitted of child abuse because both children had been unharmed. For the sake of Roger and the unborn child, Eli hates to disrupt the family by a public intervention. Besides, any public intervention, no matter how successful, will jeopardize the client-nurse relationship. What should Eli do?

The number of infants prenatally exposed to cocaine is on the rise; and it will leave in its wake children suffering from long-term effects – strokes, organ malformation, and neurobehavioral impairments. Health care providers are under increased pressure to intervene with prenatal detection and through coercive, sometimes punitive, legal sanctions. This forces health promotion nurses to examine the limits of the intervention to prevent disease. Even when unsure that answers exist, nurses can make some sense of this by examining the subissues.

OBLIGATIONS TO FETUSES

One critical ethical issue that must be addressed is the extent of the obligation of the mother to her fetus. For women who intend to deliver live-born children, strong obligations exist to promote the well-being of the developing fetuses. Regardless of one's view of the moral status of the fetus, the actions during gestation that affect the fetus may have consequences that are manifested throughout a child's life. Most people would consider parents negligent if they did not provide the elements necessary for their offspring to flourish, especially keeping them out of harm's way. Likewise, women who expect to deliver offspring but do not keep them from harm's way – feeding the fetus cocaine and alcohol – can be thought of as negligent. The freedom of the pregnant mother can be limited, among other reasons, by the existence of obligation to others, by the need to avoid personal burdens, and by legal guarantees of liberty and privacy.

THIRD-PARTY INTERVENTION

Another ethical subissue, separate from that of the pregnant woman who fails to promote the interest of the developing fetus, is the issue of whether a third party, such as the nurse or the state, should intervene, and if so, how far? Wide agreement exists that not every act of personal irresponsibility requires outside interference, otherwise most fallible humans would have excessive intervention in their lives. Intervention is sometimes warranted after an appraisal of the burdens and benefits of different courses of action. A rule of thumb is that intervention is more justifiable when the action produces little burden and great benefit to the parties involved. Less justifiable are actions that have grave burdens and minuscule benefit.

In Eli's case, she must first evaluate what harms and benefits will result from nonintervention and from intervention. If Eli continues with the present health education, is it likely to be effective? Is there any evidence that the fetus will be born with health problems even if the education strategy is tried? If Ms. Smith is imprisoned, for example, will it stop her drug use? Will incarceration stop the damage to the fetus, or might the damage already be done?

A second step of ethical analysis must identify the burdens and benefits associated with the values in conflict. For example, overriding her autonomy and liberty rights, including the right to informed refusal for treatment, counts as a burden for Ms. Smith if she is incarcerated. At the same time, while incarceration seems severe, protecting the health of a potential person might be considered a benefit. In this case, it is factually indeterminate whether there will be harm to the fetus or the harm may have already occurred. Therefore, the warrant for intervention – especially the punitive kinds – seem to have less justification than the warrant for refraining.

Case 4: Protecting Innocent Children

In a large East Coast city, public health nurses responsible for the ongoing immunization of children for measles, mumps, and rubella are experiencing terrible resistance from parents in poor sections of the inner city. A recent measles outbreak has claimed the lives of five children and placed another four in the hospital. The deaths affected families who belong to a religious congregation that does not believe in any medical treatment. The pastor preaches divine healing based on the Book of James, which reads, "The prayer of the faithful shall save the sick and the Lord shall raise him up." The parents are asserting that it is their right to practice their religion and raise their children as they see fit. The most pressing problem is whether to force immunization on the small group of unimmunized children who have not yet been exposed to measles.[16,17,22,31] The larger problem is devising a strategy to deal with the growing number of families who, for religious reasons, refuse to have their children immunized.[68,83] The nurses responsible for providing immunization have called a special meeting to discuss the ethical issues involved. What are they, and how would you resolve them?

Nurses at the meeting immediately identified three questions that had to be asked. What are parental rights, and do they extend to refusing immunization for their children? If parents refuse to immunize their children, when, if ever, should a third party intervene? Is refusal of life-sustaining treatment for children on religious grounds justifiable? The first two questions, it should be noted, are not new to health promotion, as evidenced from the previous case of Eli and Ms. Smith's maternal-fetal conflict. The first question concerning parental rights is an extension of the issue of parental responsibility for their offspring. There is broad agreement that parents have the responsibility to provide their children with what is necessary to flourish. At a minimum, that includes keeping children out of harm's way, especially when to do so creates little burden for the parents and great benefit for the child. The complicating matter in this case is a claim of "rights" on the part of the parents.

RIGHTS LANGUAGE

Rights language in health care ethics has been a source of controversy, in part because of the overlegalized tone of the language that tends to preempt extensive ethical discussion. For some, whether the right is provided by law is the only factual determination to be made, and ethical discussion grinds to a halt. One way to think about rights language is to understand corresponding responsibilities of others. One person's right to autonomy and self-determination is another person's responsibility to avoid trammeling liberties by respecting the person as a person. Rights of this kind are called "liberty" rights. More controversial is the concept of "entitlement" rights. A person's right to minimum education or health care can be seen as an entitlement, where the responsibility to provide it devolves on others, on the Golden Rule principle that any of us might find ourselves in need of this basic help some day.

PARENTAL RIGHTS

Parental rights should not be confused with property rights. Parents do not own children in the way that they own chattels. Rather, parental rights confer responsibilities on parents to protect the liberties of children and to ensure that the children receive the basic health care that all persons would want for themselves.[13] Of course, in the continuing battle over the right to health care, the amount of care due to each of us is hotly contested; but there is a broad consensus that health service that is cheap and effective and significantly prolongs life prospects (as is the case with immunization) must be part of a guaranteed minimum. In this case, therefore, there is good reason to maintain that parents who claim the parental right to deny their children basic health care are doing so with weak moral justification, if any at all.[68,83]

STATE INTERVENTION

The second question the nurses explored is when, if ever, a third party should intervene in cases of refusal to immunize. As discussed in the case of Eli and Ms. Smith, not every act of negligence on the part of individuals deserves intervention. As a general rule, if intervention creates little burden for the parents and great benefit for the child, it is warranted; but grave burden to parents and little benefit to the child prohibits action. The nurses must still ask whether the intervention would actually bestow the benefit on the children or could be safely forgone? Although measles immunization might be clearly effective, the nurses agreed that the efficacy of an intervention must be determined before overriding parent's wishes.

Case 5: Sex Education for Teenagers

Marion works as a nurse health promoter for a large school district in a midwestern state that neither requires nor encourages the teaching of prevention of pregnancy or of sexually transmitted disease. Marion realizes that her district is not alone, with nearly one third of states and one fifth of large school districts omitting to teach sex education. She is alarmed because the United States has one of the highest adolescent pregnancy rates in the Western world – each year more than one million teenagers become pregnant, and 50% of these pregnancies resulted in live births.[78]

Marion has raised the possibility of an education program on contraception. A principal at one school she serves emphatically stated that she was not to consider developing a program or even providing teenagers with information about pregnancy prevention. Parents at the school have made it clear: the issue shall not be raised and shall be handled only by parents at home. Marion is most concerned about minority teenagers at this school because they have twice the pregnancy rate of white teenagers.

Marion is torn. On the one hand, professionally she wants to comply with the school district, and as a parent she always fought to retain control over the education of her two children. On the other hand, she understands the consequences of early childbearing. The younger the mother, the greater the likelihood that both mother and child will experience health complications as a result of later prenatal care and other lifestyle factors. Teenage mothers are at greater risk of socioeconomic disadvantage, lower intellectual and academic achievement, and other behavior problems. Given the seriousness of the issue, Marion wonders whether the circumstances dictate that she ignore the wishes of both principal and parents and provide both contraceptive information and, under rare circumstances, contraceptives to teens at risk.

WHAT ARE THE ETHICAL ISSUES?

As Marion begins to sort out the ethical issues, it is important for her to identify the questions that must be answered. Who should ultimately decide what information an adolescent is to receive – the parent, the nurse, the government, or the teenager? What criteria should be used to balance the health interests of the adolescent with the right of the parents to raise a teenager as they see fit? To what extent, if ever, should the common good of society prevail over the interests of the parents?

DECISION MAKING BY MINORS

After Marion has determined parental views and gathered and assessed the relevant facts, such as the effectiveness of various education programs, then she must name and characterize the values at play in this issue. Her first ethical dilemma concerns who should make the final decision about providing information on contraceptives. Marion knows the general ethical consensus about autonomy and informed consent, which implies that competent people can do with their bodies as they please, within the limits imposed by the interests of others. She is perplexed as to whether teenagers are competent to give informed consent. She knows, for example, that the law admits exceptions for emancipated minors and for those who marry before reaching the age of majority. As she searches for a standard to judge who should make the decision, she realizes that the features that characterize informed consent sharpen her ability to analyze the situation. For example, informed consent requires, among other things, that the client be free of coercion and able to understand and appreciate the risk and benefits of all the options.[63] Marion's desire to have a program on contraception has been thwarted by social powers beyond her control, but she believes that some teenagers can make the decision, although at this point in the moral analysis she is not sure she would provide information on contraception.

OVERRIDING PARENTS' WISHES

A second question she must examine has to do with the criteria for balancing teenagers' health interests with the parents' interests. If she refrains from any health intervention, the burden for the teenager is a potential pregnancy or the risk of contracting a sexually transmitted disease – one of which, AIDS, is fatal. If she provides the information, the real (not potential) burden is that of overriding parents' interest. Another point to consider is the harm to the teenagers if the intervention fails and pregnancy or venereal disease occurs. Marion realizes that she is uncertain whether her intervention will actually accomplish the prevention of pregnancy or disease. If she could know with certainty that the intervention would actually benefit the adolescent rather than merely hold out the potential for benefit, she would know she had greater justification. At the moment she is uncertain and looks for more clarity about her dilemma.

THE COMMON GOOD

The last question Marion asks is this: To what extent, if ever, should the common good of society prevail over the interests of parents? Marion is aware of the measles immunization case, and she understands that parental interests or rights stop at the point where they fail to provide the basic health care all children need – otherwise the children would be unfairly disadvantaged from participating in society. She is uncertain, however, whether information about avoiding of venereal disease and pregnancy counts as a basic service to which all people are entitled, including children. Given the protracted conflict in society over sex education, she is not likely to find a consensus on this issue soon. But Marion feels that she must act now. What is she to do with the uncertainty of each of the questions she has examined?

Answered separately, no question points to any clear direction or strategy. Taken together, the answers bring more lucidity to the moral dilemma. For example, if the teenagers asking for information are, in her judgment, able to make informed decisions, if Marion is aware that requesting teenagers are actually or likely to be sexually active, and if no other social means are available to provide a health service, then she would have stronger moral justification to provide information, and perhaps contraceptives under limited circumstances.

This analysis demonstrates that moral questions are usually a set of subissues. Each subissue, alone or together, might go far in resolving the entire moral dilemma, or, like most of life, they might only point in a faint yet perceptible direction. At the completion of the analysis, a nurse might feel ambiguous about the rightness or wrongness of the course of action. However, if nurses have systematically examined the facts, the values, and the methods of ethics, then they can be more assured they have made a morally adequate analysis.

SUMMARY

Perhaps the most crucial theme confronting nurses throughout the ethical issues and decision processes is also the single most serious cause of professional burnout: the perception that nurses, although they have tremendous power over the individual client, over the most intimate details of the client's life, and at times even over life and death, have little power over the health care system to effect changes in the client's best interests.

The nurse has the ethical responsibility to enforce principles of ethics by addressing and acting against injustices in the system and educating peers, clients, legislators, and society in general about changes needed to improve the quality of health care in a cost-effective manner.

A second theme is the day-to-day value conflicts with physicians and health care administrators. As client advocates, nurses are required to challenge, for example, a physician's or administrator's analysis of a client situation, if in their professional judgment the analysis is potentially lethal, dangerous, or counter to the client's best interest. Nurses need to know exactly what to do within and beyond the agency if the conflict with the physician or administrator is irreconcilable. In the end, nurses are ethically and legally responsible for their actions, despite the power of others, including physicians, administrators, and legislators.

Nursing is the study of the whole person and the application of this study in the person's care. The humanization of the whole person is considered by the discipline of ethics. The nurse's level of sensitivity and ability to implement basic ethical principles through the roles of educator, advocate, and enforcer determine the proper approaches to the study and care of the whole person developing higher levels of health.

References

1. American Nurses' Association: *Code for nurses with interpretive statements,* Kansas City, Mo, 1985, The Association.
2. American Nurses' Association: *Human rights guidelines for nurses in clinical and other research,* Kansas City, Mo, 1975, The Association.
3. American Nurses' Association: *Standards of nursing practice,* Kansas City, Mo, Mo, 1972, The Association.
4. Aroskar MA: Community health nurses: their most significant ethical decision-making problems, *Nurs Clin North Am* 24:967-975, 1989.
5. Ashley B, O'Rourke K: *Health care ethics,* St Louis, 1989, Catholic Hospital Association.
6. Bader D, McMillan E: *AIDS – ethical guidelines for healthcare providers,* St Louis, 1987, The Catholic Health Association of the United States.
7. Bai K: *Deontological theories.* In Reich W, editor: *Encyclopedia of bioethics, vol 1,* New York, 1978, Free Press.
8. Bandman E, Bandman B: *Nursing ethics through the lifespan,* ed 2, Norwalk, Conn, 1990, Appleton-Lange.
9. *Basic HHS policy for protection of human research subjects,* Washington, DC, 1981, US Government Printing Office.
10. Beauchamp T, Childress J: *Principles of biomedical ethics,* ed 3, New York, 1989, Oxford University Press.
11. Benjamin M, Curtis J: *Ethics in nursing,* ed 3, New York, 1992, Oxford University Press.
12. Bok S: *The tools of bioethics.* In Reiser S, et al, editors: *Ethics in medicine,* Cambridge, 1977, Massachusetts Institute of Technology.
13. Boyle PJ: AIDS education and parental rights, *SLU Pub Law Rev* 8:45-54, 1988.
14. Braaten C, Braaten L: *The living temple: a practical theology of the body and the foods of the earth,* New York, 1976, Harper & Row.
15. Catholic Hospital Association: *Religious aspects of medical care,* St Louis, 1975, The Association.
16. Clark R: Measles abating, but city might still seek inoculations, *Philadelphia Inquirer,* Feb 23, 1991.
17. Copeland L: Shots urged in warning on measles, *Philadelphia Inquirer,* Dec 7, 1990.
18. Curran C: Theology and genetics: a multi-faceted dialogue, *J Ecumenical Studies* 7:61, 1970.
19. Dauner CD: The race to universal health coverage (summary of 1990 Gallup health poll), *Federation Am Health Systems Rev,* Sept/Oct 1990.
20. Davis A, Aroskar M: *Ethical dilemmas and nursing practice,* ed 3, Norwalk Conn, 1991, Appleton-Lange.
21. Davis A, Krueger J, editors: *Patients, nurses, ethics,* New York, 1980, Ameri-

can Journal of Nursing Publications.
22. Diaz IM: City measles-vaccine plan targets those at highest risk, *Philadelphia Inquirer*, Feb 21, 1991.
23. Downe RS, Fyfe C, Tannahill A: *Health promotion models and values*, New York, 1990, Oxford University Press.
24. Doxiadis S, editor: *Ethical issues in preventive medicine, behavioral and social sciences, no 26*, Dordrecht, The Netherlands, 1985, Martinus Nijhoff.
25. Durham J, Cohen F: *The person with AIDS*, ed 2, New York, 1991, Springer Publishing.
26. Dworkin G: *Paternalism*. In Reiser S, et al, editors: *Ethics in medicine*, Cambridge, 1977, Massachusetts Institute of Technology.
27. Dyck A: *On human care: an introduction to ethics*, Nashville, 1977, Abingdon.
28. Faden R, Beauchamp T: *A history of informed consent*, New York, 1986, Oxford University Press.
29. Feldman D: *Abortion: Jewish perspectives*. In Reich W, editor: *Encyclopedia of bioethics, vol 1*, New York, 1978, Free Press.
30. Fenner K: *Ethics and law in nursing professional perspectives*, New York, 1980, Van Nostrand Reinhold.
31. Fitzgerald S: Epidemic looms, so Philadelphia plans to accelerate measles vaccination, *Philadelphia Inquirer*, Nov 29, 1990.
32. Fitzpatrick FJ: *Ethics in nursing practice: basic principles and their application*, London, 1988, The Linacre Centre.
33. Fletcher J: Ethical aspects of genetic controls, *N Engl J Med* 285:776, 1983.
34. Fletcher J: *The ethics of genetic control*, Buffalo, NY, 1988, Prometheus Books.
35. Frankena W: *Ethics*, ed 2, Englewood Cliffs, NJ, 1973, Prentice Hall.
36. Fry S: Accountability in research: the relationship of scientific and humanistic values, *Adv Nurs Sci* 20:32, 1981.
37. Gibbons W, editor: *Pacem in terris—encyclical letter of His Holiness Pope John XXIII*, New York, 1963, Paulist Press.
38. Glaser J: Conscience and the superego, *Theological Studies* 32:30, 1971.
39. Gong V, Rudnick N: *AIDS—facts and issues*, New Brunswick, NJ, 1991, Rutgers University Press.
40. Gray B: *Human subjects in medical experimentation: a sociological study of the conduct and regulation of clinical research*, New York, 1981, John Wiley & Sons.
41. Gula R: *What are they saying about moral norms?*, New York, 1982, Paulist Press.
42. Gustafson J: *Genetic engineering and the normative view of the human*. In Williams PN, editor: *Ethical issues in biology and medicine*, Cambridge, 1978, Schenkman.
43. Haering B: *Medical ethics*, Notre Dame, Ind, 1973, Fides.
44. Hauerwas S: *Toward an ethics of character*. In *Vision and virtue*, Notre Dame, Ind, 1974, Fides.
45. Jakobovitz I: *Jewish medical ethics*, ed 2, New York, 1975, Bloch.
46. Jonas H: *Philosophical reflections on experimenting with human subjects*. In Reiser S, et al, editors: *Ethics in medicine*, Cambridge, 1977, Massachusetts Institute of Technology.
47. Ladd J: *The task of ethics*. In Reich W, editor: *Encyclopedia of bioethics, vol 1*, New York, 1978, Free Press.
48. Lanik G, Webb AA: Ethical decision making for community health nurses, *J Community Health Nurs* 6:95-102, 1989.
49. Lauer E, Mlecko J: *A Christian understanding of the human person*, New York, 1982, Paulist Press.
50. Leininger M: *Ethical and moral dimensions of care*, Detroit, 1990, Wayne St University Press.
51. Levine C, Bayer R: Screening blood: public health and medical uncertainty, *Hastings Center Report* 15:8, 1985.
52. McCormick R: Notes on moral theology: the abortion dossier, *Theological Studies* 35:312, 1974.
53. McLeroy KR, Gottlieb N, Burdine J: The business of health promotion: ethical issues and professional responsibilities, *Health Educ Q* 14:91-109, 1987.
54. Munhall P: Nursing philosophy and nursing research: an apposition or opposition, *Nurs Res* 31(3):40, 1982.
55. Murphy C, Hunter H: *Ethical problems in the nurse-patient relationship*, Boston, 1982, Allyn & Bacon.
56. Nuremberg Code, Readings, Hastings & Hudson Institute of Society, Hastings on Hudson, NY, 1948, Ethics & Life Sciences.
57. Ozonoff V, Ozonoff D: On helping those who help themselves, *Hastings Center Report* 7:7-10, 1977.
58. Paltrow LM: When becoming pregnant is a crime, *Criminal Justice Ethics* 9(1): 41-49, 1990.
59. Pence T, Cantrall J: *Ethics in nursing: an anthology*, New York, 1990, National League for Nursing.
60. Perkins R: Perspectives on the public good, *Am J Public Health* 71:3, 1981.
61. President's Commission for the Study of Ethical Problems in Medicine and Biomedical and Behavioral Research: *Making health care decisions: the ethical and legal implications of informed consent in the patient-practitioner relationship, vol 1*, Washington, DC, 1982, US Government Printing Office.
62. President's Commission for the Study of Ethical Problems in Medicine and Biomedical and Behavioral Research: *Report: 1982, making health care decisions, vol 1*, Washington, DC, 1982, US Government Printing Office.
63. President's Commission for the Study of Ethical Problems in Medicine and Biomedical and Behavioral Research: *Securing access to health care: the ethical implications of differences in the availability of health services, vol 1*, Washington, DC, 1983, US Government Printing Office.
64. Ramsey P: *Genetic therapy: a theologian's response*. In Hamilton MP, editor: *The new genetics and the future of man*, Grand Rapids, Mich, 1972, Eerdmans.
65. Ramsey P: *Parenthood and the future of man*. In *Fabricated man*, New Haven, Conn, 1970, Yale University Press.
66. Rawls J: *Justice as fairness*. In Reiser S, et al, ediitors: *Ethics in medicine*, Cambridge, 1977, Massachusetts Institute of Technology.
67. Reich W, editor: *Encyclopedia on bioethics*, New York, 1978, Free Press.
68. Religious exemptions to child neglect laws still being passed despite convictions of parents, *JAMA* 264(10):1226-1233, 1990.
69. Robertson J: *Reproductive theologies: legal aspects*. In Reich W, editor: *Encyclopedia of bioethics, vol 4*, New York, 1978, Free Press.
70. Ruthmann M: Celebrating leisure today, *Review of Religions* 23(2):37-41, 1973.
71. Shaw A: *Dilemmas of informed consent*. In Hunt R, Arras J, editors: *Ethical issues in modern medicine*, ed 2, Palo Alto, Calif, 1988, Mayfield.
72. Shilts R: *And the band played on*, New York, 1987, St Martin's Press.
73. Shinn R: *Gene therapy: ethical issues*. In Reich W, editor: *Encyclopedia of bioethics, vol 2*, New York, 1978, Free Press.
74. Silverman M, Silverman D: AIDS and the threat to public health, *Hastings Center Report* 15:19, 1985.
75. Smith SA, Davis AJ: Ethical dilemmas: conflicts among rights, duties, and obligations, *Am J Nurs* 80:1463, 1980.
76. Spector R: *Cultural diversity in health and illness*, ed 3, New York, 1991, Appleton-Century-Crofts.
77. Stanley B, et al: The functional competency of elderly at risk, *Gerontologist* 28(suppl):53-58, 1988.
78. *Teenage sexual and reproductive behavior, facts in brief*, Albany, 1990, Alan Guttmacher Institute.
79. Vatican Congregation for the Doctrine of the Faith: *Instruction on respect for human life in its origin and the dignity for its procreation*, Feb 22, 1987.
80. Veatch RM, Fry ST: *Case studies in nursing ethics*, Philadelphia, 1987, JB Lippincott.
81. Watson G: Helmet use, helmet use laws, and motorcyclist fatalities, *Am J Public Health* 71:3, 1981.
82. Wold J: AIDS testing, an ethical question, *J Neuroscience Nurs* 22:258, 1990.
83. Young R: *In the interests of children and adolescents*. In Aiken W, LaFollette H, editors: *Whose child? Children's rights, parental authority and state power*, Totawa, NJ, 1980, Littlefield, Adams.

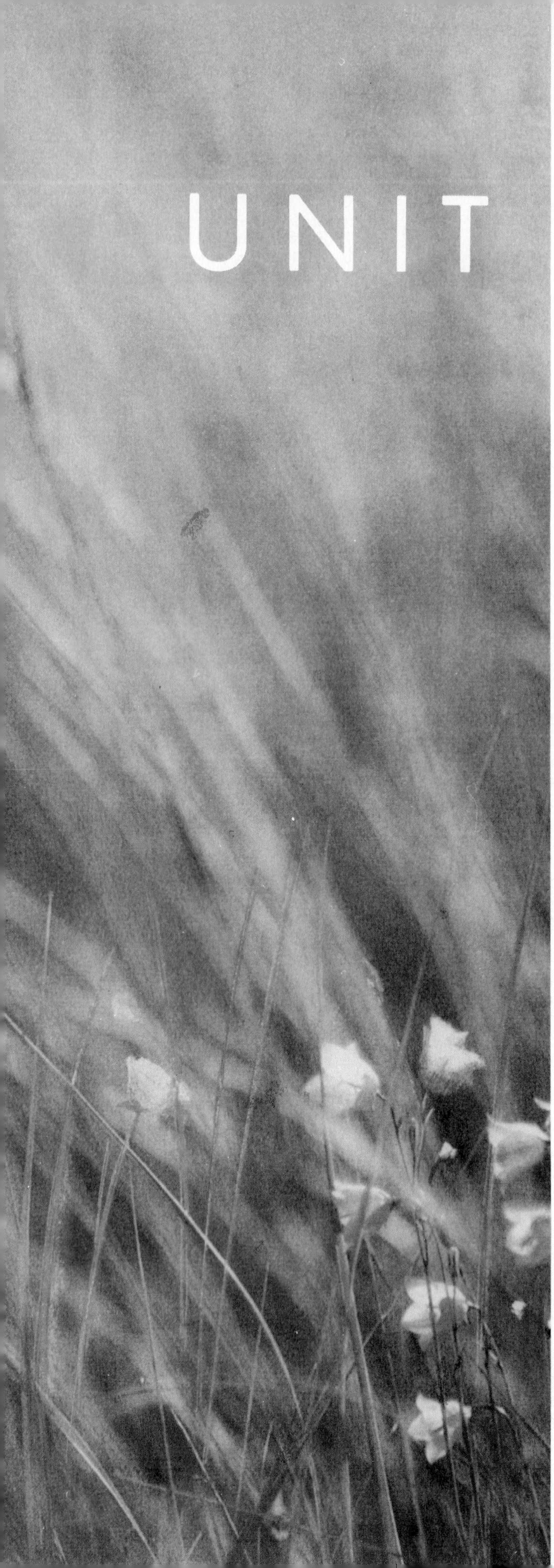

UNIT TWO

Assessment for Health Promotion

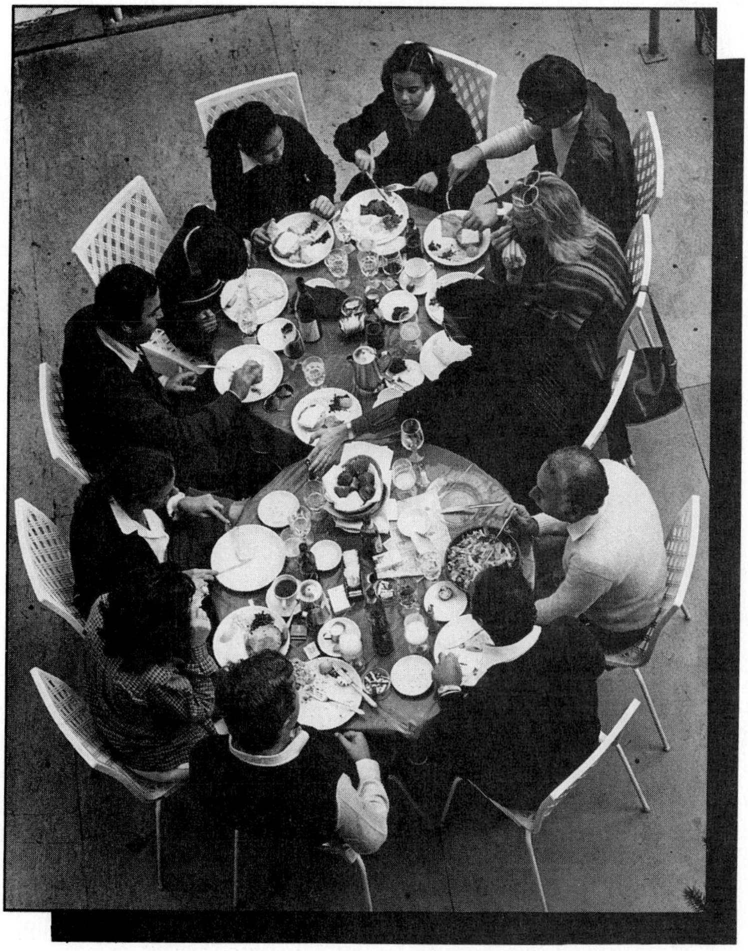

CHAPTER

7

Health Promotion and the Individual*

Carol Lynn Mandle

Rosemary Gruber-Wood

Objectives

After completing this chapter, the nurse will be able to

- *Define the framework of functional health patterns as described by Gordon.*
- *Describe the use of the functional health pattern framework in assessing the individual throughout the lifespan.*
- *Give examples of the clinical data to be collected within each health pattern.*
- *Give examples of the following categories of behavioral changes within the health patterns: (1) functional, (2) potentially dysfunctional, and (3) actually dysfunctional.*
- *Describe aspects to consider while identifying the risk factors or etiologic factors of actually or potentially dysfunctional health patterns.*
- *Discuss planning, implementing, and evaluating nursing interventions in health promotion with the individual.*
- *Develop a specific health-promotion plan based on an assessment of an individual, nursing diagnosis, and contributing risk or etiologic factors.*

This unit presents patterns of behaviors displayed by individuals, families, and communities and provides guidelines for health assessment in multiple practice arenas. The determination of growth and development within each behavioral pattern is introduced in this unit but is fully expanded and specified to each developmental phase within the chapters of Unit Four.

Although the nurse's role has evolved over time, a central unifying theme links all definitions, philosophies, and frameworks of nursing. From Nightingale's belief that the laws of health and nursing are the same and pertinent for both the well and the sick individual to current conceptual frameworks for nursing, health promotion continues to be an integral component.[39] The American Nurses' Association (ANA) defines the practice of nursing as the performance of services using the nursing process in (1) promoting and maintaining health; (2) case finding and managing illness, injury, or infirmity; (3) restoring optimal functioning; or (4) helping the patient achieve a dignified death.[2,4] Although this definition was designed to provide a model for state nursing practice acts, the familiar terminology in the ANA social policy statement is more concise: "Nursing is the diagnosis and treatment of human responses to actual or potential health problems."[2,3,59] These responses are delineated into health-restoring responses (reactions to health problems, as illness) and health-supporting responses (concerns about potential

*Sections of this chapter are adapted from the curriculum for the Adult Health Masters Program, Boston College, Chestnut Hill, Mass; and Gordon M: *Nursing diagnosis: process and application,* ed 2, New York, 1987, McGraw-Hill.

health problems, as susceptibility to illness).[2]

Based on such a definition, primary prevention is a crucial element of nursing and includes generalized health promotion as well as specific protection against disease. This concept of health promotion connotes an active process involving specific protection (immunizations, occupational safety, environmental control) along with a lifestyle, value and belief system, and a set of behaviors that enhance health. Chapter 1 describes the health of any individual, family, or community as a sustainable balance involving complex responses between internal physiologic and psychologic systems and the external environment. The nurse needs a framework to assess this interaction among a person's biophysical state, psychosocial makeup, and the environment.

With health promotion serving as the underlying theme, this chapter focuses on the nursing assessment of the individual. The framework used for assessment is the functional health patterns described by Gordon, as mentioned in previous chapters and redefined here. This same framework is used throughout this unit to demonstrate assessment approaches to the family and community as well (Chapters 8 and 9). This chapter also discusses components of the nursing process as they relate to health promotion for the individual. This is possible only through a clear understanding of the functional health pattern framework.

ASSESSMENT OF THE INDIVIDUAL

Nursing assessment aims at determining the health status of the client. Table 7-1 demonstrates the aspects common to a "good" nursing assessment. Assessment here refers to collection of data only, although an artificial component separation – diagnosis or problem identification – is considered separately for clarity. This follows guidelines proposed by Bloch[8] and used in the ANA Standards of Care.[4] Assessment of health status must consider not only physiologic parameters, but the entire biopsychosocial being interacting with the environment. Patterns of behaviors, beliefs, perceptions, and values are essential components of a health (nursing) assessment if the maximal health potential of the individual is to be realized. Understanding patterns is basic to understanding the health of an individual.[12,57,58,67]

Gordon has taken a set of health-related behaviors, that have been traditional concerns of nursing* and developed an assessment framework of 11 functional health patterns.[30] Functional patterns interact to make up an individual's lifestyle. The nurse, using such a framework, combines assessment skills with subjective and objective data to construct patterns reflective of that lifestyle.

*References 1, 6, 42, 47, 53, and 73.

***Table 7-1.* Aspects of a nursing assessment**

Definition	Deliberate and systematic data collection
Components	Subjective data: health history—subjective reports and client perceptions Objective data Observations of nurse Findings of physical examination Information from health record Results of clinical testing
Function	Description of client's health status
Structure	Organization of interdependent parts describing health, function, or patterns of behavior that reflect the "whole" individual and environment
Process	Interview, observation, and examination
Format	Systematic but flexible; individualized to client, nurse, and situation
Goal	Nursing diagnosis or problem identification To identify areas of strengths, limitations, alterations, responses to alterations and therapies, and risks

This section expands on functional health patterns assessment as a framework and the assessment process using this framework. Each pattern is presented and includes

1. Definition of the pattern
2. Significance of the pattern to the individual's lifestyle, including developmental focus and environmental influences when appropriate
3. Assessment objectives
4. Assessment parameters for the health history
5. Pattern indicators within the physical examination
6. Implications for practice, including specific examples for clarification

Functional Health Pattern Framework

The wholeness of the person and the totality of the person's interactions with the environment are the philosophic foundations of this textbook. They are also the perspective of Gordon's typology of 11 functional health patterns, which provide a mechanism for data collection that encompasses the entire person and all the life processes. By examining the specific functional patterns and the interaction between patterns, the nurse can accurately determine and diagnose actual or potential problems, intervene more effectively, and achieve outcomes that promote health and well-being.[28-31] In addition to providing a framework for assessing individuals, families, and communities, the functional health patterns provide a diagnostic framework. (See box on pp. 87-88 in Chapter 4.)

***Table 7-2.* Typology of 11 functional health patterns**

Pattern	Description
Health perception and health management	Client's perceived health and well-being and how health is managed
Nutritional and metabolic	Food and fluid consumption relative to metabolic need and indicators of local nutrient supply
Elimination	Excretory function (bowel, bladder, skin)
Activity and exercise	Exercise, activity, leisure, and recreation
Sleep and rest	Sleep, rest, and relaxation
Cognitive and perceptual	Sensory-perceptual and cognitive patterns
Self-perception and self-concept	Self-concept pattern and perceptions of self (body comfort, body image, feeling state)
Role and relationship	Role engagements and relationships
Sexuality and reproductive	Client's satisfaction and dissatisfaction with sexuality; reproduction
Coping and stress tolerance	General coping pattern and effectiveness in stress tolerance
Value and belief	Values, beliefs (including spiritual), or goals that guide choices or decisions

Adapted from Gordon M: *Nursing diagnosis: process and application,* ed 2, New York, 1987, McGraw-Hill; and Gordon M: *Manual of nursing diagnosis: 1993-1994,* St Louis, 1993, Mosby.

DEFINITION

Functional health patterns are an interrelated group of behavioral areas that provide a view of the whole individual. The typology of 11 patterns serves as a useful tool to collect and organize the assessment data and creates a mechanism for verifying information with the client or relaying it to other nurses and members of the health care team.

Each pattern, briefly described in Table 7-2, is a biopsychosocial expression of the whole person. Client reports and nursing observations provide the data for describing the patterns. As a framework for assessment, functional health patterns provide an effective means for the nurse to perceive and record the complex interactions of a person's biophysical state, psychologic makeup, and relationship to the environment.

CHARACTERISTICS

Functional health patterns are characterized by the focus. Four areas of focus have been identified: pattern, client-environmental, developmental, and functional.

Pattern focus implies that the nurse explores patterns or sequences of behavior over time. Gordon's use of the term *behavior* encompasses biophysical, psychologic, sociologic, and any other classification of behavior.[29] The recognition of a pattern by the nurse is a cognitive process that occurs during information collection. As information is collected, a pattern emerges that represents historic and current behavior over time. This is easiest when behavior or information is quantifiable, as with blood pressure, and is facilitated when baseline data are available for the individual. Patterns within patterns are developed and assessed. Blood pressure, for example, is a pattern within the activity and exercise pattern. The individual baseline and subsequent readings may present a pattern within expected norms. Erratic blood pressure measurements indicate absence of pattern; this lack of pattern forms a type of pattern in itself. The categories of functional health provide a structure for analyzing a factor *within* a category (blood pressure: activity pattern) and also provide a structure to focus the search for causal explanations, usually *outside* the category (excess sodium intake: nutritional pattern).[30]

The concept of *client-environmental focus* can be demonstrated by food intake. According to systems theory, anything external to the individual is considered environment. Although reference is made within many patterns to environmental influence, it often refers to the physical environment. Common to each functional health pattern are environmental influences such as family values and society mores. Food intake of the individual is governed by personal preference, knowledge of food preparation, and ability to consume and retain food, as well as by cultural and family habits, financial ability to secure the food, and crop availability. For many, especially children, nutritional intake is governed by another who secures, prepares, and serves the food, such as the mother or father.

Human growth and a *developmental focus* are reflected in each pattern. The previous discussion of health addressed the complex interaction between biopsychosocial systems of the individual and the environment. One of the main influences on this dynamic interaction is the development of the person. Fulfillment of developmental tasks increases the complexity of the components and interactions of health. These tasks, however, also provide learning opportunities for the individual to maintain and improve health. Bruhn and others[13] have suggested specific health tasks for the individual to accomplish at each developmental phase of the life cycle, as identified by Erikson[25] and Havighurst[34] and presented in Table 7-3. The learning of these tasks begins at birth and continues to the end of

***Table 7-3.* Relationship between selected developmental tasks and wellness tasks for each stage of life cycle**

Erikson's eight life stages[25]	Havighurst's developmental tasks[34]	Examples of minimal wellness tasks for each developmental stage[13]
1. Infancy (trust versus basic mistrust)	Learning to walk Learning to take solid foods Learning to talk Learning to control elimination of body waste	Acquiring ability to perform psychomotor skills Learning functional definition of health Learning social and emotional responsiveness to others and to physical environment
2. Early childhood (autonomy versus shame and doubt)	Learning sex difference and sexual modesty Achieving physiologic stability Forming simple concepts of social physical reality Learning to relate emotionally to parents, siblings, and others Learning to distinguish right and wrong and developing a conscience	Learning about proper foods, exercise, and sleep Learning dental hygiene Learning injury prevention (safety belts and helmets, sunscreen, smoke detectors, poisons, firearms, swimming)
	Learning physical skills necessary for ordinary games	Refining psychomotor and cognitive skills
3. Late childhood (initiative versus guilt)	Building wholesome attitudes toward self as a growing organism Learning to get along with peers	Developing self-concept Learning attitudes of competition and cooperation with others Learning social, ethical, and moral differences and responsibilities
4. Early adolescence (industry versus inferiority)	Learning appropriate masculine or feminine role Developing fundamental skills in reading, writing and calculating Developing concepts necessary for everday living Developing conscience, morality, and scale of values Achieving personal independence Developing attitudes toward social groups and institutions	Learning that health is important value Learning self-regulation of physiologic needs—sleep, rest, food, drink, and exercise Learning risk taking and its consequences (injury prevention)
5. Adolescence (identity versus role confusion)	Achieving new and more mature relations with peers of both sexes Achieving masculine or feminine social role Accepting physique and using body effectively Achieving emotional independence of parents and other adults Achieving assurance of economic independence Selecting and preparing for occupation Preparing for marriage and family life Developing intellectual skills and concepts necessary for civic competence Desiring and achieving socially responsible behavior	Learning economic responsibility Learning social responsibility for self and others (preventing pregnancy and sexually transmitted diseases) Experiencing social, emotional, and ethical commitments to others Accepting self and physical development Reconciling discrepancies between personal health concepts and observed health behaviors of others (use of alcohol, drugs, tobacco, firearms, violence) Learning to cope with life events and problems (suicide prevention) Considering life goals and career plans and acquiring necessary skills to reach goals Learning importance of time to self and world
6. Early adulthood (intimacy versus isolation)	Selecting, learning to live with mate Starting a family; managing a home Taking on civic responsibility	Committing to mate and family responsibilities Selecting a career Incorporating health habits into lifestyle
7. Middle adulthood (generativity versus stagnation)	Accepting, adjusting to physiologic changes Achieving adult social responsibility Maintaining economic standard of living Assisting teenage children	Accepting aging self and others Coping with societal pressures Recognizing importance of good health habits Reassessing life goals periodically

Continued.

***Table 7-3.* Relationship between selected developmental tasks and wellness tasks for each stage of life cycle – cont'd**

Erikson's eight life stages[25]	Havighurst's developmental tasks[34]	Examples of minimal wellness tasks for each developmental stage[13]
8. Maturity (ego integrity versus despair)	Adjusting to decreasing physical strength and health Adjusting to retirement and reduced income Adjusting to death of spouse Establishing an explicit affiliation with own age group Establishing satisfactory physical living arrangements	Becoming aware of tasks to health and adjusting lifestyle and habits to cope with risks Adjusting to loss of job, income, and family and friends through death Redefining self-concept Adjusting to changes in personal time and new physical environment Adjusting to previous health habits to current physical and mental capabilities

Adapted from Bruhn J, et al: *J Comm Health* 2:215-217, 1977; *Guide to clinical preventive services. An assessment of the effectiveness of 169 interventions.* Report of the US Preventive Services Task Force, Baltimore, 1989, Williams & Wilkins; and *Healthy people 2000: national health promotion and disease prevention objectives*, US Department of Health and Human Services Pub No PHS 91-50213, 1992, Public Health Service.

the lifespan. Developmental focus and influence is included in the pattern areas to follow. Unit Four explores each of these developmental tasks and the related learning and practice of these health behaviors resulting from appropriate nursing interventions for health promotion.

The last area of focus, *functional focus,* refers to the individual's functional level, a traditional area of concern to nursing. Other disciplines examine functional patterns, but the assessment data vary. Genitourinary functions for medicine imply frequency or voiding patterns, and characteristics of urine such as color, odor, and laboratory analysis. In addition to these factors, nursing assesses how the particular voiding pattern affects the person's lifestyle, especially the effect of frequency on sleep patterns and the ability to carry out desired activities such as shopping or socialization patterns. Additional concerns might include whether the individual is able to walk or climb stairs to the bathroom or manage such activities safely at night.

RATIONALE FOR USE

As evidenced in the discussion of characteristics, the focus is certainly *health oriented.* The patterns themselves may be categorized under classifications of behavior familiar to nurses.

The biologic and physiologic classification includes (1) nutritional and metabolic patterns, (2) elimination patterns, (3) activity and exercise patterns, and (4) sleep and rest patterns. The psychosocial classification encompasses (1) role and relationship patterns, (2) self-perception and self-concept patterns, (3) coping and stress-tolerance patterns, and (4) value and belief patterns. Still other patterns may represent a combination of both physiologic and psychosocial aspects: (1) health perception and health management pattern, (2) sexuality and reproductive pattern, and (3) cognitive and perceptual pattern.

The importance of this basic information to health promotion has long been established. The results of a study by the Commission on Chronic Illness indicate areas or components of healthful living,[18] as listed in the box on p. 159. Beland and Passos add "a system of values that serves as a guide to action" (value and belief) to the list.[7]

Despite the classification of data elicited, the information collected is *basic.* Various theoretic or conceptual frameworks of nursing collect the same data, variations exist in the interpretation of the data and the interventions used to achieve the desired outcomes. Thus, the assessment structure (functional health pattern framework) is relevant to all conceptual models.

A distinct advantage in the use of functional health patterns is that they are concise and easily learned. Whereas repeated use facilitates learning, the nurse who is just beginning to use functional health patterns for assessment may find an acronym (Schrevsnacs) or mnemonic sentence ("However, Never Expect Anticipated Solutions," Cautioned Sister Rose, "Since Cooperation Varies") useful. Once the 11 terms are committed to memory, they serve as a guideline for assessment and for retrieving from memory the specific items to be assessed in each area.

Other advantages of a functional health pattern framework specific to the practice of nursing include the following:

1. The structure provides a means of collecting, organizing, presenting, and analyzing data to arrive at a nursing, not a medical, diagnosis, as well as providing a consistent nursing focus.
2. The format is flexible and can be tailored to the client, the situation, or the nurse.
3. The information collected is suitable to any arena of practice, whether in the home, clinic, or institution and whether assessing the individual (adult or child), family, or community.

Theoretic components of nursing (education and research) are also facilitated with use of functional health patterns. The student or researcher is able to

❑ ❑ COMPONENTS OF HEALTHFUL LIVING

Nutrition—adequate, safe, and well-distributed food supplies as well as appropriate levels of personal nutrition. (Nutritional and metabolic)

Mental hygiene—beginning at an early age, it is important that the individual develop an equanimity in the face of the natural and inevitable frustrations of living, an appreciation of the values of family life, and an acceptance of self and limitations. (Coping and stress tolerance, role and relationship, self-perception and self-concept)

Adequate housing—proper safeguards against accidents for persons of all ages, particularly safeguards for children, the aged, and the handicapped. (Health management)

Moderate and well-balanced personal habits—restraints in use of alcohol and tobacco, sufficient rest and appropriate amount of exercise, careful attention to personal hygiene. (Health management, sleep and rest, activity and exercise, elimination)

Useful and productive role in society. (Role and relationship, sexual and reproductive)

General education and education specifically for health. (Cognitive and perceptual)

Recreation—access to recreational opportunities and facilities and proper balancing of recreational activities against satisfying work. (Activity and exercise, role and relationship)

Sense of personal security—related to access to health services, legalized provisions for minimum wages and some sort of job security, and provision for income maintenance during illness or following retirement. (Health perception and health management, self-perception and self-concept, role and relationship)

Adapted from Commission on Chronic Illness: *Chronic illness in the US, vol 1, Prevention of chronic illness*, Cambridge, 1957, Harvard University Press.

NOTE: Associated functional health patterns are in parentheses.

- Organize clinical knowledge in a way relevant to the nursing diagnosis
- Gain advanced knowledge of client problems amenable to nursing care and of diagnosis-specific interventions and outcomes
- Identify areas in which knowledge in nursing requires expansion

Note that medical science is incorporated into but is not the focus for organizing clinical knowledge.

The Patterns

Each pattern is a biopsychosocial expression of the individual and should reflect lifestyle or life processes from both the client's and the nurse's perspective. In addition, it should reflect (1) a pattern or sequencing of behaviors, (2) the role of the environment (physical environs and family, societal, and cultural influences), and (3) any influences of a developmental nature.

The assessment of each pattern as functional, dysfunctional, or potentially dysfunctional should include an indication of the client's satisfaction with the pattern. Any problems reported should be further assessed to include the client's explanation of the problem, remedial actions taken, and the perceived effect of these actions.

A major goal in assessing each pattern is to determine the client's knowledge of health promotion, the ability to manage health-promoting activities, and the value the individual ascribes to health promotion.

This section develops each pattern in sufficient detail to allow the nurse to use a functional health pattern framework for assessment and diagnosis in the clinical practice of nursing. Since it is also helpful to understand the role each pattern plays in the individual's life and the nurse's practice, there will be a discussion of individual significance and nursing implications.

HEALTH PERCEPTION AND HEALTH MANAGEMENT

This pattern provides an overview of the client's health status and health practices employed to reach the current level of health or wellness. The focus is on the perceived health status and the importance placed on health, along with the client's level of commitment to maintaining health. While eliciting information of this sort, it is likely that areas will be introduced that need further exploration under another functional health pattern. For example, if a client says it is no longer possible to mow the lawn without becoming short of breath or suffering severe back pain, this information is stored and retrieved when assessing the activity and exercise pattern or the cognitive perceptual pattern.

The importance of this pattern area to individuals is apparent. If clients do not perceive that health problems are present, are unaware of necessary health promotion in the absence of problems, or feel that they are capable of managing their own health or that any activity on their part is useless in promoting health, their lifestyles and ability to function will most certainly be affected. Health-promoting activities (adequate nutrition, activity and exercise, sleep, and rest), routine professional examinations, self-examinations, immunizations, and safety precautions (auto safety restraints, locked medicine cabinets) have been shown to be instrumental in improving or maintaining an optimum quality of life.

The objective in assessing the health perception and health management pattern is to obtain data about perceptions, management, and preventive health practices.[30] Clues may lead to tentatively identifying potential health hazards, noncompliance to a prescribed medical or nursing regimen, or inability to manage health effectively.* Along with these, the nurse should not overlook unrealistic health and illness perceptions and expectations.

Specific assessment parameters assessed during the history include the health and safety practices of the individual, previous patterns of adherence or compliance, and use of the health care system – knowledge of the availability of health services, patterns indicating at what point health care is sought, and accessibility to health care through financial resources, health insurance, and transportation factors.

Besides methods of health management, the nurse explores health perception as the client describes current health, perception of past problems, and anticipation of future problems associated with health or health care. Expectations are indicative of health beliefs, locus of control, and realistic understanding of health state and any health problems.

The nurse always takes a medication history, including use of prescription and nonprescription drugs; use of cigarettes, alcohol, and caffeine; and drug allergies. An important point to remember is that whereas the past medical history performed by the physician describes only accurate and verifiable data, the nursing assessment of this pattern is specifically concerned with the client's perception and level of understanding.

Examination of the individual provides only limited clues within this pattern, since its basis is the client's perception rather than the actual health status. The general appearance may provide some indication of true health status, but actually the entire health assessment, including history and examination, is the best indicator of whether the client's perception is accurate. General appearance and condition may reveal evidence as to when the client actually seeks health care or may reveal multiple bruises or cognitive and perceptual disturbances that would be risk factors for injury. An inspection of the home environment might uncover additional risk factors.

The significance of this pattern to nursing cannot be overstressed. Health perceptions influence data collection and provide direction for all future planning of care. Clients' health beliefs, also discussed under the value and belief pattern, directly influence their participation in care. Clients are less apt to engage in self-care or preventive measures if they (1) believe it is the responsibility of health team members to keep them healthy, (2) do not recognize nor acknowledge their susceptibility to an impending health problem, or (3) believe that fate rather than their actions governs their future.

Health management in the past served as a predictor of future health management. If there was previous lack of adherence to a prescribed regimen, it will likely occur again unless the nurse is able to identify and remedy related causes. To illustrate such a situation, consider an individual with high blood pressure. In the past, the client failed to keep follow-up appointments, often "forgot" to take medication, and ate foods with high sodium content. It is important to determine whether this evident noncompliance is based on a conflict within the value system of the individual (health beliefs); inaccurate information; misunderstanding; decreasaed ability to learn, retain, or retrieve information (knowledge deficit); or denial of illness (health perception). Variables such as transportation difficulties, nutritional preferences, daily activities (individual and family patterns), and ability to read written instructions (literacy, visual acuity) may have affected the individual's behaviors.

The kinds and amount of information collected within the health perception and health management pattern depend on the purpose of data collection and the client population. Often, problems within this area may not be apparent until other patterns are assessed.

NUTRITION AND METABOLISM

This pattern describes nutrient intake relative to metabolic need.[29] The focus then includes not only the client's description of food and fluid consumption (history) but also the nurse's observations and perceptions regarding the adequacy of nutrition (physical examination). The nurse should also elicit the client's satisfaction with current eating and drinking patterns, including restrictions, and the client's perception of problems associated with eating and drinking, growth and development, skin condition, and healing processes.

All body functions and the lifestyle of the client are governed by adequate intake and supply of nutrients to tissues and organs. Sufficient food and fluid intake is necessary to provide the needed energy for performance of all activities, both the internal physiologic functioning of the body organs and the external gross body movements. Any interruption in the acquisition or retention of food or fluids will offset this balance and significantly alter the person's daily lifestyle. Nutrition and metabolism also govern the rate of individual growth and development.

The assessment objective is to collect data about a typical pattern of food and fluid consumption, adequacy of this pattern of consumption, and as with all patterns, any perceived problems associated with nutritional intake. Specific clues may point to a client who is overweight, underweight, overly hydrated, dehydrated, or experiencing difficulties in skin integrity, such as breakdown or delayed healing. Or, individuals may be at risk for developing these problems.

Parameters for assessment fall into two broad categories: (1) those that evaluate nutrient intake and (2) those that evaluate metabolic demands. Nutrient intake may be

*The use of the terms *cues* or *clues* to problems within this chapter section refers to the presence of defining characteristics identified by the North American Nursing Diagnosis Association and found in Kim and Moritz.[39]

assessed with 24-hour recall of food and fluid consumption; a listing of diet restrictions, food allergies, vitamin supplements, caffeine and alcohol ingestion (if not included in medication history); and a time schedule of eating and drinking patterns. Assessment includes screening for problems associated with swallowing or chewing.

If problems seem apparent, the focus assessment might include patterns of food preference, feelings about present weight, and a detail of eating habits. Eating may be affected if the individual eats alone rather than with a family unit. Frequent dining out may be indicative of problems in this or other functional patterns. If the diet consists of fast foods, the consumption pattern may uncover a deficit of essential vitamins or minerals. If appropriate, the nurse assesses areas pertinent to obtaining food. Who purchases it? Is shopping preplanned, as with a grocery list? Are there adequate financial resources and a food budget? Is food stored properly? Who prepares the food? In what manner are most foods prepared (fried, broiled, steamed, boiled, baked)?

Metabolic demands vary from individual to individual and within the same individual in times of illness, stress, growth, high activity levels, healing, or recovery. Both developmental and environmental conditions may alter the metabolic demands. Appetite and reported changes in weight, skin integrity, and general healing ability are the parameters elicited during the interview or health history. The client may also note a decreased tolerance in hot and cold weather.

The observations and perceptions of the nurse play a vital role in assessing the nutritional and metabolic pattern. The physical examination allows assessment of both the nutrient supply to the tissue and the metabolic needs of the individual. Objective findings serve as indicators to measure the reliability of the subjective reports concerning nutrient intake.

Gross metabolic indicators include temperature, height, and weight. The physical examination also focuses on skin, bony prominences, dentition, hair, and mucous membranes. Skin and mucous membranes, in particular, utilize nutrients rapidly and thus provide excellent indices for evaluating adequacy of nutrient supply. Assessment of the skin includes color, temperature, turgor, and a description of any skin lesions, areas of dry or scaly skin, rashes, pruritus, or edema. The mucous membranes are also examined for color, integrity, moisture, and lesions. Dentition is evaluated for structure (Are teeth erupted at normal stages of development? Are teeth firmly implanted? Are dentures fitting properly?), decay, and evidence of oral hygiene. Healing is assessed if there is evidence of injury at the time of examination.

In assessing the individual, the nutritional and metabolic pattern should naturally follow the health perception and management pattern. Nutritional intake is often mentioned when describing health practices. By referring again to the client's initial discussion of "three meals a day," the nurse can direct the interview into more specific details of nutritional intake. Another useful method of leading from one pattern into another without causing disjointedness is to assess drug history at the end of health perception and management, adding caffeine and alcohol intake and thus beginning fluid consumption evaluation. If the nurse prefers to begin with food consumption, a question discussing the use of vitamin supplements bridges the gap between the two patterns. Regardless of the response, the nurse can then ask, "Why do you find that (un)necessary?" A description of nutritional intake generally follows with little additional prompting.

Several points need to be emphasized at this time. No matter the purpose of the particular assessment – initial screening, follow-up visit, or yearly checkup – the assessment of nutrition versus metabolic need should be a continuing process. Any internal altered chemical state expresses itself outwardly. Pregnancy, for example, may result only in increased appetite or possibly weight changes as well. Appetite and weight changes along with physical indicators may also be apparent in the nonpregnant, healthy woman. The nurse should note these changes, checking other patterns that may be the cause, such as decreased activity (activity and exercise) or increased stress (coping and stress tolerance). Decreased mental alertness or confusion may be caused by inadequate nutrition (fluid and electrolyte disturbances). Although problem identification occurs following assessment of all 11 functional health patterns, a problem in any one area serves as a clue to the possibility of other dysfunctional patterns. Assessment of the pattern is facilitated by synthesizing and analyzing data collected in the other 10 functional health patterns. Nutrition and metabolism are especially significant in patterns of health management, elimination, activity, sleep, cognition, roles, and stress tolerance. The value and belief system may significantly alter all other functional patterns. Sociocultural values and ethnic backgrounds play a major role in determining an individual's pattern of eating.

It is particularly important to note how patterns of nutrient supply and demand vary over the lifespan, as well as eating habits and food preferences. Raw fruits and vegetables may be fun "finger food" for the toddler, but the older adult, especially one with loose dentures or arthritis of the temporomandibular joint (jaw), may find it impossible to eat such foods.

Implications for practice include a strong focus on educational needs. Assessment aims not only to disclose dysfunctional or potentially dysfunctional patterns but also to demonstrate functional patterns. If good nutrition is part of the health promotion activities of the individual, this should be considered a strength. Health promotion in this pattern may provide a stepping stone for such activities in the other patterns. For example, if a balanced nutritional intake is seen to improve functional level, then that individual may also learn relaxation techniques to decrease the effect of stress. An understanding of the balance of food and fluid intake to body requirements will assist the individual to adjust caloric intake as growth decreases and to prevent overweight problems in the adult years.

Proper education can prevent potential problems. Although an individual may follow the prescribed no-salt diet and demonstrate an understanding of which foods contain significant amounts of sodium, it is vital to assess if the client also understands why this is important. Potential problems with compliance might be avoided several years later if the nurse includes this education in the plan of care.

ELIMINATION

This pattern is designed to describe the function of the bowel, bladder, and skin in the excretion of wastes. The nurse measures the regularity, quality, and quantity of stool and urine according to the client's subjective reporting, assessing aids used to achieve regularity or control and any pattern changes or perceived problems. Skin is considered here only in terms of excretory function – the amount of perspiration and associated odor control.

The significance of elimination pattern to the whole person may vary on an individual level. Many clients view regularity of elimination as a measure of their health and as a sensitive indicator of proper nutrition and stress level. The client's perceptions are all important in determining if the pattern is problematic and dysfunctional, and assessment is based on what is "normal" for each individual. Many misconceptions about regularity exist, especially in the area of bowel function. More than many other areas, this is one in which individual clients often treat themselves when problems are perceived; it is important to collect data about treatment methods used.

Any difficulty in control of exreta has many culturally based implications. If any lack of control exists, it frequently alters body image (self-perception), and altered modes of elimination may also affect feelings of sexuality. Both lack of control and altered modes of elimination impinge on the activity level of the individual, decrease socialization, and even affect sleeping patterns.

Developmental levels direct the line of questioning. Assessment of children is geared to toilet-training methods, whereas regularity is more often a concern of the adult. Besides constipation, the older adult may begin to develop problems of control. Women past childbearing age are particularly prone to stress incontinence.

The assessment objective is to collect data about regularity and control of excretory patterns.[30] The nurse investigates clues suggesting constipation patterns, diarrhea, or any form of incontinence through focus assessment. Changes in elimination pattern, pain or discomfort, and any perceived problems are also assessed, and data collection includes an explanation of the problem, methods of self-treatment, and perceived results.[29]

Pattern parameters are data such as quantity, quality (color, odor, consistency), and frequency or regularity of stool, urine, and perspiration. The nurse assesses excretory mode, time patterns, and control of stool and urine, exploring changes in pattern, perceived problems, and elimination habits with the client. Examination includes gross screening of specimens, with the nurse noting amount, consistency, color, and odor. Any drainage from wounds or fistulas should be noted as skin is assessed.

The transition from nutrition to elimination pattern often occurs naturally. Roughage level in the diet affects bowel elimination patterns, and urinary elimination problems are frequently linked to fluid intake. Even skin integrity may herald questioning about drainage and lead to discussion of additional elimination patterns.

Many individuals do not consider laxatives as they discuss current medication. The nurse must ask specific questions about any remedial actions taken if constipation is a problem. A perceptive nurse will note discrepancies between dietary intake and reported regularity of bowel movements. Assessment may disclose a dependency on laxatives, suppositories, or enemas and may indicate that the client has a knowledge deficit regarding bowel elimination. Health education in areas of normal bowel function, nutritional guidelines to assist the individual in elimination, or an exercise program may significantly alter the elimination pattern.

Urinary frequency may also demand further health education. Research that indicates that delayed time between urination is associated with increased incidence of urinary tract infections guides the nurse in helping the client establish a more suitable elimination routine.

As mentioned earlier, assessment is a cognitive process that systematically collects and organizes data. As the assessment continues, the nurse constructs a pattern from data in all 11 functional health patterns. Detailed exploration of areas are indicated whenever a problem is suspected.

Although the client claims perspiration is not a problem, further assessment is necessary if the client obviously exhibits an odor control problem. An activity intolerance may exist that prevents the previously necessary daily shower, or toileting facilities may not be readily available. Recent life events may have resulted in depression and decreased interest in self-care and hygiene. On the other hand, if the client says daily activities include four showers or baths, the nurse must be alert to the possibility of an elimination problem even if no problem is evident or determine if the pattern merely indicates personal values or frequent vigorous exercising. If excess perspiration and odor control are problems, there could be a metabolic disturbance that may need medical evaluation.

Although any area perceived to be a problem by the client is a problem, the nursing assessment is also designed to evaluate patterns of dysfunction or potential dysfunction of which the client is unaware. The nurse then shares the analysis of the data with the client, basing the care plan on mutually shared goals.

ACTIVITY AND EXERCISE

This pattern describes the client's activity level, exercise program, and leisure activities. The nurse assesses movement capability, activity tolerance, and self-care abilities, as well as use of assistive devices, changes in pattern, client satisfaction with activity and exercise patterns, and any perceived problems.[30]

Limitations within the client's movement capabilities or ability to perform activities of daily living significantly alter the client's lifestyle and may in turn affect every other functional health pattern. The importance of movement and independent functioning in self-care is an almost universally accepted value. Child-rearing practices demonstrate this value; parents boast of their infant who walks early, their toilet-trained toddler, and their preschooler who dresses without assistance. The "devastation of paralysis," even in the older adult, signifies the value society places on independent movement and function.

The activity and exercise pattern provides a good indicator of the individual's commitment to health promotion and preventive care. The importance of exercise to health status has been well documented, and public awareness has grown tremendously in recent years. The number of individuals who jog or walk as part of a regular fitness routine has certainly increased, as can clearly be seen at nearly every public park in metropolitan areas. The growing number of health spas demonstrates increased membership, and those involved in selling exercise programming to group consumers (businesses, church and social groups, housing complexes) claim increasing participation.

Besides examining exercise and mobility levels, this pattern provides an indication of energy expenditure levels and activity tolerance levels. Leisure activities provide a clue to the individual's value system. The American work ethic and competitive nature of many occupations may create a void in leisure or recreational activities. The nurse directs the client's focus to as many aspects of health promotion as possible; unless this is brought to the client's attention, he or she may be too busy to realize there is no time for recreation.

Since the ability to move and perform activities of daily living directly affect the ability to control the immediate environment, an obvious link exists between the activity and exercise pattern and the individual's health. Environment also affects mobility; individuals living alone in a high crime area may limit activity to the home because they are afraid to leave. The elderly client may be too far away from public transportation to do grocery shopping; in the past, this walk may have been the major mode of exercise. The number of stairs the client must negotiate with a cane may restrict activities. Weather may also play a role in altering exercise. For individuals with any neuromuscular or perceptual disturbances, the environmental barriers may be a major handicap. Only recently has legislation faced issues concerning access to public buildings for the handicapped.

The objective of this assessment is to determine the client's pattern of activities that require energy expenditure. Components reviewed are daily activities, exercise, and leisure activities.[30] The nurse seeks clues to uncover strengths and weaknesses within the pattern. Decreased energy levels, changes within the patterns of activity and exercise, the associated explanation of such changes, perceived problems, and coping strategies to overcome difficulties are important clues that demand in-depth exploration. In general, any client with respiratory or cardiac disease warrants an in-depth assessment, and focused assessment is necessary for individuals with neuromuscular, perceptual, or circulatory impairments.

Although many medical conditions may affect the client's activity and exercise pattern, the nursing goals are designed to help find alternate solutions to limitations, improve activity tolerance levels through planned exercise programs, and prevent further dysfunction by prescribing activities to ensure maximal functioning. Assessment within this area may indicate the need for further medical evaluation to diagnose suspected disease or monitor current disease progression.

Dimensions described and assessed include daily activities, leisure activities, and exercise. Daily activities include (1) occupation (position, hours of work or school, amount of physical exercise versus cognitive or sedentary activities), (2) self-care abilities (feeding, bathing, grooming, dressing, toileting), and (3) home management (cooking, cleaning, shopping, laundry, outdoor activities). Problems within any of these areas require further explanation: Is it a problem of energy expenditure, mobility limitations, or decreased motivation caused by depression, grieving, or incongruent values?

Leisure activities focus on recreational activities, which may be classified according to degree of energy expenditure and level of socialization. Breen[10] describes activities on four levels: (1) active social (organized sports, backyard softball, golf), (2) active isolate (jogging, walking, gym workout), (3) sedentary social (bingo, cards, lecture and discussion groups), and (4) sedentary isolate (reading, knitting, coin or stamp collecting). Although not all activities fall into any one category, these can help the nurse assess recreational activities. The information elicited should include type and frequency of the activity along with the value the client places on it. The data may prove useful once goals are established, and an area of particular interest might be incorporated into the client's plan of care. For example, a particularly despondent individual who at one time was an avid follower of classical music may again be remotivated if this information is properly used. Feelings of self-worth or esteem are closely associated with recreational activities, especially in the older individual.

Exercise parameters include type, frequency, duration, and intensity of the client's regular exercise. The nurse should also assess the importance of exercise to the client and his or her feelings about exercise.

A 24-hour recall of the previous day's activities provides an initial picture of the pattern; specifics are then addressed as described for each major component. A weekly log is particularly useful for follow-up visits and whenever a problem is suspected. In addition to the weekly log, a focus assessment includes such details as mode of transportation most often used. Does the individual go everywhere in a car? Is public transportation used, and if so, how far away is the route? Are elevators used rather than climbing a flight of stairs?

Factors interfering with exercise or mobility include dyspnea, fatigue, muscle cramping, neuromuscular or perceptual deficits, chest pain, and angina. As with other patterns, feelings of satisfaction or client perception of problems always provide valuable indications of dysfunctional or potentially dysfunctional patterns.

The nurse carefully evaluates subjective reporting of complaints, such as dyspnea, by noting any client difficulty during the interview and physical examination. Components of the examination assess circulatory, respiratory, and neuromuscular indictors. The nurse measures and records skin color and temperture, heart rate (apical and radial measurement), and blood pressure; and notes respiratory rate, rhythmicity, depth of inspiration, and effort involved. Ambulation is observed, and a record is made of gait, posture, and balance. Muscle tone, strength, and coordination, along with range of motion, may provide useful clues to validate client reports of activity and exercise. The use of assistive devices or prostheses is evaluated in terms of proper use, proper fit, and degree of assistance or support provided.

The history and examination are closely linked. Examination alone may not disclose early morning pain and stiffness of the joints, and this subjective reporting is invaluable. When appropriate, the nurse may request the client to climb stairs, or perform self-care activities, which is useful in assessing level of impairment. Various instruments have been designed to quantify level of ability or disability. Gordon uses an adapted version of work by McCourt[50] to assess self-care activities and physical mobility. For some clients, a metabolic activity index, in which each activity is measured according to kilocalories of energy expended per minute, may be a helpful "quantifier" in assessing and planning care.

Developmental norms have been established for the infant and toddler. Childhood development is carefully monitored through such milestones as sitting, crawling, walking, running, and hopping. However, the nurse must remember that some degree of activity is needed regardless of age or health status. Careful assessment of ability, limitations, and interests will guide the nurse in establishing improved patterns of activity and exercise after the whole individual is assessed; the nurse is again cautioned to reserve problem identification until all patterns have been constructed. Useful clues within this pattern may guide the interview in the other pattern areas, but premature closure is dangerous. At this point only tentative hypotheses are possible, and often the explanation of the problem lies in still another functional health pattern. For example, if the individual expresses inability to perform exercise on a routine basis, is it because it is not valued, associated with knowledge deficit, personal or family value system, or overriding priorities? Is it because of general fatigue caused by inadequate or decreased sleep time, associated with anxiety, nocturia, pain, or infant waking every 3 hours for feeding? Is it because of responsibilities associated with the care of several preschoolers and inadequate financial resources to secure a babysitter? The assessment's purpose is to narrow the scope of possible explanations.

SLEEP AND REST

Perhaps the single most important factor that is assessed in this pattern is the perception of adequacy of sleep and relaxation. Subjective reports of fatigue or energy levels provide some indication of client satisfaction.

Because of the assumed role that sleep and rest play in preparing the individual for the required or desired daily activities, it becomes extremely important when these patterns are perceived to be insufficient to promote rest and provide energy. Although the exact function of sleep has not been clearly identified, it seems to serve a restorative function in most individuals. Sleep deprivation studies provide vivid demonstrations of the need for different types of sleep: light, deep, dream, or rapid eye movement (REM).

Once again, problems within this pattern may cause problems in other patterns. A person who has difficulty with sleep may be tense and irritable, unable to tolerate stress, more prone to infectious processes, and incapable of health-promoting relationships. It is likely that alterations in appetite, elimination difficulties, and activity intolerance will also be experienced. Some degree of cognitive dysfunction generally occurs.

Interestingly, sleep researchers note that although one can fool other people and often even one's self, sleep patterns are remarkably accurate indicators of stress tolerance. Groen states that "during times of anxiety, sleep is absent or disturbed."[32] The inability to initiate or maintain sleep provides clues to other dysfunctional patterns. Sleep problems may be related to physical discomfort, family stress, role or work stress, conflict in the values of the individual or family, nutritional intake (caffeine), activity levels (inactivity, daytime boredom), fears, fluid intake or urinary elimination patterns (nocturia), and schedule of activities associated with role responsibilities (mother and nighttime feedings, 24 hours on call for work, frequent shift changes). Any change in environment or habit will affect sleep patterns, as does the individual value placed on sleep.

Research studies have linked many variables to sleep disturbances. Age, sex, temperament, individual circadian rhythm, state of mind or emotional state, health status, degree of fatigue, physical condition or comfort, nutritional intake, and many drugs (prescription or over-the-counter as well as nicotine, caffeine, and alcohol) may cause differences in sleep patterns. The quantity and quality of recent sleep obtained as well as different forms of exercise govern the amount and type of sleep. However, the single most important determinant of a person's sleep pattern is age.[78] Environment, including noise, lighting, temperature, and barometric pressure, also plays a role in the person's ability to sleep.

The objective in assessing a sleep and rest pattern is to describe the effectiveness of the pattern from the client's perspective. The wide variation in sleep time – from 4 hours to more than 10 hours – does not necessarily affect functional performance; different individuals require different amounts of sleep. Pertinent information includes data suggestive of difficulties with sleep onset, sleep interruptions, and awakening. The nurse also evaluates such disturbances as dreaming and nightmares, sleepwalking, nocturnal enuresis, and penile tumescence. Counseling, institution of safety measures, or medical referral may be necessary.

In addition to sleep, the nurse assesses rest and relaxation according to the client's perceptions. Activities of the sedentary isolate type, such as reading or crocheting, may be very relaxing for some individuals.[10] Passive involvement, as with television viewing, may provide the only source of relaxation for the client. Daily naps or various forms of relaxation exercises (meditation, yoga, breathing exercises) may also be a part of this pattern.

Assessment parameters of the dimension of sleep are divided into sleep quality and sleep quantity. Sleep quality assesses the client's perception of sleep adequacy, performance level, and physical and psychologic state on awakening.

Sleep quantity, besides being the hours slept each day, is used to disclose a schedule of sleep times. The nurse assesses time of retiring, time of awakening, and additional periods of sleep throughout the day for regularity. Sleep onset and number of and reasons for awakenings provide clues to possible problems. If a problem exists, focusing may evaluate the efficiency of time spent in bed for sleep compared to actual sleeping time.

The dimensions of rest and relaxation include the parameters of type, frequency or regularity, and duration. The perceived effectiveness of methods used to promote rest is also assessed.

The value attributed to sleep by the client will largely affect his or her motivation and ability to achieve it. Individuals are conditioned to sleep under certain circumstances, and maintaining their bedtime rituals is a distinct advantage in sleep promotion. A person expecting to sleep most often will, providing that established patterns are maintained. Thus, the nurse should also assess changes in schedule and routines associated with bedtime. When assessing bedtime routines, the nurse includes rituals along with other aids to sleep, such as natural ones (warm milk) or medications (prescription and nonprescription).

Physical examination by the nurse includes the client's general appearance as well as behavior and performance changes.

As with pain, sleep is a subjective experience. Comprehensive examination may be performed – for example, with the polysomnograph – but this is beyond the scope of nursing. Research indicates that subjective reporting of sleep quality and measures of sleep time closely approximate electroencephologographic findings.[37] The large percentage of difficulties associated with sleep are amenable to nursing therapies.

Nursing implications focus on the need to be alerted to evidence of sleep disturbances so that proper interventions can be made before sleep deprivation occurs. The nurse concentrates on subjective reports of difficulties or feelings of not being well rested. Care is taken not to interpret isolated findings; every person has experienced at least one poor night's sleep.

Frequent awakenings do not necessarily imply sleep interruption. Many individuals may awaken innumerable times during the night but return to sleep within seconds. This may be especially true of elderly individuals, who generally spend most of the night in stages of light sleep. Since their normal developmental pattern does not include deep sleep, awakenings may not affect the sleep cycles and resultant feelings on awakening in the morning. More commonly, however, the elderly client experiences difficulty returning to sleep because of discomfort, fears, or other variables.

Gaining a sense of the client's biologic rhythm and peak performance time may be helpful to the nurse in planning return visits or health education. Individuals commonly refer to themselves as "morning people" or "night owls"; the patterns of retiring and arising may provide such clues.

Patterns or schedules of sleep and rest in conjunction with subjective reports regarding physical and mental well-being help determine appropriate interventions.

COGNITION AND PERCEPTION

Cognitive patterns include the ability of the individual to understand and follow directions, retain information, make decisions, solve problems, and use language appropriately. Sensory and perceptual patterns describe auditory, visual, olfactory, gustatory, tactile, and kinesthetic sensations and perceptions. Pain perception, as well as pain tolerance, is described within this pattern area.[29]

Thinking and perceiving are major components by which capacity for independent functioning of the individual is measured. Any difficulties in cognitive or perceptual patterns must somehow be compensated for to ensure the individual's safety. The balance between the individual and the environment necessary for health is clearly important; decreasing levels of cognition or perception require increasing levels of environmental control. Sheltered work environments and group living arrangements for the mentally or sensory impaired individual are examples of this.

Developmental stage plays a significant role in cognitive and perceptual abilities. Vision and hearing do not reach full potential until school age; 20/30 vision is normal for the preschooler. The ability to problem solve and conceptualize is also marked by developmental stages.[65] As the adult reaches maturity, declines in visual acuity, hearing, touch, and even taste begin and continue through the later years.

The interrelationships between the individual, the developmental stage, and the environment are extremely important. The 20-year-old male who dropped out of high school at age 16 and is employed in a factory as an assembly-line worker and the 20-year-old male who is a second-year premed student at a competitive university will in all probability exhibit different behavior patterns. The cognitive functioning of the individual must be evaluated within the context of the environment.[30] The complexity of the environment chosen by the individual results in different levels of functioning, and the nurse's expectations should reflect this difference.

In addition to the environmental complexity level, the level of sensory input within the environment and the individual's capacity to perceive this input play key roles in determining problem areas. Basic orientation of the individual to the environment is instrumental in determining functional level. Just as a person on vacation often cannot remember the date or the day of the week, it is not unusual to see a client who recently changed office location having difficulty concentrating. The likelihood of this complaint is at least doubled if the lights flicker or the noise level is significantly different in the office.

The objective in assessing the client's cognitive and perceptual pattern is to describe the adequacy of language, cognitive skills, and perception relative to desired or required activities.[30] The nurse collects and assesses clues that may indicate potential problems, especially those indicating sensory deficits, sensory deprivation or overload, and ineffective pain management. Cognitive dysfunction may result in impaired reasoning, knowledge deficits related to health practices, and memory deficits.[9,69,72]

A number of assessment parameters are available. All clients should be questioned regarding sensory perceptual problems. Subjective reporting includes whether the client has been routinely tested for hearing and vision and when. Any changes noted in the sensation or perception of the individual are noted. Besides decreased ability or acuity in hearing, vision, smell, and taste, the nurse evaluates other perceptual disturbances, such as vertigo; increased or decreased sensitivity to heat, cold, or light touch; and visual or auditory hallucinations or illusions. Use and perceived effectiveness of assistive devices, such as hearing aids, glasses, and contact lenses, are noted.

Any discomfort or pain is evaluated further. Useful tools have been designed to record and quantify changes in pain perception.[38,51] Specifically, the location, type, degree, and duration of pain provide indicators of possible causes or sources. Relief measures used to control pain (medication, heat, cold applications, relaxation) and the effectiveness of each provide additional data and possible areas in which health education may be useful. For all individuals it is appropriate to explore tolerance to pain: Do you feel you are particularly sensitive to pain? What level of pain is associated with your cut (sprain, broken bone, labor contractions)?

Areas of cognitive patterning to be explored at this point include educational level, recent memory changes, ease or difficulty in learning, and preferred method of learning. Even if no problems are apparent or suspected, the nurse may assess this in more detail if health teaching plans are to be made.

Objective data are accumulated throughout the entire interviewing or assessment process. This data collection begins with the nurse's perception of the client's general appearance – hygiene and grooming, proper use of clothing as well as neatness and appropriateness of dress, and indication that these are appropriate to the client's developmental stage. Language and vocabulary use, ability to relate an idea with words or with actions if speech is impaired or not yet developed, and even grammatic correctness provide clues to cognitive functioning. Amplitude and quality of speech, affect and mood, and attention and concentration are all indicative of the individual's mental status. For many individuals this information is sufficient to relay a sense of the level of understanding, memory, and mentation. Problem-solving abilities can generally be determined as the client is asked to relate any perceived problems, explanation of the problems, actions taken to solve the problems, and results of those actions. Since this is a basic assessment in each functional health pattern, the nurse already has an idea of whether thought processes are logical, coherent, and relevant for that individual. The fund of information is generally apparent, at least in regards to health promotion, even as the nurse assesses health perception and management patterns.

If the nurse perceives no apparent problems within the cognitive realm, the information is recorded as part of the objective data or findings of the physical examination. Data to be noted include language; vocabulary; attention span; and grasp of ideas; as well as level of consciousness; orientation to person, place, and time; language spoken and whether primary or secondary; and behavior during the interview and examination, including posture, facial expression, and general body movements.

If, however, a problem is apparent or even suspected because of age, hereditary factors, or any inconsistencies in the assessment data, a focus assessment is essential. Coma scales or functional dementia scales[37,38,55] may be utilized when appropriate. More commonly a mental status examination is performed to assess orientation, registration, attention and calculation, language (ability to name objects, repeat abstract ideas, and follow commands), and recall (immediate, short-term, and long-term memory). The client should also read, write, and copy a design.[26]

The examination of sensory perceptual pattern evaluates hearing, vision, and areas of pain at a screening level; comprehensive examinations are available and may be indicated. A full neurologic assessment is warranted if specific sensory deficits are reported following the examination.

Although these assessment areas may seem overwhelming, the time required is generally less than in most other pattern areas, perhaps because more information relevant to cognition and perception patterns is available as each pattern is assessed. Transition into the cognitive and perceptual pattern from any other pattern might be facilitated by referring to a problem already described, with the nurse asking, for example, "Do you generally find it easy to solve problems effectively?" The self-perception follows the cognitive pattern particularly well, since any measure of mental status includes feelings and perceptions of the individual regarding self. Mood, affect, and such responses to the interviewer as eye contact are further indications of the client's level of esteem. The relationship between cognitive and perceptual ability and the ability to function (self-care) or manipulate within the environment (activity, exercise) is overwhelming.

The placement of each of the patterns in a sequence suitable to each nurse and each client or situation has already been discussed. However, if there is reason to suspect that the client's cognitive and perceptual pattern may be dysfunctional and that the client is an unreliable historian, it is wise to incorporate this pattern into the assessment immediately after the health perception and management pattern or as soon as reasonable doubt exists as to the client's ability to describe a pattern. This will save valuable time and permit the nurse to identify a more reliable pattern.

The nurse should also remember that every person has at one time experienced temporary memory lapses. These alone should not be sufficient for the nurse to make a judgment. Sequence of behaviors along with clustering of appropriate signals (defining characteristics) are necessary to any nursing diagnosis. Just as important is the need to assess all pattern areas before data analysis and problem identification.

Cognitive data along with sensory abilities guide the nurse in planning care. This is especially apparent in health teaching. The formulation of the health teaching plan should reflect the client's preferred method of learning, taking into account information storage and retrieval abilities, compensatory mechanisms for sensory deficits, neuromuscular and sensory levels necessary for skills development, and the demonstrated developmental level. Goals and short-term objectives should demonstrate an individually tailored plan. Although the end goal for the newly diagnosed diabetic person would be self-care, the appropriateness of the plan reflects different expectations for the adult than for the child and for the surgeon than for the automobile mechanic.

SELF-PERCEPTION AND SELF-CONCEPT

This pattern includes client's sense of personal identity, goals, emotional patterns, and feelings about himself or herself. Self-image and a sense of worth stem from the client's perception of personal appearance, competencies, and limitations. It includes the client's self-perception as well as others' perceptions. The nurse assesses both verbal and nonverbal cues.

The significance of the sense of "self" to the whole person is best exemplified by personal experiences. If you feel good about yourself, it shows in the way you look and act. Likewise, if you feel unable to accomplish anything worthwhile, it leads to changes in eating, sleeping, and activity patterns.

The individual's developmental level affects and is affected by this pattern. Erikson identifies eight stages of human development, proposing that with each stage a central task or crisis must be resolved before healthy growth can continue.[25] According to Erikson, early childhood is the time to develop a sense of autonomy versus shame and doubt. If this is appropriately achieved or resolved, the child can then develop initiative during the next stage. One of the tasks Havighurst[34] identifies during this later phase is building wholesome attitudes toward oneself (self-esteem), whereas Bruhn and colleagues[13] refer specifically to developing self-concept. Delays or a failure to develop a concept of self will affect future development and the ability to accomplish subsequent tasks (see Table 7-3).

Environmental influences on the self-concept pattern are largely caused by the family climate and relationship pattern. Combining the developmental tasks of Erikson and the appropriate stages of the family life cycle (see Chapter 8) clearly demonstrates the family's role in the individual's development.[23]

Besides family, all persons closely associated with the client affect that person's concept of self-esteem. Most persons care what others think of them, and the support of significant others affects the self-perception and self-concept pattern.[56]

It is vital for the individual to achieve a sense of "I" versus "we." A sense of "I" as a person apart from the roles that the person may assume is equally important – "me" versus roles as mother, daughter, son, student, or nurse.

The assessment objective in this pattern area is to describe the client's patterns and beliefs regarding general self-worth and feeling states.[30] The nurse looks for clues that indicate identity confusion, altered body image, disturbances in self-esteem, and feelings of powerlessness. Anxiety, fear, and depression are states that can be identified and are responsive to nursing interventions.

Erikson's framework is helpful in describing a sequential and healthy developmental pattern as related by the client. The accomplishment of the wellness tasks may be apparent in other functional health patterns and provide additional indications of developmental level (see Unit Four).[13]

In addition to assessing the client's developmental level and pattern, feelings about himself or herself are elicited. The nurse must determine what knowledge the client has of individual strengths and limitations along with his or her attitude toward these. The client is asked to describe his or her personal appearance and capabilities in the cognitive, affective, and psychomotor domains. This provides evidence of a sense of identity and worth, as well as self-image and body image.

A description of emotional patterns or a general feeling state concludes the history if no problems are indicated. When necessary, a focused assessment may use specific tools to measure body image,[48] anxiety,[81] or depression.[5,80]

The nurse notes general appearance and affect, which may have been assessed as part of a formal mental status examination. A lowered self-esteem may be indicated by head and shoulder flexion, lack of eye contact, and mumbled or slurred speech. Anxiety or nervousness might reveal extraneous body movements, such as foot shuffling or tapping, facial tension or grimace, rapid speech, voice quivering, twitches or tremors, and general restlessness or shifts in body position. Any such indicators demand further exploration to determine underlying problems.

Self-concept or lack of it alters the nurse-client interaction. Assessment within this pattern is particularly difficult because of its personal nature. Once a client shares this sort of information with the nurse, which can be facilitated if the nurse possesses strong communication skills and a caring attitude, the client will be more involved in goal planning and more open to nursing interventions.

ROLES AND RELATIONSHIPS

This pattern describes the roles assumed and the relationships engaged in by the individual. As part of the assessment, the client's perception is the major component and should include his or her level of satisfaction with roles and relationships.

The need for relationships with other persons is a universal need for each individual.[63] In high-level wellness, basic needs for communication and fellowship along with love have been identified by Dunn.[22] Similarly, Maslow's hierarchy of needs includes a sense of love and belonging.[45,46]

The ability to communicate with other persons in a meaningful way greatly affects the whole person. The balance necessary for health between the individual and the environment – anything external to or separate from the individual – is indicative of the major role that relationships with others play in health status.[14,27,57,58]

The role of development is apparent in Erikson's stages of ego development. This system of hypotheses about readiness proposes that attainment of each stage is regarded as necessary for progression toward a later stage. For example, a person can become immersed in a relationship of genuine intimacy only after self-identity has been stabilized.[25]

Certain developmental tasks for family development have been similarly identified by Duvall (see Chapter 8).[23] The emphasis here is on the role of the individual within the family as well as within the larger context of society.

The objective of the role and relationship pattern assessment is to describe a client's pattern of family and social roles along with the associated responsibilities. The client's perception of satisfaction or dissatisfaction with the established relationship is a component of this area.[30] Loss, change, or threat produce the major problems within this pattern. Clues indicative of impaired verbal communication, social isolation, alterations in parenting, independence-dependence conflicts, dysfunctional grieving, and potential for violence are important.[52,61,62]

The assessment focuses on the role and relationships of the individual in regard to family, work, and community. Within the family, assessment parameters include the structure, roles, dynamics (decision making and power and authority, division of labor, communication patterns), and social support systems.

Student and employee roles and relationships assess the specific occupation or position, along with work responsibilities and work environment (stress, safety, and health factors). Financial concerns, job security, and retirement plans are elicited. Time commitments allowing for leisure and level of physical exercise in regard to work have previously been assessed with activity pattterns.

Community roles and relationships assess the individual's involvement within the neighborhood and other social groups. Specifically, the nurse elicits the level of socialization and amount of social support available.

Within all three components – family, work or school, and community – the client is asked to describe his or her level of satisfaction with the present roles and relationships. The nurse should explore parenting or marital difficulties and any abuse.

Specific attention is paid to any threat of change or actual changes or loss. Grieving is evaluated as to appropriateness. The nurse also evaluates the relationship between role components. Family or work roles alone may not cause stress, but combining them together at the same time may result in difficulties, as with the working mother or traveling husband and father.

Unless the nurse sees the individual in the company of

significant others, as with a home visit, objective data is not available. When possible, the family interaction and communication pattern is noted. Cognizant of the importance of family and meaningful relationships, the nurse is especially alert to potential problems with the college student away from home, the individual who travels or moves frequently, and sole family survivors (elderly persons often outlive many of their family members and friends).[52,61,62]

Maslow's hierarchy of needs is an important consideration for health promotion. Unless basic physiologic needs and security are met, the individual is not able to participate and benefit from health teaching in the role and relationship pattern.[28] A parent who cannot financially feed the children concentrates efforts on securing food and not on more effective means of discipline.

The relationship between the different functional health patterns is clearly apparent in the light of developmental stages. If one has difficulties within the self-concept pattern, that person almost certainly will have difficulties with relationships.[25,56] Since relationships affect the whole person, problems in the role and relationship pattern may be exhibited in other areas, such as difficulty in sleeping and altered appetite.

SEXUALITY AND REPRODUCTION

This pattern describes the individual's sexual self-concept, sexual functioning and methods of intimacy, and reproductive areas. It combines subjective data, nursing observations, and physical examination in the collection of data. Normal development and perceived satisfaction are crucial elements.

Sexuality is the behavioral expression of sexual identity. The importance of this pattern area to the individual's life and health are closely related to the self-perception and the relationship patterns. Body image, self-concept, and role and gender identity are linked to sexual identity. This concept of sexual self, along with the individual's relationship pattern, results in the level of sexual functioning achieved and the perceived satisfaction of same. Sexual functioning involves, but is not limited to, sexual relations with a partner.

Reproductive patterns are equally significant both to this pattern assessment and to the whole individual, as well as the family and community (see Chapters 8 and 9).

Developmental influence includes the individual's development of reproductive capacities (secondary sex characteristics, genital development) and of ego integrity[25] and the family life-cycle stage,[23] as previously discussed.

The role of the environment is instrumental in the expression of a person's sexuality and reproductive pattern. Culture and family norms regulate expression of sexuality and combine with other factors, such as the family's financial stability, to influence reproductive patterns. The various norms within society may create problems in gender identity (sexual self-concept), as well as in acceptable expressions of sexuality (sexual functioning).

An objective of assessment in this pattern is to describe behavioral problems or difficulties.[30] Equally important is assessing the individual's knowledge of sexual functioning and preventive health practices (breast and testicular self-examinations, Pap smear, effective contraceptive use) for prevention of infection. Clues are evaluated for any potential or actual sexual dysfunction.

The parameters assessed include (1) sexual self-concept, which may be derived from information collected in self-perception and role-relationship pattern; (2) sexual functioning, with the nurse noting evidence of some form of intimacy, the level of sexual activity or libido, and the effect of health or illness on sexual expressions; and (3) reproductive patterns, in which the nurse collects data pertinent to menstruation (onset, duration, frequency, last menstrual period, discomfort and feelings related to male and female menopause), reproductive stage (gravida, para, use of birth control methods), and health-promotion factors (preventive practices, knowledge of sexual functioning).

The nurse assesses the client's level of satisfaction with sexual self-concept, sexual functioning, and reproduction. Problems or difficulties (ineffective or inappropriate sexual performance, discharges, infections, venereal disease, discomfort, history of abuse) are further evaluated. Additional information is collected if sexual dysfunction or trauma is probable.[36,77]

The physical examination evaluates the development of genital organs and secondary sex characteristics. The nurse may observe forms of intimacy, such as holding hands and hugging, between client and partner.

There are nursing implications for both approach and health teaching as the sexuality and reproductive pattern is assessed. Discussions relating to this pattern area may be threatening to the client: depth of exploration should in part be governed by the client's wishes. If problems relative to the client's life processes are influenced or related to sexual or reproductive patterns, the nurse encourages discussion, perhaps at a later time, once a firmer and more trusting relationship is established.

Health promotion is facilitated by a clear picture of the individual's knowledge and practice of preventive practices. Although sex education is most often associated with school programs, education on sexual functioning should be provided for adults. Such education should be a key element in preparation for parenthood classes. Improved understanding of sexual functioning can only lead to discovering improved methods of sexual performance and a greater satisfaction level.

COPING AND STRESS TOLERANCE

Gordon[29] describes this pattern as a description of the individual's general coping pattern and the effectiveness of the pattern in terms of stress management. The pattern includes the individual's (1) ability to handle life crises and resist factors that disrupt the self-integrity of the ego, (2) mode of conflict resolution, and (3) accessibility to necessary resources.

The ability to manage stress effectively within life is a learned behavior. Some stress is a necessary part of life; without it, there is no motivation to grow. Stress is a problem only if the ability to tolerate it is not strong enough, leading to interference with daily activities.[20,66]

Most stress comes not from great tragedies but rather from an accumulation of minor irritations. Stress is not as inherent in the event but in individual perception of the event. Whereas one individual is "stressed" because of missing the bus and can only think of being 10 minutes late, another will consider it an opportunity to spend 10 minutes reading the newspaper. This difference in perception may represent a different set of values used in identifying sources of stress or an effective strategy for dealing with the stress.

For purposes of assessing this pattern, coping, or the individual behavior response to stress, includes both problem-solving ability and use of defense mechanisms. Coping is viewed not as a single act but as a process incorporating many behaviors. The function of coping is to deal with the threat or emotional distress of an event. The effectiveness of coping is assessed from the client's perspective and from the nurse's observation of the client's ability to function in the presence of actual or potential stressors within the environment.

The perception of stress and the ability to manage stress depend on personal development, amount of stress previously experienced, the current level of stress within the environment, and the available sources of social support. Although an elderly client may have experienced many stresses during life and managed them effectively, he or she may no longer be able to cope because of trying to deal with too many stresses – physical incapacitation, fixed income, fear of illness or injury, and lack of transportation – or because a social support system is no longer available.[63]

The objective in assessment is to determine the client's stress tolerance and past coping patterns. The nurse evaluates clues to difficulties in handling past and current stressors and changes in the effectiveness of a coping pattern to determine personal coping capacity.[70]

The assessment parameters include (1) the coping task, including the physical, psychologic, and socioeconomic stimuli with which the individual must cope; (2) coping style, or the tendency to use a specific style, such as approach oriented, avoidance oriented, or nonspecific; (3) coping strategy, including specifics; and (4) coping effectiveness.

Coping strategy or mode of coping may be divided into information seeking, direct action (fight or flight), inhibition of action, or use of social support. Modes of conflict resolution may be divided into problem solving or other use of such defense mechanisms as denial or eating, smoking, drinking, and sleeping and use of medication such as Valium. Girdano and Eberly[27] offer specific strategies of problem solving: (1) social engineering strategies, such as time management or planned change; (2) personality engineering strategies, such as assertiveness training or cognitive rehearsal; and (3) altered states of consciousness, such as meditation or relaxation. The nurse is alert to the use of any of these strategies while assessing all functional health patterns to help determine a coping pattern.

Coping effectiveness is best assessed by eliciting the individual resources – variety of coping mechanisms used by the client, flexibility of these mechanisms, and health-promotion value associated with each mechanism – and the client's functional level.

Stress-tolerance patterns elicit the amount of stress effectively handled in the past. The use of anticipatory coping is assessed, along with whether the individual knows how to cope but does not (production deficit), or simply does not know how to cope (skill deficit).

Other indicators of value within this pattern area are discussed under the self-perception pattern. The objective data include physical signs of restlessness, irritability, and nervousness (increased heart rate and blood pressure, perspiration).

The nurse must be aware that evidence of coping ability and tolerance to stress is found in every other functional health pattern. Evidence of stress also affects the other patterns (insomnia, weight loss, decreased concentration).[24,60]

Health promotion can be greatly assisted by early intervention. Holmes and Rahe[35] have found a significant relationship between perceived stressful life events and subsequent illness. Coping patterns and stress tolerance in the past may uncover unhealthy behavior, such as smoking and drinking, that needs to be replaced by alternative coping strategies. Stress-reduction workshops would be helpful for most of the population, since it can be predicted with certainty that the future will include stress, some of which may be overwhelming without coping strategies.

VALUES AND BELIEFS

This pattern describes values, beliefs, and goals of the individual and thus includes one's perception of what is right and what is good for oneself and any conflicts that one's beliefs and values may present.

Each pattern has addressed the value system of the individual and society. Life is governed by what the individual believes or values, and these values and beliefs are developed over time, reflecting personal experiences as well as family and societal influences.[11,21,33]

The objective in assessing this pattern is to understand the basis for the client's health-related decisions and actions.[30] The client's health beliefs influence his or her behavior in seeking health care, practicing preventive measures, participating in planning health goals, and undertaking self-care.[33] Rosenstock[68] suggests that an individual will engage in preventive health behavior according to whether a threat to wellness or health status exists. Several other health belief models expand on this concept by including other motivations, such as personal values and environmental influences. The nurse assesses clues to conflicts within the client's value system or between his or her value system and that of the family or society.

Dimensions of assessment include the client's values, beliefs, or goals that guide choice or decisions that are health related. The nurse collects this information while exploring each pattern and includes it in this pattern to summarize, clarify, or secure any additional information. Specifically, the values and beliefs about self, relationships, and society are assessed. The nurse discusses the client's beliefs, goals, and purposes of life along with any conflicts the client perceives as existing between his or her philosophies and those of the family, culture, and society. The client's source of strength, such as God or significant individual practices, is elicited; religious beliefs and preference are included.

Past goals and expectations are assessed through the client's satisfaction. The nurse must identify the client's goals and expectations concerning health; these must be clear to help the client achieve them. Health-promotion interventions are based on the individual's value system and health beliefs, as previously discussed.[33,40,41,64,75]

The brevity of this discussion is no indication of the importance the value and belief pattern plays in the assessment of the individual. The development of each pattern indicates the role of individual values.

Assessment Process

Chapter 4 discusses the assessment process. The purpose of this section is to present information about skills needed, types of data collected, and format used as it specifically relates to functional health-pattern assessment of the individual. In addition, guidelines reviewing crucial issues are presented along with examples of methods available for the assessment of individuals' functional health patterns.

SKILLS

The *communication* skills outlined in Chapter 5 are all necessary if a thorough and accurate health assessment is to be obtained. Listening cannot be overemphasized; it is particularly important to avoid missing cues that may indicate a dysfunctional or potentially dysfunctional pattern. Fig. 7-1 provides an example of basic data to be collected within the functional health patterns.

The use of open-ended questions allows for pattern

Health perception–health management pattern

1. History
   a. How has general health been?
   b. Any colds in past year? If appropriate: absences from work?
   c. Most important things you do to keep healthy? Think these things make a difference to health? (Include family folk remedies if appropriate.) Use of cigarettes, alchohol, drugs? Breast self-examination?
   d. Accidents (home, work, driving)?
   e. In past, been easy to find ways to follow things doctors or nurses suggest?
   f. If appropriate: What do you think caused this illness? Actions taken when symptoms perceived? Results of action?
   g. If appropriate: Things important to you in your health care? How can we be most helpful?
2. Examination
   a. General health appearance.

Nutritional-metabolic pattern

1. History
   a. Typical daily food intake? (Describe.) Supplements (vitamins, type of snacks)?
   b. Typical daily fluid intake. (Describe.)
   c. Weight loss/gain? (Amount.) Height loss/gain? (Amount.)
   d. Appetite?
   e. Food or eating: Discomfort? Swallowing? Diet restrictions?
   f. Heal well or poorly?
   g. Skin problems: Lesions, dryness?
   h. Dental problems?
2. Examination
   a. Skin: Bony prominences? Lesions? Color changes? Moistness?
   b. Oral mucous membranes: Color, moistness, lesions.
   c. Teeth: General appearance and alignment. Dentures? Cavities? Missing teeth?
   d. Actual weight, height?
   e. Temperature

Fig. 7-1. Adult assessment of functional health patterns. (Adapted from Gordon M: *Nursing diagnosis: process and application*, ed 2, New York, 1987, McGraw-Hill; and Gordon M: *Manual of nursing diagnosis: 1993-1994*, St Louis, 1993, Mosby.)

Continued.

Elimination pattern

1. History
   a. Bowel elimination pattern. (Describe.) Frequency? Character? Discomfort? Problem in control? Laxatives etc.?
   b. Urinary elimination pattern. (Describe.) Frequency? Problem in control?
   c. Excessive perspiration? Odor problems?
   d. Body cavity drainage.
2. Examination
   a. If indicated: Examine excreta or drainage color and consistency.

Activity-exercise pattern

1. History
   a. Sufficient energy for desired/required activities?
   b. Exercise pattern? Type? Regularity?
   c. Spare-time (leisure) activities? Child: play activities.
   d. Perceived ability (code for level) for:

Feeding	______	Dressing	______	Cooking	______
Bathing	______	Grooming	______	Shopping	______
Toileting	______	General mobility	______		
Bed mobility	______	Home maintenance	______		

Functional level codes:

Level 0:	Full self-care
Level I:	Requires use of equipment or device
Level II:	Requires assistance or supervision from another person
Level III:	Requires assistance or supervision from another person and equipment or device

2. Examination
   a. Demonstrated ability (code listed above) for:

Feeding	______	Dressing	______	Cooking	______
Bathing	______	Grooming	______	Shopping	______
Toileting	______	Bed mobility	______		
General mobility	______	Home maintenance	______		

   b. Gait _____ Posture _____ Absent body part? (Specify) _____
   c. Range of motion (joints) _____ Muscle firmness _____
   d. Hand grip _____ Can pick up a pencil? _____
   e. Pulse (rate) _____ (rhythm) _____ Breath sounds _____
   f. Respirations (rate) _____ (rhythm) _____ Breath sounds _____
   g. Blood pressure _____
   h. General appearance (grooming, hygiene, energy level)

Sleep-rest pattern

1. History
   a. Generally rested and ready for daily activities after sleep?
   b. Sleep onset problems? Aids? Dreams (nightmares)? Early awakening?
   c. Rest-relaxation periods?
2. Examination
   a. If appropriate: Observe sleep pattern.

Cognitive-perceptual pattern

1. History
   a. Hearing difficulty? Hearing aid?
   b. Vision? Wear glasses? Last checked? When last changed?
   c. Any change in memory lately?
   d. Big decision easy/difficult to make?
   e. Easiest way for you to learn things? Any difficulty?
   f. Any discomfort? Pain? If appropriate: how do you manage it?
2. Examination
   a. Orientation.
   b. Hears whisper?
   c. Reads newsprint?
   d. Grasps ideas and questions (abstract, concrete)?
   e. Language spoken.
   f. Vocabulary level. Attention span.

Fig. 7-1, cont'd. Adult assessment of functional health patterns.

Self-perception–self-concept pattern

1. History
   a. How describe self? Most of the time, feel good (not so good) about self?
   b. Changes in body or things you can do? Problem to you?
   c. Changes in way you feel about self or body (since illness started)?
   d. Things frequently make you angry? Annoyed? Fearful? Anxious?
   e. Ever feel you lose hope?
2. Examination
   a. Eye contact. Attention span (distraction).
   b. Voice and speech pattern. Body posture.
   c. Nervous (5) or relaxed (1); rate from 1 to 5.
   d. Assertive (5) or passive (1); rate from 1 to 5.

Role-relationship pattern

1. History
   a. Live alone? Family? Family structure (diagram)?
   b. Any family problems you have difficulty handling (nuclear/extended)?
   c. Family or others depend on you for things? How managing?
   d. If appropriate: How family/others feel about illness/hospitalization?
   e. If appropriate: Problems with children? Difficulty handling?
   f. Belong to social groups? Close friends? Feel lonely (frequency)?
   g. Things generally go well at work? (School?)
   h. If appropriate: Income sufficient for needs?
   i. Feel part of (or isolated in) neighborhood where living?
2. Examination
   a. Interaction with family member(s) or others.

Sexuality-reproductive pattern

1. History
   a. If appropriate to age and situation: Sexual relationships satisfying? Changes? Problems?
   b. If appropriate: Use of contraceptives? Problems?
   c. Female: When menstruation started? Last menstrual period? Menstrual problems? Para? Gravida?
2. Examination
   a. None unless problem identified or pelvic examination is part of full physical assessment.

Coping-stress tolerance pattern

1. History
   a. Any big changes in your life in the last year or two? Crisis?
   b. Who's most helpful in talking things over? Available to you now?
   c. Tense or relaxed most of the time? When tense, what helps?
   d. Use any medicines, drugs, alcohol?
   e. When (if) have big problems (any problems) in your life, how do you handle them?
   f. Most of the time, is this (are these) way(s) successful?
2. Examination: None

Value-belief pattern

1. History
   a. Generally get things you want from life? Important plans for the future?
   b. Religion important in life? If appropriate: Does this help when difficulties arise?
   c. If appropriate: Will being here interfere with any religious practices?
2. Examination: None

Other concerns
   a. Any other things we haven't talked about that you'd like to mention?
   b. Any questions?

Fig. 7-1, cont'd. Adult assessment of functional health patterns.

construction. A nonjudgmental attitude is vital in establishing rapport with the client. It may directly affect the subsequent amount and type of information the client is willing to share as well as data reliability. Many individuals know the "right" answers (types of food to be eaten, recommended amount and frequency of exercise), but knowing does not necessarily imply practicing. A nonjudgmental attitude will allow any answer to be the "right" answer.

In addition to skill in communication, *observation* and

The depth of exploration is determined by the situational context and the presence or absence of significant cues. Situational context includes the setting (private office or curtained cubicle), the physiologic and psychologic comfort of the client (individual in pain or one concerned that the results of the health assessment may result in loss of job) and the purpose of the assessment (data base; problem-focused assessment; emergency assessment; or follow-up, time-lapsed reassessment).[30]

examination skills are essential. The clinical expertise of the nurse directs the assessment of each pattern as cues are probed further *(branching)* and the range of possibilities is narrowed *(focus assessment)*.[30,31] This is discussed later, since this sort of diagnostic skill is a major variable in the diagnostic process.

DATA COLLECTION

Essential elements of data collection include the method of collection, the nature of the data, and the depth of exploration. Data are collected through subjective reports and objective nursing observations. The subjective data are obtained through reports of the client (primary source) whenever possible. In assessment of the individual, secondary sources (parents, relatives) are used only when absolutely necessary, as deemed by age or cognitive functioning ability of the client, such as a child or a confused individual. This is further discussed as it relates to the type of data being collected (see the section on cognitive-perceptual pattern earlier in this chapter.)

The nature of the data collected may be uncertain in many of the human sciences. It will be assumed to be reliable, except as previously noted, or when the nurse has reason to believe otherwise. It is possible to corroborate the subjective reports with objective measures in some instances. For example, if the client reports a nutritional intake appropriate to metabolic demand and still gains considerable weight in the absence of any medical condition, the nurse is alerted to the possibility of unreliable data.

Using nutritional intake again as an example demonstrates the type of data available. Listing foods prepared for each meal or packed for lunch is not a valid indicator of foods consumed; the school-age child's report of eating all the foods packed may not always be reliable and may need to be verified by a teacher or classmate. Past as well as current data are necessary for pattern construction. Foods eaten in the past compared with foods being eaten at present provide a more accurate picture of current health status.

Obviously, some patterns are easier to evaluate than others. Corroboration of subjective reports in an area such as self-perception is more difficult. Nursing observations should include verbal as well as nonverbal cues; body language (posture, gestures), eye contact, and displays of emotion (crying, fist slamming) should be noted.

Cues that may indicate the possible presence of problems are significant when they (1) represent an unexpected change in the client's usual patterns, not a result of developmental norms or previously instituted therapies; (2) deviate from appropriate population norms; or (3) represent a behavior that results in nonproductivity for the individual.[30] Other cues govern the depth of the assessment and are representative of the characteristics of functional health patterns. Pattern areas are explored at least until a pattern emerges, environmental and developmental influences are apparent, and functional ability is demonstrated. The presence of defining characteristics for a specific diagnosis directs further assessment.[29,30,37] Pattern construction continues until sufficient evidence (cluster of cues) exists to identify a problem (nursing diagnosis) and propose interventions based on contributing etiologic factors.

FORMAT

The specific sequencing of patterns in collecting and recording information gathered during a functional health pattern assessment is flexible. However, the method of recording should be systematic and consistent. It is usually advantageous to first interview the client and then perform the physical examination. *It is vital for clarity that subjective and objective data be separately recorded*. The subjective data are recorded in phrases, and each pattern is separately labeled. Information is recorded in concise language and should probably include at least some direct quotes of the client. The objective data may follow functional health patterns or a systems ("head-to-toe") approach. (See Fig. 7-1 and Nursing Assessment Database in Chapter 4.)

A distinct advantage in the format is the openness of each pattern. In-depth exploration in some areas may be included, whereas screening information may be appropriate in other patterns. The important thing is not to collect irrelevant data. The same information is not necessary for all clients, and forms to be filled in for initial data bases generally do not include this option. Likewise, checklists and predesigned formats with questions do not provide space for all pertinent data. The functional health pattern format records all information pertinent to a particular pattern, even when collected following the initial visit. This prevents important assessment data from being lost amidst the progress notes.

GUIDELINES

The development of each pattern in the following section provides dimensions and parameters for assessment. These dimensions and parameters are not inclusive but provide a base for initial assessment in the absence of problems. The nurse, using his or her knowledge of the situation and perception of whether problems exist, directs the line of questioning to an appropriate depth. A complete physical examination should be performed in the usual manner, either by the physician or the nurse, as governed by the situation or institutional guidelines.

A method of data collection, 24-hour recall, is mentioned in several patterns as a way of describing the client's normal pattern. Obviously this is of value to such aspects as nutritional intake or daily activities. The nurse may use another version, the weekly log, when problems are apparent or when further description is necessary. A weekly log is helpful in determining such patterns as nutrition, elimination, sleep, and activity and may also be used to discuss self-perception, role and relationships, or coping with stress. As an example, the client may be quested to record every time he or she encounters a stressful situation. The client is asked to list feelings or factors preceding and following the stressful event, explain why he or she perceived the event as stressful, what he or she did about it, and the effects of such action. Such a process is helpful in assessing coping and stress-tolerance patterns and promotes improved understanding by the client and the nurse. This understanding is helpful in mutually setting goals and planning appropriate interventions.

Two concepts are crucial elements in discussing the process of assessment. The first is that all patterns need to be assessed before forming any diagnosis. Although a tentative diagnosis may occur during the collection of data regarding nutrition, it is not definitive until the nurse assesses the other 10 areas. The problem of nutrition alteration, more than body requirements (exogenous obesity), may be related to overindulgence, knowledge deficit regarding proper nutrition in relation to health promotion, inadequate exercising, depression, self-image, family eating habits, or the value placed on eating by the client, or the client's family, culture, and community. It is clearly apparent that unless the reason or probable cause is discovered, nursing interventions cannot be focused, and evaluation of nursing interventions may demonstrate that none of the outcomes has been achieved.

When potential problems are suspected within any pattern, the nurse may use this suspicion as a guide to direct and complete the assessment. The pattern then is determined to be (1) functional, indicating the client's strengths and high-level wellness; (2) dysfunctional, indicating the client's limitations and actual health problems; or (3) potentially dysfunctional, indicating presence of risk factors and potentially problematic areas.[25,30]

The second concept crucial to assessment is that it be a continual process. Data collection continues during all nurse-client interactions. The same is true of the overall diagnostic process.[30] The collection of data is only the first step in the process of collecting, interpreting, and clustering information and then naming the cluster through the nursing diagnosis. More important, "the specific delineations (of the components of the nursing process) are not intended to imply that practice consists of a series of discreet steps, taken in strict sequence, beginning with assessment and ending with evaluation, but rather that the processes are used concurrently and recurrently."[4]

INDIVIDUAL HEALTH PROMOTION THROUGH THE NURSING PROCESS

The nursing process – the systematic approach to reduce or eliminate the client's problem – is accomplished by first collecting necessary data. The nurse in turn analyzes the data, identifies nursing diagnosis, projects outcomes, prescribes interventions, and evaluates effectiveness. Reassessment, reordering of priorities, new goal setting, and revision of the plan continues as part of the process toward outcome attainment.[4] Little and Carnevali[44] describe the nursing process as helping clients and their families cope more effectively with demands of daily living and their desired life activities and lifestyle in the face of actual or potential challenges to their health.

This section demonstrates the nursing processes used to promote the health of the individual. Since many components of the nursing process are discussed in the previous section on functional health patterns, this discussion further exemplifies that the steps are used concurrently and recurrently.[4]

Collection and Analysis of Data

The assessment is a systematic technique for learning as much as possible about the client.[79] The main purpose in collecting data from a new client is to see whether health problems exist and to identify the client's health goals.[30]

The data collection includes necessary biographic data, such as age and sex and the purpose of the visit. This is followed by the assessment of the previously outlined 11 functional health patterns. Subjective reporting, nursing observations and perceptions, and the physical examination are assessed and recorded. The remaining discussion focuses on nursing diagnosis.

PROBLEM IDENTIFICATION

Although the concept of problem identification has been debated in the past, most nurses now have distinguished *nursing diagnosis* as the problem label. Diagnosis is a careful examination and analysis of the facts in an attempt to explain something. Nursing diagnosis is the naming of a client response to actual or potential health problems/life processes.[15,30,43,71] "Nursing diagnoses provide the basis for selection of nursing interventions to achieve outcomes for which the nurse is accountable."[16] The North American Nursing Diagnoses Association (NANDA) has provided leadership in developing standardization of the descriptions of human responses that nurses treat. The most recent revision of this taxonomy contains 99 nursing diagnoses approved for clinical testing and has been endorsed by the ANA.[16,17,49]

Gordon[29] proposed the accepted format of nursing diagnosis, PES, that lists the problem, etiology, and signs and symptoms, or defining characteristics for each diagnosis accepted for clinical testing.

In discussions of problems, it must be clearly demonstrated what is meant by a "problem." The concept as used here refers to Gordon's proposition that a health problem is defined as a dysfunctional pattern and that nursing's major contribution to health care is in prevention and treatment of such patterns.[30] A pattern is dysfunctional if it represents a deviation from established norms or from the client's previous condition or goals. (Normative behavior is further discussed in Unit Four.)

Gordon goes on to say that a dysfunctional pattern is a problem when it generates therapeutic concern on the part of the client, others, or the nurse and when it is amenable to nursing therapies. Therapeutic concern, as defined by Taylor,[74] refers to a client's desire to receive treatment and a nurse's desire to provide it.

As patterns are assessed, the nurse proposes several hypotheses regarding functional or dysfunctional labeling. At the completion of the assessment, conclusions must be drawn. It is possible that all patterns are functional, that some are functional, and that others are dysfunctional or potentially dysfunctional.

Functional refers to wellness and optimum health. Dysfunctional patterns, indicating some health problem, may be present in the absence of disease. In other words, nursing care may be needed for health promotion and health maintenance, not health restoration. The history of Frank Thompson in Chapter 1 effectively illustrates the mutliple nursing care needs of an individual who is not ill.

In potentially dysfunctional patterns, sufficient evidence exists or enough risk factors are present to indicate that a pattern dysfunction will probably occur if interventions are not made. This early identification of potential problems is possible through systematic data collection and analysis.

PROBLEM ETIOLOGY

To plan care, the nurse must first determine to the best of his or her ability what has caused the actual or potential health problem, or its contributing etiologic factors. The etiologic factors of most dysfunctional patterns lie within another pattern or patterns. Although etiology is never an absolute within human sciences, the projection of outcomes or goals must be based on some probable cause(s). Interventions then focus on mediating or resolving the probable cause(s). Most often multicausal factors are involved, and problems are said to "relate to" rather than be caused by these factors.

Since potential problems are not actual problems but risk states, they have no etiology and are identified when risk factors are present. Intervention is directed toward risk reduction through education (classes, brochures) to improve nutrition, prevent accidents, and so on. Risk estimate theory and potential health problems are further developed in Chapters 8 and 9 and Unit Four.

DIAGNOSTIC VARIABLES

The ability to arrive at an accurate diagnosis, even if all the appropriate information is available, is governed primarily by the nurse's clinical skills. Experience improves the technique if nursing is performed as a scientific process. Nursing requires gathering information, interpreting it on the basis of normative values, organizing and grouping inappropriate findings, identifying the problem, and then attempting to plan appropriate goals and interventions.

Difficulties are encountered when there are no available norms, which occurs frequently in the psychosocial assessment components. The use of the 11 interdependent functional health patterns helps to solve such difficulties. By focusing on each of these areas, it is easier to see if a problem does or does not exist. Any change within the pattern may be a sign of dysfunction as well as an unhealthful but stabilized behavior. This might include a 2-year-old who is still not walking – developmental growth is a major factor in activity patterns of infants, toddlers, and children.

The use of physiologic parameters clearly demonstrates the idea of a stabilized dysfunctional pattern, but equal care must be given to psychologic development. Evidence of a 26-year-old gentleman who lives with his mother and gives no indication of independent decision making should certainly be further explored.

It should be apparent that assessment information primarily comes from the initial contact with the client and the database; this is generally the case in health-promotion activities. In any acute situation or emergency, however, quick assessment of the major problems are given priority on a hierarchy-of-needs basis, and the full nursing assessment is temporarily postponed.

For further understanding of the nursing diagnosis, the nurse is referred to books discussing the development of diagnoses, the diagnostic process, and specific details of each accepted diagnosis.[15-17,28-31,39]

Planning of Care

Planning in the nursing process is the proposal of diagnosis-specific treatment to assist the client toward the goal of optimal health. It is based on the client's goals and the determined nursing diagnosis. The clarity of the goals and diagnoses are critical to the development of an effective plan of care.

Yura and Walsh[78] identify the following purposes of the planning phase: (1) to assign priority to the problems diagnosed; (2) to specify the behavioral outcomes or goals with the client, including the expected time of achievement; (3) to differentiate client problems that could be resolved by nursing intervention, those that could be handled by the client or family member, and those that would have to be handled with or referred to other members of the health team; (4) to designate specific actions, the frequency of these actions, and the immediate, intermediate, and long-term results; and (5) to list client problems (nursing diagnosis) and nursing actions (frequency, expected outcomes or goals) on the nursing care plan or blueprint for action. This plan provides the direction for client and nursing activities and is the guide for the evaluation.

Implementing the Plan

Implementing is the completion of the actions necessary to fulfill the goal(s) toward optimal health; it is the enactment of the nursing care plan toward the behaviors described in the proposed client outcome. The cognitive, affective, and psychomotor behaviors of both the client and the nurse may be demonstrated.[19]

> The selection of a nursing intervention depends on several factors . . .: 1) the desired patient outcome, 2) the characteristics of the nursing diagnosis, 3) the research base associated with the intervention, 4) the feasibility of successfully implementing the intervention, 5) the acceptability of the intervention to the client, and 6) the capability of the nurse.[14,49]

The Nursing Interventions Classification is being developed.[49] As discussed in Unit One, a critical component of effective communication is the accurate interpretation of client information. This feedback process continues throughout all phases of the nursing process; the nurse continues to collect data to modify as needed and does not blindly implement the care plan. As discussed in Unit Three, the most frequently used nursing interventions in health promotion are screening, educating, counseling, and crisis intervention. All these require strong communication abilities from the nurse.

Evaluating the Plan

The process of analyzing changes experienced by the client occurs in the evaluation phase of the nursing process, with the nurse examining the relationships between nursing actions and the client's goal achievement. Yura and Walsh[78] emphasize that evaluation is always considered in terms of how the client responded to the planned action. As already discussed, the nursing diagnosis or health problems and the goal, or expected outcome, guide the evaluation of the nursing care plan.

> Many variables influence outcomes: the interventions prescribed by the health care providers, the health care providers themselves, the environment in which the care is received, the patient's own motivation and genetic structure, and the patient's significant others. The task for nursing is to define which patient outcomes are sensitive to nursing care, that is, to identify for each patient the expected and attainable results of nursing care.[14]

SUMMARY

Data relevant to the health-promotion activities of the individual focus primarily on the assessment of the current health status so that the nurse can identify problem areas, or areas of dysfunction, within the individual's health and lifestyle pattern. This is a fundamental first step and precedes all other components of the nursing process. Without a clear picture of the problem, nursing activities are fruitless.

Gordon's functional health pattern framework provides the framework for the individual assessment.[30] The focus of each pattern includes the developmental influences exerted, the environmental role played, and the functional ability displayed, along with the behavioral patterns specific to each individual. The interaction between internal mechanisms and the environment is assessed through these 11 functional health patterns.

When assessing each pattern, the nurse must understand the pattern definition, the significance of the pattern to the whole individual, the developmental influences, the environmental role, the assessment objectives, the assessment parameters and indicators, and the nursing implications. Assessment is essential to all components of the nursing process in health promotion for the individual.

References

1. Abbey J: *Fancap: what is it?* In Riehl J, Roy C, editors: *Conceptual models for nursing practice*, ed 2, New York, 1980, Appleton-Century-Crofts.
2. American Nurses' Association: *The nursing practice act: suggested state legislation*, Kansas City, Mo, 1980, The Association.
3. American Nurses' Association: *Scope of nursing practice: a social policy statement*, Kansas City, Mo, 1980, The Association.
4. American Nurses' Association: *Standards of clinical nursing practice*, Kansas City, Mo, 1991, The Association.
5. Beck A: Screening depressed patients in family practice, *Postgrad Med* 52:81, 1972.
6. Beckness E, Smith D: *System of nursing practice*, New York, 1975, FA Davis.
7. Beland L, Passos J: *Clinical nursing: pathophysiological and psychosocial approaches*, ed 3, New York, 1975, Macmillan.
8. Bloch D: Some crucial terms in nursing – what do they really mean?, *Nurs Outlook* 22:689, 1974.
9. Boss BJ: The neuroanatomical and neurophysiological basis of learning, *J Neuroscience Nurs* 18(5):256-264, 1986.
10. Breen L: *The adult years – a report prepared for the Bartholomew County Retirement Foundation*, Lafayette, 1961, Department of Sociology, Purdue University.
11. Brink JP: Value orientation as an assessment tool in cultural diversity, *Nurs Res* 33(4):198-203, 1984.
12. Bromwell L: Use of life history in pattern identification and health promotion, *Adv Nurs Science* 7(1):37-44, 1984.
13. Bruhn J, et al: The wellness process, *J Comm Health* 2:215-217, 1977.
14. Bulechek G, McCloskey J: *Nursing interventions classification: taxonomy of nursing interventions*, St Louis, 1993, Mosby.
15. Carpenito L: *Nursing diagnosis: application to clinical practice*, ed 4, Philadelphia, 1989, JB Lippincott.
16. Carroll-Johnson RM: *Classification of nursing diagnoses: proceedings of the ninth conference*, Philadelphia, 1991, JB Lippincott.
17. Carroll-Johnson RM: Reflections on the ninth biennial conference, *Nurs Diagnosis* 1:50, 1991.

18. Commission on Chronic Illness: *Chronic illness in the US, vol 1, Prevention of chronic illness,* Cambridge, 1957, Harvard University Press.
19. Cox CL: An interaction model of client health behavior: theoretical prescription for nursing, *Adv Nurs Science* 5(1):41-56, 1982.
20. Dixon J, Dixon J, Spinner J: Preceptors of life pattern disintegrity as a link in the relationship between stress and illness, *Adv Nurs Science* 11(2):1-11, 1989.
21. Downing CK, Kuckelman Cobb A: Value orientation of homeless men, *Western J Nurs Res* 12(5):619-629, 1990.
22. Dunn H: *High level wellness,* Arlington, 1972, Beatty.
23. Duvall E, Miller B: *Marriage and family development,* ed 6, New York, 1984, HarperCollins.
24. Engel GL: The clinical application of the biopsychosocial model, *Am J Psychiatry* 137(5):535-544, 1980.
25. Erikson E: *Childhood and society, 35 anniv ed,* New York, 1986, WW Norton.
26. Folstein M, Folstein S, McHugh A: Mini mental state, *Psych Med* 10:125, 1982.
27. Girdano S, Eberly N: *Controlling stress and tension: a holistic approach,* ed 2, Englewood Cliffs, NJ, 1986, Prentice Hall.
28. Gordon M: *Manual of nursing diagnosis: 1993-1994,* St Louis, 1993, Mosby.
29. Gordon M: Nursing diagnosis and the diagnostic process, *Am J Nurs* 76:1299, 1976.
30. Gordon M: *Nursing diagnosis: process and application,* ed 2, New York, 1987, McGraw-Hill.
31. Gordon M: Toward theory-based diagnostic categories, *Nurs Diagnosis* 1:5-11, 1990.
32. Groen J: *The measurement of emotions and arousal in the clinical physiological laboratory and in medical practice.* In Levi L, editor: *Emotions: their parameters and measurements,* New York, 1975, Raven Press.
33. Harvey RM: The relationship of values to adjustment in illness: a model for nursing practice, *J Adv Nurs* 17:164-167, 1992.
34. Havighurst R: *Developmental tasks and education,* ed 3, New York, 1972, David McKay.
35. Holmes T, Rahe F: The social readjustment rating scale, *J Psychosomatic Res* 11:213, 1967.
36. Holmstrom L, Burgess A: Assessing trauma in the rape victim, *Am J Nurs* 75:1288, 1975.
37. Jones C: Glasgow coma scale, *Am J Nurs* 79:1551, 1979.
38. Jones D, Lepley M: *Assessment across the lifespan,* New York, 1992, McGraw-Hill.
39. Kim M, Moritz D: *Classification of nursing diagnoses, proceedings of the third and fourth national conference on classification of nursing diagnosis,* New York, 1981, McGraw-Hill.
40. Kleinman A: *The illness narratives,* New York, 1988, Basic Books.
41. Lau RR, Hartman KA, Ware JE Jr: Health as a value: methodological and theoretical considerations, *Health Psychology* 5(1): 25-43, 1986.
42. Lawton M: The functional assessment of elderly people, *J Am Geriatric Society* 19:465, 1971.
43. Lindsey AM: Identification and labeling of human responses, *J Prof Nurs* 6(3):143-150, 1990.
44. Little D, Carnevali D: *Nursing care planning,* ed 2, Philadelphia, 1976, JB Lippincott.
45. Maslow A: *The farthest reaches of human nature,* Magnolia, Mass, 1983, Peter Smith.
46. Maslow A: *Motivation and personality,* ed 3, New York, 1987, Harper & Row.
47. McCain F: Nursing by assessment – not intuition, *Am J Nurs* 65:82, 1965.
48. McClosky J: How to make the most of body image theory in nursing, *Nursing* 6:68, 1976.
49. McClosky J, et al: Classification of nursing interventions, *J Prof Nurs* 6:151-157, 1990.
50. McCourt A: *Measurement of functional deficit in quality assurance: quality assurance update,* Kansas City, Mo, 1981, American Nurses' Association.
51. Meinhart N, McCaffrey M: *Nursing management of the patient with pain,* East Norwalk, Conn, 1983, Appleton-Century-Crofts.
52. Meleis A: Role insufficiency and role supplementation: a conceptual framework, *Nurs Res* 24:264-271, 1975.
53. Mitchell P: *Concepts basic to nursing,* ed 3, New York, 1981, McGraw-Hill.
54. Monroe L: Psychological and physiological differences between good and poor sleepers, *J Abnormal Psychol* 72:255, 1967.
55. Moore J, et al: *A functional dementia scale, presented at 35th annual meeting of Gerontological Society of America,* NIA Grant No K07 AG00102, Boston, 1982.
56. Muhlenkamp AF, Sayles JA: Self esteem, social support and positive health practices, *Nurs Res* 35(6):334-338, 1986.
57. Newman M: *Health as expanding consciousness,* St Louis, 1986, Mosby.
58. Newman M: *Nursing's emerging paradigm: the diagnosis of pattern.* In McLane AM, editor: *Classification of nursing diagnosis proceedings of the seventh conference,* St Louis, 1987, Mosby.
59. New York State Nurses' Association: *Report on the special committee to study the nurse practice act,* Albany, NY, 1970, The Association.
60. Nightingale F: *Notes on nursing: what it is and what it is not,* London, 1969, Harrison & Sons.
61. Norbeck JS: Social support: a model for clinical research and application, *Adv Nurs Science* 3(2):43-59, 1981.
62. Norbeck JS, et al: The development of an instrument to measure social support, *Nurs Res* 30:264-269, 1981.
63. Norbeck JS, Lindsey AM, Carrieri V: Further developmental of the Norbeck social support questionnaire: normative data and validity testing, *Nurs Res* 32(1): 4-9, 1983.
64. Pender NJ: *Health promotion in nursing practice,* Norwalk, Conn, 1987, Appleton & Lange.
65. Piaget J: *Intelligence and affectivity: their relationship during child development,* Palo Alto, 1981, Annual Reviews (Translated by Brown T, Kaegi C).
66. Pollock SE: The stress response, *Crit Care Q* 6(4):1-14, 1984.
67. Rogers M: *An introduction to the theoretical basis of nursing,* Philadelphia, 1970, FA Davis.
68. Rosenstock I: The health belief model and preventative health behavior, *Health Educ Monog* 2:354, 1974.
69. Roy C Sr: *Alterations in cognitive process.* In Mitchell PH, et al, editors: *AANN's neuroscience nursing,* Norwalk, Conn, 1988, Appleton & Lange.
70. Scott DW, Oberst MT, Dropkin MJ: A stress coping model, *Adv Nurs Science* 3(1):9-23, 1980.
71. Shoemaker J: In Kim M, Moritz D: *Classification of nursing diagnoses,* New York, 1981, McGraw-Hill.
72. Slater MC: *Altered levels of consciousness: impaired thought processes.* In Snyder M, editor: *Neurological and neurosurgical nursing,* New York, 1983, Wiley.
73. Smith D: A clinical nursing tool, *Am J Nurs* 68:2384, 1968.
74. Taylor F: A logical analysis of the medico-psychological concept of disease, part I, *Psych Med* 1:356, 1971.
75. Tompkins ES: Nurse/client values congruence, *Western J Nurs Res* 14(2): 225-236, 1992.
76. Williams R, Karacan I, Hursch C: *Sleep disorders: diagnosis and treatment,* ed 2, New York, 1988, John Wiley & Sons.
77. Woods N: *Human sexuality in health and illness,* ed 3, St Louis, 1984, Mosby.
78. Yura H, Walsh M: *Human needs and the nursing process,* ed 5, New York, 1988, Appleton-Century-Crofts.
79. Yurick A, et al: *The aged person and the nursing process,* New York, 1980, Appleton-Century-Crofts.
80. Zung W: From art to science: diagnoses and treatment of depression, *Arch Gen Psychiatry* 29:328, 1973.
81. Zung W: A rating instrument for anxiety disorders, *Psychosomatics* 12(6):271, 1971.

CHAPTER

8

Health Promotion and the Family

Nancy Curro McCarthy

Objectives

After completing this chapter, the nurse will be able to

- *Describe the use of the functional health pattern framework in assessing families throughout the lifespan.*
- *Give examples of the clinical data to be collected in each health pattern at the different family developmental phases.*
- *Give examples of the following behavioral changes within the health patterns of families: (1) functional, (2) potentially dysfunctional, and (3) actually dysfunctional.*
- *Describe developmental and cultural characteristics of the family to consider while identifying risk factors or etiologic factors of potentially or actually dysfunctional health patterns.*
- *Discuss planning, implementing, and evaluating nursing interventions in health promotion with families.*
- *Develop a specific health promotion plan based on a family assessment, nursing diagnosis, and contributing risk or etiologic factors.*

The primary approach to health promotion and disease prevention is through the family. It is in families that children and adults are nurtured, provided for, and taught about health values by word and by example. It is in families that an individual first learns to make choices that promote his or her own physical and emotional health.

Healthy People 2000: National Health Promotion and Disease Prevention Objectives[13] from the U.S. Department of Health and Human Services has identified families as the bedrock of our society. The document goes on to report that families have been formally defined as a group of two or more people related by birth, marriage, or adoption and residing together in a household.

Nursing has fostered the concept of health as a systemic view that is applicable to families. Anderson and Tomlinson[1] have written on the family health system as an emerging paradigm. Their definition of family health links family structure, function, and health variables (including both wellness and illness), incorporates the biopsychosocial and contextual system aspects of nursing, specifies the paradigm view, and addresses the levels of family interaction. Anderson and Tomlinson maintain this definition suggests a paradigm shift in that it embraces more than the health of individuals as part of a family but recognizes the family health system as the central phenomenon of study.

The family seen as a living open system was developed by Fawcett[7] using Rogers'[23] Life Process Model. Fawcett[8] has continued her research using the concept of the family as an integral, unified whole characterized by a unique and ever-changing pattern and organization. The continuous alterations in pattern and organization reflect the mutual and simultaneous interaction between the family system and the environment. In Fawcett's research, pregnant and postpartal women and their husbands represent the open family system, pregnancy-related experiences represent pattern and organization, and strength of identification represents mutual and simultaneous interaction.

Kristjanson and Chalmers[14] in a pilot study of community health nurse-client interaction found five major content areas that were identified: maternal health, growth and development of children, focused health concerns, health screening, and social and environmental health concerns. Health promotion was a theme in all the various categories, and preventive health teaching was an element in every nursing exchange.

Luker and Chalmers[17] in a study done to explore the concept of gaining access to clients as it emerged from an in-depth qualitative study of health-visiting practice identified three components of the Pender and Pender[21] health-promotion model that facilitated access to clients: clients who place a high value on health; clients who perceive that control over their personal health is primarily related to their own actions, actions of others, or a matter of chance; and the clients' definition of health.

Zerwekh[26] has identified four strategies intrinsic to encouraging family self-help: (1) believing in the clients' ability to make choices and helping families believe in themselves, (2) listening to what the family wants and starting there, (3) expanding the family's vision of options, and (4) feeding back reality to help the family see the patterns of their lives and the implications of unhealthy choices.

Gillis[10] writing on family nursing presents nine challenges regarding family nursing research, theory, and practice. Paramount among the challenges is open dialogue about the field. In addressing accumulated knowledge about families and nursing practice as one of the nine challenges, Gillis states there are few reviews that consider family and health. In the reviews that were examined by Gillis, there were several summative documents that were mentioned. The reviews of Feetham,[9] Gillis and others[11] accumulated research in nursing and catalogued the work according to focus, design, and methods. Gillis states nursing needs to specify what we know about families and how to care for them in health and illness.

This chapter uses system theory, developmental theory, and risk estimate theory to guide the nursing process with families. The 11 functional health patterns, as described in Chapters 4 and 7 are used for posing questions to obtain assessment data. The analysis phase of the nursing process categorizes these data into stages of family development, and from the analysis a nursing diagnosis is formulated. A family's health status is considered functional, potentially dysfunctional (potential problem), and dysfunctional (actual problem). The planning with the family states the goals and objectives for measuring behavioral change. Implementation of the nursing plan can be carried out by the nurse, the family, or other health professionals. Four types of interventions are discussed for health promotion and disease prevention. Various roles the nurse may assume through stages of family development also are listed. Evaluation considers outcomes that are specific, objective, and measurable and that rely on the family's subjective interpretation of success and the nurse's observation of changes in family functioning.

NURSING PROCESS AND THE FAMILY

The nursing process with the family begins when the nurse and the family meet for the purpose of enhancing wellness or solving a problem or a potential problem. Although this encounter may occur in several settings, the home is a natural environment for families. Members of different age groups – infants, children, and the elderly – are apt to be more readily available in the home. The nurse also can observe firsthand the physical environment during the home visit (e.g., detecting household items that may present a safety hazard). The nurse can see the whole family as a unit, observing mealtime rituals, roles of family members, and interpersonal interactions. Generally the nurse telephones the family and sets up an appointment for the visit. Including each member of the family in the visit will provide the nurse with a broader perspective than will interviewing an isolated member. During the visit the nursing process is carried out *with* the family and not for the family; the family becomes a partner with the nurse in all phases of the process. Guidelines for the home visit are presented in the box on p. 181.

Several factors influence the assessment phase of the nursing process: the nurse's perception of what constitutes a family; knowledge of theories, norms, and standards; and ability to put the family at ease during visits. In addition to factors that pertain to the nurse, familial factors also influence the assessment phase: cooperation from family members, mutual agreement to work toward a desired goal, and the family's ability to see the relevance of nursing actions regarding their needs and wants.

The assessment phase of the nursing process identifies and seeks information from the family about its activities in health promotion and disease prevention. To obtain this information, the nurse must know the family's progress through its developmental tasks and its ability to generate low-risk-taking behaviors associated with disease prevention. Approaches considered in this chapter are the developmental framework and the risk factor estimate. Developmental norms, as proposed by Duvall,[5] and risk factor estimates, as proposed by the surgeon general's report,[14] are used to guide the nurse through the steps of the nursing process.

❑ ❑ GUIDELINES FOR HOME VISIT TO PROMOTE HEALTH AND PREVENT DISEASE

Planning the Visit

Make arrangements with family.
Study information regarding family from agency record, referral forms, and other sources of information.
State purpose of visit.
Obtain appropriate supplies and teaching aids for visits.

Making the visit

Introduce self and explain purpose of visit.
Place nurse's bag in appropriate place.
Include all family members in discussion.
Identify family's request for assistance.
Understand the situation from the family's perspective.
Identify appropriate activities for health promotion and disease prevention.
Identify how the home visit is to be financed.
Make a contract with the family that states specific goals and objectives the family wants to reach.
Terminate the visit with specific instructions and information on the next visit: when it will occur, what will happen, who will be present, and what the family needs to accomplish before then.

NURSE'S ROLE

Working with the family from a systems perspective, the nurse understands how family members interact, what family norms and expectations are, how effectively members communicate, how the family makes decisions, and how the family deals with needs and expectations. The nurse's role in health promotion and disease prevention includes the following tasks:

1. To become aware of family attitudes and behaviors toward health promotion and disease prevention
2. To serve as role model for the family
3. To collaborate with the family in assessing, improving, enhancing, and evaluating their current health practices
4. To assist the family in growth and development behaviors
5. To assist the family in identifying risk-taking behaviors
6. To assist the family in decision-making regarding choices of lifestyle
7. To provide reinforcement for positive health-behavior practices
8. To assist the family in learning behaviors that promote health and prevent disease
9. To serve as a liaison for referral or collaboration between community resources and the family

How the nurse works with families to assist them with health promotion and disease prevention will depend on the framework used to guide, observe, and classify the situation. Table 8-1 presents nursing roles for families in various stages of development.

THE FAMILY FROM A SYSTEMS PERSPECTIVE

The family can be defined as a set of interacting individuals who are related by blood, marriage, cohabitation, or adoption and who are interdependent in carrying out relevant functions through roles. Relevant functions of the family include values and practices placed on health. Health is seen as any activity undertaken by the family for the purpose of health promotion and disease prevention. The effective execution of health-related functions is based on the way in which the family progresses through its developmental tasks and its ability to generate low-risk-producing behaviors associated with disease prevention. Choices regarding health-promotion and prevention behaviors determine the potential for the family to enhance health practices in its members.

Systems theory perceives patterns of living among the people who make up the family system.[7] Behaviors and responses of family members are seen as influencing the family's pattern and life. Meanings and values are vital components of the family system and provide motivation and energy. Every family has a unique culture, value structure, and history. Values, the means of interpreting events and information, are passed down from generation to generation and are subject to change by continuing interaction with the environment. The family processes information and energy exchange with the environment through values; the values identify the meaning of the information for the family's use.

Systems have boundaries that separate the family system from the rest of the environment and control the flow of information, energy, and matter between the system and the surrounding environment to maintain the system. This becomes the family's psychic energy and internal manager, made up of interactions and relationships of members with each other and with those outside the family system. The family is considered more as a unified whole than the sum of its parts – an integrated system of interdependent functions, structure, and relationships that reacts as a single whole. Living systems are open systems. As a living system, the family must be open to constantly exchanging energy and information with the environment; the greater the openness of the family, the greater the changes possible. Change in one part or member of the family results in changes in the family as a whole. Change requires adaptation of every member within the family as roles and functions take on new meanings. Once the family has made the change, it does

***Table 8-1.* Nurse's roles in health promotion and disease prevention through stages of family development**

Stage	Nursing role	Stage	Nursing role
Couple	Counselor on sexual and marital role adjustment Teacher and counselor in family planning Teacher of parenting skills Coordinator for genetic counseling Facilitator in interpersonal relationships	Family with adolescents	Teacher of risk factors to health Teacher in problem-solving issues regarding alcohol, smoking, diet, and exercise Facilitator of interpersonal skills with teenagers and parents Direct supporter, counselor, or referrer to mental health resources Counselor on family planning Referrer for sexually transmittable disease Participant in community organizations on disease control
Childbearing family	Monitor of prenatal care and referrer for problems of pregnancy Counselor on prenatal nutrition Counselor on prenatal maternal habits Supporter of amniocentesis Counselor on breastfeeding Coordinator with pediatric services Supervisor of immunizations Referrer to social services	Family with young or middle-aged adults	Teacher in problem-solving issues regarding lifestyle and habits Participant in community organizations for environmental control Case finder in the home and community Screener for hypertension, Pap smear, breast examination, cancer signs, mental health, and dental care Counselor on menopausal transition for husband and wife Facilitator in interpersonal relationships among family members
Family with preschool and school-age children	Monitor of early childhood development; referrer when indicated Teacher in first-aid and emergency measures Coordinator with pediatric services Counselor on nutrition and exercise Teacher in problem-solving issues regarding health habits Participant in community organizations for environmental control Teacher of dental care hygiene Counselor on environmental safety in home Facilitator in interpersonal relationships	Family with older adults	Referrer for work and social activity, nutritional programs, homemakers' services, and so on Monitor of exercise, nutrition, preventive services, and medications Supervisor of immunization Counselor on safety in the home

not revert back to its former state; the change is incorporated as part of the system.

Families are composed of both structural and functional components. *Structure* refers to the family's roles and relationships, whereas *function* is the process of continuous change in the system as information and energy are exchanged between the family and the environment.

DEVELOPMENTAL FRAMEWORK

Building on Erikson's theory of psychosocial development,[6] Duvall[5] has identified stages of the family life cycle and critical family developmental tasks. Although Duvall's classification has been criticized for its middle-class homogeneity and lack of diversity in family forms, it is useful in assessment of families because it provides a way for anticipating what to expect. By knowing the composition of the family, how the members are related, and the family's particular life cycle, the nurse can predict somewhat reliably the overall pattern of the family's activities, what significant elements to look for, and what forces probably will be found. The box on p. 183 lists tasks essential to the family's survival and continuity. In general, Duvall maintains that all families have these basic tasks as long as they exist, with each performing them in its own way. The nurse collects data to ascertain how the family is meeting each task. In addition to the general tasks of survival and continuity, each family has stages of developmental and specific tasks related to each stage. A specific task is a growth responsibility that arises at a certain stage in the life of a family. Failure in the tasks may lead to disapproval by society (child abuse or neglect) and possible intervention by police, welfare, health department, or other agencies. Failure early in the life cycle may lead to difficulty with later developmental tasks.

As the family enters each new stage of its development, a critical role transition occurs. Events such as being married, bearing children, releasing members as teenagers and young adults, and continuing as a couple or single person through the "empty nest" and aging years move the family into and through new stages in its history.

❑ ❑ TASKS FOR FAMILY SURVIVAL AND CONTINUITY

- Providing shelter, food, clothing, health care, and the like for its members
- Meeting family costs and allocating such resources as time, space, and facilities according to each member's needs.
- Determining who does what in the support, management, and care of the home and its members.
- Ensuring each member's socialization through the internalization of increasingly mature roles in the family and in society.
- Establishing ways of interacting, communicating, and expressing affections, aggression, sexuality, and so on within limits acceptable to society.
- Bearing (or adopting) and rearing children, then incorporating and releasing family members appropriately.
- Relating to school, church, work, and community life, and establishing policies for including in-laws, relatives, guests, friends, mass media, and so on.
- Maintaining morale and motivation, rewarding achievement, meeting personal and family crises, setting attainable goals, and developing family loyalties and values.

Adapted from Duvall EM: *Marriage and family development,* ed 6, New York, 1985, Harper & Row.

Each new developmental stage requires adaptations and new responsibilities. At the same time each developmental stage opens up new opportunities for the family to realize its fullest potential. As the family enters each new stage, the nurse is alerted to what may be expected and to an approximate timetable for anticipating change. Each new stage then becomes an opportunity for health promotion and intervention.

The stages of family development, although reflective of the traditional nuclear family and extended family networks, can be applied to other family configurations. For example, the couple who marries and brings to the union children of various ages from a previous marriage must accomplish the developmental tasks of the couple stage, as well as specific family stages of the children. The couple and the children bring values and beliefs from past unions that the existing group must integrate and share. In situations where there are no children, individual development is integrated into the lives of the couple. The childless couple obviously presents a different set of developmental tasks than those proposed for the couple with children.

In assessing a family's developmental stage and its performance of the tasks appropriate to that stage, the nurse uses a guideline for analyzing family growth and health-promotion needs. Table 8-2 summarizes the family developmental tasks during critical stages.

***Table 8-2.* Selected developmental tasks of the family at critical stages**

Stage	Positions in family	Developmental tasks
Couple	Wife Husband	Establishing mutually satisfying marriage Relating to kin network Planning to have or not to have children
Childbearing family	Wife-mother Husband-father Infant daughter or son or both	Having and adjusting to infant and supporting needs of all three family members Renegotiating marital and extended family relationships
Family with preschoolers	Wife-mother Husband-father Daughter-sister Son-brother	Adjusting to predictable and unexpected costs of family life Adapting to critical needs and interests of preschool children in stimulating, growth-promoting ways Coping with energy depletion and lack of privacy as parents
Family with school-age children	Wife-mother Husband-father Daughter-sister Son-brother	Adjusting to growing children's activity Promoting joint decision making of children and parents Encouraging and supporting children's educational achievement
Family with adolescents	Wife-mother Husband-father Daughter-sister Son-brother	Maintaining open communication between family members Strengthening marital relationship Supporting ethical and moral values within family Balancing freedom with responsibility with teenagers as they mature and emancipate themselves
Family with young adults	Wife-mother-grandmother Husband-father-grandfather Daughter-sister-aunt Son-brother-uncle	Releasing young adults with appropriate rituals and assistance Reestablishing marital relationship as couple Maintaining supportive home base

Adapted from Duvall EM: *Marriage and family development*, ed 6, Philadelphia, 1985, JB Lippincott. Reprinted by permission. Harper & Row.

Continued.

***Table 8-2.* Selected developmental tasks of the family at critical stages – cont'd**

Stage	Positions in family	Developmental tasks
Family with middle-age adults	Wife-mother-grandmother Husband-father-grandfather	Preparing for retirement Maintaining kin ties with older and younger generations
Family with older adults	Widow/widower Wife-mother-grandmother Husband-father-grandfather	Adjusting to retirement Adjusting to loss of spouse Closing family home or adapting its elderly members

RISK FACTOR ESTIMATE

Traditionally, epidemiology has used levels and trends of mortality and morbidity (death and illness) rates as indirect evidence of health. Data such as infant mortality rates, stillbirth rates, and leading causes of death have long been used as indicators of the collective health of a community. Healthy family functioning links the stages of the family life cycle and specific risk factors together. Epidemiology often describes a disease association in terms of risk. Risks to health can be physiologic, many of which are genetic in origin, or psychologic, which can result from a low self-image. Risks may arise from the environment, including the physical environment and socioeconomic conditions. As a pivotal part of the environment, the family is deemed the most important of the naturally occurring social support systems in the lowering of risks in its members.

A risk estimate is derived by comparing the frequency of deaths, illnesses, or injuries from a specific cause in a group having some specific trait or risk factor with the frequency in another group not having that trait or in the population as a whole. Some diseases may occur more frequently in certain families, such as sickle cell anemia in black families and Tay-Sachs disease in Jewish families. Such high-risk families are not difficult to identify because of the hereditary association with these diseases.

Other diseases, however, are not linked so clearly to heredity and are much more difficult to attribute to specific causes. The natural history of chronic disease, for example, may predispose individual members to greater risk, but the specific cause may be difficult to identify. Leppink[16] identifies six progressive stages in the natural history of chronic diseases:

1. No-risk stage: period in an individual's life when no risk exists of developing the disease, varying from a few to many years.
2. Risk stage: one or more of the causative agents or factors become part of the host's environment.
3. Infiltration stage: causative agent or agents are active in the individual even though no symptoms or sign of overt disease can be detected by any known diagnostic means.
4. Critical stage: signs are present. This is the transition from wellness to illness. If the risks had been eliminated before this stage, the disease process could have been reversed or significantly decelerated. The client probably is unaware that a disease process is underway. It may still be possible to arrest or reduce the seriousness of the disease and enhance longevity.
5. Symptom stage: the client is now aware of problem and seeks help from the health care system. Diagnosis may still be elusive. Any behavioral change is likely to have no significant effect on the course of the disease.
6. Overt disease stage: evidence is seen and a definitive diagnosis can be established readily. Some degree of disability exists, and little can be done to effect reversal or regression of anatomic changes.

With cancer of the lung, for example, the stages of the natural history of chronic disease indicate that the client may be at no risk until starting to smoke. At some point the dysplasia of the epithelial cells of the bronchi will indicate the disease is active. Intervention at stage 3 will prevent the disease, and anatomic changes can be reversed.

This model can be used with such chronic diseases as cervical cancer, cerebrovascular accident (stroke), and heart disease. Prevention or reduction of morbidity usually is possible by changing some behavior or activity during the first three stages of the disease.

Throughout the family's life cycle, probabilities of risk change depend on the family's activities in health promotion and disease prevention. The stages of family development are used to classify risk factors (Fig. 8-1). The age-specific developmental stage and the age-specific health problems appear on Table 8-3 and represent periods when the family may be most vulnerable or sensitive to certain risk factors as well as the time when health promotion and disease prevention can be enhanced. Many of the health problems listed are related to excesses: smoking, drinking, faulty nutrition, overuse of medications, fast driving, and relentless pressure to achieve. Excesses may be caused by habits learned in the family setting. Of the 10 leading causes of death listed in the surgeon general's[13] report, at least seven could be substantially reduced if the family improved just five habits: diet, smoking, lack of exercise, alcohol abuse, and stress.

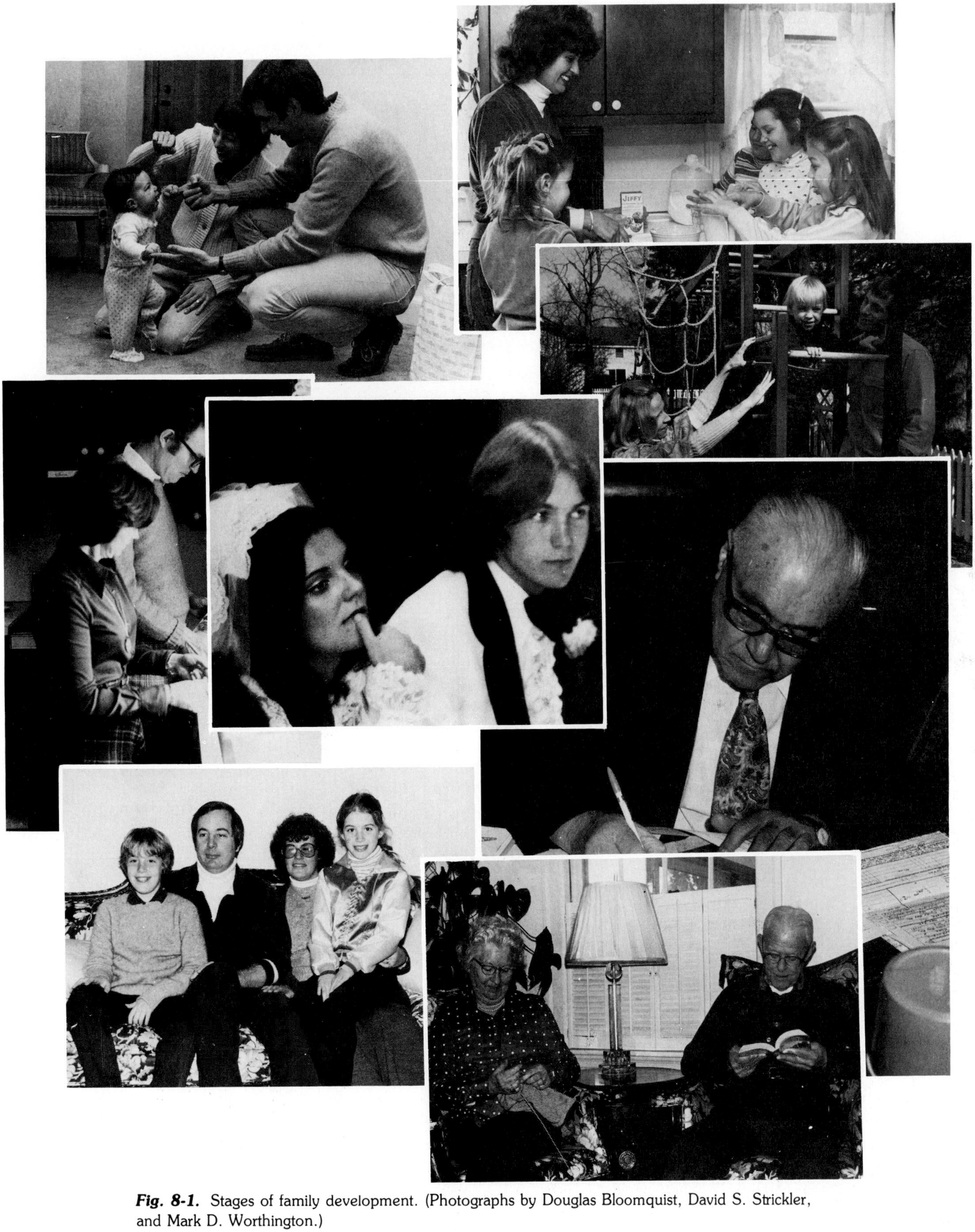

Fig. 8-1. Stages of family development. (Photographs by Douglas Bloomquist, David S. Strickler, and Mark D. Worthington.)

***Table 8-3.* Family stage-specific risk factors and related health problems**

Stage	Risk factors	Health problems
Beginning childbearing family	Lack of knowledge concerning family planning Teenage marriage Lack of knowledge concerning sexual and marital roles and adjustments Underweight or overweight Lack of prenatal care Inadequate nutrition Poor food habits Smoking, alcohol, drug abuse Unmarried status First pregnancy before age 16 or after 35 History of hypertension and infections during pregnancy Rubella, syphilis, gonorrhea, and autoimmune deficiency syndrome (AIDS) Genetic factors present Low socioeconomic and educational levels Lack of safety in the home Home unsafe	Premature baby Unsuccessful marriage Low birth-weight infant Birth defects Birth injuries Accidents Sudden infant death syndrome (SIDS) Respiratory distress syndrome (RDS) Sterility Pelvic Inflammatory disease (PID) Fetal alcohol syndrome (FAS) Mental retardation Child abuse Injuries Birth defects
Family with school-age children	Home unstimulating Working parents with inappropriate use of resources for child care Poverty environment Abuse and/or neglect of children Generational pattern of using social agencies as a way of life Multiple closely spaced children Low family self-esteem Children used as scapegoat for parental frustration Repeated infections, accidents, hospitalizations Parents immature, dependent, and unable to handle responsibility Unrecognized or unattended health problems Strong beliefs about physical punishment Toxic substances unprotected in the home Poor nutrition (overeating and undereating)	Behavior disturbances Speech and vision problems Communicable diseases Dental caries School problems Learning disabilities Cancer Injuries Chronic diseases Homicide Violence
Family with adolescents	Racial and ethnic family origin Lifestyle and behavior patterns leading to chronic disease Lack of problem-solving skills Family values of aggressiveness and competition Socioeconomic factors contributing to peer relationships Family values rigid and inflexible Daredevil risk-taking attitudes Denial behavior Conflicts between parents and children Pressure to live up to family expectations	Violent deaths and injuries Alcohol and drug abuse Unwanted pregnancy Sexually transmitted diseases Suicide Depression
Family with middle-aged adults	Hypertension Smoking High cholesterol Diabetes Overweight Physical inactivity Personality patterns related to stress	Cardiovascular disease, principally coronary artery disease and cerebrovascular accident (stroke) Cancer Accidents Homicide

Adapted from *Healthy people 2000: national health promotion and disease prevention objectives,* US Department of Health and Human Services, Public Health Service 91-50212, Washington, DC, 1990, US Government Printing Office.

Table 8-3. **Family stage-specific risk factors and related health problems – cont'd**

Stage	Risk factors	Health problems
Family with middle-aged adults	Genetic predisposition	Suicide
	Use of oral contraceptives	Abnormal fetus
	Sex, race, and other hereditary factors	Mental illness
	Geographic area, age, occupational deficiencies	
	Habits (diet with low fiber, pickling, charcoal use, broiling)	
	Alcohol abuse	
	Exposure to certain substances (sunlight, radiation, water or air pollution)	
	Social class	
	Residence	
	Depression	Periodontal disease and loss of teeth
	Gingivitis	
Family with older adults	Age	Mental confusion
	Drug interactions	Reduced vision
	Depression	Hearing impairment
	Metabolic disorders	Hypertension
	Pituitary malfunctions	Acute illness
	Cushing's syndrome	Infectious disease
	Hypercalcemia	Influenza
	Chronic illness	Pneumonia
	Retirement	Injuries such as burns and falls
	Loss of spouse	Depression
	Reduced income	Chronic disease
	Poor nutrition	Elderly abuse
	Lack of exercise	Death without dignity
	Past environments and lifestyle	
	Lack of preparation for death	

The risks that are family related can be inferred from (1) lifestyle (habits of overeating, drug dependency, high sugar intake, high-cholesterol diets, smoking), (2) biologic factors (genetic inheritance, congenital malformation, mental retardation), (3) environmental factors (work pressures leading to stress; anxieties; tensions; air, noise, and water pollution), (4) social and psychologic dimensions (crowding, isolation, rapid and accelerated rates of change), and (5) the health care system (overuse, underuse, or inappropriate use of accessibility).

The family's role in reducing risk factors focuses mainly on influencing health behaviors in its members. Families are induced to make personal lifestyle choices in a society that glamorizes many hazardous behaviors through advertising and the mass media when health consequences may not be immediately visible. Families can be influential in assisting their members to weigh the consequences of risk-taking behavior. Awareness of risk factors may prompt families to make an extra effort to reduce risks more directly under their control and thus lessen overall risk of disease and injury. Healthy behavior, including judicious use of preventive health care services, is a significant area of family responsibility for the personal health of its members.

FUNCTIONAL HEALTH PATTERNS

The typology of 11 functional health patterns provided by Gordon[12] helps organize the collection of basic assessment information. The structure of the pattern represents a standardized assessment format that can be integrated into the developmental and risk factor approach. Information obtained in the 11 functional patterns is judged against family developmental norms and age-specific risk factors. When a problem in one pattern is diagnosed, the etiologic factors may be found in that pattern and in one or more of the other patterns as well. Problems in one pattern are reflected in other areas because the patterns are interdependent (see Chapter 7).

Problems in functional patterns are identified as a dysfunctional health pattern, not disease; a potential dysfunction is predicted when risk factors are present. A developmental risk and a risk of change toward a less functional health pattern are types of risk states. If risk factors are present, a family is said to be susceptible to or at risk for a problem (see Table 8-3).

Gordon interprets a risk state as a potential problem, which indicates the presence of factors that predispose a family to a dysfunctional health pattern. To formulate a nursing diagnosis, the nurse names the problem and etiologic factor. Causality may result from probable causes logically related to the problem or may precede or occur with a problem. The nurse must identify etiologic factors to plan care, then direct intervention toward the causal factors that can be changed and are predicted to have an impact on the problem. Risk factors are the signs indicating a potential problem; in a sense, they are the cause. Since this potential state is predicted and is not an actual state with an actual cause, etiology may be nonspecific. Intervention in this case is directed toward reducing risk factors.

The sequence of patterns in the history begins with the family's health perception and health management. This pattern gives an overview that can be used to predict where problems may exist in other patterns and may require in-depth assessment. It starts the history taking from the family's perspective and helps the family to define the situation. The role and relationship pattern define the family structure and function. Lifestyle indicators are assessed through the remaining nine patterns.

Health Perception and Health Management

This pattern identifies characteristics about the family's general health perceptions and management and preventive practices. Pratt[22] has identified six healthy characteristics of families: (1) members facilitate an interaction process, (2) members enhance individual development, (3) role relationships are structured effectively, (4) members actively attempt to cope with problems, (5) members promote healthy home environments and lifestyle, and (6) members establish regular links with the broader community.

Health practices vary from family to family, each identifies and carries out health-maintenance activities related to what members believe is healthy and what they think is feasible, as demonstrated in their lifestyle practices.

Questions the nurse asks on assessment include the following:

What is the family's philosophy of health? Does each family member believe the same? Does the family practice what they believe?

What behaviors or lifestyle practices, such as smoking, alcohol, and drug abuse, does the family engage in?

What behaviors are the family exhibiting that point to chronic disease?

Does the family engage in health-related behaviors, such as eating three meals a day at regular times, eating breakfast every day, exercising a minimum of 2 or 3 days a week, sleeping 7 to 8 hours each night, and abstaining from smoking?

Are risk factors present for infections, such as lack of immunization, lack of knowledge of transmittable diseases, and lack of personal hygiene?

Are there risk factors that point to body injury, accidents, unprotected drugs, and chemicals in the home in easy reach of children?

Do elderly members know what medications they are taking and what they are for?

Are there medications in the home that are not being used and should be discarded?

Is nutrition adequate to maintain adequate energy levels?

Are any unattended health problems present?

Is there a history of repeated infections and hospitalizations? Is safety lacking in the home?

Is the home unstimulating or overstimulating?

Where does the family go for health and illness care?

Is the family engaged in a dental program?

Describe the family's previous experience with a nurse and other health professionals.

Roles and Relationships

This pattern identifies characteristics of family roles and relationships. Structural and functional aspects are assessed.

Structural aspects of the family include each member's name, role (mother, aunt, sister), age, sex, education, and occupation. The family's origin (ethnic, cultural) and genetic heritage completes what generally is considered family identification data. Traditionally, families have been described as nuclear (husband, wife, children) and extended or family of orientation (aunts, uncles, grandparents, cousins).

The prevalence of the traditional nuclear family has been influenced by societal changes, such as the women's movement, employment of mothers, marriage, divorce, and remarriage. This has resulted in greater recognition of other family structures, such as those that are listed in Table 8-4. Numerous questions and unresolved issues are related to the specific effects of different family structures on childrearing and individual growth and development and pose a challenge to the nurse in health promotion and disease prevention.

Spradley[24] has classified divergent family structures as falling into three types that are of particular relevance to the nurse. The first type is the growing numbers of adolescent unwed mothers whose own developmental needs and lack of parenting skills pose particular challenges for the nurse. The second type refers to those couples who after widowhood or divorce have remarried and merge two families. Merged families, according to Spradley, require considerable adjustment and relearning of roles, tasks, communication patterns, and relationships. The third type identified by Spradley is made up of elderly

***Table 8-4.* Variety of family forms**

Configurations	Positions in family
Single parent (separated, divorced, widowed)	Mother or father Son(s), daughter(s)
Unmarried single parent (never married)	Mother or father Son(s), daughter(s)
Unmarried couple	Two adults
Unmarried parents	Mother and father Son(s), daughter(s)
Commune family	Mothers and fathers Shared son(s), daughter(s)
Stepparents	Mother and father Son(s), daughter(s) from previous marriages
Adoptive parents	Mother and father Son(s), daughter(s) adopted

couples, or elderly individuals (mostly women) living alone. This group of people often need assistance in understanding the functions and developmental tasks that would help them adjust and experience positive aging.

Culkin Rhyne,[3] in writing about understanding and supporting families in the process of divorce, states that it is important to understand divorce as a series of events involving a period of transition. The process is complex and multifaceted, requiring the disintegration of one family structure and the reorganization of another. The developmental levels of the children, their individual temperaments, and the quality of their environmental support will all play a role in how the children respond. Supporting the children may be difficult for the parents who are at the same time experiencing an adjustment to each other. How parents handle the situational crisis and accomplish the organization of the family in the postdivorce period is a significant variable in long-term individual and family adjustment.

Dietz-Omar[4] studied family coping with stepfamilies and traditional nuclear families during pregnancy. Stepfamilies emerged as "evolving" new families, and thus the author suggested they more than likely needed assistance in working out roles, rules, bonding, and boundary issues within their family structures. Traditional nuclear families, on the other hand, were experiencing a pregnancy other than a first one with their spouse and may have felt more capable of adding another child. The author notes that these established families may have acquired satisfactory levels of adaptability and cohesion through negotiation of behavioral and emotional involvement within the family structure.

The family's ability to perform health-promotion and disease-prevention functions may be influenced by the way it is organized. For example, a single parent without an extended family network support may be in need of community resources to help raise the children. A two-parent family living near its extended family may have all the support needed to raise children but may need to become aware of growth and development stages and immunization schedules.

The same individual may experience different family forms in a lifetime. A person may be part of a nuclear family as an infant, a single-parent family after parents are divorced, a stepparent family when the mother remarries, and an unmarried-couple family when the person is one of two adults who share a household. The person brings to each new family configuration values and beliefs regarding disease prevention and health promotion practiced in previous unions. The nonshared values can result in divergent expectations unless they are integrated into a shared set of values and beliefs with the new union. Shifting family forms have affected individuals in ways that could well determine the future viability of the family and the direction of the health care system.

GENOGRAM

A useful way of viewing the family from identification data is to draw a genogram, or family diagram, depicting each member of the family and showing connections between generations. Genetically related diseases with family members and extended family are identified. If relevant, data are gathered on maternal and paternal grandparents, including aunts and uncles and their children. The extent of the family genogram depends on the clues leading to familial history of disease. It may be necessary to name the genetically linked diseases, since individuals often forget what they are called.

Fig. 8-2 depicts a genogram of the three-generation Foley family. The nuclear family consists of Mr. and Mrs. Foley and their daughter, age 2. The extended family of Mr. and Mrs. Foley consists of grandparents, parents, aunts, and uncles. The genogram shows a history of chronic diseases on both sides of the family and should alert the nurse to risk factors (see Table 8-3) that are associated with the chronic diseases of cerebral vascular accident (CVA), cardiovascular disease (CVD), chronic obstructive pulmonary disease (COPD), tuberculosis (TB), cancer (CA), diabetes, and arthritis. Being overweight is a risk factor associated with CVD, hypertension, diabetes mellitus, and cancer.

ASSESSMENT QUESTIONS

The nurse should consider questions in assessing the family's health patterns. Data collected in the 11 functional patterns give clues to the family's health-promotion and disease-prevention practice (see box on pp. 192-193 for assessment questions in the 11 functional health patterns).

Risks to healthy family functioning may be identified in

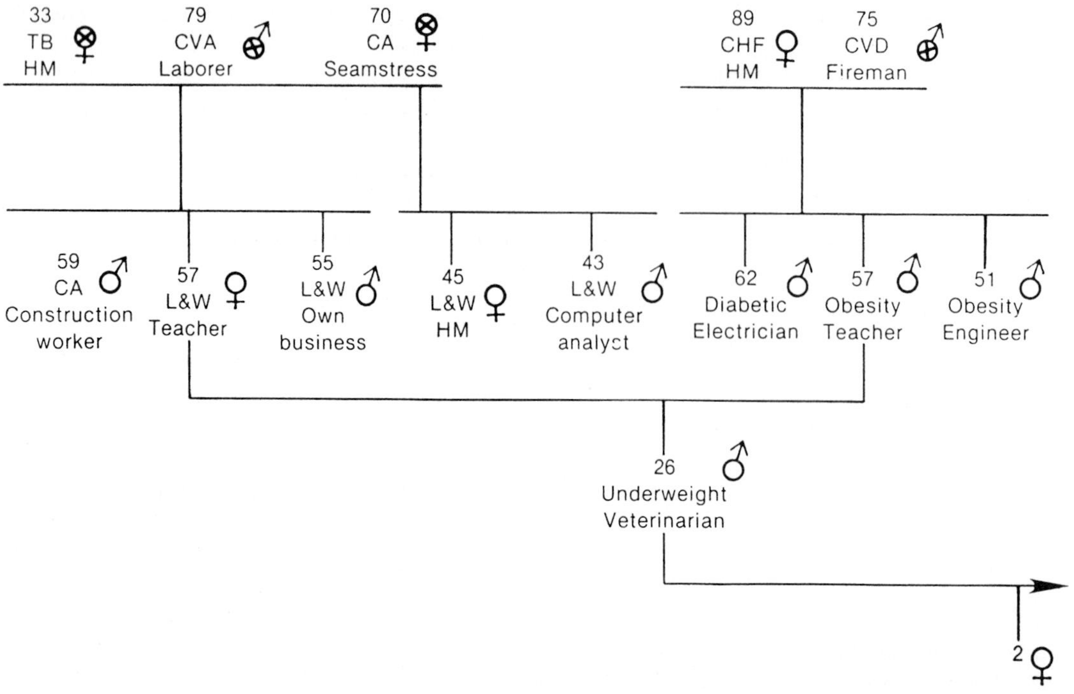

Fig. 8-2. Genogram of Foley nuclear family. *CA,* cancer; *CHF,* congestive heart failure; *COPD,* chronic obstructive pulmonary disease; *CVA,* cerebrovascular accident; *CVD,* cardiovascular disease; *HA,* heart attack; *HM,* homemaker; *L&W,* living and well; *TB,* tuberculosis. Numbers indicate ages.

each pattern, and some risk factors may be found in one or more areas. Air pollution from cigarette smoking, for example, could be identified easily as an environmental factor (home). The family's reaction to smoke pollution, however, will determine the extent of the family's susceptibility (genetics). If the family has a high incidence of chronic obstructive lung disease in the nuclear extended family or in past generations, and all adult members of the family smoke (health perception and health management), ignoring the warnings of research (cognitive), then several pattern areas may indicate risk factors present. The point, however, is that the nurse must recognize and identify not only the risk factor but the interrelationships of risks and their effects on each other.

ANALYSIS AND NURSING DIAGNOSIS

After completing the data collection, the nurse compares the information to documented norms of health promotion and disease prevention. Norms or expected values can be derived from the family's baseline information of 11 functional pattern areas, knowledge of growth and development for all age groups and the family as a whole, and risk factor estimate and population norms.

Population norms specify a range of normal limits for particular groups. For example, age is associated with various risk factors; some disorders are so common that they are called childhood diseases and diseases of the elderly. Age-specific risks to communicable diseases, such as chickenpox (varicella) or pertussis, exemplify this. In certain other diseases, such as lung cancer, a long period is associated with long-term exposure. When risk increases with cumulative exposure, the frequency of the disease increases with age. Sex also is related to various risk factors (e.g., breast cancer in women and heart attacks in men).

Analysis of data on values, beliefs, self-perception, or role relationships with general population norms may not be so easy; the nurse also must consider cultural, ethnic, and religious factors. Analysis may have to be based on whether the family perceives the situation to be a problem or a potential problem. Thus, the family's baseline information is important, since it provides comparative criteria in the analysis. Reviewing previous records of the family also might be useful in obtaining this data. If no previous record exists, the information taken on first contact provides criteria for subsequent measurement of progress.

From the analysis of the data the nurse formulates a nursing diagnosis, which is a statement of the family's health status as applicable to nursing intervention. A family's health status can be diagnosed as functional (successful coping experience, extended family network, financially solvent, open communication), potentially dysfunctional (rigid rules, undefined roles, inadequate housing), and

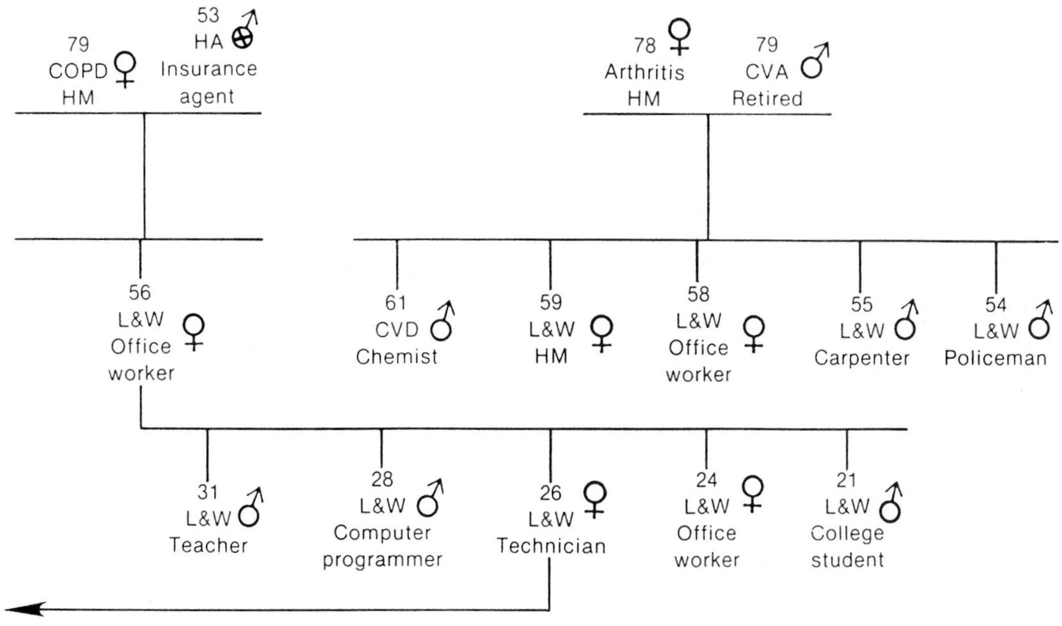

Fig. 8-2, cont'd. Genogram of Foley nuclear family.

dysfunctional (alcohol and drug abuse). Indicators that make the family dysfunctional are clarified and identified as a health problem.

After making a judgment about the family's health status, the nurse then can identify a nursing need that will solve the problem. Validating the potential or actual health problem with the family is important; only when the nurse and family agree on the situation can cooperation occur. If the family does not agree, further assessment or negotiation may be needed. The family and the nurse also must agree on the sequence of the problem resolution.

Analyzing Data

Analysis of data is accomplished by using the three approaches to the family: systems theory, developmental theory, and risk estimate theory.

From a systems approach the family is evaluated as open or closed, with permeable or rigid boundaries in terms of change. The systems approach includes the structural and functional components of family as a system. The 11 functional patterns are used to obtain baseline data on assessment.

The developmental theory approaches the family from tasks and stages of progression through its life cycle. The nurse analyzes data collected for cues that identify the stages of the family life cycle as well as the tasks that need to be accomplished for successful family function. The nurse then notes the family's developmental needs.

Specific cause in risk estimate theory, mentioned earlier, may be difficult to isolate, as in the leading causes of death in the United States today. For example, at least five known risk factors are associated with heart disease: high blood pressure, obesity, high blood lipids, heredity factors, and smoking. Family-related risks can be inferred from lifestyle, biologic factors, environmental factors, and sociopsychologic dimensions. The purpose of risk analysis is to provide the family with realistic health threats, currently known or estimated, to which they are particularly vulnerable before they develop signs or symptoms of dysfunction (see Table 8-3).

The stages of family development are used as a guide to categorize and analyze the baseline data. If the nurse finds gaps, missing data, or conflicting information, plans are made to obtain the necessary information on the next visit.

COUPLE FAMILY

The first stage may or may not begin with marriage. In today's society legal marriage may not be the basis for the relationship, and the adults may define themselves as a family unit. Married or not, two individuals move from their family of orientation to an unfamiliar couple relationship. Analysis of critical family developmental tasks include establishment of a mutually satisfying adult relationship that fits into the kinship network. The major adjustment for the couple is learning how to mesh two personalities, two life histories, and two aspirations of growth. Major decisions in this stage include whether the two partners both work, how money (making, spending, saving) is handled, where they are going to live, how they are go-

❑ ❑ 11 FUNCTIONAL HEALTH PATTERNS ASSESSMENT GUIDELINES FOR FAMILY

Family Assessment

The 11 functional health pattern areas are applicable to the assessment of families. Families are the primary client in community health nursing. In some cases, a family assessment may be indicated (1) in the care of an infant or child whose development is influenced by family health patterns or (2) when an adult has certain health problems that can be influenced by family patterns. The following guidelines provide information on family functioning:

1. *Health-perception–health-management pattern*
   History:
   a. How has family's general health been (in last few years)?
   b. Colds in past year? Absence from work/school?
   c. Most important things you do to keep healthy? Think these make a difference to health? (Include family folk remedies, if appropriate.)
   d. Members' use of cigarettes, alcohol, drugs?
   e. Immunizations? Health care provider? Frequency of checkups? Accidents (home, work, school, driving)? (If appropriate: Storage of drugs, cleaning products, scatter rugs, etc.)
   f. In past, been easy to find ways to follow things doctors, nurses, social workers (if appropriate) suggest?
   g. Things important in family's health that I could help with?
   Examination:
   a. General appearance of family members and home.
   b. If appropriate: Storage of medicines, cribs, playpens, stove, scatter rugs, hazards, etc.
2. *Nutritional-metabolic pattern*
   History:
   a. Typical family meal pattern/food intake? (Describe.) Supplements (vitamins, types of snacks, etc.)?
   b. Typical family fluid intake? (Describe.) Supplements: type available (fruit juices, soft drinks, coffee, etc.)?
   c. Appetites?
   d. Dental problems? Dental care (frequency)?
   e. Anyone have skin problems? Healing problems?
   Examination:
   a. If opportunity available: Refrigerator contents, meal preparation, contents of meal, etc.
3. *Elimination pattern*
   History:
   a. Family use of laxatives, other aids?
   b. Problems in waste/garbage disposal?
   c. Pet animals waste disposal (indoor/outdoor)?
   d. If indicated: Problems with flies, roaches, rodents?
   Examination:
   a. If opportunity available: Examine toilet facilities, garbage disposal, pet waste disposal; indicators of risk for flies, roaches, rodents.
4. *Activity-exercise pattern*
   History:
   a. In general, does family get a lot of/little exercise? Type? Regularity?
   b. Family leisure activities? Active/passive?
   c. Problems in shopping (transportation), cooking, keeping up the house, budgeting for food, clothes, housekeeping, house costs?
   Examination:
   a. Pattern of general home maintenance, personal maintenance.
5. *Sleep-rest pattern*
   History:
   a. Generally, family members seem to be well rested and ready for school/work?
   b. Sufficient sleeping space and quiet?
   c. Family find time to relax?
   Examination:
   a. If opportunity available: Observe sleeping space and arrangements.
6. *Cognitive-perceptual pattern*
   History:
   a. Visual or hearing problems? How managed?
   b. Any big decisions family has had to make? How made?
   Examination:
   a. If indicated: Language spoken at home.
   b. Grasp of ideas and questions (abstract/concrete).
   c. Vocabulatory level.
7. *Self-perception–self-concept pattern*
   History:
   a. Most of time family feels good (not so good) about themselves as a family?
   b. General mood of family? Happy? Anxious? Depressed? What helps family mood?
   Examination:
   a. General mood state: nervous (5) or relaxed (1); rate from 1 to 5.
   b. Members generally assertive (5) or passive (1); rate from 1 to 5.
8. *Role-relationship pattern*
   History:
   a. Family (or household) members? Member age and family structure (diagram).
   b. Any family problems that are difficult to handle (nuclear/extended)? Child rearing? If appropriate: Spouse ever get rough with you? The children?

11 FUNCTIONAL HEALTH PATTERNS ASSESSMENT GUIDELINES FOR FAMILY—cont'd

Family Assessment

c. Relationships good (not so good) among family members? Siblings? Support each other?
d. If appropriate: Income sufficient for needs?
e. Feel part (or isolated) from community? Neighbors?

Examination:

a. Interaction among family members (if present).
b. Observed family leadership roles.

9. *Sexuality-reproductive pattern*

History:

a. If appropriate (sexual partner within household or situation): Sexual relations satisfying? Changes? Problems?
b. Use of family planning? Contraceptives? Problems?
c. If appropriate (to age of children): Feel comfortable in explaining/discussing sexual subjects?

Examination: None

10. *Coping–stress-tolerance pattern*

History:

a. Any big changes within family in last few years?
b. Family tense or relaxed most of time? When tense what helps? Anyone use medicines, drug, alcohol to decrease tension?
c. When (if) family problems, how handled?
d. Most of the time is this way(s) successful?

Examination: None

11. *Value-belief pattern*

History:

a. Generally, family get things they want out of life?
b. Important things for the future?
c. Any "rules" in the family that everyone believes are important?
d. Religion important in family? Does this help when difficulties arise?

Examination: None

From Gordon M: *Manual of nursing diagnosis: 1993-1994,* St Louis, 1993, Mosby.

ing to relate to in-laws and other family members, and if and when to have children. Other decisions, consciously or unconsciously made, are the sharing of the work load tasks of cooking, washing, cleaning, shopping, and so forth.

Integrating health practices and habits into the lifestyle of the couple is a health-related developmental task that needs consideration in analysis. Health behavior constitutes those actions taken toward promotion of health and prevention of disease; for example, following hygienic practice, participating in well-balanced programs of rest, exercise, and a balanced diet; attending smoking-cessation classes; wearing seat belts; and directing activities toward the attainment of self-actualization. Each individual brings values and beliefs from the family of origin and develops other values and beliefs from personal experiences. Consciously working out health practices that are going to be part of the couple's lifestyle will promote health as a value at the beginning of the family life cycle.

Achieving a mutually satisfying relationship depends on the way the couple is able to handle conflicts and differences. If the method the couple uses to solve problems is congruent with one another, they will be able to make adjustments that will prove satisfying to both partners. If one individual is in the habit of solving problems by avoiding conflict at any price, then problem solving will tend to be ineffective.

If the decision to adopt or give birth to a child is made, then commitment to long-term responsibilities becomes a focus of family development and a primary health need. The nurse, in analyzing learning needs of the pregnant couple, should consider all aspects of the couple's decision and motivations that may be involved with the pregnancy. With single-parent families becoming increasingly common, through divorce, death, adoption, or the choice to have a child out of wedlock, the analysis of data must consider the special needs of these family forms.

The free attitudes and practices in society regarding sexuality have given rise to risks of sexually transmitted diseases such as genital herpes, gonorrhea, and syphilis. Autoimmune deficiency syndrome (AIDS), one of the more recent sexually transmitted diseases, was first described in 1981. It is a disease with a unique set of problems that poses a threat to the young adult and, therefore, to the family and society. The human immunodeficiency virus (HIV) can be transmitted through heterosexual and homosexual sexual intercourse, direct contact with infected blood, shared needles during intravenous drug use, and perinatal transfer from infected mothers to their infants. Prevention of HIV transmission requires either abstinence from or modification of relevant behaviors and adherence to safety precautions for health care workers handling infectious bodily fluids.[25]

Risk factors associated with sexuality include lack of knowledge regarding "safer sex," anatomy and physiology of the reproductive system, personal hygiene, lack of prenatal care, pregnancy before age 16 and after age 35, history of hypertension and infection during pregnancy, and unplanned or unwanted pregnancy.

Risk factors for premature pregnancies and unsatisfying marriage are lack of knowledge concerning family planning, age of bride and groom (teenage pregnancies more at risk, persons in late 20s less at risk), and lack of knowledge concerning sexual and marital roles and adjustments. In unplanned adolescent pregnancies, the parents place an undue biologic risk on their developing child. Lack of knowledge concerning prenatal care, birthing, and child-rearing practices compounds the risks for both the mother and child. The parents unable to carry out the role functions of parenting are at risk for an unsatisfying marriage, breakdown in relationships, and inappropriate developmental growth at the beginning stage of the family life cycle.

If the couple decide to remain childless, then their learning needs may focus on available methods of contraception.

CHILDBEARING FAMILY

The birth of a baby is the beginning of a new unit. All members of the family must learn new roles while the unit expands in functions and responsibilities. The way the triad develops will be influenced by the parents' past history as a dyad and their past experiences in other groups, particularly their families of origin.

The family may be thrown into disequilibrium while the couple is exploring ways to accommodate the new member into the group. As a group, the three explore ways to meet each other's needs, to minimize differences, and to work together. First-time parents often feel a lack of emotional support during the first few months of parenthood. The first few days at home from the hospital may be especially trying if the couple have no network of family or friends on which they can depend for support. Analysis of needs during this critical time can be effective in helping the new parents. Parents may be proficient in caring for the baby's needs but may be lacking in the ability to feel any self-growth in the parenting role. If the wife has been working, she may find the routines of baby care and being in the house all day boring. The husband may be anxious about one income being adequate to support the family and may increase his work schedule. Neither may be able to offer the other emotional support if neither has been prepared to find satisfaction in parenthood. As the childbearing family struggles to adapt to a new member, the family of origin or other support systems (self-help groups, neighbors, friends) may be called for assistance.

Some parents thrive during the period when the infant needs almost total and constant care and nurturance. They are able to find support in each other and in a network of family and friends. The couple who find satisfaction in parenthood seem to realize that parental influence begins at birth and is the single most important factor on the child's physical, emotional, and cognitive development; they are ready to assume the responsibility. The parents' ability to assume responsibility depends largely on their own maturity; how they were cared for as children; their feelings about self, culture, social class, and religion; their relationship with each other; their values and philosophy of life; their perceptions of and experiences with children and other adults; and the life stresses they have experienced. A direct relationship has been found between the degree of emotional health of children and the degree to which the relationship between the parents was positive.

In analyzing child-rearing needs of the family, the nurse considers these factors as well as the family's developmental task of providing for the physical health, economic support, and nurturing actions vital to the child's learning and social development. In analyzing the couple's needs during this stage, the nurse must be aware of the interactions between the triad. Observing the way decisions are made concerning needs will demonstrate how the family functions, what roles each member has, and how effectively the family meets the needs of all its members.

Risks associated with role relationships include working parents with inappropriate use of resources for child care, abuse or neglect of children, multiple closely spaced children, low family self-esteem, children used as scapegoats for parental frustration, immature parents who are dependent and unable to handle responsibility, and strong beliefs about physical punishment or obedience.

FAMILY WITH PRESCHOOL CHILDREN

This family may have more than one child, each growing and developing at an individual pace. Preschool children place great demands on the family; the family must adjust to each new member that comes into the group and must provide space and equipment for expansion.

The home environment must be adapted to the critical needs and interests of preschool children. In analyzing data about the home, the nurse observes whether the child has stimulation-promoting opportunities to experience and explore. The home should be made safe and at the same time allow for exploration by the child. Instead of keeping children away from the kitchen or garden, ways to include the child into a cooking or planting activity will provide learning experiences for the child. Other environmental influences that will affect the child's rate and style of development include religious practices, ethnic background, education, and disciplinary techniques.

Increasing evidence shows that onset of ill health is linked strongly to environmental influences. In the home environment, contamination of air, water, and food increases health risks. For example, lead poisoning, a preventable disease that continues to affect thousands of children, can be the result of lead paint and other factors in the home. Although lead-based paint has been restricted to the exterior of homes in the United States, many homes still have it on interior walls. Both the home and the automobile should be considered as possible sources of exposure to the poisonous agent, carbon. The nurse also reviews data for safety in the home.

Developmental tasks for the family include adjusting to an energy depletion in the couple while they are responding to the demands of parenthood and each other. The nurse may be asked to explore alternate means of finding relief from parenting for the couple. They need time for themselves and at the same time need to know the children are safe with a responsible person; economic restraints may make this difficult.

The family with preschoolers must be aware of the health-promotion habits of proper foods, exercise, sleep, and dental hygiene. Through their example, the routines they provide for the children, and their use of positive reinforcement, the parents can do much in teaching the preschooler about health.

FAMILY WITH SCHOOL-AGE CHILDREN

The family with children in school may have reached its maximum size in numbers and interrelationships. The parents' major problem during this stage is the dichotomy between self-interest and finding fulfillment in rearing the next generation. The family's developmental tasks revolve around the major goals of reorganization to prepare for the expanding world of school-age children. Promoting school achievement is one of the critical tasks in socialization of children. Viewing social and educational goals in terms of family culture and the parent's own defined goals is particularly important in this stage of development. For example, many opportunities for health education exist in schools for influencing children to develop desirable health habits and to acquire healthy health beliefs. Yet, because of parental pressure, health education in the school is oriented toward problems such as smoking, drugs, and alcohol abuse. Thus, the message given is that health is problem and crisis oriented, when the children should be learning the positive aspects of healthy behaviors. As a result, neither the school nor the home may be providing the school-age child with skills that involve developing values about health and making decisions about risk-taking behaviors and their consequences. During this period of development the family can be very influential at home and in school in teaching children how to assess risks for engaging in certain behaviors and what benefits to look for when practicing other behaviors.

Another important developmental task during this stage for both parents and child is letting go as activity broadens inside and outside the home. Parents are likely to be involved in community groups such as the Parent-Teacher Association, scout groups, sports teams, and other volunteer organizations. The mother may enter the work force or renew educational opportunities. Parents can foster a positive self-concept in their children by encouraging them to join in the family discussions and planning in establishing policies and making decisions. The group's position on health practices is included in family policies and decisions.

In this stage, the family is vulnerable to such risk factors as an unsafe and unstimulating home, repeated infections, abuse and neglect of children, poverty environment, and low family self-esteem. Children exposed to an unstimulating and unsafe home environment are at risk for behavior disturbances, school problems, and learning disabilities. Parents who cannot manage their children in growth-promoting ways soon experience depletion of energy and may turn to unorthodox ways of finding relief from parenting. I know one woman who knew the exact symptoms to describe to the emergency room staff that would ensure hospitalization for her three children so that she could have a free weekend now and then.

FAMILY WITH ADOLESCENTS

Families with adolescent members may experience a "change-in-life pregnancy," which may mean the parents must care for an infant while other children in the family are in school. Having a new member enter the family at this stage may be a source of joy or a source of frustration to the family. The overall goal with adolescent members is loosening family ties to allow greater responsibility and freedom in preparation for releasing young adults. While each member of the family is working through individual developmental tasks in the midst of social pressures, the family as a whole has tasks to accomplish. Strengthening the marital relationship to build a foundation for future family stages is a critical task during this time.

Open communication, a critical developmental task at this stage, may be difficult between parents and adolescents, since there is often mutual rejection by parents and adolescents of each other's values and lifestyle. Family values and standards are questioned and challenged. Although mother and father clearly hold the balance of power in deciding who will do what, who uses the family car, and how the family money is spent, adolescents may want to do what their friends do, have their own car, and make their own money to spend how they see fit. Parents who give adolescent members opportunities to experience social, emotional, and ethical situations with others are providing learning opportunities for enhancing a sense of autonomy and responsibility.

Families must deal with the developmental task of balancing freedom with responsibility as adolescents mature and emancipate themselves. Health problems in this age group include violent deaths, injuries, and alcohol and drug abuse. Contributing risk factors are lack of problem-solving skills, family values of aggressiveness and competition, socioeconomic factors contributing to peer relationships, rigid and inflexible family values, daredevil risk-taking attitudes, and conflicts between parents and children. The family, although not in complete control and totally responsible for these risk factors, may have little control over such risks as low socioeconomic variables. The family also cannot readily decrease many environmental risks to violent deaths and injuries; some responsibility lies with the highway system, automobile manufacturers, and the legislature regarding standards of safety. The family must rely largely on the efforts of public health officials and others to reduce these environmental risks.

However, the family can be a supportive force for adolescents in this stage of development, such as including them in the decision-making process by allowing them to choose alternate behaviors and experience the resulting positive and negative consequences. Having made a choice, a commitment to the chosen behavior will follow. Family values of winning and not losing, aggressiveness, and competition may need to be reexamined during this period; the adolescent may decide they are no longer applicable. The change in values in the adolescent may produce conflict and pose a threat to the family, which may respond by placing an undue amount of pressure on the adolescent to conform to family values. In matters of life and death, parents need to be firm and take a stand; for example, "No driving when drinking!"

This stage of family development may be viewed as an identity crisis in the adolescent, the adults, and the family itself. The child is moving from childhood to adulthood, while the adult is passing from parent to nonparent. The adolescent is struggling to find identity independent of and yet connected to the family. Adults are in midlife and must come to terms with their own adolescent fantasies and decide who they are and who they will be for the rest of their lives.

FAMILY WITH YOUNG ADULTS

This family is seen as a launching center because children begin to leave home. In letting their children go, parents are relinquishing 20 years or so of the parenting role and returning to their original marital dyad. The couple build a new life together, while maintaining relationships with aging parents, children, grandchildren, and in-laws.

A couple may find it difficult to redefine their relationship. For the woman, her role as mother is changing because the children no longer need her in the same way. If she has devoted the past 20 years to raising children, she may feel unneeded and lacking in purpose. She may decide to enter the work force for the first time and may need help in the transition. The husband-father may be at the peak of his career or may realize he will not progress further. In addition to individual changes occurring between the couple, the family with young adults may experience other pressures. Aging parents in the extended family may need assistance, and children may need financial and emotional support in leaving home for college, marriage, or work. Financial and emotional responsibilities with other members of the family may prevent the couple from focusing on themselves and their marital relationship during this developmental phase.

Health-promoting activities that can be enhanced during this stage are coping with pressures of social and occupational responsibilities and mobility, recognizing the importance of good health habits and practices, accepting aging in self and in marital partner, and reassessing life goals.

FAMILY WITH MIDDLE-AGED ADULTS

This family may consist of only two members; thinking of self and enhancing self-concept and the marital relationship typically occur at this time. Usually the children have all left home, and the parents are experiencing a new freedom and well-being. Some marriages, having lasted to this stage, have a certain amount of security and stability; the couple have reached an understanding about meeting each other's needs. The pressures of parenting have lifted, and the couple can enjoy the accomplishments of their children and grandchildren. The couple probably have lived in a neighborhood long enough to have acquired a network of friends. Long-time acquaintances seek their participation in neighborhood rituals and events. Economic security and personal self-esteem may be at their peaks for the couple.

On the other hand, some marriages that have lasted to this stage may be in trouble. The last child departing from home may create the "empty nest syndrome." If the couple have not prepared themselves for this stage, they might look elsewhere for opportunities to enhance self-concept. The husband, feeling his father role no longer necessary, may look for a younger wife with whom to begin a new family. The wife, no longer feeling needed by her children or husband, may turn to alcohol, drugs, or other self-destructive behaviors. Both husband and wife may be experiencing problems particular to their sex and may be unable to turn to each other for the necessary support.

Health tasks in this developmental stage require a new awareness because of the susceptibility or vulnerability to illness and disease in this age group. The couple must become aware of the risks to health and adjust lifestyle and habits to cope with them. Losses at this stage also may result in health problems; the couple may need to cope with the deaths of family and friends and a declining income. If the husband or wife has developed a physical or mental illness, the other may have to adjust to the current physical and mental capabilities. A redefining of self-concept may be necessary.

Middle-aged families are susceptible to a host of risk factors leading to the three most prevelant causes of death: heart disease, cancer, and CVA (stroke). The family lifestyle may help to decrease risks by placing a high value on physical activity, not smoking, maintaining adequate but sound nutritional habits, and consuming moderate amounts of alcohol. Lifestyle habits that are transmitted through role modeling have a greater impact on the younger members of the family than any verbal edict. If possible, middle-aged members can be instrumental in choosing an environment that is free or low in water and air pollution and free from crippling stress factors such as excessive noise, traffic, and overcrowding. Family members also can apply pressure on key persons in the community to decrease risks in the environment.

FAMILY WITH OLDER ADULTS

Adjustment to retirement is one of the crucial tasks of the family with older adults. Retirement affects many aspects of a person, including relationships with others. Besides a loss of work, retirement also means a sharp reduction in income for most people. Adjusting living standards to retirement income and being able to supplement this income with wage-earning activity is a task of the aging family. Other tasks during this stage include adjusting the home environment to be safe and comfortable and adjusting to the loss of a spouse, which may require the surviving member to look to the family for support and satisfaction. The loss of lifelong friends may create further dependence on family members.

Health promotion during this stage is directed toward maintaining functional ability, limiting the effects of disabling conditions, and maintaining the quality of life. The elderly fear being helpless and useless and unable to care for themselves. In analyzing risk factors in the aging family, the nurse looks at the couple's ability to function well enough to carry out normal roles and responsibilities. As with all persons, older adults hope for a state of well-being that will allow them to perform at their highest functional capacity of physical, psychologic, and social levels. Many elderly persons remain in their own homes, and the majority are vigorous and completely independent. Only 5% reside in institutions, and many of these are temporary residents who are recovering from illness and expect to return to the community.

Ego integrity (the union of all previous phases of the life cycle) is the challenge in this stage and demands successful aging through continued activity. Having gone through the various stages of family development, the couple accept what they have done as their own. At this time they may pursue other interests or maintain former activities to feel needed and useful.

Formulating Family Nursing Diagnosis

The purpose of writing a family nursing diagnosis is to help the family promote health through the life cycle and prevent disease through low-risk-taking behaviors. The nurse derives the diagnosis from inferences of assessed validated data and from perceptions. A concise summary statement of a problem or potential problem, the diagnosis provides direction for goals, objectives, and interventions by identifying the negative health state and the factors that must be changed to alleviate or prevent it. Andrews[2] provides the following guidelines for the nursing diagnosis:

1. Must be concise and clear.
2. Must be client centered.
3. Must be specific and accurate.
4. May be a descriptive statement.
5. May be expressed as an etiologic statement.
6. Must provide direction for nursing intervention.
7. May be implemented by nursing intervention.
8. Must reflect the client's current health status.

These guidelines are used in Table 8-5, which provides examples of family nursing diagnoses using developmental and risk factor approaches.

***Table 8-5.* Examples of family nursing diagnoses**

Theoretic model	Stage	Health status	Pattern	Problem
Developmental	Family with adolescents	Potential alteration in parenting	Role and relationship	Value systems of parents and adolescent members in conflict
	Family with preschoolers	Potential for physical injury	Health management	Medications and poisonous cleaning substances within reach of children
	Family with older adults	Grieving	Role and relationship	Loss of spouse
Risk factors	Young couple	Compromised and ineffective	Coping	Teenage marriage Pregnancy before age 16
	Middle-aged adults	Reactive and situational depression	Self-perception and self-concept	Feelings of failure Inability to relate to spouse and children Alcohol and drug abuse

PLANNING WITH FAMILY

A plan of intervention is designed on completion of the assessment, analysis, and nursing diagnosis. The purpose of the plan is to bring about some behavioral change in the family that will promote health or prevent dysfunctioning. As in the assessment phase, the family is an active participant in the planning process; the degree of responsibility the family assumes for personal health status is important to the success of behavior change outcomes. The planning process involves several steps, with the nurse and family identifying

1. Order of priority for problems or potential problems
2. Items that can be handled by the nurse and the family and those that must be referred to others
3. Goals and objectives to resolve the problem
4. Actions and expected outcomes

The planning phase is completed with the nursing plan, which in turn provides direction for implementation of the plan and the framework for evaluation.

As mentioned earlier, a family's health status can be diagnosed as functional, potentially dysfunctional, or dysfunctional. If the family's health status is considered functional, the nurse verifies the situation, and a plan for periodic reevaluation of the family's health status is formulated jointly. Plans to continue healthy living behaviors are reinforced, and specific information the family requests or needs is given, such as immunization schedules, growth and development milestones, and recommended dietary allowances. The family is instructed to seek further assistance if necessary. In working with health families, the nurse controls the assessment and analysis phases of the nursing process. If the health status is judged functional, the planning of health education materials, the scheduling of periodic examination, and the accessibility of the nurse are professional responsibilities. The implementation and evaluation of the health promotion activities are the family's responsibilities.

In setting priorities in health promotion and disease prevention, a life-threatening situation rarely is encountered. However, if the family's data reveal such a situation, the identified problem receives the first priority of intervention. For other identified potential or actual problems, the nurse relies on the family to decide which problem or potential problem to approach. Maslow's hierarchy of needs[19] is useful in designating priorities of physical, safety, love, esteem, and self-actualization; the nurse should remember that safety needs must be fulfilled before approaching esteem needs. Once the ordering of priorities is established, the family and nurse determine who will work on the problem.

Problems or potential problems that can be resolved by the nurse are identified separately from those that need referral or the family's intervention. Problems that the family can handle or is already involved with are considered strengths and should be acknowledged and supported by the nurse. For example, if there is consistency among values and actions, physical fitness, weight management, and ability to cope with stress, the family is already taking informed and responsible action in these areas. The extent to which family members can provide their own health promotion and prevention will depend on their knowledge, skills, motivation, and orientation toward health.

Problems that need medical, legal, or social attention should be referred to appropriate agencies. The nurse should have a directory of available resources in the community to consult when referrals are needed.

Problems that need nursing interventions must be stated in nursing actions that are clear, purposeful, moral, capable of being accomplished, and adapted to the particular life situation, beliefs, and expectations of the family.

Goals

A goal is a statement describing a desired outcome. Included in the goal is what is expected of the family, under what circumstances the behavior will be demonstrated, and the criteria to determine when and how behavior will be performed. Health promotion goals reflect a desire to function at a higher level of health and to grow beyond maintaining health or preventing disease, as illustrated by these examples.

Nursing diagnosis	Goal
Family coping; potential for growth hindered by inadequate understanding of response to stress	Each family member will observe and record own reactions in tense situations for 1 week.

Nursing diagnosis	Goal
Potential alteration in parents' busy schedules	All family members will participate in a recreational activity together once a week.

Health promotion goals reflect a desire to change a health habit that indicates a potential problem before signs and symptoms appear.

Nursing diagnosis	Goal
Inadequate coping skills to handle smoking cessation	Family will support member who enrolls in a smoking-cessation program.
Alteration in nutrition: potential obesity, excessive caloric intake	Family will reduce caloric intake by 500 calories per day.
Knowledge deficit of meditation skills	Family will read *Relaxation Response* by Herbert Benson.

Both the nurse and the client are partners in goal formation. The nurse contributes knowledge and understanding of the various implications of the nursing diagnosis; the client brings motivation and the family's unique perspective to the problem. Together their contributions determine the goal outcome and thus increase the family's level of health.

Objectives

Once goals are established for the appropriate diagnosis, objectives are developed that specify how to reach the goal. Usually a number of objectives are written for each goal, since several goals may exist for each nursing diagnosis. For example:

Nursing diagnosis	Goals	Objectives
Potential for health management deficit because of sedentary lifestyle	Decrease risk for hypertension.	Take brisk walk 4 times a week for 45 minutes.
		Buy blood pressure cuff and learn to take own blood pressure.
		Have blood pressure checked at clinic every 3 months.
	Maintain desired weight of 190 pounds.	Keep 24-hour recall of food for 1 week.
		Cut calories to lose 1 pound every 2 weeks for 6 months.
		Plan exercise regimen and calorie intake to maintain weight.

IMPLEMENTATION

Implementation is putting the nursing plan into action. The implementation phase is not to be considered unchangeable; as the nurse and family work together, new information is used to adapt and change the plan as necessary. Nursing interventions are aimed at assisting the family in carrying out functions it cannot perform for itself. In health promotion and disease prevention, the nurse assists the family in improving its capacity to act in its own behalf.

Families may know they are taking risks by smoking, drinking, and engaging in a stressful lifestyle. As the nurse explains the rationale behind proposed changes, the family may choose to deny they are jeopardizing their future health and continue with their risk-taking behaviors. Such a situation will test the nurse's ingenuity; the family's resistance may be caused by factors the nurse has not considered. For example, the family may have more pressing basic needs, such as food, clothing, and housing. Health promotion and disease prevention may not have been part of the family's life experiences, giving the nurse the educational task of trying to change attitudes and values so the family will be more open to health needs.

In health promotion and disease prevention, four types of nursing interventions are found: (1) increasing knowledge and skills, (2) increasing strengths, (3) decreasing exposure, and (4) decreasing susceptibility.

Increasing *knowledge and skills* so families can improve their capacity to act on health promotion and disease prevention behaviors may be the primary strategy. Inherent in this strategy is assisting families to make informed choices about healthful lifestyle behaviors and to eliminate harmful environmental influences that affect their health. The first step is creating awareness, which is accomplished in the first three steps of the nursing process as the nurse and family work together to uncover actual or potential problems. The second step is to recognize those families at risk; the third step offers families at risk the benefits of nursing knowledge about motivating and supporting behavioral change.

Family *strengths,* as defined by Otto,[19] are those factors or forces that contribute to family unity and solidarity and that foster the development of inherent family potential. These include

- Physical, emotional, and spiritual factors
- Healthy child-rearing practices and discipline
- Meaningful and clear communication
- Support, security, and encouragement
- Growth-producing relationships and experiences
- Responsible community relationships
- Growth with and through children
- Self-help and acceptance of help
- Flexibility in family functions and roles
- Mutual respect for individuality
- Crisis as a means for growth
- Family unity and loyalty and intrafamily cooperation
- Adaptability of family strengths

Families with strengths may need to learn new, unfamiliar skills for mastering a specific technique, such as meditation, and to apply new tools for decision making. These families rarely require the ongoing supervision or support of sustained interventions aimed at changing their coping patterns, communication, or role behavior. They may be highly capable of seeking and utilizing information. Assisting functional families may involve simply providing information in terms that can be understood and offering them opportunities to ask questions and clarify information.

Reducing *exposure* to risk factors may include making parental behaviors more in tune with the child's behaviors.

In homes with less-educated parents, the parents respond differently to the child's attempt to communicate and in their behavior toward the child. This may lead to significant differences later in the child's intellectual ability. For example, using adequate restraints in automobiles and protecting the toddler from wandering into dangerous streets or places conducive to falls are means of reducing exposure to fatal accidents.

No substitute can be found for continuous supervision of a child. Homes can be made less hazardous by educated attempts to remove common hazards from children's reach. This includes putting all cleaning solutions and medications beyond their reach; erecting barriers in front of exposed heaters, high windows, and stairways; keeping pots and pans turned inward on the stove and out of reach; fencing in a yard or a swimming pool; and teaching them to avoid dangerous areas. Becoming aware of peeling paint and toxic chemicals that parents might carry home from the job on their clothing also can protect the child.

Reducing *susceptibility* means educating the family about the principles of prevention. The family must realize how diseases are spread from person to person; through hair, water, and food; and by insects and the rodents on which insects live. The role of personal hygiene and cleanliness in avoiding infections also must be recognized. The family must know which signs and symptoms need medical attention and learn how to take care of minor illnesses.

Pender[20] cites several research studies that support the importance of perceived susceptibility as a predictor of preventive behavior. Perceived susceptibility is the family's own estimated subjective probability that it will encounter a specific health problem. Family perceptions of health risks and their susceptibility will determine how they change their behavior. If the overweight family believes obesity to be a threat to their health and if the nurse works with them in changing their eating habits to reduce weight and maintain weight norms, the family is likely to act positively to the change. If nurses introduce threat as a motivator to action, they are morally obligated to reduce the threat by meaningful and purposeful interventions. (See Table 8-1 for various nursing roles used in the implementations stage.)

EVALUATION

The purpose of evaluation is to determine how the family responded to the planned interventions and if these were successful. Goals and objectives stated in specific behavioral terms will make evaluation much easier than if they are given in general terms. Specific criteria used to evaluate interventions, such as weight changes, increased lung capacity from an exercise program, and lower pulse rate as a result of relaxation exercises, are simple to measure. Other factors of health promotion and disease prevention are not so easy to measure but must be considered in the evaluation step of the nursing process. As stated earlier, when considering such factors as values, beliefs, self-perceptions, or role relationships, the nurse may have to base evaluation on whether the family indicates the interventions were successful. In addition, the family's baseline data are used as comparative criteria in evaluation. The nurse reassesses the situation and compares the new information with the information on the original assessment to determine if change has occurred.

Leavitt[15] identifies five measures of family functioning that can be used to determine effectiveness of interventions:

1. Changes in interaction patterns
2. Effective communication
3. Ability to express emotions
4. Responsiveness to needs of members as individuals
5. Problem-solving ability

Using these measures, the nurse returns to the original assessemnt of the family's functioning and compares current observations with previous data in the evaluation.

If the planning phase of the nursing process has identified the criteria (norms, standards, and so on) for the desired outcomes, these outcomes are the basis of evaluation. Data from the family describing their behavior relative to the desired outcomes determine whether the nursing care was successful. With the criteria stated, the goals and objectives outline how the family can demonstrate a successful outcome and the behavior change expected to result from nursing intervention. The more objective and measurable the desired outcome, the more reliable are the results of evaluation.

Once the goals and objectives are reached, the problem no longer exists. If evaluation shows the nursing actions did not achieve goals or objectives, the nurse must review the nursing process to determine if there were gaps in the assessment data, errors in analysis or nursing diagnosis, or alternate interventions that might have been considered. The nurse also needs to review the process with the family to determine if they have contributed to outcome failure. Finally, the agency employing the nurse may be another factor; if intervention is costly or a shortage of staff exists, health promotion and disease prevention may have low priority.

SUMMARY

The family's learning of health promotion and disease prevention begins at birth, with the family providing the stimulus for incorporating health in the value system of its members. From a systems perspective, the family has both structure and function; relevant functions include values and practices placed on health. The effective execution of health-related functions involves the family's progression, through its developmental tasks and its ability to generate low-risk-producing behaviors associated with disease prevention.

Developmental and risk estimate theories can be applied effectively to the nursing process of the family. The nurse uses functional patterns, an inherent part of both theories, to collect data for assessment. After organizing information on family life cycle stages for analysis, the nurse writes the nursing diagnosis, plans with the family, and then implements and evaluates the interventions used to promote health and prevent disease in the family.

References

1. Anderson KH, Tomlinson PS: The family health system as an emerging paradigmatic view for nursing, *Image* 24:57-63, 1992.
2. Andrews PB: *Nursing diagnosis.* In Griffith-Kenney JW, Christensen PJ: *Nursing process,* ed 2, St Louis, 1986, Times Mirror/Mosby College Publishing.
3. Culkin Rhyne M: Understanding and supporting families in the process of divorce, *Nurse Practitioner,* 37-51, 1986.
4. Dietz-Omar M: Couple adaptation in stepfamilies and traditional nuclear families during pregnancy, *Appl Nurs Res* 4: 31-33, 1991.
5. Duvall EM, Miller B: *Marriage and family development,* ed 6, New York, 1985, Harper & Row.
6. Erickson E: *Childhood and society,* New York, 1963, WW Norton.
7. Fawcett J: The family as a living open system: an emerging conceptual framework for nursing, *Int Nurs Rev* 22:113, 1975.
8. Fawcett J: Spouses; experiences during pregnancy and the postpartum: a program of research and theory development, *Image* 21:149-157, 1989.
9. Feetham S: *Family research: issues and direction for nursing.* In Werley H, Fitzpatrick J, editors: *Annual review of nursing 2,* New York, 1984, Springer-Verlag.
10. Gillis CL: Family nursing research, theory and practice, *Image* 23:19-22, 1991.
11. Gillis CL: *Family research in nursing.* In Gillis CL, et al, editors: *Toward a science of family nursing,* Menlo Park, Calif, 1989, Addison-Wesley.
12. Gordon M: *Nursing diagnosis: process and application,* ed 2, New York, 1987, McGraw-Hill.
13. *Healthy people 2000: national health promotion and disease prevention objectives,* US Department of Health and Human Services, Public Health Service 91-50212, Washington, DC, 1990, US Government Printing Office.
14. Kristjanson L, Chalmers K: Nurse-client interactions in community-based common ground, *Public Health Nurs* 7:215-223, 1990.
15. Leavitt MB: *Families at risk: primary prevention in nursing practice,* Boston, 1982, Little, Brown.
16. Leppink H: *Health risk estimation.* In Faber MM, Reinhardt AM: *Promoting health through risk reduction,* New York, 1982, Macmillan.
17. Luker KA, Chalmers KI: Gaining access to clients: the case of health visiting, *J Adv Nurs* 15:74-82, 1990.
18. Maslow AH: *Motivation and personality,* ed 2, New York, 1970, Harper & Row.
19. Otto HA: *A framework for assessing family strengths.* In Reinhardt AM, Quinn MD, editors: *Family centered community nursing, vol 2,* St Louis, 1980, Mosby.
20. Pender NJ: *Health promotion in nursing practice,* ed 2, Norwalk, Conn, 1987, Appleton-Century-Crofts.
21. Pender NJ, Pender AR: Attitudes, subjective norms and intentions to engage in health behaviors, *Nurs Res* 35:15-18, 1986.
22. Pratt L: *Family structure and effective health behavior: the energized family,* Boston, 1976, Houghton Mifflin.
23. Rogers ME: *An introduction to the theoretical basis of nursing,* Philadelphia, 1970, FA Davis.
24. Spradley BW: *Community health nursing concepts and practice,* ed 3, 1990, Glenview, Ill, Scott, Foresman/Little, Brown.
25. Talashek M, et al: The AIDS pandemic: a nursing model, *Public Health Nurs* 6: 182-188, 1989.
26. Zerwekh JV: A family caregiving model for public health nursing, *Nurs Outlook,* pp 213-217, 1991.

CHAPTER

9

Health Promotion and the Community

Nancy Curro McCarthy

Objectives

After completing this chapter, the nurse will be able to

- *Describe several theoretic frameworks of community nursing practice.*
- *Discuss the scope of nursing practice in the community.*
- *Identify community sources of health information.*
- *Develop a plan for assessing a community using the functional health pattern framework.*
- *Give examples of the data to be collected in each health pattern of the community.*
- *Give examples of the following behavioral changes within the health pattern of the community: (1) functional, (2) potentially dysfunctional, (3) actually dysfunctional.*
- *Describe characteristics of the community to consider while identifying risk factors or etiologic factors of potentially or actually dysfunctional health patterns.*
- *Propose three ways to organize community health assessment data.*
- *Distinguish unfreezing, changing, and refreezing phases and health strategies of planned change in the community.*
- *Discuss planning, implementing, and evaluating nursing interventions in health promotion with communities.*
- *Develop a specific health promotion plan based on community assessment, nursing diagnosis, and contributing-risk or etiologic factors.*

Several trends in society over the last two decades have sparked the interest of the public in health promotion and disease prevention activities. The landmark document published by the surgeon general in 1979,[9] the subsequent documents in 1980[18] and 1986,[16] and most recently *Healthy People 2000*[12] have been helpful in changing the focus of health care from a reactive stance focused on the treatment of disease to a proactive stance emphasizing prevention of disease and promotion of health. By stating national health objectives in relation to age-specific risks to good health, the documents set a course to reduce the percentages of risk factors and thereby reduce the incidence of disease.

Another trend has been the changing population in the United States. The U.S. Census Bureau estimates that 60 million people, 20% of the American population, will be over age 65 by the year 2025. Older people tend to have more chronic diseases and thus consume a larger portion of health care services than other age groups. It is also anticipated that the aging population will require more home health care and nursing home services than previous generations because of their increasing longevity and the chronic nature of their illnesses. A growing number of articles in the literature propose that the major improvements in the population's health will be derived from self-care, health promotion, and disease prevention–not from medical services and technology.

Health promotion and disease prevention have a long history in public health nursing. As far back as Florence Nightingale, community health nurses included the client in the decision-making process and put the emphasis on health rather than disease. The "community as client" concept includes the community and health professionals in decisions concerning, for example, the allocation of scarce resources. To begin to resolve such dilemmas, a database identifying the specific needs for health promotion and protection activities is needed. In this chapter a database guide is presented as a format for retrieving information about the health status of a community.

Understanding the dynamic and complex nature of communities and being able to gather certain facts about them are important prerequisites for effective planning, delivery, and coordination of health promotion and protection activities. Nurses can collect certain information about their communities and use it in planning and implementing nursing actions to promote and protect community health. Because health needs and concerns vary in each community, the type of health promotion and protection activities will also vary. As knowledge is gained about the community, the nurse is better able to address a wide range of health-related responses observed in the community. Those responses can be reactions to actual health-related problems such as disease or to potential health problems. Community responses are frequently multiple, continuous, and fluid and tend to vary. Many potential health concerns are discrete, or individually distinct.

This chapter focuses on the application of the nursing process to a community as client within a systems framework. Community as client is first defined with emphasis on characteristics of space, interaction, and population. The focus on population and community as client and the roles of the community nurse also are described. An overview of selected theories, frameworks, and principles is presented as background to the nursing process.

The application of the nursing process to a community as client is arranged in a systematic manner to reflect the steps of the process. Gordon's typology[7] of 11 health-related pattern areas provides the structure for the assessment of the community client. An example of a data collection guide is presented to facilitate comprehension, synthesis, and application of observation, interviews and measurement data necessary for planning community health promotion and protection activities. Examples of community health data analysis and planning also are given to assist in understanding comprehension and application of this information.

DEFINITION OF COMMUNITY

The term *community* is used in various contexts with varied meanings, depending on the frame of reference. In this text community is a specific population living in a geographic area under similar regulations and having common values, interests, and needs. The important concept is that community has geographic and interactional aspects. Also, people are assumed to share the need for and use of resources in their environment. These resources are influenced by the passage of time and the environment in which they are located.

Important to any concept of community are people, the living systems who give it shape, character, and form. An individual's health is reflected in the community through the person's contribution to its statistical rates as well as to its cultural and psychologic makeup. Conversely, the community is reflected in the individual through similar modes of expression.

COMMUNITY HEALTH NURSING

Community health nursing practice is a synthesis of nursing practice and public health concepts applied to promoting the health of populations.[1] It is not limited to any particular individual or groups of individuals. Since the client is the community, the concerns of these nurses are the community's responses to existing and potential health-related problems, including such health-supporting responses as monitoring and teaching population groups. The nurse may supply a community at risk with education needs to inform and help develop health-oriented skills, attitudes, and related behavioral changes.[2] Community nursing practice directed toward individuals, families, and groups contributes to total community health.

Community health nursing is also concerned with the relationships essential in accomplishing its health-related mission. The complexity and dynamic nature of communities and increasing public involvement in health and health policy highlight the importance of the human interactions inherent in community nursing's responses to the potential community health problems, needs, and expectations. Nursing practice therefore requires a broad knowledge base derived from the natural, behavioral, and humanistic sciences, as well as application of intellectual, interpersonal, and technical skills through the nursing process.

The scope of community nursing is general and comprehensive; nursing roles are independent, interdependent, and dependent and frequently overlap. Independent nursing functions include assessing, analyzing and diagnosing, planning, implementing, and evaluating nursing activities such as health promotion and health education. Interdependent functions include collaboration and interdisciplinary team work–functions recognized as crucial to effective community nursing. Dependent functions include implementing therapeutic treatment plans of team members.

The three nursing roles applied in the community are enhanced by the use of the nursing process. Various theoretic frameworks also are used to help the nurse effectively carry out nursing functions and thereby give credence to the community nurse's activities.[25]

THEORETIC FRAMEWORKS FOR COMMUNITY NURSING

Nursing authors, especially those writing community health textbooks–including Roy,[21] Rogers,[19] Johnson,[11] Orem,[17] Neuman,[15] and King[12]–have addressed various nursing theories and frameworks and how each might be used to direct the nursing process and its application to the community as client. Clark,[3] for example, in *Nursing in the Community* demonstrates how some of these approaches can be used with the individual, family, and community. Neuman,[15] a nurse theorist, has developed a health care systems model for assessing and understanding clients. An adaptation of the model has been suggested in applying the nursing process to population-focused practice.

Other theories and frameworks from different disciplines can also be used to direct the nursing process and its application to the community as client. These include systems theory, developmental theories, and risk-factor theories derived from epidemiology. Systems theory provides a useful overall framework broadly applicable to the nursing process. Developmental theories and risk factors, which provide support in a more specific way, are especially important in analyzing community data and providing a rationale for interventions.

The frameworks selected for use in community nursing practice and described in this chapter are not all-inclusive; many theoretic approaches are available and relevant. The frameworks described here can serve as a guide for the nurse applying the nursing process to the community as client.

Systems Theory

Systems theory provides an overall framework in which otherwise unconnected parts can be integrated. A system can be viewed as an entity composed of interrelated, interacting parts or components within a boundary that filters both the type and rate of input and output.[23] A community viewed as a system implies that it has both structure and function. These aspects of a specific population living in a geographic area are determined in a community assessment.

STRUCTURE

The structure of a community system or subsystem can be seen as the formal or informal arrangement of its parts at a given time, including both animate and inanimate properties. The population, schools, fire department, and health resources are examples of structural parts. Nursing, which operates within the context of the health system, also can be considered a component of a community system.

The parts within a community also are viewed as subsystems, each of which is in itself a system. The suprasystem, often a county or state, is the larger system of which the community is a part. Fig. 9-1 shows a hierarchic arrangement of a community system.

The arrangement and organization of a community system's parts, such as the age distribution of the population and types of health promotion and protection programs and their availability and accessibility, can change over time. The parts also may remain relatively stable for long periods, based on the state of the environment and processes occurring within and between the parts and the larger environment.

The existence, arrangement, and assimilation of a community's parts play a major role in providing direction to both health promotion and health protection activities. Therefore, the nurse must consider the various community parts or systems as they relate to health when conducting an assessment. Viewing the community structure as a collection of persons (population) and considering the arrangement of the community's health care parts, such as existing health services, are especially important.

The study of population is referred to as *demography*. Demography provides information on the population with respect to characteristics such as size, age distribution, sex ratio, racial composition, marital status ratios, nationality, language, religious grouping, and educational and occupational distributions.

Obtaining demographic data of a population living in

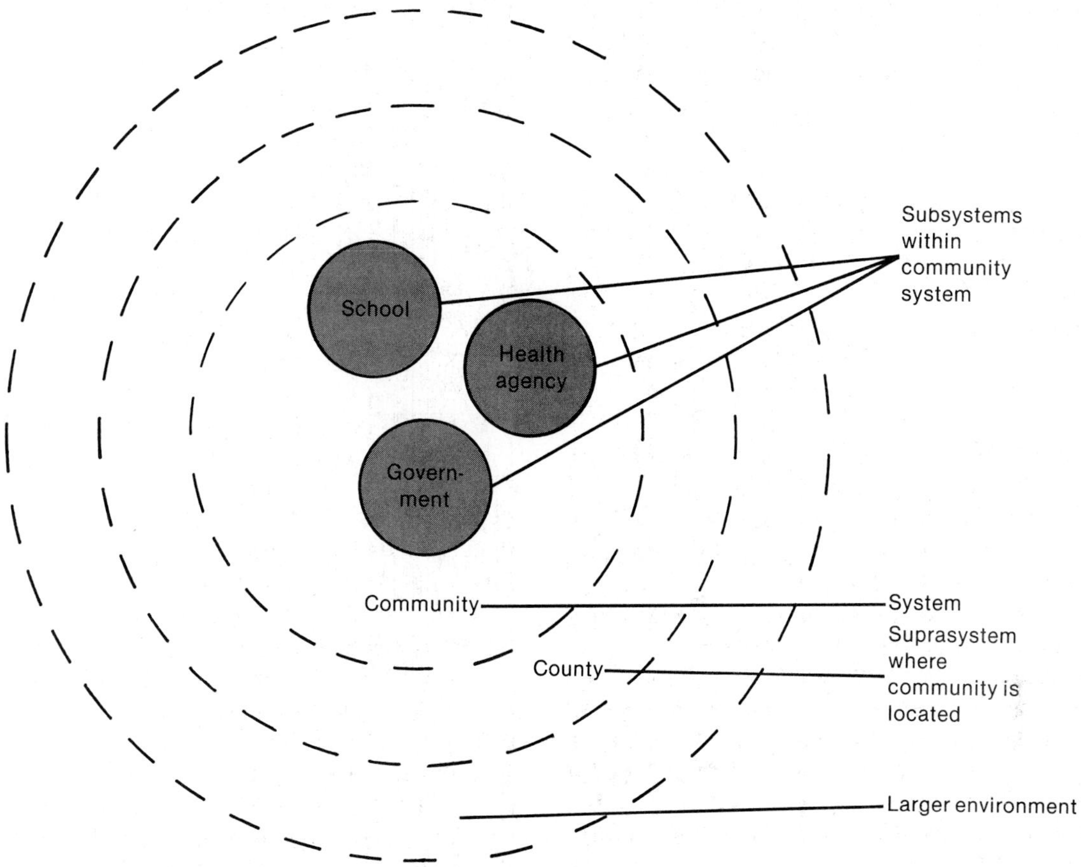

Fig. 9-1. Hierarchic nature of community system.

a specific area provides an important basis for analysis and a means for identifying developmental concerns of various population groups who might be at risk. Such information also can provide clues for the direction of health strategies. For example, an examination of the age distribution over the past several years reveals important population shifts and a need for additional health promotion activities; the large increase in the population over age 65 may require changes in community health priorities to reflect this group's needs. Demographic information is so vital that it generally is considered first in a community assessment.

Comparison statistics about population characteristics, which also need to be considered in community structure, enable the community nurse to make inferences about the community. Tables 9-1 and 9-2 are examples of comparisons made among three systems: the *town,* a part of the county; and the *county,* a part of the larger system, the *state.* Comparisons typically are made between communities of similar population size.

FUNCTION

The function of a community refers to the process of dynamic change or adaptation in the system's parts, as well as the way the community system and its sub-

Table 9-1. **Family income: number and percentage of families in various brackets at town, county, and state levels**

	Town		County		State	
Income	**No.**	**%**	**No.**	**%**	**No.**	**%**
Under $3000	150	2.0	14,862	10.4	89,343	6.4
$3000-$4999	295	4.3	16,076	11.3	100,670	7.2
$5000-$9999	1291	18.9	48,861	34.4	420,972	30.2
$10,000-$14,999	1767	25.8	36,456	25.7	429,883	30.9
$15,000+	3316	49.0	25,764	18.2	349,924	25.1
Median income	$14,728		$9133		$10,981	

Table 9-2. **Births: age, number, and percentage of unmarried mothers at town, county, and state levels**

	Town		County		State	
Income	**No.**	**%**	**No.**	**%**	**No.**	**%**
Less than 15	0	0	39	94.9	87	95.4
15-19	28	40.9	2247	57.4	7749	45.2
20-24	94	11.7	5842	19.8	20,420	14.2
25-29	258	0.4	8100	6.5	24,131	4.8
30-34	242	0.4	4818	4.9	1194	4.1
35-39	54	–	1270	6.3	2929	5.7
40-44	1	–	226	7.5	548	6.2
44+	0	–	11	9.1	30	6.7

systems interact. How community members make decisions and allocate health promotion and protection resources are important considerations.

Strategies are processes through which decisions are made to obtain compliance from another system or subsystem. Schaller[22] has identified four general approaches to effect change: (1) coercion, which uses force; (2) cooptation, in which one item is offered for another; (3) conflict, which serves to clarify issues but may have a negative effect; and (4) cooperation, which obtains compliance with persuasion. Because cooperation requires skill in communications and interpersonal relations, it can be very time consuming; but it also can effectively produce change that is accepted. With the exception of coercion, the least desirable strategy for change, each of these approaches can be effective. The four strategies are discussed further in the community assessment section of this chapter.

INTERACTION

Interaction is an important concept in systems theory. Through dynamic interaction with the environment a system exchanges matter, energy, and information in such communication forms as verbal and behavioral and uses information to make decisions. Interaction is also important if the community system is to survive, protect, and promote the health of its members. Through environmental interactions, a community system uses mechanisms of adaptation. The community nurse must determine how the community applies these mechanisms toward health services.

Various psychologic, physiologic, and environmental health-related patterns also emerge from these interactions. For example, certain human activity patterns can alter the natural environmental patterns negatively, which in turn influences human health patterns. Gordon's assessment framework[7] focuses on 11 health-related functional patterns; community-environment interaction is assumed in each. The approach used in assessing these patterns is dictated by the framework used, such as the systems theory just described.

Developmental Framework

A developmental framework can be used to identify existing or potential health problems for a particular age group in a community. A population group is defined as an aggregate of persons who share similar personal or environmental characteristics. Since community nurses are interested in the total community population, they use a developmental, age-correlated approach to identify health promotion and protection activities for all age groups.

At each stage of life, age-related risks[12] can be identified and different steps taken to maximize well-being and promote health as a lifelong concern. For example, adolescent single mothers with infants are at high risk both emotionally and physically and require help with parenting skills. Since accidents are the greatest threat to children's health, accident prevention activities are a priority for this age group. Many age-related risk factors associated with individuals and families discussed in Chapters 7 and 8 can be extended to include community groups.

Risk Factor Framework

Risk factors are associated with a community's disease, illness, and death rates.[10] A risk factor does not necessarily play a causal role in these rates but simply helps predict the likelihood of a particular adverse health condition developing.

Risk factors may include a combination of demographic, psychologic, physiologic, or environmental characteristics or only one. For example, age, sex, race, geographic location, consumption pattern, or lack of health services may be considered risk factors, since one or more may contribute to disease or death and thus put the population sharing them at risk. The degree of influence of various risk factors differs from person to person and group to group because of genetic makeup, geographic location, lifestyle patterns, resources, socioeconomic status, level of education, or environmental variations. Some groups may be at high risk from a single risk factor such as insufficient immunizations or exposure to asbestos. However, synergism does operate. A combined potential for adverse health effects exists when many risk factors are present, since they interact in different ways and can even multiply each other. [10] As a result, communities can experience substantial variability in both incidence and susceptibility to adverse health conditions. Thus the risk factor concept is based on disease, and conversely health, being multifactorial in genesis; the essential cause frequently cannot be attributed to any single risk factor. For example, risk factors such as air pollution, smoking, and forms of radiation in various combinations may be related to high rates of lung cancer, emphysema, and bronchitis in a community. The potential to control many or just a few risk factors and to have relevant health-related resources available is the basis of health promotion and protection activities.

Nursing Process and the Community

The nurse initiates the nursing process by collecting basic information about the community in a systematic way. In the preassessment phase, consideration is given to data that will enable the nurse and community to identify either strengths and problems or concerns relating to health promotion and protection. The first step is stating measurable outcomes of the assessment process by identifying

- populations at risk
- actual and potential community health concerns
- community strengths
- gaps in community health-protection and health-promotion resources,
- mismatches between the status quo and community-oriented health-related goals

The next step is to establish a database from which to plan health promotion and protection services and plan community-health-related responses. To achieve these objectives effectively, the community nurse must employ cognitive skills, objectivity, critical thinking, and perceptual capabilities–the tools used to collect and analyze community data.

TYPES OF ASSESSMENT

In collecting community data, the nurse considers several factors. The first is the nature of the information available; certain characteristics of community information influence both how it is collected and how it is used.

A second influencial factor is the context in which information is collected. Because of the complexity, size, and number of community characteristics, the nurse is unlikely to obtain a totally comprehensive data collection. A comprehensive assessment involves obtaining all possible information about a community, is generally carried out over an extended period, and usually calls for a large interdisciplinary team approach. Community nurses, however, often participate in aspects of a comprehensive assessment.

A familiarization assessment is the type most widely used and is necessary for nurses working in a community. This assessment uses existing information about a community, such as published population data and health-related information, in addition to obtaining specific information from key community persons. Health promotion and protection resources also are identified.

Data collection activities should not be done in isolation; ideally they should represent a combined effort by all groups working within the community. Health professionals, key community figures, and residents can provide much necessary and pertinent information. The collected data are shared with interested community persons.

METHODS

The nurse obtains community assessment data through observation, interview, and measurement. These three methods most frequently are used in various combinations to ensure the validity of the information.

Obtaining data through *observation*–often referred to as the "windshield survey" approach to assessment–includes the use of the senses–sight, touch, hearing, smell, and taste–to determine community appearances, such as the type and state of residential dwellings; the people; and the physical and biologic characteristics, such as animal and plant life, temperature, transportation, sounds, and odors. Some communities have an observable characteristic "flavor." The community's physical characteristics can influence health. What type of space is observed? Children need space to run and play; young and middle-aged adults require space for recreation and exercise. What spatial barriers are noted? The community nurse can obtain a great deal of subjective data by just walking or riding around a community and using the senses. The data obtained by observation can provide important clues about the community, its actual or potential health problems, and its strengths. When observation data are analyzed, hypotheses can be generated that are assessed further using interview and measurement data.

The second method, the *interview,* is probably the most common approach for collecting information from persons. Interview data include any verbal statement from community residents, key community officials, health care personnel, or various community agency staff people. This method is a useful way to obtain information about how members perceive their community. Key community leaders can provide important information about community health concerns, needed health resources, and community strengths. Particular health beliefs and community health goals also can be ascertained.

Community residents also can provide useful information regarding their perceptions of health, health concerns, and needs; and the availability, accessibility, and acceptability of health services. Health agency personnel can provide data on available health resources, whom they serve, and when they are available, as well as their perceptions of concerns and needs. Developing a basic set of questions in advance will enhance the relevance of interview data.

Measurement, the third method, uses instruments to quantify data in information collection. Measurement data include population statistics, pollution indices, morbidity and mortality rates, census statistics, and epidemiologic data. These data can be found in community libraries, health departments, environmental protection agencies, schools, police and fire departments, and local health system agencies, as well as town, city, or state planning offices. Publicly supported agencies are required by law to share their information with interested persons, and community nurses should not hesitate to request such data.

SOURCES OF COMMUNITY INFORMATION

Census information found in libraries and public agencies is the most complete source for population information. Because the U.S. census is completed once every 10 years at the beginning of the decade, the data for most communities becomes less accurate as the decade progresses. Community agencies such as the chamber of commerce and local planning commissions work with census data to develop projection statistics and developmental trends, which the nurse can use to gain an understanding of population patterns and dynamics. Health data usually are available from town, city, or state public health departments and community health-related organizations.

Environmental measurement data can be obtained from the local branch of the U.S. Environmental Protection Agency (EPA). The sanitation department of the local health department is generally in charge of monitoring water supplies, food, and sanitation of a community. School health information is available from the health department, school nurse, or school administration.

Information regarding land use, boundaries, housing conditions, utilities, and community services generally is available from the town, city, or county administration. Community newspapers can provide an excellent source of information regarding community dynamics, health-related concerns, cultural activities, and those who make community decisions. Recording community observation, interview, and measurement data is approached in the same manner that data are recorded for an individual or family. A triple-column format separating data from each method can facilitate recording.

Assessment

The functional health patterns assessment guidelines (see box on pp. 209-210) uses Gordon's 11 functional health patterns to assess the community. Observation and interview are used to collect data from questions posed. The data guide is designed for flexibility. The examples of assessment questions can be modified, augmented, or deleted to adapt to the unique aspects of the community. As noted in previous chapters, information obtained in one pattern can become an important factor in pursuing information in another area because the patterns are interrelated.

Risk and developmental age factors also influence health patterns. For example, a health concern might be identified in one pattern area, such as an increase in an age-related factor of teenage pregnancy (sexuality and reproduction), and data from other areas might reveal the containment of sex education in the home (coping and stress tolerance) and the unacceptability of sex education in the school curricula because of parental nonsupport (values and beliefs). Limiting sex education in the home and ignoring it in the school may be factors that young females of childbearing age share in the community, placing them at risk for unwanted pregnancies. Factors from several pattern areas may form a cluster that has the potential for placing certain groups at risk. Each pattern forms a database for the community assessment as defined in the following section.

ENVIRONMENTAL PROCESSES

Environment encompasses everything external to community members and includes three broad areas: physical (inanimate), biologic, and social. Alterations in environmental processes can threaten the health and integrity of a community, necessitating health promotion and protection activities. The health-related patterns previously discussed all are influenced by the environment; the environment in turn is influenced by a community's patterns.

Physical (Inanimate) Agents. The nurse assesses this

❑ ❑ THE 11 FUNCTIONAL HEALTH PATTERNS ASSESSMENT GUIDELINES FOR COMMUNITIES

Communities develop health patterns. In some practice settings the community is the primary client. In other cases an individual client or a family may have, or be predisposed to, certain problems that require an assessment of certain community patterns. The following are guidelines for a comprehensive community assessment, but selected patterns can also be assessed, depending on the focus of care delivery:

1. *Health-perception–health-management pattern*
   History (community representatives):
   a. In general, what is the health/wellness level of the population on a scale of 1 to 5, with 5 being high? Any major health problems?
   b. Any strong cultural patterns influencing health practices?
   c. Do people feel they have access to health services?
   d. Is there demand for any particular health services or prevention programs?
   e. Do people feel fire, police, safety programs are sufficient?
   Examination (community records):
   a. Morbidity, mortality, disability rates (by age group, if appropriate)?
   b. Accident rates (by district, if appropriate)?
   c. Currently operating health facilities (types)?
   d. Ongoing health promotion–prevention programs; utilization rates?
   e. Ratios of health professionals to population?
   f. Laws regarding drinking age?
   g. Arrest statistics for drug use/drink driving by age group?
2. *Nutritional-metabolic pattern*
   History (community representatives):
   a. In general, do most people seem well-nourished? Children? Elderly?
   b. Food supplement programs? Food stamps: Rate of use?
   c. Is cost of foods reasonable in this area relative to income?
   d. Are stores accessible for most? "Meals on Wheels" available?
   e. Water supply and quality? Testing services (if most have own wells)? (If appropriate: Water usage cost? Any drought restrictions?)
   f. Any concern that community growth will exceed good water supply?
   g. Are heating/cooling costs manageable for most? Programs?
   Examination:
   a. General appearance (nutrition, teeth, clothing appropriate for climate)? Children? Adults? Elderly?
   b. Food purchases (observations at food store checkout counters)?
   c. "Junk" food (machines in schools, etc.)?
3. *Elimination pattern*
   History (community representatives):
   a. Major kinds of wastes (industrial, sewage, etc.)? Disposal systems? Recycling programs? Any problems perceived by community?
   b. Pest control? Food service inspection (restaurants, street vendors, etc.)?
   Examination:
   a. Communicable-disease statistics?
   b. Air pollution statistics?
4. *Activity-exercise pattern*
   History (community representatives):
   a. How do people find the transportation here? To work? For recreation? To health care?
   b. Do people (senior, others) have/use community centers? Recreation facilities for children? Adults? Seniors?
   c. Is housing adequate (availability, cost)? Public housing?
   Examination:
   a. Recreation/cultural programs?
   b. Aids for the disabled?
   c. Residential centers, nursing homes, rehabilitation facilities relative to population needs?
   d. External maintenance of homes, yards, apartment houses?
   e. General activity level (e.g., bustling, quiet)?
5. *Sleep-rest pattern*
   History (community representatives):
   a. Generally quiet at night in most neighborhoods?
   b. Usual business hours? Are industries round-the-clock?
   Examination:
   a. Activity/noise levels in business district? Residential?
6. *Cognitive-perceptual pattern*
   History (community representatives):
   a. Do most groups speak English? Bilingual?
   b. Educational level of population?
   c. Schools seen as good/need improving? Adult education desired/available?
   d. Types of problems that require community decisions? Decision-making process? What is best way to get things done/changed here?
   Examination:
   a. School facilities? Dropout rate?
   b. Community government structure; decision-making lines?
7. *Self-perception–self-concerpt pattern*
   History (community representatives):
   a. Good community to live in? Going up in status, down, or about the same?
   b. Old community? Fairly new?

Continued.

❑ ❑ THE 11 FUNCTIONAL HEALTH PATTERNS ASSESSMENT GUIDELINES FOR COMMUNITIES—cont'd

   c. Does any age group predominate?
   d. People's mood, in general: Enjoying life, stressed, feeling "down"?
   e. People generally have the kinds of abilities needed in this community?
   f. Community/neighborhood functions? Parades?

   Examination:
   a. Racial, ethnic mix (if appropriate)?
   b. Socioeconomic level?
   c. General observations of mood?

8. *Role-relationship pattern*

   History (community representatives):
   a. Do people seem to get along well together here? Places where people tend to go to socialize?
   b. Do people feel they are heard by the government? High/low participation in meetings?
   c. Enough work/jobs for everybody? Are wages good/fair? Do people seem to like the kind of work available (happy in their jobs/job stress)?
   d. Any problems with riots, violence in the neighborhoods? Family violence? Problems with child/spouse/elder abuse?
   e. Does community get along with adjacent communities? Do people collaborate on any community projects?
   f. Do neighbors seem to support each other?
   g. Community get-togethers?

   Examination:
   a. Observation of interactions (generally or at specific meetings)?
   b. Statistics on interpersonal violence?
   c. Statistics on employment, income/poverty?
   d. Divorce rate?

9. *Sexuality-reproductive pattern*

   History (community representatives):
   a. Average family size?
   b. Do people feel there are any problems with pornography, prostitution, or other?
   c. Do people want/support sex education in schools/community?

   Examination:
   a. Family sizes and types of households?
   b. Male/female ratio?
   c. Average maternal age? Maternal mortality rate? Infant mortality rate?
   d. Teen pregnancy rate?
   e. Abortion rate?
   f. Sexual violence statistics?
   g. Laws/regulations regarding information on birth control?

10. *Coping–stress-tolerance pattern*

   History (community representatives):
   a. Any groups that seem to be under stress?
   b. Need/availability of phone help lines? Support groups (health-related, other)?

   Examination:
   a. Statistics on delinquency, drug abuse, alcoholism, suicide, psychiatric illness?
   b. Unemployment rate by race/ethnic group/sex?

11. *Value-belief pattern*

   History (community representatives):
   a. Community values: What seem to be the top four things that people living here see as important in their lives? (Note health-related values, priorities.)
   b. Do people tend to get involved in causes/local fund-raising campaigns? (Note if any are health-related.)
   c. Are there religious groups in the community? Churches available?
   d. Do people tend to tolerate/not tolerate differences or socially deviant behavior?

   Examination:
   a. Zoning/conservation laws?
   b. Scan of community government health committee reports (goals, priorities)?
   c. Health budget relative to total budget?

From Gordon M: *Manual of nursing diagnosis: 1993-1994,* St Louis, 1993, Mosby.

aspect of the environment to obtain data about the geologic, geographic, and climatic or meteorologic aspects of the community. Certain population groups are particularly susceptible to acute respiratory disease and aggravated asthmatic episodes when the air quality is particularly poor. What is the quality of the air? How are residents informed when air quality is poor?

Water quality also is related to health. Water systems that are not fluoridated may suggest the need for oral prevention methods for children. Bacteria and noxious chemicals in the water supply can be potentially harmful. What is the quality of the water? Are high sodium levels evident? How are residents informed when water quality is poor?

The geographic location of a community and major waterways, highways, or mountains located within it can act as barriers to health facilities. Community nurses frequently identify various populations who are at risk for potential health problems because of the inaccessibility of health care services; these nurses have been instrumental in providing health promotion services to such groups. What barriers are observed in the community? Is it rural and isolated or a densely populated urban area?

Knowledge of the community's climatic conditions, although obvious to many, can provide clues to a population's susceptibility to illness related to temperature or humidity conditions.

Biologic Agents. The objective of assessing the biologic environment is to obtain data about living things, such as plants, animals and their waste products, disease agents, microbial pathogens, and toxic substances that can be potentially hazardous to health. Are rats and rodents evident? Are deforestation or defoliation activities evident? Obtaining such information can provide clues to population groups who might be at risk.

Social Processes. Industrialization, urbanization, and highly developed social and political systems have important implications for health, such as providing the community with environmental sanitation, health promotion and protection services, and facilities for education. Poorly developed and typically agrarian communities are correspondingly deficient. Assessing the social environment also includes a study of the role and relationship pattern.

Roles and Relationships. The nurse assesses this area to obtain information about community communication patterns and formal and informal relationship patterns. Community nurses are particularly concerned with roles and relationships that affect the community's ability to realize its health potential. Patterns of official communication are important to know so that health promotion activities can be publicized; major communicators can help make or break a health-related program. Key community leaders may not always be easily identified; community members can help the nurse in this area.

Use of the media and other mass information programs can increase communication, the flow of health information, and the numbers of community members reached. What communication and interaction patterns does the community use? Are there neighborhood or community newspapers, newsletters, fliers, or radio announcements? Who are the residents observed on the streets? Are there women with small children, adolescents, or adults? Do residents seem friendly? Are they willing to stop and talk, or do they ignore you and walk away? Is there evidence that residents isolate themselves from outside communities? Where do the elderly reside?

What are the informal patterns of relationships? Where do persons meet: bars, laundromats, street corners, meeting halls, parks? Are particular groups highly mobile or transient? The formal organizational structure of the community can provide evidence of the locus of power. Are key community leaders available and easily accessible to community residents?

❑ ❑ ❑

Communities have many similarities: people, social systems, and psychologic, physiologic, and environmental patterns. The health-related patterns can provide a useful framework for collecting observation, interview, and measurement data. Table 9-3 presents an assessment guide according to collection methods and the health patterns. The health-related patterns the nurse chooses for an assessment depends on the community setting, the focus of the assessment, and the nurse's preference. Assessing all pattern areas provides a basic set of data that then can be analyzed, as well as used for comparison purposes in evaluation.

Analysis and Community Diagnosis

Analysis refers to the categorization of data and the determination of patterns. Once information about a community is obtained, the data must be sorted out, organized, and synthesized in a meaningful way to ascertain patterns of health activities and trends. Decision making and judgment, inherent in the nursing process, are particularly significant during the analysis and diagnostic phases. Community data can be grouped and organized in several ways.

ORGANIZATION OF DATA

Data can be synthesized through the use of various techniques, such as charts, figures, and tables. Graphic presentations of population distributions, morbidity and mortality data, or vital statistics can be most effective in pinpointing significant community concerns and actual or potential health problems. The data can then be compared with the community health-related responses to these concerns.

Mapping is another valuable technique that facilitates data analysis. Data changing with time, for example, can be followed with a series of maps; several variables that may be spatially identical and contiguous can be analyzed simultaneously, such as the location of environmental hazards, of densely populated areas, or of health promotion services and major highways. Poor environmental conditions; the distribution of illness, disease, and death rates; and the accessibility of health protection and health promotion activities for the population can be determined at a glance with dotted scatter maps. When maps are used, the population base of the community must be identified. For example, a less-populated geographic area might have fewer health facilities for its residents than another area; one community might have fewer neonatal deaths than another because it has fewer women of childbearing age.

The use of theoretic frameworks and the 11 pattern areas will also facilitate the organization and analysis of community data. Several guidelines are presented to help the community nurse analyze community client data. Analysis often supports the need for further data collection.

DATA ANALYSIS GUIDELINES

Check for Missing Data. Because of the complexity, size, and number of community characteristics, the

Table 9-3. **Example of data analysis and synthesis with the community as client**

Data clues	Health pattern application	Strength and concerns	Nursing diagnosis
Population structure			
Total population	10,400		
Age	0-4 5-14 15-19 20-44 45-65 65+		
Total no. in age group	1000 3000 800 2000 3000 600		
Males	600 2000 3000 750 1000 200		
Females	400 1000 5000 1250 2000 400		
Health perception pattern			
Community residents are concerned about adolescent drinking problem police officials report daily disturbances in parks and town parking lots where young adults congregate to "party" in late evening.	Interview data	Concern	
Mortality rate in motor-vehicle accidents in past year	Measurement data 75 died in car accidents, 28 deaths under age 19, 9 within a 6-week period.	Concern	
Value and belief pattern			
Parents of deceased teenagers have formed group and believe "something should be done about driving and drinking."	Interview data	Strength	
Role and relationship pattern			
Community newsletter High school has radio station and includes community announcements and health briefs prepared by community nurses.	Media use Circulation: 9000	Strength	
Coping and stress-tolerance pattern			
Health education, driving education, and driving safety programs are not available in high school.	Interview data	Concern	
Community has attempted to improve road conditions in areas of highest fatalities; trees have been removed, but road is in despair with large holes.	Observation data		Potential for increasing incidence of premature death in the high-school population related to drinking and driving and absence of health teaching and driving safety programs in school, poor road conditions

community nurse cannot obtain all the possible facts about the health-related pattern areas. However, missing or insufficient data that indicate areas in need of further assessment should be identified. Additional assessment may be necessary to determine specific approaches or a particular community diagnosis. Missing data in a community assessment might include pollution indices, links between health resources and population groups, accessibility to resources, or morbidity statistics, all of which may be necessary to determine actual or potential health concerns. Census data may not be current, and this should be noted. Missing data generally are indicated under a nursing diagnosis.

The nurse also should examine community data for incongruities; it is not uncommon to obtain conflicting information. For example, a key community official might deny the existence of pollutants in the water supply, whereas newspaper reports of water analysis findings of the health department indicate otherwise. The nurse must validate such inconsistencies before identifying existing or potential health concerns.

Identify Patterns. The subjective and objective data of the assessment are examined for clues to determine whether patterns emerge or clustering of information occurs. During this stage the community nurse makes decisions and begins to formulate ideas and tentative judgments, "diagnostic hypotheses," about possible health concerns, possible community groups at risk, and probable etiologies and relationships. This activity further directs the search for additional clues in the data to confirm, reject, or revise the hypotheses generated. Judgments or hypotheses are being generated constantly in the selection of clues that could form patterns in the data or relationships. The community nurse, in obtaining interview data, for example, may have generated certain hypotheses that directed the search for additional information or may determine the need for education programs within the community.

Community nurses can easily become overwhelmed with the data collected. Thus they must narrow down the multitude of possible community health promotion and protection concerns. One approach is to formulate broad problem statements based on the health-related pattern areas.[7] For example, does the community have an elimination problem (noxious chemicals evident), a coping and stress tolerance problem (inability to obtain a particular health education program), or a health perception and health management problem (high teenage mortality rate from motor vehicle accidents)? Asking such broad questions will help direct the community nurse to clues in the database.

Apply Theories, Models, Norms, and Standards. Analyzing community data requires a broad knowledge of developmental age-related risks and theories and concepts of nursing, public health, and epidemiology. This base enables the nurse to search for additional clues in the health-related patterns to develop community nursing diagnoses amenable to nursing interventions.

The developmental approach can be used as a basis for identifying groups with potential health concerns. Because different age-groups vary in susceptibility, the nurse must examine the community's resources to determine if they are directing services to highly susceptible groups. For example, community data may indicate an increase in live births among older women, which may indicate a need for additional health promotion services for this group. If community data show an increasing number of aging citizens, the nurse should explore the existing health services available and accessible to them.

Data also are analyzed for population groups according to common personal or environmental characteristics. For example, the nurse may identify select groups at risk based on a shared health concern such as substance abuse, lack of immunizations, unsafe housing conditions, high exposure to asbestos or noxious chemicals, or inadequate health services. A shared characteristic such as race may provide clues to susceptible groups in need of particular screening activities; a black population may need hypertension screening if such services are lacking, and children may be susceptible to dental caries and require screening if fluoridated water systems are lacking.

Other groups may have illiteracy in common. The literacy of a community is critical in health promotion activities, since it determines the methods used by nurses in establishing programs for specific health education.

Various standards are also used in analyzing data. For example, community data regarding air can be compared with state or national ambient air-quality standards to determine health concerns.[14] The term *ambient* in this context refers to outside air in a town, city, or other defined region. Continuous air-monitoring stations are generally located in various urban and rural areas within each state.

Model Standards: Guidelines for Community Attainment of the Year 2000 National Health Objectives[8] presents a framework for communities to establish a realistic timetable for reducing or preventing the principle health problems in a community. The use of model standards emphasize

- health outcomes
- flexibility
- focus on the entire community
- use of government as residual guarantor
- use of negotiation with professionals and lay people
- use of standards to provide uniform objectives to assure equity and social justice
- guidelines emphasizes local discretion for decision making
- accessibility of services
- character of programs

In using the model standards with health perception and health management patterns, the nurse uses outcome and process objectives compatible with both local priorities and the *Healthy People 2000* objectives. For example: By the year 2000, increase to at least 75% the proportion of people aged 10 and older who have discussed issues related to nutrition, physical activity, sexual behavior, tobacco, alcohol, other drugs, or safety with family members on at least one occasion during the preceding month. (Baseline data available in 1991). The indicator for meeting this objective is the percentage discussing issues with family in the past month (p. 102). In this way, the nurse can compare the baseline data to the outcome data in determining if the objective has been met.

The nurse should explore the data concerning the health perception and health management pattern and then determine what available community resources are directed toward preventing problems such as high infant mortality, motor-vehicle accident, or high childhood disease rates. In this way gaps in health promotion and protection services can be identified more readily.

Identify Community Strengths and Health Concerns. Community data are analyzed and interpreted in light of community strengths and concerns, within obtainable limits of certainty. This requires making judgments and inferences about the community's health, responses to health situations and conditions, and population needs. One approach is to assume health concerns exist unless the assessment data indicate otherwise.[7]

To make a diagnosis, the community nurse first summarizes the data and then makes one or more of the following judgments:[25]

1. No problem exists, but a potential health concern may be offset by providing health promotion or protection services. For example, "a potential for increased sexually transmitted disease in the high-school population" could be offset by providing health education in the high school.
2. A problem exists but is recognized by community members or health-related professionals and is being effectively handled.
3. A problem exists that has been recognized by the community, but resources are inadequate or the community has not responded. Assistance is needed.
4. A problem exists that the community recognizes but cannot deal with at this time, for example, a lack of fluoridated water systems. Dentists, nurses, and nutritionists could be assigned to assist the community in resolving a potential problem of dental caries.
5. A problem or potential health concern exists that needs further study.

A community may have many strengths. Identifying these is important because they can be integrated into plans for health promotion and protection activities. For example, a community may have many nutritional feeding programs for its elderly, women, and children. However, few community members may know about such resources because of poor community communications. Examples of community strengths and concerns are shown in the box on this page.

Identify Etiologies and Risk Factors. In this step the data are examined for those factors or characteristics that contribute to the list of the identified potential and existing health-related concerns. The nurse makes inferences about various population groups, identifying factors that place them at risk. For example, "Children entering elementary school may be at risk for rubella and mumps related to inadequate health protection services in the community" (a health management deficit in the community). The identification of the risk factors gives direction to community nursing actions. Some risk factors may signify an immediate health concern for a population group, such as polluted water supplies; others may indicate a potential health problem if they are not altered, such as a lack of knowledge regarding childhood disease protection.

❑ ❑ EXAMPLES OF COMMUNITY STRENGTHS AND CONCERNS

Strengths	Concerns
Well-child clinic available	Unavailable
Elderly feeding program accessible	Inaccessible
Sex education in schools acceptable	Unacceptable
Family planning services accessible	Inaccessible
Fluoridated water system	Nonfluoridated
Open communication	Dysfunctional communication
Interagency cooperation	Dysfunctional transactions
Adequate kitchen and plumbing facilities	Inadequate
High interest of key leaders in health promotion	Disinterest

In identifying risk factors, the community nurse also must consider those risk factors that have the potential for being altered, eliminated, or controlled through nursing actions. Some factors, such as age, race, and sex of a population, cannot be altered; others, such as lack of health education programs, can be altered to lower a particular group's risk to potentially harmful health situations or conditions.

COMMUNITY NURSING DIAGNOSIS

A community assessment, as previously described, culminates in a nursing diagnosis or diagnoses. The process of determining a community diagnosis includes: (1) a community situation or state within a population or population group(s); (2) data collection using some combination of observation, interview, and measurement; (3) a framework; (4) existing or potential health concerns; (5) appropriate risk factors related to the health concerns; and (6) a requirement for nursing actions. A diagnosis becomes the basis for planning and implementing interventions and nursing actions and for making evaluative judgments about health concerns.

A community diagnosis is stated in a clear and concise manner to facilitate communication among community health professionals, team members, and lay persons. Lists of community diagnostic categories specific to populations are beginning to be developed. Community health nurses need to continue to develop diagnostic statements that are community and population centered, specific, accurate, and amenable to nursing interventions.

The diagnosis may be written or stated according to the structural and functional aspects of a community.

Structural aspects include those related to the population, such as the demographic characteristics of groups who have similar characteristics–preschool children, adolescents, a high school population, and so on. The functional aspects include those related to the psychologic, physiologic, or environmental health patterns, such as decision-making (cognitive and perceptual pattern) or communication links among health care resources (role and relationship pattern). Information about health concerns and risk factors are obtained from the 11 functional health patterns.

The structural and functional aspects of the community provide a framework from which diagnostic statements can be made and should include the three elements of *who, what,* and *why:*

1. The "who" is the identification of the specific population group at risk (childbearing population, children, elderly, adolescents).
2. The "what" is the identification of the existing or potential health concern (accidents, drug abuse).
3. The "why" is the probable etiologic or risk factors believed to be related to the existing or potential health concern.

Table 9-3 gives an example of how community data are categorized and synthesized. The first column indicates community data as categorized by the appropriate health patterns. The second column lists the relevant health patterns applied and consists of supporting data and sources of data. The third column indicates community strengths and concerns. The fourth column states the nursing diagnosis. The community diagnosis is formulated after synthesizing all the data. Interview, observation, media, and measurement data are indicated as appropriate means for data collection.

Planning

The community health planning phase begins with the nursing diagnosis. The desired goals are expected to resolve existing or potential health concerns. For example, if a high rate of childhood diseases in the community is the problem, decreasing the rate is the goal. The identification of the specific or potential health concern, together with planned actions to achieve the desired outcome, become the framework and data for evaluation. Health planning therefore can be viewed as a problem-solving approach that has several purposes.

PURPOSES OF COMMUNITY HEALTH PLANNING

The four major purposes of the planning phase are

1. To prioritize the problems diagnosed from the assessment phase.
2. To differentiate problems that nursing actions can resolve from those that others can best handle.
3. To identify immediate, intermediate, and long-term goals; behavior objectives oriented to community behavior and derived from the goals; and the specific actions to achieve the objectives.
4. To write the problems, actions, and expected behavior outcomes on a community nursing care plan.

The planning phase culminates in a nursing plan that provides the framework for evaluation. Once developed, the plan is implemented.

The cost to deliver health services, the kinds of personnel involved, and the financial resources available will influence the priority given to health concerns, as will community values and the nurse's philosophy about persons, health, the community, and nursing. Examples of problems given high priority in some communities include infectious agents, sexually transmitted disease, alcohol and drug use, smoking, inadequate nutrition, inadequate infant and child care, high death rate from motor-vehicle accidents, and unwanted teenage pregnancies.

Community participation in health planning is essential to help assign priorities. As recipients of health-related services, members also can help to ensure that the services being planned are of reasonable cost and high quality. Community residents can help to ascertain the benefits sought by groups in need and whether the planned health services will be responsive to the needs and concerns of the population for whom they are intended. If community members and the nurse differ in setting priorities, mutual communication and a statement of the reasons for designating a particular priority can help resolve the difference.

When planning, the nurse must differentiate those problems that nursing intervention can resolve from those community health concerns that could be best handled by community members, referred to health-related professionals, or handled with community suppression of rodents, poor sanitation conditions, or absence of community recreational facilities should be referred to appropriate community leaders or agencies.

Developing goals as well as measurable behavioral outcomes or objectives and designating those actions that will achieve the expected outcomes are important nursing activities. Ways to write outcomes or measurable objectives are discussed in Chapter 11. Outcomes are projected before actual implementation of planned actions and are stated in terms of the client behaviors expected to result from nursing actions. Thus the effectiveness of nursing actions can be evaluated.

Health planning emphasizes promoting and protecting the health of population groups within the community; problems, solutions, and actions therefore are defined on this level. Community nurses who plan and implement health plans for one community population group, such as school-age children, help the community to begin developing health promotion services to all residents. Nurses frequently act as agents of change by taking responsibility in influencing and changing existing and potential health patterns and behavior. Decisions and plans for health interventions are based on the community nurse's awareness and understanding of human behavior and principles of planned change.

Planned Change. Planned change is the result of specific efforts by individuals or groups and involves fundamental shifts in their behavior.[22] Individuals can be the agents of their own health conditions; health often is determined more by what the person does than by what some outside germ or infectious agent can do. Some important community health objectives partly depend on individuals deciding to change their lifestyle–for example, by reducing their alcohol consumption or giving up smoking.

Efforts to influence and reinforce changes in community health behavior are the central focus if risk reduction programs are to be effective. Any change effort by community nurses and groups can be viewed as a three-phase process: unfreezing, changing, and refreezing (Fig. 9-2).[10]

Unfreezing is a stage of preparing a situation for change and involves disproving existing attitudes and behaviors to create a desired need for something new or a dissatisfaction with the status quo. Developing a *need* for change regarding particular health concerns in a community is thus critically important. A community already may have recognized the existence of a health concern and realized a change is needed to rectify it. Through lack of knowledge, planning, or inertia, however, strategies to eliminate the problem have not been implemented.

Unfreezing is facilitated by social and environmental pressures, recognition of a health concern, and an awareness of a better way to maintain, promote, or protect health. Involving community members is essential, since they can help increase consumer awareness of what constitutes health behavior, and can change attitudes or misconceptions about health activities.

Changing involves the actual efforts in influencing or modifying residents, tasks, structure, or technology. Many communities attempting change enter this phase of planning prematurely, are too quick to change things, and are apt to end up creating resistance to change in a situation that is inadequately unfrozen.

The *refreezing* stage of planned change involves maintaining the momentum of a change and includes such tactics as providing both positive reinforcement of desirable outcomes and support. Evaluation also can be considered during this step, since it provides the necessary information to make constructive modifications. Inadequate or improper refreezing can result in changes that are abandoned.

Many studies have tried to explain why some groups of people participate in certain health programs while others reject them. The early health belief model proposed by Rosenstock[29] and more recent models developed by Cox[5] and by Walker, Sechrist, and Pender[24] (among others) identify concepts critical to understanding how individuals undergo a change in health behavior. In Rosenstock's model, the following steps are identified:

1. Perceiving the behavior as a threat to health in terms of susceptibility and seriousness.
2. Believing the behavior is a threat to health.
3. Taking action to adopt preventive health.
4. Reinforcing the new behavior.

In this model the consumer at first takes on a passive role; the transition from passive to active occurs between steps 2 and 3, belief to action. If the ultimate goal is to improve the health of a community through risk-reduction programs, community members need to be influenced so they assume more responsibility for their health and become more "active" in adopting healthy lifestyles and behaviors. In planning health promotion activities, the nurse therefore must consider effective strategies to motivate and support the community's transition from a passive to an active state.

Once the plan is developed, it becomes a guide to nursing actions. The nurse must make additions and changes based on the community's problems, resources, and resolution of these problems to keep the plan viable.

The data summarized in Table 9-4 suggest an inability of the community to contain its mortality rates from auto accidents and also suggest a health management deficit regarding its teenage population. The inferred nursing diagnosis pinpoints two risk factors: (1) alcohol abuse and driving and (2) absence of health education in the school. Table 9-5 gives an example of a community-oriented health promotion plan based on the goals recommended by the surgeon general's report on health promotion and disease prevention. As shown, several specific objectives have been derived from a broad goal. The objectives' direction is based on the nursing diagnosis, which includes risk factors that can be altered.

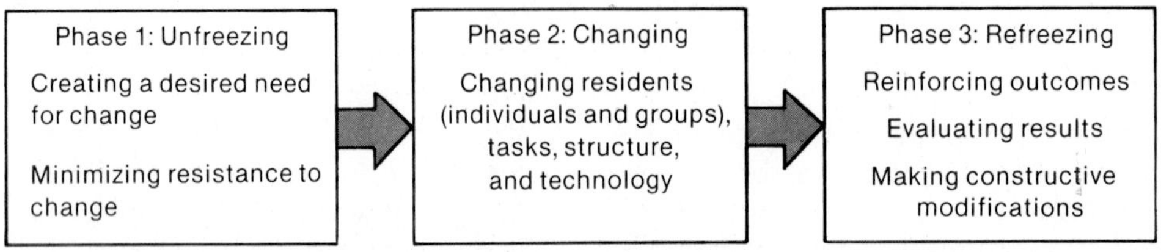

Fig. 9-2. Three phases of change.

***Table 9-4.* Implementation of community health plan, with objectives and rationale**

Nursing diagnosis: **Potential for increasing incidence of fatal motor-vehicle accidents in high-school population related to alcohol use and driving.**
Goal: **North High School population will have reduced incidence (at least 20%) of fatal motor vehicle accidents related to alcohol abuse and use by December 1995.**

Objectives	Plans	Rationale
1. Community will have access to information regarding incidence of fatal motor vehicle accidents and drunken driving arrests of its high-school population for last 5 years by March.	Interview local police regarding incidence of fatal auto accidents and substance abuse in community. Interview parents of deceased high-school students, students, teachers, physicians, and clergy, emergency room personnel, regarding incidence of problem and suggested measures for decreasing problem; suggest interviews be broadcast over high-school radio station. Have several persons write to community newspaper commenting on broadcast and problem.	*Unfreezing:*[13] for change to occur, community has to become dissatisfied with status quo and sense need for change. *Empiric-rational strategy:* persons are rationale; discussion of facts can bring about support for change.[22] Important elements for preventing problem include educating public; having key community leaders discuss their views and concern lends credibility and is necessary for action. Persons tend to listen to those with informal power.[6] Keeping problem issue before community can raise consciousness.[10]
2. Community will take action to inform population at risk about responsible driving and drinking by June.	Suggest to school principal and school board creation of task force of community residents to plan health program on individual responsibility and alcohol use in high school. Task force to include teachers, students, parents, clergy, police, nurse, and physician. Task force to examine ways to determine Examine ways to determine and teach content Integrate into curricula Recommend community members, such as nurse, be involved in teaching content.	*Changing:* moving to a new level; community involvement will influence acceptability of changes.[13] Community residents like to be involved in decision making.[6] It is important to establish trust and collaboration between community groups; this opens communication channels between adolescents and health community.[6] Community involvement facilitates acceptance of change.[6]
3. Community will implement educational program to its high-school population related to use of alcohol and individual responsibility by November.	Implement educational plan.	*Refreezing:* moving to level of change[13] brought about by community forces. Educational strategies built around concept of individual responsibility are essential elements in promoting health of young adults.[6]

Examples of various rationales show how the nurse can incorporate major concepts of planned change into a community-based health promotion plan.

Communicating the plans to other health professionals, community members, and key officials should not be overlooked; this is an essential aspect of planning. An article describing the educational plan can be published in local newspapers and bulletins, and school officials can send letters to students' parents.

Other community-based actions the nurse may become involved in to attack alcohol abuse in the community are listed in the box on p. 218. The various plans have been categorized according to the health patterns to show that a community problem can be approached from many directions. Plans that are feasible and well formulated help prepare for implementation.

Implementation

Once the plan for health promotion and health protection activities has been developed, the implementation of the nursing process begins. The plan may be implemented by the community nurse alone or together with team members and community residents and tested for viability. Its success or failure will depend on the nurse's intellectual, interpersonal, and technical skills, as well as the plan's acceptability to community members.

***Table 9-5.* Potential sources of resistance to health promotion programs, with agent responses**

Source of resistance	Response
Lack of communication regarding the implementation of program	Communicate through community newsletter, newspapers, high-school radio station, and posters
Misinformation regarding time and place of health activity	Disseminate valid information
Fear of unknown	Inform and encourage
Need for security	Clarify intentions and methods
No desired need to change behaviors	Demonstrate opportunity for change
Cultural, religious beliefs, or vested interests threatened	Enlist key community leaders in change planning
Inaccessibility	Focus activities near largest potential target population and in area accessible to public transportation

Resistance to change usually should be overcome for the planned intervention to be successful. However, resistance to new health promotion and protection activities is feedback that can be used constructively. In general persons resist change when they are defending something important that appears threatened by the change attempt.[4] Table 9-5 lists several factors identified as deterrents to community participation in health programs. An informed nurse can take steps to deal with such factors to help ensure the successful implementation of the plan. The nurse must recognize that community members may resist the type of planned activities or the individuals promoting them. Others resist changing their own attitudes or lifestyle behaviors.

Community nurses implement health promotion and protection plans in a variety of community settings, including schools, industry, public and private health agencies, and ambulatory care settings, where various population groups are relatively healthy. The simplicity or complexity of implementing health actions will vary from one community or population group to another. As the nursing plan is implemented, however, nurses also learn more about the community and their own responses, strengths, limitations, and abilities to cope and adapt.

Although the implementation phase has an action focus, it also includes assessment, planning, and evaluation activities to monitor the actions taken to resolve, reduce, eliminate, or control the health concern.

❑ ❑ PLAN OPTIONS FOR COMMUNITY-BASED ACTION: ALCOHOL ABUSE

Coping and stress-tolerance pattern

Identify available community alcohol treatment resources.

Regulation and enforcement: develop local alcohol control laws oriented toward prevention of abuse; develop consistent state regulation and control laws.

Role and relationship pattern

Increase communication between community control agencies, the school, residents, and health-related agencies.

Restrict community advertisements for alcohol in community newsletters and newspapers.

Evaluation

Evaluation is the phase of the nursing process in which the community nurse learns whether the actions designated in the nursing plan actually achieved the desired outcomes. The client's progress or lack of progress toward goal achievement is determined by the client and the nurse.[1] The nurse is responsible for the evaluation data, even though community members or health team members may participate in the process. For example, if a reduction in the incidence of fatal motor-vehicle accidents is expected to result from nursing actions, the nurse is responsible for obtaining the community's behavioral outcomes, which should show that a reduction occurred and that nursing actions helped bring about these outcomes.

As previously noted, the nursing plan, which includes the nursing diagnosis and expected outcomes, provides the framework for evaluation. The community is the focus; its goals and objectives define what is evaluated and are considered in terms of how the client responded to the actions planned. For example, if a reduction in particular childhood disease rates is expected following nursing actions, the nurse compares client responses before with those after nursing actions. This also determines whether nursing actions are effective, partly effective, or ineffective in achieving the desired goal.

Evaluation is an ongoing process and is approached in a purposeful, goal-directed manner. Determining the effect of nursing actions during and after implementation are important elements in evaluating the degree to which goals are achieved. The frequency of evaluation will depend on the situation, the changes expected, and the objectives. For example, a bleeding client may need to be evaluated every 15 minutes for signs of change, whereas evaluation of behavioral changes in community groups is not so immediate. In any population group, existing or potential health problems will be resolved or controlled within different intervals. Because evaluation is determined by immediate, intermediate, and long-range goals, the process is continued until the goals are realized.

The results of evaluating the community nursing plan

are also important, since they may indicate the need to reassess, revise, or modify the plan. Community planning and nursing actions are not always effective in achieving the goals related to the health concerns and needs of the community; as noted, resistance to change may play an important role. As a result, the community nurse reassesses the situation and plans a new approach, then implements and evaluates the revised plan. Thus the nursing process is a continuous cycle.

Equally important is the community nurse's self-evaluation to determine strengths and weaknesses or how the nursing plan might have been implemented more effectively or efficiently. The quality of health promotion and protection services to a community depends on the professional qualities of those providing the services and their effective use of the nursing process.

SUMMARY

Illness, disability, and disease are not inevitable events experienced equally among a community's members. Understanding the dynamic and complex nature of communities is an important function of the community nurse if the planning, delivery, and coordination of health promotion and protection activities for high-risk populations is to be effective.

The nurse uses various theoretic frameworks to assess the community's health-related patterns, health concerns, and health action potential and to implement the nursing process. Community data must be collected and analyzed so that subpopulations at risk can be identified. The community nurse identifies populations at risk or aggregate at risk so that specific health promotion and protection services can be directed most profitably. These activities can be enhanced through the nursing process.

Many communities have obvious deficiencies in health services that warrant health planning action. Community nurses play a significant role in health planning directed toward reducing risks associated with disease, premature death, and injury and promoting the health of community members. Principles of planned change also are used to increase the community's awareness of health, healthy behavior, and participation in preventive health services.

The simplicity or complexity of applying the nursing process with a community as client will vary from one community or geographic area to another. Community nurses must research the relation of particular health promotion actions to specific community phenomena to provide the necessary scientific evidence of the benefits of nursing actions.

References

1. American Nurses' Association: *Nursing: a social policy statement,* Kansas City, Mo, 1981, The Association.
2. American Nurses' Association: *Standards of community health nursing practice,* Kansas City, Mo, 1986, The Association.
3. Clark, M: *Nursing in the community,* Norwalk, Conn, 1992, Appleton & Lange.
4. Cottrell LS: *The competent community.* In Kaplan BH, Wilson RN, Leighton AH, editors: *In further explorations in social psychiatry,* New York, 1976, Basic Books.
5. Cox CL: The health self-determinism index, *Nurs Res,* vol 34, 1985.
6. Goeppinger MJ, Shuster GF: *Community as client: using the nursing process to promote health.* In Stanhope M, Lancaster J: *Community health nursing: process and practice for promoting health,* ed 3, St Louis, 1992, Mosby.
7. Gordon M: *Nursing diagnosis: process and application,* New York, 1987, McGraw-Hill.
8. *Healthy communities 2000 model standards: guidelines for community attainment of the year 2000 national health objectives,* ed 3, Washington, DC, 1991, American Public Health Association.
9. *Healthy people: the surgeon general's report on health promotion and disease prevention,* Health and Human Services, Washington, DC, 1979, US Government Printing Office.
10. *Healthy people 2000: national health promotion and disease prevention objectives,* Health and Human Services, Washington, DC, 1990, US Government Printing Office.
11. Johnson DE: *The behavioral system model for nursing.* In Riehl JP, Roy C, editors: *Conceptual models for nursing practice,* New York, 1980, Appleton-Century-Crofts.
12. King I: *A theory for nursing: systems, concepts, process,* New York, 1981, John Wiley & Sons.
13. Lewin K: *Field theory in social science,* New York, 1951, Harper.
14. Massachusetts Department of Environmental Protection: *Massachusetts environmental law reports,* Boston, Mass, 1990, Atlantic Legal Publishers.
15. Neumar B: *The Neuman systems model: application to nursing education and practice,* Norwalk, Conn, 1982, Appleton-Century-Crofts.
16. *The 1990 health objectives for the nation: a midcourse review,* Health and Human Services, Washington, DC, 1986, US Government Printing Office.
17. Orem D: *Nursing concepts of practice,* ed 3, New York, 1985, McGraw-Hill.
18. *Promoting health: objectives for the nation,* Health and Human Services, Washington, DC, 1980, US Government Printing Office.
19. Rogers ME: *Nursing: a science of unitary man.* In Riehl JP, Roy C, editors: *Conceptual models for nursing practice,* New York, 1980, Appleton-Century-Crofts.
20. Rosenstock I: The health belief model and preventive health behavior, *Health Educ Monog* 2:354, 1974.
21. Roy C: *Introduction to nursing: an adaptation model,* ed 2, Englewood Cliffs, NJ, 1984, Prentice Hall.
22. Schaller LE: *The change agent.* In Brooten DA, Hayman LL, Naylor MD: *Leadership for change: an action guide for nurses,* ed 2, Philadelphia, 1988, JB Lippincott.
23. Von Bertalanffy L: *General systems theory,* New York, 1968, George Braziller.
24. Walker SN, Sechrist KR, Pender JJ: The health-promoting lifestyle profile: development and psychometric characteristics, *Nurs Res* 36:76-81, 1987.
25. Yura H, Walsh MB: *The nursing process: assessing, planning, implementing, evaluating,* ed 5, Norwalk, Conn, 1988, Appleton & Lange.

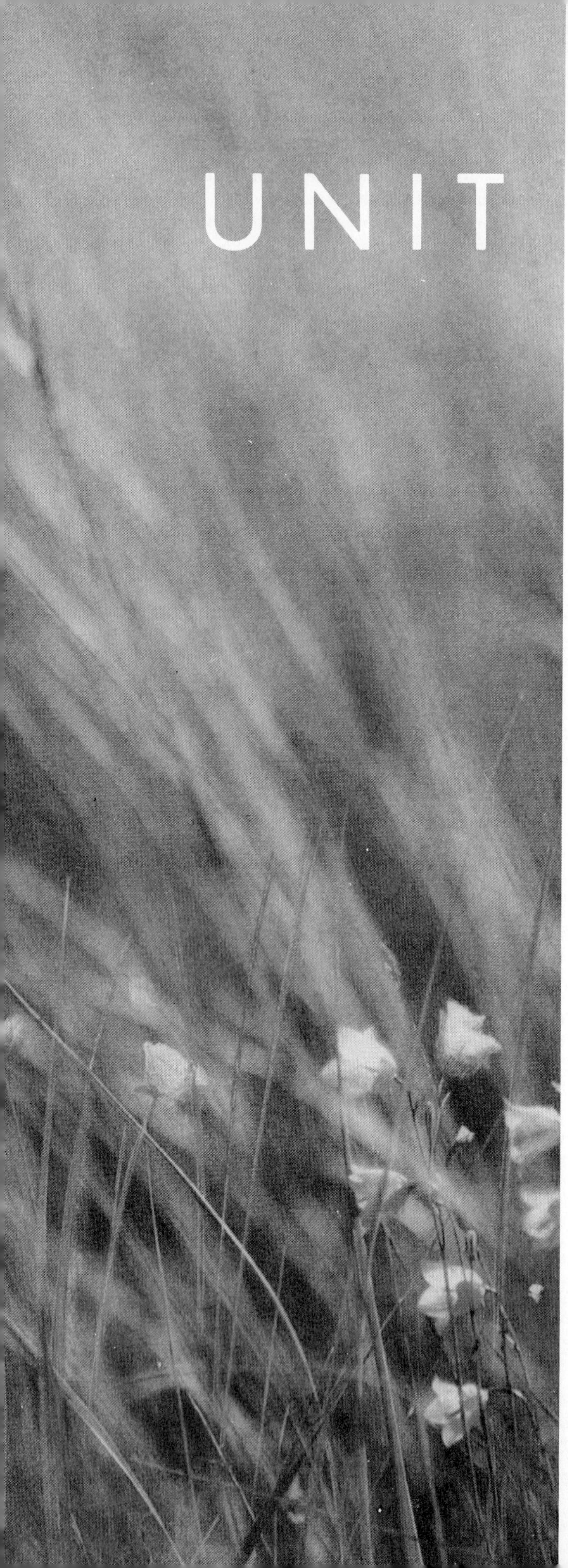

UNIT THREE

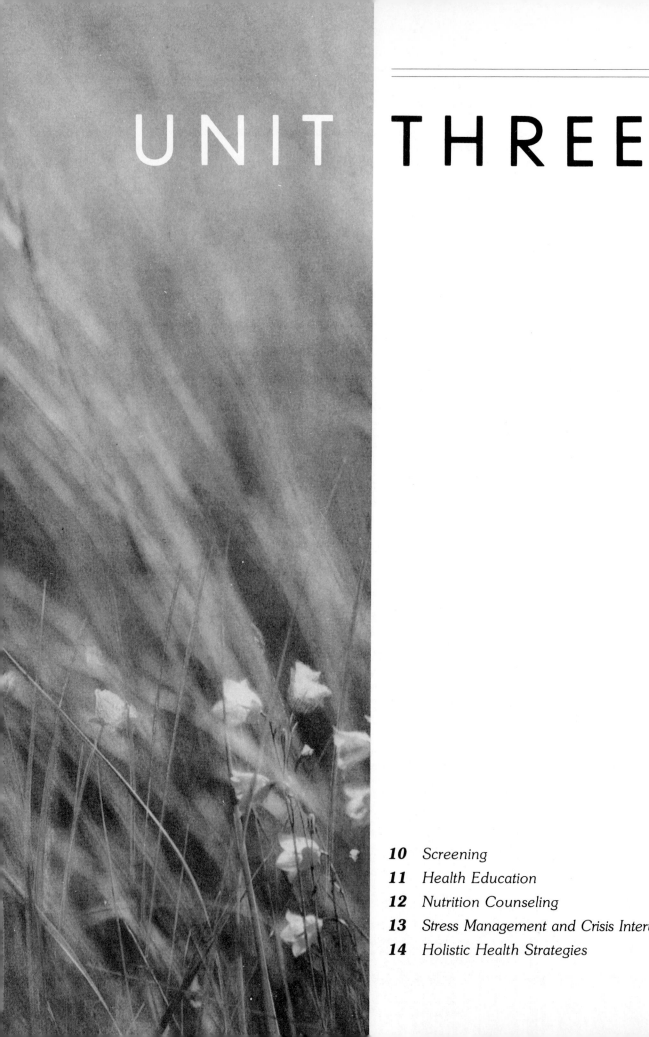

Interventions for Health Promotion

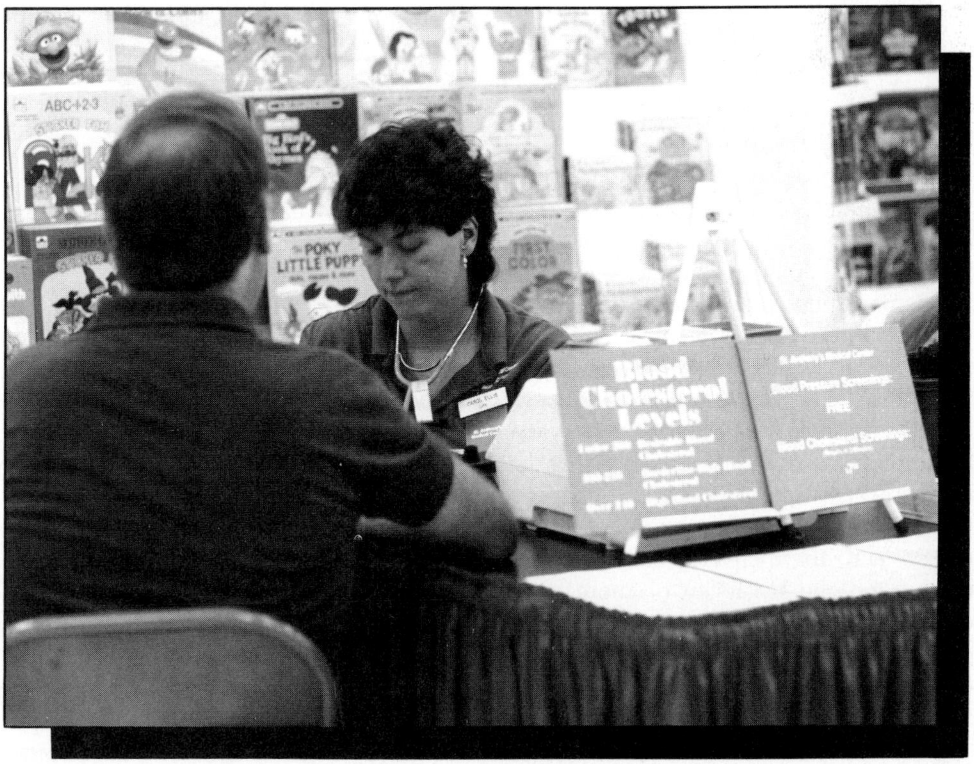

CHAPTER

10

Screening

William Martimucci

Krishan Gupta

Objectives

After completing this chapter, the nurse will be able to

- *Define screening and its relation to preventive health care intervention.*
- *Identify the advantages and disadvantages of the screening process.*
- *Define the disease specific criteria that determine a screenable disease.*
- *Discuss the medical and economic issues related to the screening process that result in ethical implications.*
- *Explain sensitivity and specificity as they relate to the efficacy of screening.*
- *Identify the broad range of community resources included in and affected by the screening system.*
- *Describe the nursing role in the screening process.*
- *Examine various health maintenance examination protocols.*

Screening is receiving growing recognition as a valuable tool for health care professionals, particularly as health care delivery moves more towards preventive interventions. Although health education about screening comes under the rubric of primary prevention (see Chapter 1), the actual process of screening is a form of secondary prevention. The primary objective of screening is the detection of a disease in its early stages in order to treat it and thus deter its progression. The basic assumption guiding this process is that detection during the early, asymptomatic period allows treatment at a time when the disease's course can be altered significantly. With the increasing knowledge of disease processes and the avilability of more sophisticated and effective remedies, screening is becoming possible for a growing number of disorders. A secondary, but equally important, objective of screening is to reduce the costs of treating the disease by avoiding the more vigorous intervention required during its later stages. The added attraction of a cost-conscious approach to health care mandates that health care professionals at all levels acquire a basic understanding of the screening process and its application.

This chapter describes the screening process, as well as the strengths and weaknesses common to its implementation. The presentation is designed as a checklist that allows the nurse to (1) analyze the screenability of a particular disease and (2) determine the means of implementing a screening program specific to the population, the disease, and the system of health care delivery.

DEFINITION, ADVANTAGES, AND DISADVANTAGES

The screening concept is based on the principle that disease is preceded by a period of asymptomatic pathogenesis (disease development) when risk factors predisposing a person to the pathologic condition are building momentum toward manifestation of the disease. Screening takes advantage of the early pathogenic state. The administration of often simple tests during this stage identifies specific variables that distinguish between individuals who most likely do have the condition and those who do not. Screening is not considered a diagnostic measure; it is seen as a preliminary step to direct a physician in assessment of the ostensibly healthy individual's chances of becoming unhealthy. The ultimate goal could be curative, but more often it is to prevent further development of the disease or to ameliorate the possible outcomes.

Formally stated by the World Health Organization, screening is "the presumptive identification of unrecognized disease or defect by the application of tests, examination or other procedures which can be applied rapidly. Screening tests sort out apparently well persons who have a disease from those who probably do not."[16]

Milio[20] implies several advantages of screening: "It is a service component which appears to be expanding on the assumption that it is *not* characteristic of the (health) system as a whole. In other words, it is relatively *not* expensive, is readily deployable, is often relatively simple and non-specialized, and is preventive in nature and thereby health-promoting." Although exceptions exist, screening tests are most often simple and inexpensive and frequently can be administered by a trained technician. The simplicity of the screening procedure decreases the time and the cost of health care personnel involved and enables lesser-skilled technicians to administer the test, which again reduces costs and permits the more appropriate use of highly skilled, costly professionals at the definitive diagnostic stage.

Another advantage is the ability to apply the screening process to both individuals and large groups. Combined with the relatively low cost of one screening test, such flexibility makes it adaptable to all levels of the health care delivery system.

The disadvantages associated with screening stem largely from the imperfection of modern science, which results in a margin of error for most instruments and tests produced. In screening, when program effectiveness depends on the test's ability to distinguish between those who probably do have the disease and those who do not, the margin of error can precipitate serious consequences. Some individuals who *do not* have the condition will be referred for further testings, and some who *do* have the disease will not. Those incorrectly referred suffer needless anxiety while awaiting more definitive diagnostic procedures. They also must bear the burden of the cost of follow-up visits and the time lost and inconvenience encountered.

More important, however, are the effects on those whose disorders have been missed. These individuals leave with a false sense of a healthful state that will at some point be shattered. They also lose the opportunity to receive early treatment that could prevent irreversible damage. The difficulty of balancing the benefits to some against the losses to others is an ethical issue encountered in most screening programs. Because the significance of this disadvantage can vary, it should be assessed for each project, disease, and population.

SELECTION OF A SCREENABLE DISEASE

The selection of a screenable disease goes beyond examination of the disease alone. The selection process often must encompass less tangible factors, such as the emotional and financial impact of the disease's detection on the screened population. Even after gathering data and reviewing the critical issues, the final decision "to screen or not to screen" must often be reached with incomplete data or with answers that raise highly ethical issues. The potential uncertainties confounding the decision emphasize the need to conduct an exhaustive analysis of available material to enable as objective and scientific a decision as possible.

The answers to three questions provide a basis for designating a disease as screenable or not:

1. Does the *significance* of the disorder warrant its consideration as a community problem?
2. *Can* the disease be screened?
3. *Should* the disease be screened?

As simplistic as these questions may appear, the answers or lack of answers not only exposes numerous complex issues but ultimately enables a well-informed decision to be made on screenability.

Significance

The significance of a disease refers to the level of priority the disease is assigned as a public health concern. Although the opinions of political and public interest groups may enter into the evaluation of significance, it is generally determined by the *quantity* and *quality* of life affected by the disorder. The greater the physical and psychologic harm experienced by the population, the greater the need to designate the disease as a priority health problem. The first step in assessing screenability is evaluation of this significance to decide if the disorder warrants the time, effort, and funds that must be allocated to a screenable disease.

Estimating the quality of life affected by a disease presents a problem: the perception of quality is subjective, and individual evaluations may differ. For example, not all persons equally perceive the disability resulting from a disease; some adapt, whereas others cannot.

Those who cannot would be more likely to say that the quality of their lives is significantly lower than that of others around them.

By contrast, measures of the quantity of life affected by the disease are more readily obtainable. Disease-specific mortality rates present one picture of this effect, whereas prevalence and incidence rates provide another. Prevalence defines the number of *old and new* cases during a specific time; incidence examines only the *new* cases during a specified period. Thus long-term chronic conditions usually are measured by their prevalence, whereas seasonal, sporadic, infectious conditions often are assessed by their incidence.

In this day of cost-conscious health care, a new dimension has been added to the evaluation of significance; the cost required to treat the disease. In some cases, the prevalence of the disorder may not be great, but the problem requires disproportionate amounts spent on maintenance or treatment after the condition is fully expressed. For example, with phenylketonuria (PKU), the incidence is not significant, but the cost of an undetected case at birth is lifetime institutionalization. Given the costly outcome if undetected and the reasonable price of the test to detect the disorder, the cost of screening all newborns is a nominal fee.

Can the Disease Be Screened?

With the relative significance of the disease established, the next step is to determine if health professionals *can* screen for the disease. Do well-documented *diagnostic criteria* for the disorder exist? Is there a *screening instrument*? Are sufficient *community resources* available to support a screening program?

DIAGNOSTIC CRITERIA

Detection of a disease requires knowledge of characteristics that clearly indicate its presence or, as in screening, its early pathogenic, asymptomatic state. Selected diagnostic criteria should be well documented, not merely accepted or commonly used indicators. Clearly, the impact of uncertainty in detecting disease is amplified when considering application of the screening design. Some diseases are defined by the presence or absence of a single, isolated factor, as in sickle cell anemia. Other conditions are indicated by measurement of statistically derived, numeric values for which a "normal" range has been set. Disagreement concerning the parameters of the normal range, combined with contentions that what is abnormal for one client is not abnormal for another, makes these conditions more controversial to designate as screenable disease. Hypertension and glaucoma, discussed later in this chapter, fall into this group.

SCREENING INSTRUMENTS

The next step is to determine if methods exist to detect the disease during early pathogenesis. If instruments are available, a careful analysis should determine if any fulfill the requirements for the screening process: safe, preferably inexpensive, and most important, accurate. Ultimately the question is how well the instrument can distinguish those individuals who probably do not have and will not develop the condition from those who are likely to develop it. The two variables that aid in instrument evaluation are reliability and validity.

Reliability. Reliability is an assessment of the reproducibility of the test's results when the test is performed by different individuals with the same level of skill during different periods and under different conditions. If the same result emerges from two individuals performing the test, *interobserver* reliability is shown. If the same individual is able to reproduce the results various times, *intraobserver* reliability is shown. Testing for instrument reliability can therefore yield data on (1) the accuracy of the test, (2) the variability of the observer's results, and (3) the variance of the factor being measured by the test.[1]

From these data the health professional can determine the amount of training required of the health care technicians or personnel who will administer the test. For example, if interobserver reliability is low, additional training might be required to work toward a more consistent method of delivering the test. This is frequently necessary in hypertension screening. If intraobserver reliability is low, the health professional might surmise that the instrument and not the individual is at fault.

Validity. Validity measures the test's ability to correctly distinguish between diseased and nondiseased clients. In a controlled setting, validity is evaluated by testing the instrument on a group consisting of a *known* proportion of individuals who have positive or negative test reactions. The ideal result is to have the instrument pick out 100% of the diseased persons (positive reactions) and 100% of the nondiseased individuals (negative reactions). Because such accuracy rarely occurs in practice, the measure of validity has been divided into two components, sensitivity and specificity, to quantify the margin of error in the screening instrument.

Sensitivity. This measures the test's ability to identify diseased persons by comparing *true positives* (TP)–persons the test picked who were diseased–with the known prevalence (P) of the condition in the validation group:

$$\text{Sensitivity} = \frac{TP}{P}$$

The prevalence can be expressed as the true positives added to the *false negatives* (FN)–persons the test identified as disease-free who were actually disease-laden–so that the following formula for sensitivity emerges:

$$\text{Sensitivity} = \frac{\text{TP}}{\text{TP} + \text{FN}}$$

For example, if the instrument detected 85 persons with cancer, missing 15 of the 100 cancer cases known to exist in the population, the sensitivity would be:

$$\frac{85 \text{ TP}}{85 \text{ TP} + 15 \text{ FN}} = \frac{85 \text{ TP}}{100 \text{ P}} = 85\% \text{ sensitivity}$$

To some this would appear to be a highly sensitive and useful instrument; to others, such as the 15 individuals who would miss the benefits of an early diagnosis of cancer, the instrument may appear inaccurate and useless.

Specificity. Specificity measures the test's ability to recognize negative reactions or nondiseased individuals. It is represented by a ratio of true negatives (TN) to the total of known negative reactions, which can be broken down into true negatives (TN) plus false positives (FP):

$$\text{Specificity} = \frac{\text{TN}}{\text{TN} + \text{FP}}$$

Assume that the instrument identified only 90 of the individuals who *did not* have syphilis while missing 10 of the known 100 syphilis-free cases. The resulting specificity would be:

$$\frac{90 \text{ TN}}{90 \text{ TN} + 10 \text{ FP}} = \frac{90 \text{ TN}}{100 \text{ known negative reactions}} = 90\% \text{ specificity}$$

The percentage again seems favorable, except to the 10 confused and anxious individuals who have been mislabeled with this socially unacceptable and potentially fatal disease.

Application of sensitivity and specificity data to the actual outcome of the program raises some interesting points. Consider the issues a public health nurse must face when given a newly developed test for abdominal cancer with low specificity and moderate sensitivity.

Low specificity means few true negatives and more false positives. The nurse and other health professionals then must consider (1) the cost, inconvenience, and psychologic stress experienced by the persons with false-positive reactions during the period following their incorrect screening test and (2) the additional referrals that will be made unnecessarily and the ability of the existing follow-up services to meet these needs.

With only a moderate level of sensitivity, a moderate number of false negatives could occur, sending away individuals with abdominal cancer who perhaps could benefit from treatment. The issue raised here is ethical: Should a screening program be implemented knowing that individuals who could benefit from treatment will be sent away? How positive must the benefits be to some to justify the losses to others?

The issues emerging from investigation of the screening instrument demonstrate the significant effect it has on the entire screening process. Data on the reliability and validity of the screening test provide valuable information to evaluate, anticipate, and ideally control these effects, enabling the program to work effectively toward its goal.

COMMUNITY RESOURCES

Implementing a screening program depends first on available appropriate community resources, such as funds, health care workers, follow-up and treatment sources, and administrative personnel, and second on their judicious organization. Knowledge of the disease's characteristics and the screening instrument are useless without the financial and human support to apply it.

A community assessment provides an individualized, systematic method of data collection to evaluate the quantity and quality of available resources. In the case of screening, however, evaluation must also determine the compatability of the screening program's needs with the community's ability and willingness to allocate these resources.

A tool that puts into perspective the numerous variables encountered in a community assessment is *systems theory,* which breaks a program, a business, or an environment into different functional components while defining the relationship between each component (Fig. 10-1). *Input* is channeled through a *processor,* which converts the input into the desired *output.* Within the processor, a *control* defines the manner in which processing is performed. External to these components are *constraints,* other systems that affect the operation of the central system. The last component is the *feedback loop,* which demonstrates that the success or failure of the final product will influence the function of the system at all points.

In terms of a screening design, the following elements emerge from the development of a system diagram: the community or high-risk population as the input; the health care professionals as the processor; a sponsoring group as the control; and referred or nonreferred individuals as the two output categories. Constraints affecting the operation of a screening program are financial concerns, political issues, and follow-up/referral services. A systems approach not only identifies the necessary community resources but defines how these resources interact. Using this added dimension,

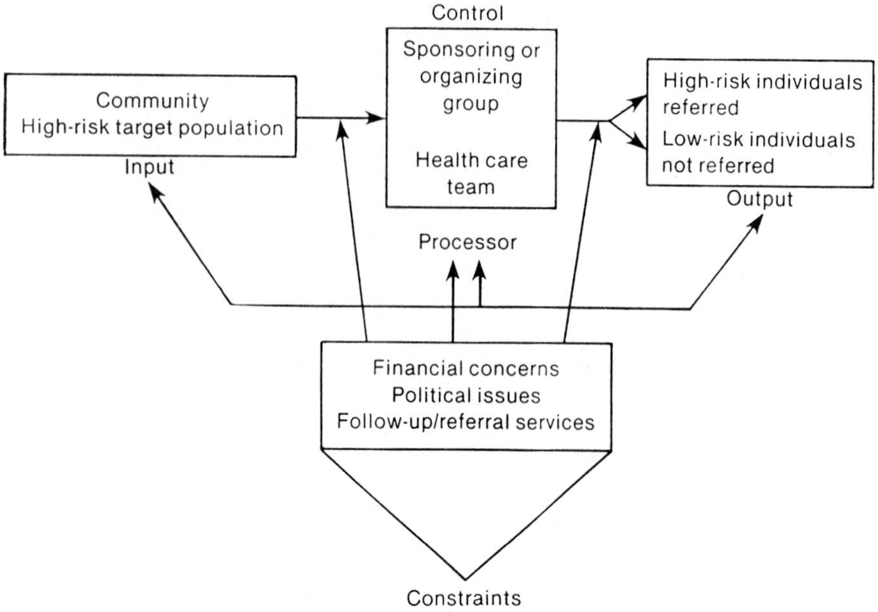

Fig. 10-1. System diagram of components and interaction of screening program.

administrators can assess problem areas that could interfere with the screening program's success.

The *input* or response from the community is affected partly by experience with other screening porgrams and the positive or negative feedback. Did controversial issues surround either the condition screened or the allocation of funds for it? Were there political issues associated with the sponsoring group (constraints)? Additional factors that will influence community participation are the means used to inform them, the accessibility of the program's location, the availability of transportation, and the convenience of the program's hours. Defining each of these factors is the responsibility of the program's sponsoring group.

As the screening system's *control,* the sponsoring group develops and conducts the delivery of the program. The group must both contract and organize necessary community resources and design the method of moving the target population smoothly into and out of the system. For example, the selection of a site could involve contacting churches, community centers, and schools. More than one location might be advisable to ensure accessibility to all. Transportation could require organization of volunteer drivers, negotiations with taxi companies, and so on. The problems and the methods of solving these problems are as numerous as the screening programs developed. The primary rule is never to assume that what was appropriate and effective for one community will be the same for another.

The origins of the sponsoring group vary from a community-service organization to the local public health department responding to a mandate from the state. Regardless of its origin, the group must perform a self-evaluation to compare its levels of expertise with those required to implement the screening effort successfully. Early identification of the group's strengths and weaknesses allows effective use of talents and compensation for weaknesses.

As the *processor,* the health care team operates the screening system. The team's responsibilities consist of rapidly and effectively administering the screening test and then designating the appropriate output category of the participants. Several considerations are relevant in organizing health care professionals. Even in communities where such professionals are abundant, their willingness to participate could be influenced by the success or failure of previous efforts to effect a positive health outcome and to handle the additional demands made on these professionals in the aftermath of referrals. Elaborating plans to control each can therefore enhance the credibility of future efforts and increase future participation.

For communities with few care facilities, health professionals may be scarce, necessitating development of a contract for service with professionals in other cities and escalating the cost of screening. At the other extreme, more densely populated areas may offer many available personnel, so that rotation of staff could reduce the number of hours required by each and make donated time possible.

Financial support of the screening program is a *constraint* that can influence all points in the system. Although some programs are delivered entirely on a voluntary basis, other program organizers must submit grant proposals to local, state, or even federal departments when consideration of medical and economic ethics is involved. Planners must look beyond the screening day and investigate financial resources for follow-up care. Assistance expected from federal, state, and private third-party groups, as well as special arrangements negotiated by or arranged through the screening program, should be made available to the screening participants.

Another constraint of the screening system design is follow-up medical service. In addition to financial accessibility, follow-up medical services should be accessible in terms of convenient locations and open hours. For example, an evening clinic may compensate for those who are reluctant or financially unable to miss work. Development of an efficient referral system links the follow-up resources to the screening program, providing continuity of care. Ideally a method is devised to encourage and check on compliance with referrals. Public health nurses can make home visits or telephone calls for this purpose.

The capability of existing follow-up facilities to handle the influx of referred individuals must be questioned. Will this unjustly affect the availability of health care professionals for others in the community? A survey could investigate a less active period at the follow-up facilities, with the screening program scheduled during this time.

Identification and organization of community resources is the most complex step in the screening design because it requires investigation and integration of numerous constituents. Systems theory is only one approach to analyzing community resources and their effect on disease screenability.

Should the Disease Be Screened?

Having determined that the disease is *significant* and *can* be screened, the final step in identifying a screenable disease is to establish if health professionals *should* screen for the disorder. What influences the success or failure of a screening program? Which factors can be controlled and which cannot? Which are mandatory for success? Where can compromises be made? A review of three additional subjects–natural history, treatment, and ethical issues (discussed in the next section)–begins to answer these questions.

NATURAL HISTORY

Since screening is based on the disease's asymptomatic period, adequate information must exist on the natural history of the condition specifying the optimum time for screening as well as how intervention during this time affects the prognosis. Without this knowledge, health care professionals are unable to explain how the consequences of the detected disease differ from those of the undetected. Thus they can neither evaluate nor explain the health benefits to be derived through participation in the screening program.

In a screening program the issue relating to a disease's natural history usually centers around the adequacy and scientific credibility of available data, not simply the presence or absence of information. For example, in the most common form of hypertension, essential hypertension, the etiology is unknown. Although research supports an association between hypertension and cerebrovascular disease, not all individuals who have hypertension develop cerebrovascular disorders. Also, what is "increased" blood pressure or hypertension for one person, may be "normal" for another.

The absence of any curative effect can be almost as detrimental as the presence of adverse effects. Not only has the program misled the screened population that a health benefit will result from their efforts, but detection and treatment used both personal and community funds that as yet have not altered the course of the disease. However, in the United States the efforts to control hypertension have led to a significant decrease in morbidity and mortality during the past 20 years.

TREATMENT

Compliance with a therapeutic regimen is the key role of the individual in a screening design. The first step, compliance with the postscreening referral, depends on the accessibility of the follow-up clinic, the hours it may be open, and the cost. Controlling these factors through efficient use and organization of community resources can increase compliance at this level.

The next step is compliance with the prescribed regimen, such as drug therapy. Evaluation of an expected rate of compliance may include a review of the literature discussing former success or failure in compliance with the drug and identification of treatment characteristics that impair compliance, such as cost or inconvenient side effects. Side effects present an interesting problem, since the confounding factor is often the subjective significance attributed to them. For example, hypertension may be successfully detected, but some individuals may find the inconvenient side effects of diuretic therapy intolerable, resulting in noncompliance.

Undoubtedly the most difficult variable to control in screening, the rate of compliance does determine the ultimate effectiveness of treatment and consequently of the screening effort. Thus serious consideration must be given to factors that could enhance compliance. For example, nurses can provide ongoing education about the drug and its importance, help clients develop medication schedules more suited to their lifestyles, and detect early signs of side effects that can be resolved before noncompliance begins.

Safety of the treatment is a particular concern when

considering the widespread application of a remedy following a screening program. Risks or harmful side effects can be costly in terms of both human health and increased medical care needed to correct the *iatrogenic* condition (resulting from medical intervention). The medical team must decide if these risks significantly diminish the success of the treatment and finally weigh the benefits to be derived from the treatment against the harm of its side effects.

ETHICAL CONSIDERATIONS

Any step taken toward improving health usually is deemed a just and moral act within the medical system's values. However, when approaching medical practice with a more critical eye and realizing that not all the results of the well-intended practice are beneficial, the need to balance the benefit against the detriment becomes an issue. The resulting decision process becomes a value judgment–an ethical decision.

Although the majority of ethical issues surrounding screening are applicable to both individual and mass screening programs, they are more evident when viewed in relation to a group. For this reason, the following discussion focuses on issues emerging from such a setting.

Medical Ethics

A screening program is unlike the normal mechanism of the health care system. Instead of receiving those who have performed a self-assessment and elected to enter the system, a mass screening program invites unsuspecting, apparently well individuals to be tested for unwellness. The request for participation *implies* that a health benefit will be derived, although at this stage nothing is said about what it will be or what the consumer must do to obtain it. Program planning that attempts to clarify this implication and inform participants of the issues develops the basis for an ethically sound project and enhances the screenability of the disease.

Because most screening programs are called "hypertension" screening or "diabetic" screening, it is not surprising that participants enter assuming the results received are diagnostic and will classify them as disease free or disease laden. This is untrue, since the screening goal is only identification and referral of high-risk individuals. Thus the initial presentation of and contact with the program imply a benefit not being delivered. To alleviate this problem, the planning committee should develop a method of informing participants of the meaning and limitations of the results. Participants need to know whether the ultimate benefit is preventive, ameliorative, or curative and, most important, what responsibility they must assume to secure this outcome. Some screening programs, such as those for glaucoma or hypertension, distribute a card containing test results and a qualifying remark:

> This pressure is within/not within the accepted norm. Having the test results of ____________ today does not mean that you do or do not have the condition or that you could not develop it in the future. If your pressure was in the accepted norm:
>
> - You should still be screened again when the opportunity is available.
>
> If your pressure was not in the accepted norm:
>
> - You are identified as at high risk of having or developing the condition.
> - You should seek further medical advice very soon.

Such a card is useful to clarify the results and inform the person of the next step. Although some always will classify themselves as disease free or disease laden, the goal is to minimize this misinterpretation.

Of even greater ethical concern than human misperception is the misinterpretation made by the screening instrument. As the information on sensitivity and specificity indicates, false positives and false negatives occur with any screening instrument. One of the more difficult ethical issues in screening is to evaluate whether the benefits received by those correctly screened are worth the problems experienced by those incorrectly screened. What obligation does the project have to incorrectly screened individuals? What is an acceptable number of persons with false-negative test results, all of whom will both miss the benefit of early treatment and be misled about the need for tests in the near future? What will be the response of an individual who has a false-positive reaction? Answers to these questions are generally value judgments that vary according to the disease.

Evidence suggests, however, that an individual given a false positive result would react to being labeled with a condition. In a significant controlled study by Haynes and others,[12] workers, after being told they had "hypertension," had a significantly higher absentee rate from illness than they had during a comparable period immediately before screening. Labeling an individual with a disease not present can result in behavioral changes.

Two other side effects of labeling, or especially mislabeling, are the *stigmatization* resulting from a socially or personally unacceptable disorder, such as venereal disease, and the *anxiety* of the incorrectly screened individual awaiting further testing. The degree of both vary with the disease and the individual perception. For many, the relief of finally learning that they are disease free may soften the blow. Since a screening test that is 100% sensitive and 100% specific is rare, some individuals who do not have the disease will suffer the long-term effects of the incorrect screening test, adding the inconvenience and cost of treatment to the anxiety and stigmatization. Ethically the situation presents a difficult problem that must be resolved by focusing on the benefit to be gained by those who have the disease compared with the detriment to those mislabeled. The most explicit example is screening for HIV infection.

Two issues that contribute to either clarifying or further confounding the medical ethics of screening are *cutoff* points for the screening instrument and *borderline* cases. How precisely do the instrument's numeric values define the high-risk disease state? The goal of a screening program, identifying individual as high risk or not, depends on this numeric value. When the parameter for this distinction is not clear, a cutoff point is set. Above this point the person is seen as disease positive; below, disease negative. Consequently, readjusting the cutoff point becomes a highly controversial issue, since it controls the percentage of positive and negative results. If the disease is potentially life-threatening, an increase in false-positive results (lower cutoff point) would be preferred to missing individuals who may have the disease. Also, if a disease is relatively benign in terms of potential stigmatization, anxiety, and problems with treatment, lowering the cutoff point could again be safe and ethical. On the other hand, if the disease does not satisfy these characteristics, raising the cutoff point would be the answer, referring fewer people but increasing accuracy and eliminating some of the false-positive results.

A problem closely related to a cutoff point is defining a policy for borderline cases. Hypertension is a common disease in which a variance of 5 to 10 mm Hg can make the difference in labeling a person as high risk or not. A more sophisticated approach may be taken to discriminate between a borderline case that should be referred and one that should not. The health professional can specify other risk factors associated with hypertension, such as family history, diet, and smoking, as criteria contributing to the decision to refer an individual. With the increasing interest and knowledge of risk factors, the effectiveness of this method should improve.

The medical ethics of screening will continue to demand review of the same questions and issues; however, the answers may change as more is discovered about the various conditions and their treatments. Thus an updated literature review is imperative before reviewing these issues in relation to a particular screenable disease.

Economic Ethics

Associating a monetary value with health care outcomes is generally against the nature and idealistic approach of most health care professionals. The tendency is to place no limits on the cost of promoting a healthy, disease-free or disease-controlled status, resulting in a philosophy that all care should be given to all persons at all costs. This philosophy is especially present among nurses, who until recently were rarely expected to consider the cost of treatment and materials. Today, because of the greatly increasing cost of health care, setting priorities in planning and financing health programs becomes as important as it is in developing a nursing care plan. Assessing the feasibility of a screening program, in which community funds allocated to the program could mean a lack of funds for other projects, illustrates this point. The persons benefiting from a screening test will be countered by those suffering from a lack of service for other medical or social needs. These trade-offs result in ethical decisions, demanding careful analysis by the screening administration.

Screening can be a costly project for both organizers and consumers. Initial operational costs must be considered, including (1) buying or renting the screening instruments, (2) renting floor space (if none is freely donated), (3) engaging professionals or technicians to administer the tests, and (4) interpreting the results.

These costs again are encountered when persons are referred for further evaluation. *Consumer* costs include follow-up medical visits and treatment, as well as the time, and therefore income, lost while complying with each. Given the combined operational and consumer costs, the major question is: "Do the costs result in the desired health outcome to the individual, group, or community?" In other words, are the benefits reaped worth the expenditures required? The answer is determined partly by what values *other than monetary* ones are attributed to the benefit, such as saving a life. However, a strictly economic approach generally eliminates the intangible variables, demanding the use of more objective data for decision making.

When alternative program designs are being considered along with screening, three major approaches may be employed to direct a thorough evaluation of the economic resources affected: (1) cost/benefit, (2) cost-effectiveness, and (3) cost-efficiency analyses. Once far from the thoughts of health care workers, the current relevance and use of such concepts require a basic understanding of their role in the selection of a screenable condition. Although presented here in successive fashion, they are entirely separate methods, and are most frequently used independently of each other.

COST/BENEFIT

Cost/benefit analysis is performed first because it allows comparison of various outcomes in monetary terms. This comparison is necessary in health planning when the initial consideration is which health outcome (reduction of cardiovascular disease, decreased infant mortality, reduction of visual problem) will be of *most benefit* to the community *at the most reasonable cost.*

Benefit here is divided into two types: *direct,* such as reduced hospital days and reduced cost of treatment; and *indirect,* such as the maintenance of a healthy, productive individual in the work force. These benefits are quantified through the use of sophisticated mathematics to present values in cost/benefit ratio. (Admittedly, quantification can be difficult in health care; benefits are often those intangible variables defying monetary value.) For example, a program to reduce cardiovascular disease costing $2000 to deliver and yielding $10,000 in benefits has a cost/benefit ratio of $2000 \div 10{,}000 = 0.2$. Comparing it with a program to reduce infant mortality, which costs $6000 and yields $12,000 in benefits and has a cost/benefit ratio of $6000 \div 12{,}000 = 0.5$, one finds the cardiovascular program a more proficient means of improving one aspect of the community. (The ratio also may be expressed as benefit/cost, in which case the larger the number, the better the program.)

COST EFFECTIVENESS

After choosing reduction of cardiovascular disease as the desired outcome, the next step is a cost-effectiveness analysis, which determines the optimum use of available resources to reach a predetermined, constant end point–the desired health outcome. The outcome remains the same; the best method of deriving it is the issue. For example, considering the selected health outcome, reduction of cardiovascular disease, the alternative methods might be (1) screening for hypertension, (2) taking electrocardiograms on all persons age 25 or older who are admitted to the hospital, (3) an antismoking campaign, or (4) nutrition counseling. Implementation of all would be ideal, but with limited resources a choice must be made.

Since cost effectiveness does not require assessment of the dollar value of health or life, the comparative value used to compare these methods could be the cost to reduce mortality (cost per eliminated death). The program with the least cost to eliminate one death, such as $200 per eliminated death, would be the most cost effective. Detailed explanation of the methods used to derive these figures is not within the scope of this chapter. The important difference is the type of information made available to the decision-making process.

COST EFFICIENCY

The last approach to help put the economic resources into perspective is cost-efficiency analysis. The purpose is to budget a limited amount of money toward achieving as much of the preselected desired outcome as possible. The funds are the central issue, not the health benefit. The result could be cutbacks in quality, equipment, or personnel, which in a screening program could mean poor accuracy and poor effectiveness. A means of assessing programs that could be implemented without limiting their quality goes back to use of the cost/benefit ratio. For example, with a $10,000 budget, a program costing $9000 with cost/benefit ratio of 0.2 would be selected over a program costing $10,000 with a ratio of 0.6. For the amount of money invested, the resulting benefits are greater.

OTHER ISSUES

The three economic approaches just discussed provide careful examination of alternate outcomes and programs before the screening design is selected. They provide objective data that can help justify selection of a screening program but unfortunately do not eliminate other ethical issues surrounding its implementation. When does the cost of screening and identifying those at high risk warrant channeling monies away from those who already have the condition and who could benefit from curative intervention? A cost-effectiveness analysis could compare the cost of a curative treatment program with that of a screening program.

A screening program is affected by additional issues related to economic ethics:

1. If the specificity of the screening instrument is low, increased false positives will occur, resulting in increased expenditures for unnecessary follow-up examination and wasted professional time.
2. If sensitivity is low, false negatives will occur, resulting in increased costs for treatment when the condition finally is detected in a more advanced stage.
3. Cases detected may be past the treatable or curable stage, resulting in costs for palliative care.

Although prohibiting a screening program based solely on these issues is difficult, their impact should be considered along with the other factors affecting disease screenability.

SOME IMPORTANT SCREENING CRITERIA

In spite of the fact that periodic medical examination and check-ups have been urged since the early part of this century, continuing controversy as to the exact value of screening has led to a somewhat disappointing response. Indiscriminate screening programs may lead to a gross waste of resources with little return. The benefits of an early detection program depend upon the characteristic of the disease, the specific group of individuals with potential health problems, and the specific tests employed. The features in the box on p. 231 are known to influence the outcome of a screening program.[9]

❑ ❑ CRITERIA FOR SCREENING

1. The disease must have a significant effect on the longevity or the quality of life.
2. The disease must have a sufficiently high prevalence rate to justify the cost of the screening program.
3. The disease must have been shown to have better therapeutic results if detected in the early stage and worse results with delayed detection and treatment.
4. The disease must have a significant asymptomatic period allowing an opportunity for detection and treatment that will reduce the rate of morbidity and mortality.
5. The disease must have an acceptable method of treatment.

SELECTION OF A SCREENABLE POPULATION

Selection of a screenable population is as important as selection of a screenable disease. The objective is to identify a high-risk group that, when tested, will yield a significant number of diseased persons. With such results, the effort and cost put into screening the population are minimized, and the health benefit received is maximized. The main criterion used to define an appropriate population is the definitive presence of risk factors related to the disorder. To ensure a thorough examination of possible risk factors, both host-dependent and agent-dependent factors should be reviewed.

Person-Dependent Factors

One characteristic related to the person, *age*, is increasingly important, since its distribution changes throughout the population (Tables 10-1 and 10-2). Accepted practice always has placed a high priority on screening the vulnerable, high-risk infant population, partly because health professionals are soon faced with the results of negligence affecting children's growth and development. As the average lifespan increases, however, the effects of longer-range risk factors are becoming apparent, making certain prevalent and costly chronic conditions equally important to control. Ideal populations for screening therefore can be found in

***Table 10-1.* Recommended women's guide to health tests and screenings**

Test	Purpose	Age	Frequency
Routine physical exam	General checkup for *healthy* persons	Birthing-2	As directed by pediatrician
		2-20	Every 1-2 years
		21-40	Every 1-3 years
		40 +	Annually
Breast exam	To detect changes in the breast that could go unnoticed by you	20-40	Every 3 years
		40 +	Annually
Pap smear	To detect uterine abnormalities, including cancer	18 +	Annually
Mammogram	To detect changes in breast tissue that are too small to be felt	40	First mammogram
		40-50	Every 1-2 years or as directed by physician
		50 +	Annually or as directed by physician
Electrocardiogram	To test heart function	40	One baseline
		41 +	
Colorectal exam	To detect traces of blood in stool – an early sign of colorectal cancer	40-50	Every 2 years
		50 +	Annually
Cholesterol test	To check serum cholesterol – a major factor in heart disease	Birth-15	As directed by physician
		15 +	Once every 5 years if levels are within normal range
Breast self-exam	To detect changes in breast tissue or appearance	18-Menopause	Monthly; 1 week after onset of period
		Postmenopause	Monthly; first day of every month
Blood pressure	To detect hypertension – a major risk factor for cardiovascular disease	5 +	Annually if blood pressure is normal
			As directed by physician if blood pressure is abnormal
Tuberculosis skin test	To detect presence of tuberculosis bacteria	5 +	Every 2 years
Tonometry	To check for signs of glaucoma	40 +	Every 2-3 years or annually if indicated by family history

***Table 10-2.* Recommended men's guide to health tests and screenings**

Test	Purpose	Age	Frequency
Tuberculosis skin test	To detect presence of tuberculosis bacteria	5 +	Every 2 years
Tonometry	To check for signs of glaucoma, an eye disease which can lead to permanent vision loss	40 +	Every 2-3 years, or annually if indicated by family history
Testicle exam	Self-exam: To check for testicular cancer Professional exam: To check hard lumps	15 +	Self-exam: Monthly Professional exam: Upon detection of of lumps or to correct undescended testicle
Routine physical exam	General checkup for health maintenance	Birth-2	As directed by physician
		2-20	Every 1-2 years
		21-40	Every 5 years
		41 +	Every 2-3 years, or as directed by physician
Prostate exam	To detect prostate cancer, a common but highly treatable disease	40 +	Annually
Electrocardiogram	To see if heart is functioning properly	35	One baseline
		36 +	As directed by physician
Colorectal exam	To check for signs of colorectal cancer, a common disease that is highly treatable with early detection	40 +	Annually
Cholesterol test	To see if cholesterol content of blood is too high – a major factor in heart disease	By age 20	Every 3 years if indicated by family history
		25 +	Every 3-5 years if levels are normal
Blood pressure	To detect hypertension, a major risk factor for cardiovascular disease	5 +	Annually if blood pressure is normal As directed by physician if blood pressure is abnormal

senior-citizen housing projects or elderly day-care settings. Middle-aged adults are also being recognized as a screenable group for certain conditions; breast cancer, glaucoma, and heart disease commonly appear during this period.

Sex has obvious implications for screening programs, most of which tend to be biased toward one *sex*. For example, women are tested for two commonly screened conditions, breast cancer and cervical cancer.

A population representing a particular *race* of people can sometimes be appropriate for screening. For example, blacks are screened at birth for sickle cell anemia with increasing regularity. Another condition, Tay-Sachs disease, is found mainly in Jewish children.

Income level has repeatedly been associated with the presence or absence of a healthful state. Lower-income groups demonstrate a susceptibility to a variety of illnesses. In view of the concentration of disease in low-income areas, this population is often appropriate for a multiphasic screening project in which numerous diseases are screened during one program.[20] However, because a screening project is effective only when treatment of discovered illnesses is guaranteed, special consideration should be given to financial and community resources when applying the screening design to a poor community.

Personal characteristics related to *lifestyle*, could suggest the need to screen a group for diet-related problems, such as hypercholesterolemia or obesity. Individuals with particular sexual habits could also provide a potential source for screening.

Once screening is completed, health care providers bear a responsibility to educate individuals as to the next step in the evaluation of their potential condition. Those being screened also bear a certain responsibility to seek treatment and follow through if the effect of screening is to be meaningful.

Environment-Dependent Factors

Environment-related risk factors relevant to the screening design are those *environmentally* and *occupationally* derived. Both fields are relatively new, with limited information on the natural history and treatment of respective disorders. Although the current lack of information reduces the credibility of developing a screening program, the growing significance of these factors demands special consideration.

In occupational health a legitimate population for screening is the high-risk work area, where harmful chemicals, airborne particles, or high-decibel machinery put the worker at risk of cancer, respiratory conditions, or auditory problems. At the other extreme is the sedentary executive work life, in which stress and all of its by-products are prevalent. The use of an occupational health nurse to provide individual screening for such problems is being recognized as an integral role of both health and business.

The environment has long been associated with the presence or absence of certain conditions. Urban industrialized areas are associated with an increased incidence of bronchitis, emphysema, and respiratory tract infections. Other areas are subject to the effects of carcinogenic wastes in rivers, acid rain in the air, or even nuclear radiation. Primary prevention would be the preferred mode of treatment; however, with the shortsightedness of present society, secondary prevention appears to be the current preferred alternative. Screening therefore must focus on the short-term results of certain environmental conditions and monitor for the development of chronic trends.

TYPES OF PROGRAMS

The design of the screening program is influenced by the combined characteristics that make the disease and the population screenable, such as the availability of professional, financial, and community resources and the types of risk factors represented. Examination of alternative screening designs reveals two approaches. The first examines the program's contact with the population, resulting in (1) individual and (2) group screening programs. The second approach evaluates the disease to be screened and results in (1) one-test disease-specific and (2) multiple-disease screening programs. Four combinations, such as individual disease-specific and individual multiple-disease screening, can be made.

Individual Screening

In an individual screening program, one person is tested by a health professional who has designated the individual as high risk. The practitioner can make this selection independently, the institution or clinic can define a specific policy, or a legislative body can require the screening by law, as with phenylketonuria (PKU), which many state laws require be screened in all newborns.[25] The Papanicolaou (Pap) smear for cervical cancer is another common example of individual screening. In some clinics, the standard gynecologic examination might also include a gonococcus smear for individuals who are within a ceratin age group or who have a certain lifestyle.

Depending on the screening instrument, individual screening can be performed in office, home, or institution. For example, a public health nurse with a sphygmomanometer can screen family members for hypertension while on a health promotion visit (see Fig. 10-2).

Group or Mass Screening

Group or mass screening is more common than individual programs. A target population is selected on the basis of (1) an increased incidence of a condition: (2) a recognized element of high risk within the group, such as lower-income populations or numerous factory workers; or (3) a significant prevalence of the condition, as with hypertension. This target population may be invited to a central location on a designated day (or sometimes several days) to be tested for the selected disorder.

Since group screening consists of rapid application of the screening test to many individuals, it offers an efficient design for disease detection and is accepted as an economic alternative. Mass screening, however, is also more prone to ethical complications. The effects of labeling and stigmatization are apparent more rapidly, and the economic issue of allocating funds to detect instead of cure disease is more prominent in the public eye.

One-Test Disease-Specific Screening

One-test disease-specific screening is the administration of one test in search of a specific characteristic indicating high risk of developing a disorder, such as a blood pressure reading to evaluate the risk of hypertension, a blood sugar test to check for diabetes, or a tonometric pressure reading for glaucoma.

Multiple-Test Screening

Multiple-test screening is using two or more tests to detect more than one disease. In some cases the same sample can be used to evaluate the possibility of several conditions, saving time and money and thus making the process efficient and economic. A blood sample, for example, can be evaluated for both elevated sugar and cholesterol levels.

PERIODIC HEALTH MAINTENANCE EXAMINATION

The periodic health maintenance examination is an examination of an apparently healthy person by a

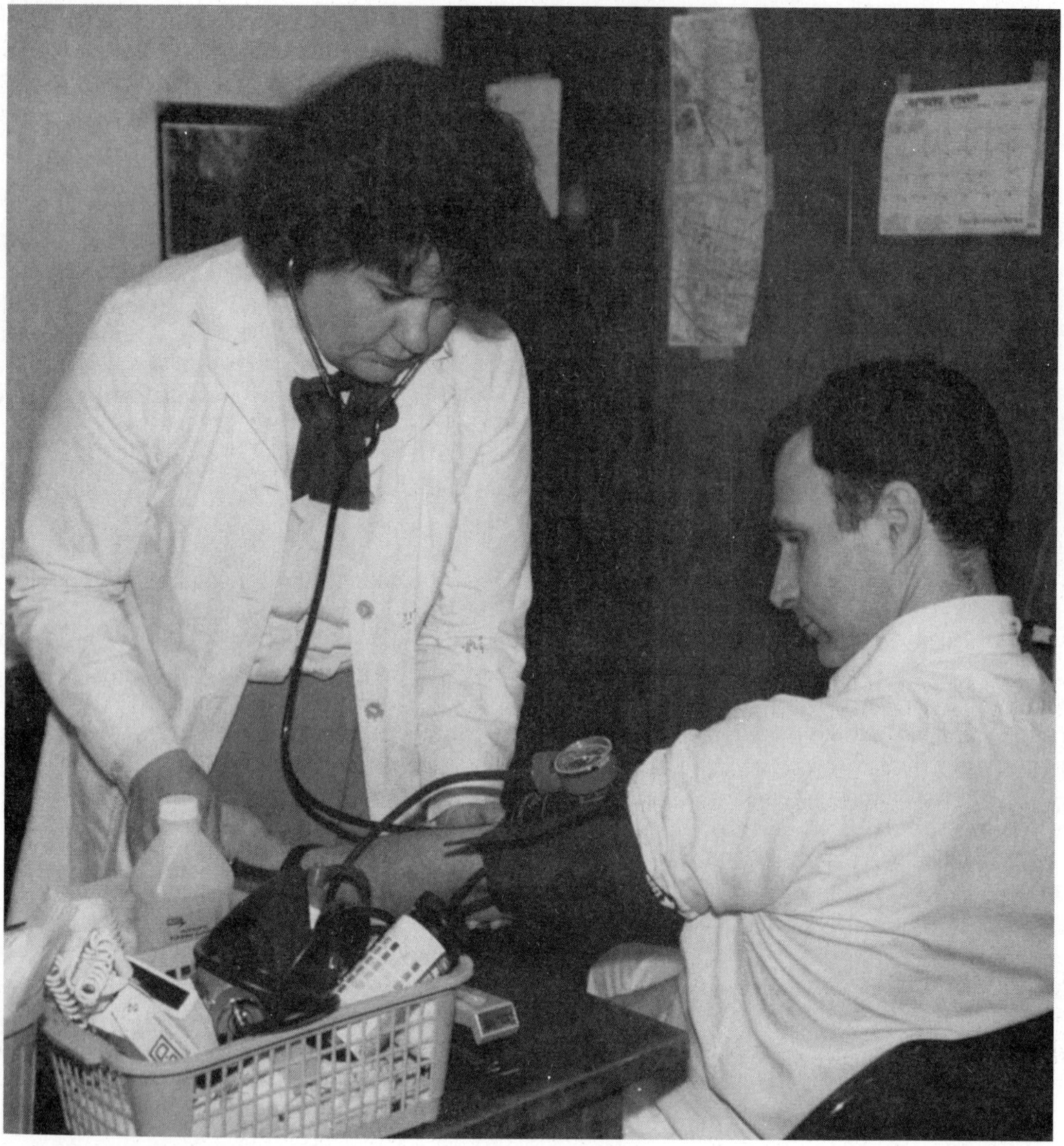

Fig. 10-2. A nurse may screen for hypertension while making health promotion visits to families. (From Bullough B, Bullough V: *Nursing in the community*, St. Louis, 1990, Mosby.)

physician, repeated at regular intervals. Periodic health examination involves the following:

- Obtaining a careful history
- Thorough physical examination
- Appropriate laboratory investigation
- Health counseling and referral

Since the purpose of the screening is to detect the disease in the asymptomatic period, the history is often found to be of limited help in the absence of any specific symptoms. The physical examination may reveal some abnormal findings, for example, an irregular pulse, organomegaly, abnormal neurologic signs, and so on. The exact interpretation of some of these physical signs may present difficulties. Simple examination techniques, such as blood pressure measurements, tonometry, and digital rectal examination and sigmoidoscopy, are helpful in the early detection of hypertension, glaucoma, and rectal tumors repectively. Although the complete examination is a time-consuming process, it has been argued that up to 60% of previously undetected disease is discovered during the physical examination: Laboratory tests and special procedures may account for the diagnosis of no more than 30% of unsuspected disease; and the remaining 10% of new disease is detected from a history alone.[14] It is important to note that for screening purposes, even if the physical examination itself fails to provide any positive findings, the periodic examination remains incomplete without appropriate laboratory and other screening tests, since during the asymptomatic period these may be the only way to detect a disease.

Several recent studies have tried to evaluate the ex-

❑ ❑ **REASONS FOR REJECTION OF ANNUAL PHYSICAL EXAMS**

1. Difficulties in meeting the needs of different age groups.
2. Undue repetition of annual tests and procedures; in many cases longer intervals have been found to be equally effective.
3. Affordability of annual physical examination only by an affluent segment of the population because of its high cost.
4. Failure of insurance companies to reimburse the cost of annual physical exams.

act role of periodic health maintenance examinations.[8,24,27,29] These studies seem to favor only selective examination at appropriate intervals for selected diseases (incurring minimum cost and discomfort for the client) based on objective evidence that early intervention offered better results in the areas of morbidity and mortality. The Canadian Task Force on the periodic health examination also rejected the idea of comprehensive annual examinations and favored a selective approach dependent on age, sex, and degree of risk.

The practice of doing an annual physical examination has been rejected by most authorities for one or more of the reasons listed in the box above.

CONSIDERATION OF COMMONLY SCREENED CONDITIONS

A number of disorders commonly screened presumably meet the criteria for a screenable disease. The following section reviews six of these to demonstrate the complexity of issues that can surround screening of diseases already analyzed for their screenability. Other screenings that are not discussed in this chapter, but that are of value, are scoliosis screening, hearing screening, vision screening, occupational health screenings, and sexually transmitted disease screenings.

Given the rapid pace of medical research, some of the weaknesses presented, but it is hoped none of the strengths, already may be outdated.

Phenylketonuria

Phenylketonuria (PKU) is a condition characterized by the genetically determined lack of phenylalanine hydroxylase, an enzyme necessary to metabolize an important amino acid, phenylalanine. In its absence blood levels of the phenylalanine increase, causing irreversible damage to the brain and central nervous system, resulting in severe mental retardation. The significance of PKU lies not so much in the incidence of the condition (1:10,000 newborns)[6] but more in the economic burden of institutionalizing the child if the condition is not treated.

Knowledge of PKU's natural history defines an optimum time to administer the test: 2 to 3 days after birth to as long as 4 to 5 weeks, after which brain damage occurs. Some controversy created by the British policy of testing children at 6 to 14 years of age and the resulting documentation of fewer false-negative reactions surrounds the timing of the test.[24] Some believe that other factors, such as a more effective laboratory control and a better compliance with follow-up, influenced these results.[26]

The effective screening method is an individually administered, disease-specific blood sample test for evaluation of phenylalanine. This sample is often used to test for other conditions, reducing the cost of detecting PKU. Dietary control of phenylalanine intake is a safe, effective treatment for PKU. With this diet, individualized according to the infant's rate and point of growth and development, mental retardation can be avoided. PKU therefore fulfills the basic law of screening: early intervention can affect a disease's progress. Medically and economically, PKU screening is almost a model screenable disease.

Breast Cancer

Breast cancer is one of the more commonly screened cancers, partly because it represents a significant cause of mortality in women 35 to 54 years old.[19] In her lifetime a woman has a 7% chance of developing the condition.[12]

The natural history of breast cancer has not been clearly defined. At present the disease is indicated by a lesion in the breast; severity is based on size of the lesion and length of time it has been present. Screening for asymptomatic cases and finding unnoticed and presumably smaller masses permit more successful and conservative treatment because of the less severe stage.

The diagnostic criterion for identification of cancerous breast lesions is the presence of malignant cells in the excised lesion. The accuracy of histologic interpretation is usually good, although it has been diminished by the detection of some lesions that cannot be classified as either benign or malignant. The problems and uncertainties related to classifying lesions and defining appropriate treatment raise serious concern about the potential for unnecessary mastectomies.[21]

Breast cancer accounts for 18% of female cancer deaths. The American Cancer Society recommends that all women make monthly breast examinations and receive regular clinical exams. A baseline mammogram has been recommended for women between the ages of 35 and 40, with follow-up tests every 2 years until age 50, and tests annually thereafter (see Fig. 10-3). In addition, the American Cancer Society recommends that women over the age of 65 have mammograms performed every 2 years at least until the age of 80. Departure from more standardized recommendations in the elderly population is reasonable if the physician, together with patient and her family, take into account individual circumstances, such as life expectancy and medical or physical condition.[5]

Breast cancer still remains a dreadful disease, with an estimated 100,000 new cases per year and approximately 35,000 deaths per year. Unfortunately, the incidence of breast cancer has been on the rise for the last 30 years, with almost 1 in 7 women developing the disease. Since the prognosis is much better if the cancer is detected at an early stage, (85% 5-year survival rate for stage 1), screening becomes essential, especially in the high-risk group.[4]

Nulliparous women (women who have never had children) run a high risk of breast carcinoma, women who had their first child before the age of 20 constitute the lowest risk group. Women who start menstruating at an earlier age and reach menopause in their later years are also known to be a somewhat higher risk, as are those who bore their first child in their late 30s. Bilateral ovarectomy (removal of both ovaries) before menopause seems to provide some protection against breast carcinoma. Women with fibrocystic disease of the breast, an otherwise benign condition, are also considered to be in the high-risk category.

The nurse is often the health care provider who teaches a woman how to do self-breast examination. Self-breast examination should be encouraged. In many cases this practice has proved to be lifesaving through early detection of a potentially lethal cancer. However, self-breast examination alone contains some pitfalls, as cited in the box on this page.

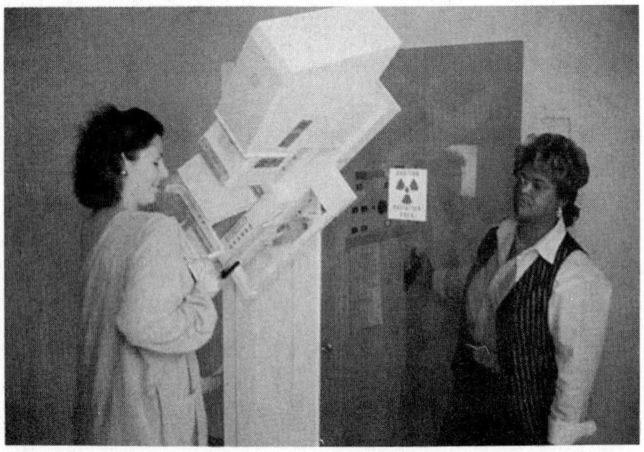

Fig. 10-3. Mammography is used to screen women at high risk for breast cancer. (From Edge V, Miller M: *Women's health care*, St Louis, 1994, Mosby.)

❑ ❑ PITFALLS OF USING SELF-BREAST EXAMINATION ALONE

1. Early lesions are difficult to palpate.
2. Pendulous breasts are difficult to examine.
3. Cancer cure rate is poorer, compared with that of early detection through mammography. Mammography, which has been shown to be a much more sensitive test than self-examination, can detect cancers of less than 1 centimeter in diameter. Physical examination by a physician is helpful in most cases if the tumor is over 2.5 cm in size.

Although the safety of mammography has been questioned periodically, the risk of radiation exposure from mammography remains minimal. Furthermore, mammography remains the most sensitive investigative tool available for early detection. Because of its high sensitivity, however, mammography presents a problem with specificity. Only about 25% of the masses detected by mammography prove to be cancerous. The economics of the unnecessarily high number of biopsies has been used by some as an argument against the "overuse" of mammography. However, if smaller and localized masses without distant metastases are to be detected at an early stage, there does not seem to be any choice but to accept the recommended schedule of mammography.[5]

Colorectal Cancer

Colorectal cancer, the second leading cause of cancer deaths in men, is also one of the most common malignancies if both sexes are considered. Colorectal cancer accounts for 15% of all cancers and approximately 50% of all tumors of the gastrointestinal tract. There are over 61,000 deaths each year due to these cancers in the United States alone, with over 150,000 new cases diagnosed every year.[20] Both males and females are affected almost equally, with the risk of this type of cancer rising gradually with advancing years, and peaking in incidence in those around age 60.[5]

A campaign for early detection of colorectal carcinoma has been widely publicized by the American Cancer Society in recent years. Early detection of colorectal cancer is associated with a better outcome in both morbidity and mortality; the 5-year survival rate is over 90% for patients with a localized disease. Unfortunately, in over 55% of cases the disease is found to have extended either locally or distantly, resulting in a poor outcome.[5]

The American Cancer Society recommends proctosigmoidoscopic examination for colorectal cancer at 3 to 5 year intervals after the age of 50, provided negative examinations have been recorded for 2 consecutive years. Annual stool guaiac testing has been recommended for persons over the age of 50 (previously over the age of 40). Annual digital examination is still urged after the age of 40, although most colorectal malignancies are beyond the reach of the examining finger.[9] Sigmoidoscopy is of great help in the detection and removal of polyps–potentially malignant growths–particularly those over 2 centimeters in size and those that are villous. Although sigmoidoscopy is a major tool used in the early detection of these tumors, the high cost of the procedure, the associated discomfort and complications, and the fact that some polyps are inaccessible are some of the reasons why sigmoidoscopy is not always an easily acceptable procedure to an otherwise asymptomatic person. However, flexible sigmoidoscopy has been shown to detect an average of three times as many polyps and cancers and to be more acceptable to clients than was rigid proctosigmoidoscopy.

Stool guaiac testing is inexpensive, readily available, and recommended annually after the age of 50. However, correct interpretation of stool guaiac results requires that the nurse be aware of the significant number of both false positive and false negative results.

All high-risk groups of clients need frequent digital examinations, stool guaiacs, and colonoscopic examinations. High-risk groups for colorectal cancer include familial polyposis coli, family history of colorectal cancer, cancer family syndrome. Clients with a past history of ulcerative colitis; adenomatous polyps; previous colorectal cancer; or endometrial, ovarian, or breast cancer have a higher risk of developing colorectal cancer de novo.[23]

Prostate Cancer

The American Cancer Society has estimated about 165,000 new cases of prostate cancer for 1993.[7] There are nevertheless still controversial issues relating to screening. The American Cancer Society recommends annual digital rectal examination in men 40 years old and older.[23] Now there are two available tools for the detection of prostate cancer–prostate-specific antigen (PSA) and transrectal ultrasonography. The use of these new tests for screening purposes, however, has not been well defined.[10] PSA is a tumor marker, a simple blood test that becomes elevated in prostate cancer. Because it also will be elevated in benign prostatic hypertrophy, it cannot be used as a sole criterion for diagnosis. Transrectal ultrasonography helps determine mass, size, and consistency of the prostate. Combined use of the prostate specific antigen, transrectal ultrasonography, and digital rectal examination are useful in the evaluation of suspecting prostate cancer; but their combined use in screening is not recommended.

Cholesterol Levels

Through extensive research, educational programs, and media attention our knowledge and understanding of the implications of cholesterol levels have increased dramatically. The public now seeks out screening because of increased awareness of the role of cholesterol in a healthy lifestyle. However, the need to continue the public health programs to further develop this awareness is still evident and necessary for underserved populations. The National Heart, Lung and Blood Institute (NHLBI) continues to issue recommendations on screening.[22] The National Cholesterol Education Program (NCEP), launched by NHLBI, consists of guidelines for adults with high blood cholesterol levels. These guidelines are listed in the box below.

In addition to adult screening, initiatives for children have been developed by the American Academy of Pediatrics. Cholesterol screening is recommended on an elective basis for children over 2 years old or those with a family history of hyperlipedemia or early MI.[3] Some groups recommend universal cholesterol screening for all children. Clear guidelines for frail elderly patients have not yet been determined.

The reduction in cardiovascular morbidity and mortality has been clearly shown by a series of studies including the World Health Organization Cooperative Trial,[27,28] The Lipid Research Clinics Coronary Primary Prevention Trial,[17,18] and the Helsinki Heart Study.[11]

Hypertension

As one of the most prevalent chronic conditions, hypertension is believed to affect more than 60 million persons in the United States today. Research has proved that it "significantly impairs life expectancy; the higher the blood pressure, the greater the reduction of longevity."[13] Detecting high blood pressure is precritical sec-

❑ ❑ NATIONAL CHOLESTEROL EDUCATION PROGRAM GUIDELINES

Cholesterol level	Frequency of test
<200 mg/100 ml	Repeat every 5 years
200 to 239 mg/100 ml	Repeat test, take average of both tests
240 mg/100 ml and over	Further testing (lipid profile) and treatment

ondary prevention in relation to hypertension, but it is primary prevention for (1) coronary heart disease, (2) cerebrovascular disease, and (3) peripheral vascular disease.

In certain forms, such as renal hypertension, the precipitant and natural history are known; however, for the most prevalent form, essential hypertension, these factors are unknown. Diagnostic criteria vary as to the systolic and diastolic pressure indicative of a hypertensive state. Development of such criteria is complicated by the increasing mean blood pressure with age. In addition, what has been found hypertensive for one individual appears to be normotensive for another. In screening the lack of specific criteria necessitates setting a cutoff point and determining a borderline category and related policy.

The standards for such cutoff points related to hypertension presently are taken from an extensive, prospective study by NHLBI in 1971. They have defined mild hypertension as a diastolic blood pressure (DBP) of 90 to 104 mm Hg, moderate hypertension as 104 to 114 mm Hg, and severe hypertension as 1151/3 mm Hg. This is the pressure found in the person's right arm while in a sitting position.[24]

Policies toward borderline cases vary according to the screening programs. The pressure may be repeated after a set period, or a public health nurse may be asked to make a home visit to check the person's pressure in a less stressful setting. The sphygmomanometer is a rapid, safe, and effective means of evaluating blood pressure in the hospital, clinic, or home. The major limitation of this screening instrument is low interobserver reliability.

NHLBI recommends blood pressure measurements at least once every two years for a person with diastolic levels 85 mm Hg and a systolic level 140 mm Hg. Annual blood pressure measurements are needed for individuals with a diastolic of 85 to 89 mm Hg, and those with higher levels require more regular monitoring.[15]

Hypertension is treated effectively with antihypertensive medications, including diuretics, beta blockers, calcium channel blockes, and ACE-inhibitors. The prescribed regimen may vary from physician to physician, since studies have yet to establish an acceptable standardized treatment based on levels and ranges of pressure.[13]

Implementation of a hypertension screening program therefore raises these primary concerns:

1. Lack of knowledge of the condition's natural history
2. Effect of varying diagnostic criteria
3. Implications of setting a cutoff point
4. Unstandardized treatment regimen and its side effects

Nonetheless, when hypertension is effectively treated, it has important long-term implications for decreased mortality and morbidity because of diminished end organ effects. It should therefore be a part of any comprehensive screening program.

Glaucoma

Glaucoma is the third leading cause of blindness in the United States,[16] with a prevalence of 2%. It is most significant in the population over age 65, 17% of whom experience impaired vision secondary to glaucoma.[16]

Three diagnostic criteria exist for glaucoma: (1) an increase in intraocular pressure (IOP), as measured by a tonometer; (2) damage to the optic nerve, which is subjectively assessed through ophthalmoscopic evaluation of the optic nerve; and (3) visual field loss, as measured by a visual field examination. Although the presence of all three is diagnostic of glaucoma, experts disagree over which variable alone is indicative of the condition. Although the exact cause of glaucoma is not known, the natural history currently is explained by the increased IOP, which results from an obstruction of the outflow of aqueous humor from the eye's interior and damages the optic nerve, causing loss of vision.

Consistent with the present theory of natural history, treatment of glaucoma focuses on decreasing IOP. Recent literature, however, suggests that this treatment mode may not be correct, since an increased IOP is not always associated with visual field loss. To complicate matters, other studies show that what has traditionally been defined as "normal" pressure is not an appropriate guideline for all; some subjects showed optic nerve damage with pressures only slightly above the norm. These data suggest that in some individuals the optic nerve is inherently weak and more susceptible to glaucoma–characteristics believed to increase with age.[2] Because of the indecision over an acceptable normal or abnormal pressure, a cutoff point usually must be set.

Depending on the diagnostic variable measured, a choice of screening instruments is available. For measuring IOP, three types of tonometers are available; the applanation, the air puff, and the Schiotz. The applanation tonometer is highly accurate and safe. In some states it can be administered by technicians and other nonphysician eye professionals, whereas in others this is prohibited because a law forbids nonphysicians to administer the needed topical anesthetic. The air-puff tonometer is accurate and safe, can be administered by a technician, and does not require medication. The Schiotz tonometer, a small, hand-held instrument frequently used in screening programs, is less accurate than the other tonometers and has a side effect of potential corneal abrasions. Nonphysician health care personnel can administer it.

Again, if optic nerve damage and visual field loss were included in screening criteria, ophthalmoscopic examinations and visual field testing would be included in the screening program. Each additional test would increase the screening time and the health professionals needed.

Inclusion of the ophthalmoscopic examination also could impose a political, territorial issue on the screening project. Both ophthalmologists (physicians who are eye specialists) and optometrists (eye professionals with graduate-level training) would like to see this examination included in screening because of the sensitivity added to detection. However, ophthalmologists consider optometrists inadequately trained and with limited experience to perform this assessment. On the other hand, optometrists believe their mandate is referral of abnormal findings, which precisely fits the screening design, and they find their training and experience adequate to perform this evaluation. These conflicting views complicate the decision to include an ophthalmoscopic examination in the screening program and also make choosing the professionals to perform the screening a politically volatile issue.

The issues surrounding glaucoma screening are

1. Uncertain combination of diagnostic criteria and screening instruments
2. Questionable association of increased IOP with visual field loss
3. Implications of setting a cutoff point
4. Political repercussions of selecting one group of eye professionals over another

Screening for HIV

HIV (Human immunodeficiency virus) disease is the single most important epidemic in the world during the waning years of this century. The need for HIV screening is a controversial topic that crosses tissues on confidentiality, insurance administration, job security, and personal rights.

Because this infectious disease can be transmitted to others by varying routes, screening should be offered to high-risk individuals, as well as to contacts of known HIV-positive clients. Although there is no effective treatment at this time, early institution of AZT *may* diminish some of the complications of the disease and therefore improve quality of life. The education of public health and research communities in the epidemiology of the disease is an important factor in considering screening for HIV.

The U.S. Preventive Screening Task Force recommends screening for HIV disease for persons seeking treatment for sexually transmitted disease; IV drug abusers; homosexual and bisexual men; people with a history of prostitution or multiple sexual partners; women whose past or present sexual partners were HIV infected, bisexual, or IV drug abusers; persons with long-term residence or birth in an area with high prevalence of HIV infection; and persons with a history of transfusions between 1978 and 1985. All individuals tested require pretest and posttest counseling, regardless of positive or negative results.[23]

Screening for HIV disease may prove to be important for individuals infected, in that early interventions can be sought out. There interventions could be aimed at improving quality of life and decreasing complications with the development of AIDS. In addition, the significant benefit in potentially diminishing the spread of the disease is also a consideration.

NURSE'S ROLE

The potential and need for nursing involvement exist at all levels of a screening program. As nurses become more involved in decision making in hospital and community health policy, they will be faced with the question: Should this condition be screened or not? In this role as decision maker and planner, the nurse is responsible for reviewing all the issues concerning a screenable disease: (1) criteria specific to the disease, (2) medical and economic ethics, and (3) community resources affected. A thorough literature review may be necessary to supplement and update knowledge of the condition. The nurse must also carefully consider the significance of incomplete data and its effect on the project's success. The last step, if the choice is to screen, is the planning and development of an efficient referral system to enhance continuity of care and to ensure compliance with the recommended referral.

Nurses have long been in the *screener* role, giving tuberculin tests and Snellen eye tests or checking blood pressures. As in any nursing intervention, adequate knowledge of the method of administration and the potential side effects is needed. Teaching clients the meaning and limitation of the test results is an important element of this role, as is informing them of their part in obtaining the implied benefit.

This combined *health educator-screener* component also means the nurse should continue to evaluate clients for additional risk factors and teach them means of altering or improving these risks, as through such lifestyle factors as diet, exercise, alcohol intake, or smoking. The nurse is practicing primary prevention interventions, but in coordination with secondary preventive role.

A new and perhaps controversial screening role for nurses may emerge if the periodic health examination becomes an accepted, integrated component of health care delivery. Given that the screening tests and their frequency and timing are predetermined and, as with the Canadian Task Force's product, may be detailed in an extensive chart format, the following questions arise. Where does the responsibility of the nurse begin and end with this examination? Which health professional consistently flags the client as being either at risk or at the age appropriate for the specified screening? Who instigates or orders and performs the appropriate examination and follows up results to distinguish those who probably have the problem from those who probably do not?

The nurse's role has long included identifying and reporting abnormal findings, which the physician then pursues. Therefore, in principle the periodic health examination fits into the current state of nursing practice and particularly into the expanded role of nursing. Whether this major screening role becomes accepted nursing practice will depend not only on the evolution of preventive medicine and of the physician's role in preventive care, but also on the desire of the nursing profession to move into this direction and assume the far-reaching responsibility for health maintenance of the population.

SUMMARY

As a method of precritical, secondary prevention, screening is the rapid administration of a simple test to delineate individuals who probably have a condition from those who probably do not. It can be an effective, efficient tool in preventive medicine if used for conditions applicable to the screening model and directed toward a high-risk population. A unique characteristic and significant advantage of screening is that it can be applied to individuals or groups.

Three major questions provide a means of analyzing the screenability of a disease:

1. Is the condition *significant*?
2. *Can* the condition be screened?
3. *Should* the condition be screened?

These questions act more as *guidelines* for selection of a screenable disease; as the section reviewing specific diseases shows, screening often occurs without full compliance with these criteria.

Screening programs are not appropriate for all conditions or all communities. Alternate methods of reaching the desired health outcome should always be considered. Screening in health care presents numerous roles for nurses and provides them with a valuable preventive tool in their care for healthy individuals.

References

1. Abdel R: *Community medicine in developing countries,* New York, 1974, Springer Publishing.
2. Allen PT, Avorn J: *Screening for glaucoma in the elderly,* unpublished case study, 1979, Harvard University School of Public Health.
3. American Academy of Pediatrics: Indications for cholesterol testing in children, *Pediatrics* 83:141-142, 1989.
4. American Cancer Society: Update January 1992: the American Cancer Society guidelines for the cancer related checkup, *CA* 42:44-45, 1992.
5. American Cancer Society: Guidelines for the cancer-related health checkup: recommendations and rationale, *CA* 30:194-240, 1980.
6. Bailey E, et al: Screening in pediatric practice, *Pediatr Clin North Am* 21(1):126, 1974.
7. Boring CC, Squires TS, Tong T: Cancer statistics, 1993, *CA* 43:7-26, 1993.
8. Breslow L, Somers AR: The lifetime health monitoring program: a practical approach to preventive medicine, *N Engl J Med* 296:601, 1977.
9. Caldroney RD: The periodic health examination, *Hosp Pract* 22(7):203, 1987.
10. Cupp MR, Oesterling JE: Prostate-specific antigen, digital rectal examination and transrectal ultrasonography: their roles in diagnosing early prostate cancer, *Mayo Clin Proc* 68:297-306, 1993.
11. Frick MH, et al: Helsinki heart study: primary prevention trial with genfibrozilin middle-aged men with dyslipidemia: safety of treatment, changes in risk factor and incidence of coronary heart disease, *N Eng J Med* 317:1237-1245, 1987.
12. Haynes RB, et al: Increased absenteeism from work after detection and labelling of hypertensive patients, *N Engl J Med* 299(14):741, 1978.
13. Hypertension Direction and Follow-Up Program Cooperative Group: Five-year findings of the hypertension detection and follow-up program, *JAMA* 242(23):2562, 1979.
14. Kessler II: *Case findings and mass screening in early detection of disease.* In Spittel JA Jr, editor: *Clinical medicine, vol 1,* Philadelphia, 1984, Harper & Row.
15. Lappe M, Roblin RO: Newborn genetic screening as a concept in health care delivery: a critique, ethical, social and legal dimensions of screening for human genetic disease, 10:2, 1974.
16. Leske MC, Rosenthal J: Epidemiologic aspects of open-angle glaucoma, *Am J Epidemiol* 109(2):250, 1979.
17. The Lipid Research Clinics Coronary Primary Preventive Trial Results I: Reduction in incidence of coronary heart disease, *JAMA* 251:351-364, 1984.
18. The Lipid Research Clinic Coronary Primary Preventive Trial Results II: The relationship of reductions in incidence of coronary heart disease to cholesterol lowering, *JAMA* 251:365-374, 1984.
19. Mahoney LJ, et al. The best available screening test for breast cancer, *N Engl J Med* 301(6):315, 1979.
20. Milio N: Ethics and the economics of community health services: the case of screening, *Linacre Q* 348:350, 1977.
21. Miller AB: Risk benefit in mass screening for breast cancer, *Semin Oncol* 5(4):352, 1978.
22. National Heart, Lung and Blood Institute: *Recommendations regarding public screening for measuring blood cholesterol: summary of national heart, lung, and blood institute worksheet,* Bethesda, Md, 1988, National Heart, Lung and Blood Institute.
23. Report of US Preventive Screening Task Force: *Guide to clinical preventive screening: an assessment of the effectiveness of 169 interventions,* New York, 1989, Williams & Wilkins.

24. Sackett DL, Holland WW; Controversy in the detection of disease, *Lancet,* p 358, 1975.
25. Sepe SJ, et al: An evaluation of routine follow-up blood screening of infants for phenylketouria, *N Engl J Med* 300:608, 1979.
26. Starfield B, Holtzman NA: A comparison of effectiveness of screening for phenylketonuria in the United States, United Kingdom, and Ireland, *N Engl J Med* 293:118, 1975.
27. Task Force to the Conference of Deputy Ministers of Health Examination: Report of a task force to the conference of deputy ministers of health, Health and Welfare of Canada, 1980.
28. World Health Organization: Cooperative trial on primary prevention of ischaemic heart disease with clofibrate to lower serum cholesterol: final mortality follow up, *Lancet,* 2:600-604, 1984.
29. Yankauer A: The ups and downs of prevention, *Am J Public Health* 71(1):6-9, 1981.

CHAPTER

11

Health Education

Carol L. Wells-Federman

Lea Edwards

Objectives

After completing this chapter, the nurse will be able to

- *Define health education.*
- *Describe the aims of health education.*
- *Discuss learning principles that affect health education.*
- *Describe the health belief model and behavior change process.*
- *Use basic concepts of marketing to plan health education programs.*
- *Describe a system for planning health education programs.*
- *Identify steps to administering health education programs.*
- *Identify steps in preparing a teaching plan.*
- *Select content and learning strategies appropriate to the health learning needs of a target audience.*
- *List ways to evaluate student progress.*
- *Set personal plans for developing teaching skills.*

The mandate of *Healthy People 2000* brings health education strategies and interventions to the forefront of health promotion and patient care in the 1990s.[20] Behavioral research indicates that people can make choices that will increase both quality and quantity of life. What some people need to know are the facts that will guide them to healthy choices. Many need motivation through positive influences in their lives. Some people need help to change health-risking habits or situations. Still others need the support to escape victimization and move forward.[46]

Nursing with its unique contribution to patient care represents a significant professional resource that can help to facilitate these changes through health education strategies. Nurses, in partnership with other health care professionals, can be the link between the philosophy of *Healthy People 2000* and the people who need to hear its messages and act upon those messages.

The average life expectancy of the American population as a whole has increased.[11] However, recent morbidity and mortality data point to the continuing need for better understanding of how to implement healthy behavior change strategies, prevention, and health-promotion interventions for this population. Louis W. Sullivan, Secretary of Health and Human Services, in a recent article in the *American Journal of Health Promotion* calls upon the leadership of health care professionals to disseminate and use the information about combating the leading preventable diseases, causes of violence, and health-related problems.[46] He emphasizes a move toward self-empowerment of people to enable them to make and sustain these health-promoting behavior changes. The nurse, using health education principles, can assist the client in achieving these goals in a way that is consistent with their personal lifestyle, values, and beliefs.

NURSING AND HEALTH EDUCATION

The Professional Nurse and Health Education, published in 1975 by the American Nurses' Association (ANA), states that the professional nurse's responsibility includes "teaching the patient and family relevant facts about specific health-care needs and supporting appropriate modification of behavior."[2] In the ANA's *Model Nurse Practice Act* of 1979 patient education is defined as a component of the registered nurse's practice.[1] The rights of individuals to know about their health problems and treatments have invariably been upheld through the courts. Patient education is a professional requirement and the legal duty of professional nurses.[22,44]

Nurses usually function as health care coordinators for their clients. Depending on the interest and needs of the client, they establish a partnership to guide the client in the selection and use of relevant health services. Health education provides the nurse with specific strategies and tools for assessing an individual's readiness for their health, conveying technical information, and helping them to practice health care techniques at home. These strategies also help the nurse to facilitate behavior change while satisfying the person's right to relevant health information and to the freedom to make decisions about his or her health. Health education encourages self-care, self-empowerment, and ultimately greater independence of the health care system.

Sometimes nurses specialize in public health education. This means that they take on the full-time role of coordinating the educational services provided by a health agency or institution. As a *health education specialist,* the nurse may use marketing strategies to enhance the effectiveness of health education programs focused on certain target populations. The health education specialist helps other nurses and health professionals to improve their skills in developing and delivering teaching plans.

Definition

Health education is defined as "any combination of learning experiences designed to facilitate voluntary adaptations of behavior conducive to health."[24,43] This definition, developed by Lawrence Green and others at the Johns Hopkins University School of Public Health, includes several key concepts. First, health education involves the use of teaching-learning strategies. Second, learners maintain voluntary control over decisions to make changes in their actions. Third, health education focuses on behavior changes currently found to improve health status.

Health education facilitates development of health knowledge, skills, and attitudes through the application of behavioral and social learning theories.[37,41] These theories will be discussed later in this chapter. Generally, health education strategies help to ensure that clients–or consumers–of health services are satisfied and have received health care most relevant to their problems. From a public health perspective, health education programs should serve to improve the effectiveness of medical treatment plans and the individual's ability to make lifestyle changes that promote wellness and prevent disease and disability.[23]

The following is an example of a nurse-client situation in which a health education approach may be used to meet the client's health needs.

Sada Thompson, a 21-year-old university senior, visits university health services because she wants to change her method of birth control. She has had side effects to the birth control pill she has been taking for the past year and knows little about other options. She has recently started dating John after breaking up with Steven 3 months ago. Last weekend, John began pressing her to have sex with him. Sada is feeling uncertain about what she needs to do to take care of herself and how to discuss this with John. She is aware of all the talk about AIDS on campus, and she knows John has been very popular and has dated several other girls in school. This concerns her.

Sada needs to learn new information, may need to acquire new skills, and must clarify any feelings or attitudes that affect her decision to use a new birth control method and ensure her continued safety. After recording her medical history and arranging for a gynecologic examination and laboratory tests, the nurse develops a teaching plan. Selecting one or more strategies for helping Sada review all the birth control options, the nurse establishes an environment in which Sada may choose voluntarily to try a new method or request a change in her prescription for oral contraceptives. Together they identify actions Sada can take to properly use the method. They also anticipate and identify ways she can solve problems in adjusting to the new method.

The nurse answers Sada's immediate questions about safe sex, gives her several pamphlets written for college students about this topic, and suggests she participate in the peer counseling night on sexually transmitted diseases (STDs) that will be held on campus in 2 weeks. The peer counseling hotline number and drop-in hours were given to her, and the nurse explained that these students are trained to help other students talk about and deal with this important issue. The nurse invites

Sada to call or come back to the office for additional help and information as well as more problem-solving discussion.

This example illustrates that educational interventions, in addition to direct health services, are necessary to meet the client's goal. Although physicians and nurses prefer that clients choose to take actions that will promote rather than detract from health, the client controls the at-home application of medical recommendations. In this example, the client receives educational assistance from the nurse to solve a health problem.

Goals

The goal of health education is to help persons achieve by their own actions and initiatives, optimum states of health. Health education should facilitate an individual's ability to improve personal living conditions; make informed decisions about personal, family, and community health practices; and utilize health services appropriately.[8,23,26,28,50]

Health education encourages the practice of healthy lifestyle behaviors found to prevent acute and chronic disease, decrease disability, and enhance wellness. It is not merely information distribution, an activity used to increase awareness; rather it involves guiding persons through stages of problem solving and decision making.[17] The result of health education should be voluntary behavior changes based on the analysis of past and new knowledge, attitudes, personal skills, and environmental conditions.

Health education is one of three categories of activities aimed at the promotion of health and the prevention of disease. Other categories include health protection (environmental health and safety control measures) and preventive health services (primary preventive services, such as family planning, pregnancy, and infant care).[23] In the community, all three categories of activity must be integrated to improve health and social conditions.

Health education and health counseling are mutually supportive activities. Health educators often use one-to-one and group counseling techniques as strategies for active health learning. Counselors may refer clients to health education resources or assist them in acquiring health information pertinent to solving a health problem. The following example helps to illustrate the goals of health education.

Kate Hanson, 22 years old, visits the local family health center with the complaint of fatigue and flu-like symptoms. During the assessment with the nurse, Kate discloses that she has missed her last two periods.

The physician's exam and the laboratory tests confirm her suspicions of pregnancy. Psychosocial evaluation reveals that Kate works part-time as a secretary for a temporary agency, and lives in an apartment with her recently unemployed husband Jim. Further interviewing reveals that she has minimal knowledge of prenatal care, has a diet of take-out food high in fat, sodium, and sugar with infrequent consumption of fresh fruits or vegetables and has three to four beers on the weekends. Kate has never taken vitamins, leads a sedentary lifestyle, and is obviously overwhelmed by the news that she is pregnant.

The nurse first takes steps to create a safe and trusting atmosphere in which Kate can feel free to share her concerns and apprehensions. Finding that Kate needs counseling about telling her husband of the pregnancy, the nurse discusses this with her. Kate is then taught the importance of taking a multiple vitamin with an iron supplement daily, to discontinuing the use of any medications or alcohol, and making time for more rest during the day. Sensing that this was all that could be acted upon at this time, the nurse gave Kate two pamphlets on prenatal care and made an appointment for her to return in a week with her husband. Kate acknowledged that she understood the instructions, and the nurse documented the teaching and recommendations in Kate's chart.

At the next visit, the nurse met with Kate and her husband and explored the meaning of the pregnancy in their lives and helped them to identify actions they will need to take. The recommendations that were made during Kate's first visit were reviewed and reinforced. The nurse then detailed specifics of dietary changes and the need for proper rest and exercise and helped them to problem solve as they adjust to these new responsibilities. Most importantly, the nurse gave them information on the clinic's weekly prenatal classes and explained that since the classes are partially covered by local community funding, the charge would be minimal. The classes include information such as proper diet, physical and psychologic changes during pregnancy, labor and delivery, the newborn, and the postpartum period. The classes are conducted by the nurse practitioner at the clinic and are given in a group format to facilitate social support and problem solving among expectant parents.

The nurse gave them several other pamphlets to read at home, made an appointment for Kate to see the doctor in a couple of weeks, and encouraged her to call if she had questions or concerns in the meantime. A schedule of the prenatal classes was reviewed, and a date for the next session identified. They were also encouraged to meet with the social worker to explore their financial needs and options due to Jim's recent layoff. Kate and her husband acknowledged that they understood what they needed to do, and the nurse documented what was taught and discussed in Kate's chart.

This example illustrates the goals of health education to help individuals achieve, by their own actions and initiative, optimum health and well-being. Through

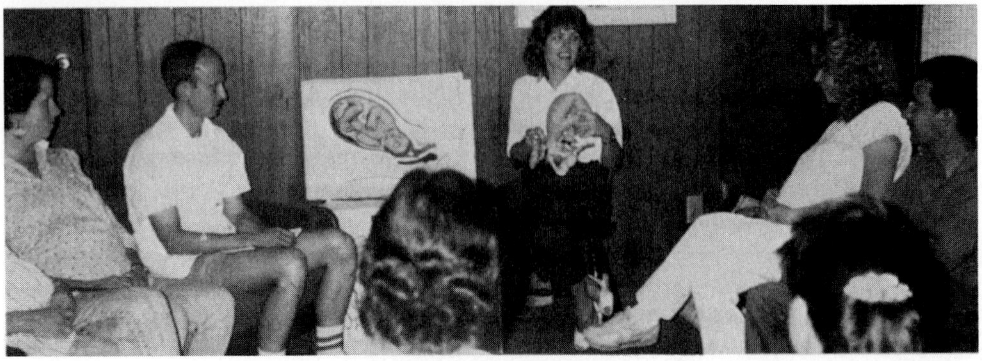

Fig. 11-1. Example of an educational group. The nurse uses a model and pictures to illustrate labor delivery to a group of expectant parents. (From Cookfair JM: *Nursing process and practice in the community,* St Louis, 1991, Mosby.)

health education, individuals can learn to make informed decisions about personal and family health practices and to utilize health services in the community. The client in this example receives educational assistance from the nurse that will promote better health and well-being for herself and her baby (Fig. 11-1).

Learning Assumptions

Factors to consider when teaching different age groups and the characteristics of the learners to be considered when developing a teaching plan are addressed in individual chapters in this text. The following, however, are a few assumptions about learning that tend to be recognized throughout public health education literature as fundamental to the planning of health education programs. These assumptions come from the general field of educational philosophy.[20,25,34]

1. Persons at all ages have the potential to learn, with some learning faster than others. Age may or may not affect a person's speed of learning, and individuals vary in ways they like to learn.
2. The individual experiencing a change process is likely to feel stress and confusion. Some anxiety often increases motivation to learn, but too much anxiety may cause fatigue, inability to concentrate, resentments, and other barriers to learning. Learning is more comfortable and effective when the environmental conditions support open exchange, sharing of opinions, and problem-solving strategies. The atmosphere should foster trust and acceptance of different ideas and values.
3. In the classroom, an instructor facilitates learning by incorporating students' experiences, observations of others, and personal ideas and feelings. Exposure to varied behavior models and attitudes helps learners to clarify actions and beliefs that will aid in meeting their own learning goals.
4. The depth of long-term learning may depend on the extent to which learners try to analyze, clarify, or articulate their experiences to others in their family, work, or social groups. The depth of learning increases when new concepts and skills are useful in meeting current needs or problems. This allows for immediate application of theory to a practical situation.
5. An educational program or intervention may only provide one step in an individual's progress toward acquiring new health-promoting behaviors. The adoption of a new behavior depends on many factors. Some conditions *predispose* an individual to take a particular action, such as former knowledge and attitudes. Availability and access to resources, such as exercise facilities, may *enable* a person to carry out new plans of action. Other environmental conditions and family characteristics help to *reinforce* or hinder behavior changes.[24]
6. Learning improves when the learner is an active participant in the educational process. When selecting among several teaching methods, it is best to choose the method that allows the learner to become most involved. Using varied methods of teaching helps the learner maintain interest and may help to reinforce concepts without being repetitious.

In recent years, teachers have found that many principles of adult learning also apply to children and adolescents. For example, children prefer learning experiences that are participatory; they learn faster when new concepts are useful in their present as well as future lives. The role of an educator for the young or elderly persons is to assess the audience's interests, current skills, and aims. This information then guides the structuring of a learning atmosphere and selection of methods most satisfying and effective for the learners.

Health Behavior Change

The process of health education leads persons toward voluntary changes of their health behaviors. This section covers: (1) the use of the health belief model to analyze the probability that a person will make changes for improving health or preventing disease, (2) the application of social learning theory to clarify environmental and social factors that affect the learning of new health behaviors, and (3) a review of four phases of the behavior change process that guide selection of educational interventions. Green and others[24] give the following pertinent definitions:

belief Statement or sense, declared or implied, intellectually and/or emotionally accepted as true by a person or group

attitude Relatively constant feeling, predisposition, or set of beliefs directed toward an object, person, or situation

value Preference shared and transmitted within a community

behavior Action that has a specific frequency, duration, and purpose, whether conscious or unconscious

behavioral diagnosis Delineation of the specific health actions that most likely can effect a health outcome

health belief model Paradigm used to predict and explain health behavior based on value-expectancy theory

Beliefs, attitudes, and values, as well as information, all contribute to motivation and behavior and are underlying components in making any decision to change behavior. Health behaviors are any activities that an individual who feels healthy undertakes to enhance health, prevent disease, or detect and control the symptomatic stage of a disease. Illness behaviors include actions that an individual who feels ill takes to obtain a diagnosis of a problem, to prevent complications, and to restore health.[9,40] To differentiate between behavioral and nonbehavioral causes of a health problem, consider the following example.

John is a black American, age 47. His father died at age 64 of a cerebrovascular accident (stroke). John's blood pressure is moderately elevated (150/92), and he is 20 pounds overweight. He quit smoking a year ago. Both his mother and his wife are beginning to change their family meal-planning habits. They were accustomed to preparing foods high in fats and cholesterol; lately the family eats more fish and poultry, which is baked rather than fried. Food portion sizes are smaller, and all family members try to use less salt at the table.

John is a marketing specialist for a computer software company and works long hours. By the time he arrives home, he is too fatigued to exercise. Once every couple weeks he swims at a local pool. John discovered his blood pressure problem 3 months ago when he had a physical examination; it had been 5 years since his last one. The physician suggested several lifestyle changes for John that would probably help to decrease his blood pressure. If John can make these changes, he may avoid taking medication.

Nonbehavioral factors possibly contributing to John's health problem of elevated blood pressure include family history of circulatory disease, age, gender, and ethnic tendency toward high blood pressure. Behavioral factors that may contribute to the elevated blood pressure include overeating; prolonged work stress; lack of exercise; and eating foods high in salt, cholesterol, and fats.

Some behaviors that should help to decrease John's blood pressure include continued avoidance of smoking; continued eating of foods low in salt, cholesterol, and fatty acids; decreased food portion sizes; increased regular aerobic and relaxation exercises, such as walking after dinner and bicycling on weekends; and actions to manage and decrease work time and work-related stress.

Treatment behaviors for John include regular blood pressure checks, making informed decisions with the physician about medications, and taking prescribed medications regularly. John will also be taught to take his own blood pressure, monitor it several times a week, and record the readings on a chart he will bring to his regular visits. He will also be encouraged to take a stress-management course given at the local hospital. The course meets in a group setting once a week for 5 weeks, and participants learn relaxation techniques and cognitive behavioral strategies to manage stress.

This is another example of a client whose needs must be met primarily by a health education approach. Lifestyle behaviors the client has control over must be clear to the client and all health professionals involved. These changeable behaviors should be the focus of teaching plans.

Identifying and teaching clients about lifestyle behaviors that need to be changed, however, is only the first step in the process of assisting clients to move from knowledge to action (Fig. 11-2). The nurse will need to utilize the health belief model and social learning theory as the next steps in formulating an action plan that meets the needs and capabilities of the client in making healthy behavior changes.

HEALTH BELIEF MODEL

The health belief model (HBM) that follows is a paradigm used by health education specialists to analyze factors that contribute to a client's perceived state of health or risk of disease and to the client's probability of taking appropriate health plans of action.[9,30,31,41] To assess a person's perceived state of health or threat of disease, the nurse considers the following:

1. Individual perceptions or readiness for change
    a. The value of health to the individual compared to other aspects of living
    b. Perceived susceptibility to a disease and to complications
    c. Perceived seriousness of the disease level threatening achievement of certain goals or aims

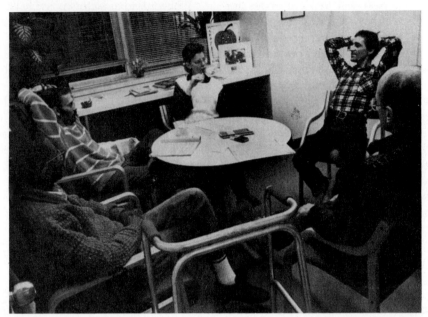

Fig. 11-2. Changing lifestyle behaviors that need to be changed is the first step in the process of assisting clients to move from knowledge to action. Many support groups exist to help people with AIDS. (From Denney NW, Quadagno D: *Human sexuality,* ed 2, St Louis, 1992, Mosby.)

   d. Belief in the diagnosis and therapy plan
2. Modifying factors about the person
   a. Demographic variables (age, sex, and so on)
   b. Socioeconomic variables, such as family and peer group characteristics, income, and education
   c. Previous experience with the disease
   d. Risk factors to a disease attributed to heredity, race, medical history, and so on
   e. Level of participation and satisfaction in regular health care
   f. Actual extent of changes necessary
   g. Personal aspirations in life, valued social and vocational activities, and so on
3. Motivating and environmental factors (cues to action)
   a. Exposure to advertising
   b. Advice from others
   c. Reminders from health professionals
   d. An illness of family member or friend
   e. Perceived benefits to comply with a treatment plan
   f. Previous success at changing behaviors

To assess a person's likelihood of taking preventive health actions, the nurse compares this picture of "perceived threat of disease" with

4. Client-provider transaction factors
   a. Past use of medical services
   b. Perceived benefits of preventive action
   c. Perceived barriers to preventive action
   d. Continued reassessment of the treatment plan between client and provider

The HBM does not specify the interventions that will influence an individual's likelihood of taking action. The HBM explains the role of values and beliefs in predicting treatment outcomes and adherence and generates data that can guide nurses in choosing effective educational strategies. The development of the most appropriate interventions for a particular client must be negotiated between the client and the health care professional.

SOCIAL LEARNING THEORY

Social learning theory (SLT) adds yet another model by which we can explain, predict, and influence behavior change.[41] Bandura's social learning theory (SLT),[5,7] which he has most recently renamed social cognitive theory (SCT),[6] holds that behavior is determined by expectancies and incentives. Rosenstock[41] delineates expectancies and incentives in this way:

1. Expectancies. These may be divided into three types:
   a. Expectancies about environmental cues (i.e., beliefs about how events are connected–about what leads to what).
   b. Expectancies about the consequences of one's own actions (i.e., opinions about how individual behavior is likely to influence outcomes). This is termed outcome expectation.
   c. Expectancies about one's own competence to perform the behavior needed to influence outcomes. This is termed efficacy expectation (i.e., self-efficacy).
2. Incentives. Incentive (or reinforcement) is defined as the value of a particular object or outcome. The

outcome may be health status, physical appearance, approval of others, economic gain, or other consequences. Behavior is regulated by its consequences (reinforcements) but only as *those consequences are interpreted and understood by the individual.* Thus, for example, individuals who value the perceived effects of changed lifestyles (incentives) will attempt to change if they believe that

a. Their current lifestyles pose threats to any personally valued outcomes, such as health or appearance (environmental cues).
b. Particular behavioral changes will reduce the threats (outcome expectations).
c. They are personally capable of adopting the new behaviors (efficacy expectations).

Two important contributions have been made by social cognitive theory to explain health behavior change.[41] The first is on the informative and motivational role of reinforcement and on the role of observational learning through modeling (imitating) the behavior of others. Opportunities to observe others performing the behavior in question such as in a local "Y" risk-factor-reduction program, where individuals exercise together and report on healthy behavior changes of smoking cessation and eating a low-fat diet, can enhance one's expectations of mastery. For modeling to affect a person's self-efficacy (an individual's perception of confidence in his or her ability to perform a specific behavior), however, the model must be similar to the observer in characteristics such as age and sex and be seen as overcoming difficulties through a determined effort rather than with ease.[21]

The concept of self-efficacy (efficacy expectation) as distinct from outcome expectation is the second major contribution of SCT.[5,6,7,45] The concept of outcome expectation (a person's estimate that a given behavior will lead to a particular outcome) is very similar to the HBM concept of "perceived benefits." Distinguishing between outcome and efficacy expectations is significant because both are required for behavior change. Fig. 11-3, Bandura's diagram, shows this relationship.[7] For example, in order for a person to begin an exercise program (behavior) for health reasons (outcome), he or she must believe both that exercise will benefit his or her health (outcome expectation) and that he or she is capable of exercising (efficacy expectation).[41]

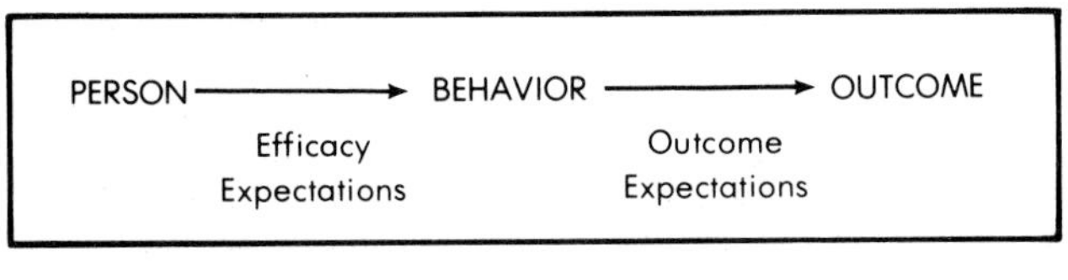

Fig. 11-3. Diagram of self-efficacy concept. (From Bandura A: *Social learning theory,* Englewood Cliffs, NJ, 1977, Prentice Hall. Reprinted with permission of the American Psychological Association.)

Regardless of our best methods of assessment and educational strategies, research in the area of health education indicates that people do not always make the choices recommended to them by health professionals.[39] We often label them "noncompliant," a term that suggests the individual has not followed our instructions–has not obeyed us. It is natural for health professionals to want people to choose the recommended course of action; however, each individual has the right to choose not to follow our advice. It is important to enlist the individual's partnership or cooperation rather than compliance.

Attempts to influence a person's behavior through education are not always carried out. It can be discouraging and sometimes futile to attempt to persuade a person to change behaviors we feel certain would make them, as well as their friends and family, healthier. Obstacles or barriers that may prevent us from influencing behavior change may be attributed to an individual's values, beliefs, and life stresses. Effective health education requires a comprehension of the factors that influence the person in decision making: values, beliefs, attitudes, current life stresses, religion, previous experiences with the health care system, and life goals.

Many health professionals tend to view a person's cooperation with the medical regimen as a single choice when in fact this cooperation often involves many choices every day. To follow a low-fat, low-cholesterol diet, for example, involves constant (often inconvenient) choices throughout the day. The expectation is that the client will do this every day for the rest of his or her life, even though we cannot guarantee freedom from angina, myocardial infarctions, or other complications.

Ultimately, we must respect a person's right to choose. We can, however, increase an individual's motivation and capabilities to change by

- involving the client in planning and goal setting
- giving information that is understandable and acceptable
- coaching the client in building new skills for mastery

The bottom line is that individuals know about their ability to shape their "health futures." After this is the imperative that they accept responsibility for making a difference in their lives and, by doing this, in the lives of their families, friends, neighbors, and community.[46] This is effectively stated by Green and Kreuter[23] in "Health Promotion as a Public Health Strategy for the 1990s."

> The overwhelming weight of evidence from research and experience on the value of participation in learning and behavior indicates that people will be more committed to initiating and upholding those changes that they helped design or adapt to their own purposes and circumstances.

After clarifying behaviors that need to be changed, the nurse can use the following set of questions evolved from SCT to assist in constructing effective educational and motivational interventions for behavior change:[37,47]

- What is the nature of the physical and social environment in which the behavior occurs?
- What are the characteristics of the situation when the behavior occurs?
- What factors tend to reinforce existing behaviors? What rewards or praise would help a person make behavioral changes?
- Are there appropriate social models in the environment from whom the person might learn new behaviors vicariously?
- What opportunities exist for the person to manage personal rewards?
- Does the person have the skills or capabilities needed to make changes?
- What does the person expect to happen as a result of these changes?
- What does the person value as outcomes to practicing new behaviors?
- Will the person be able to monitor his or her behavior and control the reinforcers in the environment?
- Does the person believe in a personal sense of competence to achieve new behaviors?
- In what ways will the environment be influenced by the person's new behaviors?

The information collected by answering the SCT questions forms the basis on which to design educational interventions appropriate to phases of the behavior change process. This description of the process is adapted from the four phases of the behavior change process developed by Parcel and Baranowski[37] and based on SCT.

1. Pretraining
   a. Becoming aware of a health concern, problem, or need
   b. Analyzing the concern, obtaining some information, weighing the pros and cons, and beginning to determine what should be done
   c. Assessing learning needs and emotional coping abilities
2. Training
   a. Entering a change program
   b. Developing a partner relationship with a health educator (nurse or other health professional)
   c. Acquiring information and skills (behavioral capabilities) that enable a behavior to be performed
   d. Reassessing expectations and desired learning outcomes
3. Initial testing phase
   a. Trying out new behaviors
   b. Implementing reinforcement strategies that support self-efficacy
   c. Monitoring results
   d. Identifying ways to maintain the behavior
   e. Solving problems
4. Continued performance
   a. Setting ongoing criteria for performance
   b. Establishing a monitoring system
   c. Establishing self-rewards
   d. Analyzing changes in the environment that result from the new behavior

Theories of health behavior change are the "heart" of health education. The theories presented in this section only help the practitioner to "get started." The goals of teaching plans will differ, depending on the client's stage in the behavior change process. Ongoing health education courses and programs in the community, school, and worksite will also differ in strategy and style, depending on these phases. The next section includes an example of a person working through these phases with educational interventions from a health professional.

Interventions

Interventions are defined as "the part of a strategy, incorporating method and technique, that actually interacts with a patient or population."[24] For health education, interventions take the form of teaching methods and strategies. The health educator or nurse selects a particular teaching method, depending on the health behavior involved and the client's (student's) progress through the behavior change process. Consider the following example.

Mrs. Pat Taylor, a recent widow at age 69, takes several regular medications–a diuretic, potassium tablets, and a high-dose vitamin. Recently she had dental work, after which the dentist gave her a prescription for empirin compound with codeine. Now she has symptoms of a winter cold and is about to decide whether to take a cold capsule, some aspirin, or cough syrup. She has always been somewhat confused as to how to select and schedule regular medications, her diet, and over-the-counter drugs, but she has never had a drug reaction. This time she decides to call her physician's office for advice.

The office nurse, Barbara Crandall, realizes that Mrs. Taylor gradually will be needing various medications; without a support person at home, she especially will need to develop safe habits of taking different medications. This phone call provides an opportunity for her to learn preventive behaviors for both her current symptoms and future conditions. After handling Mrs. Taylor's medical questions according to office protocol and determining that her client is interested in learning more about safe uses of prescription medications and over-the-counter drugs, Barbara begins the pretraining phase.

During the pretraining phase the nurse brings information to the client that builds awareness of the health issue and that expands the client's options for alternate plans of action. The client may select interventions such as audiovisual aids, pamphlets, magazine articles, or short presentations (lecturettes). To help the client analyze options, the health professional may facilitate a question-and-answer discussion or lead value-clarification exercises. The result of the pretraining phase should be a statement of goal(s) and a list of learning needs developed mutually between the client and nurse or health educator.

Barbara Crandall and the internist with whom she works periodically run educational programs for many of their elderly clients. Barbara invites Mrs. Taylor to participate in a session on medication safety. Through the use of slides and one or two group exercises, they help the members to assess their own level of knowledge on the subject and their behavior patterns. The goals of the session are to improve decision-making habits about medications and to identify changes to make in the environment and activities of daily living that will ensure safety in medication use.

Health risk appraisal is another useful strategy during the pretraining phase and is popular among middle-aged adults. It is "both a method and a tool that describes a person's chances of becoming ill or dying from specific diseases. The procedure generates a statement of probability, not a diagnosis."[38] The tool used for health risk appraisal should be well tested so that the client receives an accurate estimate of risk for the current major causes of death and disability. The appraisal tool serves to personalize health risk information in the media and helps the client to list specific behaviors causing a health risk. As a health education method, health risk appraisal helps participants to narrow the focus of their learning needs.

During the training phase the client decides that he or she is ready to enter a change program. Programmed learning strategies are appropriate for learning facts and concepts. Skill practice sessions with return demonstration by the participants are effective for developing motor skills. Group discussion and role-play methods help participants to develop problem solving, a sense of self-confidence, and emotional control skills. During this phase, the nurse also helps clients observe their own learning progress and reassess learning needs.

Mrs. Taylor's group decides to meet again to help each other solve problems they have identified about taking medications. They have asked Barbara for information about combinations of medications they should be careful about and for a list of books on the subject. After the second session, Barbara identifies that each group member will need to set personal objectives to practice the new behaviors at home. The group may not meet again. Barbara, however, will be able to follow up on their new experiences in several ways.

The initial testing phase is characterized by the trial of new skills or behaviors, usually in a setting common to the individual's lifestyle. Community diet-control programs, fitness clubs, and self-help groups are examples of programs in which the participant has continued group support while going through this tri[illegible] Educational strategies that facilitate the initi[illegible] phase include guided practice, contracting, and self-monitoring,[37] as well as continued problem solving, value clarification, and role-playing sessions.

Contracting refers to the establishment of verbal or written agreements to try or practice a specific action within a time frame. The contract is negotiated by the client with the health professional or other support person. At the end of the initial testing phase, individuals should be well aware of their "records" of performance, problems that cause barriers to performance, and aspects of their environments that promote or reinforce the desired behavior, such as rewards and social benefits.

When each group member returns for the next regular visit, Barbara Crandall asks about what each of them learned during the sessions on medications, what changes each has tried, and what were the outcomes. This information she records (without names) in a log maintained for evaluating the effectiveness of her group sessions. Depending on the needs of each client, she may suggest different ways to solve problems and monitor medication use.

The end of the behavior change process occurs as the participant performs the desired behavior(s) on a regular basis. Intervention strategies during this phase tend to take the form of helpful consultation sessions, periodic reporting of progress, and provision of rewards. Some methods used during the pretraining phase might be repeated to demonstrate progress and assess new learning needs. Tests of the participant's knowledge with verbal or written quizzes, as well as skill practice and demonstration sessions, do not determine whether a person eventually will perform a behavior regularly. In client-oriented health education, however, these evaluation techniques do serve to provide feedback and improve the client's awareness of progress.

Ethics

The practitioner of health education should strive to uphold democratic principles, such as respect for human dignity and the right to self-determination. When selecting health education interventions, however, nurses experience several ethical dilemmas.

Although the focus of health education may be on the behavior change process, the nurse must be sure that tactics of coercion, persuasion, or manipulation have not been used to effect the changes.[4,10,19] The role of the nurse is rather to facilitate a communicative environment in which persons can exercise their right to make informed free choices. Individuals need to participate in the decision-making process when their lives may be influenced by a change.

It can be frustrating to realize that each person's state

of health affects family members as well as the community. In a democratic society, however, individuals are responsible for their own health maintenance. Health professionals must accept and welcome individual differences in meeting that responsibility. By selecting interventions that create an environment of open communication and risk taking, individuals can better develop the problem-solving skills to direct their growth and development.

Another challenge for health professionals is to apply health education strategies with persons from varied cultural backgrounds, those who do not speak English as their native language, and those who cannot read at elementary levels. More time must be taken by the health professional to assess cultural beliefs that influence social and health practices, and more effort must be spent in analyzing educational interventions acceptable and satisfying for the audience. Marketing processes discussed in the next section help to identify characteristics, interests, and concerns of target populations.

MARKETING AND HEALTH EDUCATION

When nurses begin to teach groups of people, they automatically enter a program-planning and administrative process. When an organization wants to offer an ongoing health education program for specific target populations, *marketing* provides the strategies and techniques for reaching members of the group and implementing a service that will satisfy them as consumers. Combining marketing and health education strategies enables a health agency to improve its image and ability to cost-effectively serve certain populations.[33,42,48]

The marketing process and nursing process are comparable. Both involve data gathering and analysis; determination of needs and problem statements, goals, and action plans; and evaluation strategies. The nursing process usually is applied to developing a care plan for one client. Marketing involves the same type of process for meeting the needs and problems of larger target audiences. Moreover, marketing helps to clarify what combination of preventive health services, health-protection activities, and health education programs are the best interventions to solve a public health problem.

Definition

Many definitions of marketing are found in the literature. The following definition "elements" are adapted from Kotler's[32] definition of marketing for nonprofit organizations. Marketing is

- The descriptive analysis of target audiences
- The identification of value exchanges: services, products, and benefits the target audience views as valuable
- The strategic use of this information for planning and implementing programs to achieve the organization's objectives

First, marketing focuses on understanding the needs and preferences of consumers. Frequently the priorities of health professionals do not match the health and social services priorities of the public; services may be offered that a population does not recognize as useful. The location may be inaccessible, the price may be too low, or the registration procedure may be too long. The promotional flyers may not emphasize the message that is most appealing to the target population. The more information available about a target audience, the better are the chances of planning a service or product that the consumer will view as worth the cost.

As a system, marketing tends to be most effective when the consumer has a high degree of choice among competing services, products, or ways to spend time. Preventive health care and health promotion involve a great deal of voluntary consumer participation. Often the need for health habit changes is not apparent, and the less apparent the need, the harder it is to convince persons to buy. The nurse must keep in mind why a client would want to purchase a preventive health service or health education program.

Second, marketing focuses on the identification of potential exchanges between the provider and consumer. From the consumer's viewpoint, what does an organization have that will be beneficial? How much will it cost in terms of time, inconvenience, money, and long-range commitment?

Third, marketing provides the viewpoint of the consumer or receiver of service from which to plan, organize, and implement a project. Nurses and other health professionals should base decisions about the delivery of health services and programs on what consumers believe is important to their lives and health.

Marketing and assessment of community needs are closely allied.[13] Needs assessment provides a health professional with information about local population groups, existing services, and gaps in services. Marketing research may result in similar information as well as a more detailed profile of target audiences, the benefits they desire, and alternative approaches to filling service gaps. Any information about the target audience generated by marketing strategies will improve the nurse's ability to develop effective educational interventions.

ADMINISTERING HEALTH EDUCATION PROGRAMS

Many operational problems of implementing health education programs exist, such as lack of promotion, a confusing registration system, low funding for administrative support, or difficulty in finding a classroom with an appropriate learning climate. Nurses draw from the fields of organizational management and public health administration for systematic steps in delivering health education programs.[14,16]

Two models–the Precede-Proceed and the OPT/Evaluate–provide a sequence of steps for administering health education programs. The steps allow for the two-way communication between provider and consumer necessary for maintaining consumer satisfaction and for contributing to the reduction of public health problems by health behavior change.

The Precede-Proceed Model

The Precede-Proceed model is a comprehensive planning guide for the administration of health education programs developed by Green and Kreuter.[24] The first step is to decide whether an educational intervention will contribute to reducing a public health or medical problem. The Precede framework looks at the multiple factors that shape health status and guides the planner to arrive at a highly focused subset of factors as targets for intervention. Precede helps to generate specific objectives and criteria for evaluation. The Proceed framework gives additional steps for developing policy and initiating the processes of implementation and evaluation. They work in tandem, providing a continuous series of steps or phases in planning, implementation, and evaluation. Precede guides the planner in identification of priorities and setting of objectives and provides the objects and criteria for policy, implementation, and evaluation in the Proceed phases.

To develop an overview of the model, study Fig. 11-4, focusing first on the right-hand side. As an exercise, work through the following phases using a familiar community health-promotion project.

PHASE 1: SOCIAL DIAGNOSIS

The nurse lists indications of the *quality of life* from individuals and families in the target audience, including social, economic, communication, or spiritual problems. Involving the people in a self-study of their needs and aspirations is the best way to accomplish this. Situations

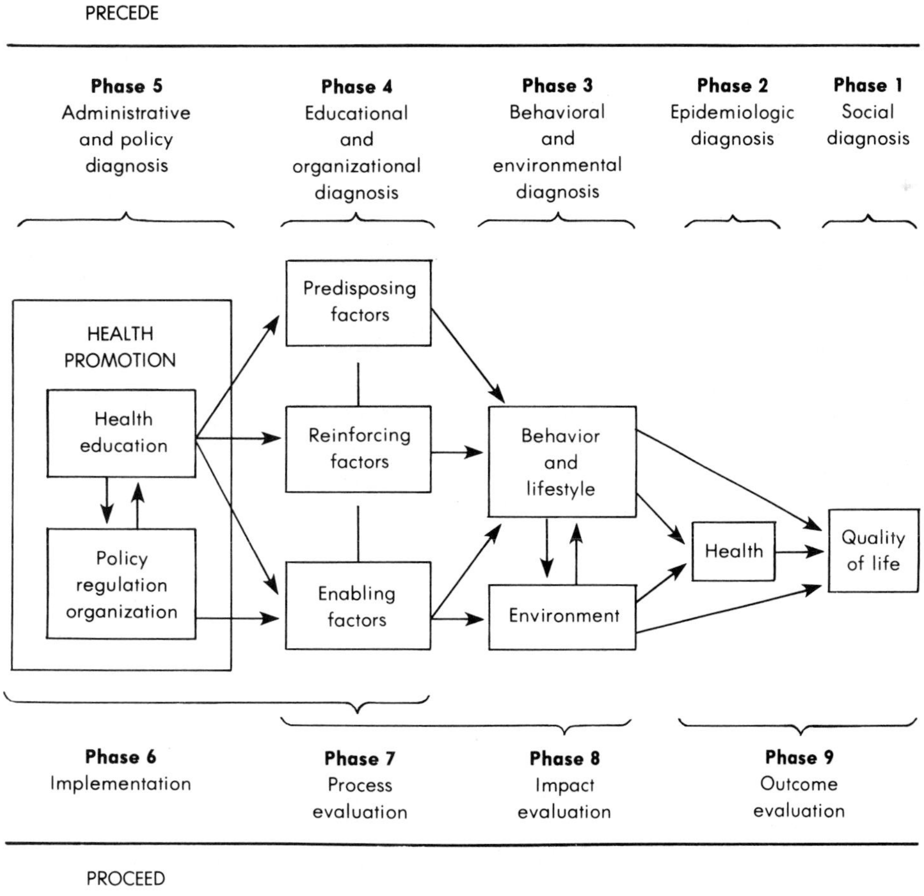

Fig. 11-4. The Precede-Proceed model for health-promotion planning and evaluation. (From Green L, Kreuter M: *Health promotion planning: an educational and environmental approach,* ed 2, Palo Alto, Calif, 1991, Mayfield Publishing. Reprinted with permission of Mayfield Publishing.)

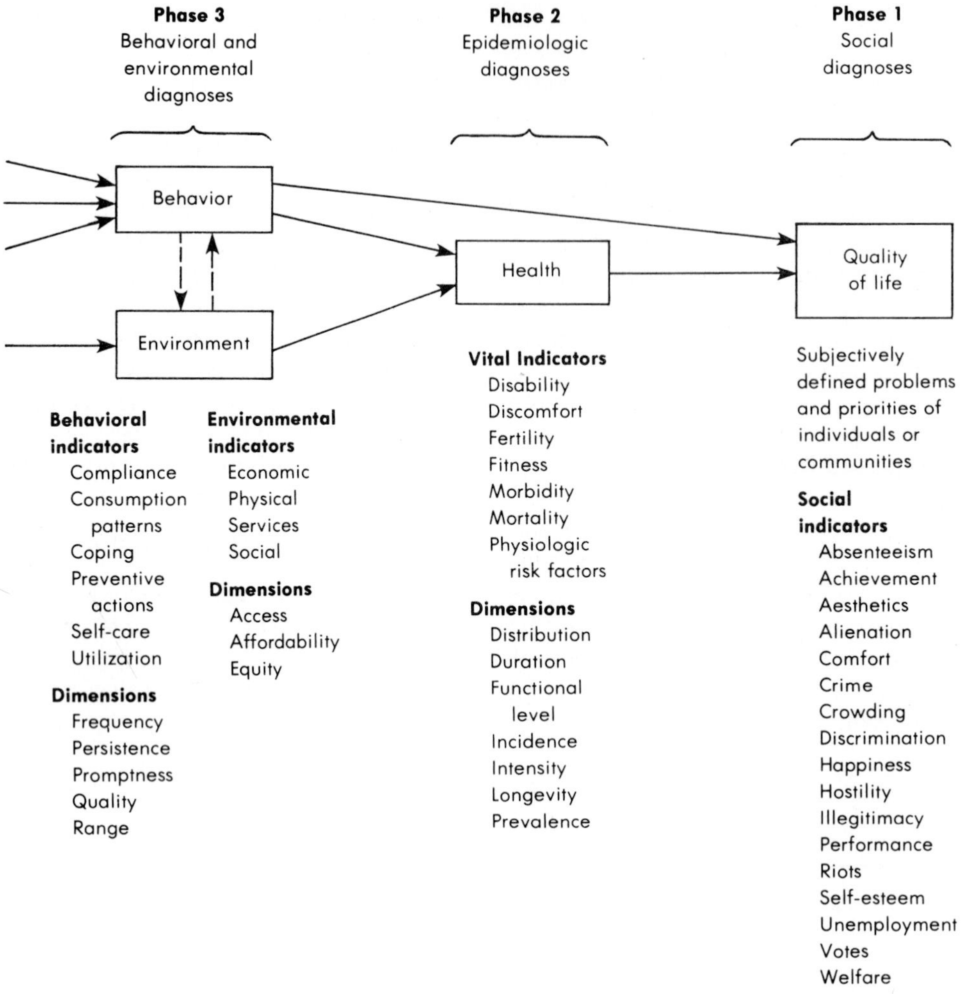

Fig. 11-5. Relationships, indicators, and dimensions of factors that might be identified in Phases 1, 2, and 3 of the Precede diagnostic process or evaluated in the extension of Proceed. (From Green L, Kreuter M: *Health promotion planning: an educational and environmental approach,* ed 2, Palo Alto, Calif, 1991, Mayfield Publishing. Reprinted with permission of Mayfield Publishing.)

that involve unemployment, loneliness or isolation, crowded conditions, or crime often have health-related causes; yet, health is often a value secondary to social concerns or benefits. Relating health problems to social problems helps both provider and consumer to expand the rationale or justification of a health education or promotion project. Community needs assessment information is especially useful for completing Phase 1. Marketing profile information provides subjective indications of the target audience's quality-of-life concerns.

PHASE 2: EPIDEMIOLOGIC DIAGNOSIS

The task of Phase 2 is to identify specific health problems that may be contributing to the problems in Phase 1. Using data from the needs assessment in Phase 1, the planner ranks the several health problems and selects the specific health problem most deserving of scarce educational and promotional resources. Examples of vital indicators or physiologic measures of health factors on which to measure these are shown in Fig. 11-5.

The nurse differentiates between health problems and nonhealth factors that contribute to the social problem(s). Epidemiologic data such as morbidity and mortality statistics suggest health problems of a target population. Data sources may include health insurance and worker's compensation statistics, local and federal public health statistics, and health service plans. These statistics indicate such problems as alcoholism, communicable and chronic diseases, infant mortality, and child abuse. Nonhealth factors include educational or income level, industrial layoffs, and climatic conditions. Analysis of the health problems facilitates ability to prioritize programs by using rates of prevalence, cost, and so forth. This step also suggests the most appropriate organizations or professional groups for helping to resolve the problem. Program goals and objectives indicate the expected impact of a health education project on the prevalence of a health problem.

PHASE 3: BEHAVIORAL AND ENVIRONMENTAL DIAGNOSIS

The nurse determines the behavioral risk factors that contribute to the health problems. Some behaviors increase the risk of several diseases. For example, smoking increases the chances of heart disease and cancer. Overeating may contribute to diabetes, high blood pressure, and obesity. The change of one health behavior, therefore, can help to reduce the risk of several diseases.

Nonbehavioral causes of a health problem are those that are not modifiable; they cannot be changed by the individual. A person cannot change age, sex, or ethnic tendencies. Environmental conditions may affect a health problem but may not be solved by the individual's behavior change. Environmental problems often need to be solved by community organization or legislation.

Some categories of changeable behaviors include lifestyle health habits; use of health care facilities; compliance with prescribed treatment plans; accident-prevention behaviors; communication and educational style between consumers and providers; and personal changes in home, work, and recreational environments. After determining the behavioral causes of a health problem, the nurse should select several priority behaviors for further analysis with the Precede model.

PHASE 4: EDUCATIONAL AND ORGANIZATIONAL DIAGNOSIS

The nurse lists factors that cause health behaviors in three categories: predisposing, enabling, and reinforcing (Fig. 11-6). *Predisposing* factors include a person's characteristics (values and attitudes, knowledge, age, sex, family heritage) that influence the tendency to practice a particular behavior. *Enabling* factors include the resources available to an individual to take certain health actions, such as personal problem-solving skills, physical abilities, and community resources. *Reinforcing* factors are aspects of a person's social environment

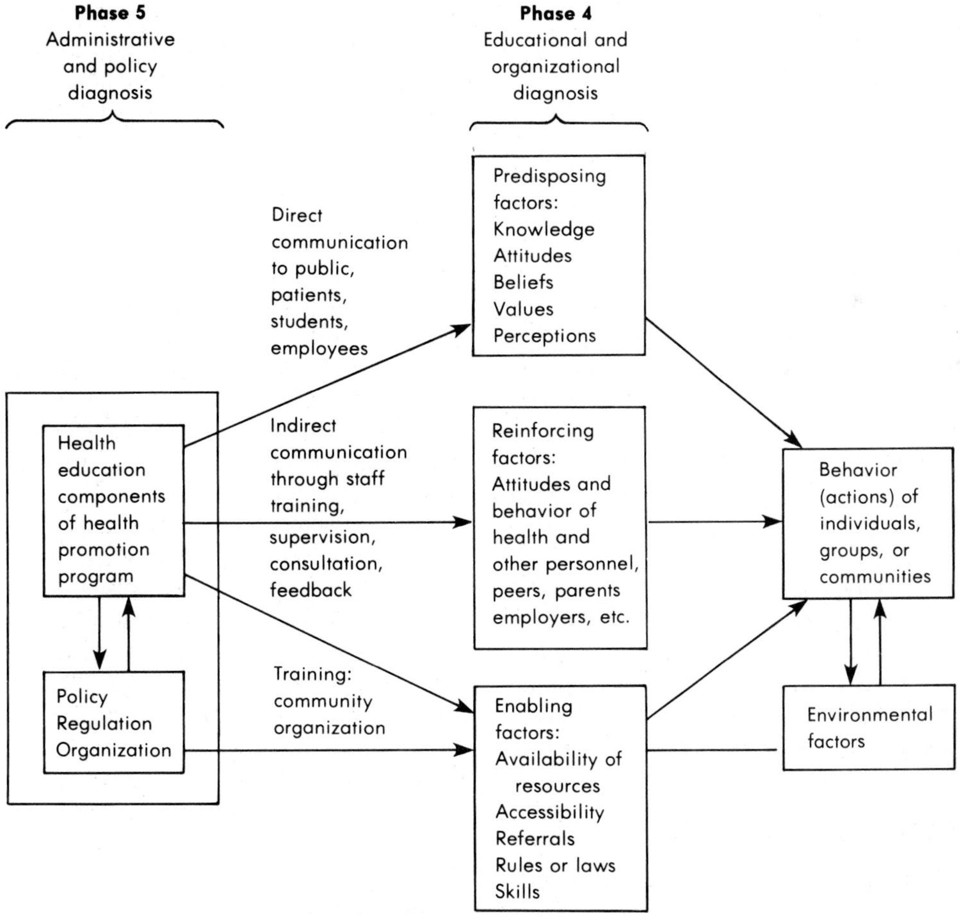

Fig. 11-6. Phases 4 and 5 of Precede address the strategies and resources required to influence the predisposing, reinforcing, and enabling factors influencing or supporting behavioral and environmental changes. (From Green L, Kreuter M: *Health promotion planning: an educational and environmental approach,* ed 2, Palo Alto, Calif, 1991, Mayfield Publishing. Reprinted with permission of Mayfield Publishing.)

that support or inhibit behavior change, such as family attitudes and behaviors of health professionals. From the list of factors, the nurse can select those factors most appropriate for a health education program. This constitutes an educational diagnosis.

PHASE 5: ADMINISTRATIVE AND POLICY DIAGNOSIS

Prepared with diagnostic information the nurse is ready for the assessment of organizational and administrative capabilities and resources for the development and implementation of a program. The nurse selects educational strategies suitable for facilitation of voluntary changes in behavior. Assessing organizational problems in implementing the health education program, the nurse develops alternate evaluation strategies and instruments.

PHASES 6, 7, 8, AND 9: PROCEED

The nurse generates a list of action steps established from the goals and objectives of the program for organizing, promoting, teaching, and evaluating. The implementation is carried out followed by the evaluation of the program. It is misleading to list evaluation as the last phase, however, for evaluation becomes an important and continuous part of working with the entire model from the beginning. The criteria for evaluation fall naturally from the objectives defined in the corresponding steps in Precede during the diagnostic process.

There are two fundamental propositions emphasized by the Precede-Proceed model: (1) health and health risks are caused by multiple factors; and (2) because health and health risks are determined by multiple factors, efforts to effect behavioral, environmental, and social change must be multidimensional or multisectoral.

ADVANTAGES

The advantages of using a planning model such as the Precede-Proceed model include the ability (1) to connect health and social problems with appropriate and effective educational strategies, (2) to develop a broad perspective about all the factors influencing health behavior and the interaction among the factors, and (3) to select evaluation techniques tailored to assess the achievement of behavioral learning objectives. This process improves the chances that an educational intervention will meet the concerns of a target audience, the consumer group.

OPT/Evaluate: A Delivery Model

The OPT/Evaluate model "consists of four groups of tasks to consider when planning the actual implementation of a health education program."[18] The four groups are organize, promote, teach, and evaluate. The model, developed by Edwards,[18] includes an action step checklist (see box on pp. 257-258) useful to the nurse who is new to organizing and teaching health education programs.

The OPT/Evaluate model is intended to help in the application of businesslike strategies for delivering health education. It provides a framework for discussing administrative aspects of health education with managers and community leaders unfamiliar with the definitions and purposes of health education and promotion.

Organize refers to the steps taken by an individual or agency for the initial coordination of the health education project. *Promote* applies to the market research, networking, and advertising steps that provide the information necessary to make organizing decisions. Such preparation should solicit support from other community health care and health-planning agencies and ensure an adequate number of participants to conduct the program. *Teach* refers to the steps necessary in preparing to conduct the class. *Evaluate* refers to the steps necessary to assess how the program objectives were met, and whether the learning objectives were realized.

The planning and organizing process must be considered before promoting a program. Several marketing-type steps are listed under the "Promote" groups, which should provide information for making both organizational and promotional decisions (see box on p. 257). Therefore, the first six steps in planning promotion should be completed before writing a basic project description or proposal (see "Organize," step 9). In addition, "Evaluate" steps 1 to 5 must be considered before completing step 13 of "Organize."

The words "organize, promote, teach, and evaluate" thus indicate functional rather than chronologic groupings. It is logical, however, that organizing precedes promoting, and promoting precedes recruiting enough participants to teach. All aspects of program administration need evaluation to develop recommendations for improving or expanding the next project.

It takes teamwork to administer a health education program. Rarely does one person have all the marketing, administration, and health teaching skills to deliver this service, even in small community settings. A steering committee, coordinated at the beginning of a project, helps ensure that at the teaching stage the resources are collected and the participants are prepared appropriately for a successful program.

TEACHING PLAN

Preparation for teaching one or more group programs, such as a seminar or course, begins after the marketing and administrative plans are well underway. These activities ensure that there are enough participants for the program and provide the structure for developing the

❑ ❑ ACTION STEP CHECKLIST FOR OPT/EVALUATE MODEL

Organize

1. Review the aims and policies of the agency.
2. Clarify the health areas for consideration.
3. Initiate a project committee.
4. Identify audience characteristics, interests, health problems, and health needs.
5. Design program goals and objectives.
6. List program options.
7. Identify criteria for program feasibility.
8. Assess all systems necessary for successful program implementation, such as
   a. Personnel orientation and instructor preparation
   b. Equipment, materials, and classroom facilities
   c. Curriculum design
   d. Promotion and scheduling
   e. Support services (transportation, babysitting)
   f. Registration, fees, and accounting
   g. Record keeping and evaluation
9. Write a basic project description or proposal.
10. Develop the budget.
11. List action steps.
12. Develop a schedule.
13. Establish evaluation questions, standards, and strategies.
14. Establish funding source(s) and an accounting system.
15. Make staff assignments and plan for supervision and performance reviews.

Promote

1. Define primary and segmented population groups.
2. Identify agencies and government offices that are serving the same population and providing related health services or educational programs.
3. Collect existing information about audience characteristics, interests, health problems, and health needs through health planning agencies, public health departments, United Way, and so on.
4. Develop interagency communication networks and understandings.
5. Identify possible areas of service duplication.
6. Identify service delivery questions that need to be answered by survey of target population, such as convenient locations, dates, and times.
7. Coordinate a promotion subcommittee, as needed.
8. Survey the target population to clarify general interests, life concerns, cultural values, and level of motivation to attend self-help education programs.
9. Identify the best avenues of communication with the target population.
10. Design promotional themes and symbols.

Promote—cont'd

11. List materials needed for advertising, such as schedules, registration forms, fact sheets, flyers, posters, press releases, newsletter announcements, radio spots, and television spots.
12. Establish procedure for collecting registration fee.
13. Schedule program dates and times.
14. Arrange for classrooms.
15. Write a promotion plan and calendar for meeting media deadlines.
16. Design a system for determining which promotion strategies are most successful.
17. Delegate specific tasks for developing materials.
18. Arrange for writing, artwork, layout, and printing of advertising materials.
19. Complete promotion plans according to the calendar.
20. Evaluate effectiveness of promotional activities in recruiting the anticipated number of participants.

Teach

1. List participant interests, characteristics, and health needs already determined by community needs assessment and survey.
2. Identify specific health learning needs.
3. Collect sample teaching curricula, audiovisual aids, flyers, and materials appropriate for the class.
4. Establish learning objectives.
5. Finalize lesson plans, including content, methods, and evaluation strategies.
6. Develop a checklist of and collect equipment, audiovisual aids, handouts, workbooks, and other materials.
7. Check that participants are registering.
8. Send response letters to confirm registration (may include an agenda, questionnaire, and so on).
9. Phone participants one day before class, if necessary.
10. Arrive early and arrange classroom furniture and equipment.
11. Conduct classes according to lesson plans with flexibility for meeting special learning needs and interests of the group.
12. Complete record-keeping evaluation and recognition procedure.
13. Plan all teaching steps with the coinstructor when team teaching.
14. Follow the same steps (1 to 3) when preparing new instructors, remembering that instructor candidates are a different population group with different learning needs.

Continued.

❑ ❑ ACTION STEP CHECKLIST FOR OPT/EVALUATE MODEL—cont'd

Teach—cont'd

15. Observe new instructors in practice teaching or in their first teaching experience to ensure that the project standards are met.

Evaluate

1. List questions about the program to be evaluated, considering the categories of
   a. Project organization
   b. Program promotion
   c. Instructor performance
   d. Participant learning
   e. Participant satisfaction
2. Check whether the program objectives and participant learning objectives are stated in measurable terms. Are the expectations of the participants clear?
3. Establish standards and/or evidence of successful completion of the objectives.
4. Identify methods of obtaining feedback on each evaluation category.
5. Select times and situations during the schedule of project implementation when data may be collected easily.
6. Design the evaluation tools and procedures.
7. Have evaluation tools reviewed by persons with expertise in testing, evaluation design, and statistics.
8. Establish the record-keeping procedures.
9. Orient the individuals who will collect the data to the recording and reporting procedure.
10. Tally the results according to the project schedule.
11. Hold program committee meetings as needed to interpret the results of each evaluation phase.
12. Finish reports, including recommendations for future projects.
13. Encourage self-assessment and continuing professional development by assisting individuals to set personal goals for the next project.
14. Recognize all staff contributing to the project.

From Edwards L: Delivering health education programs: a model, *Health Values* 6(6):13, 1982.

teaching plan–the program objectives, time available, human and material resources, and so on. When the marketing and administrative functions have been provided by others and when developing educational strategies for one client at a time, the nurse may be able to concentrate efforts on developing the teaching plan.

A health teaching plan may emphasize a phase of the behavior change process related to the client's medical or health problems. The plan may also follow the sequence of that process from pretraining to continued performance of behavior that helps to resolve a medical or health problem. The written teaching plan represents a "package" of educational services provided to a consumer, or "student." The plan, therefore, should be written from the student's viewpoint.

The process of generating a teaching plan helps the nurse to recognize and use methods of learning that involve the client as an active participant. The plan should include a list of specific actions or abilities that the client may perform at intervals during the educational intervention and at the end. Teaching plans help nurses to clarify what they expect clients as students to *do* when the educational intervention is over.

When preparing a teaching plan for one client in a primary care setting, the nurse may find background information about the client from that person's record and any agency reports that include descriptions of the client's population group. Often nurses agree to teach health classes that others have organized. In this case it is important to ask for any project reports that (1) provide marketing and needs assessment information about students expected to attend the classes and (2) indicate the steps taken to administer the whole educational program.

Nurses might approach the "exercise" of preparing a teaching plan in stages. The reader can simulate this by doing the following:

1. Review the chapter subsections that follow, and jot down ideas and information about a real or hypothetic teaching project for each subsection.
2. Make a list of information resources or human resources needed to complete the teaching plan.
3. When those resources are collected or consulted, draft a teaching plan. Use any structure for the plan that identifies the educational goal, behavioral objectives, content topics, learning methods, and evaluation strategies.
4. Review the written plan with a focus on whether the plan is an adequate tool from which to manage the educational intervention.

Assessing Learning Needs

The assessment of learning needs is important in developing health education programs for individuals, families, communities, or organizations. This involves answering five questions:

1. What are the characteristics and learning capabilities of the client?
2. What are the learner's needs for health promotion, risk reduction, or health problems?
3. What does the client already know, and what skills can he or she already perform relevant to his or her needs?
4. Is the learner motivated to change any unhealthy behaviors?
5. What are the barriers and facilitators to healthy behavior change?

CHARACTERISTICS

Activities to help the nurse identify characteristics of the learner include (1) consideration of the client's age and developmental stage in his or her lifestyle; (2) consideration of the client's level on Maslow's hierarchy of basic human needs: survival, safety, love and belonging, self-esteem, and self-actualization; and (3) review of marketing profile descriptions of the client's population segment: demographic, geographic, and psychographic characteristics. The reader is asked to refer to the individual developmental chapters in this text for further information on developmental characteristics.

HEALTH PROBLEMS

Resources of information about the health problems of a population group are epidemiologic reports, community needs assessment reports, insurance statistics, and incident reports. Nursing and medical texts often provide lists of concepts or skills a client might need to learn about a health problem to comply with a treatment plan.

CURRENT KNOWLEDGE AND SKILLS

Methods for assessing current knowledge and skills include: individual or group interviews, questionnaires or pretests, skill demonstrations, and observation of problem-solving behaviors and competencies. Health risk appraisals and other tests help the client to be an active participant in assessing learning needs.

MOTIVATION

The health belief model helps to assess a client's perception of his or her health problems and the factors that indicate the likelihood of his or her desire to take preventive actions. If a client seems unmotivated to change, the nurse looks for environmental issues, lack of knowledge or skills, or social stimuli or false incentives that may be inhibiting the person's readiness. One aim of the pretraining phase of the behavior change process is to create a learning climate that encourages the client to make decisions for health behavior change.

BARRIERS AND FACILITATORS

From the Precede model already discussed, the predisposing, enabling, and reinforcing factors that create health behaviors also provide cues to program promotion and teaching techniques that may inhibit or enhance the learning process (see Fig. 11-4). The teaching plan, to the extent possible, should incorporate activities found to facilitate learning for the client or target population. Readiness to learn new concepts, skills, or attitudes often depends on whether the educational intervention is timed appropriately. Clients may need time to research information, discuss the topic, or even identify the consequences of *not* changing before they are ready to learn new material. The time of day and sequence of learning activities may also affect readiness.

Determining Expected Learning Outcomes

To determine the expected learning outcomes of a health education intervention, the nurse should answer the following questions:

1. What are the broad public health and social goals that guide the proposed educational program?
2. What are the participant's learning goals?
3. What must the learner know, do, and believe to progress through the behavior change process?

PROGRAM GOALS

The program goal of a health education project should reflect the aim to influence improvement in some health problem or social living condition, as is indicated in Phases 1 and 2 of the Precede model (see Fig. 11-4). Program goals suggest a level of aspiration and are usually qualified. They do not indicate what combination of interventions will solve the health and social problems.[49]

LEARNING GOALS

Learning goals are best established jointly between the client and nurse. These goals reflect the health behaviors or health status change that the client will have achieved by the end of an educational intervention. Learning goals should relate to the program goal.

LEARNING OBJECTIVES

Learning objectives indicate steps to be made by the client toward meeting the learning goal. They may involve the development of knowledge or a skill or a change in attitude. Objectives are most useful when stated in behavioral terms and contain the following elements: an *action verb* that indicates the task to be done, the *person(s)* doing the task, the *conditions* that affect how the task is done, and a *measure* of the extent of results desired.[35] Learning objectives guide the selection of content and methods and help narrow the focus of a teaching plan to more achievable steps. They also aid in setting standards of performance and suggesting evaluation strategies.

Selecting Content

To select appropriate content for a health education program, the nurse considers these questions: What information, skills, and attitudes need to be taught? and What is the level of learning to be achieved?[29]

THREE DOMAINS OF LEARNING

Content is commonly divided into three domains: cognitive, psychomotor, and affective. *Cognitive* learning refers to the development of new facts or concepts, building on or applying past knowledge to new situations. *Psychomotor* learning pertains to the development of physical skills, from simple to complex actions. *Affective* learning alludes to the recognition of values, religious and spiritual beliefs, family interaction patterns and relationships, and personal attitudes that affect decisions and problem-solving progress.

To learn or change a health behavior, a person may need to acquire new information, practice some physical techniques, and clarify ways the new behavior may affect relationships with others. The nurse's role is to select a combination of content from the three domains appropriate to meet the behavioral objective. To find samples of content for a teaching plan, the nurse researches resource materials, such as books, teaching guides, journal articles, and pamphlets and flyers printed by nonprofit agencies and professional organizations. The nurse should be careful about using materials with technical vocabulary too complex for the client or group.

LEVEL OF LEARNING

The level of learning to be achieved depends on how it is anticipated for the content to be used. According to Bloom's taxonomy,[12] levels of learning are identified from simple to complex. For example, in the cognitive domain, levels of learning include

Knowledge–client recalls facts and the concept
Comprehension–client understands meaning of concept
Application–client uses the concept
Analysis–client can examine or explain the concept
Synthesis–client integrates the concept with other learning
Evaluation–client judges or compares the concept

The nurse preparing a teaching plan should differentiate between what the client *must* know and do with what would be *helpful* for the client to know and do to fulfill a learning objective. That process provides cues to what the level of learning should be. As the level of learning to be achieved becomes complex, the educational strategies and methods selected should involve the clients in more active application and analysis of the content.

Designing Learning Strategies

Designing the learning strategies for an educational intervention means selecting the methods and tools and structuring the sequence of activities. The teaching plan so far provides the foundation on which to base the activity selection and sequence. The following questions should guide the design of learning strategies:

1. What are some basic considerations for selecting teaching methods for health education programs?
2. How does the nurse, as instructor, establish and maintain a learning climate?
3. What actions can the nurse perform to increase the effectiveness of learning methods?
4. What are appropriate methods for each learning domain?
5. What methods tend to promote behavior change?

CONSIDERATIONS FOR SELECTING METHODS

First, the nurse should consider setting an environment and using methods that encourage *self-directed learning,* which implies that the client develops skills in assessing his or her learning needs and deciding how he or she wants to proceed through the learning process. The self-directed learner can participate in establishing standards of performance and gradually is able to monitor progress.[15,23] It follows that greater learning usually is achieved when the learner is an active participant in the learning situation. Whenever in doubt as to which method to choose, usually it is more effective for the nurse to choose the more *experiential* or participative method.[23]

Persons tend to prefer learning in different ways. The larger the group, the more important it is to vary the methods frequently. This increases attention spans and gives all clients a sense of an individualized educational approach.

Continuity of significant concepts or principles must also be threaded through the sequence of learning methods. This allows the nurse to reinforce and build concepts verbally, visually, and with activities as the program proceeds. The nurse must be careful, however, not to be repetitious, since this could become a barrier to learning. The flow or order of content and methods should be from simple concepts and skills to the more complex, from known material toward the less known. The nurse should avoid dealing with content that causes anxiety for the learner at the program's end or during periods when fatigue is high. Usually it is best to present standard or generalized concepts first and then indicate variations or exceptions to avoid confusion.

LEARNING CLIMATE

Several categories of activities are available when a nurse tries to establish an environment conducive to health behavior change. First are those activities that create a sense of preparedness and organization; the physical facilities are appropriate, with chairs and tables in place. Participant materials are ready to be handed out, and the audiovisual aids and equipment are hooked up. The instructor's appearance should convey comfort for the learner as well as credibility.

The second category for setting a learning climate involves communicating to the clients where they are, where the bathroom and other building facilities may be found, how breaks are scheduled, and any other logistic information. This information helps the participant relax and get ready to learn.

The third category involves any activities the nurse uses to assess individual and group learning needs, such as questions and discussion about learner interests, concerns, and problems and preprogram questionnaires. The participants should develop the feeling at this point that the educational intervention will be relevant or applicable directly to their lives. At this point the instructor should look for and reinforce the signs of motivation to participate in the experience.

Once the learning climate is set, the fourth category involves activities to maintain motivation, the sense of individualized attention and ongoing progress. Periodically the nurse should "check in" with the participants by asking, "Is this material useful, helpful? Is this what you expected? How could the program be more relevant for you?" For some groups, the instructor might lead a short discussion about how to use the information at home.

Finally the nurse works with a group jointly to maintain the learning climate. This category of activities involves observing group interactions, helping individuals to participate, intervening to help a group deal with controlling its members, and remaining cognizant of any dynamics in the group process that will facilitate or inhibit learning.

INSTRUCTOR EFFECTIVENESS

Regardless of the educational method, nurses can perform several functions to increase an intervention's effectiveness. For example, bridging concepts from one class or method to the next tends to build cognitive learning. Probing for depth of learning helps the instructor recognize what the participants are learning and how they are applying the material. When developing a teaching plan, the nurse periodically should try to construct questions that call for participants to apply, analyze, or evaluate new concepts.

When a client or group loses track of the subject or does not seem to be progressing toward meeting a learning objective, the nurse might "refocus" on the topic or "focus on the process" occurring at the moment. The latter helps clients build their own skills in becoming aware of group or family dynamics.

Other instructor functions include clarifying concepts and definitions, acknowledging individual or group contributions and progress, and using silence to communicate student responsibility for continuing the learning process. In the beginning, the nurse structures the learning experience; at the end the nurse should also wrap up or summarize the learning achieved.[39]

Especially important in health education is the instructor's role as a model. Students tend to watch closely as to whether instructors' personal actions match the recommendations they are making. Since instructors are also "human" and usually working on their own health behavior change goals, it is better not to present oneself as an "expert." The nurse tends to be more effective when assuming a partner or facilitator role to form a "helping" relationship.

TEACHING FOR EACH LEARNING DOMAIN

Methods appropriate for developing cognitive information include lecturettes (short lectures), reading assignments with study guides, self-monitoring, audiovisual aids, computer-assisted learning, and self-paced programmed learning. Quizzes help the teacher and student to assess cognitive learning.

Methods for building psychomotor skills include demonstration (in person or on film), guided practice, and on-site or on-the-job apprenticeship. To evaluate performance of skills, the nurse might observe client practice sessions; videotaping helps the student pinpoint problems. Job descriptions, with a list of specific competencies, help clients to evaluate their level of performance and set personal objectives for continuing education.

Methods for clarifying values and attitudes include group discussion and brainstorming opinion, questionnaires, voting exercises, prioritizing or rating scales, role play, and case studies. The aim of the affective learning domain is to increase a client's exposure to many alternate values and attitudes. Then the nurse provides opportunities to explore the pros and cons of varied positions and courses of action, encouraging clients to make their own informed choices. One way to help clients assess learning in the affective domain is to ask them whether certain prized attitudes or values are causing problems in their life at home, at work, in school, with relationships, or in personal health. The nurse then encourages continued exploration of these problems.

STRATEGIES THAT PROMOTE BEHAVIOR CHANGE

During the initial testing phase of the health behavior change process, nurses might use strategies, such as modeling, self-appraisal and goal setting, contracting with the client to try out a new behavior and report back; mutually developed reminders and cues; record keeping of trials and problems; reinforcement and reward strategies; and self-monitoring. During this period, the client may need individual or group assistance for problem solving and reestablishing goals. This helps to promote self-efficacy and positive behavior change.

Evaluating Progress

A few strategies for evaluating clients' progress in each learning domain already have been suggested. To plan a comprehensive evaluation of an educational intervention, however, the nurse might use these questions:

1. What tools or strategies can be incorporated in the teaching plan for observing significant learning outcomes?
2. How can feedback be obtained about the instructor's performance?
3. How can implementation factors that may have influenced the effectiveness of the educational intervention be identified?[3]
4. Is it possible to measure the extent to which this educational program affected the original program goal?

TOOLS FOR OBSERVING LEARNING OUTCOMES

The learning objectives guide a nurse in selecting tools and strategies to evaluate clients' performance; the instructor should be able to observe the student performing the task identified in the objective. Evaluation methods might include tests and quizzes, completed study sheets, student comments during class exercises and discussion, skill practice observation, small group tasks, opinion surveys, problem-solving exercises, and competency rating scales. Often a participatory teaching method also provides a nurse with evaluative information. Both nurse and client must anticipate or predict certain actions or behaviors that would fulfill an objective.

INSTRUCTOR PERFORMANCE FEEDBACK

The nurse can incorporate into the teaching plan written, verbal, and nonverbal techniques for obtaining feedback about his or her teaching performance. Postprogram questionnaires are the usual method for obtaining written feedback. The nurse may ask for verbal feedback at various times from the group, from individual students, and from observers of the class. Nonverbal communication cues from participants may indicate their satisfaction, fatigue, or frustration with the educational intervention.

IMPLEMENTATION FACTORS

The procedures used to organize and promote an educational program may affect its ultimate success. The instructor (or a program administration committee) should record activities such as advertising, registration, fee collection, and availability and repair of equipment and materials. This evaluative information then can be used to improve the next program. Surveys by telephone or by postprogram questionnaire help to obtain the consumer's opinion about these implementation procedures. Word-of-mouth referrals to future programs and support from other community agencies and professionals also may indicate that persons approve of the way the program is offered.

PROGRAM IMPACT

Sometimes the nurse is asked to justify a health education program in terms of its impact on the community's public health goals or social problems. Since health promotion involves health-protection activities, preventive health services, and health education programs combined, it would be difficult to draw a direct correlation between an educational intervention and the statistical improvement of the health problem.

By working through the Precede model, nurses often can describe the theoretic impact of an educational intervention on health behaviors, health problems, and social problems. It is important, however, to keep such statistics as the number of persons served each year, the percentage of the target population reached, the number of service providers used, the number and cost of programs, and so on. As these statistics change over time, the data will provide cues to program success and problems.

Referring Clients to Other Resources

The end of a teaching plan should include resources for students to use for continuing education, counseling, peer support, and health services. Nurses should encourage clients to see health education as a lifelong learning process. Each person has different developmental needs and health concerns through the life cycle. Moreover, any one educational intervention may only help a person move from one phase of the behavior change process to the next. Also, many variables besides learning may exist that influence a person's health practices.

TEACHING AND ORGANIZING SKILLS

To develop teaching and organizing skills in health education, the nurse must often learn new behaviors.[36] The four phases of the behavior change process provide a systematic guide for learning these professional skills.

To get started, the nurse should seek self-assessment opportunities. For example, the nurse can review the OPT/Evaluate checklist of action steps previously given (see box on pp. 257–258), placing a 1 beside those that are first-priority learning needs, a 2 beside second-priority needs, and a 3 beside those that are not priority learning needs at present. Using the list, the nurse begins to identify resources available for reading, instructor training, and practice teaching. Working on steering committees or group project teams offers opportunities to develop program-organizing skills. The nurse then drafts an initial set of learning goals.

A formal college course or continuing education workshop provides opportunities to learn the cognitive information, affective attitudes, and psychomotor skills appropriate for teaching health education programs in schools, at worksites, in health service settings, and at other community locations. The instructor training course may include practice teaching sessions. A college program may assign students to form a team to organize and teach a health program. If no formal courses are available, working with an experienced health instructor to establish an apprenticeship relationship may be helpful.

When starting to teach the first few group programs, the nurse should avoid both groups that are too large (more than 20) and those that are too small (less than five). These situations do not provide an optimum learning environment. After selecting the target audience and the general topic, the nurse works through the Precede model as a planning stage, then uses the OPT/Evaluate model to guide program organization, promotion, and the development of a teaching plan. The nurse must identify other persons or a project team available to help.

After implementing the educational intervention, the nurse sets time aside to discuss what happened. Did the program go as planned? What changes were made in the teaching plan? What would you change for next time? The nurse reviews the self-developed learning goals and determines new ones.

As the nurse teaches additional programs on either an individual or group basis, he or she will be able to clarify those instructor teaching and organizing skills that come naturally. These skills tend to improve a program's effectiveness and enable the logistics to run smoothly. The teacher is first a learner; this is as true in health education as it is in any form of education.

SUMMARY

Compared with other health professionals, nurses spend the greatest amount of time in direct contact with clients. They have many opportunities to recognize readiness to learn new information and behaviors. Nurses also often coordinate group programs. The more accurate the analysis of the educational aspects of a health promotion program and the assessment of characteristics and learning needs of the target audience, the more effective an educational intervention will be in influencing health behaviors.

The principles of health education form a generic basis for implementing a variety of health topics: accident prevention and first aid, expectant parent education, high blood pressure education, nutrition and fitness, stress management, substance abuse, and sex education, as well as patient education in areas such as diabetes and arthritis. Three scenarios described in this chapter provide insights into the nurse's role in conducting educational interventions about family planning, high blood pressure, and medication safety.

Differences exist in planning to teach one person versus a group. One-to-one interventions tend to follow a more counseling or problem-solving approach. Group interventions may range from guided discussion on concerns that evolve from the group to a more structured learning experience involving presentation, skill practice, and attitude-awareness exercises. The range of health education strategies provide nurses and all health professionals with techniques and methods applicable in health service settings, schools, worksites, and other community facilities.

References

1. American Nurses' Association: *Model nurse practice act* pub code NP-52M5/76, Kansas City, Mo, 1979, The Association.
2. American Nurses' Association: *The professional nurse and health education,* Kansas City, Mo, 1975, The Association.
3. American Red Cross: *Instruction specialist supervisor manual,* Washington, DC, 1982, American Red Cross.
4. Andrews L: *Legal issues in teaching self-care courses,* Manhattan, Kan, 1979, Free University Network.
5. Bandura A: Self-efficacy: toward a unifying theory of behavioral change, *Psychol Rev* 84:191-215, 1977.
6. Bandura A: *Social foundations of thought and action,* Englewood Cliffs, NJ, 1986, Prentice Hall.

7. Bandura A: *Social learning theory,* Englewood Cliffs, NJ, 1977, Prentice Hall.
8. Bates I, Winder AE: *Introduction to health education,* Palo Alto, Calif, 1984, Mayfield Publishing.
9. Becker MH, et al: The health belief model and personal health behavior, *Health Educ Monogr* 2(4):49, 1974.
10. Birch DA: Clarifying bioethical issues through health education activities, *Health Educ* 17(6):40, 1986.
11. Blendon R: Satisfaction with health systems in ten nations, *Health Affairs,* pp 185-195, 1990.
12. Bloom B: *Taxonomy of educational objectives,* New York, 1969, Longman-Green.
13. Bonaguro JA, Miaoulis G: Marketing: a tool for health education planning, *Health Educ* 14(1):6, 1983.
14. Bruess CE, Poehler DL: What we need and don't need in health education–1986, *Health Educ* 17(6):32, 1986.
15. Cheren M: *The self-director educator,* Columbia, Md, 1979, Council for the Advancement of Experiential Learning.
16. Dignan MB, Carr PA: *Program planning for health education and health promotion,* ed 2, Philadelphia, 1992, Lea & Febiger.
17. Duryea EJ: Decision making and health education, *J School Health* 53(1):29, 1983.
18. Edwards L: Delivering health education programs: a model, *Health Values* 6(6):13, 1982.
19. Faden R, Faden A: The ethics of health education as public health policy, *Health Educ Monogr* 6(2), 1978.
20. Farlow H: *Publicizing and promoting programs,* New York, 1979, McGraw-Hill.
21. Fitzgerald ST: Self-efficacy theory: implications for the occupational health nurse, *AAOHN J* 39(12):552-557, 1991.
22. Goldstein AS, et al: *The nurse's legal advisor: your guide to legally safe practice,* Philadelphia, 1989, JB Lippincott.
23. Green L, Kreuter M: Health promotion as a public health strategy for the 1990s, *Ann Rev Public Health* 11:319-334, 1990.
24. Green L, Kreuter M: *Health promotion planning: an educational and environmental approach,* ed 2, Palo Alto, Calif, 1991, Mayfield Publishing.
25. Grubel MF: Group dynamic practices applied to health education, *J School Health* 23(12):656, 1981.
26. *Healthy people: the surgeon general's report on health promotion and disease prevention,* US Department of Health and Human Services, (PHS) Pub No 79-55071, Washington, DC, 1982, US Government Printing Office.
27. Reference deleted in proofs.
28. Hyner GC, Melby CL: *Priorities for health promotion and disease prevention,* Dubuque, Iowa, 1987, Eddie Bowers Publishing.
29. Insel PM, Roth WT: *Core concepts in health,* ed 6, Mountain View, Calif, 1991, Mayfield Publishing.
30. Janz NK, Becker MH: The health belief model: a decade later, *Health Educ Q* 11(1):1-47, 1984.
31. Kolbe L, et al: Propositions for an alternate and complimentary health education paradigm, *Health Educ* 12(3):24, 1981.
32. Kotler P, et al: *Marketing for health care organizations,* Englewood Cliffs, NJ, 1986, Prentice Hall.
33. MacStravic RE: Health care marketing needs rational, ethical approach, *Hosp Prog* 56:60, 1980.
34. Mager RF: *Preparing instructional objectives,* ed 2, Belmont, Calif, 1984, Lake Publishing.
35. Means RK, Nolte AE: Fifty years of health education in AAHPERD: a chronology, 1937-1987, *Health Educ* 18(1):21, 1987.
36. National Task Force for Preparation and Practice of Health Educator, Inc: A guide for the development of competency based curricula for entry level health educators, New York, 1983.
37. Parcel GS, Baronowski T: Social learning theory and health education, *Health Educ* 12(3):14, 1981.
38. Parkinson RS, et al: *Managing health promotion in the workplace,* Palo Alto, Calif, 1982, Mayfield Publishing.
39. Rankin SH, Stallings KD: *Patient education: issues, principles, policies,* ed 2, Philadelphia, 1990, JB Lippincott.
40. Richardson GE, Perry NF: Strength intervention: an approach to lifestyle modification, *Health Educ* 18(3):42, 1987.
41. Rosenstock IM, Becker NH: The social learning theory and health belief model, *Health Educ Q* 15:175, 1988.
42. Rubright R, MacDonald D: *Marketing health and human services,* Germantown, Md, 1981, Aspen.
43. Saunders RP: What is health promotion?, *Health Educ* 19(5):14, 1988.
44. Smith CD: Patient teaching: it's the law, *Nursing,* pp 67-68, 1987.
45. Strecher VJ, et al: The role of self-efficacy in achieving health behavior change, *Health Educ Q* 13:73-92, 1986.
46. Sullivan LW: Partners in prevention: a mobilization plan for implementing health people 2000, *Am J Health Promot* 5(4):291-297, 1991.
47. Timmreck TC, et al: Health education and health promotion: a look at the jungle of supportive fields, philosophies and theoretical foundations, *Health Educ* 18(6):23, 1987.
48. Weiss EH, Kessel G: Practical skills for health educators on using mass media, *Health Educ* 18(3):39, 1987.
49. Williamson FE: *Health education and health planning analysis of health systems plans, focal points,* Washington, DC, 1980, US Department of Health and Human Services.
50. World Health Organization: *Expert committee on health education of the public, first report,* Tech Rep series No 89, Geneva, 1954.

CHAPTER

12

Nutrition Counseling

Arlene Spark

Objectives

After completing this chapter, the nurse will be able to

- *List the Department of Health and Human Services' nutrition objectives for the Year 2000.*
- *List the leading nutrition-related causes of death in the United States and identify the dietary factors associated with each.*
- *Contrast and compare the basic four food groups and the food guide pyramid.*
- *Discuss U.S. food aid programs for the poor and the elderly.*
- *Outline the FDA's new regulations governing food labels.*
- *Plan a 1-day menu that is consistent with recent dietary guidance for a person at any stage of the life cycle from the preschool period to older adulthood.*

NUTRITION TODAY

Food and nutrition have always been vitally important to health. Until as recently as the 1940s, many nutrient-deficiency diseases–rickets, pellagra, scurvy, beriberi, xerophthalmia, and goiter–were still prevalent in the United States. Today, although these conditions (summarized in Table 12-1) do persist in developing countries, they have virtually disappeared from developed areas of the world. An abundant food supply, fortification of some foods with critical trace nutrients, and better methods of determining and improving the nutrient contents of foods have contributed to the decline in these micronutrient-deficiency diseases in technologically advanced countries.

The introduction of iodized salt in the 1920s, for example, contributed greatly to eliminating iodine-deficiency goiter as a public health problem in the United States. Similarly, pellagra disappeared after the discovery that it is caused by inadequate niacin. Today, nutrient deficiencies are rarely reported in the United States. The few cases of protein-energy malnutrition listed annually as causes of death generally occur as secondary results of severe illness or injury, premature birth, child neglect, the problems of the homebound aged, alcoholism, or some combination of these factors.[33]

Although undernutrition still occurs in some groups of people in the United States, including those who are isolated or economically deprived, these once-prevalent diseases have been replaced by another dietary problem.

Dietary Excess and Imbalance

The diseases of nutritional deficiency have been replaced by diseases of dietary excess and imbalance. Problems resulting from overconsumption now rank among the leading causes of illness and death in the

***Table 12-1.* Summary of nutrient deficiency diseases**

Key nutrient involved and deficiency disease	Typical disease symptoms	Major dietary sources for the nutrient
Protein		
Kwashiorkor, protein-calorie malnutrition (PCM)	Growth failure in children (60% to 80% weight-for-age), edema, fatty liver, changes in hair texture, apathy, anorexia	Egg white, beef, fish, poultry, milk, cheese, legumes, nuts
Thiamin		
Beriberi	Nerve degeneration, poor muscle coordination, enlarged heart, abnormal heart rhythms	Pork, sunflower seeds, dried beans, wheat germ
Niacin		
Pellagra	The 3 D's (diarrhea, dermatitis, dementia), anorexia	Wheat bran, beef, mushrooms, salmon, tuna
Vitamin C		
Scurvy	Impaired wound healing, bleeding gums and skin, frequent infections	Citrus fruits, broccoli, strawberries, cabbage
Vitamin A		
Xerophthalmia	Blindness, poor growth, increased infections, cracks in teeth	Liver, fortified milk, sweet potatoes, pumpkin, mustard greens
Iron		
Iron-deficiency anemia	Poor growth, reduced resistance to infections, reduced learning ability in children	Red meats, oysters, clams, tofu (soybean curd), spinach
Iodine		
Goiter, cretinism	Enlarged thyroid gland, weight gain, mental and physical retardation in infants	Seafood, crops grown in iodine-rich soil (coastal areas), iodized salt

United States. Table 12-2 lists the major killers. Four of the leading causes of death in the United States are directly associated with diet–coronary heart disease, some types of cancer, stroke, and diabetes mellitus. Four more–accidents, cirrhosis of the liver, suicide, and homicide–are associated with excessive alcohol intake.[39]

Almost two thirds of U.S. deaths every year are caused by heart disease, cancers, or stroke. Figs. 12-1, 12-2, and 12-3 illustrate the 1989 death rates for these three diseases, according to race and sex.

Encouraging healthy choices in diet, exercise, and weight control is one of the major themes of *Healthy People 2000.* Dietary factors contribute substantially to the burden of preventable illness and premature death. *Healthy People* is aimed at bringing American dietary patterns into line with dietary recommendations based on the *Dietary Guidelines.*[32,34]

Year 2000 Objectives

The 22 priority areas contain 300 specific national health promotion and disease prevention objectives targeted for achievement by the year 2000. The nutrition area contains 21 of the *Healthy People* objectives; they are listed in the box on p. 268.[31] Year 2000 nutrition objectives are emphasized throughout this chapter.

***Table 12-2.* The 10 leading causes of death in the United States, 1990**

Rank	Cause of death	Percentage of total
1*	Heart diseases	34
2*	Cancers	23
3*	Strokes	17
4†	Unintentional injuries	9
	Motor vehicle accidents	2
	All other accidents	2
5	Chronic obstructive lung diseases	4
6	Pneumonia and influenza	4
7*	Diabetes mellitus	2
8†	Suicide	1
9†	Homicide and legal intervention	1
10†	Chronic liver disease and cirrhosis	1
	All causes	100

Source: NCHS statistics for 1990, cited in Wardlaw GM, Insel PM: *Perspectives in nutrition,* ed 2, St Louis, 1993, Mosby.

Note: Acquired immunodificiency syndrome (AIDS) is ranked 11.

*Cause of death in which diet plays a part.

†Cause of death in which excessive alcohol consumption plays a part.

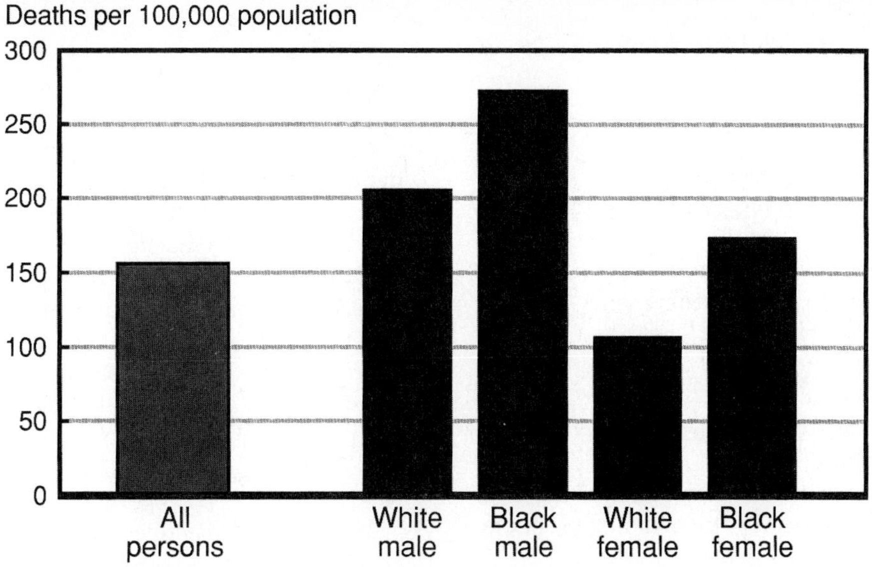

Fig. 12-1. Death rates for heart disease, according to race and sex, United States, 1989. (*Source:* National Center for Health Statistics, National Vital Statistics System.)

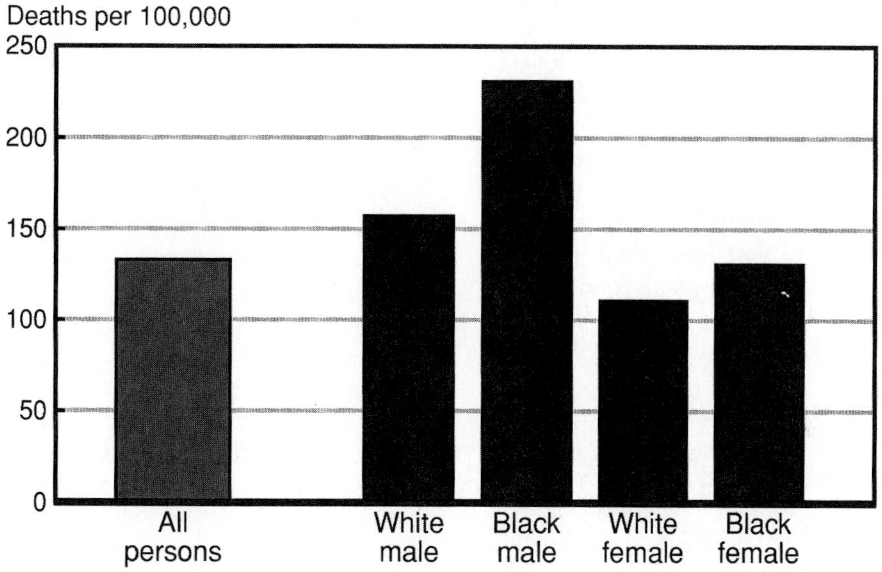

Fig. 12-2. Death rates for cancer, according to race and sex, United States, 1989. (*Source:* National Center for Health Statistics, National Vital Statistics System.)

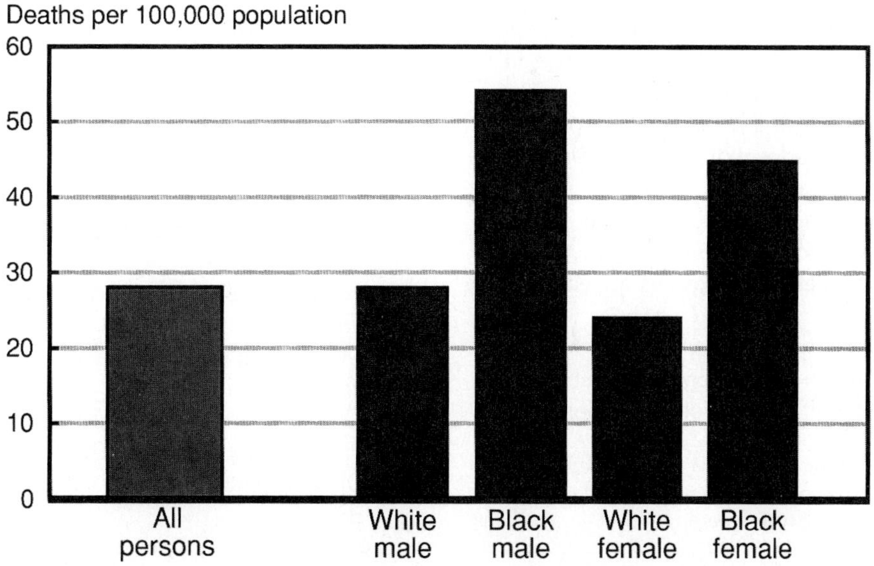

Fig. 12-3. Death rates for stroke, according to race and sex, United States, 1989. (*Source:* National Center for Health Statistics, National Vital Statistics System.)

NUTRITION OBJECTIVES FOR HEALTH PROMOTION AND DISEASE PREVENTION

- Reduce coronary heart disease
- Reverse the rise in cancer deaths
- Reduce overweight
- Reduce growth retardation
- Reduce dietary fat intake
- Increase complex carbohydrate and fiber-containing foods
- Increase sound dietary practices combined with regular physical activity to attain appropriate body weight
- Increase calcium intake
- Decrease salt and sodium intake
- Reduce iron deficiency
- Increase the number of mothers who breastfeed their babies
- Increase the number of patients and care givers who use feeding practices that prevent baby-bottle tooth decay
- Increase the use of food labels to make nutritious food selections easier
- Achieve useful and informative labeling for all processed foods and most fresh meat, poultry, fish, fruits, vegetables, baked goods, and ready-to-eat or carry-out foods
- Increase the availability of reduced-fat processed foods
- Increase the number of restaurants and institutional food service operations that offer identifiable low-fat, low-calorie food choices consistent with the dietary guidelines for Americans
- Increase the number of school lunch and breakfast services and child care food services with menus consistent with the nutrition principles in the dietary guidelines for Americans
- Increase the receipt of home food services by people aged 65 and older who have difficulty in preparing their own meals or are otherwise in need of home-delivered meals
- Increase the number of the nation's schools that provide nutrition education from preschool through twelfth grade
- Increase the number of work sites with 50 or more employees that offer nutrition education and weight management programs for employees
- Increase the number of primary care providers who offer nutritional assessment and counseling and referral to qualified nutritionists or dietitians.

Source: US Department of Health and Human Services: *Healthy people 2000: national health promotion and disease prevention objectives,* Washington, DC, 1991, Public Health Service.

HEART DISEASE

Although there has been a dramatic decline in heart disease mortality in the past two decades, about seven million Americans are still affected by coronary artery disease. Despite reductions in the major risk factors for heart disease (high blood pressure, high blood cholesterol, and smoking), this condition continues to be the leading cause of death for both men and women in the United States.[3] In 1989, as Fig. 12-1 illustrates, almost three quarters of a million people died from diseases of the heart. The age-adjusted death rate was 155.9 per 100,000 people for the United States population as a whole.[11]

Year 2000 Objective: Reduce coronary artery disease deaths to no more than 1000 per 100,000 people.

Heart disease is a special problem in the black population. In 1989, black males were about one-third more likely than white males to die from heart disease, with a death rate of 272.7 per 100,000 people, compared with a rate of 205.9 for white males. Black women were about 60% more likely to die from heart disease than white women, with a death rate of 172.9 per 100,000, compared with a rate of 106.6 for white women.[11]

Year 2000 Objective: Reduce coronary artery disease in Blacks to no more than 115 per 100,000.

Elevated serum cholesterol is one of the risk factors for coronary heart disease. The National Cholesterol Education Program (NCEP) offers recommendations for nutrient intake intended to lower average population levels of blood cholesterol in people over two years old living in the United States.[12,36] In 1976-1980, diets of U.S. adults provided 36% of calories from total fat and 13% of calories from saturated fat.[31] Similarly, preliminary data from 1987-1988 indicate that U.S. children have an average dietary intake of 35% to 36% of calories from total fat and 14% of calories from saturated fat.[36] The NCEP recommends a low-saturated fat, low-cholesterol eating pattern in order to lower the

NCEP RECOMMENDATIONS

- Total fat–an average of no more than 30% of total calories
- Saturated fatty acids–less than 10% of total calories
- Polyunsaturated fatty acids–up to 10% of total calories
- Monounsaturated fatty acids–remaining total fat calories
- Carbohydrates–about 55% of total calories
- Protein–about 15% to 20% of total calories
- Dietary cholesterol–less than 300 mg per day.[12,36]

average population levels of blood cholesterol in children over the age of two, adolescents, and adults (see box on p. 268).

Energy (calories) should be adequate to support growth and development and to reach and maintain desirable body weight (in children)[36] and to maintain desirable weight (in adults).[12]

These dietary guidelines should be met by eating a wide variety of foods. Table 12-3 lists the recommended number of servings from each food group to provide

***Table 12-3.* Step-one diet: an example of how nutrient recommendations can be translated into servings per day for different age groups**

	Age (years)						
	Child 2-3	Child 4-6	Child 7-10	Male 11-14	Female 11-14	Male 15-18	Female 15-18
Food group							
Meat, Poultry, and Fish (oz)	2	5	6	6	6	6	6
Eggs (per week)*	3	3	3	3	3	3	3
Dairy Products (servings)	3	3	4	4	4	4	4
Fats and Oils (servings)	4	5	5	7	5	10	5
Breads and Cereals (servings)†	5	6	7	9	8	12	8
Vegetables (servings)	3	3	3	4	3	4	3
Fruits (servings)	22	3	3	3	3	5	3
Sweets and Modified Fat Desserts (servings)‡	1	2	2	3	2	3	2
Nutrients							
Recommended Dietary Allowance (RDA) for Energy (cal)	1,300	1,800	2,000	2,500	2,200	3,000	2,200
Actual Energy (cal)	1,317	1,786	2,025	2,522	2,221	3,011	2,221
Fat (g)	46	62	70	86	73	103	73
(% cal)	(30)	(31)	(31)	(30)	(29)	(30)	(29)
Carbohydrate (g)	177	230	255	338	294	418	294
(% cal)	(52)	(50)	(49)	(52)	(52)	(54)	(52)
Protein (g)	59	87	104	114	109	125	109
(% cal)	(18)	(19)	(20)	(18)	(19)	(16)	(19)
Fatty acids§ and cholesterol							
Saturated Fatty Acids (g)	15	20	23	26	24	29	24
(% cal)	(10)	(10)	(10)	(9)	(9)	(9)	(9)
Monounsaturated Fatty Acids (g)	16	23	25	31	26	37	26
(% cal)	(11)	(11)	(11)	(11)	(11)	(11)	(11)
Polyunsaturated Fatty Acids (g)	10	14	14	20	16	26	16
(% cal)	(7)	(7)	(6)	(7)	(6)	(8)	(6)
Cholesterol (mg)	183	256	294	295	295	296	295
(mg chol/1,000 cal)	(139)	(143)	(145)	(117)	(133)	(98)	(133)
Fat-Soluble Vitamins							
Vitamin A (IU)	10,945	11,451	11,891	15,163	12,066	16,282	12,066
(% RDA)	(<100)	(>100)	(>100)	(>100)	(>100)	(>100)	(>100)
Water-Soluble Vitamins							
Vitamin C (mg)	122	148	153	184	158	233	158
(% RDA)	(306)	(329)	(339)	(367)	(316)	(387)	(316)

Source: US Department of Health and Human Services, Public Health Service, National Institutes of Health, National Heart, Lung, and Blood Institute, National Cholesterol Education Program: *Report of the expert panel on blood cholesterol levels in children and adolescents,* 1991, NIH Pub 91-2732.

*Nutrient analysis is for three eggs per week; with four eggs per week, the average dietary cholesterol increases by 30 mg/day.

†The Breads and Cereals food group includes bread, cereal, pasta, rice, starch vegetables, *and* dry beans and peas.

‡Each of these counts as 1 serving if prepared with egg whites or egg substitutes, skim milk or 1% milk, and unsaturated oil or margarine: 2 cookies; 1 slice of cake or pie; 1/2 cup pudding. Each of these counts as 1 serving: 1/2 tablespoons of sugar, syrup, honey, jam or preserves; 1 slice angel food cake; 1 fig bar; 1/2 cup fruit-flavored gelatin.

§The values for total fat are greater than the sum of saturated, monounsaturated, and polyunsaturated fatty acids since total fat includes fatty acids plus other fatty substances and glycerol.

||Values include a standard amount of salt added to foods in the meat, poultry, and fish group; vegetables group; and breads and cereals group. Values do not include salt added at the table or sodium present in the water supply.

Continued.

***Table 12-3.* Step-one diet: an example of how nutrient recommendations can be translated into servings per day for different age groups – cont'd**

	Age (years)						
	Child 2-3	Child 4-6	Child 7-10	Male 11-14	Female 11-14	Male 15-18	Female 15-18
Thiamin (mg)	1.3	1.7	2.0	2.4	2.1	2.9	2.1
(% RDA)	(188)	(190)	(196)	(184)	(195)	(196)	(195)
Riboflavin (mg)	1.7	2.1	2.5	2.8	2.6	3.2	2.6
(% RDA)	(213)	(188)	(206)	(186)	(200)	(175)	(200)
Niacin (mg)	13.4	20.9	24.2	28.1	25.9	32.9	25.9
(% RDA)	(149)	(174)	(186)	(165)	(173)	(165)	(173)
Vitamin B6 (mg)	1.6	2.2	2.5	2.8	2.6	3.4	2.6
(% RDA)	(160)	(198)	(175)	(165)	(184)	(172)	(184)
Folacin (μg)	267	316	351	431	379	537	379
(% RDA)	(535)	(422)	(351)	(287)	(252)	(269)	(252)
Vitamin B12 (μg)	3.4	4.7	5.8	6.1	6.0	6.6	6.0
(% RDA)	(492)	(472)	(415)	(307)	(299)	(330)	(299)
Minerals							
Calcium (mg)	889	948	1,190	1,287	1,226	1,380	1,226
(% RDA)	(111)	(119)	(149)	(107)	(102)	(115)	(102)
Phosphorus (mg)	1,100	1,365	1,651	1,852	1,738	2,073	1,738
(% RDA)	(138)	(171)	(206)	(154)	(145)	(173)	(145)
Magnesium (mg)	265	327	377	449	406	547	406
(% RDA)	(332)	(272)	(222)	(166)	(145)	(137)	(145)
Iron (mg)	10.8	14.5	16.5	20.3	18.1	24.7	18.1
(% RDA)	(108)	(145)	(165)	(169)	(121)	(206)	(121)
Zinc (mg)	7.8	11.6	13.8	15.2	14.4	16.9	14.4
(% RDA)	(78)	(116)	(138)	(101)	(120)	(112)	(120)
Sodium‖	2,093	2,780	3,234	3,859	3,479	4,485	3,479

diets for children that meet the NCEP goals outlined above. Tables 12-4, 12-5, and 12-6 provide sample "heart-healthy" menus for school children. The "healthier" menus are compared to the typical higher-fat foods children are currently eating.

The dietary guidelines described here apply to everyone over the age of 2 years. They are intended to help prevent the development of elevated cholesterol levels. Many children, adolescents, and adults, who already have undesirable levels of lipids in their blood, should receive nutrition counseling if their total cholesterol and LDL-cholesterol levels are elevated, as defined in Table 12-7. Initially, individualized nutrition guidance includes emphasizing the same NCEP low-saturated fat, low-cholesterol recommendations outlined above. But now, these recommendations are referred to as the step-one diet–the first step in the dietary treatment of hypercholesterolemia (see box on p. 274).

The goal of diet therapy is to lower LDL-cholesterol and total cholesterol levels. An additional goal for obese hypercholesterolemic individuals is to help them achieve and maintain healthy body weight. After the step-one diet is explained to the client, follow-up sessions are scheduled to monitor lipid levels and dietary compliance. In 3 to 6 months, if acceptable lipid levels have not been achieved, the client should be referred to a registered dietitian who will attempt a second step-one trial period before progressing to a diet limited in saturated fats to 7% of total caloric intake. This is known as the step-two diet (the second and slightly more aggressive step in the dietary treatment of hypercholesterolemia). The lipoprotein analysis should be repeated after 3 months.[12,36] For patients over 10 years of age, drug therapy is considered if diet therapy alone is not effective.[36]

STROKE

In 1989, the age-adjusted death rate for strokes in the United States was 28.0 per 100,000 people. Black males have the highest rate of stroke among all population groups (see Fig. 12-3). In 1989, their rate was 54.1 per 100,000, almost twice the 28.0 rate for white males. Black males were also 20% more likely to die from stroke than black females. Black females, with a death rate of 44.9, were about 86% more likely to die from stroke than white females, at a rate of 24.1.[12]

Year 2000 Objective: Reduce stroke deaths to no more than 20 per 100,000 people.

***Table 12-4.* Sample menus for children 7-10 with school lunch**

Typical	Step-one diet	Step-two diet
Breakfast at Home Orange juice (1/2 cup) Oatmeal w/maple and brown sugar (1 packet) Whole milk (1 cup)	**Breakfast at Home** Orange juice (1/2 cup) Oatmeal w/maple and brown sugar (1 packet) 1% milk (1 cup)	**Breakfast at Home** Orange juice (1/2 cup) Oatmeal w/maple and brown sugar (1 packet) Margarine (2 tsp) Skim milk (1 cup)
School lunch Oven fried chicken w/skin Mashed potatoes (1/2 cup) Green beans w/butter (1/2 cup) Canned pear (1/2) Whole milk (1 cup)	**School lunch** Oven fried chicken w/skin Mashed potatoes (1/2 cup) Green beans w/butter (1/2 cup) Canned pear (1/2) 2% milk (1 cup)	**Bag lunch** Ham sandwich: Bread (2 slices) Lean ham (2 oz) Mayonnaise (2 tsp) Lettuce, tomato, pickles Banana (1 med.) Skin milk (1 cup)
Snack at home Ham sandwich: Bread (2 slices) Ham luncheon meat (1 oz) Lettuce, tomato, pickle Mayonnaise (1/2 tbsp) Cola drink (1 can)	**Snack at home** Turkey sandwich: Bread (2 slices) Turkey luncheon meat (1 1/2 oz) Low-fat cheese (1 oz) Lettuce, tomato, pickle Mayonnaise (1 tsp) Cola drink (1 can)	**Snack at home** Turkey sandwich: Bread (2 slices) Turkey luncheon meat (1 1/2 oz) Low-fat cheese (1 oz) Lettuce, tomato, pickle Margarine (1 tsp) Mayonnaise (1 tsp) Cola drink (1 can)
Dinner at home Tuna macaroni casserole (1 serving) Carrots and peas (1/2 cup) Roll (1 small) Applesauce (1/2 cup) Water	**Dinner at home** Tuna macaroni casserole* (1 serving) Carrots and peas (1/2 cup) Roll (1 small) Margarine (1 tsp) Applesauce (1/2 cup) Water	**Dinner at home** Tuna macaroni casserole† (1 serving) Carrots and peas (1/2 cup) Margarine (2 tsp) Applesauce (1/2 cup) Water
Snack at home Chocolate brownie (2" x 1") Whole milk (1 cup)	**Snack at home** Oatmeal cookies, commercial (4 medium) 1% milk (1 cup)	**Snack at home** Oatmeal cookies, homemade† (4 medium) Skim milk (1 cup)
Calories: 2008	**Calories:** 2005	**Calories:** 1966
Fat, % cal: 35	**Fat, % cal:** 29	**Fat, % cal:** 29
SFA, % cal: 15	**SFA, % cal:** 11	**SFA, % cal:** 7
Cholesterol, mg: 261	**Cholesterol, mg:** 188	**Cholesterol, mg:** 126

Source: US Department of Health and Human Services, Public Health Service, National Institutes of Health, National Heart, Lung, and Blood Institute, National Cholesterol Education Program: *Report of the expert panel on blood cholesterol levels in children and adolescents,* 1991, NIH Pub 91-2732.

*Stick margarine used for food preparation.

†Tub margarine used for food preparation.

The modifiable nutrition-related risk factors for stroke include obesity, habitual high alcohol intake, and high intake of sodium. There is no certain method for identifying susceptible people or ascertaining how many of them become hypertensive as a result of excessive salt intake. The conservative preventive health approach is therefore to recommend a salt intake limited to 6 g or less per day for adults.[14] *Sodium chloride* is approximately 40% sodium by weight. Therefore, a diet with 6 g of salt contains about 2.4 g sodium. This is regarded as mild sodium restriction.

There are three major sources of sodium in our diet:

1. Salt added to food during cooking or at the table
2. Salt added as an ingredient to almost all processed foods (such as baked goods, that do not taste salty)
3. Salt that occurs naturally in foods, such as water and all animal products. Most unprocessed food is low in sodium content

***Table 12-5.* Sample menus for girls 11-14 with fast food lunch**

Typical	Step-one diet	Step-two diet
Breakfast at Home	**Breakfast at Home**	**Breakfast at Home**
Orange juice (1 cup)	Orange juice (1 cup)	Orange juice (1 cup)
Pre-sweetened cereal (1 cup)	Corn flakes (3/4 cup)	Corn flakes (3/4 cup)
Whole milk (1 cup)	1% milk (1 cup)	Skim milk (1 cup)
		English muffin (1/2)
		Margarine‡ (1 tsp)
Fast food lunch	**Fast food lunch**	**Sandwich shop**
Cheeseburger	Hamburger (1/4 lb.)	Tuna sandwich:
French fries (1 regular order)	French fries (1 regular order)	Bread (2 slices)
Catsup (3 packets)	Lettuce, tomato, onion, catsup	Tuna, water pack (3 oz)
Cola drink (1 small)	Animal crackers (1/2 box)	Tomato, celery, relish
	Cola drink (1 medium)	Mayonnaise (4 tsp)
		Pretzels (3/4-oz bag)
		Oatmeal cookies, homemade‡ (4)
		Cola drink (1 medium)
Snack at home	**Snack at home**	**Snack at home**
Ginger snaps (2 medium)	Multigrain low-fat crackers (4)	Multigrain low-fat crackers (4)
Club soda (1 can)	Low-fat cheese (3/4 oz)	Low-fat cheese (3/4 oz)
	Club soda (1 can)	Club soda (1 can)
Dinner at home	**Dinner at home**	**Dinner at home**
Fried chicken breast, breaded and fried in shortening, skin eaten	Broiled chicken, breast, no skin (3 oz.)	Broiled chicken, breast, no skin (3 oz.)
Boiled potato* (1)	Boiled potato† (1)	Boiled potato‡ (1)
Roll (1 small)	Broccoli spears† (4)	Broccoli spears‡ (4)
Margarine† (1 tsp)	Tomato (4 slices)	Tomato (4 slices)
Iced tea (1 cup)	Bread (1 slice)	Bread (1 slice)
	Strawberries (1/2 cup)	Margarine‡ (2 tsp)
	Nonfat yogurt (1 container)	Strawberries (1/2 cup)
	Water	Nonfat yogurt (1 container)
		Water
Snack at home	**Snack at home**	**Snack at home**
American cheese (3/4 oz)	Cupcake, commercial (1)	Cupcake homemade (1)
Crackers (4)	1% milk (1 cup)	Skim milk (1 cup)
Fruit drink (1/2 cup)		
Calories: 2219	**Calories:** 2240	**Calories:** 2248
Fat, % cal: 35	**Fat, % cal:** 29	**Fat, % cal:** 27
SFA, % cal: 15	**SFA, % cal:** 10	**SFA, % cal:** 6
Cholesterol, mg: 264	**Cholesterol, mg:** 188	**Cholesterol, mg:** 159

Source: US Department of Health and Human Services, Public Health Service, National Institutes of Health, National Heart, Lung, and Blood Institute, National Cholesterol Education Program: *Report of the expert panel on blood cholesterol levels in children and adolescents,* 1991, NIH Pub 91-2732.

*Seasoned with butter.

†Stick margarine used in food preparation.

‡Tub margarine used in food preparation.

Since sodium occurs naturally in many foods and is also added to most processed food, salt should be used only sparingly in home cooking and not at all at the table. Salty, highly processed salty, salt-preserved, and salt-pickled foods should be eaten sparingly.[11] Table 12-8 shows the sodium content of representative foods.

Year 2000 Objective: Decrease salt and sodium intake so that at least 65% of home meal preparers prepare foods without adding salt, at least 60% of people avoid using salt at the table, and at least 40% of adults regularly purchase foods modified to contain less sodium.

CANCER

About 20% of the deaths in the United States are caused by cancer–in 1989, almost one-half million people. Overall, cancer mortality rates have not changed much since 1950, when the age-adjusted rate

***Table 12-6.* Sample menus for 15-to-19-year-old males with fast food lunch**

Typical		Step-one diet		Step-two diet	
Breakfast at Home		**Breakfast at Home**		**Breakfast at Home**	
Orange juice (1 cup)		Orange juice (1 cup)		Orange juice (1 cup)	
Granola cereal (1/2 cup)		Presweetened corn flakes (3/4 cup)		Presweetened corn flakes (3/4 cup)	
Whole milk (1 cup)		Margarine (1 tsp)		Margarine (2 tsp)	
		Bagel (1)		Bagel (1)	
		1% milk (1 cup)		Skim milk (1 cup)	
Fast food lunch		**Sandwich shop**		**Sandwich shop**	
Hot dog on bun w/chili (1)		Roast beef sandwich		Roast beef sandwich	
Potato chips (1 oz)		Tossed salad (2 cups)		Tossed salad (2 cups)	
Cola drink (12 fl. oz)		Thousand island dressing (2 tbsp)		Thousand island dressing (3 tbsp)	
		Corn chips (1-oz bag)		Medium cola drink	
		Medium cola drink			
Snack at home		**Snack at home**		**Snack at home**	
Chocolate candy bar (2 oz)		Ham and cheese sandwich:		Turkey and cheese sandwich:	
Cola drink (12 fl. oz)		Bread (2 slices)		Bread (2 slices)	
		Low-fat ham (1 oz)		Turkey breast (1 oz)	
		Low-fat cheese (1 oz)		Low-fat cheese (1 oz)	
		Mayonnaise (2 tsp)		Lettuce, tomato, pickles	
		Lettuce, tomato, pickles		Mayonnaise (2 tsp)	
		Oatmeal cookies, commercial (4)		Pretzels (3/4-oz bag)	
		Orange juice (1 cup)		Gingersnaps (5)	
				Orange juice (1 cup)	
Dinner at home		**Dinner at home**		**Dinner at home**	
Beef lasagna (4" x 3")		Chicken cacciatore (3 oz.)		Chicken cacciatore (3 oz)	
Tossed salad (2 cups)		Green beans (1/2 cup)*		Green beans (1/2 cup)†	
Thousand island dressing (3 tbsp)		Rice, white (1 cup)		Rice, white (1 cup)†	
French bread (1 slice)		Margarine (1 tsp)		Margarine (1 1/2 tsp)†	
Brownies (2 each 2" x 1")		Bread (1 slice)		Bread (1 slice)	
Whole milk (1 cup)		Grapes (15)		Grapes (15)	
		Nonfat yogurt w/fruit flavor (1 cup)		Nonfat yogurt w/fruit flavor (1 cup)	
		Water		Water	
Snack at home		**Snack at home**		**Snack at home**	
Frozen yogurt (1 cup)		Peanut butter cookies, homemade (6)		Apple pie, homemade,† single crust (1/8 of 9")	
Cola drink (12 fl. oz)		1% milk (1 cup)		Skim milk (1 cup)	
Calories:	**2998**	**Calories:**	**3026**	**Calories:**	**2993**
Fat, % cal:	**36**	**Fat, % cal:**	**30**	**Fat, % cal:**	**29**
SFA, % cal:	**15**	**SFA, % cal:**	**9**	**SFA, % cal:**	**7**
Cholesterol, mg:	**258**	**Cholesterol, mg:**	**224**	**Cholesterol, mg:**	**157**

Source: US Department of Health and Human Services, Public Health Service, National Institutes of Health, National Heart, Lung, and Blood Institute, National Cholesterol Education Program: *Report of the expert panel on blood cholesterol levels in children and adolescents,* 1991, NIH Pub 91-2732.

*Stick margarine used for food preparation.

†Tub margarine used for food preparation.

per 100,000 was 125.3, rising to 133.0 in 1989.[11]

In 1989, black males experienced a risk of cancer 18% higher than that of white males and 41% lower survival rates. Black males had a 48% higher age-adjusted incidence of lung cancer and slightly lower survival rates than did white males. Black males also had a 33% higher incidence of prostate cancer, with 20% lower survival time than that of white males. Among females, although breast cancer incidence was 17% lower for black women than for whites, 5-year relative survival rates were 24% lower for black females than for whites. Lung cancer incidence rates were almost identical for black and for white females in 1989, but relative survival rates were 25% lower for black women.[12]

As illustrated in Fig. 12-2, the 1989 death rate for cancer for black males was higher than that for any

***Table 12-7.* Cutpoints of total and LDL-cholesterol for dietary intervention in children and adults**

	Total cholesterol (mg/dl)		LDL cholesterol		
	(age in years)				
Category	**2-20***	**>20†**	**2-20***	**>20†**	**Dietary intervention**
Acceptable	<170	<200	<110	<130	Recommend NCEP low-saturated fat, low-cholesterol eating pattern
Borderline	170-199	200-239	110-129	130-159	Diet therapy emphasizing a maximum of 10% of calories as saturated fats
High	≥200	≥240	≥130	≥160	Diet therapy emphasizing a maximum of 7% of calories as saturated fats

*US Department of Health and Human Services, Public Health Service, National Institutes of Health, National Heart, Lung, and Blood Institute, National Cholesterol Education Program: *Report of the expert panel on blood cholesterol levels in children and adolescents,* 1991, NIH Pub 91-2732.

†National Cholesterol Education Program: Report of the National Cholesterol Education Program Expert Panel on Detection, Evaluation, and Treatment of High Blood Cholesterol in Adults, *Arch Intern Med* 148:36, 1988.

other group identified by race and sex. Their death rate was 230.6 per 100,000, 47 higher than that for white males, who had a rate of 157.2; 76 higher than that for black females, 130.9 per 100,000; and more than twice as high as that for white females, 110.7 per 100,000.[11]

Year 2000 Objective: Reverse the rise in cancer deaths to no more than 130 per 100,000 people.

It is estimated that one third of cancer deaths are diet-related.[14] Some researchers believe that 40% of cancer incidence among men and 60% among women is related to diet. The associations between diet and cancer causation may be summarized as follows:

Cancer site	**Dietary factors**
Esophagus	Alcohol (especially with tobacco)
Stomach	Salt-preserved foods; low levels of fruits and vegetables
Colon, rectum	Fat (particularly saturated)
	Low vegetable intake
Liver	Alcohol
Lung	Greens and yellow vegetables appear protective
Breast	High-calorie diet (high fat and low fiber suspected)
Endometrium	Diet-related diseases (obesity, hypertension, NIDDM)
Bladder	Unknown
Prostate	High-fat diets

Year 2000 Objective: Increase complex carbohydrate and fiber-containing foods in the diets of adults to five or more daily servings for vegetables (including legumes) and fruits and to six or more daily servings for grain products. It is considered prudent for chil-

❑ ❑ RESEARCH ABSTRACT

One way of promoting a reduction in dietary fat intake is by changing the diet of family members. This study investigated the long-term effects of a low-fat dietary intervention on husbands of women who participated in the Women's Health Trial (WHT) from 1985 until the trial's completion in 1988. The WHT was a large multicentered randomized trial designed to assess a low-fat dietary intervention among women at moderately increased risk for breast cancer.

A year after the end of the WHT, a randomly selected sample of participants' husbands was sent dietary and health questionnaires as part of a follow-up study of the maintenance of low-fat diet among WHT participants.

The researchers found an absolute difference of 4 percentage points in fat intake between control husbands and intervention husbands. Husbands in the control group (n = 180) were consuming 36.9% of their calories from fat, compared with intervention husbands (n = 188) whose fat intake was 32.9% of their calories. The wife's attitude and fat intake were among the most important predictors of her husband's fat intake, indicating that the effect of the WHT intervention on the husbands of the participants was more probably attributable to their acceptance of lower-fat foods served at home than to their own overt actions.

The results of this study suggest that a dietary intervention aimed at women can have an effect on their husbands and may be a cost-effective approach to a healthy dietary change for both women and men.

From Shattuck AI, White E, Kristal AR: How women's adopted low-fat diets affect their husbands, *Am J Pub Health* 82:1244-1250, 1992.

***Table 12-8.* Approximate sodium content of foods**

Food group	High	mg Na	Low	mg Na
Grain products	English muffin	300	White rice, 1 cup	6
	Waffle, 1 frozen	275	Popcorn, 3 cups	3
	Potato chips, 10	200	Puffed rice, 2 cups	2
	White bread, 1 slice	115	Oatmeal, 3/4 cup	1
	Saltine crackers, 2	70	Wheat germ, toasted, 1/4 cup	1
Meat, poultry, fish	Herring, 3 oz smoked	5235	Codfish, 3 oz	65
	Frankfurter, 1 oz	310	Chicken, 3 oz	60
	Ham, 3 oz baked	280	Beef, 3 oz	55
	Bacon, 2 strips	275	Turkey, 3 oz	50
	Bologna, 1 slice	220		
	Scallops, 3 oz	215		
	Lobster, 3 oz	180		
	Shrimp, 3 oz	115		
Dairy products	Cottage cheese, 1/2 cup	460	Yogurt, 1/2 cup, frozen	60
	American cheese, 1 slice	405	Ricotta, 1 oz, whole milk	24
	Buttermilk, 1 cup	240	Cottage cheese, 1/2 cup dry curd	10
	Gouda cheese, 1 oz	230		
	Cheddar cheese, 1 oz	175		
	Yogurt, 1 cup lowfat	175		
	Milk, 1 cup	120		
	Butter, 1 tbsp	100		
Fruits and vegetables	Sauerkraut, 1 cup	1555	All fresh fruits	0-20
	Mushrooms, 1 cup, canned	800	Brussels sprouts, 1 cup	15
	Spinach, 1 cup canned	780	Mushrooms, 1 cup, fresh	10
	Creamed corn, 1 cup canned	670	Potato, 1 medium	5
	Tomato juice, 1 cup	500	Corn, 1 cup, fresh or frozen	2
	Tomatoes, 1 cup canned	430		
	Peas, 1 cup, canned	490		
	Corn, 1 cup, canned, whole kernel	385		
	Celery, 1 cup, diced	130		
	Orange drink, 1 cup	80		
	Lemonade, 1 cup	60		
Miscellaneous	Garlic salt, 1 tsp	1850	Peanuts, 1 cup, unsalted	8
	Dill pickle, 1 large	1430	Jam or jelly, 1 tbsp	2
	Soy sauce, 1 tbsp	1030	Vinegar, 1/2 cup	1
	Baking soda, 1 tsp	1000	Lemon juice, 1 tbsp	1
	Olives, 10 small green	685	Yeast, 1 pkg. dry	1
	MSG, 1 tbsp	490	Honey, 1 tbsp	1
	Bouillon, 1 cube	425	Garlic powder, 1 tsp	1
	Baking powder, 1 tsp	370	Vegetable oil, 1 tbsp	0
	Catsup, 2 tbsp	355		
	Margarine, 1 tbsp	135		

dren aged 2 and older and adolescents to progress toward this objective, as well.[31]

The National Cancer Institute recommends that adult diets contain between 20 and 30 grams of fiber daily (not to exceed 35 grams because of possible adverse effects). Typical diets in the United States contain only about 11. Foods high in fiber are usually low in fat. Table 12-9 lists the fiber content of some common foods. Note that the plant kingdom is the only source of fiber-containing foods.

OSTEOPOROSIS

Osteoporosis is a slowly developing condition that results in loss of bone mass and increased fractures, especially in the wrist, hip, and spine areas. Bone mass tends to decrease after the fourth or fifth decade of life.[18] In the United States, osteoporosis afflicts 24 million Americans–half the women over the age of 45 and 90 of women over 75.[14] The health costs associated with osteoporotic fractures have been estimated at 5 to 6 billion dollars annually.[6]

***Table 12-9.* Fiber in foods**

Grams	
16-20	1 cup baked beans; 1 cup chili with beans
10-15	1/3 cup All Bran with extra fiber; 1 cup fresh blackberries
8-9	1/3 cup All Bran; 1/2 cup stewed prunes; 1/4 cup dried apricots
5-7	1/4 cup shelled almonds; 1 cup lentil soup; 1/2 cup cooked spinach; 1 cup fresh blueberries; 1/2 cup homemade granola
3-4	1 small sweet potato or medium baked potato with skin; 1 medium banana, apple or nectarine; 1 cup fresh raspberries, strawberries, or pineapple chunks; 1/2 cup canned corn or peas; 1/2 cup garbanzo beans (chickpeas) or lima beans; 1/2 cup cooked broccoli or eggplant; 1/4 cup shelled peanuts; 1/2 cup bran cereal; 4 Rye Crisp crackers or 1 oz Kavli, Wasa, Finn, or Triscuit crackers; 3 cups popcorn
2-3	1 medium tomato or carrot; 1 slice whole wheat bread; 1 small orange or pear; 1/2 cup applesauce or fruit cocktail; 1/4 cup shredded coconut; 1 cup grapefruit sections; 2 tbsp peanut butter; 1/2 cup cabbage; 1/2 cup cooked brown rice; 1/4 cup sunflower seeds; 1 tbsp tahini (sesame butter); 1 cup New England clam chowder
1-2	1/2 cup cooked white rice; 1/2 cup cooked cauliflower; 2 stalks celery; 1/6 head lettuce; 10 grapes or 1 cup grape juice; 1 plum; 1 cup vegetable juice cocktail; 10 green olives; 1 cup Manhattan clam chowder
>1	1 slice white bread or 1 bagel; 1 cup pineapple juice; dill pickle; 1 cup tomato soup
0	Milk, yogurt, cheese, ice cream, meat, fish, poultry; butter, margarine, mayonnaise, oil

Osteoporosis is eight times more common among women. Besides set, the most important determinants of fractures are inherited skeletal mass, which may be related to race–Orientals and Caucasians being at the greatest risk; lack of regular weight-bearing exercise such as jogging, walking, or tennis; underweight; suboptimal calcium nutriture; and dietary excesses of fiber, caffeine, protein, or alcohol.

The relative importance of dietary calcium in bone health varies over the lifespan, and 60% of the deposition of final bone mass occurs during the prepubertal growth spurt. Calcium inadequacy during these 2 to 3 years can reduce a girl's ability to achieve her genetic potential for bone mass. Researchers have found that calcium supplementation of 1000 mg per day for 3 years in prepubertal identical twins resulted in increased bone mass at the spine, hip, and radius of supplemented twins compared to their unsupplemented sisters. From these findings, the researchers conclude that increased calcium intake during pubescence could increase peak bone mass and reduce fracture risk in later life.[10]

Data on calcium and age-related bone loss during premenopause indicate that vertebral bone mineral density is almost 7 percent higher in women consuming roughly 120 percent of the recommended dietary allowance (RDA) for calcium daily than it is among women consuming two thirds of the recommended intake.[10] Unfortunately, in the United States in 1985, only 22% of women 19 to 50 years old consumed 100 percent or more of their calcium RDA.

Since treatment for osteoporosis is limited, prevention is the key to reducing its incidence. The consensus is that optimizing development of peak bone mass will protect the skeleton and reduce the risk of fractures.[6] Food should be selected to provide adequate calcium, with special attention to adolescents, who have high mineral requirements, and adults, who are women susceptible to inadequate dietary calcium because of low caloric intake.

Women of all ages should be concerned about adequate calcium intake. Menstruating women need about 800 to 1000 mg of calcium per day; after menopause women not taking estrogen need 1500 mg.[5,19]

The mandate is clear for nursing professionals interested in preventive health. Encourage increased consumption of calcium-rich foods. Milk and dairy products deliver the most calcium of any food gruop, but they are also among the richest sources of fat in the American diet. Lowfat and fat-free milk and yogurt and low-fat cheeses are therefore the dairy products of choice. These foods are rich sources of calcium:

Sources of calcium	Approximate content (mg)
1 cup plain, lowfat yogurt	400
3 oz sardines, with bones	370
1 cup fruit yogurt, lowfat	345
¼ of 14-inch cheese pizza	330
1 cup fluid milk (whole milk, fat-free skim milk, 1% or 2% reduced-fat milk, buttermilk, calcium-fortified soy milk)	300
1 oz swiss cheese	270
1 oz cheddar cheese	200
½ cup cooked collard greens	180
1 oz American cheese	170
4 oz tofu (soybean curd)	145
1 tablespoon blackstrap molasses	140
1 5-inch stalk broccoli	100
½ cup cooked kale	100
2 oz cornbread, enriched	95

Calcium absorption is affected by the disaccharide lactose, vitamin D, and exercise. Calcium is best absorbed from dairy foods, which are a source of lactose. Vitamin D, which is also necessary for calcium absorption, is synthesized in the body when it is exposed to the ultraviolet rays of the sun and is commonly added to milk. Elderly people may be at risk for suboptimal levels of Vitamin D–especially ones who do not drink milk and those who, being housebound or institutionalized, get less exposure to the sun. Exercise enhances calcium absorption. Regular exercise, even moderate exercise such as walking, produces a decrease in the rate at which bone loss occurs and improves calcium balance.[10]

For those under 25 years of age, the calcium RDA is 1200 mg; for adults at least 25 it is 800 mg. Anyone whose intake is less than the RDA should develop strategies for increasing calcium. Children, particularly preadolescent girls, should be getting enough. Regular physical activity is important. By their actions, nurses can help themselves and their families and serve as role models for patients and others by applying the principles of prevention in their own personal behavior patterns.[38]

While maintaining a daily calcium intake through food is preferable, calcium supplements are available for those who do not get enough of the mineral through their regular diet. Calcium carbonate (40% elemental calcium), calcium citrate (24%), calcium lactate (14%), and calcium gluconate (9%) are preferred. Dolomite and bone meal are not recommended because they may be contaminated with lead.

OBESITY

As almost everyone in health care in the United States knows, a paradox exists in modern America. On the one hand, many people who do not need to lose weight are trying to do so. On the other, most who do need to lose weight are not trying, and those who try are not succeeding.[35]

Being overweight can seriously affect health and longevity. It is associated with the leading nutrition-related causes of death in the United States: noninsulin-dependent diabetes mellitus (NIDDM), cardiovascular diseases, and some cancers; it is also associated with gout and gall bladder disease. Overweight may be a factor in the development of osteoarthritis of the weight-bearing joints.[14]

Year 2000 Objective: Reduce overweight to a prevalence of no more than 20% among people aged 20 and older and no more than 15% among adolescents aged 12 through 19.

Gender. As Table 12-10 shows, nearly 25% of the men in the United States are estimated to be overweight, and 8% are estimated to be severely overweight. Among women, 27% are estimated to be overweight, and 11% severely overweight.[8]

Ethnicity. Among men, there is a modest ethnic variation in the prevalence of overweight, the greatest difference occurring between Whites and Mexican-Americans. Among women, the ethnic variation in overweight is substantial. Almost 25% of white females are overweight, but Mexican-American and Puerto Rican females have a greater prevalence of overweight than white women, and 45% of black females are overweight. Potential contributing factors to the greater propensity for adult black women to become obese include a more sedentary lifestyle, higher energy intake, earlier menarche, and earlier age at first childbirth.[4]

Education. Educational level is strongly associated with overweight in black and white adults of both sexes. Between 20 and 44 years of age, the lowest prevalence of overweight occurs among those with less than 9 years of education, while the highest occurs in those with 9 to 12 years. Prevalence among people with more than 12 years of education is intermediate in between those of the two lower-education groups. The pattern is less clear for men 45 to 74 years of age and for Hispanics of all ages. In Blacks of both sexes at 45 to 74 years, however, the prevalence of overweight among those with greater than a high school education is less than half that of those in the lower education groups.

Table 12-10. **Estimated prevalence of overweight and severe overweight for people age 20 to 74 in the United States**

	Men (percentage)		Women (percentage)	
	Overweight	Severe Overweight	Overweight	Severe Overweight
White	24.4	7.8	24.6	9.6
Black	26.3	10.4	45.1	19.7
Mexican	31.2	10.8	41.5	16.7
Cuban	28.5	10.3	31.9	6.9
Puerto Rican	25.7	7.9	39.8	15.2
Total	24.2	8.0	27.1	10.8
(in millions)	(15.4)	(5.1)	(18.6)	(7.4)

Source: National Health and Nutrition Examination Survey II (1976-1980) and the Hispanic Health and Nutrition Examination Survey (1982-1984). Adapted from Kuczmarski RJ: Prevalence of overweight and weight gain in the United States, *Am J Clin Nutr* 55:495S, 1992.

Helping Overweight Clients. In the health field, one of the most common requests heard is, "Please help me lose weight."

In 1958, Albert Stunkard summarized in just two sentences the results of the previous 30 years of efforts to control obesity by dietary means: "Most obese people will not stay in treatment for obesity. Of those who stay in treatment, most will not lose weight, and of those who do lose weight, most will regain it."[35] Unfortunately, Stunkard's observation holds true today.

In 1992, an NIH-sponsored technical support conference[35] examined the methods for voluntary weight loss and control in the United States. These features of obesity are identified in the box below.

What are the possible adverse effects of weight loss?[35]

1. Repeated weight gain and loss may have adverse psychologic and physical effects. For example, there is evidence that mildly to moderately overweight women who are dieting may be at risk for binge-eating without vomiting and purging.
2. While data on the health effects of repeated weight gains and losses, or weight cycling, are also inconclusive, weight cycling appears to affect energy metabolism and may result in faster regaining of weight.

Nurses Can Make a Difference. Nursing care can make a difference in client outcome. The nurse-client relationship provides many opportunities to encourage behavior change, to reinforce positive changes (such as improved dietary practices, increased activity, and steady weight loss), and to encourage the use of community resources through appropriate referrals to outside agencies and facilities, such as acceptable supervised or nonsupervised weight loss programs. Clients expect such advice on maintaining their health. Thus, even nurses who do not explicitly supervise weight loss clearly can play an important role in encouraging their clients and in prodding them with direction in their weight control efforts.

❑ ❑ FEATURES OF OBESITY

1. Obesity is a chronic disease.
2. It has many causes.
3. Cure is rare; palliation realistic.
4. Weight loss is slow.
5. Recidivism is common.
6. Weight regain may be slow, but it is often rapid.
7. Treatment is often more frustrating than the underlying disease.

Calculating Desirable Body Weight. The following rule of thumb is used by dietitians and nutritionists in rapidly estimating an adult's "desirable" body weight.

1. For women over the age of 25 years, allow 100 pounds for their first five feet, plus 5 pounds for each additional inch of height. For men over the age of 25 years, allow 110 pounds for the first five feet, plus 5 pounds for each additional inch of height.
2. Decrease 1 pound for each year under 25, to an age of 18 years.
3. To the body weight calculated, multiply by 110% for a large frame or by 90 for a small frame.

To illustrate, a 23-year-old woman with a large-sized frame who is 5 feet, 4 inches tall should weigh 100 pounds plus 20 pounds (120 pounds) minus 2 pounds (118 pounds) times 110% or 129.8 (i.e., 130) pounds.

Losing Weight. To quickly estimate how many calories per day an adult needs to lose weight, use these formulas. For women, multiply current weight in pounds by 10; for men, multiply current weight in pounds by 12. For every 10-pound weight loss, estimation of the calories needed will result in 100 and 120 calories less for women and men, respectively. To illustrate, using the woman described above, her desirable weight is 130 pounds. If she weighs 180 pounds, to calculate what percentage she is over her desired weight, divide her present weight by her desired weight. That is: 180 pounds/130 pounds = 38%. She currently weighs 38 percent more than her desirable weight. For her to lose weight, an intake of 1800 calories per day (present weight of 180 pounds × 10) should be reasonable.

Table 12-11 illustrates the number of servings from each of the food groups that would provide a balanced diet at varying energy levels. The 1800-calorie meal plan would be appropriate to suggest to this woman. Serving sizes for each food group appear in Table 12-12.[1,2]

DIABETES

The nutritional requirements of people with diabetes are essentially the same as those for the general population. Restricting total caloric intake in order to achieve a healthy body weight is the primary dietary intervention recommended for NIDDM. Adhering to an NCEP diet (restricting fat intake to ≤30% calories) is also advised because of the very high rate of mortality from atherosclerosis among those with NIDDM.[13]

Total incidence of diabetes was 28 per 100 in 1989; the year 2000 target is 25 per 1000. Prevalence of diabetes fell from 28 per 1000 in 1987 to 25 in 1990 for the total population. For American Indians and Alaska Natives and for Blacks, the prevalence of diabetes fell from 69 (1987) to 67 (1989) and from 36 (1987)

***Table 12-11.* Diet patterns for different energy levels**

Exchange	Energy level (kcal)					
	1200	1500	1800	2000	2600	3000
Starch/bread	4	6	8	9	13	15
Vegetable	3	3	4	5	6	6
Fruit	3	3	4	4	5	6
Meat	5	5	5	6	7	8
Milk	2	3	3	3	3	3
Fat	4	5	6	7	10	12

***Table 12-12.* Energy and nutrient content of foods in the six exchange lists**

List	Portion size	Carbohydrate (g)	Protein (g)	Fat (g)	Energy* (kcal)
Starch/bread†	1 slice	15	3	Trace	80
Vegetable‡	1/2 cup	15	2	–	25
Fruit	1 portion	15	–	–	60
Meat	1 oz				
lean		–	7	3	55
medium fat§		–	7	5	75
high fat‖		–	7	8	100
Milk	8 oz				
nonfat		12	8	Trace	90
low fat		12	8	5	120
whole		12	8	8	150
Fat	1 tsp	–	–	5	45

Sources: American Dietetic Association and American Diabetes Association: *Exchange Lists for Meal Planning*, 1986; American Dietetic Association and American Diabetes Association: *Exchange Lists for Weight Management*, 1989.

*The energy value for each exchange list represents an approximate average for the group. It does not reflect the precise number of grams of carbohydrate, protein, and fat. For example, an ounce of lean meat contains about 7 g protein (about 28 calories) plus about 3 g fat (about 27 calories) – which is approximately 55 calories.

†In addition to grain products – bread, pasta, and cereals – this list contains starchy vegetables – potatoes, corn, and lima beans.

‡This list contains nonstarchy, low-calorie vegetables.

§This list contains lowfat cheeses such as cottage cheese and ricotta.

‖This list contains peanut butter and high-fat cheeses.

to 35 (1990), respectively.[11] *The year 2000 targets for Blacks, American Indians, and Alaska Natives are for 25, 62, and 32 per 1000, respectively.*

Diabetes-related deaths remained at the 1986 baseline of 38 per 100,000 people in 1989. For Blacks, diabetes-related mortality rose from 65 per 100,000 (1986) to 68 (1989), and for American Indians and Alaska Natives, it increased from 54 (1986) to 63 (1989). The CDC notes that these increases might reflect improved documentation on death certificates of diabetes-related deaths.[34] *The year 2000 targets for Blacks, American Indians, and Alaska Natives are 34, 58, and 48 per 100,000, respectively.*

Diet and Prevention

In any assessment of the role diet may play in the prevention of heart disease, cancers, stroke, and other diseases, it must be understood that they are caused by a combination and interaction of environmental, behavioral, social, and genetic factors. The exact proportion that can be attributed directly to dietary factors is unknown. While some researchers suggest that dietary factors overall are responsible for at least a third of all cases of cancer and coronary heart disease, these estimates are based on interpretations of research studies that cannot completely distinguish dietary factors from genetic, environmental, and behavioral causes.

Many dietary components are involved in diet and health relationships. Chief among them is the disproportionate consumption of foods high in fats, often at the expense of foods high in complex carbohydrates and dietary fiber that may be more conducive to health.

FOOD AND NUTRITION RECOMMENDATIONS

The kinds and amounts of food needed to obtain the necessary energy and nutrients are defined in four recent U.S. government publications. They are

- The Recommended Dietary Allowances[7]
- Diet and Health: Implications for Reducing Chronic Disease Risk[14]
- Nutrition and Your Health: Dietary Guidelines for Americans[24]
- The Food Guide Pyramid[23]

These four sets of food and nutrition guidelines are discussed in the next part of this chapter. The goal for this section is to heighten nurses' interest in food and nutrition so much that they will want to start adopting the recommendations presented here in order to improve their own diets. Modifying behavior to incorporate these guidelines will benefit the nurses as well as the clients. If nurses believe that eating right promotes health, if they are convinced that "preventive nutrition" can reduce disease risk, if they change their own behavior in ways that enhance health, then not only they, but their families, significant others, and clients will benefit from their personal commitment to food, nutrition, and healthful dietary practices.

The Recommended Dietary Allowances

The RDAs are defined as the level of intake of essential nutrients that the Food and Nutrition Board of the National Research Council (FNB/NRC) on the basis of scientific knowledge, judges to be adequate to meet the known nutritional needs of virtually all healthy people in the United States.[7]

Specifically, in addition to protein, RDAs are set for the vitamins A, C, D, E, K, thiamin, riboflavin, niacin, B_6, B_{12}, and folate; the minerals calcium (Ca), phosphorous (P), and magnesium (Mg); and trace mineral iron (Fe), zinc (Zn), iodine (I), and selenium (Se). Nutrients are separated from the main RDAs because there is less information for them on which to base allowances.

It is important to understand that *the RDAs are not daily necessities.* Nor are they *minimum requirements.*

RDAs are time-averaged goals to be achieved over at least a 3-day period and, for some nutrients such as Vitamins A and B_{12}, over periods for as long as several months.

The RDAs include a safety factor specific to each nutrient. Except for their recommendations for energy, the RDAs exceed the actual nutrient requirements for most people. Anyone who consumes less than the RDA of any particular nutrient is not necessarily getting an inadequate amount of that nutrient. But as the percentage of the RDA consumed decreases, the risk of inadequate nutrient intake begins to increase.

"Should I take a nutrient supplement?" is a question the nurse is asked often. A large proportion of people in the United States take dietary supplements, but not necessarily because of nutrient needs. While the adverse effects of large doses of certain nutrients (such as Vitamin A) have been recognized for years, there are no documented reports that daily vitamin and mineral supplements that supply up to the RDA of a particular nutrient are either beneficial or harmful for the general population. "Low-dose" supplements that contain the RDAs for micronutrients (vitamins and minerals) appear to be generally safe. While the desirable way for the general public to obtain recommended levels of nutrients is by eating a variety of foods, those who do take dietary supplments should avoid taking them in excess of the RDA on any given day.[14]

Diet and Health: Implications for Reducing Chronic Disease Risk[14]

This report is a comprehensive review of the relationships of dietary patterns and nutrient intake to the risk of diet-related chronic diseases that affect Americans. On the basis of the evidence, dietary changes are recommended that can improve health prospects for many. Of highest priority among these changes is to reduce intake of foods high in fats and to increase intake of foods high in complex carbohydrates and fiber. Shown in the upper box on p. 281 are the nine recommendations for maintaining health that were developed, based on the conclusions drawn from this extensive review of the scientific literature.

Nutrition and Your Health: Dietary Guidelines for Americans[24]

In contrast to the RDAs, which are quantitative recommendations for *nutrient* intakes, the *Dietary Guidelines* (see box on pp. 281-283) are recommendations for *food* intakes. The guidelines focus on obtaining a diet that is sufficient in protein and the vitamins and minerals addressed in the RDAs, without the excesses that are prevented by following advice given in *Nutrition and Health.*

The guidelines were first issued in 1980 in response to the public's desire for authoritative, consistent guidance on diet and health.[22] They were revised in 1985.

❑ ❑ THE NINE DIETARY RECOMMENDATIONS OF THE COMMITTEE ON DIET AND HEALTH, 1989

1. **Fats and cholesterol.** Reduce total fat to 30% or less of calories. Reduce saturated fatty acid intake to less than 10% of calories. Reduce the intake of cholesterol to less than 300 mg daily.
2. **Fruits and vegetables.** Eat 5 or more servings of a combination of fruits and vegetables every day. Also increase intake of starches and other complex carbohydrates by eating at least 6 servings daily of a combination of breads, cereals, and legumes
3. **Protein.** Maintain protein intake at moderate levels, i.e., less than twice the RDA for all age groups, which is 1.6 g/kg body weight for adults.
4. **Body weight.** Balance food intake and physical activity to maintain appropriate body weight.
5. **Alcohol.** Alcohol consumption is not recommended, but for those who do drink alcoholic beverages, limits consumption to the equivalent of less than 1 ounce of pure alcohol in a single day. That is the equivalent of 2 cans of beer, 2 small glasses of wine, or 2 average cocktails. Pregnant women should avoid alcoholic beverages.
6. **Salt.** Limit salt (NaCl) intake to 6 g or less daily. Limit the use of salt at the table. Salty, highly processed salty, salt-preserved, and salt-packed foods should be consumed sparingly.
7. **Calcium.** Maintain adequate calcium intake.
8. **Supplements.** Avoid taking dietary supplements in excess of the RDA in any one day.
9. **Fluoride.** Maintain an optimal intake of fluoride, particularly during the years of primary and secondary tooth formation and growth.

Source: National Research Council. Committee on Diet and Health: *Diet and health: implications for reducing chronic disease risk,* Washington DC, 1989, National Academy Press.

❑ ❑ DIETARY GUIDELINES

What should you eat to stay healthy?

The Dietary Guidelines for Americans featured in this brochure help answer this question. They are seven guidelines for a healthful diet–advice for healthy Americans ages 2 years and over. These guidelines are the best, most current advice from nutrition experts.

Many American diets have too many calories and too much fat (especially saturated fat), cholesterol, and sodium. They also have too little complex carbohydrates and fiber. Such diets are one cause of America's high rates of obesity and certain diseases–heart disease, high blood pressure, stroke, diabetes and some forms of cancer. The exact role of diet in some of these is still being studied.

The foods Americans have to choose from are varied, plentiful and safe to eat. Use this booklet to help choose a healthful diet.

Eat a variety of foods

Eating a variety of foods–not a few highly fortified foods or supplements–is the best way to get the energy, protein, vitamins, minerals, and fiber you need.

No single food can supply all the nutrients in the amounts you need. For example, milk supplies calcium but little iron, meat supplies iron but little calcium. To have a nutritious diet, you must eat a variety of foods.

Any food that supplies calories and nutrients can be part of a nutritious diet. It's the content of the total diet over a day or more that counts.

Maintain healthy weight

If you are too fat or too thin you are more likely to develop health problems. Being too fat is linked with high blood pressure, heart disease, stroke, the most common type of diabetes, certain cancers, and other types of illness.

What is a healthy weight for you? There is no exact answer right now. In the meantime, use this information to help judge if your weight is healthy. A healthy weight for adults means meeting these three conditions:

1. Your weight falls within the range for your height and age in the table.

Suggested weights for adults

Height without shoes	Weight in pounds without clothes* (19-34 years)	(35 years and over)
5′0″	97-128	108-138
5′2″	104-137	115-148
5′4″	111-146	122-157
5′6″	118-155	130-167
5′8″	125-164	138-178
5′10″	132-174	146-188
6′0″	140-184	155-199
6′2″	148-195	164-210
6′4″	156-205	173-222

*The higher weights in the ranges generally apply to men, who tend to have more muscle and bone; the lower weights often apply to women, who have less muscle and bone.

Continued.

❑ ❑ DIETARY GUIDELINES–cont'd

Maintain healthy weight–cont'd

2. Your waist measure is smaller than your hip measure. Too much fat around the waist is believed to be of greater health risk than excess fat in the hips and thighs.
3. Your doctor has advised you not to gain or lose weight because of a medical problem.

If your weight is not "healthy," set reasonable weight goals and try for long-term success through better habits of eating and exercise.

Choose a diet low in fat, saturated fat, and cholesterol

Many Americans have diets high in fat, saturated fat, and cholesterol. Such diets are linked to increased risk for heart disease, obesity and certain types of cancer.

Here are the goals suggested for fat and saturated fat in American diets. Remember, these goals for fats apply to the diet over several days, not to a single meal or food.

Total fat. Your goal for fat depends on your calorie needs. An amount that provides 30 percent or less of calories is suggested. The chart below shows the upper limit on the grams of fat per day that corresponds to various daily calorie intakes:

Calories	Total fat per day (grams)	Saturated fat per day (grams)
1600	53 or less	less than 18
2200	73 or less	less than 24
2800	93 or less	less than 31

Saturated fat. An amount that provides less than 10 percent of calories is suggested. All fats contain both saturated and unsaturated fat (fatty acids). The fats in animal products are the main sources of saturated fat in most diets, with tropical oils (coconut, palm kernel, and palm oils) and hydrogenated fats providing smaller amounts.

Cholesterol. Animal products are the sources of all dietary cholesterol.

Eating less fat from animal sources will help lower the cholesterol, total fat and saturated fat in your diet.

Food Tips to Reduce Fat, Saturated Fat, and Cholesterol

- Use fats and oils sparingly in cooking.
- Use small amounts of salad dressings and spreads, such as butter, margarine, and mayonnaise. Try reduced or nonfat substitutes.
- Choose lean cuts of meat and trim visible fat.
- Take skin off of poultry.
- Have cooked dry beans and peas instead of meat occasionally.
- Moderate the use of egg yolks and organ meats.
- Choose skim or lowfat milk and nonfat or lowfat yogurt and cheese most of the time.

Food Tips to Reduce Fat, Saturated Fat, and Cholesterol–cont'd

- Check labels on foods to see how much fat and saturated fat are in a serving.
- Choose liquid vegetable oils most often because they are lower in saturated fat.

Choose a diet with plenty of vegetables, fruits, and grain products

Eat more vegetables, including dry beans and peas; fruits; and breads, cereals, pasta, and rice. A varied diet that emphasizes these foods supplies important vitamins and minerals, fiber, and complex carbohydrates and is generally lower in fat.

It's better to get fiber from foods that contain fiber naturally than from supplements. Some of the benefit of a high fiber diet may come from the food that provides the fiber, not from the fiber alone.

Use sugars only in moderation

Sugars and many foods that contain them in large amounts supply calories but are limited in nutrients. Sugar comes in many forms, such as table sugar (sucrose), brown sugar, honey, syrup, corn sweetener, high-fructose corn sweetener, molassses, glucose (dextrose), fructose, maltose, and lactose.

Use sugars in moderation–sparingly if your calorie needs are low. Diets high in sugars have not been shown to cause diabetes.

Both sugars and starches–which break down into sugars–can contribute to tooth decay. Avoid excessive snacking, brush your teeth with a fluoride toothpaste, and floss regularly to help prevent tooth decay. Check with your dentist or doctor about the need for supplemental fluoride, especially for children.

Use salt and sodium only in moderation

Most Americans eat more salt and sodium than they need. In populations with diets low in salt, high blood pressure is less common than in populations with diets high in salt. Eating less salt and sodium will benefit people whose blood pressure goes up with salt intake.

Food Tips to Moderate Use of Salt and Sodium

- Use salt sparingly, if at all, in cooking and at the table.
- Foods that tend to be higher in sodium include many cheeses, processed meats, most frozen dinners and entrees, packaged mixes, most canned soups and vegetables, salad dressings and condiments like soy sauce, pickles, olives, catsup, and mustard.
- Use salted snacks, such as chips, crackers, pretzels, and nuts sparingly.
- Check labels for the amount of sodium in foods, and choose those lower in sodium most of the time.

❑ ❑ **DIETARY GUIDELINES—cont'd**

If you drink alcoholic beverages, do so in moderation

Alcoholic beverages supply calories but little or no nutrients. Drinking them has no net health benefit, is linked with many health problems, and can lead to addiction. It is also the cause of many accidents.

Some people who should not drink alcoholic beverages are women who are pregnant or trying to conceive; individuals who plan to drive or engage in other activities that require attention or skill; individuals using medicines, even over-the-counter kinds; individuals who cannot keep their drinking moderate; and children and adolescents.

What's moderate drinking? For women, this means no more than 1 drink a day, and for men, no more than 2 drinks a day.

Count as a drink:
- 12 ounces of regular beer
- 5 ounces of wine
- 1½ ounces of distilled spirits (80 proof)

A daily food guide

Get the nutrients your body needs by eating different foods from five food groups each day. Most people should have at least the lower number of servings from each group. Some people may need more because of their body size and activity level. Young children should eat a variety of foods but may need smaller servings.

Food group/ daily servings	What counts as a serving
Vegetables 3-5 servings	• 1 cup raw leafy greens • ½ cup other kinds of vegetables
Fruits 2-4 servings	• 1 medium apple, banana, orange • ½ cup fruit, fresh cooked, canned • ¾ cup juice
Breads, cereals, rice, and pasta 6-11 servings	• 1 slice bread • ½ bun, bagel • 1 ounce dry cereal • ½ cup cooked cereal, rice, pasta

Food group/ daily servings	What counts as a serving
Milk, yogurt, and cheese 2-3 servings	• 1 cup milk • 8 ounces yogurt • 1½ ounces natural cheese • 2 ounces process cheese
Meat, poultry, fish, dry beans, and peas, eggs, nuts, and seeds 2-3 servings	• Amounts to total 5-7 ounces of cooked lean meat, poultry or fish a day • Count ½ cup cooked beans, 1 egg or 2 tablespoons of peanut butter as 1 ounce of meat.

Developed as a cooperative effort by United States Department of Agriculture, United States Department of Health and Human Services, Food Marketing Institute: *USDA's food guide,* 1991.

PROMOTING DIET AND HEALTH WITH THE DIETARY GUIDELINES

In 1991, *Improving America's Diet and Health*[21] was published. This book is closely related to the report on diet and health. It promotes the nine recommendations of *Diet and Health* (listed previously in the chapter) by proposing a series of strategies and actions to put the dietary guidelines into action. Included in the book are recommendations to

- Enhance awareness, understanding, and acceptance of dietary recommendations.
- Create legislative, regulatory, commercial, and educational environments supportive of the recommendations.
- Improve the availability of foods and meals that facilitate implementation of the recommendations.[21]

The general tactics for increasing the prevalence of healthful eating patterns include

- Altering the food supply by subtraction, addition, and substitution (for example, reducing the fat in meat and cheese, fortifying food with nutrients, and replacing some fat in margarine with water).
- Altering the food-acquisition environment by providing more food choices that help consumers meet dietary recommendations; better information, such as better food labels; advice at points of purchase, such as tags indicating a good nutrition buy in

supermarkets and cafeterias; and options for selecting healthful diets, such as better food choices in vending machines and in restaurants.
- Altering nutrition education by presenting consistent messages in education programs. Advertisements for products, and public service announcements and by broadening exposure to formal and nonformal nutrition education, such as mandating nutrition education on dietary recommendations from kindergarten through grade 12, in health care facilities, and in medical and nursing education (such as this chapter in this book).

The Food Guide Pyramid[23]

The *Food Guide Pyramid* (see box on p. 285) replaces the old "basic four" food groups on all new U.S. government nutrition education materials. The pyramid was developed as a graphic representation of the dietary guidelines to help people implement the guidelines by making appropriate food choices.

The food guide pyramid emphasizes food from the five major food groups shown in its lower sections. Each of these food groups provides some, but not all, of the nutrients recommended in the RDAs.[22] Foods in one group cannot replace those in another. No one food group is more important than another–for good health and a balanced diet, all the groups are needed.

GRAINS, FRUITS, AND VEGETABLES

At the base of the pyramid are breads, cereals, rice, and pasta-foods from grains. According to the pyramid, our diets should contain more servings of grain products each day than of any other food group. The level above the grains contains other foods from the plant kingdom–fruits and vegetables. Together, the grains, fruits, and vegetables supply fiber, vitamins, and minerals and are almost completely fat-free.

Americans eat only about three servings daily of fruits and vegetables rather than the five to nine servings recommended. A program called *5 A Day* is designed to address the goal of making Americans more aware of the way fruits and vegetables can improve their health. This program, jointly sponsored by the National Cancer Institute and Produce for Better Health Foundation, is the first national effort to focus on the positive role of fruits and vegetables in reducing the risk of cancer and other chronic diseases.

DAIRY AND MEAT

On the next level of the pyramid, above the fruits and vegetables, are foods in two more groups–dairy (milk and other dairy products such as yogurt and cheese) and the meat group (which contains meat, fish, poultry, and eggs, plus dry beans and nuts–protein-rich foods from the plant kingdom).

FATS, OILS, AND SWEETS

The tip of the pyramid shows fats, oils, and sweets. A major function of the pyramid is its focus on fat, because most American diets are too high in fat, especially saturated fat.

The fats, oils, and sweets group makes up the smallest area of the pyramid, indicating that fats and sweets should be eaten in very small quantities when compared to the amounts of foods from the other food groups. No specific recommendation is made for a number of servings from the fats and sweets group to be included in the diet daily. This group is included in its conspicuous location of the top of the pyramid both as a reminder of its importance and to illustrate the concepts of "moderation" and "proportionality."

THE PYRAMID AND THE BASIC FOUR

There are both similarities and differences between the pyramid and the basic four. Three of the pyramid's food groups are the same as those of the basic four: dairy, meat and meat alternates, and grains. Fruits and vegetables, which make up a single food group in the basic four, have been separated in the pyramid to emphasize the need for adequate consumption of each.

The recommended number of daily servings of foods in the basic four are

Dairy: 2 servings
Meat: 2 servings
Fruits and vegetables: 4 servings
Bread and cereals: 4 servings

A comparison of the numbers of servings in the basic four with those in the pyramid shows an increased reliance on the plant-based foods–grains, vegetables, and fruits. These foods are low in fat content, completely cholesterol-free, and the sole source of fiber.

SERVING SIZES

Suggested numbers of servings and suggested serving sizes are provided with the pyramid illustration for all food groups except fats, oils, and sweets. (As mentioned earlier, the primary guideline for this group is "use sparingly.") Serving sizes are shown in the pyramid box. They are the same as the suggested serving sizes used in the basic four. Keeping serving sizes in the pyramid the same should help simplify the transition from the old, familiar four food groups to the new six-food-group approach. This minimizes the number of changes nurses will need to incorporate into patient education.

The serving sizes in the pyramid are also very similar to the serving sizes used in the "exchanges" (see the box on pp. 285-287). There are two notable exceptions. Six

❑ ❑ THE FOOD GUIDE PYRAMID

What's the best nutrition advice?

It's following the Dietary Guidelines for Americans. These are seven guidelines for a healthful diet–advice for healthy Americans 2 years of age or more. By following the dietary guidelines, you can enjoy better health and reduce your chances of getting certain diseases–such as heart disease, high blood pressure, stroke, certain cancers, and the most common type of diabetes. These guidelines are the best, most up-to-date advice from nutrition experts.

- Eat a variety of foods.
- Maintain healthy weight.
- Choose a diet low in fat, saturated fat, and cholesterol.
- Choose a diet with plenty of vegetables, fruits, and grain products.
- Use sugars only in moderation.
- Use salt and sodium only in moderation.
- If you drink alcoholic beverages, do so in moderation.

What is the food guide pyramid?

The food guide pyramid is an outline of what to eat each day based on the dietary guidelines. It's not a rigid prescription but a general guide that lets you choose a healthful diet that's right for you.

The pyramid calls for eating a variety of foods to get the nutrients you need and at the same time the right amount of calories to maintain healthy weight.

Use the pyramid to help you eat better every day, the dietary guidelines way. Start with plenty of breads, cereals, rice, pasta, vegetables, and fruits. Add 2-3 servings from the milk group and 2-3 servings from the meat group. Remember to go easy on fats, oils, and sweets, the foods in the small tip of the pyramid.

Key

- Fat (naturally occurring and added)

▼ Sugars (added)

These symbols show fat and added sugars in foods. They come mostly from the fats, oils, and sweets group. But foods in other groups–such as cheese or ice cream from the milk group or french fries from the vegetable group–can also provide fat and added sugars.

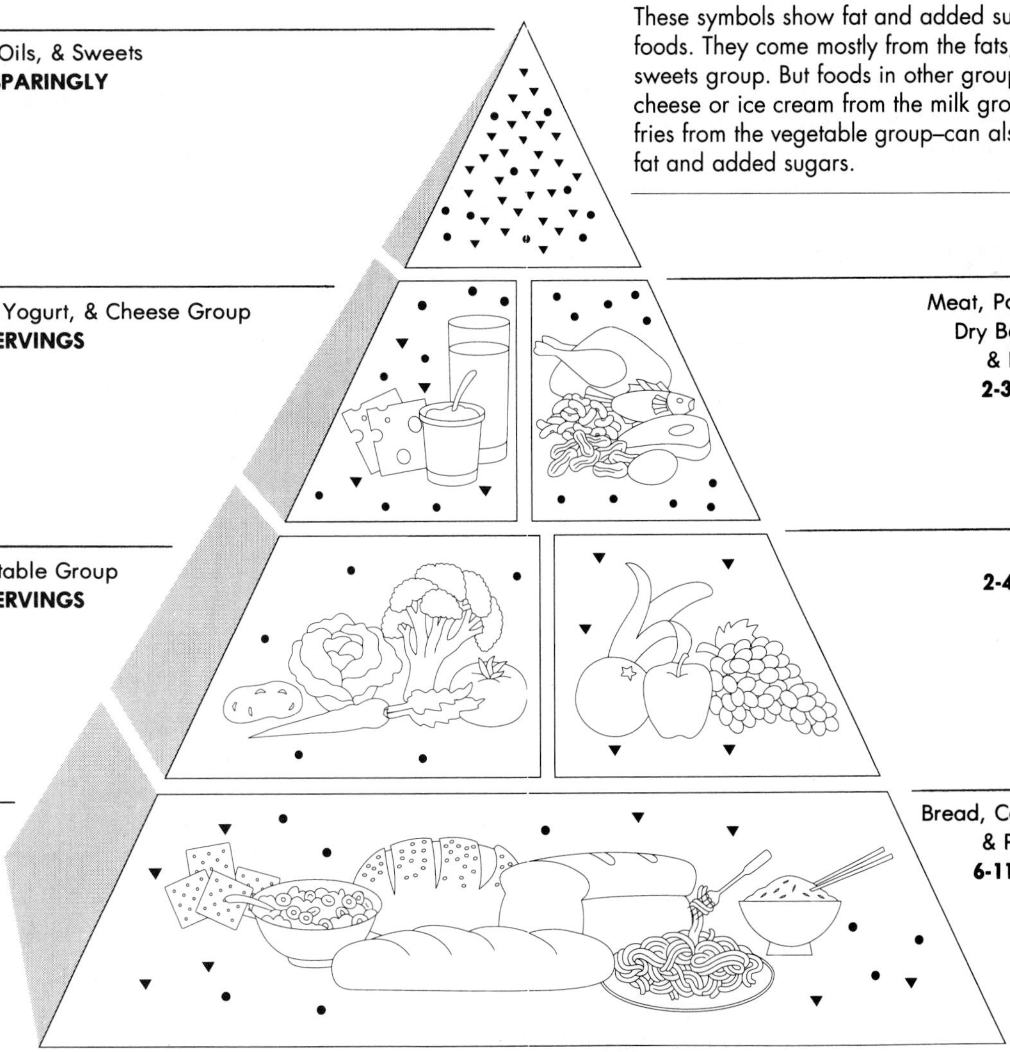

Continued.

❑ ❑ THE FOOD GUIDE PYRAMID–cont'd

Looking at the pieces of the pyramid

The food guide pyramid emphasizes foods from the five major food groups shown in the three lower sections of the pyramid. Each of these food groups provides some, but not all, of the nutrients you need. Foods in one group can't replace those in another. No one of these major food groups is more important than another–for good health, you need them all.

What counts as 1 serving?

The amount of food that counts as 1 serving is listed below. If you eat a larger portion, count it as more than 1 serving. For example, a dinner portion of spaghetti would count as 2 or 3 servings of pasta.

Be sure to eat at least the lowest number of servings from the five major food groups listed below. You need them for the vitamins, minerals, carbohydrates, and protein they provide. Just try to pick the lowest fat choices from the food groups. No specific serving size is given for the fats, oils, and sweets group because the message is use sparingly.

Food groups

Milk, yogurt, and cheese

- 1 cup of milk or yogurt
- 1½ ounces of natural cheese
- 2 ounces of process cheese

Meat, poultry, fish, dry beans, eggs, and nuts

- 2-3 ounces of cooked lean meat, poultry, or fish
- ½ cup of cooked dry beans, 1 egg, or 2 tablespoons of peanut butter count as 1 ounce of lean meat

Vegetable

- 1 cup of raw leafy vegetables
- ½ cup of other vegetables, cooked or chopped raw
- ¾ cup of vegetable juice

Fruit

- 1 medium apple, banana, orange
- ½ cup of chopped, cooked, or canned fruit
- ¾ cup of fruit juice

Bread, cereal, rice and pasta

- 1 slice of bread
- 1 ounce of ready-to-eat cereal
- ½ cup of cooked cereal, rice, or pasta

How to make the pyramid work for you

The food guide pyramid shows a range of servings for each major food group. The number of servings right for

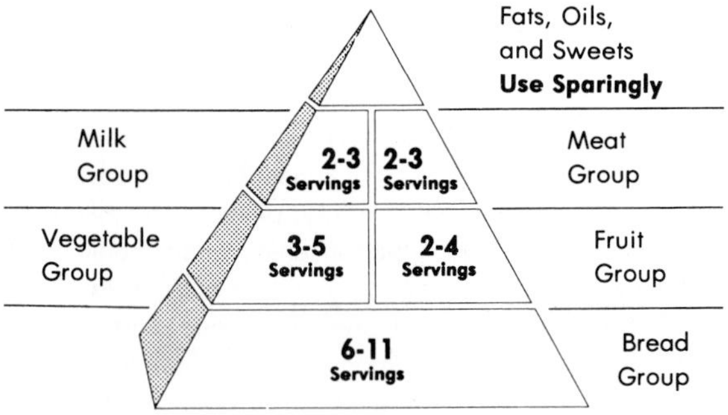

you depends on how many calories you need, which in turn depends on your age, sex, size, and level of activity. Almost everyone should have at least the lowest number of servings in the ranges.

Now take a look at the table below. It tells you how many servings of each major food group you need for your calorie level. It also tells you the total grams of fat recommended for each calorie level: the dietary guidelines recommend that Americans limit fat in their diets to 30 percent of calories. This includes the fat in the foods you choose as well as the fat used in cooking or added at the table.

How many servings do you need each day?

	Many women, older adults	Children, teen girls, active women, most men	Teen boys, active men
Calorie level*	about **1,600**	about **2,200**	about **2,800**
Bread group servings	6	9	11
Vegetable group servings	3	4	5
Fruit group servings	2	3	4
Milk group servings	2-3†	2-3†	2-3†
Meat group servings	2, for a total of 5 ounces	2, for a total of 6 ounces	3, for a total of 7 ounces
Total fat (grams)	53	73	93

*These are the calorie levels if you choose low fat, lean foods from the 5 major foods groups and use foods from the fats, oils, and sweets group sparingly.

†Women who are pregnant or breastfeeding, teenagers, and young adults to age 24 need 3 servings.

❑ ❑ THE FOOD GUIDE PYRAMID–cont'd

Pyramid pointers: selection tips for building a better diet

The most effective way to moderate the amount of fat and added sugars in your diet is to cut down on "extras"–foods in the sixth food group (fats, oils, and sweets). Also choose lower fat and lower sugar foods from the other five food groups often. Here are some tips:

Fats, Oils, and Sweets (Use Sparingly)

- Go easy on fats and sugars added to foods in cooking or at the table–butter, margarine, gravy, salad dressing, sugar, and jelly.
- Choose fewer foods that are high in sugars–candy, sweet desserts, and soft drinks.

Vegetable Group (3-5 Servings)

- Different types of vegetables provide different nutrients. Eat a variety.
- Include dark-green leafy vegetables and legumes several times a week–they are especially good sources of vitamins and minerals. Legumes also provide protein and can be used in place of meat.
- Go easy on the fat you add to vegetables at the table or during cooking. Added spreads or toppings, such as butter, mayonnaise, and salad dressing, count as fat.
- Use lowfat salad dressing.

Bread, Cereal, Rice, and Pasta Group (6-11 Servings)

- To get the fiber you need, choose several servings a day of foods made from whole grains.
- Choose most often foods that are made with little fat or sugars, like bread, English muffins, rice, and pasta.
- Go easy on the fat and sugars you add as spreads, seasoning, or toppings.
- When preparing pasta, stuffing, and sauce from packaged mixes, use only half the butter or margarine suggested; if milk or cream is called for, use lowfat milk.

Fruit Group (2-4 Servings)

- Choose fresh fruits, fruit juices, and frozen, canned, or dried fruit. Go easy on fruits canned or frozen in heavy syrups and sweetened fruit juices.
- Eat whole fruits often–they are higher in fiber than fruit juices.
- Count only 100 percent fruit juice as fruit. Punches, ades, and most fruit "drinks" contain only a little juice and lots of added sugars.

Milk, Yogurt, and Cheese Group (2-3 Servings)

- Choose skim milk and nonfat yogurt often. They are lowest in fat.
- 1½ to 2 ounces of cheese and 8 ounces of yogurt count as a serving from this group because they supply the same amount of calcium as 1 cup of milk.
- Choose "part skim" or lowfat cheeses when available and lower fat milk desserts, like ice milk or frozen yogurt. Read labels.

Meat, Poultry, Fish, Dry Beans, Eggs, and Nuts Group (2-3 Servings)

- Choose lean meat, poultry without skin, fish, and dry beans and peas often. They are the choices lowest in fat.
- Prepare meats in lowfat ways
  –Trim away all the fat you can see.
  –Remove skin from poultry
  –Broil, roast, or boil these foods instead of frying them
- Nuts and seeds are high in fat so eat them in moderation.

Developed as a cooperative effort by United States Department of Agriculture, Human Nutrition Information Service, 6505 Belcrest Road, Hyattsville, MD 20782; and Food Marketing Institute, 800 Connecticut Avenue, NW, Washington, DC 20006.

ounces (3/4-cup) of fruit juice counts as a serving of fruit in the new pyramid, whereas only 4 ounces of juice counts as one fruit in the diabetic exchange system. In the pyramid, a serving of meat is a 2- to 3-ounce portion of lean meat, while in the diabetic system, one meat exchange weighs 1 ounce.

FOOD LABELS

To be of most use to consumers, food labels must be easy to read and understand and consistent with recent dietary recommendations, such as the dietary guidelines.

How should food labels be designed to help people

select nutritious foods? Labels need to contain information most important for consumers to know–useful and accurate facts about serving size and calories. Labels would carry information on food components such as calcium and iron that have a protective effect on health and need to be encouraged in many people's diets. Labels would also disclose information on food components, such as sodium, both total and saturated fats, and cholesterol, that many people need to consume more moderately.

Background: The "Old" Food Label[17]

From 1975 through 1993, food labels in the United States followed a uniform sequence and format prescribed by the Food and Drug Administration (FDA). Information about amounts of protein, vitamins and minerals per serving appeared on labels expressed as a percentage of the U.S. recommended dietary allowances. The FDA developed the U.S. RDAs by taking the highest level of the National Research Council's 1968 seventh edition of the *Recommended Dietary Allowances* for each nutrient and making it the standard for expressing nutrient levels. Although the RDAs were updated in 1974, 1980, and 1989, the U.S. RDAs, which were phased out of use by mid-1984, were never updated.

In general, FDA's regulations for the "old" food labels mandated the following, in the order indicated: (1) serving size for the food, (2) the number of servings in the container, (3) the number of calories per serving, (4) the amount of protein (in grams) per serving, (5) the amount of fat (in grams) per serving, (6) the amount of protein expressed as a percentage of the U.S. RDA, and (7) for one serving, the percentage of the U.S. RDA of each of seven nutrients (Vitamin A, Vitamin C, thiamin, riboflavin, niacin, calcium, and iron). Sodium was treated somewhat differently. The listing of sodium in milligrams was optional. However, rules adopted in 1984 required sodium content to be declared. The FDA's regulations also allowed a manufacturer to list any of a dozen other vitamins and minerals, in terms of percentage of the U.S. RDA, in a serving.

Food Label Reform

Criticism of the way food labels listed nutrition content grew intense in the 1980s, spurred by four related developments. First, scientific studies had convincingly shown important linkages between dietary habits and the prevalence of chronic disease, most notably cardiovascular disease, cancer, stroke, diabetes, and obesity. Second, food consumption surveys revealed that Americans' diets were excessively abundant in such components as calories, fats, cholesterol, and sodium–the very factors associated with the leading chronic diseases. Third, American consumers became increasingly attentive to the health benefits of foods. Food producers and manufacturers responded to this consumer interest in "healthy" foods (products richer in fiber content, and lower in sodium, total and saturated fat, cholesterol, and sugar) by developing foods with a composition, that could be promoted as reflecting this new interest in nutrition and health (see Fig. 12-4). Fourth, *The Surgeon General's Report* recommended reforms of nutrition labeling in the United States. Thus, the National Label Education Act (NLEA) mandating the new food labels was passed in 1990.[15] The box on labeling contains a detailed summary of the new regulations.

The New Label

New labels started to appear on the foods in grocery store aisles late in 1993. Effective in mid-1994, they are required to replace all the seriously dated labels used since the 1970s. The purpose of the food-labeling reform currently under way is to help consumers choose more healthful diets and to offer an incentive to food companies to improve the nutritional qualities of their products. A sample label is shown in Fig. 12-4.

- Adding to the justification for the new food label are two year 2000 nutrition objectives: (1) increase to at least 85% the proportion of people aged 18 and older who use food labels to make nutritious selections (up from 74% in 1988); (2) achieve useful and informative nutrition labeling for virtually all processed foods (up from 40% in 1988) and at least 40% of fresh foods and ready-to-eat carry-away foods (no baseline data available).[31]
- Almost all foods will carry nutrition labels. Previously, nutrition labeling was voluntary, except for products enriched or fortified or when a nutritional claim was made. Only about 60% of food products carried nutrition labels in the past.
- New labels contain information on the amount per serving of saturated fat, cholesterol, dietary fiber, and other nutrients that are of major health concern to today's consumer. Excluded from labels will be a requirement for information on thiamin, riboflavin, and niacin.
- Replacing the U.S. RDAs are nutrient reference values, expressed as percentages of daily values (DVs), designed to help consumers see how a food fits into an overall daily diet. The DV comprises two new sets of dietary standards: daily reference values (DRVs) and reference daily intakes (RDAs). To make label reading less confusing, only the daily value term appears on

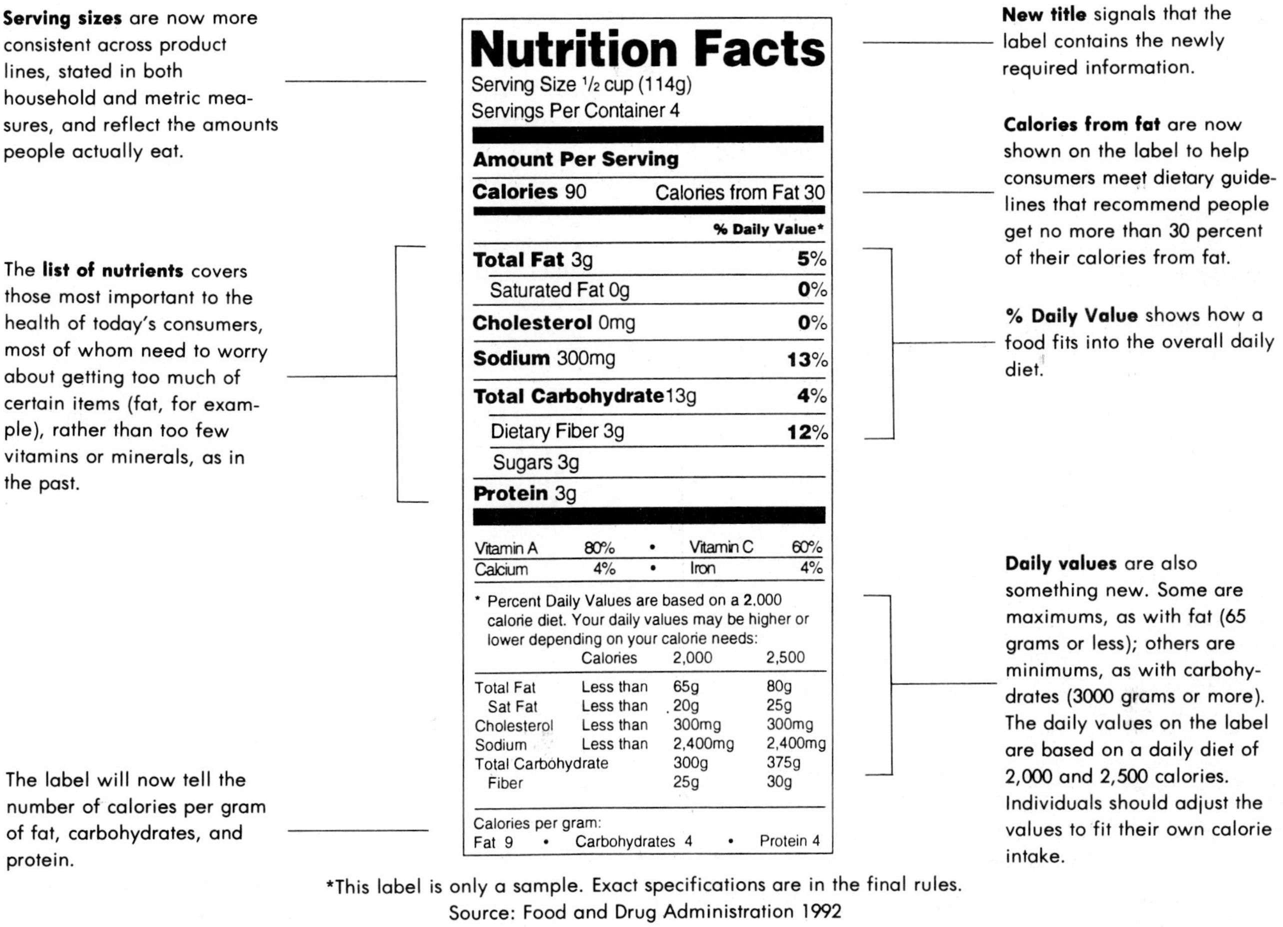
Serving sizes are now more consistent across product lines, stated in both household and metric measures, and reflect the amounts people actually eat.
The list of nutrients covers those most important to the health of today's consumers, most of whom need to worry about getting too much of certain items (fat, for example), rather than too few vitamins or minerals, as in the past.
The label will now tell the number of calories per gram of fat, carbohydrates, and protein.
Nutrition Facts
Serving Size 1/2 cup (114g)
Servings Per Container 4
Amount Per Serving
Calories 90
Calories from Fat 30
% Daily Value*
Total Fat 3g 5%
Saturated Fat 0g 0%
Cholesterol 0mg 0%
Sodium 300mg 13%
Total Carbohydrate 13g 4%
Dietary Fiber 3g 12%
Sugars 3g
Protein 3g
Vitamin A 80% • Vitamin C 60%
Calcium 4% • Iron 4%
* Percent Daily Values are based on a 2,000 calorie diet. Your daily values may be higher or lower depending on your calorie needs:
Calories 2,000 2,500
Total Fat Less than 65g 80g
Sat Fat Less than 20g 25g
Cholesterol Less than 300mg 300mg
Sodium Less than 2,400mg 2,400mg
Total Carbohydrate 300g 375g
Fiber 25g 30g
Calories per gram:
Fat 9 • Carbohydrates 4 • Protein 4
New title signals that the label contains the newly required information.
Calories from fat are now shown on the label to help consumers meet dietary guidelines that recommend people get no more than 30 percent of their calories from fat.
% Daily Value shows how a food fits into the overall daily diet.
Daily values are also something new. Some are maximums, as with fat (65 grams or less); others are minimums, as with carbohydrates (3000 grams or more). The daily values on the label are based on a daily diet of 2,000 and 2,500 calories. Individuals should adjust the values to fit their own calorie intake.
*This label is only a sample. Exact specifications are in the final rules.
Source: Food and Drug Administration 1992

Fig. 12-4. The new food label at a glance. The label, carrying up-to-date nutrition information, is required on most packaged foods (compared to about 60 of products before 1994). The new food label serves as a key to help in planning a healthy diet. (*Source: FDA Backgrounder:* The new food label, Dec 10, 1992.)

the label. As a part of the new regulations, DRVs are being introduced for macronutrients that are sources of energy–fat, carbohydrate (including fiber), and protein–and for cholesterol, sodium, and potassium which do not contribute calories. DRVs for the energy-producing nutrients are based on the number of calories consumed per day. A daily intake of 2000 calories has been established as the reference. This level was chosen because it is believed to have the greatest public health benefit for the nation.

- Uniform "descriptors" for a food's nutrient content may be used on the new label. Terms such as *light, low-fat,* and *high-fiber* will mean the same for any product on which they appear. The FDA has set specific definitions for the following terms; *free, light, more, high, low, good source, reduced,* and *less.* For meat, fish, and poultry, the "descriptors" *lean* and *extra lean* may be used where applicable.
- Serving sizes are standardized on the new labels, making it easier to compare the nutritional value of similar products.
- The new labels may carry claims about the relationship between a nutrient and a disease, to help consumers who are concerned about eating foods that may help them keep healthier longer. For a health claim to be made on a package, the FDA must first determine that the diet-disease link is supported by scientific evidence. At this time, the FDA is allowing claims about seven relationships between food components and food, and disease risks:

Food component/food	Disease risk
Fat	Cancer
Fiber in grain products, fruits, and vegetables	Cancer
Fruits and vegetables	Cancer
Cholesterol	Heart disease
Soluble fiber in fruits, vegetables, and grains	Heart disease
Calcium	Osteoporosis
Sodium	Hypertension

❑ ❑ THE NEW FOOD LABEL REGULATIONS

Nutrient panel–content

The new food label features a nutrition panel headed with the title "Nutrition Facts." The following dietary components appear on the panel in the order they are listed here. Those in *italics* are mandatory.

total calories	soluble fiber
calories from fat	insoluble fiber
calories from saturated fat	*sugars*
total fat	sugar alcohol
saturated fat	other carbohydrate
polyunsaturated fat	*protein*
monounsaturated fat	*Vitamin A*
cholesterol	*Vitamin C*
sodium	*calcium*
potassium	*iron*
total carbohydrate	other essential vitamins and minerals
dietary fiber	

If a claim is made about any of the optional components or if a food is fortified or enriched with any of them, nutrition information for these components then becomes mandatory.

The required nutrients were selected because they address today's health concerns. The order in which they must appear reflects the priority of current dietary recommendations. Vitamins like thiamin, riboflavin, and niacin are not required because deficiencies are no longer considered of public health significance. However, they may be listed voluntarily.

Nutrient panel–format

Food components–such as fat, cholesterol, sodium, carbohydrates, and protein–are declared as a percentage of their daily value. The amounts of these substances in grams and milligrams are listed to the right. A column headed "% Daily Value" appears, as does a footnote to help consumers place their individual nutrient needs with respect to the daily values used on the label.

Requiring these food components to be declared as a percentage of the daily value is intended to prevent misinterpretations that arise with quantitative values. For example a food with 140 mg of sodium could be mistaken for a high-sodium food because 140 is a relatively large number. In actuality, 140 represents less than 6% of the daily value for sodium, which is 2400 mg.

Serving sizes

The serving size is the basis for reporting each food's nutrient content. However, unlike the past practice of leaving the serving size up to the discretion of the food manufacturer, serving sizes are now more uniform to reflect the amounts that people actually eat. Serving sizes are also expressed in both common household units and metric units.

Daily values–DRVs

The label reference value, daily value (DC), comprises two sets of dietary standards: daily reference values

Daily values–DRVs–cont'd

(DRVs) and reference daily intakes (RDIs). To make label reading less confusing, only the daily value term appears on the label.

There are DRVs for the macronutrients fat, carbohydrate, protein, and fiber; cholesterol; and sodium and potassium. DRVs for carbohydrate, fat, and protein are based on the number of calories consumed per day. A daily intake of 2000 calories has been established as the reference. This level was chosen because it was felt to have the greatest public health benefit for the nation. DRVs for the macronutrients are calculated as follows:

Fat based on 30% of calories
Saturated fat based on 10% of calories
Carbohydrate based on 60% of calories
Protein based on 10% of calories
Fiber based on 11.5 g of fiber per 1000 calories

Because of current public health recommendations, DRVs for the following food components represent the uppermost limits considered desirable:

Total fat: less than 65 g
Saturated fat: less than 20 g
Cholesterol: less than 300 mg
Sodium: less than 2400 mg

Daily values–RDIs

The RDI replaces the old "U.S. RDA" that was used on food labels from 1973 through 1993. However, the values for the new RDIs will be the same as the U.S. RDAs for the time being. In 1994 the FDA is expected to propose new RDI values.

Content descriptors

Regulations for nutrition labels spell out what terms may be used to describe the level of a food factor in a food and how these terms may be used. These are the core terms:

Free. This term means that a product contains no amount, or a trivial amount, of one or more of fat, saturated fat, cholesterol, sodium, sugars, and calories. Descriptors for these food factors are defined as follows:

Low fat: 3 g or less per serving
Low saturated fat: 1 g or less per serving
Low sodium: less than 140 mg per serving
Very low sodium: less than 35 mg per serving
Low cholesterol: less than 20 mg per serving
Low calorie: 40 calories or less per serving

Lean and extra lean. Terms that may be used to describe the fat content of meat, poultry, seafood and game meats.

Lean: less than 10 g fat, less than 4 g saturated fat, and less than 95 mg cholesterol per serving and per 100 g

Extra lean: less than 5 g fat, less than 2 g saturated fat, and less than 95 mg cholesterol per serving and per 100 g

❑ ❑ THE NEW FOOD LABEL REGULATIONS–cont'd

Content descriptors–cont'd

High. This term can be used if the food contains 20 percent of more of the DRV for a particular nutrient in a serving.

Good source. This term means that one serving of a food contains 10% to 19% of the DRV for a particular nutrient.

Reduced. This term means that a nutritionally altered product contains 25 less of a food factor or calories than the regular or reference product. However, a "reduced" claim cannot be made if its reference food already meets the requirement for a "low" claim.

Less. This term means that a food, whether altered or not, contains 25% less of a food factor or of calories than the reference food. For example, this claim can be carried by pretzels that have 25% less fat than potato chips.

Light. This descriptor can mean three things:

1. A nutritionally altered product contains one-third fewer calories or half the fat of a reference food. If the food derives 50% or more of its calorie from fat, the reduction must be 50% of the fat.
2. The sodium content of a low-calorie, low-fat food has been reduced by 50%. In addition, "light in sodium" may be used of foods in which the sodium content has been reduced by at least 50%.
3. The term *light* can be used to describe physical characteristics such as color or texture.

More. This term means that a food contains at least 10% more of the DRV of a nutrient than the reference food.

Fresh. This term can be used only on a food that is raw, has never been frozen or heated, and contains no preservatives, although irradiation at low levels is permitted. "Fresh frozen," "frozen fresh" and "freshly frozen" must be used for foods frozen while still fresh. Blanching (brief scalding) is allowed.

Other definitions

The regulations also address other claims.

Percent fat free. A product making this claim must be low-fat or fat-free. In addition, the claim must accurately reflect the amount of fat present in 100 g of the food. thus, for a food containing 5 g fat per 100 g, the claim would be "95 percent fat free."

Healthy. FDA is issuing a proposal to define "healthy." Under the proposal, healthy could be used to describe a food low in fat and saturated fat, with no more than 480 mg sodium and 60 mg cholesterol. A final rule was expected in 1993.

Ingredient labeling

The ingredient declaration appears on all foods that have more than one ingredient.

When appropriate, the ingredient list includes FDA-certified color additives, sources of protein hydrolysates, and declaration of caseinate as a milk derivative in the ingredient list of foods that claim to be nondairy, such as coffee whiteners. The main reason for these requirements is that people allergic to additives will be better able to avoid them.

Beverages that claim to contain juice must declare the total percentage of juice on the information panel.

Health claims

Claims for seven relationships between a food factor and a food and the risk of disease or health-related condition are allowed.

Calcium and osteoporosis. To carry this claim, a food must contain 20% or more of the DV for calcium (200 mg) per serving, have a calcium content that equals or exceeds the food's content of phosphorous, and contain a form of calcium that can be readily absorbed and used by the body. The claim must name the target group most in need of adequate calcium intake (teens and young adult white and Asian women) and state the need for exercise and a healthy diet. A product containing 40% or more of the DV for calcium (400 mg) must state that a total dietary intake greater than 200% of the DV for calcium has no known benefit.

Fat and cancer. To carry this claim, a food must meet the descriptor requirements for "low-fat" or, if fish or game meats, for "extra lean."

Saturated fat and cholesterol and coronary heart disease (CHD). This claim may be used if the food meets the definition for "low saturated fat," "low cholesterol," and "low-fat" or, if fish or game meats, for "extra lean."

Fiber-containing grain products, fruits, and vegetables and cancer. To carry this claim, a food must be or must contain a grain product, fruit, or vegetable and meet the descriptor requirements for "low-fat" and (without fortification) be a "good source" of fiber.

Fruits, vegetables, and grain products that contain fiber and risk of CHD. To carry this claim, a food must be or must contain fruits, vegetables, and grain products and meet the descriptor requirements for "low-fat," "low saturated fat," and "low-cholesterol" and contain (without fortification) at least 0.6 g fiber per serving.

Sodium and hypertension (high blood pressure). A food meeting the descriptor requirements for "low-sodium" may carry this claim.

Fruits and vegetables and cancer. This claim may be made for fruits and vegetables that meet the "low-fat" descriptor requirements and (without fortification) be a "good source" of at least one of the following: fiber, Vitamin A, or Vitamin C.

Adapted from *FDA backgrounder,* The new food label, Dec 10, 1992.

FOOD, NUTRITION, AND POVERTY

Hunger represents one extreme of the dichotomy of excess versus deprivation. At a time when many people are being encouraged to eat moderately, those who do not have enough to eat must also be considered. Concern for the hungry is primarily focused on the quantity of food they eat, because sufficient caloric intake to support growth in children and maintain a healthy body weight in adults is the first concern in feeding programs. But when caloric sufficiency is achieved, the nutritional quality of the diet becomes the paramount issue. Nutrient adequacy is as essential as caloric sufficiency in combating hunger and its long-term effects.

Satisfying hunger is an immediate need. Stopgap measures to ease its pain are justifiable. However, without long-term solutions, the hunger will only return to demand another quick fix. The impact of hunger goes well beyond the immediate suffering it causes. Hunger compromises the ability to learn. Hungry children have significantly higher absentee rates; and on the days they spend in school, their powers of concentration are greatly reduced. So hunger is more than simply an issue of compassion for those who do not have enough to eat. It is an issue of failed beginnings for children–the future of our planet.

In addition, the high prevalence of chronic diseases among the disadvantaged must not be overlooked. Care must be taken to ensure that efforts directed to eliminating hunger do not result in the consumption of diets that exacerbate the incidence of heart disease, stroke, and some types of cancers–the leading causes of death in the United States.

Recognizing the need to help provide poor people with enough food to eat, the United States spent nearly $29 billion for food assistance in 1991. Almost all of that budget was used to fund the programs described in this section: Food Stamp Program ($18.8 billion), Child Nutrition Programs ($5.9 billion), WIC ($2.4 billion), and the Feeding Program for the Elderly ($0.5 billion).

Poverty and Income Distribution

For most people in the United States, income has risen over time, providing more options for personal consumption expenditures, including expenditures on food. Inflation-adjusted household income increased for every income group from 1970 to 1990 (income groups are defined as each quintile in the income distribution). However, growth in income has not increased for all households equally. Poverty still exists in the United States.

According to official poverty statistics, in 1990, 13.5% of the population lived below the "poverty level"–a level of income set annually by the government for use in determining eligibility for various types of government programs, such as those discussed in this section. As can be seen from Table 12-3, the poverty level in 1992 was an annual income of $13,400 or less for a family of four. Nonmetropolitan populations generally experience a higher poverty rate than populations living in metropolitan areas.

Groups with particularly high poverty rates include

- Children: approximately one in five children live in poverty in the United States today (see Fig. 12-5)
- People living in families headed by women: families headed by single women have a poverty rate of over one third and account for one half of all poor children
- People living alone or with nonrelatives
- Blacks

Food Assistance for the Poor

For those who are poor, obtaining a nutritious diet without assistance can be a challenge. Federal, state, and local governments, as well as private charitable organizations, help to mitigate this problem by providing literally billions of dollars annually in food and nutrition. Overall, the bulk of food aid in the United States is financed at the federal level by the Department of Agriculture (USDA). One in six people in the United States receives government-sponsored food assistance

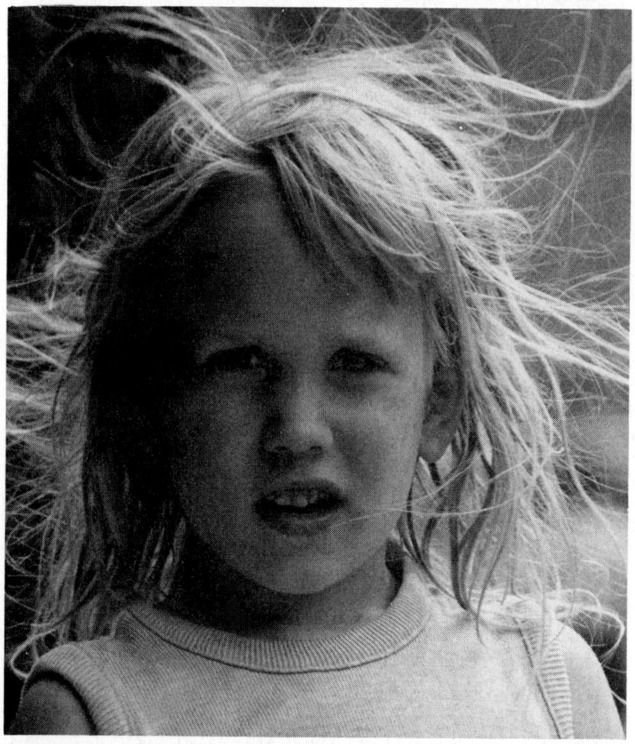

Fig. 12-5. Approximately one in five children lives in poverty in the United States today. Half these children live in families headed by women. (Photograph by Philip Leonard.)

at some point every year. The major programs that provide domestic food and nutrition assistance are described here. Their combined budget for 1991 was about $28 billion.

THE NATIONAL SCHOOL LUNCH PROGRAM[27]

NSLP is a federally assisted meal program that provides balanced, low-cost or free lunches to about 24 million children each school day. The program is usually administered by the state education agency, which provides school lunches through agreements with local schools. At the federal level, the program is administered by the Food and Nutrition Service (FNS), a USDA agency.

Schools that choose to take part in the lunch program are provided with cash subsidies and donated commodities by the USDA. Donated foods include meats, canned and frozen fruits and vegetables, fruit juices, vegetable shortening, peanut products, vegetable oil, and flour and other grain products. In return for this financial and food support, the schools must serve free or reduced-price lunches to children that meet the federal minimum pattern requirements.

- Children from families with incomes at or below 130% of the poverty level are eligible for free meals.
- Children from families between 130% and 185% of the poverty level are eligible for reduced-price meals.
- Children from families over 185% of poverty pay a regular price for the subsidized meals.

Lunches must provide one third of the RDAs and, to the extent possible, be consistent with the dietary guidelines recommendations for reducing sugar, salt, and fat intake.[20]

Year 2000 Objective. At least 90% of school lunch and school breakfast menus should be consistent with the nutrition principles in the dietary guidelines.

Calories are reduced when fat is reduced. Despite the almost universal recommendation to lower fat content of diets eaten in the United States, meals served in schools must remain nutritionally adequate with regard to calories in order to support the growth and developmental needs of children.[10]

THE SCHOOL BREAKFAST PROGRAM[29]

Assistance to states is provided by the School Breakfast Program to initiate, maintain, or expand nonprofit breakfast programs in eligible schools and residential child-care institutions.[20] The program is administered by the FNS. Any child attending a participating school may receive a free, reduced price, or full-price breakfast based on the same income criteria the SLP uses. In 1991, a daily average of 4.1 million children participated.

THE SPECIAL SUPPLEMENTAL FOOD PROGRAM FOR WOMEN, INFANTS, AND CHILDREN[30]

Popularly known as WIC, this grant program administered by the FNS provides supplemental foods, as well as health care referrals and nutrition education, at no cost. Low-income pregnant or postpartum women and children younger than 5 years at risk nutritionally are eligible for WIC. The income eligibility level is <185% of the poverty level, as illustrated in Table 12-13. Nutritional risk is determined by federal guidelines. (The health screening for WIC eligibility determination is performed at no cost to applicants to the program.) Three major types of nutritional risk are recognized:

1. High-priority medically based risks: anemia, underweight, low maternal age, history of pregnancy complications.
2. Diet-based risks such as inadequate dietary patterns determined by 24-hour recall, food frequency questionnaire, or diet history.

Table 12-13.* Poverty guidelines in the United States, 1991-1992

Household size	Poverty guidelines (100% poverty)	Free meal eligibility (130% poverty)	Reduced-price eligibility (185% poverty)
1	$6,220	$8,606	$12,247
2	8,880	11,544	16,428
3	11,140	14,482	20,609
4	13,400	17,420	24,790
5	15,660	20,358	28,971
6	17,920	23,296	33,152
7	20,180	26,234	37,333
8	22,440	29,172	41,514
For each additional family member add:			
	2,260	2,938	4,181

Source: US Department of Agriculture, Food and Nutrition Service: The national school lunch program, *Food Program Facts,* Oct 1991.
*Annual income guidelines for the continental United States from July 1, 1991 through June 30, 1992.

3. Conditions such as alcoholism or drug addiction that predispose people to medically based or diet-based risks.

WIC participants receive coupons redeemable for foods rich in protein, calcium, iron, vitamin A, and vitamin C. Included are iron-fortified infant formula and infant cereal, iron-fortified adult cereal, fruit or vegetable juice rich in vitamin C, eggs, milk, cheese, and peanut butter or dried beans. Special therapeutic formulas are provided when prescribed by a physician for a specific medical condition. Each WIC participant is designated to receive one of six different food packages: infants from birth through 3 months, infants from 4 months through a year, women and children with special dietary needs, children 1 to 5 years old, pregnant and breastfeeding women, and nonbreastfeeding postpartum women. More than 1.5 million infants participate in WIC, almost one third of the babies born in the United States.

NUTRITION PROGRAM FOR THE ELDERLY[28]

The NPE is administered by the U.S. Department of Health and Human Services (HHS); the USDA contributes commodities and cash to HHS programs for the elderly. The HHS programs provide elderly people with nutritionally sound meals (one third of the RDAs) through home-delivered meals (popularly known as meals-on-wheels) or in senior citizen centers and similar settings. The meals provide the focal points for activities that have the dual objective of promoting better health and reducing the isolation that may occur in old age. Age is the only factor in determining eligibility for NPE. People age 60 or older and their spouses regardless of age are eligible. Indian tribal organizations may select an age below 60 for defining an "older" person for their tribes. There is no income requirement to receive meals under NPE: each participant may contribute as much as he or she wishes toward the cost of the meal. Meals are free to those who cannot make a contribution. In 1991, on the average, over 900,000 meals were served every day.

THE FOOD STAMP PROGRAM[26]

Food coupons or food stamps, as they are known, are used to supplement the food-buying power of eligible low-income households. The program provides monthly allotments to low-income households to help purchase a nutritionally adequate diet. There is no requirement, however, that food stamps must be used to purchase food that is healthful. Households can use food stamps to buy any food or food product for human consumption, as well as seeds and plants for use in home gardens and to produce food. Among the items households cannot buy with food stamps are alcoholic beverages, tobacco, hot ready-to-eat foods, lunch-counter items, foods to be eaten in the store, vitamins, medicines, and pet foods.

The program is administered nationally by the FNS and locally by state welfare agencies. In 1991, the average monthly benefit per person was almost $64.00. Half of food stamp recipients are children, and 8% are elderly. To qualify, households must meet eligibility criteria that includes a gross income at or below 130% of the federal poverty guidelines (see Table 12-13). Most able-bodied adult applicants must also meet certain work requirements. Households may own certain resources. In addition to income, the food stamp allotment is also based on family size. In 1992, the maximum allotment levels based on household size were

Household size	Allotment level
1	$111
2	203
3	292
4	370
5	440
6	528
7	584
8	667
Each additional member	83

Source: US Department of Agriculture, Food and Nutrition Service: The food stamp program, *Food Program Facts,* p 3, Oct 1991.

Nutrition Screening for the Poor

Nutrition screening is the process of discovering characteristics or risk factors known to be associated with dietary or nutrition problems. Its main purpose is to identify individuals–such as the elderly and the poor–who are potentially at high risk because of complex and involved problems that touch upon nutrition. To serve this purpose, screening criteria must be simple, relatively straightforward, and easy to administer. Screening is also helpful in establishing priorities for the most efficient use of available and valuable time and money.[16]

Although developed to be used primarily with the elderly, the screening tool *Determine Your Nutritional Health,* which appears in Fig. 12-6, may be adapted for use with any age group starting with adolescents. The goal of this short, easy-to-read, self-administered, screening device is to raise consciousness about the importance of nutrition to an individual's health.

Determine Your Nutritional Health consists of two brief parts.[6] The first is a self-assessment that helps people identify aspects of their eating habits and lifestyles–such as eating fewer than two meals a day or having three or more drinks of beer, liquor, or wine almost every day–that may place them at nutritional risk.

DETERMINE YOUR NUTRITIONAL HEALTH

The Warning Signs of poor nutritional health are often overlooked. Use this checklist to find out if you or someone you know is at nutritional risk.

Read the statements below. Circle the number in the yes column for those that apply to you or someone you know. For each yes answer, score the number in the box. Total your nutritional score.

	YES
I have an illness or condition that made me change the kind and/or amount of food I eat.	2
I eat fewer than 2 meals per day.	3
I eat few fruits or vegetables, or milk products.	2
I have 3 or more drinks of beer, liquor or wine almost every day.	2
I have tooth or mouth problems that make it hard for me to eat.	2
I don't always have enough money to buy the food I need.	4
I eat alone most of the time.	1
I take 3 or more different prescribed or over-the-counter drugs a day.	1
Without wanting to, I have lost or gained 10 pounds in the last 6 months.	2
I am not always physically able to shop, cook and/or feed myself.	2
TOTAL	

Total Your Nutritional Score. If it's —

0-2 **Good!** Recheck your nutritional score in 6 months.

3-5 **You are at moderate nutritional risk.** See what can be done to improve your eating habits and lifestyle. Your office on aging, senior nutrition program, senior citizens center or health department can help. Recheck your nutritional score in 3 months.

6 or more **You are at high nutritional risk.** Bring this checklist the next time you see your doctor, dietitian or other qualified health or social service professional. Talk with them about any problems you may have. Ask for help to improve your nutritional health.

These materials developed and distributed by the Nutrition Screening Initiative, a project of:

AMERICAN ACADEMY OF FAMILY PHYSICIANS

THE AMERICAN DIETETIC ASSOCIATION

NATIONAL COUNCIL ON THE AGING

Remember that warning signs suggest risk, but do not represent diagnosis of any condition. Turn the page to learn more about the Warning Signs of poor nutritional health.

Fig. 12-6. Determine your nutritional health. (*Source:* The Nutrition Screening Initiative, Washington, DC, 1992.)

Continued.

The Nutrition Checklist is based on the Warning Signs described below. Use the word <u>DETERMINE</u> to remind you of the Warning Signs.

DISEASE

Any disease, illness or chronic condition which causes you to change the way you eat, or makes it hard for you to eat, puts your nutritional health at risk. Four out of five adults have chronic diseases that are affected by diet. Confusion or memory loss that keeps getting worse is estimated to affect one out of five or more of older adults. This can make it hard to remember what, when or if you've eaten. Feeling sad or depressed, which happens to about one in eight older adults, can cause big changes in appetite, digestion, energy level, weight and well-being.

EATING POORLY

Eating too little and eating too much both lead to poor health. Eating the same foods day after day or not eating fruit, vegetables, and milk products daily will also cause poor nutritional health. One in five adults skip meals daily. Only 13% of adults eat the minimum amount of fruit and vegetables needed. One in four older adults drink too much alcohol. Many health problems become worse if you drink more than one or two alcoholic beverages per day.

TOOTH LOSS/ MOUTH PAIN

A healthy mouth, teeth and gums are needed to eat. Missing, loose or rotten teeth or dentures which don't fit well or cause mouth sores make it hard to eat.

ECONOMIC HARDSHIP

As many as 40% of older Americans have incomes of less than $6,000 per year. Having less--or choosing to spend less--than $25-30 per week for food makes it very hard to get the foods you need to stay healthy.

REDUCED SOCIAL CONTACT

One-third of all older people live alone. Being with people daily has a positive effect on morale, well-being and eating.

MULTIPLE MEDICINES

Many older Americans must take medicines for health problems. Almost half of older Americans take multiple medicines daily. Growing old may change the way we respond to drugs. The more medicines you take, the greater the chance for side effects such as increased or decreased appetite, change in taste, constipation, weakness, drowsiness, diarrhea, nausea, and others. Vitamins or minerals when taken in large doses act like drugs and can cause harm. Alert your doctor to everything you take.

INVOLUNTARY WEIGHT LOSS/GAIN

Losing or gaining a lot of weight when you are not trying to do so is an important warning sign that must not be ignored. Being overweight or underweight also increases your chance of poor health.

NEEDS ASSISTANCE IN SELF CARE

Although most older people are able to eat, one of every five have trouble walking, shopping, buying and cooking food, especially as they get older.

ELDER YEARS ABOVE AGE 80

Most older people lead full and productive lives. But as age increases, risk of frailty and health problems increase. Checking your nutritional health regularly makes good sense.

The Nutrition Screening Initiative, 2626 Pennsylvania Avenue, NW, Suite 301, Washington, DC 20037

© The Nutrition Screening Initiative is funded in part by a grant from Ross Laboratories, a division of Abbott Laboratories.

A5944/MARCH 1992

***Fig. 12-6,* cont'd.** Determine your nutritional health.

The second part has two purposes. The first is to provide basic education on nutritional risk factors and indicators. The second, using the mnemonic d-e-t-e-r-m-i-n-e, is designed to remind both the general public and health professionals about the warning signs of poor nutritional health. *Determine*–part of the title *Determine Your Nutritional Health*–stands for

Disease
Eating poorly
Tooth loss or mouth pain
Economic hardship
Reduced social contact
Multiple medicines
Involuntary weight loss or gain
Needs assistance in self-care
Elder years above age 80

SCREENING FOR MALNUTRITION

The single largest demographic group at disproportionate risk of malnutrition are the elderly. Nutrition screening holds a tremendous preventive health potential for older adults. Any individual, however, young or old, needs attention if he or she has been identified with warning signs from the *determine* checklist.

The nurse should provide nutrition counseling or refer to a dietitian if the client has food-related problems. A dietitian or community nutrition program may be appropriate if any of the following are identified in the individual:

- Inappropriate, inadequate, or excessive food intake
- Problems complying with a specialized diet
- Need for nutrient-specific counseling or counseling related to a specific disease
- Weight at more than 120% of what is desirable
- Serum cholesterol at more than 240 mg/dl
- Functionally dependent for eating or for food-related ADL

The nurse should refer the client to a physician if body wight is 20 percent above or below the desirable weight or if there has been an involuntary decrease in weight of more than 10 pounds in the past 6 months. Additional anthropometric measurements suggesting malnutrition include

- Triceps skinfold thickness <10th percentile
- Midarm, muscle circumference <10th percentile
- Serum albumin <3.5 g/dl
- Evidence of osteoporosis or mineral deficiency (indicated by a history of bone pain or fractures, particularly in housebound elderly females)
- Evidence of vitamin deficiency (indicated by inadequate fruit and vegetable intake; angular stomatitis, glossitis, or bleeding gums; pressure sores in the bedridden).

Year 2000 Objective: Increase to at least 75% the number of primary care providers who provide nutritional assessment and counseling or referral to qualified nutritionists or dietitians. In 1988, physicians provided diet counseling for an estimated 40% to 50% of their patients.[31]

SOURCES OF INFORMATION ABOUT FOOD AND NUTRITION

Nurses interested in food and nutrition need to know where to find reliable information. Local resources include registered dietitians (RDs) at local hospitals or in private practice; professors of nutrition, biochemistry, and foods and nutrition at nearby colleges and universities; local newspaper food editors; extension agents; and public health nutritionists who work at department of health or WIC centers.

There are excellent sources of nutrition information in print. Among them are the books, journals, and newsletters. Reputable information is also available from government (tax-supported) agencies, professional associations, and voluntary and for-profit organizations. Many of these organizations provide their publications lists on request.

SUMMARY

This chapter has introduced a wide range of subjects, including the year 2000 nutrition objectives, the most current diet recommendations to reduce the risks of developing nutrition-related diseases, FDA regulations for the new 1994 food labeling, and government food aid programs for the poor and the elderly. Together, these topics form the basis of what is known as *preventive nutrition,* a requisite for the promotion of the public's health. The nurse should share with everyone, including family, friends, and clients. The nurse should also become a role model for healthy living by eating well. The most effective nutrition educators practice what they teach.

References

1. American Dietetic Association and American Diabetes Association: *Exchange lists for meal planning,* Chicago, 1986, American Dietetic Association.
2. American Dietetic Association and American Diabetes Association: *Exchange lists for weight management,* Chicago, 1989, American Dietetic Association.
3. American Heart Association, Council on Cardiovascular Nursing. Cholesterol Education Program for Nurses Task Force: *Nurses' cholesterol education handbook,* Dallas, 1990, American Heart Association.
4. Burke GL, et al: Correlates of obestiy in young black and white women: the CARDIA study, *Am J Public Health* 82:1621, 1992.
5. Cummings S, et al: Epidemiology of osteoporosis and osteoporotic fractures, *Epidemiol Rev* 7:178, 1985.
6. Dwyer J: *Screening older Americans' nutritional health: current practices and future possibilities,* Washington, DC, 1991, The Nutrition Screening Initiative.
7. Food and Nutrition Board: *Recommended dietary allowances,* ed 10, Washington, DC, 1989, National Academy Press.
8. Kuczmarski RJ: Prevalence of overweight and weight gain in the United States, *Am J Clin Nutr* 55:495S, 1992.
9. Johnston C, et al: Calcium supplementation and increases in bone mineral density in children, *N Engl J Med* 327:82, 1991.
10. Lytle L, Snyder MP: School food service for the 1990's: advancements and challenges, *Food & Nutrition News* 65:7, 1993.
11. National Center for Health Statistics: *Prevention profile: health, United States, 1991,* Hyattsville, Md, 1992, Public Health Service.
12. National Cholesterol Education Program: Report of the national cholesterol education program expert panel on detection, evaluation, and treatment of high blood cholesterol in adults, *Arch Int Med* 148:36, 1988.
13. National Institutes of Health: *Diet and exercise in noninsulin-dependent diabetes mellitus. National Institutes of Health Consensus Development Conference Statement, vol 6,* National Institute of Arthritis, Diabetes and Digestive and Kidney Diseases and the Office of Medical Applications of Research, Bethesda, Md, 1986, US Department of Health and Human Services.
14. National Research Council. Committee on Diet and Health: *Diet and health: implications for reducing chronic disease risk,* Committee on Diet and Health, Food and Nutrition Board, Commission on Life Sciences, National Research Council, Washington, DC, 1989, National Academy Press.
15. Nutrition Screening Initiative: *Nutrition screening manual for professionals caring for older Americans,* Washington, DC, 1991, The Nutrition Screening Initiative.
17. Porter DV, Earl RO, editors: *Nutritional labeling: issues and directions for the 1990s.* Report of a study by the committee on the nutrition components of food labeling. Food and Nutrition Board, Institute of Medicine, National Academy of Sciences, Washington DC, 1990, National Academy Press.
18. Ramazzotto LJ, et al: Calcium nutriture and the aging process: a review, *Gerontology* 5:159, 1986.
19. Snow-Harter C: Exercise, calcium and estrogen: primary regulators of bone mass, *Contemp Nutr* 17:1, 1992.
20. Statewide Training Network for School Food Service Workers. The State Education Department: *Good nutrition–better forever,* Albany, NY, University of the State of New York.
21. Thomas PR, editor: *Improving America's diet and health: from recommendations to action.* A report of the committee on dietary guidelines implementation. Food and Nutrition Board, Institute of Medicine, National Academy of Sciences, Washington, DC, 1991, National Academy Press.
22. Welsh S, Davis C, Shaw A: A brief history of food guides in the United States, *Nutr Today* 27:6, 1992.
23. US Department of Agriculture: *The food guide pyramid.* Home and garden bulletin no 252, Washington, DC, 1992, US Government Printing Office.
24. US Department of Agriculture and US Department of Health and Human Services: *Nutrition and your health: dietary guidelines for Americans,* Home and garden bulletin no 232, Washington, DC, 1990, US Government Printing Office.
25. US Department of Agriculture and US Department of Health and Human Services: United States country paper. Presented in Rome, Italy, Dec 1992, International Conference on Nutrition.
26. US Department of Agriculture, Food and Nutrition Service: The food stamp program, *Food Program Facts,* pp 1-7, Oct 1991.
27. US Department of Agriculture, Food and Nutrition Service: The national school lunch porgram, *Food Program Facts,* pp 1-4, Oct 1991.
28. US Department of Agriculture, Food and Nutrition Service: Nutrition program for the elderly, *Food Program Facts,* pp 1-2, Oct 1991.
29. US Department of Agriculture, Food and Nutrition Service: The school breakfast program, *Food Program Facts,* pp 1-3, Oct 1991.
30. US Department of Agriculture, Food and Nutrition Service: The special supplemental food program for women, infants, and children (WIC), *Food Program Facts,* pp 1-3, Oct 1991.
31. US Department of Health and Human Services: *Healthy people 2000: national health promotion and disease prevention objectives,* Washington, DC, 1991, Public Health Service.
32. US Department of Health and Human Services: *Promoting health/preventing disease: objectives for the nation,* Washington, DC, 1980, US Government Printing Office.
33. US Department of Health and Human Services: *The surgeon general's report on nutrition and health,* DHHS (PHS) Publ no 88-50210, US Department of Health and Human Services, Public Health Service, Washington, DC, 1988, US Government Printing Office.
34. US Department of Health and Human Services. Public Health Service: diabetes and chronic disabling conditions, *A Public health service progress report on healthy people 2000,* Washington DC, US Department of Health and Human Services.
35. US Department of Health and Human Services. Public Health Service, National Institutes of Health: *Methods for voluntary weight loss and control.* National Institutes of Health Technology Assessment Conference, March 30 to April 1, 1992, Bethesda, Md, 1992, National Institutes of Health.
36. US Department of Health and Human Services. Public Health Service. National Institutes of Health. National Heart, Lung, and Blood Institute. National Cholesterol Education Program: *Report of the expert panel on blood cholesterol levels in children and adolescents,* 1991, NIH Pub no 91-2732, Washington, DC, 1991, US Government Printing Office.
37. US Department of Health, Education, and Welfare: *Healthy people: the surgeon general's report on health promotion and disease prevention,* Washington, DC, 1979, Public Health Service.
38. Wallace R, et al: Inventory of knowledge and skills relating to disease prevention and health promotion, *Am J Prev Med* 6:51, 1990.
39. Wardlaw GM, Insel PM: *Perspectives in nutrition,* ed 2, St Louis, 1993, Mosby.

CHAPTER

13

Stress Management and Crisis Intervention

Katherine Smith Detherage

Sally Stark Johnson

Carol Lynn Mandle

Objectives

After completing this chapter, the nurse will be able to

- *Define stress and stressors.*
- *Discuss the nurse's roles in stress management.*
- *Differentiate crisis from stress.*
- *Describe situational and developmental crises.*
- *Describe the phases of a crisis.*
- *Identify the factors that affect the outcome(s) of stress.*
- *Define crisis intervention and identify its goals.*
- *Discuss the nurse's roles in primary prevention of crises.*
- *Describe the normal grieving process.*
- *Identify the factors that influence the outcome of mourning.*
- *Discuss nursing interventions for clients who are mourning.*

Stress is part of living. Individuals frequently encounter biologic, physical, mental, psychologic, social, or environmental events–stressors–that require change or adaptation. These stressors can range from the activities of daily living–caring for children, meeting work deadlines, and cleaning or repairing the house–to events like taking a crucial examination, losing a relative by death, losing possessions in a fire, losing a job, or getting married. Some persons manage successfully to get through the stressful event in a healthy manner by using appropriate problem-solving abilities and familiar coping behaviors that have worked in other stressful situations. Here is a case example:

Martha is a single, 24-year-old computer programmer who had been employed by a small manufacturing company for 6 months. Four days ago the company's president notified the employees that because of decreased sales over the last three quarters, the company would lay off half its employees; if sales did not increase, the company would close.

Martha learned today that she was one of three employees in her department to be laid off. Her immediate reaction was, "Why me?" She became very angry and told her immediate supervisor that there were other less-qualified people in her department who should be laid off rather than she herself. She also accused top-level officials of bad fiscal management. For the rest of the day Martha was preoccupied, her concentration was inadequate, and she said little to her fellow workers.

On awakening the next morning after a restless night, Martha was tired, her head ached, and generally she did not feel well. She decided to call in sick and spent the day in bed. Throughout the day Martha mulled over the events of the past 4 days. She knew that she had been a good employee, yet she was being laid off. Why? Mentally going through the other people in her department, she realized that the three people being laid off, herself included, had less seniority than the other employees.

Martha felt much better about the situation. She knew that it would be difficult to manage without a job, but she had some savings and knew she could move in temporarily with her parents. She also realized that computer programmers were currently in demand. Martha decided to call her friend, Betty, who might have some information on possible job openings for programmers within her company.

Martha handled the stressful event of job loss by using coping behaviors that had worked for her in the past. Specifically, she ventilated her anger at her supervisor, withdrew by calling in ill, and sought the help of a friend. Although she has not resolved the stressful situation completely, Martha's behavior demonstrates a healthy coping mechanism.

Others are not as successful in managing a stressful event. With these persons, the causes of stress are so overwhelming that their usual methods of coping are ineffective, as in this example:

John Smith, age 42, had been employed at the local electronics firm since high school. He is married, the father of six children, ranging in age from 18 months to 14 years. His wife Virginia remained at home with the youngest children but derived a small income from selling cosmetics by telephone. The family raised their own chickens and planted a garden each spring to offset the high cost of feeding a family of eight.

John worked hard at his soldering machine in the plant and established a reputation as a good worker. He was conscientious and tried to maintain a high quality of production. He averaged 20 hours of overtime a week on second shift to supplement his full-time wage.

John was concerned about the extra needs of his family. They had a meager savings account, with little money to rely on. His daughter Sarah needed braces, and it was possible the family car would not pass inspection. He would have liked to be closer to his family, especially the boys; but by day's end he was exhausted. He would snap at the children for their noise or only eat and fall asleep.

John was paid by piecework; he received a rate for every piece but something was deducted for each incorrectly soldered one. Recently he had tried to speed his rate of production to earn some extra money for the car and Sarah's braces. A few months ago John began to experience some pains in his chest. He decided it was heartburn and started to chew antacid tablets, although they really did not help. One time the pains became so severe that he could not even lift his arms and had to sit down to catch his breath. He was afraid to tell his supervisor for fear he would be sent to the health clinic. If the doctor found something wrong, he believed he would no longer be able to provide for his family. He could not afford to lose any time from work with a family that depended on him.

Last night John arrived home after a 12-hour shift, looking very pale. He skipped dinner because his heartburn was bothering him and went straight to bed. Awakening in the middle of the night gasping for breath, John staggered to the window to get more air. The pain in his chest was viselike, radiating down both arms. His wife awoke from the cold breeze entering the room and found John slumped on the floor.

John's resulting heart attack not only caused him physical crisis but also created a psychologic and economic crisis for both him and his family.

Many life events can lead to stress (see the box to the left on p. 301 for symptoms of stress). Every day, nurses see persons who are stressed and are either at risk for crisis or in crisis. All types of nurses become involved: the nurse who works for an industrial company facing massive layoffs; the community health nurse who works in a neighborhood with substandard housing, poor health care, and a high crime rate; the nurse who works in student health services at a large university; and the nurse who works triage in the emergency department of a metropolitan hospital. Whatever the locale, nurses soon realize that their clients are at risk, some more than others, for undergoing a crisis. (See the box to the right on p. 301 for strategies for managing stress.)

The universality of stress and crisis requires nurses to understand stress and crisis theories. These theories provide the nurse with theoretic frameworks to systematically guide interventions when working with individuals, families, and communities faced with potential or actual stressful events.

This chapter presents stress, stress management, crisis, and crisis interventions as they relate to the primary prevention framework. Some events, such as those that are part of the process of growth and maturity, can be anticipated. Primary planning for these situations will assist the client to make a smoother transition from one developmental stage to the next. Other situations are unexpected and require immediate intervention to prevent further personal disorganization. The nurse who has helped the individual, family, or community to attain their maximum level of physical and mental health functioning will find these persons better able to cope

❑ ❑ SYMPTOMS OF STRESS

Physiologic/Behavioral

Increased heart rate
Rise in blood pressure
Dryness of mouth and throat
Sweating
Tightness of chest
Headache
Nausea/vomiting
Indigestion
Diarrhea
Trembling, twitching
Grinding of teeth
Insomnia
Anorexia
Fatigue
Slumped posture
Pain, tightness in neck and back muscles
Urinary frequency
Missed menstrual cycle
Reduced interest in sex
Accident proneness
Startle reaction
Hyperventilation

Affective

Irritability
Depression
Angry outbursts
Emotional instability
Poor concentration
Uninterest in activities
Withdrawal
Restlessness
Anxiety
Increased use of sarcasm
Tendency to cry easily
Nightmares
Suspiciousness
Jealousy
Decreased involvement with others
Bickering
Complaining, criticizing
Tendency to be easily startled
Increased smoking
Use of alcohol and drugs

Cognitive

Forgetfulness
Poor judgment
Poor concentration
Reduced creativity
Less fantasizing
Errors in arithmetic and grammar
Preoccupation
Inattention to details
Blocking
Reduced productivity

❑ ❑ STRATEGIES FOR MANAGING STRESS

- Evaluate sources of stress at work and attempt to change them.
- Learn to manage time effectively.
- Limit overtime.
- Discuss and try to solve problems with co-workers.
- Try not to personalize criticisms. Remember, it is often the situation that is the problem, although you may be the target of their emotions.
- Rotate assignments of those who are difficult to care for.
- Recognize the symptoms of stress in yourself and seek the help of an objective party to assist you in discussing and managing your feelings.
- Learn techniques for controlling your response to stress (e.g., deep breathing, repeating a saying in your mind that helps you stay calm, counting to 25).
- Withdraw from the situation and seek help when you feel you may lose control.
- When you feel "burned out" or as though you cannot cope, talk to your supervisor about scheduling time off.
- Instead of coffee and cigarette breaks, enjoy breaks in which you do short relaxation exercises, recline in a quiet area, or listen to relaxation tapes.
- Eat a well-balanced diet; avoid junk foods.
- Exercise regularly.
- Do something for yourself to unwind between work and home.
- Take naps; allow ample time for sleep.
- Schedule leisure activities into your life; develop a hobby.
- Do not rely on cigarettes, alcohol, or drugs to assist in relaxation.
- Learn about meditation and relaxation exercises and attempt to build them into your life.

with unanticipated events. Primary prevention does not imply prevention of stress, for it is neither practical nor feasible to suggest that nurses should or could prevent all stress from occurring. Rather, the nurse's role in primary care is to maximize the client's level of wellness so he or she can deal most effectively with problems. For the client experiencing stress, the nurse's role is to intercede to prevent further physical or psychologic breakdown resulting from the stressful event and to strengthen the client's future coping behaviors, minimizing the probability of stress-related illnesses and crises.

HISTORICAL PERSPECTIVE

Although stress events and crisis situations have always occurred, only in the past 30 to 40 years have they been viewed as a phenomenon for study, and only more recently have stress management and crisis intervention gained recognition as appropriate therapeutic tools. What has occurred in our society to cause such an awakening?

Consider Tevye, the main character in *Fiddler on the Roof,* who states

> A fiddler on the roof. Sounds crazy, uh? But here in our little village of Anatevka, you might say every one of us is a fiddler on the roof, trying to scratch out a pleasant, simple tune without breaking his neck. It isn't easy.
>
> You may ask, "Why do we stay up here if it is so dangerous?" We stay because Anatevka is our home. And how do we keep our balance? That I can tell you in one word. Tradition.
>
> Because of our traditions we've kept our balance for many, many years. Here in Anatevka we have traditions for everything–how to sleep, how to eat, how to work, how to wear clothes. For instance, we always keep our heads covered and wear little prayer shawls. This shows our constant devotion to God. You may ask, "Why did this tradition get started?" I'll tell you. I don't know. But it's a tradition. And because of our traditions every one of us knew who he was and what God expects him to do.*

For Tevye life was based on tradition. His life role was predetermined, from his work as a farmer to his relationship with his wife and children. If he ever felt confused about his purpose in life, he simply consulted the local rabbi for advice and support. The ebb and flow of this life created a peaceful existence within his small Russian community. He had achieved homeostasis, or balance, between himself, his surroundings, and his beliefs.

Although this is a fictional situation, it represents life before the technologic age. Most people lived in small communities, sharing a common occupation. Families lived for many generations either in the same house or close to a central home. As the children grew and married, they remained at home, joining the family business. All family members shared in daily work assignments, passing their social, cultural, and religious beliefs to succeeding generations. This coexistence of the extended family fostered a family identity, a psychologic and economic network of support for each family member.

The age of technology shifted economy from its agrarian origins; producing goods without machines was no longer economically viable. Large families were no longer needed for labor-intensive tasks. Family units became smaller, usually consisting of parents and unmarried children. The extended family began to dissolve, as younger members moved to the city. Urbanization required that families' attempt to create a new network of supports from new friends, neighbors, and coworkers.

Urban life today is not conducive for families to find such networks of support as existed in Anatevka. Our highly mobile society implies that coworkers are transferred, and neighbors from many different ethnic and cultural backgrounds may not necessarily share the same values, beliefs, and interests, making it difficult to form a network of persons that could be considered a surrogate extended family.

In addition, technology and urbanization have created new changes and problems. Advanced air and space travel, rapid communication systems, more accessible education, and a higher standard of living for some also have brought more stress to life, as has the competition to "keep up" or "get ahead" at home, school, or work. Inflation, high tax rates, increased crime, and indiscriminate use of drugs have pressured individuals and families to foster a sense of unity in a society that has displaced the extended family, thus creating fewer supportive mechanisms that individuals and families need in times of change and stress.

Every individual and family is faced with certain inevitable life stresses, such as the addition of a new family member through birth or adoption, children entering or finishing school, marriage, retirement, illness, and death. Everyone also passes through developmental stages. Both the passage to maturity and the situational stresses create a temporary imbalance. Its outcome depends on the person's ability to cope with the new situation. Equilibrium is restored if the individual is able to cope in a positive manner. If not, the stress leads to disorder and possible dysfunction, crisis ensues, and chaos may result.

Nurses can use their knowledge, understanding, and application of stress and crisis theories to assist individuals and families to cope more effectively, not only with the demands of normal growth and development, but also with the stressful demands of our highly urbanized and technical society.[41]

Differentiating between Stress and Crisis

The terms *stress* and *crisis* are often used interchangeably, but they denote separate phenomena.

Stress is a specific reaction to a life event. The event, called a *stressor,* may be a change in the economic, environmental, political, or social-cultural forces that affect our lives. The person reacting to the stressor is said to be in a *stress state.* How the person copes with

*From *Fiddler on the Roof,* copyright 1964 by Joseph Stein. Used with permission.

the stressor will determine whether the event leads to a state of crisis. In addition, the person's perception of the stressor will also determine if the event will lead to crisis. Change may be viewed as positive, called *eustress,* or negative, called *distress.* For example, one man may perceive losing his job as blocking his life's goals *(distress),* where another person may see it as a welcome opportunity for growth with a different company *(eustress).*

Much of our understanding of the stress reaction comes from the work of Hans Selye.[45] His endocrinology research described the combination of hormonal and nervous system changes that trigger the "fight or flight" response. The body's physiologic response to a stressor is the same whether the change is positive, such as anticipating a date, or negative, such as anticipating a court appearance. This response is designed to ready the body's defenses for action. Unfortunately, unlike animals, humans today cannot always use this response to escape from stressors. Social norms exclude us from fleeing stressful situations or fighting back in a physical way. While animals return to a state of homeostasis following a fight-or-flight response, people frequently internalize their responses, allowing the stress response to continue.

Stress–whether stemming from life events, chronic strain, or environmental pressures–is associated with biologic changes contributing to emotional, cognitive,[28] and behavioral dysfunctions (such as chemical abuse, suicide, or violence) and if chronic, to pathologies such as migraine headaches, hypertension, gastrointestinal disorders, and arthritis.[3,47]

In contrast, crisis is a self-limiting state, usually lasting from 1 to 6 weeks. Caplan[7] observed an identifiable beginning, middle, and end to crisis. Intervention for crisis usually occurs around the fourth week and lasts from 1 to 12 weeks.

Dynamics of Stress and Crisis

The word *crisis* is derived from the Greek word *krisis,* meaning decision. Adopted from early medicine, crisis meant "typical of pneumonia" and was seen as a turning point or a point of no return; that is, the person would either return to a state of health or die.

Today, the many definitions of crisis reflect an author's particular style or theoretic foundation. Some authors deal only with individual crisis; others include families and population in their definitions. Some use psychoanalytic terminology, whereas others choose the language of general systems theory. Most persons working in crisis intervention refer to the studies by Caplan[7] and Lindemann.[29]

Rapoport[39] views crises as "turning points–as points of no return," and "an upset in a steady state." Blondis and Jackson[4] see crisis as "a dramatic change in one's life." Parad[34,35] states that "crisis consists of a hazardous circumstance of stress which constitutes a threat for individuals and families because (a) the stress jeopardizes important life goals such as health, security, and ties of affection and (b) the problems posed cannot be immediately solved by the immediate resources of the ego, thereby generating a high level of uncertainty, anxiety and tension."

This chapter uses Caplan's definition of crisis: "Crisis occurs when a person faces an obstacle to important life goals that are for a time insurmountable through the customary methods of problem solving. A period of disorganization ensues, a period of upset, during which many abortive attempts at solution are made."[4]

Individuals, as open and living systems, interact consciously and unconsciously with their internal and external environments to maintain a steady state or equilibrium. When a situation, such as an illness or a threat of danger, produces a disturbance to equilibrium, the person activates problem-solving abilities and coping mechanisms to restore equilibrium. If the stress is such that it pushes the person beyond the ability to restore equilibrium, crisis will result.

The epidemiologic model of Leavell and Clark shows the interaction of host, agent, and environment in maintaining a state of equilibrium (see Chapter 1). The triangle will remain in balance as long as it is not confronted with stressors beyond its ability to adapt. Minor imbalances can be tolerated by triangle adjustment. However, when the usual problem-solving abilities and coping mechanisms of a family, person, or community are unsuccessful, a major triangle imbalance occurs, increasing the risk of dysfunction. Crisis ensues when the risk of dysfunction to the triangle no longer can be tolerated, eventually resulting in exhaustion.

Generally, three types of solutions exist for any problem. First, the person can tolerate the problem. Tolerance, usually a temporary situation, often leads to one of the other solutions because the problem still remains, continuing to stress and leading to a state of disequilibrium. Changing the situation is the second solution; the person takes charge of the stressful situation and adapts to it, restoring a steady state. In the chapter's first case study, Martha realized that she could not avoid her job loss and called a friend to inquire about other prospective employment opportunities. This action demonstrates her ability to adapt to her problem and attempt to resolve it. The third solution is to escape the situation. Although also a temporary solution, escape may provide time to restore the ability to cope.

Unfortunately none of these solutions works to achieve equilibrium in crisis, since the usual coping mechanisms are ineffective in a crisis. According to Caplan[7] and to Lindemann,[29] when a person or family is in crisis, the internal equilibrium is off balance, and the usual psychologic resources are overtaxed, creating a risk for further breakdown. Rapoport[38] noted three interrelated factors that can produce a state of crisis:

1. There is a hazardous event that poses a threat.
2. A threat to instinctual need is linked symbolically to earlier threats and leads to vulnerability or conflict.
3. There is an inability to respond with adequate coping mechanisms.

These observations are not intended to present a bleak picture for the person in crisis; primary intervention may prevent crisis, whereas intervention at the secondary level of care will identify families at the onset of the problem to prevent further breakdown.

Balancing Factors Affecting Consequences of Stress

Specific reasons explain why a stressor will lead an individual or family into one crisis but not into another. Occurring between the initial stressful event and the resolution of the problem are balancing factors:[1]

1. Ability to perceive the event realistically, that is, to understand the relationship between the stressor and stress reaction. Once the situation is identified, the individual must actively seek information to resolve the problem.

   Caplan[7] observed the phases that characterized the reaction to a stressful event. In the initial phase tension rises in response to the stressor; the person attempts to cope with the stressful event by using previous problem-solving approaches. If these approaches are ineffective, the second phase develops when the tension level rises and the person becomes more upset and institutes emergency problem-solving measures. During the third phase the tension level continues to rise, and the problem is either solved, redefined, or avoided. If the problem remains unsolved, the person enters the final and fourth phase of disorganization. This lack of ability to solve problems under stress will lead to a rise in stress and personal disorganization.
2. Presence of situational supports. Human beings are social animals who need other persons to help them solve problems. They must develop the ability to seek and use help when confronted with a task or with feelings that affect equilibrium. If they think they have no interpersonal or institutional resources for situational help, disequilibrium will result, possibly leading to crisis.
3. Presence of adequate coping mechanisms. Everyone has a unique pattern of behavior that allows him or her to reduce the tension level and maintain equilibrium. Usually the individual manages by being aware of personal thoughts and feelings and expressing them verbally or by using other forms of behavior to decrease tension and master the stressful situation. If the person is not able to do this, tension levels continue to rise and may result in crisis.

The nurse must assess the individual or family for these balancing factors before beginning to plan a strategy for intervention. Once the initial assessment is completed, the nurse can help the individual or family to supplement personal strengths to avoid a crisis state and future health consequences. A paradigm that outlines the balancing factors in effect during a stressful event is presented in Fig. 13-1. This diagram should help the nurse to visualize a stressor's effect during a state of equilibrium and the factors that lead to or prevent crisis and longer-term health consequences.

An Assessment for Persons at Risk for Stress and Crisis: Social Readjustment Rating Scale

In 1949 at the University of Washington School of Medicine, Holmes and Rahe[20-22] initiated a method of correlating life events with illness. Their research investigated the relationship between social readjustments, stress, and the susceptibility to illness. From this research, the Social Readjustment Rating Scale (SRRS) was developed, a weighted assessment of 42 life events that require individual adaptation and adjustment (Table 13-1).

To use the scale, the person checks off the events that have happened within the last year, then totals the score. The total equals the number of life change units (LCUs) for that year. A score less than 150 LCUs per year would indicate little or no change, roughly a 50% chance for illness. Scores of 150 to 199 place the individual at risk for mild health change. At 200 to 299 the person would experience moderate risk of health changes, whereas a score of 300 or more LCUs signify major change, with the chance of illness at almost 90%.[20-22]

The events listed in the scale are common to everyone. Many are pleasurable changes, such as finishing school, getting married, or becoming pregnant. Rather than the adversity of the event, the biologic and psychologic reaction to the change creates the stress. Selye[45] applied the term *distress* to excessive stress that results from prolonged stress or frustration. Some stress is beneficial; the distress is what damages. The key is to find optimum stress levels, with enough to generate energy into the system without overtaxing adaptive capabilities.

Although the development of the SRRS was a landmark contribution to the study of human stress, there are many well-recognized deficiencies in both its content

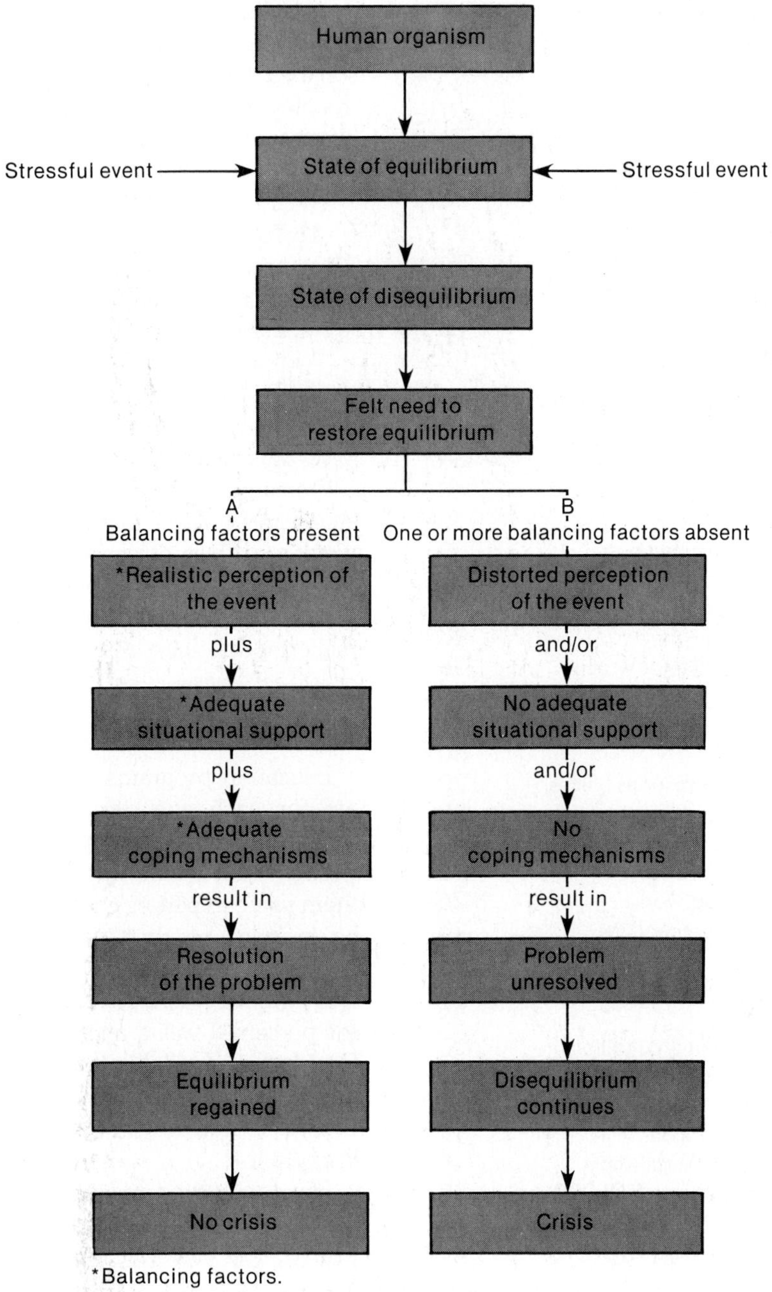

Fig. 13-1. Paradigm of effect of balancing factors in stressful event. (From Aguilera DC: *Crisis intervention: theory and methodology,* ed 6, St Louis, 1990, Mosby.)

and its applications. For example, several very stressful life events (e.g., death of one's child) are not included. Also, the literature now demonstrates that not everyone experiences adverse effects when exposed to a specific number or combination of stressful life events. Reversal characteristics–including developmental phase, environmental factors, and coping repertoires–appear to be mediators within the potential stress response and longer-term health consequences.[36] Research is needed to study these interactions, especially using longitudinal methods to explore health consequences.

SRRS STUDY

A study conducted by Schwartz and Schwartz[43] demonstrates one use of the SRRS for primary preventive intervention. The purpose was to investigate the similarities and differences of LCUs between mothers of full-term infants and mothers of premature babies during the 2 years preceeding the pregnancy and during the

***Table 13-1.* Social readjustment rating scale (SRRS)**

Rank	Life event	Life change unit (LCU) value
1	Death of spouse	100
2	Divorce	73
3	Marital separation	65
4	Detention in jail	63
5	Death of a close family member	63
6	Major personal injury or illness	53
7	Marriage	50
8	Termination of employment	47
9	Marital reconciliation	45
10	Retirement from work	45
11	Major change in health of family	44
12	Pregnancy	40
13	Sexual difficulties	39
14	Addition of new family member	39
15	Major business adjustment	39
16	Major change in financial state	38
17	Death of close friend	37
18	Changing to different line of work	36
19	Major change in arguments with wife	35
20	Mortgage or loan over $10,000	31
21	Mortgage foreclosure	30
22	Major change in work responsibilities	29
23	Son or daughter leaving home	29
24	In-law troubles	29
25	Outstanding personal achievement	26
26	Wife starting or ending work	26
27	Start or end of formal schooling	26
28	Major changes in living conditions	25
29	Major revision of personal habits	24
30	Trouble with employer	23
31	Major change in working conditions	20
32	Changing to new school	20
33	Change in residence	20
34	Major change in recreation	19
35	Major change in church activities	19
36	Mortgage or loan less than $10,000	17
37	Major change in sleeping habits	16
38	Major change in family get-togethers	15
39	Major change in eating habits	15
40	Vacation	13
41	Christmas	12
42	Minor violations of the law	11

Reprinted with permission from Holmes TH, Rahe RH: The social readjustment rating scale, *J Psychosom Res* 11:21(4), 1967. Copyright 1967, Pergamon Press.

pregnancy itself. The hypothesis was that mothers of premature infants would have higher SRRS scores. Fifty women were studied; 25 mothers of full-term babies and 25 mothers of infants born at less than 37 weeks of gestational age.

The study found a statistically significant difference in lifestyles between the two groups. The mothers with greater life changes gave birth to more premature infants. The LCUs most frequently observed were personal injury or illness; marital separation; in-law troubles; gain in the number of family members; and changes in finances, arguments, and social and eating habits. The findings supported the hypothesis.

The implications of this study noted by the authors are

1. To identify mothers with high LCUs preceding and during pregnancy.
2. To increase personnel to support the psychologic needs of the mother and the physical and emotional needs of the infant.
3. To expand existing mother-infant programs for high-risk patients to determine the infant mortality and morbidity rate.

Premature infants are at a higher level of risk for abuse and neglect than full-term infants. Primary prevention with mothers before childbirth will help to prevent child abuse and can be accomplished by a number of methods. Nurses are in an ideal position to make the following resources available.

FAMILY RESOURCES

Education programs on child development appropriate for each age group could be held for students throughout the educational process. This would provide needed information to all potential parents and give them some experience with child care. Boys should also be included so they can learn the importance of a fathering role and their contribution to a stable family life. Without essential information, physical punishment for perceived willful acts by the infant would continue. Punishment for "children" activities pervades all social classes. Teaching as many persons as possible the process of normal growth and development is therefore important.

Family planning and birth control information must be available to prospective parents and women of childbearing age. Children often may be abused because they are not wanted; availability of help for prospective parents would lessen this danger.

Another area for family education is our legal system. Many judges are reluctant to break up a home, even when documentation shows that a child has central nervous system trauma and musculoskeletal damage from abusive treatment. Health professionals need to rethink the risks involved to a child returning to an abusive home without a family assessment or support system for the parents. Natural parents may not always be the best parents for the child, but each case must be evaluated individually to provide fair treatment for all.

The support systems of the community may relieve a stressful situation at home. The community provides several services, such as homemakers, friendly visitors, and religious and civic organizations, that offer time, supervision, and transportation. Each community has developed its own resource network and is an important area the nurse can help the family assess and use.

Potential for Positive Growth

Many believe stress has growth-promoting potential. Prompt therapeutic intervention allows the individual, family, or community to acquire new coping patterns, which may lead to a higher level of mental health than in the precrisis state. Typically, stress will also reactivate any previously unresolved problems. This phenomenon provides individuals with new opportunities to deal with their past problems while resolving the current situations. Within each situation are risk factors that involve the host, agent, and environment. With this epidemiologic triangle, the risk factors affecting the host are ego strength; previous coping patterns; past experiences; perceptions of the event; and intervention by family, friends, or professionals. Environmental risk factors consist of community resources, education, financial status, religion, and cultural ties.

These risk factors affect the outcome so that the individual, family, or community either

1. Acquires new coping mechanisms, resolves past conflicts, and achieves a higher level of mental health;
2. Adapts and returns to a previous level of functioning; or
3. Responds with maladaptive behavior.

STRESS MANAGEMENT

Healthful behaviors, such as good nutrition; adequate sleep, rest, and exercise; and supportive social relationships may help strengthen an individual's resources against stress.[47,48] Developing positive approaches to stress has also been shown to be effective. For example, the studies by Kobassa have shown that stress-hardy workers have a decreased incidence of illness and absenteeism in the workplace. She defined the characteristics of stress hardiness to be (1) a sense of commitment (rather than alienation) to work, home, and family; (2) viewing stress as a challenge, an opportunity for growth; and (3) having a sense of control in making decisions and influencing one's own life events.[26]

Because people with low stress hardiness appear to be at greater risk for crisis and longer-term health consequences of stress, interventions are directed at increasing their resources and coping (physical, emotional, and problem-solving) skills through education and social support. In addition, prayer, meditation, biofeedback, guided imagery, therapeutic touch, yoga, hypnosis, and other relaxation-response techniques are useful in preventing and alleviating stress responses.[3,5,24]

These techniques (as further discussed in Chapter 14 and throughout the developmental chapters) are offered in a variety of locations–play groups, child and senior day-care centers, schools, universities, community centers, churches or temples, fraternal organizations, employee assistance programs, hospitals, and television or video programs–to reach all age, occupational, and cultural groups.

Individuals are taught to pause and observe their stressors and physical, emotional, cognitive, and behavioral responses to them. Based primarily on the studies by Beck[2] and Burns,[6] cognitive therapy helps individuals work with their thoughts, beliefs, feelings, and physical experiences toward healthier, more effective outcomes.

Many techniques are used to cope with stressful situations. "Coping is the art of finding a balance between acceptance and action, of letting go and taking control."[3] Individuals are encouraged to choose and develop a variety of coping strategies for the varying stressors in their lives.[30] Examples of coping strategies include creating affirmative (e.g., "I'm making the right change for me" or "I can handle it"), distraction, direct action, reframing (looking at a situation from a different perspective), communicating, social support, spirituality,[16] emotional catharsis (e.g., crying), journal writing,[15] and time management.[3,5,23-25,42]

Types of Crisis

The two main types of crisis are developmental and situational. Developmental crises are periods of disorganization that occur at times of role transition during normal growth and development. Situational crises result from external events perceived as hazardous.

DEVELOPMENTAL CRISIS

Each of us is constantly growing and maturing, physically, psychologically, and socially. The state of dynamic equilibrium proceeds along an upward path, propelling us from birth to death. As we try to maintain our balance, we are faced with certain inevitable changes in our lives that must be confronted and resolved to continue the process of normal growth.[13] Rapoport[38,39] described these critical transition points–birth, school, marriage, and death–as normal and expected development, but she notes that each of these experiences is novel for everyone. If these developmental crises are resolved, equilibrium is maintained, and growth continues. If the stress created by the crisis is not handled effectively, past conflicts may return or new conflicts may arise, leading to a poorer state of mental health.

Erikson[12] described human development as a series of crises that must be coped with by using maturational and social experiences. These crises evolve over time and may require changes in behaviors and thought processes. As in any crisis, a person may feel out of balance and tense but unable to identify the problem. A series of vignettes adapted from the case records of Howard King, a pediatrician, are presented in the following section. Each study describes an aspect of developmental crisis within the Erikson framework and demonstrates the nursing interventions undertaken to assist the client in resolving his or her crisis. These examples are provided to help the nurse relate Erikson's theoretic framework to the crisis events of selected populations.

The following vignette is an example of the crisis encountered in Erikson's second stage, autonomy versus shame and doubt. The critical task during this developmental period is to view the self as separate from the environment. The mother in this case had identified this problem in her son David.

During a routine health appointment, Mrs. Brown expressed her concern about her son David's dependence on his pacifier. Although he did not use a pacifier during the day, she stated, "It makes a big difference when he goes to bed." David has four of them "stashed away" in different parts of the house. She saw this as a major difficulty for her son, age 18 months.

The nurse elicited a more detailed family history. This information revealed that Mrs. Brown had sucked her thumb until she was a teenager, despite numerous attempts by her parents to coat her thumb with an unpleasant-tasting solution. Mrs. Brown's parents, as well as her in-laws, were either overt or closet alcoholics. Her parents also were heavy smokers, as was Mrs. Brown.

The nurse pointed out that Mrs. Brown had described three generations of family who had oral coping strategies. She suggested that David would cope with the loss of his pacifier and not transfer it to his thumb, at least not for any lengthy period, if other events in his and his parents' lives were stable. His parents had to be ready to cope with his temporary grieving over the loss of the pacifier. The nurse expressed to Mrs. Brown that it was unfortunate that her parents had not given her the opportunity to do the same. Both Mr. and Mrs. Brown were comfortable helping David cope with that loss once they realized they were passing on their anxiety from one generation to another.

Often an issue raised about a child reflects the multiple problems within a family. In the next case the nurse became aware of a marital conflict and prolonged depression in a father who was a physician by following up a mother's complaint that her 3-year-old son tended to reject the neighborhood children. A problem that seemed to center on Erikson's third stage, initiative versus guilt, actually represented a larger family problem. In this situation Mrs. Jones unconsciously identified her son Bobby with her husband.

Dr. and Mrs. Jones had moved recently to the Boston area. Although the nurse's first contact with Mrs. Jones was because of her new infant, the nurse inquired as to how 3-year-old Bobby was doing. Mrs. Jones mentioned that he was coming into their bed at night. The nurse suggested that she and her husband try to set limits to that activity. Mrs. Jones also noted that he tended to be very clingy and did not like other children. She said her husband was very happy in Boston, but that she still missed their former home.

The next visit was specifically for Bobby. Mrs. Jones again mentioned his rejection of the neighborhood children. She said, "He's always been that way . . . it's embarrassing . . . he says to other people, 'When are you going to leave.' I thought it would change." She asked if she should be concerned. The nurse agreed and asked her to discuss it further.

A family history revealed that Bobby's birth had been a difficult breech delivery. During his first year he cried a great deal, and his motor development had been slow. He had not been near any peers during his first 2 years, and there had been several moves before coming to Boston. His parental history showed that Mrs. Jones, an older sibling, also was isolated and moody growing up. Therapy had helped her to overcome her sense of isolation. In contrast, her husband, an only child, was exceptionally close to his mother and abandoned by his father, a workaholic who was rarely at home. Dr. Jones's mother had died about the time of Bobby's birth, but since there was no funeral, Dr. Jones's father had discouraged him from coming home. It appeared to Mrs. Jones that her husband was becoming more like his father: "He's not home much . . . rarely plays with the children . . . we have little social life." She noted her husband had little energy and that their sex life was almost nonexistent. Mrs. Jones evidently was speaking about her husband when she spoke about Bobby's moodiness and alienation from his peers.

Nursing interventions evolved over three meetings. During the first meeting the nurse shared Mrs. Jones's grief and mourning over leaving her former home, friends, and support systems. The nurse indicated her interest in the whole family and offered specific help with the need for limit setting for Bobby. In the second visit the nurse confronted Bobby's antisocial behavior and elicited a more detailed family history. Several accomplishments occurred during the final visit: (1) Bobby's functioning was surveyed, and a list of his strengths was made; (2) the correlation was made between the family history and Bobby's problem; and (3) Dr. Jones's uncompleted state of mourning for his mother was discussed.

Mrs. Jones agreed that Bobby's isolation needed to be separated from her own history and her husband's present problem. The nurse supported her decision to seek marital counseling.

The final case history demonstrates the life crisis of adulthood, Erikson's generativity versus stagnation. Alienation, the most frequent crisis observed in adults, is similar to the crisis associated with maternal deprivation. Problems arise from the lack of intimate connections with the social environment that sustains a person's sense of identity. The study of Mrs. Smith illustrates how an emerging postpartum depression and the potential for serious child abuse was averted by listening, clarification, and support during the first few months of life. In this situation a new mother, Mrs. Smith, identified her infant both with her hated mother and with her own despised self.

The nurse encountered Mrs. Smith soon after the delivery when she talked about her new son as follows: "I feel I'm depressed . . . he's so fragile he makes me nervous . . . I'd like to leave him here . . . I had a horrible pregnancy . . . I'm more afraid of him than he is of me . . . I feel like I'm going to drop him on the floor . . . I feel like jumping out the window." The nurse acknowledged Mrs. Smith's feelings and encouraged her to talk about her own childhood.

Mrs. Smith was the youngest of four siblings, conceived just before her father's death. She had a horrible relationship with her own mother, an unrecovered alcoholic who believed she was cursed the day she gave birth to Mrs. Smith. She would say to her daughter, "You're no good . . . a louse." Mrs. Smith's father had been an alcoholic, as were her mother's father and mother. Her mother's parents had died when Mrs. Smith's mother was an adolescent. Seeking the parents she missed, her mother married a man 20 years her senior, at the price of developing alcoholism.

The nurse met with Mrs. Smith twice during her hospitalization and after hospitalization during scheduled well-child visits and supported her in many ways, encouraging her to express her negative feelings toward her baby, reassuring her of the normality of these feelings, and pointing out the difference between feelings and actions. The nurse encouraged Mrs. Smith to discuss her feelings about her mother's impending visit and supported her decision to ask her not to come until Mrs. Smith felt more confident with the infant. The nurse further helped Mrs. Smith to begin to mourn the loss of her own father and helped her to identify other sources of support among her family and friends by listening to her and counseling her when appropriate.

Finally they began to outline Mrs. Smith's mother's own tragic life, allowing Mrs. Smith to understand that her mother's hatred was not directed toward her daughter as a person but represented a displacement of her own personal history. By separating the personalities involved, the nurse gradually was able to help Mrs. Smith view her own children in more realistic terms and to become a genuinely nurturant parent.

As these case studies demonstrate, developmental crises are not easily recognized. They do not stand out distinctly but are interwoven in a complex jumble of life events. Life itself is a tangle of situations and relationships that form the fabric of one person or family. It is important to be aware of the complexity of events that seemingly cover the true health problem of developmental crises.

SITUATIONAL CRISIS

Much of the theory for therapeutic intervention with persons in situational crisis was initiated by Lindemann[29] after his work with the bereaved victims of the Coconut Grove Fire in Boston in 1942. The Coconut Grove was a famous dinner club and lounge that was consumed in a flash fire, killing 490 people. Lindemann originally was interested in designing an approach for positive mental health maintenance and preventing community emotional disorganization. After his work with the bereaved, he continued to research the concept of emotional crisis and described certain inevitable life events as hazardous.

Situational crises are caused by sudden unexpected external events over which the person has no control. They are unpredictable and unplanned: a mother gives birth to a handicapped child; fire destroys a family's home; an elderly woman loses her apartment because of condominium conversion. Each of these situations produces stress, with the person's ability to adapt leading to either mastery of the new situation or failure, with impairment of future functioning. Aguilera[1] states, "Although such situations create stress for all people who are exposed to them, they become crises for those individuals who by personality, previous experience, or other factors in the present situation are especially vulnerable to this stress and whose emotional resources are taxed beyond their usual adaptive resources."

Phases of Crisis

Regardless of the type of crisis, situational or developmental, a person experiences certain predictable patterns of behavior. These phases of a crisis are shock, defensive retreat, acknowledgment (renewal stress), and adaptation and change.[14]

SHOCK

The shock phase begins when the person initially is faced with the crisis event, such as receiving a diagnosis of cancer, going through a divorce, or reaching retirement age. The person can perceive the nature of the event, but its impact is not fully realized. These feelings of unreality usually last anywhere from minutes to hours. When full realization of the impact of the event occurs, the person perceives a real danger and feels overwhelmed and helpless. Anxiety increases, often to a point of panic. Confused and bewildered by the event, the person is unable to decide in which direction to turn. Attempting to solve the problem, the person finds usual methods of coping are ineffective. At this phase the person is most open to help and suggestions from others.

DEFENSIVE RETREAT

This second phase of crisis typifies a fight-or-flight response. The person's main goal is to reduce the sense of overwhelming stress. Unable to tolerate the stressful feelings, the individual attempts to "shut out" the imposed threat. Denial and wishful thinking are typical reactions to the flight response; for example, parents who refuse to believe that their newborn baby is mentally retarded or the man who believes that his wife will not seek a divorce.

Typical reactions of the fight response include blaming others and anger: the man who blames the supervisor for losing his job or the family angry with the fire department for failure to quench the fire that destroyed their home. These avoidance mechanisms are necessary for a time so the person can maintain a sense of "self" or equilibrium. When denial, wishful thinking, and anger occur over a prolonged period, however, they become unhealthy and may lead to physical and emotional illness.

ACKNOWLEDGMENT

During the third phase of crisis the person acknowledges the reality of the situation. For continued normal growth and development, the person must face reality and no longer use denial. The person must admit that a change in life has occurred. Stress arises again at this point, and a sense of loss ensues with feelings of depression and confusion. The person begins to reorganize thought perceptions toward the crisis events and begins to formulate planned actions for future goals. These actions may take several directions. If the person is too withdrawn or depressed, suicidal thoughts may emerge. If the individual is apathetic, thoughts of retreating and giving up may dominate plans. The most constructive direction to take is for the person to recognize the strengths of personal systems and the ability to cope with the present situation.

As previously mentioned, suicide intentions and feelings of depression occur during this phase. If suicide occurs or if a psychotic depression develops, then the person obviously is unable to enter the final phase of crisis.

ADAPTATION AND CHANGE

In the final phase, adaptation, the person regains a new sense of self and decides that life is worth living and hope exists for the future. Feelings of anxiety and tension decrease, and the individual views the problem in a more realistic manner, more openly talking about the crisis event. The person begins to recognize strengths and a sense of self-worth and tests them against the vicissitudes of reality. External resources are used more freely during this adaptation phase.

Usually the person becomes a much stronger individual after the crisis has resolved, having been able to cope and to learn new coping abilities. These abilities will benefit and prepare the individual for possible future crisis.

CRISIS INTERVENTION

An individual, family, or community in a state of crisis needs immediate help to solve the crisis, with the focus on what is happening here and now. Although other long-standing, deep-rooted problems may affect how the person copes with the crisis, the aim of intervention is not to delve into the person's background to find the basis for solving them. Crisis intervention is a short-term mode of therapy for assisting individuals and families to cope with current crisis events. Psychotherapy is necessary to prevent crisis in those who have deeper problems.[34,35]

Parad and Resnick[34,35] define crisis intervention as "the active entering into the life situation of an individual, family or population to (1) cushion the impact of a stress that throws the person (or persons) off balance and (2) help mobilize the resources of those affected directly by the stress." This definition implies that the nurse is responsible for two areas of crisis intervention: (1) to become actively involved with the client to help restore equilibrium, and (2) to obtain the help of the client's significant others to assist in solving the immediate crisis.

Goals

According to Parad and Resnick,[34,35] the two main goals of crisis intervention are

1. To reduce the impact of the stressful event.
2. To use the crisis situation to help those affected deal with present problems and to the extent possible learn new and more effective ways of coping with subsequent crises.

As mentioned, the ultimate goal of crisis intervention is assisting persons to function at a higher level than their precrisis state.

Nursing Interventions

The steps in crisis intervention follow those of the nursing process: assessment, planning, intervention, and evaluation (anticipatory planning). Aguilera[1] has identified key nursing interventions during each phase of the process.

ASSESSMENT

After obtaining the essential demographic data, such as name, age, address, and next of kin, the nurse determines the reliability of the client as a historian. Is he or she in contact with reality, or is there confusion and disorientation? If the client is confused, the nurse obtains information surrounding the crisis event from a relative or significant other who may have accompanied the client. After assessing the lethality of the situation, the nurse may also make a referral to another health care provider or setting, such as a psychiatrist in an inpatient setting if the client's condition warrants more intense, prolonged therapy. If the client is not confused, the nurse proceeds to interact directly with him.

Initially the focus is on the problem or crisis event. What happened that made the client seek help today? When did the event occur? Was it sudden, or has it been developing over a time? How has this event affected him and his significant others? What has been his response to the event? Then the nurse determines the client's perception of the event. What does this event mean to him and to his significant others? Have there been drastic changes in his life because of this event? Have life goals been affected? Is the client perceiving the crisis in a realistic manner?

The nurse also identifies external resources available to the client for support: family, friends, clergy, or community agencies. It is important to determine which supports are most meaningful to the client and which ones will be most appropriate and helpful when planning for intervention.

Next the nurse assesses the client's coping abilities. Has the client experienced similar stressful situations in the past? If so, what techniques were used to relieve this stress? Did these techniques work? If they did not work, why not? The nurse should ask the client what he thinks he could do to relieve his present stressful situation.

Finally the nurse ascertains if the client is homicidal or suicidal, using a clear and direct approach and asking such questions as: Do you have plans to kill yourself or others? If so, when and how will you do this? If the client is suicidal or homicidal, the nurse makes a referral to a psychiatrist to protect the client or his potential victim.

Fig. 13-2 presents a form that may be used to organize the assessment data for crisis intervention.

During the assessment phase, the nurse also observes the nonverbal behaviors of the client; he may be saying one thing while his nonverbal behavior indicates something different. Assessing the client's ego functioning (memory, judgment, problem solving, perceptions), mood (happy, sad, depressed), and level of anxiety will guide the nurse in planning for intervention.

PLANNING

Planning for nurse intervention is based on the assessment data previously obtained. However, the nurse does not plan interventions alone or attempt to solve the problem for the client. Intervention is planned mutually with the client; if possible, his significant other shares in the entire process.[14]

The nurse analyzes the assessment data to determine the client's strengths and weaknesses as a guide for the plan for care, considering the client's age, state of health, ego functioning, mood, level of anxiety, and the presence or absence of the balancing factors (perception of the event, situational supports, adequate coping mechanisms). Variables such as the client's sociocultural status and religious affiliation also are investigated.

The type of crisis that has occurred, situational or developmental; the phase of crisis the client is in; and how the crisis has affected the client (Is he ill? Able to work?) also determine and guide the plan of care.

Once the assessment data have been clarified and analyzed, the nurse and client work together to identify goals and develop the plan of care. The plan must be realistic and must focus on alleviating or minimizing the effects of the immediate crisis. Examples of plans that can be formulated are (1) planning for the provision of the client's immediate physical needs, such as food, clothing, shelter, or health care; (2) identifying community agencies that can assist the client; (3) identifying what coping mechanisms are most useful for the client; and (4) identifying significant others who can help the client.

INTERVENTION

Nursing intervention is a deliberative, collaborative, and ongoing process until client goals have been reached. The crisis may be resolved completely or the effects of the crisis on the client may be minimized.[17-19]

At each visit with the client the nurse restates the problem, identifies the goals and the plans formulated to achieve them, and determines how well goals are being met. If the crisis effects have decreased or if the plans are not working, new goals or plans have to be redefined. The nurse assesses the client's level of anxiety, ego functioning, mood, and nonverbal behaviors. Specific, mutually agreed actions the client should be taking

Date ________

Name ________
Age ________
Address ________
Telephone no. ________
Reliable historian
Yes ________
No ________

Next of kin ________
Address ________
Telephone no. ________
Information obtained from:
Client ________
Next of kin ________
Other ________
Name ________
Address ________
Telephone no. ________

1. Identification of problem or crisis event
   Reason for seeking help:

   Time event occurred:
   Sudden onset ________
   Gradual onset ________

   Effects of crisis on client:

   Effects of crisis on client's significant others:

   Response to crisis event:

2. Perception of crisis event
   Meaning of crisis to client:

   Meaning of crisis to client's significant others:

   Changes in client's life because of the crisis:

   Effects of crisis on client's life goals:

   Is client perceiving crisis in realistic manner?

3. Identification of external support resources available to client (Note supports that are most meaningful to client.)
   Family:

   Friends:

   Clergy:

   Community agencies:

   Others:

4. Coping abilities
   Usual methods of coping:

   Coping behaviors that can be used to relieve present crisis:

5. Is client homicidal? ________ If yes, give details:

6. Is client suicidal? ________ If yes, give details:

Fig. 13-2. Sample form for obtaining assessment data before crisis intervention.

7. Ego functioning
   Memory:

   Judgment:

   Problem-solving ability:

   Perceptions:

8. Mood (happy, sad, and so on)

9. Level of anxiety
   Mild _______ Moderate _______ Severe _______

Fig. 13-2, cont'd. Sample form for obtaining assessment data before crisis intervention.

are identified, clarified, and evaluated. Clarification and understanding of the goals and plan of care allows the client to know where he is going and how he will get there.[17-19]

These have been general interventions to identify the overall scheme of nursing intervention for crises. However, more specific kinds of interventions are necessary, and the following are offered as guidelines.[11,22,32]

1. *Communicate effectively and openly with the client.* Effective communication is the basis for the nurse-client relationship and the key factor in implementing the nursing process. Ineffective communication will both hinder the development of the relationship and impede the progress of meeting the client's needs and goals. (See Chapter 5 for a review of the helping relationship and communication theory.)
2. *Allow for expression of feelings.* Emotions increase during times of crisis, and often the client is afraid or unwilling to express them openly. The client may have feelings of anger, hostility, rejection, helplessness, or hopelessness. Ventilation of feelings can be an emotional catharsis for the client. The nurse should offer opportunities for their expression, such as: "This must be difficult for you. Tell me how you are feeling now." Whatever feelings the client expresses, the nurse communicates understanding of such feelings under the given circumstances.
3. *Assist the client to perceive the crisis and its effects realistically.* During a crisis the client's anxiety may be at such a high level that he is viewing the crisis unrealistically. For example, a recently divorced woman's self-concept may be so low that she thinks she is unattractive and will never again be able to meet another man. In this instance the nurse assists the client in recognizing that the loss of her husband in no way diminishes her role as a woman or as a sexual being.
4. *Encourage the client to talk about the crisis.* Reliving and retelling the event will both reduce tension and allow the client to perceive the crisis more realistically.
5. *Promote more effective coping behaviors.* The nurse should explore with the client specific coping behaviors that have worked for him in the past and those that may work for him now and in the future. The nurse can ask such questions as, "What would you like to do now to help solve the problem? Do you know anyone who has had a similar problem? If so, what did they do to solve it?" Mutually finding new coping behaviors for the client may be a slow problem-solving process, but once one is tried and found successful, the client will have the courage to try others. The nurse must discourage the client from blaming others for the crisis; this avoids the truth and removes the responsibility of crisis resolution from the client. This is a flight response and, if continued unabated, it will delay crisis resolution. The nurse responds to this behavior by actively listening to the client, then raises doubts by questioning his remarks.
6. *Encourage the client to accept help from others.* As mentioned earlier, the client in crisis needs help: from the nurse, other health professionals or agencies, friends, family, or community organizations. Clients in a crisis are usually more willing to accept help that is offered. However, in some instances the client may have to be encouraged to receive assistance, especially when help is needed for activities of daily living or to meet his basic physical needs.
7. *Encourage the client to establish personal and social relationships.* The lack of personal and social supports puts a person at a higher risk for crisis. During the crisis event the client is more amenable to intervention and may be willing to explore ways to meet and socialize with other persons. Those who

are alone because of the crisis event, such as an elderly widower, can find support and gratification from contact and interaction with others and also may find them to be a source of help in possible future crises.

EVALUATION

Evaluation is ongoing throughout the nursing process, but its final phase is to identify (1) if the crisis is resolved, (2) if the client's goals are met, and (3) how effective were the interventions. Also, the nurse plans with the client in this step to learn what worked best for his crisis resolution and how to deal with such situations if they should arise again.

The nurse discusses with the client his present level of functioning. Is it at the same level of precrisis functioning or is it at a higher level? The client may have developed new coping behaviors that were effective or found new sources of support from a religious affiliation or a community agency. The nurse assists the client to explore how he can use the new behaviors or support groups to prevent or minimize the effects of possible future crises. The client should also develop realistic goals for the future and realistic plans to achieve them.

Primary Prevention

The phrase *primary prevention of crisis* implies preventing the crisis from occurring. With both situational and developmental crises, this is not always possible or even desirable. The person does not know when a situational crisis will occur, such as when a tornado will strike or a divorce will ensue, nor can the person prevent the biologic changes that occur from one developmental period to another.[8]

The nurse should remember that a stressful event does not constitute a crisis; the client's perception of and response to the event determine if a crisis will occur. A tornado, old age, retirement, or death of a loved one may be viewed as crises, but they may not constitute crises for those individuals, groups, or populations who do not perceive the event as such and who manage to resolve the event by using their usual coping behaviors and situational supports. Therefore, the emphasis of primary prevention for crisis is not to prevent the stressful event per se, but to prevent it from becoming a crisis by minimizing its effects on the client, group, or population through the interventions of health promotion and specific protection.

HEALTH PROMOTION

Physically, psychologically, and spiritually healthy persons are better equipped to cope with what life offers than those who are unhealthy in these areas. They usually display more effective coping behaviors, have significant others with whom they interact, and have access to or belong to social or community organizations. The physical and psychologic resources of healthy people equip them with a reserve that can be called upon in the crisis event to alleviate or diminish its effects. Thus the promotion of healthful behaviors, such as yearly physical examinations, good nutrition, and health education, are major deterrents in the prevention of crises.[37,46]

SPECIFIC PROTECTION

Anticipatory planning is intervention that may specifically protect clients, groups, or communities from crisis events. It provides opportunities for them to try out new behaviors and to plan for the future before a crisis ensues. During a precrisis state, anxiety levels are low and learning can occur more readily.

Anticipatory planning is especially helpful to those individuals, groups, or communities considered at high risk for crisis. When these persons are identified early, primary prevention is most effective in either preventing a crisis or minimizing crisis effects.

Parad and Resnick[34,35] identify risk factors for crisis including many interrelated problems (see the box below). Use of the previously described Social Readjustment Rating is another method of identifying persons at risk.

The goals of primary prevention of crisis are to promote health and healthy behavior and to identify persons, groups, or communities at risk for crisis. Inter-

❑ ❑ RISK FACTORS FOR CRISIS

Difficulty in learning from experience
History of frequent crises, ineffectively resolved because of poor coping ability
History of mental disorder or other serious emotional disturbances
Low self-esteem, which may be masked by provocative behavior
Tendency toward impulsive "acting out" behavior (doing without thinking)
Marginal income
Lack of regular, fulfilling work
Unsatisfying marriage and family relations
Heavy drinking or other substance abuse
History of numerous accidents
Frequent encounters with law enforcement agencies
Frequent changes in address

vention should be directed toward encouraging them to use appropriate coping behaviors and assisting them in identifying external resources that may help to avert the crisis or minimize its effects.[9,40]

The following two case studies are examples of how primary prevention of crisis can be initiated for individuals. The first case illustrates a developmental crisis; the second, a situational crisis. For each case the following areas are included:

1. Description of the crisis events
2. Discussion of the reactions to the events by the participants
3. Assessment of the events
4. Health promotion activities
5. Specific protection activities
6. Early diagnosis and prompt treatment

CASE STUDY: DEVELOPMENTAL CRISIS OF FACING DEATH

Until recently Americans have sheltered themselves from the process of dying. Death has been considered an unwelcome stranger, feared by most and removed from our thoughts until we are confronted by its reality. We avoid dealing with our mortality by delaying our "grief work" until our later years. When that time arrives, we must then answer the questions deferred from earlier life, such as, "What meaning has my life had?" and "When death comes, will I be prepared?" These questions can be unsettling, especially for the elderly who sense their proximity to death and may perceive an inability to rectify their previous life deeds. This is the crisis of ego integrity versus disgust and despair, as identified by Erikson.[12]

Why is death a stranger to us? Certainly each of us has been involved with the loss of a loved one or object: as children providing funerals for birds and animals, and as adults mouring the loss of friends and relatives. These situations may touch us briefly, but we neglect to use these opportunities to gain insight into our feelings of our own death. We hide the dying behind closed hospital doors and whisk the deceased away in stretchers that hide the body from view; we expect the bereaved to keep reign of their emotions; we cover graves with artificial grass to keep them neat and clean, devoid of emotion and reality. These actions help us to protect ourselves from the pain of the current loss and the pain of dealing with our own inevitable death.

George is about to retire from his job with the telephone company. An employee for 35 years, George was hired after World War II and worked his way from linesman to a supervisory position.

He and his wife are looking forward to his retirement. They have made plans to travel across the country and visit their children and grandchildren, then settle into their former summerhouse on the lake. After they sell their present house, they anticipate more leisure time for golf and fishing. George has saved some money and has a good pension from the phone company.

As his last day at work approaches, George finds himself plagued with new fears. Suddenly leaving work seems bleak. "It's not just retiring from work," he thinks. "It's like retiring from life." "I've worked all my life, now what do I do, just wait to die? I'm not ready for that. If I leave now, I'll lose everything I've worked for. Who will remember me when I'm gone?"

Discussion. George's retirement has triggered his developmental crisis of ego integrity versus disgust and despair. He is leaving his life of work and entering the world of retirement. To him, leaving this known for the unknown is symbolic of his death. It is a loss, he states, for which he is not prepared.

As George examines his life, he fears that his deeds do not measure up to his standards. This life event review is normal for an older person trying to find meaning to existence. If one believes the pros do not outweigh the cons, the task is especially difficult.

Although George has done some planning for his retirement, he had not considered the emotional component of retiring. He needs help in reviewing his life events to find an acceptable answer for the meaning of his life and to accept his mortality.

Assessment. By using the epidemiologic model of Leavell and Clark (see Table 1-1), the nurse can identify the characteristics of host, agent, and environment that are creating this crisis situation. The host, George, is an older citizen experiencing a recent loss of status. The agent is his retirement from his job and the lack of planning for his final stage of growth. The environment is a society in which the topic of death remains a social taboo. Once these factors are identified, the nurse can complete a detailed assessment of George and his community, then begin to plan and implement an intervention.

Health Promotion Activities. Primary prevention activities for George could have begun much earlier in his life. The opportunity for a health education program at work for all employees could have been initiated by the occupational health nurse or through a contract between the company and the public health nurses for the community. Many persons are not aware of the process of growth and development and how it affects their families and themselves. A program combining mental and physical health, including a section on psychosocial human growth, would benefit all employees and would have helped George to prepare for his final stage of growth.

The U.S. elderly population is expanding; in some cities and towns substantial percentages of the population are over age 65. Nurses cannot ignore this group, for they are active and contributing members of society who need nursing help. Nursing support can be demonstrated at town meetings by voting for continued funding of elderly activities such as community centers, health care, and a council on aging. By demonstrating concern for the needs of senior citizens, nurses can help to promote a healthy transition to an elderly life. Nurses also can become advocates for the elderly, speaking out for issues or writing to legislators on behalf of this age group.

The media, television, radio, newspapers, and magazines have helped to create public awareness of the need to discuss death and dying and have provided insight into alternate care for the dying. They have responded to the need for a forum for these topics with articles and programs on hospital care and support systems for care of the dying at home, as well as exposés on the need to face emotions and talk out feelings about death. This coverage reaches many people and should receive nursing support, both verbal and financial. The articles and programs can also form the basis for topic discussion in schools, religious groups, and health promotion seminars.

Specific Protection Activities. The occupational health nurse at the telephone company placed George in touch with the council on aging and its senior center before his retirement and also gave him information for applying to the American Association of Retired Persons. The latter offers a bimonthly magazine and monthly newsletter for and about the elderly, provides discounts on prescriptions and group health insurance, and is a lobbying representative for persons over age 55. Workers at the senior center gave George the opportunity to share his leadership expertise and love of the outdoors by joining their foster grandparent program, an outreach project for children who need special attention. George found that his work with children placed him in contact with a new group outside his peers and helped him to increase his sense of self-worth. These activities gave him some insight into the impact his life had on others. He began to regain his confidence and shed his feelings of hopelessness and isolation.

The occupational health nurse contacted the community health nurses to provide further counseling for George. During her home visits, the community nurse met with George and his wife to explore their feelings about retirement and their future together. After an initial interview they identified problems to be discussed and agreed to a short-term period of home visits to begin to resolve the crisis of retirement. The nurse introduced George to a discussion group on death and dying at the church and supported his attendance.

The nurses' awareness of the need for early planning for retirement helped George to make the transition more smoothly. The contact with the council on aging and his work with the children helped him to maintain his dignity; his involvement with the church group helped him to verbalize and examine his feelings and philosophy about death; and the home visits provided him with a consistent health care model to coordinate his transition.

Early Diagnosis and Prompt Treatment. The public health nurse in George's community recognized the crisis potential of retired workers based on her community assessment and use of the epidemiologic triad. The nurse arranged a meeting with key community figures to foster a support network for senior citizens and to find individuals who could use their services. The members of the support network included religious leaders of the community, the director of the council on aging, and representatives from local civic organizations.

Working together, they targeted several community members, including George, who recently had retired and were exhibiting symptoms of withdrawal and social isolation. The nurse visited George and assessed his unrealistic perception of his self-worth and dying and his lack of adequate situational supports. Together they worked through his feelings to clarify his perceptions, while he began to establish contact with social organizations to develop new contacts and continue his growth as an individual. In this way the nurse helped George to resolve his developmental crisis.

CASE STUDY: SITUATIONAL CRISIS OF DIVORCE

Divorces in the United States are growing in alarming numbers. Approximately three out of five marriages will end in divorce.[33] The consequences of this phenomenon for the family and its individual members are far reaching, and many adverse effects can occur.

Divorce causes changes and losses for all involved. It can cause relocation and loss of a familiar home and surroundings, a change in economic and social status, and a change in a person's self-perception. Whatever effects a divorce causes, the involved persons have to cope with the necessary adjustments and attempt to forge for themselves a new life outside the confines of an intact family. Divorce, as a stressful event, can easily become a crisis if the individuals involved do not have adequate coping behaviors or situational supports to help them resolve the event in a healthy manner.

Joyce was stunned when her husband Bob arrived home from work and bluntly announced, "I don't like being married anymore, I want a divorce." Taken by surprise, Mrs. Parks could barely get out the only word that she uttered: "Why?" That same evening Bob packed his clothes and left.

Joyce, age 31, and Bob, age 33, grew up in a small New England town where their families had known each other for years. Without waiting to graduate from high school, Joyce and Bob married when they both were juniors. Bob eventually returned to and graduated from high school and, by working days and attending college at night, received his college diploma. In the meantime three children had been born. Joyce did not return to school.

Two years ago, Bob was offered a job in a small electronics firm in the south. Because of the attractiveness of the offer and the chances for advancement, the Parks moved with the blessings of both families. After the move Joyce stayed home more with the children: Bob Jr., age 13; Ted, age 8; and Mary, age 5. Bob enjoyed his job; Joyce, however, was homesick for her family. She missed the companionship of her sisters-in-law; and because she didn't know anyone, she rarely left the house except for shopping and, whenever it rained, driving the boys to school. Bob did not take her out and frequently told her, "You have nothing in common with my friends." Eventually Joyce became close friends with her next-door neighbor.

About a year after they moved, Joyce learned that her father had cancer and was undergoing treatment at the local hospital. The news was depressing for Joyce, since her mother died of cancer 4 years before and the only person to care for her father was his widowed sister. Bob and Joyce decided that when school was out, Joyce and the children would return to New England for the summer. Bob would stay 1 week and would return to pick them up 2 weeks before school started.

Joyce and the children enjoyed their summer. She spent a great deal of time with her father, who was responding well to the treatments. Joyce knew that the treatments did not eliminate the cancer and that this series would be his last. She was pleased, however, with the care her father received from his sister.

Bob returned for Joyce and the children 1 week before school was to start. The day after their return, Bob broke the news of wanting a divorce. After he left the house that night, Joyce went next door to tell her neighbor what had happened. She was distraught, questioning over and over again, "What happened? What did I do wrong? Why did it happen to me? What am I going to do? How can I manage without him?" In addition to these unanswered questions, Joyce expressed feelings of loss and inadequacy as a woman, thinking she had failed to keep her marriage intact.

Discussion. Joyce's impending divorce has caused feelings of helplessness and confusion. Married before graduating from high school, Joyce has spent her adult life with her husband and subsequent children, never having had the opportunity for living alone, having a job, or making decisions that did not include her husband or children. Now she is being faced with the disintegration of her family unit.

Joyce's life had not prepared her for divorce, she had not developed situational supports outside her family unit. In addition, she already had experienced several losses in the past, such as her mother and family and friends because of relocation, and would be experiencing future losses, including her father and husband. Joyce needed help in coping with the impending divorce and subsequent losses and in planning for the future as a single parent.

Assessment. Again the nurse can assess the characteristics of the host, agent, and environment that comprise the triangle of this potential crisis situation. The host is Joyce, who is facing an impending divorce with seemingly few coping abilities and situational supports. The agent is an impending divorce that is unexpected and thereby unplanned. The environment is a society that views the intact family of husband, wife, and children as its basic unit. By making a detailed assessment of each component, the nurse can plan and formulate appropriate interventions that will assist Joyce to cope successfully with the potential crisis of divorce.

Health Promotion Activities. Health promotion activities for Joyce should have started during high school. The nurse at Joyce's high school could have initiated classes for both sexes on sex education, marriage and the family, and normal growth and development. The content of such classes could have included topics such as the roles and responsibilities of a husband and wife, the concept of parenting, budgeting, and other financial information.

Marriage and family life are integral mainstays of our society, yet young persons frequently are not instructed on how to deal with the role changes and the responsibilities that marriage and family bring. If Joyce and Bob had been provided with such information during their high school years, they might have refrained from marriage at such an early age. Also, Joyce could have finished high school; this would have helped her to seek employment after the divorce. Nurses, as health care providers and citizens, can support the introduction of classes on marriage, the family, and other related topics in the school system. Young persons need this information to make rational decisions when confronting life changes related to normal growth and development.

Other health promotion activities also could have been implemented earlier for Joyce. She could have become involved in groups outside her family, such as the local parent-teacher association, a bridge club, or a tennis club. Whatever the mode of activity, everyone needs an outlet for personal expression and affiliation with others to develop as a social being and to enhance self-esteem.

Specific Protection. With the help of her neighbor, Joyce made appointments with a lawyer and with the local mental health center. At the center Joyce was assigned to a mental health nurse who would work with her throughout the divorce proceedings. An assessment of the situation was made by the nurse, and in collaboration with Joyce, goals and plans for intervention were discussed. The goal was to assist her in adjusting to the divorce and to minimize its crisis effects. The nurse would see Joyce on a weekly basis.

The nurse encouraged Joyce to ventilate her feelings about her husband and the impending divorce. Joyce expressed anger and frustration and often questioned why she had not suspected Bob's divorce plans. She continued to receive support from her neighbor and finally expanded her friendship to two other neighborhood women.

The nurse arranged weekly counseling sessions for the entire family during which the psychologist saw the family as a group, the children alone, and then Bob and Joyce together. These sessions allowed each member to express their feelings about the divorce and to explore tentative plans for the future.

With the nurse's help, Joyce investigated ways to finish high school. She enrolled in night classes at the local high school to qualify her to take the equivalency examination. This action was the first step in acquiring basic skills to increase her chances for meaningful employment. In the meantime Joyce was able to obtain a part-time job as a sales clerk in the neighborhood shoe store, which enabled her to feel less dependent on her husband and gave her a sense of accomplishment and self-esteem. She was able to meet new persons and joined a bowling team.

With the help of Joyce's lawyer, the nurse found a support group affiliated with the local church for separated and divorced persons. Joining this group helped Joyce see that others were experiencing similar problems and that they managed successfully to cope with them. Her feelings of helplessness and confusion began to abate when she discovered that she, too, could make rational decisions about her future goals.

The crisis effects of divorce were minimized for Joyce by early interventions. The personal and situational supports mentioned enabled Joyce to cope more effectively with her divorce and also gave her the opportunity to try out new behaviors to assist her with future potential crisis events.

❑ ❑ ❑

A succinct listing of primary preventions for the crises presented in these two case studies is presented in Table 13-2.

***Table 13-2.* Primary preventive interventions for selected crises in the case studies**

Problem	Individual intervention	Group (educational intervention)	Community (environmental intervention)
Divorce	Help develop effective coping behaviors Provide individual counseling Prepare for meaningful employment Identify personal and situational supports Encourage formulation of future plans	Provide premarital counseling and health education classes 1. Marriage and family life 2. Parenting 3. Normal growth and development 4. Childrearing 5. Husband and wife roles Establish support groups	Establish classes for high school students of both sexes 1. Normal growth and development 2. Sex education 3. Marriage and family
Retirement	Help develop effective coping behaviors Assist in planning for future activities Maintain physical and psychologic health Provide individual counseling	Establish support groups Increase awareness of community resources and programs Council on aging Community centers Legal services Housing Health services Support advocacy groups Gray Panthers National Council of Senior Citizens	Provide preretirement counseling for employees Encourage memberships in the American Association of Retired persons Support federal programs SCORE (Service Corps of Retired Executives) RSVP (Retired Senior Volunteer Program) Volunteers in Service to America (VISTA) Senior Companion Program Foster Grandparents Peace Corps
Death	Help develop effective coping mechanisms Provide individual counseling Support planning for final stage of growth	Support hospice care Establish support groups	Create public's awareness through media of television, radio, newspapers, and magazines Establish discussion groups Schools Community organizations Religious affiliations

GRIEF AND MOURNING AS RESPONSES TO LOSS

Lindemann[29] described an acute grief syndrome with psychiatric and somatic components after his work with bereaved victims mentioned earlier. He studied a group of 101 clients by direct interview and through respiratory, gastrointestinal, and metabolic studies. After analyzing the data by observation of changes in mental status and the subjective reporting of symptoms experienced, he concluded that there was a normal process of grieving.

The syndrome may either appear directly following a situational or developmental crisis or occur later. It may be exaggerated or seemingly absent. The process also may be distorted, but with proper intervention techniques these distortions can be corrected to allow a normal grieving process to occur.

The Mourning Process

Grieving is usually preceded by a loss. Because nurses come in contact daily with persons experiencing losses, they must understand the dynamics of grief and mourning for proper intervention.[9]

Why do people mourn a loss? Engel[10,11] contends that during the course of normal growth and development, a person becomes dependent on a variety of external objects to provide a basis for self-concept; to varying degrees these become necessary for effective ego functioning and for the continued and sustained sense of intactness, fulfillment, success, and hope. This dependence accounts for a person's vulnerability to loss or threat of loss and the compensation for such loss through the process of mourning. The meaning a psychic object (home, job, antique automobile) has for one person may be different for another, depending on the detail of his or her life experiences.

A loss refers to an external object suddenly being made no longer available or accessible to the person. Engel outlines several classifications of object loss:

1. Loss of body parts or functions, including amputation, paralysis, loss of body strength, menopause, impotence, and decline in intellectual capacity
2. Loss of membership or status in social, political, professional, military, or religious groups
3. Failure of plans or ventures
4. Changes in way of life and living
5. Loss of home, house, personal possessions, valued gifts, and mementos
6. Loss of job, profession, or occupation
7. Loss of pets

Each loss throughout life builds on successive losses; how a person progresses through the mourning process usually depends on how well previous losses have been resolved. The cumulative effect of a loss is reflected in the work of Holmes and Rahe[20,21,22] (see Table 13-1). Thus it is important for the nurse to assess not only the meaning of the current loss to the client but also the number of previous losses. Engel's classification illustrates that the feeling of loss is experienced whether the separation is from another person; by death, divorce, or illness; from a body part; or from an object such as a car, job, home, or pet.

Identification of all previous losses and changes based on the Social Readjustment Rating Scale (Table 13-1) helps the nurse to understand the client's previous coping mechanisms and increases the nurse's awareness of his potential for personal illness or crisis. The plan of intervention depends on this information; once it is known, the nurse can begin to assist the client experiencing the loss with his grief work.

GRIEF

According to Engel,[10,11] "grief refers more to what is felt or experienced, and mourning to the responses involved." Grief work is the process of resolving a loss and renewing life without the lost person or object. The term usually is associated with death but encompasses the mourning and resolution that occurs with any loss.[9]

Much of Lindemann's and Engel's work is the result of studies of persons experiencing loss through death; their terminology reflects this work with the bereaved. The nurse must remember that the feelings of loss, grief work, and consequent nursing interventions are the same regardless of the object lost.

Lindemann[29] described the following symptoms as characteristics of grief reactions. Bodily symptoms of somatic distress occur when the deceased is mentioned during visits or when sympathy is extended to the bereaved. These episodes occur in waves that last from 20 minutes to an hour and are so intense that normally a person will avoid the syndrome at any cost. The most pronounced symptoms are the need for sighing, a lack of muscular power, exhaustion, and digestive problems, such as a feeling of tightness in the throat, choking with shortness of breath, and an empty feeling in the abdomen. Another symptom is described subjectively as tension or mental pain. The survivors in the Lindemann study related their intense preoccupation with the image of the deceased and described feelings of unreality and an altered sensorium, which is typical of the behavior associated with anxiety. As tension rises, the ability to attend to other matters is reduced. Strong feelings of guilt preoccupy grieving persons who reconstruct past events and search their memory for evidence of failure to do right for the deceased. Typically they accuse themselves of negligence and exaggerate minor omissions of deeds.

In addition, feelings of hostility are directed toward others. Bereaved persons find themselves alienating friends and relatives, persons who normally provide comfort. The anger is dispersed widely and not targeted to any specific group or individual. Finally the daily pattern of conduct is lost. Grieving persons describe themselves as wandering from room to room trying to carry on their usual activities. They find it difficult to organize themselves for any task, usually picking things up and putting them down.

According to Lindemann,[29] "The duration of grief reaction seems to depend upon the success with which the person does the "grief work,'" that is, achieving emancipation from the bondage to the deceased, readjusting to the environment from which the deceased is missing, and forming new relationships.

STAGES OF MOURNING

Engel[11,12] describes three stages of the mourning process, using as a prototype a bereaved person who has lost a loved one by an unexpected death. These stages are shock and disbelief, a developing awareness of the loss, and restitution.

Shock and Disbelief. The initial response when hearing of an unexpected death is shock and disbelief; the person cannot accept the reality of the event. Feelings of numbness follow as the survivor attempts to block out or escape this reality. Bereaved persons may try desperately to carry on normal activities or may become motionless or dazed. Often they appear disoriented, making it difficult to get their attention.

The main defense mechanism used during this phase is denial, which protects the bereaved from the intense stress and overwhelming feelings caused by the death. This state lasts from a few minutes to hours or sometimes days.

Awareness of the Loss. The second stage involves admitting the reality of the death. When the thoughts of death come to conscious awareness, an acute feeling of sadness occurs, followed by feelings of anxiety, helplessness, and hopelessness. Anger may be directed toward those bereaved persons think might be responsible for the death or toward themselves if they feel responsible or believe they could have prevented the death.

Crying is a natural reaction and often is necessary to release pent-up emotions. In some instances the person is unwilling to cry in the presence of others, either because of stoicism or cultural practices, and therefore will cry in privacy. The inability to cry is a serious matter, usually caused by guilt or ambivalent feelings toward the deceased person.

Restitution. The ceremonial rites that surround the funeral are a necessary beginning to the resolution of the death. The funeral symbolizes unequivocally the finality of the relationship with the deceased. The bereaved person is able to give to and receive support from other family members and friends who share in grieving for the deceased.

The work of grief continues for the mourner after the funeral ceremonies. The person accepts the loss of the loved one and attempts to fill the painful void by turning to family and friends. Increased awareness of the body occurs, and the bereaved often experiences bodily sensations and pains similar to those experienced by the deceased.

The person spends much of this phase of mourning in talking about the deceased, retelling over and over incidents and anecdotes and their relationship together. Often the deceased is idealized, with the mourner glossing over any defects and emphasizing only the good aspects. Idealization usually results when the mourner develops an intellectual memory of the deceased and identifies consciously and unconsciously by taking on certain admired qualities and attributes of the deceased.

Eventually the person is able to seek out others besides family and past friends for sources of gratification and for replacement of the broken ties caused by the loss. The bereaved lifts the self-imposed ban on pleasure and enjoyment, allowing himself once again to feel joy and be happy.

The work of mourning usually lasts 6 to 12 months. Its resolution is complete when the mourner can remember realistically, without intense pain, both the pleasures and the disappointments of the lost relationship.

Factors Influencing Satisfactory Acceptance of Loss

Certain factors impinge on the bereaved person and influence the success and time spent in resolving losses. Engel[11,12] has identified these factors as follows:

1. *Importance of the deceased as a source of support.* The more dependent the mourner on the deceased, the more difficult to resolve the loss.
2. *Degree of ambivalence toward the deceased.* The presence of unresolved anger, hostility, and guilt toward the deceased hinders the progression of resolution.
3. *Age of the lost object and the mourner.* It is more difficult to resolve the loss of a child than that of an aged relative. Also, children as mourners have fewer capabilities for loss resolution than do adults.
4. *Number and nature of previous grief reactions.* Losses build on each other, and any unresolved loss is revived during subsequent ones, making the work of mourning more difficult.
5. *Degree of preparation for the loss.* Anticipatory grieving by the mourner may occur when a person is terminally ill; but unexpected death leaves no room for such preparation.
6. *Physical and psychologic health of the mourner.* The stronger the physical and psychologic health

of the mourner at the time of the loss, the greater the capacity to cope with the loss.

Nursing Process and Mourning

ASSESSMENT

Obtaining a detailed health history from the mourner to plan nursing interventions is unnecessary. The nurse needs only the information that directly relates to the loss. Initially the nurse determines the relationship between the mourner and the lost object or person. What did the object or person mean to the mourner? How dependent was the relationship? Will the absence alter the mourner's future life goals?

The nurse then identifies the typical coping patterns of the mourner. Has the client experienced similar losses in the past? If so, how was the loss resolved? If these coping behaviors worked for the client before, they may be useful in the resolution of the present loss.

The nurse also should identify the mourner's religious, social, and cultural milieu and his attitudes toward death, if the lost object was a person. Does the mourner believe in a life after death? What are the cultural rituals that surround the death event? Does the mourner's culture allow for expressions of feelings? The nurse then determines the client's external resources that may help in coping with the loss. Are there family and friends from whom he can obtain help? Does he have a clergyman he can turn to for support and advice? Are there community agencies that can assist him while resolving the loss?

Finally, the nurse identifies the absence or presence of factors that influence the process of mourning. Some of this information may have been obtained previously, such as the client's age, the importance of the lost object as a source of support, and the quantity and quality of other relationships. The nurse determines the mourner's degree of ambivalence toward the lost person or object. Were there simultaneous feelings of love and hate? The client's degree of preparation for the loss is also established: Was it sudden or gradual? The nurse determines the physical and psychologic health of the mourner as well. Is the client in good health? Does he have physical disabilities? Has he been known to have a mental disorder in the past?

Fig. 13-3 presents a form to organize the assessment data for persons who have experienced a loss. Once the assessment data are obtained, the nurse proceeds to the planning phase.

Planning. The planning phase of the nursing process for intervention in mourning generally follows the guidelines described previously in crisis intervention. The problem is clarified, and goals and plans for meeting them are formulated. The problem-solving approach is used throughout the process.

Name ________________ Date ____________
Age __________

1. Nature of the lost object (or person)
2. Meaning the lost object (or person) had for the mourner
3. Mourner's typical coping patterns
4. Mourner's social and cultural milieu
5. Mourner's attitude toward death (if applicable)
6. Special resources (support systems) the mourner possesses for coping with the loss
7. Factors that influence the mourning process:
   Importance of the loss object (or person) as a source of support
   Degree of ambivalence toward the lost object (or person)
   Age of the deceased (if applicable)
   Quantity and quality of other relationships
   Degree of preparation for the loss, which was
   Sudden _____
   Gradual _____
   Mourner's physical health
   Mourner's psychologic health

Fig. 13-3. Sample form for obtaining assessment data about persons experiencing a loss.

Intervention. The crisis intervention and primary preventive interventions of crisis previously described are equally applicable in nursing interventions with the mourner.[8,31]

Wishing to delay "grief work" to avoid both the acute discomfort of the grieving process and the necessary expression of emotion is normal. The nurse can persuade those involved to yield to the process and accept the discomfort. By working through the stage of shock and disbelief, the person can begin to accept emotionally what has happened.

Emotional acceptance takes time, work, and much discomfort. It is a necessary process, since avoiding the pain will result in distorted grief reactions later. The nurse who desires to protect bereaved persons should be aware of the necessity of allowing them to express their feelings of discomfort and loss. By maintaining an accepting attitude and sharing in the grief work, the nurse can facilitate the grieving process, encouraging crying and verbalization of guilt feelings, reviewing the relationship with the deceased, and encouraging the mourner to seek help from family and friends. By understanding normal grief reactions, the nurse can anticipate and accept anger and rage. The religious and cultural differences of the bereaved person are respected. The nurse discourages maladaptive means of coping with loss, such as heavy use of alcohol and other drugs, promiscuity, or prolonged denial. It is often best that the mourner not make any drastic moves or changes during the mourning process, such as relocating, quitting a job, or remarrying. Grief work, as mentioned earlier, lasts from 6 to 12 months, and its process is usually facilitated if the mourner remains in the environment shared with the deceased until the loss is resolved.

Evaluation. Adaptation to a loss is evaluated throughout the mourning process using the steps previously described in evaluating crisis intervention.[44]

An example of an evaluation of grief work follows.

ASSESSMENT

Mrs. Jones, age 59, in good health, lives alone in a high-rise apartment for the elderly. Husband of 34 years died 6 months ago. Daughter and son live in same city. Talks little of husband but cries readily when she does.

Planning

Long-term goal: in two months Mrs. Jones will discuss freely her husband, their life together, and his death. Arrange half-hour visits weekly with Mrs. Jones.

Intervention

Establish helping relationship.
Use appropriate communication techniques.
Encourage Mrs. Jones to discuss husband, their life together, and his death.
Listen attentively, maintaining accepting attitudes.
Allow the retelling of events, even if heard many times.
Encourage and support Mrs. Jones's need to cry and the ventilation of other feelings.
Clarify and summarize what occurred at each visit.
Inform Mrs. Jones of next visit and last visit at each session.

Evaluation. Evaluate at each visit if goal is being met. Is Mrs. Jones talking about her husband and their life together? Is the amount of crying decreasing? Once the goal is met, nursing interventions are complete. According to Kübler-Ross,[27] "The ultimate goal of the grief work is to be able to remember without emotional pain and to be able to reinvest emotional surpluses."

Distortions and Normal Grieving

Abnormal reactions to the normal grieving process are manifested by delayed and distorted reactions. Delayed reactions are caused by the person's involvement with important tasks or the need to maintain the morale of others. Grieving may be postponed, with no obvious reaction to the death for weeks or years. The process may occur after a time through a deliberate effort by the bereaved person or spontaneously at a specific point. For example, grieving may begin when a son reaches the same age as his father at the time of his death.

SUMMARY

Each of us is touched by crisis in our lifetime. Both unexpected situational crises and developmental crises occur.

Lindemann's initial work with bereaved victims studied the process of grieving; and Fink and Caplan have outlined the phases of crisis, shock, defensive retreat, acknowledgment, and adaptation and change. The goal of intervention is twofold: to reduce the impact of the immediate stressor and to use the crisis situation to achieve a higher level of mental health functioning. This may be accomplished by the acquisition of new, more effective coping mechanisms.

Active involvement with the client(s) to help restore equilibrium and to mobilize the resources of those affected by the stress is necessary because of the short-term nature of crisis intervention. This can be best accomplished by the organization offered in the nursing process: assessment, planning, intervention, and evaluation. Key components of the nurse-client relationship for crisis resolution are open and effective lines of communication, freedom to express feelings, the realistic perception of the crisis event, effective coping behaviors, and the presence of social support systems.

Although not all crises can be avoided or prevented, some may be averted by primary preventive activities. A complete community assessment to identify health problems and community resources will assist the nurse in establishing relevant prevention programs. The epidemiologic model of Leavall and Clark also provides the nurse with a tool for early identification and assessment of persons at risk for crisis.

Crisis intervention for nurses is a challenge, intellectually, personally, and professionally. After implementing crisis theory, the nurse often is rewarded by seeing clients functioning at a healthier level than before the crisis event occurred–the ultimate goal of crisis intervention.

References

1. Aguilera DC: *Crisis intervention,* St Louis, 1994, Mosby.
2. Beck A: Cognitive therapy: a 30 year retrospective, *Am Psychol* 46(4):368-375.
3. Benson H, Stuart EM: *The wellness book: the comprehensive guide to maintaining health and treating stress-related illness,* New York, 1992, Carol Publishing.
4. Blondis MN, Jackson BE: *Nonverbal communication with patients, back to human touch,* New York, 1977, John Wiley & Sons.
5. Borysenko J: *Minding the body–mending the mind,* Reading, Mass, 1987, Addison Wesley.
6. Burns DD: *Feeling good handbook: using the new mood therapy in everyday life,* New York, 1989, William Morrow.
7. Caplan G, Caplan RB: *Mental health consultation and collaboration,* San Francisco, 1992, Jossey-Bass.
8. Constantino RE: Comparison of two group interventions for the bereaved, *Image-J Nurs Scholarship* 20, 83-87, 1988.
9. Crowles KV, Rodgers BL: The concept of grief: a foundation for nursing and practice, *Res Nurs Health* 14:119-127, 1991.
10. Engel G: Grief and grieving, *Am J Nurs* 64:93-98, 1964.
11. Engel GL: Is grief a disease: a challenge for medical research, *Psychosom Med* 23:18-22, 1961.
12. Erikson E: *Childhood and society,* New York, 1993, WW Norton.
13. Field P, McCabe-Schneiderman N: *Stress and coping across development,* Hillsdale, NJ, 1988, Erlbaum.
14. Fink S: *Crisis management: planning for the inevitable,* Watertown, Mass, 1986, American Management Association.
15. Francis ME, Pennebaker JW: Putting stress into words: the impact of writing on physiological, absentee and self reported emotional well-being measures, *J Health Promotion* 6:280-287, 1992.
16. Frankl V: *Man's search for meaning,* Boston, 1963, Beacon Press.
17. Gilliand B: *Crisis intervention strategies,* ed 2, Pacific Grove, Calif, 1993, Brooks/Cole Publishing.
18. Greenstone JL: *Elements of crisis intervention: crisis and how to respond to them,* Pacific Grove, Calif, 1993, Brooks/Cole Publishing.
19. Hoff LA: *People in crisis: understanding and helping,* ed 3, Redwood City, 1989, Addison Wesley.
20. Holmes T, David E: *Life change events research 1966-1978 an annotated bibliography of the periodical literature,* Westport, Conn, 1984, Greenwood.
21. Holmes T, David E: *Life change, life events and illness: selected papers,* Westport, Conn, 1989, Greenwood.
22. Holmes TH, Rahe RH: The social readjustment rating scale, *J Psychosom Res* 11:213-218, 1967.
23. Jeffers S: *Feel the fear and do it anyway,* San Diego, 1987, Harcourt Brace.
24. Kabat-Zinn J: *Full catastrophe living: using the wisdom of your body and mind to face stress, pain and illness,* New York, 1990, Delacorte Press.
25. Kabat-Zinn J, Massion A, Kristeller J: Effectiveness of a mediation-based stress reduction program in the treatment of anxiety disorders, *Am J Psychiatry* 149:936-943, 1992.
26. Kobasa S, Maddi S, Kahn S: *Hardiness and health: a prospective study, J Personality Social Psychology* 42:168-177, 1982.
27. Kübler-Ross E: *Death: the final stage of growth,* Englewood Cliffs, NJ, 1975, Prentice Hall.
28. Lazarus R, Folkman S: *Stress appraise and coping,* New York, 1984, Springer Publishing.
29. Lindemann E: Symptomatology and management of acute grief, *Am J Psychiatry* 101:52, 1944.
30. Martelli M, Auerbach S, Alexander J: Stress management in health care setting: matching interventions with coping styles, *J Consulting Clinical Psychology* 55:201-207, 1987.
31. Murphy SA: Preventive intervention following accidental death of a child, *Image-J Nurs Scholarship* 22:174-179, 1990.
32. Murray R, Zentner J: *Nursing assessment and health promotion strategies through the lifespan,* ed 5, East Norwalk, Conn, 1993, Appleton-Lange.
33. Neely R: *The divorce decision,* New York, 1984, McGraw-Hill.
34. Parad H: *Crisis intervention: selected readings,* Ann Arbor, 1984, Books Demand.
35. Parad H, Parad L: *Crisis intervention: the practitioners' sourcebook for brief therapy,* Milwaukee, 1990, Family International.
36. Pellitier KR: *Mind as healer, mind as slayer: a holistic approach to preventing stress disorders,* Magnolia, Mass, 1984, Peter Smith.
37. Pruitt RH: Effectiveness and cost efficiency of interventions in health promotion, *J Adv Nurs* 17:926-932, 1992.
38. Rapoport L: The state of crisis: some theoretical considerations, *Soc Service Rev* 36:211, 1962.
39. Rapoport L: Normal crises, family structure, and mental health, *Fam Process* 2:68, 1963.
40. Roberts AR, editor: *Contemporary perspectiveness on crisis intervention and prevention,* Englewood Cliffs, NJ, 1991, Prentice Hall.
41. Robischon P: *The challenge of crisis theory for nursing.* In Reinhardt AM, Quinn ME, editors: *Family-centered community nursing,* St Louis, 1973, Mosby.
42. Schafer W: *Stress management for wellness,* New York, 1987, Holt Reinhart & Winston.
43. Schwartz JL, Schwartz LH: *Vulnerable infants: a psychosocial dilemma,* New York, 1977, McGraw-Hill.
44. Scruby LS, Sloan JA: Evaluation of bereavement intervention, *Canadian J Public Health* 80:394-398, 1989.
45. Selye H: *Stress without distress,* New York, 1975, NAL Dutton.
46. Ulrich-Adcock MR, Marcus ED, Kirchnew DL: *Community health education: the development of effective program strategies.* In Lazes PM: *The handbook of health education,* ed 2, Germantown, Md, 1987, Aspen Systems.
47. US Department of Health and Human Services, Public Health Service: *Healthy people 2000: national health promotion and disease prevention objectives,* Washington, DC, 1992, US Government Printing Office.
48. Woolfolk R, Hehrer P: *Principles of stress management,* New York, 1984, Guilford Press.

CHAPTER

14

Holistic Health Strategies

Joni Cohen

Dennis T. Jaffe

Objectives

After completing this chapter, the nurse will be able to

- *Discuss the relationship between holistic health and wellness education.*
- *List several assumptions of holistic health.*
- *Discuss how personal health is an important factor in promoting wellness in others.*
- *Design a health assessment process appropriate for the individual nurse's work setting.*
- *Discuss the use of a journal to enhance psychologic self-care.*
- *List the three phases of a Personal Health Exploration.*
- *List several measures that help prevent burnout in service-oriented professionals.*
- *Define and differentiate among relaxation training, guided imagery, and biofeedback.*

AN EVOLVING DIMENSION OF NURSING PRACTICE

A comprehensive perspective on health and a set of techniques for clinical practice has been given the name *holistic.* Holistic health is an expansion of the idea of the person as a biopsychosocial being. Nursing has always been oriented to a client having multiple needs that impact on his health and well-being. Holistic health focuses on the interactions and offers a model and various techniques to return responsibility for health back to the client.

In the last decade, there has been a significant shift in the acceptance of a holistic health perspective by clients and health care professionals. Many of the philosophic viewpoints and alternative methods advocated by a holistic health approach are no longer seen as experimental or alternative but have been widely incorporated into current health-care practice. In 1990, the U.S. Public Health Service published *Healthy People 2000,* which includes an emphasis on health promotion strategies and focuses upon the importance of personal health choices as having a powerful impact on an individual's health.[37] More health care professionals are approaching health care as a partnership with clients, and involving them in their own healing process. In addition, standard holistic health techniques such as relaxation training, biofeedback, and guided imagery are included in what might be considered a more traditional treatment approach. The rise in wellness programs is another indication of a growing incorporation of the ideas and practices of holistic health.

One of the motivating forces for the emergence of holistic health is the failure of traditional medical practices to treat many prominent diseases of today effectively. These diseases, both major and minor, chronic and catastrophic, mental or physical, all seem to some degree to result from misdirected responses to stress. Over time our bodies are placed under undue strain and, unless the tension is alleviated, break down in some way.

Understanding the risk factors that contribute to illness and modifying the client's attitudes, behaviors, and environment can promote well-being, enhance the healing process, and ideally prevent serious illness. Nurses are in a key position to help the client and themselves become healthier.

Holistic nursing is becoming more widespread. The nursing literature has shown an increase in the number of articles on holism and a holistic viewpoint of health.[22] Holism has even been proposed as nursing's paradigm.[22,23] A recent review of seven nurse theorists' definition of health shows a high congruence with the concept of holism. These include Orem's Self-Care Deficit Theory, The Neuman System Model, Roy Adaptation Model, Roger's Science of Unitary Beings, Parse's Human Becoming Theory, Newman's Theory of Health, and Watson's Theory of Caring.[6] In addition, a positive construct of health has been defined by nurses which involves knowledge, attitudes, and behaviors related to fostering health behavior at the individual and community level; exuberant well-being, becoming, and growing are seen as aspects of health.[29]

This chapter gives an overview of the development of the holistic health model and current trends in holistic health care. Health assessment techniques, along with tools for holistic nursing care, are delineated. The health of the nurse as an essential ingredient in holistic nursing also is discussed.

Historical Perspective

Approaching health care in a holistic way is becoming more accepted in today's health care scheme, as evidenced by the emergence of the self-care model; however, the philosophy behind the holistic perspective is quite old. The word *holistic* comes from the Greek word *holos,* which means the entirety or completeness of a thing in its wholeness.[1] Hippocrates believed that the body could be understood only if perceived as a whole and that phsyicians should work to heal the whole and not just the parts.[9] The systematic scientific study of health, focusing on a particular part of the body, led away from this view of treating the whole person.

The concept of holism emerged again in modern times when Jan Smuts, a prime minister of South Africa, wrote *Holism and Evolution* in 1926.[46] According to Smuts, holism is a creative force within each person, and this force moves toward synthesis. As entities grow and develop, they evolve into a new level of being, a new whole; and this whole becomes greater than the sum of the parts. Smuts was followed by others from many different disciplines, and a new holistic health model has evolved. A summary of the major ideas in the holistic health model is given in the box on p. 326.

Based on these concepts, the Association for Holistic Health[1] has developed working definitions:

> Holistic health is more than the absence of illness; it is defined as the individual realization of continually higher expressions of health in body, mind, and spirit.
>
> Holistic health is an ongoing state of wellness which involves taking care of the physical self, expressing emotions appropriately and effectively, using the mind constructively, being creatively involved with others and becoming aware of higher levels of consciousness. . . . Central to the concept of holistic health is the premise that only the individual can heal himself by developing healthy life patterns and attitudes and by becoming the director, effector, and evaluator of his own uniquely designed wellness program. Holistic health does not stand in opposition to traditional health care methods, but serves instead as a bridge between traditional and alternative methods.

The popularity of the holistic health approach also may be viewed as a reaction against certain trends in current medical practice. Although the focus on biomedical science, crisis medicine, and high technology has brought many advances to clients and vastly increased our understanding of the physiologic functioning of the human body, it has neglected other aspects of the client and of healing.[28] Today, care for chronic health problems eats up health care dollars. Behavior and environment create disease that modern technologic medicine often can do little to alleviate. Depersonalization and increasing costs of medical care have left clients feeling worse, uncared for, and helpless.

Holistic health arrived to reverse this tide. The goal of holistic health is not to cure but to empower. Therefore, holistic health practices are as relevant to use with terminal clients as with a healthy newborn baby. This holistic perspective can be seen as a reversal of some of the dysfunctional aspects of the traditional medical model that emerged from the last part of the 19th century. Holistic health also can be seen as a return to aspects of health and healing that were common before the advent of modern medical science.

The traditional medical model of the 19th century emphasizes the separation between mind, body, and spirit. Illness is seen as external to the person and caused by invading organisms. An unequal relationship exists between the patient and physician; the physician is seen as the powerful, learned one, and the patient is expected to obey without question. In contrast, the holistic perspective emphasizes the unity among mind, body, and spirit. A sense of partnership exists between the physician and the client. Illness is recognized as the

❑ ❑ ASSUMPTIONS OF HOLISTIC HEALTH[1,2,11]

1. Holistic health is wellness oriented and directed toward maintaining and improving existing health or wellness, rather than focusing on disease and illness.
2. Health implies a state of unity among all aspects of the individual. It is a harmonious interrelationship and interdependency among the physical, mental or intellectual, emotional, spiritual, social, and environmental aspects. Lifestyle, ecosystem, social responsibility, sense of community, and relationships also are considered. The emphasis is on the functional interrelationships among these various dimensions.
3. Health is on a continuum, with wellness on one end and death on the other. Internal factors include genetic predisposition, nutritional state, and attitudes. External factors include physical enviornment, social relationships, support system, and economic factors.
4. Human beings are open systems. Within each person is an innate organizing principle that continually guides the individual toward greater order, complexity, and self-differentiation.
5. Body and mind are connected intimately and are interdependent. A person's attitudes, beliefs, values, and perceptions affect health in positive or negative ways.
6. Humankind has an innate capacity for self-healing and self-evolution. The focus of health and healing exist within each individual. The responsibility for changing one's health status thus rests with the self, and one has the moral repsonsibility to change those things that one can and do everything in one's power to get well.
7. Symptoms of illness signal disharmony among the various aspects of one's being. These states can be opportunities for growth and learning. The focus is not on the symptoms but on the interruption of the body-mind-spirit harmony.
8. Holistic health is open to a variety of methods for attaining balance, using both traditional and alternate methods. It is more interested in the correction of causal factors of imbalance than in symptom amelioration.
9. Holistic death promotes positive attitudes, including love, harmony, responsibility for one's own actions, self-acceptance, forgiveness, a sense of meaning and purpose, and an intention to be of service to others.
10. The role of the nurse and other health professionals is to facilitate the client's potential for healing.

result of many factors, not only physical ones, and the treatment approach begins with an assumption of the person's own capacity for healing. The holistic perspective focuses on promoting health through preventive treatment. It also applies to persons who have recovered from an illness and wish to understand how they contributed to making themselves receptive to the illness, how they can learn to help prevent a recurrence, and what they can do to improve their future health status.[49]

It is important to understand, however, that the holistic approach to healing should not be interpreted to blame the person who is ill for that illness. As holistic health has become more widely accepted as a way of understanding and treating illness, there is a tendency–both within the healing profession and among the general population–to consider that the person who is ill has created that illness and is, therefore, responsible for it. This attitude promotes guilt in the ill person and can hamper both the treatment and the healing process.

The intent of holistic health is to empower patients to actively engage in their own healing process. Its purpose is to encourage the person to investigate whether lifestyle changes, shifts in attitude, nutrition, or other behavior can help prevent further occurrences of health problems, ease the pain associated with an illness, and improve the quality of life of the patient.

The goal of holistic health is not necessarily to make the person "get well" but, rather, to help the patient understand and be connected with what is happening in his or her body. Illness is a condition, not an indication of failure. It is, therefore, crucial for the health professional who operates within the holisitc health approach to reassure the patient and to work in a way that validates and honors the patient as a valuable person, irrespective of the presence or absence of illness.

Holistic health represents an expansion of the variables considered relevant in health and medicine, rather than a rejection of the wisdom contained in the traditional model. In many ways the new model is a revival of the ancient Hippocratic tradition of the healer and a recognition of the value of medical practice in the East, which is based on bringing the mind, body, and spirit into harmony and balance.

As seen in Chapters 12 and 13, many of the principles and areas of assessment of holistic health have been incorporated into current nursing practice. Examples of these areas are nutrition, exercise, coping strategies, and relaxation techniques. These were always part of a holistic health evaluation. *Holistic Nursing: A Handbook for Practice*[8] is an excellent resource that shows the integration of a holistic approach in nursing practice.

As current nursing practice is incorporating more of the principles and practices of holistic health, it is important to understand that holistic health is more than a focus on self-care and/or the application of holistic techniques; it is also a process which includes the aspect of the personal inquiry. This asks individuals to look at the emotional meaning of any health problems they might have and significance of those problems in light of their sense of life purpose. The heart of a holistic health perspective is the assumption that a person's mental and emotional state and that of the physical body are interwoven. Thus, it is essential to bring this interrelationship into the patient's conscious awareness in order for him or her to decide on what changes need to be made to improve health status.

The holistic health approach to illness gives preference to the most gentle forms of healing available, after evaluating time and effectiveness factors.[1] These include such alternative practices as biofeedback, vitamin-nutrient therapies, and chiropractice. Autogenics and practices from the East, including acupuncture and acupressure, are discussed later in this chapter. Traditional medicine is advocated where appropriate–for example, for acute infectious conditions, traumatic injuries, or life-threatening illnesses.

Wellness and the Active Client

One of the most important aspects of holistic health is that the role of the client shifts from a passive to an active state. This means that the client, regardless of how ill or well he or she may be, is expected to take an active role in improving his or her health status. Only through the client's own action can he or she attain full health and vitality. A basic premise of holistic health is that the client has the power to bring about his or her own healing. The health professional does not have all the power; it is given back to the client.

A holistic health treatment program might include changes in diet, exercise habits, attitudes, interpersonal relationships, and types of work. The client may be asked to reexamine his or her entire lifestyle and to gradually incorporate changes in a planned fashion, with the help of a nurse or health counselor (Fig. 14-1). The application of a self-care approach in nursing practice is explored in *Self-Care Nursing* by Hill and Smith.[14] Many of these ideas and suggested lifestyle changes are included in *Healthy People 2000,* which emphasizes health promotion and preventative health strategies.[37]

Wellness Education

Wellness education is an aspect of holistic health practice appropriate for all people, regardless of their health status. Although it was originally developed for people with no discernible physical illness but who were bored,

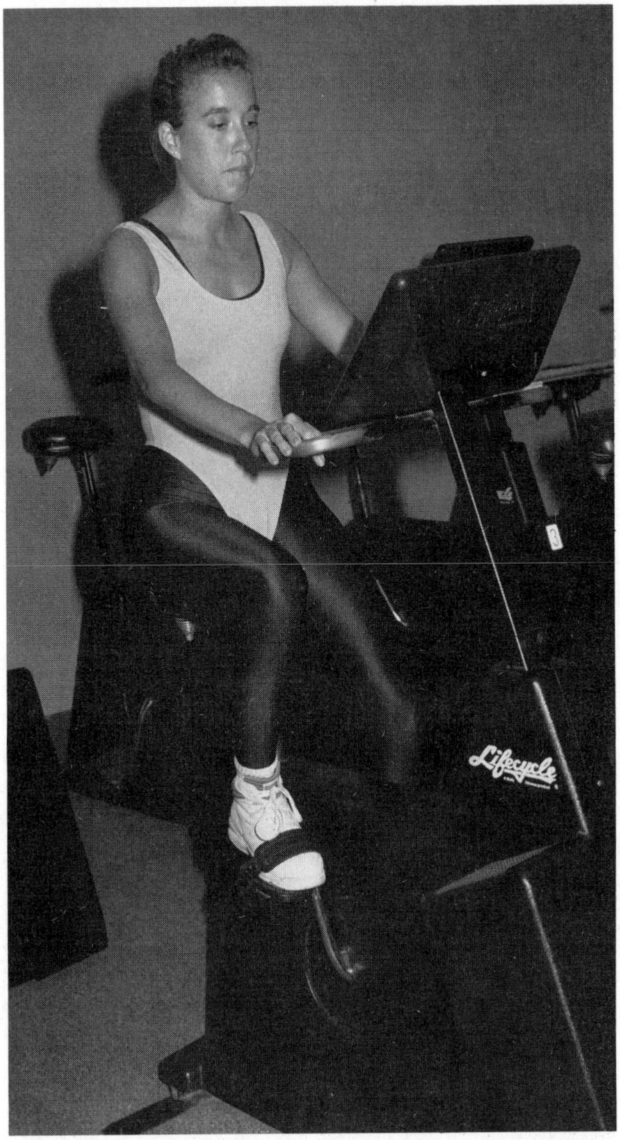

Fig. 14-1. Exercise is part of a holistic treatment program. (From Stanhope A: *Community health nursing: process and practice for promoting health,* ed 3, St Louis, 1991, Mosby.)

anxious, depressed, or in some way dissatisfied with their lives, wellness education should be included as part of any nursing intervention. Travis,[49] a pioneer of wellness education, established the Wellness Center in Mill Valley, Calif., to teach persons how to care for themselves in a healthy way.

The center's program covers four areas: physical awareness, nutrition, stress control, and self-responsibility. It is designed to help persons achieve new understanding and control of their lives (see box at the top of p. 328). At the center, clients are expected to assume responsibility for their own well-being and are given an opportunity to understand their basic physical and emotional needs and how they can change their lifestyles to have these needs met in more healthful ways.

❑ ❑ OUTCOMES OF WELLNESS EDUCATION

- Know what the client's real needs are and how to meet them.
- Act assertively.
- Relate to troublesome physical symptoms in ways that improve the condition as well as increase knowledge about oneself.
- Enjoy a basic sense of well-being, even in times of adversity.
- Know how to create and cultivate close relationships with others.
- Create the life one really wants, rather than just react to what seems to happen.
- Know the inner emotional and physical patterns and understand the signals the body sends.
- Trust that one's personal resources are the greatest strengths for living and growing.
- Experience oneself as a wonderful person and learn to love oneself.

Adapted from Travis J: Wellness education and holistic health–how they're related, *J Holistic Health* 1:25, 1975.

Medical Self-Care

Medical self-care is another facet of the client gaining power through self-knowledge. Self-care education teaches persons how to take care of themselves and how to seek out and best use the services of traditional medicine intelligently.[10] Self-care classes, which can be offered by nurses, are most useful when geared specifically to the needs and interests of the community they serve.

A major proponent of medical self-care is Sehnert,[45] a family practitioner who developed a series of 16 2-hour classes teaching laypersons how to handle common illnesses and injuries, common drugs and their effects, and a number of preventive health practices. Graduates of these self-care classes feel less anxious about health matters and have fewer visits to physicians. An example of his course for the health-activated patient is seen in the box to the right. Sehnert has trained health workers from all over the United States to teach medical self-care classes to various populations. His book, *How To Be Your Own Doctor (Sometimes)* is based on his classes and contains a self-help medical guide.

❑ ❑ SEHNERT'S EDUCATION PROGRAM

- Acquiring and using a black bag of medical tools. This includes stethoscope, blood pressure cuff, otoscope, tongue blade, high-intensity penlight, dental mirror, and oral and rectal thermometers.
- Learning to pay more attention to the body's messages, such as headache, sore throat, and good feelings.
- Gaining familiarity with drugs, including their purpose, use, and warnings.
- Doing introductory yoga.
- Maintaining a copy of one's medical record.
- Learning how to interview and rate prospective or current physicians.
- Planning a visit to the physician so as to present all the pertinent information and getting a busy physician to answer questions.
- Using decision-making flow charts (clinical algorithms) to decide what to do when confronted with certain physical symptoms.

Adapted from Sehnert F: *How to be your own doctor (sometimes)*, New York, 1975, Grosset & Dunlap.

TOOLS FOR HOLISTIC NURSING CARE

Therapeutic Touch

Therapeutic touch is a nursing practice developed by Kreiger,[26] which evolved from the ancient practice of the laying on of hands. Therapeutic touch can be used in health assessment and nursing intervention.

A nurse using therapeutic touch begins by *centering* or moving into a meditative state to get in touch with universal *prana* or energy, such as by taking three deep, easy breaths. Then, with an intent to help and with attention focused on the client, the nurse begins the assessment process. The nurse begins to move the hands symmetrically around the client 2 to 6 inches from the body, which allows their energy fields to interact. As this is done, the nurse becomes aware of various sensations: temperature variations, pressure, tingling, or pulsation.

Different practitioners may experience different sensations.[40] A sensation of pressure is often an indication of a congestion in the vital field. The nurse can "unruffle" or unclog the field by placing the hands at the area where the pressure was felt, with the palms facing away from the client's body, and then moving the hands away from the body in a sweeping gesture. Kreiger recommends either making the sweep perpendicular to the body surface or sweeping downward, following the directions of the long bones of the extremities. This unruffling facilitates the next step, which is the transfer of universal prana through the nurse to the client.

During the *transfer stage,* the nurse returns to the sites of imbalance and seeks to balance the energy so that the client's field feels "smooth" and equalized.[26] The transfer stage does not last longer than 20 minutes and may be done either in silence or with a verbal exchange. When finishing a transfer, the nurse again "centers" to renew the self with energy.[39]

The basis for this practice is the theory that each person has several interpenetrating energy *bodies* or fields–physical, vital or bioenergetic,[20] emotional, mental, and spiritual[23] (Fig. 14-2). According to Rogers' synergistic theory,[42] persons' energy fields interact, and this interaction allows therapeutic touch to work. Therapeutic touch is thought to work primarily through the *vital* field, which interpenetrates and extends beyond the physical body by about 6 inches.

Krieger,[26] using some concepts of Eastern philosophy, postulated that a healthy person has access to an overabundance of universal prana (vital energy), whereas a person who is ill has less prana. Further, an imbalance in vital energy can be perceived in the energy field before illness manifests. A client who is fairly healthy and has an intent to help can assess for energy imbalance and then direct the life force to "boost" his energy for his own healing. The goal is to bring about balance, which will speed the healing process. Ideally, if the energy is balanced, it will prevent physical illness.

In studying the interrelation between health and vital energy, Kreiger hypothesized a correlation would exist between the amount of vital energy or prana and the hemoglobin level.[26] To investigate these assumptions, Kreiger conducted a pilot study in 1971, hypothesizing that the mean hemoglobin value of an experimental group after treatment by laying on of hands would exceed their pretreatment values, whereas no significant difference should occur in the prehemoglobin and posthemoglobin values of the control group. She selected hemoglobin because she believed that prana might be related to oxygen. Oskar Estabany, a renowned healer, worked with 19 ill people in the experimental group and

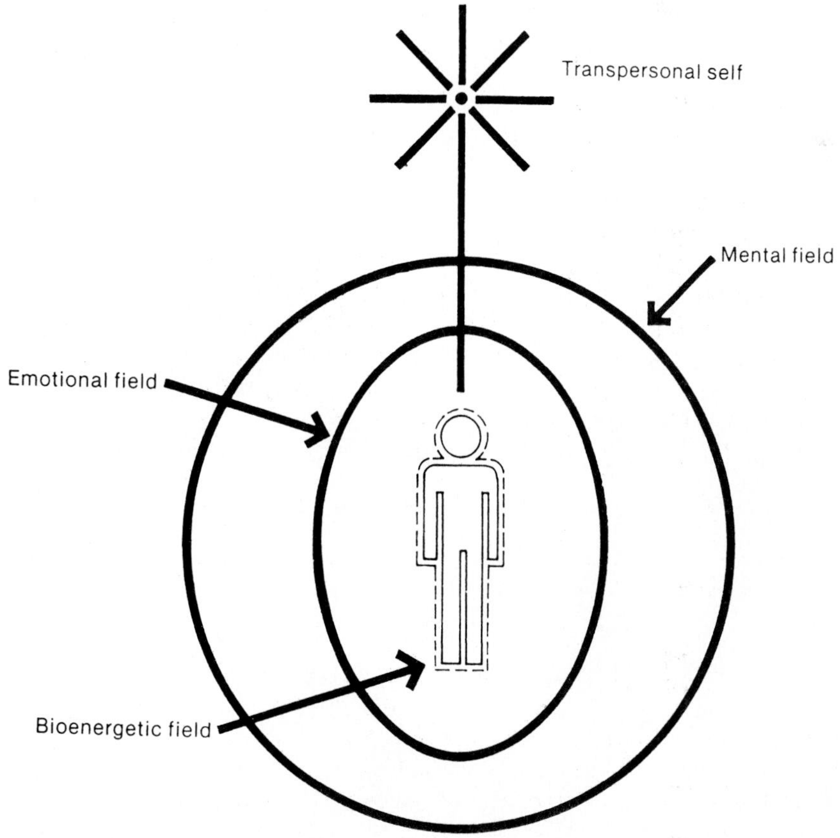

Fig. 14-2. Therapeutic touch is based on every person possessing several interacting energy fields. (Redrawn from Robert Gerard, 1977.)

nine ill people in the control group. Ages and sexes of the members were comparable. Her hypothesis was confirmed.

In 1972, Kreiger repeated the experiment using 43 ill people in the experimental group and 33 in the control group; again her hypothesis was confirmed. In 1973 she replicated the study and controlled for several intervening variables, including smoking, diet, medication, breathing exercises, meditation, and biorhythm change. There were 46 subjects in the experimental group and 29 in the control group; her hypothesis was again confirmed.[27]

Kreiger believed that the laying on of hands is a natural ability if two factors are present: (1) a strong intent to help another and (2) the person possessing a healthy body. She then undertook another study after teaching 32 registered nurses to be "healers." The experimental group consisted of 16 nurses who included therapeutic touch in caring for their patients, whereas the 16 control nurses did not. Each nurse worked on the two patients. The experimental group showed a significant increase in the mean hemoglobin level. The control group did not have a statistically significant result.[27]

Therapeutic touch seems to be particularly useful in eliciting a generalized relaxation response and promoting relief from pain[26,52] (Fig. 14-3). Heidt investigated this by using a standardized anxiety questionnaire for 90 patients on a cardiovascular ward. There were three groups: (1) the experimental group received 5 minutes of therapeutic touch; (2) another group had pulses taken in four places during 5 minutes by a nurse who remained silent; and (3) the third had a nurse who stayed and talked to them for 5 minutes but did not touch them. The patients then filled out a second questionnaire to measure anxiety, which showed that in the experimental group anxiety decreased. Anxiety also decreased in the patients who were touched but not significantly. Anxiety actually increased in some third-group members.[42]

A recent study has shown that noncontact therapeutic touch significantly increases the healing rate of full-thickness dermal wounds. The study included 44 subjects who were randomly divided into treatment and nontreatment groups. A randomized double-blind, placebo-controlled protocol was utilized. A medical doctor created a full-thickness wound under local anesthesia using a skin biopsy instrument to make a precise wound. The first treatment sessions were conducted the same day as the incision, followed by daily treatments for 16 days. Each subject came to the treatment room and put his arm through a hole which opened to an adjoining room, where the practitioner was located. Noncontact therapeutic touch was given for 5 minutes to the subjects in the experimental group only. Each subject remained in the room for 20 minutes. On days 8 and 16, the perimeter of the wounds was measured. The results showed that the treated group had a significantly smaller average wound size than the nontreated group. The study concluded that therapeutic touch enhances the

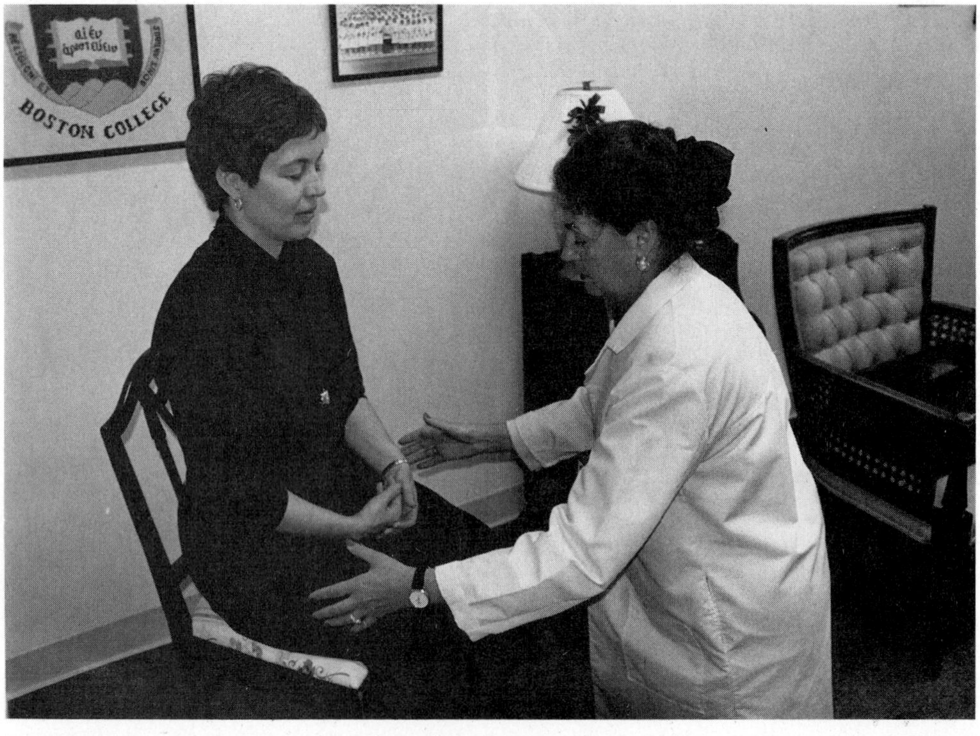

Fig. 14-3. During therapeutic touch, both the patient and the nurse experience a sense of deep relaxation.

healing of full-thickness dermal wounds.[54] Quinn has compiled a thorough review of significant recent research on therapeutic touch and suggestions for further research.[37-39]

Learning therapeutic touch involves learning how to meditate or center, acquiring experimental knowledge of energy fields, and finally practicing. Nurses wishing to learn more about his technique are directed to Kreiger's *Therapeutic Touch,*[26] which describes the basis of this modality and presents many excellent exercises to facilitate learning. Another good book is *Therapeutic Touch, A Practical Guide* by Macrae.[30] Classes in therapeutic touch are available through

Nurse Healers-Professional Associates, Inc.
175 Fifth Ave., Suite 2755
New York, NY 10010

Acupuncture

Acupuncture is an ancient form of healing used by the Chinese that seeks to balance the body's energy to promote health. Needles are inserted at specific points to stimulate or disperse the flow of energy. Use of acupuncture requires extensive training and practice and in some states official certification. At present, few nurses are educated in this practice. Fortunately, many of the benefits of acupuncture can be obtained using acupressure, which is relatively simple to learn and easily integrated into nursing practice.

Acupressure

Acupressure, as with acupuncture, is based on a theory of Oriental medicine: a life force, in the form of energy, or chi (like prana), circulates throughout the body in well-defined cycles. This chi circulates through energy pathways called *meridians.* There are 12 bilateral meridians and two central meridians, which are the main yin-yang channels (Fig. 14-4). When the chi is in balance, a person is healthy. An energy imbalance, either an excess or a deficit, is the basis of illness. The purpose of acupressure is to open congested meridians, allowing energy to balance and thus promote a healthier state. Results might include a decrease in muscle tension or pain, an increase in vitality, or a sense of emotional balance.

Several forms of acupressure exist. *Shiatsu,* which has a Japanese origin, uses a deep pressure over particular points along the meridian (*acupoints*). The practitioner works on points located symmetrically on opposite sides of the body. The *Jin Shin* forms of acupressure, *Jysitsu* and *Do,* touch-specific acupoints in prescribed sequential combinations to help reestablish a normal flow of chi along the meridians. Unlike Shiatsu, the points are not necessarily symmetric. A full acupressure session usually takes about an hour, and the effects may be short term or long term, depending on the nature of imbalance.

Although little research has been done on the effects of acupressure, studies have documented the effects of acupuncture. One result is the increased production of the body's own pain killers, *endorphins* and *encephalins,* which work at the same site in the brain as morphine. Becker, of Upstate Medical Center in Syracuse, NY, believes that the acupoints and meridians are part of a primitive data transmission and control system that has the function of sensing injury and effecting repair.[3] Thus, acupuncture and acupressure aid in stimulating the body's own healing capacity.

With acupressure, as in therapeutic touch, the practitioner begins by centering, preparing to use the universal sources of chi to facilitate balancing the energy field. Many simple, easy, and harmless acupressure "quickies" are particularly suited to primary prevention. These can be taught to clients, who can then do them on themselves (see box on p. 333 and Fig. 14-5). For example, the *pelvic release and leg opener* is particularly good for joggers and tennis or racketball players, since it reduces the chances of muscle strains and sprains. Persons on long airplane trips can avoid jet lag by a simple four-step "quickie." The *surface skin flow* relaxes the body, whereas the *bodily flow* serves to strengthen and balance the whole system.

To use acupressure, the nurse begins by making sure the client is comfortable, and finds the points as indicated (see box on p. 333). The left hand is placed on the point designated by LH, the right hand on the point designated by RH. A light yet firm touch should be applied. As the points are touched, the nurse begins to feel a very subtle sensation or pulse under the fingers. At first, the pulses at various points will be different; but as they continue to be held, they will come into synchronization, or balance. When the acupoints are balanced, the nurse gently removes the fingers. Balance of the points generally takes 1 to 5 minutes.

Touch for Health

Touch for Health is a health enhancement practice that has evolved from chiropractic and the modern practice of ancient Oriental health care disciplines. Touch for Health acknowledges the person as a structural, chemical, psychologic, and spiritual being.[48]

Thie,[48] one of the developers of Touch for Health, states that the goal is "to discover if and where the body is transmitting signaling errors, thereby reducing its ability to utilize the inherent recuperative potentials and/or health-enhancing abilities." One of the indica-

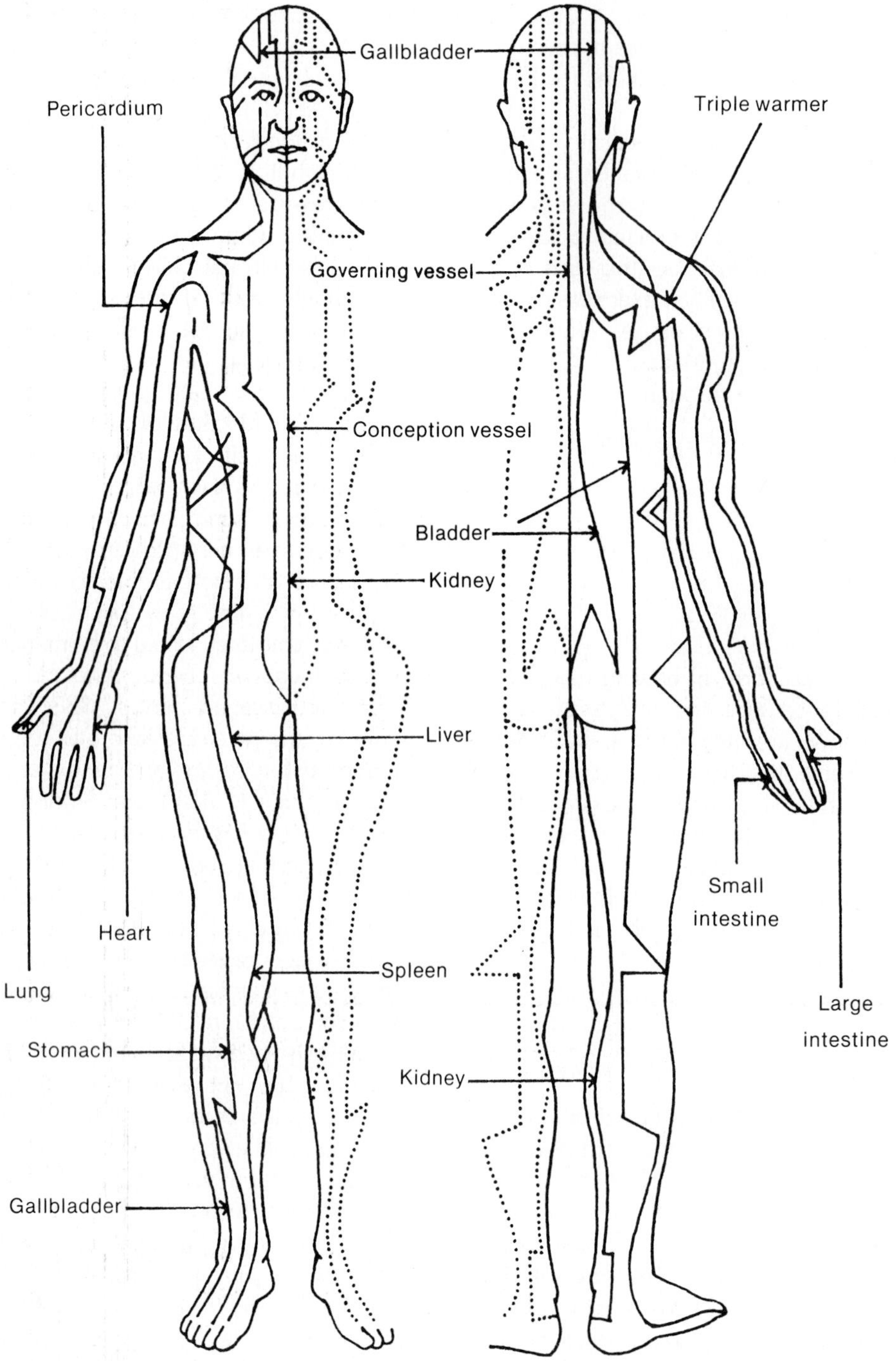

Fig. 14-4. Major body meridians, or energy pathways. Acupressure's purpose is to open congested meridians and balance energy to promote a healthier state. (Redrawn from Mann F: *The meridians for acupuncture,* London, 1974, William Heinemann Medical Books.)

tors of a *signal error* is a weakening of muscles. The techique used involves observing the person's posture and testing various muscles to assess the body's functioning and then using specific kinesiology techniques to restore muscle balance and thereby bring balance to the body. Touch for Health can help correct minor malfunctions and thus prevent some minor illnesses from developing.

Certain muscles are related to specific organs, acupuncture meridians, lymph vessels, and nutritional states. For example, the pectoralis major muscle is associated with the stomach and could be used to test for nutritional deficiencies or allergies. If this muscle tests "weak" and an appropriate food or dietetic supplement that has the missing nutrient is placed in the mouth, then the muscle will retest as strong. If the weakness continues, then some other energy imbalance is present, which might be corrected by massaging the

❑ ❑ ACUPRESSURE QUICK RELEASES

Acupressure is derived from an Oriental folk art of self-help to release stress problems within the body. It is "the way of the compassionate spirit, the art of God through compassionate man." Pressure points are illustrated in Fig. 14-5.

Pelvic release and leg opener

Muscle spasms of legs, poor circulation in legs and feet, cold feet; a runner flow

1. Pubic bone and Coccyx
2. Right (R) #6 and R #10
3. R behind buttocks and R behind knee
4. Left (L) #6 and L #10
5. L behind buttocks and L behind knee

"Feel good flow"

Bursitis, arthritis, constipation
LH behind L knee and RH behind R knee

Jet lag

1. R #19 and R behind buttocks
2. R #19 and R #6
3. L #19 and L behind buttocks
4. L #19 and L #6

Fatigue

L #19 and R #19

Diarrhea

L #21 and L of coccyx

Sore throat

#2 and opposite side #22

Mental alertness

#22, both sides

Surface skin flow

Relaxing the body, skin problems, insect bites, shock, adrenal exhaustion, sunburn
Small toe and K_1 same side

Bodily flow

(strengthens and balances whole system)
Small toe and #9 same side

Headache

Middle toe and #9 & #12 same side

Nausea

Low #13 and #12 same side

Fainting, shock

1. Surface skin flow or
2. Hold both thumbs

Sinus release

Do on opposite eye of congestion.
Use opposite hand to eye.
Use index finger to circle eye orbit; start at inside edge, and move around top.
At same time use other hand and hold at top of fifth finger and move down.
When you reach outside edge of eye orbit, continue around lower part and return to inside edge.
At same time, start at bottom of fourth finger and move up to top.

Hiccups, hyperventilation

#5, both sides and opposite side #17

Coughing, choking

#3, both sides

Calming; relieving nerves, tension

Hold ring finger and small finger 3 minutes or longer.

Increase breathing, open lungs and chest

Put thumb on ring finger nail.

Insomnia

1. Lace fingers together and place on solar plexus; or
2. R hand on top of head and L hand on tip of chin.

Constipation, headaches, dental work

Massage Hoku point.

All-over pain relief

L hand on Achilles tendon, outside edge and R hand on same #9

From Acupressure and Living Center. Used with permission.

appropriate acupressure points, meridians, or neurolymphatic points or holding the associated neurovascular points. The muscle then can be retested to see if these corrections worked.[47]

In addition to structural imbalances, Touch for Health balancing techniques can help a person recover from emotional upsets. The pectoralis major and the supraspinatus muscles are associated with emotional states.[48] After testing these muscles, the nurse lightly places the fingertips on the neurovascular points on the client's forehead while the client thinks about what was upsetting. After a few minutes, the client usually feels a sense of relief, and the related muscles will retest strong. This is an easy technique to use to help the client feel

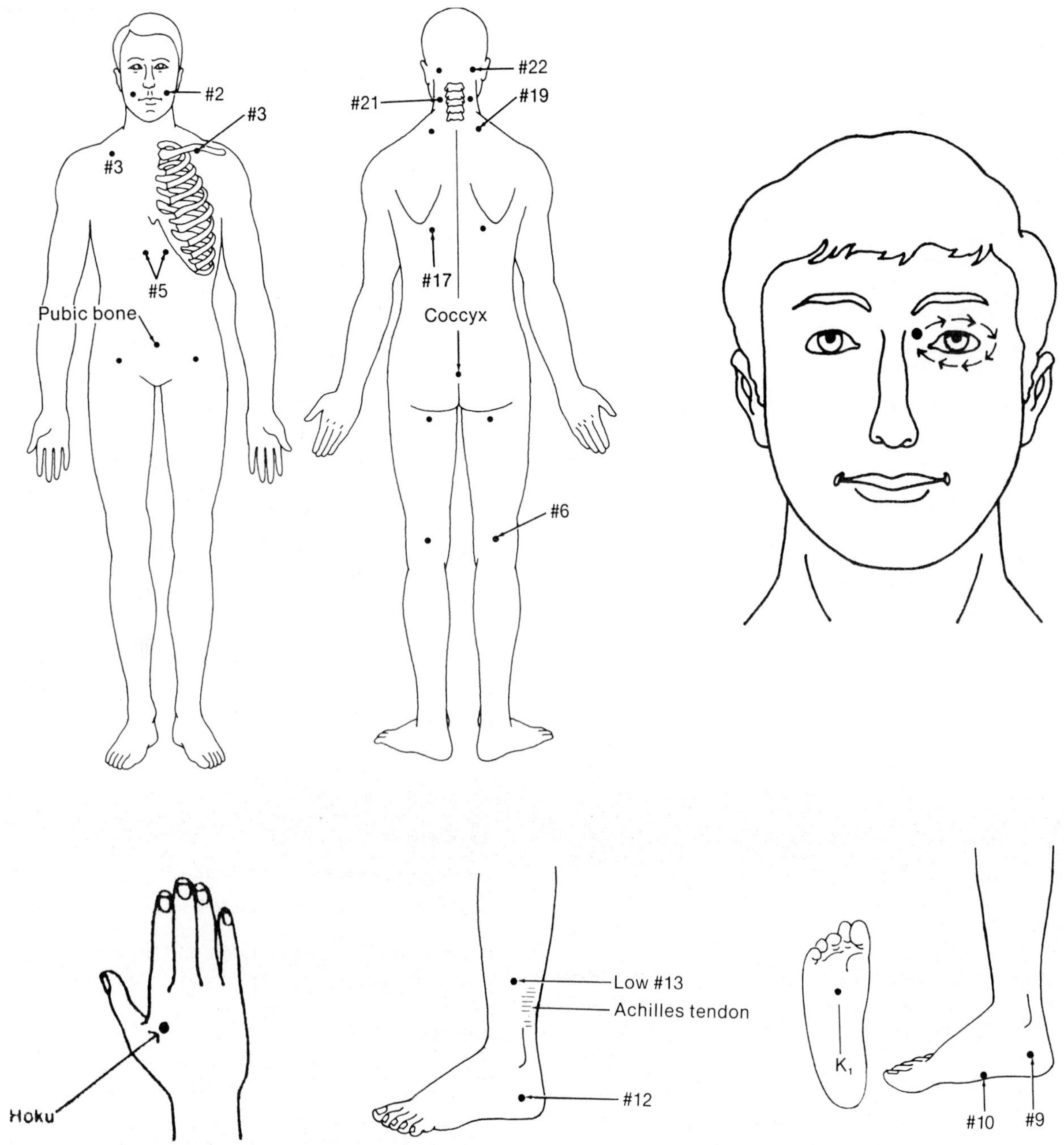

Fig. 14-5. Pressure points used in acupuncture. (Courtesy of Barbara Rapko, PhD, RN.)

calmer and can reduce the need for tranquilizers.

At present, no clinical studies in the nursing or medical literature have evaluated the effectiveness of Touch for Health. This is similar to the status of acupuncture 20 years ago; those who use Touch for Health would welcome such an evaluation. This is a fruitful area for nursing research.

Touch for Health is a tool that nurses may use as part of an assessment process as well as to evaluate the effectiveness of its treatments. On completion of a Touch for Health Instructor course, nurses could teach clients some simple Touch for Health techniques, which they then could use to monitor and improve their own, their family's, and other community members' health.

Relaxation and Self-Regulation Training

Meditation or relaxation techniques seem to activate a natural potential of the nervous system to repair and regenerate itself, with a corresponding increase in sense of personal autonomy, well-being, and many positive side effects. In addition, no professional help or cost is incurred in the use of self-regulation techniques once they are learned.

As with other holistic techniques, relaxation methods are a prophylactic measure that can be applied at any phase of health or illness. They are preventive measures helping the body bounce back and regenerate each day and can be used to ease the damage of minor physical and emotional stress symptoms and as an alternative to tranquilizers, alcohol, smoking, or overeating.[34] Relaxation techniques are increasingly being used in combination with modern medical treatments to treat high blood pressure, cardiovascular disease, chronic pain, infertility, insomnia, and some of the symptoms of cancer and AIDS.[5]

Several types and modalities are used to attain the relaxation state. All these seem to produce similar results and aim for the same general goal. The following are brief descriptions of some of the most commonly used relaxation techniques:

1. *The Relaxation Response* (developed by Benson[4]). The person turns awareness away from the outside world and focuses loosely, without forcing, on a certain object-word, a part of the body, a mental picture, a thought, or a picture. When the mind wanders, the person gently brings the focus back to the subject. This attention is called *passive awareness* or *passive attention*. The focus is on the process, not the end point (see the box to the right).
2. *Progressive relaxation.* Attention is focused on each muscle group, one by one, in each part of the body, and by tensing each one, then relaxing it, the person learns how to relax even the residual and chronic tension from each muscle.[19]
3. *Meditation.* An ancient set of practices, appearing in every religious and cultural tradition; of broadening inner awareness by stilling the usual conscious modes of thought and activity.
4. *Autogenic training (AT).* An approach used widely in Europe, consisting of the repetition of a series of specific formulas that make suggestions of physical states in the body. AT begins with the patient learning to induce a feeling of heaviness in the arms and legs and then a sensation of warmth in the hands and feet, by repeating phrases such as, "My left arm is warm," in a standard posture and manner.
5. *Self-hypnosis.* Using self-suggestion and images of relaxation and peace, the person enters the relaxation state using a variety of seed thoughts and then conditions a certain response to them.
6. *Guided imagery.* A person uses standard or invented images that suggest the end state he or she wants to produce in the body. For relaxation, the image of going to a lovely beach or vacation spot can be used. To help heal pain or symptoms, persons can picture their diseases and then imagine something happening to heal them, thereby sending a positive suggestion to the body.
7. *Biofeedback.* This uses apparatus that gives instantaneous, usually audio or visual, feedback on minute changes in physiologic states (Fig. 14-6). The most common types of biofeedback are muscle tension, temperature, and skin conductivity. Either spontaneous or learned relaxation techniques are used to produce change, usually deep relaxation, as the person receives the instant feedback.

❑ ❑ TECHNIQUE FOR EVOKING THE RELAXATION RESPONSE

1. Sit quietly in a comfortable position.
2. Close your eyes.
3. Deeply relax all your muscles, beginning at your feet and progressing up to your face. Keep them relaxed.
4. Breathe through your nose. Become aware of your breathing. As you breathe out, say the word, "One," silently to yourself. For example, breathe in . . . out, "One"; in . . . out, "One"; and so on. Breathe easily and naturally.
5. Continue for 10 to 20 minutes. You may open your eyes to check the time but do not use an alarm. When you finish, sit quietly for several minutes, at first with your eyes closed and later with your eyes open. Do not stand up for a few minutes.
6. Do not worry about whether you are successful in achieving a deep level of relaxation. Maintain a passive attitude and permit relaxation to occur at its own pace. When distracting thoughts occur, try to ignore them by not dwelling on them and return to repeating, "One." With practice the technique should come with little effort. You should wait 2 hours after any meals, since the digestive processes seem to interfere with the elicitation of the response.

Adapted from Benson H: *The relaxation response,* New York, 1975, William Morrow.

PSYCHOPHYSIOLOGIC EFFECTS

Benson was among the first to suggest that a psychophysiologic opposite to the stress response existed, which he labeled the "relaxation response." This response may be activated by a variety of techniques, ranging from meditation and religious practices to modern self-hypnosis and biofeedback training.

The outcome of all these methods is that the nervous system enters a state of parasympathetic arousal; breathing becomes deeper and slower, muscle tension

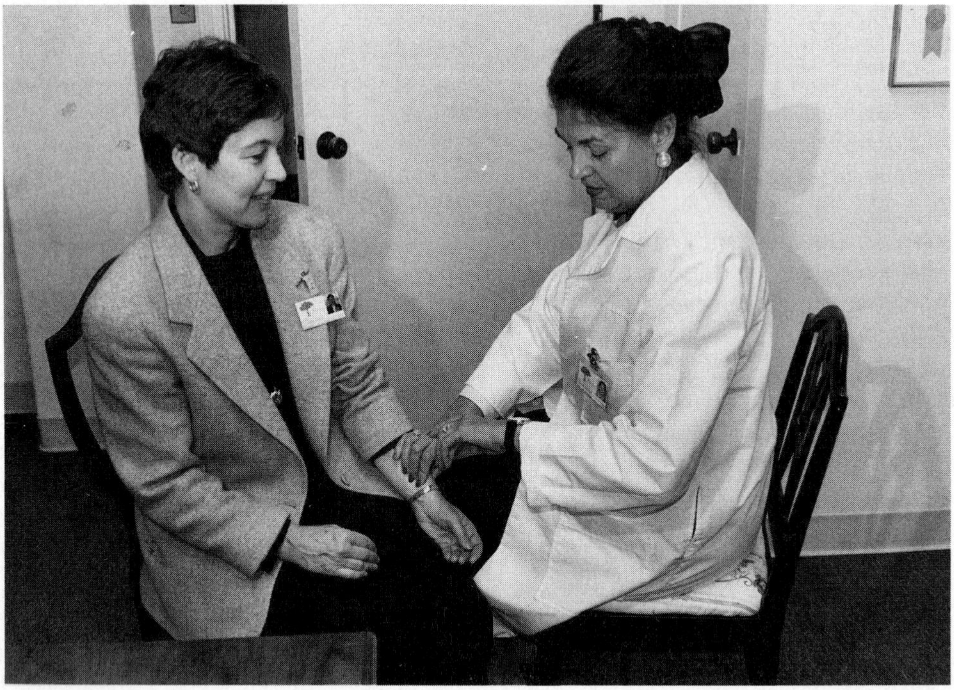

Fig. 14-6. Learning about self-regulation via biofeedback training. This has provided many clients with relief from pain and other physical symptoms.

decreases, awareness becomes global and unfocused, and a sense of peace and well-being predominates over other concerns.[53] Negative emotions such as anxiety are nearly impossible to experience in this relaxation state; and a deep, wakeful restful period of alertness, which seems to speed up and enhance all the body's natural self-healing processes, emerges. Although other common states have some of these positive qualities–for example, the rest of sleep or after heavy exertion or deep, creative involvement in a problem or task–there seems to be some unique positive qualities to the relaxation state and some clear psychophysiologic benefits for persons who enter this state regularly.[4]

Schwartz[44] found that when a person becomes more aware of internal functioning and pays attention to it, the body often becomes self-calibrating, allowing itself to move spontaneously toward greater health.

PSYCHONEUROIMMUNOLOGY

This is an emerging field of science which examines the interrelationships among psychologic, neurologic, hormonal, and immune responses and health. Research in this area is documenting that psychologic and physical stress can often inhibit immune functions while other factors such as social support many enhance immune response.[7,35] This area of science may provide the empiric evidence of the importance of a holistic health approach.

APPLICATIONS TO NURSING

A nurse is often in the best situation to teach these relaxation techniques. Even a few minutes of instruction in relaxation can have enormous impact. Most nurses can rapidly learn Benson's Relaxation Response, progressive relaxation, and some simple guided imagery techniques. AT and biofeedback require more training and supervised experience but are well within the scope of nursing practice.

Nurses are also using audiotapes to combine the techniques of relaxation and guided imagery. In a randomized controlled clinical trial, patients undergoing cholecystectomy were evaluated on three indexes of recovery. The clients in the experimental group listened to a series of four 20-minute audiotapes that utilized relaxation with guided imagery, specifically designed to augment the healing process. These were provided on the day prior to surgery and the first 3 days postoperatively. The results showed that the experimental group had significantly less state anxiety, lower cortisol levels, and less surgical wound erythema than those in the control group.[16]

The most effective teachers of relaxation techniques also use them in their daily lives. These methods not only teach a useful skill but also alter the whole perspective of the client. Relaxation is a concrete demonstration to the client that he makes a difference, and this difference cannot take place without active involvement and daily participation. The use of the technique is a model of a holistic process.

ASSESSING HEALTH AND WELLNESS

Health Assessment Process

From a holistic health perspective, health assessment is an expansion of the present nursing assessment process. One of the goals of the health assessment is to establish a healing partnership between nurse and client. Holistic health assessment also stresses that the client's attitudes toward health and healing have a profound effect on the healing process.

One of the most important aspects of the health assessment is how it is done. The process involves a helper and a client who is willing to take a great deal of initiative to explore his life and inner world.

Although sophisticated computer analyses of nutritional factors, risk factors, and stress levels might be employed, these instrumented inquires are only tools for evaluation. The most important information lies within the client: emotions, attitudes, coping style, values, and personal history. Therefore, only a portion of the health assessment can be quantified or standardized.

Types of Health Assessment

RISK FACTOR AND HEALTH PROFILE ANALYSIS

Epidemiology uses sophisticated statistic techniques to analyze health statistics and to define behavioral, environmental, and psychologic factors that influence disease statistics in large populations.[12] Epidemiologic research has enabled health professionals to learn about hazards that may subtly create illness over many years, leading to changes within the body that initially may not be directly measurable.[51] Most of what we know about nutrition, exercise, stress, and environmental pollution comes from careful analyses of disease statistics, which identifies factors causing significantly greater numbers of persons to become ill.

Robbins and Hall[41] conducted research on characteristics of persons who get heart disease, using a large number living in Framingham, Mass. This study and others similar to it indicate that certain risk factors such as smoking increase a person's chances of developing heart disease and cancer. Many other risk factors, such as hereditary characteristics, air quality, and stress level, also influence the outcome. The authors developed a computerized questionnaire for individuals to answer questions about all aspects of their lives, family health history, stressful events, diet, exercise, and other daily routines. From this study they determined the effect on lifespan of certain health habits.

Other research shows that life expectancy may be affected by factors such as using seat belts, living in neighborhoods with poor air quality, excessive use of certain foods and chemicals, and eating breakfast daily.

Many lifespan and health profiles now exist. Although there is sometimes too little definitive research to make firm conclusions about the causes of diseases such as cancer and heart disease, the use of health profiles and risk factor questionnaires is an important new aspect of health care. Today's common illnesses usually can be traced largely to personal behavior and are, therefore, preventable or postponable. Health profiles make clients aware of risk factors in their own lives, which may motivate them to change to a more healthy lifestyle.

WELLNESS ASSESSMENT

As mentioned earlier, Travis pioneered wellness education; his wellness assessment tool is now nationally used as an assessment process to help realign a client's entire conception of health and personal power and control over health. His *Wellness Workbook*[50] includes many of the risk factor and health hazard inquiries, in addition to other assessment tools. Travis asks persons to take responsibility for all things that interfere with reaching an optimum level of wellness.

Instead of simply asking whether persons engage in certain health practices, Travis believes that the process demands that they explore why they do *not* do things they know are healthy. He asks persons to note the major obstacles that prevent them from developing healthy behaviors and to make some commitments to changing.

Travis and his colleagues also ask clients to explore their values and personal life, including parenting, sexuality, life goals, achievements, loving relationships, and other factors not ordinarily linked to health and illness. Travis views everything that interferes with a rich, full, loving, rewarding life as relevant to health. He argues that there is no reason for a person not to strive to live a full, creative, expressive life.

JOURNAL THERAPY

Although most forms of psychologic self-care are not discussed in this chapter, the use of a personal journal as a tool for assessment is so important and so connected to self-awareness, self-responsibility, and self-help that it is included here among assessment tools. As devised by Progoff,[36] a Jungian psychologist, the personal journal uses Jungian methods of active imagination, internal dialogue, life planning, and meditation exercises to help persons work on their own problems, without the intervention of a therapist (Fig. 14-7). Journal therapy was devised when Progoff, looking into the ways in which persons developed self-awareness through personal journals, created a series of exercises for people to reflect on their lives, feelings, goals, and inner lives.

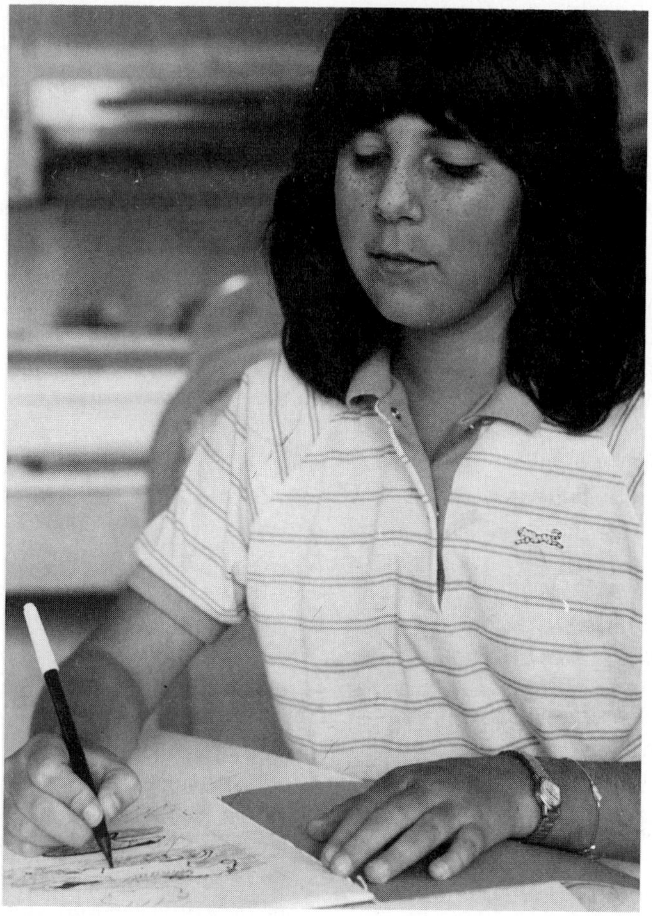

Fig. 14-7. Taking time for reflection and journal writing can facilitate the process of self-discovery and understanding. Self-awareness is a key part of holistic health.

There are journal sections for daily activities, dreams, stepping stones of personal development, and dialogues with one's inner selves, including one's body, one's aspirations, and one's relationships. The goal of the process is self-awareness, learning about hidden aspects of oneself via the dialogue process.

In holistic health, the personal journal and inner dialogue are used often to help clients discover inner connections between their health, feelings, early experiences about their body, and their current distress. When physical or emotional crises develop, these symptoms often reflect imbalances or disconnections within the whole person. For example, disowned feelings, needs, or life goals might be experienced many years later in the form of physical symptoms. The journal method is a pathway to self-awareness that respects the client's autonomy and ability to help himself or herself.

PERSONAL HEALTH EXPLORATION: A MODEL FOR HOLISTIC NURSING

One of the most important implications of the holistic model relating to nursing is the concept of disease as an ongoing process. When a person develops a stomach ulcer, chronic back pain, a heart attack, or even cancer, this dramatic physical breakdown is considered to be the final stage of a long-term, insidious process of developing illness. The holistic health approach provides a useful model for working with clients as partners, helping them explore and modify actual and potential risk factors in their physical, emotional, and interpersonal lives.

The Personal Health Exploration, developed by Dennis Jaffe, is a conscious process of counseling and education. Clients learn to become active participants in their own health process. The traditional dyad of passive client and all-knowing, all-powerful physician becomes transformed in the course of the counseling process into the new, triadic, balanced interrelationship between primary physician, activated client, and health resource guide. These work together, each with their particular responsibilities, functions, and roles, to create health.

The nurse or other health professional acts in the role of a *health resource guide,* counseling the client to look at themselves, and assisting them in creating and implementing a program to increase their health.

Many complaints brought to physicians are minor: loss of energy, vague discomforts, anxiety-related physical upsets, or pain that cannot be related to any specific disease process. The typical medical response is reassurance, often combined with pain medication or a tranquilizer.[25] The assumption is that when the symptom is taken away, so is the problem. The holistic approach is different.

A person entering a medical office for a vague complaint or for a periodic health checkup would not only be asked for a catalogue of symptoms. The health resource guide would also help the client move from the particular minor symptoms or difficulties to an exploration of all the factors in his or her life that might contribute to current or future difficulties. The most important and the most difficult theme that needs to be understood is that health is related to all aspects of life and that the type of reflection and change demanded by the program entails long and hard work daily and willingness to consider major life change.

There are three phases to a personal health exploration: (1) the personal inquiry, (2) the relaxation and self-regulation training, and (3) the development of a personal health plan. These phases are not linear but rather overlap.

Personal Inquiry

In this phase, the client is asked to look at various aspects of his life, including personality, personal relationships, health habits, particular minor or chronic symptoms or distresses of any type, and values and goals, to determine where obstacles to health might lie and also to catalogue health resources. Clients receive a Personal Health Workbook, which contains articles, explanations, outlines, self-assessment questions for the inquiry phase, and exercises for home practice (Fig. 14-8). Clients are encouraged to read some of the workbook before the initial interview.

The nursing assessment data base in Chapter 4 and the assessment of functional health patterns in Chapter 5 are other forms that can be used during the personal inquiry phase. The main difference in the personal health workbook is the intention to place symptoms or stress problems into the broader life context in which they take place to discover their personal meaning and significance.

The Personal Health Exploration begins by inquiring into current physical or psychologic symptoms or ongoing stress in the client's current life. If a symptom is chronic or recurring, patterns are examined, and what is going on before and at the moment the symptom occurs is explored. The purpose is not for secondary intervention alone but to intervene to promote health.

Triggering stresses, trauma, or events, not only for major breakdowns but for the onset of each minor symptom, usually are present. For example, clients with chronic pain such as headache often discover repressed, unexpressed, or unheeded anger, frustration or dislike, or a buildup of physical tension just before the onset. Illnesses relate to losses of job, others in the family (often parents, spouses, or children), moving out, or of meaning or pleasure in life. A woman with various minor difficulties reported that a few months previously she had suffered financial reversals and began to dread the thought of growing old without adequate financial security and always having to work at her unfulfilling job. She believed that she gave up on life as she developed more and more serious ailments. Sometimes symptoms are triggered by guilt, perhaps about sexuality. A woman developed colitis several months after an abortion; another man an ulcer soon after admitting to himself that he was gay. The triggering event very often is an unresolved emotional trauma or life change. A preventive intervention might have averted these difficulties.

Questions also are asked about the consequences of symptoms and stresses on the client, his or her sense of self and the future, and on family and work. Some secondary gain always complicates becoming optimally healthy, and psychosocial benefits to symptoms usually can be found. For example, illness is often the only allowable way to take a rest or vacation.[15] It becomes clear that illness can be a covert way for persons to compel nurturance or feel justified in asking for something for themselves. Often an illness will strike a self-denying, unselfish client who always gives to others but can never ask for oneself. Clients are asked to define one or more benefits of symptoms in their lives.

A review follows of social, family, behavioral, cognitive, and emotional systems to understand what personal dissatisfactions, conflict, self-defeating habits, trauma, past events, or changes might weaken a person's resistance to illness. The outline used is similar to the personal systems review of Ireton and Cassata.[18] The goal is to pinpoint all potential contributors to the current health status and to illuminate the person's customary responses to stress and tension (see Fig. 14-8).

Specific dysfunctional responses to stress emerge in this interview. For example, many persons suppress all their needs and responses to stressors. A woman with severe gastrointestinal disease reported that she could not express anger or make demands on her family, even though she knew that her frustration increased her gastric secretion to a dangerous level. Many persons also allow conflicts or difficulties to exist continually without feeling it is possible to resolve them. A man with severe stress symptoms believed that he was completely powerless to have his wife stop interfering in his daily affairs and checking up on him behind his back. Still others experience a continual cycle of worry or anticipatory or retrospective anxiety; they replay negative situations or imagine negative outcomes, thoughts that have the physiologic effect of arousing their stress response in the absence of an environmental threat. In every initial

SECTION I: PERSONAL HEALTH HABITS

What you put into your body—nutrition—how you take care of your body—rest, relaxation, and exercise—and your general level of awareness, love, and acceptance of your body, are the major factors important in health. To investigate your health behavior, you might keep a weekly diary of food, exercise, sleep, relaxation, and stress. In this way you create an accurate record of your behavior, which is the first step in a program of modification and change. The following pages are *aids* for that process and ask important questions about your health behavior.

1. Lester Breslow of UCLA, after observing the health and behavior of thousands of adults, has demonstrated that a person's life expectancy and health are related to the following basic health habits:
   ___ Three meals a day at regular times and no snacking
   ___ Breakfast every day
   ___ Moderate exercise two or three times a week
   ___ Adequate sleep (7-8 hours, not more or less per night)
   ___ No smoking
   ___ Moderate weight
   ___ No alcohol or only in moderation

Check off how many you observe regularly, giving yourself two checks if you are nearly perfect in that category. Statistically, each habit adds a few years to your life.

Nutrition

2. How much awareness do you have of your particular diet, and its effects on your body?
3. In a sentence or two, describe your relationship to food.
4. My favorite foods are:
5. I eat _____ meals a day.
6. My smoking habits are ______________________________
7. My drinking habits are ______________________________
8. Do you see a relationship between stress and tension, emotional upsets, and your diet or eating habits? _____ Describe.

Exercise and relaxation

A person needs to (1) exercise the body regularly to the point of sweating, (2) get adequate rest in the form of sleep, and (3) practice frequently a form of relaxation response, meditation, self-hypnosis, or related technique that elicits deep relaxation. The more stressful and demanding your life, the more you need both relaxation and exercise: the basic pair of methods of keeping the body healthy and in tune.

Exercise

9. I exercise vigorously approximately _____ hours a week.
10. The type of regular exercise in my life are:
    ___ active walking
    ___ jogging
    ___ sport (which) ______________
    ___ heavy labor
    ___ other (describe) ______________
11. Describe your exercise habits and patterns:
12. My attitude toward exercise is:
    ___ I love it
    ___ I hate it
    ___ I'll do it if I have to
    ___ other ______________
13. I would feel better about exercise, or exercise more, if ______________________________

____

Sleep

14. I average _____ hours of sleep per night.
15. My sleep is usually
    ___ restful and refreshing
    ___ fitful
    ___ interrupted
    ___ other ______________

Fig. 14-8. Personal Health Workbook. (Prepared by Dennis T. Jaffe, PhD.)

16. I most often awake feeling
    ___ refreshed
    ___ anxious
    ___ exhausted
    ___ unfinished
    ___ other ____________
17. I fall asleep
    ___ easily
    ___ with difficulty
    ___ with difficulty when I am under stress
    ___ regularly using food ___, drink ___, or medication ___
18. Are there any problems, dissatisfactions, or difficulties connected with your sleep patterns? What aspects would you like to change?

Body awareness

19. I consider my normal energy level to be
    ___ high
    ___ moderate
    ___ adequate for most of what I do
    ___ barely adequate
    ___ low
    ___ other descriptive term that seems appropriate ____________
20. I consider myself to be
    ___ tuned into my body's functioning, rhythms, special needs
    ___ unaware of my body's functioning, rhythms, special needs
    ___ other ____________
21. When I experience my body right now, what does it tell me?
22. How do I feel about my body? (Check all that apply)
    ___ I like it
    ___ I dislike it
    ___ I am proud of it
    ___ I am a little ashamed or self-conscious about it
    ___ I barely tolerate it
    ___ I have no special feelings or awareness
    ___ I am not sure I have one
    ___ other feelings and attitudes ____________
23. In a sentence, describe your relationship to your body. ____________
24. The part of parts of my body I like best are ____________
    Why, or what about them? ____________
25. What do you want to change about your body awareness or relationship to your body?
26. Draw a picture of yourself as you see or feel yourself now.

SECTION II: HEALTH HISTORY

How aware are you of your history of illness? How much do you know about what is or was going on physically in your body when you were ill with each of your illnesses? Are you aware of the parts of your body, organs, and organ systems that are weak and tend to be the first to feel the effects of the stress in your life? Each person has one or more target organs, the weak links in his or her physical chain, which are the first to break down.

Knowing your health history, knowing your illnesses and target organs, and looking for patterns can be useful in preparing your own health program. In question 27, fill in as well as you can your personal health history, including dates, severity, organ affected, treatment and also other in your family who may have had that or a similar illness (include the age at which they had it).

27. **Personal Health History** (give most recent first):

Month, year	**Diagnosis**	**Symptoms**	**Severity, duration**	**Organ affected**	**Treatments**	**Other family members with illness and age at onset**

Continued.

Fig. 14-8, cont'd. Personal Health Workbook.

SECTION III: FAMILY AND LIFE HISTORY

28. Please write something about each member of your family of origin, mentioning perhaps such things as how important they were to you, how close or distant you were, where they are now, and the quality of your relationship.
    Father:
    Mother:
    Brothers and sisters:
    Other important family members:
29. Describe the general health and/or serious illness of each of your parents. If deceased, mention when, and the cause of death.
30. Mention something about your childhood home life and family environment, including stressful or traumatic events, family crises, degree of conflict or tension, and any special memories.
31. How do you remember your family responded to illness? What do you remember about your health or illness as a child, and how your family reacted to it?
32. List the most important events, crises, transitions, changes (negative or positive), or developments in your life. Take time to do this, because hopefully it should lead to a period of reflection on your life history, and how it created you as you are today. List the events and briefly, in a sentence or two, describe what they were and their effect on you. Place an asterisk or two in front of those events that seem especially central to your life. Some of the important events will be childhood traumas, changes in the family through birth and death, important relationships or emotional changes, and so on.
33. Describe briefly your educational history.
34. Comment on its importance and meaningfulness to your life.
35. Starting with your present work or major life activity (not necessarily for profit), describe the work or jobs you have done.
36. In your life now, what is your most meaningful or central activity?
37. What are the other important jobs or activities that you do?
38. Right now, how do you feel about your work, career? What are your most common feelings about it?
39. How would you like your work or career to change?

SECTION IV: LEISURE AND SOCIAL ACTIVITIES

40. Write five things that you do to play.
41. Describe something that you laughed about during the week.
42. What things do you do that make you feel good?
43. How many people, outside your immediate family, do you see in a typical week?
44. What sort of friendships do you have? Are they especially close? Do you have few or many? Are they primarily of the same or opposite sex? Please write about your friendships.
45. Describe your present living conditions—whom you live with, how long you have lived there.
46. Please list some of the main satisfactions and dissatisfactions with your living conditions.
    Satisfactions:
    Dissatisfactions:
47. List the most important people in your life right now and indicate their relationship to you, and in a few words, describe the nature of the relationship or how it feels to you or why its important in your life.

Person	Relationship/description

Sex

48. Is sex an important aspect of your life? _____ How important, and what role, would you say sex plays in your current life?
49. Are you currently in a sexual relationship? _____ Please write something about it. How satisfying is it for you?
50. Please write something about your sexual history, attitudes and feelings about sex in your family, sexual awakening, and previous sexual relationships.
51. Did you feel particularly sexually attractive or unattractive at times in your life? _____ During what periods or times?
52. What would you most want to change about your current sexual relationships?

Fig. 14-8, cont'd. Personal Health Workbook.

Group or community

53. Every person derives meaning and identity from the human community of which they are a part. A person might identify with many communities—a neighborhood, professional group, friendship network, extended family, religious or ethnic group, political group, and so on. List, in order of their centrality to your life, your communities and affiliations and their importance to you.

Group or community	**Importance**

54. List some of the ways that you affect your environment or one of your communities. How powerful do you feel in making changes in your world?

SECTION V: LIFE STRESS AND COPING PATTERNS

Recurrent daily stresses

55. Often specific times, activities, or events are the most regular sources of stress in your life. Think about the past few weeks and which stressful situations occurred regularly, how you usually respond to them (what you did, how you felt), and how you might modify them to make them less stressful or destructive to you.

Description of stressful event	**Your response (internal and external)**	**Potential ways to modify event**

56. What seems to be your usual response to stressful situations? For example, do you blow up, withdraw, take it out on others, get sick, get anxious, cry, become afraid, avoid situations, try to forget, or some combination?
57. What situations make you feel calm, relaxed, at peace, or comfortable?
58. What situations make you feel anxious, tense, depressed, fearful, or upset?
59. When you are in such situations, how do you make yourself feel better?
60. Underline any of the following symptoms or difficulties that apply to you:

Headaches	Dizziness	No appetite
Palpitations	Stomach trouble	Insomnia
Bowel disturbances	Fatigue	Alcoholism
Nightmares	Take sedatives	Tremors
Feel tense	Feels panicky	Take drugs
Depressed	Suicidal ideas	Shy with people
Unable to relax	Sexual problems	Can't make decisions
Don't like weekends or vacations	Overambitious	Home conditions bad
Can't make friends	Inferiority feelings	Unable to have a good time
Can't keep a job	Memory problems	Concentration difficulties
Financial problems	Fainting spells	

Others:

61. Which of these symptoms cause you the most concern? Which would you be willing to work on changing?
62. Life change index (see Table 11-1, Social Readjustment Rating Scale).

For past and anticipated future life events, add up the mean values assigned to each life event listed in Table 11-1 to get your life change units for both the past year and the coming year. If your total for the past year is over 150, research suggests that you are at risk for a health change or illness, and you need to take steps to counteract the buildup of stress.

SECTION VI: PERSONALITY AND PERSONAL IDENTITY

Personality

63. Please write a few words that help to describe you and tell the kind of person you are.
64. What are the most important, or most regular, emotions in your life?
65. What emotions would you say control you?
66. Do you have trouble expressing

___ anger	___ joy	___ happiness
___ sadness	___ love	___ other (specify)
___ crying	___ sexuality	

Fig. 14-8, cont'd. Personal Health Workbook.

Continued.

67. What do you feel are your major strengths as a person, your most important personal qualities?
68. What are your weaknesses, your negative aspects?

Personal Identity

69. Who am I?

A person has many identities, which embody activities, feelings, and powers within and in the environment and personal relationships. List as many as you can of the ways that you would answer the question, "Who am I?", letting yourself respond freely to any way that you might interpret or experience an answer to that question—in terms of role; in metaphoric or feeling terms; or in terms of job, accomplishment, or way you think of yourself. Afterward, go back and rank them, starting with 1, in order of their centrality or importance to you.

SECTION VII: VALUES AND INNER LIFE

70. The external events in your life are intimately affected by your inner world, beliefs, and world view. In the first column, write one of the 10 things that you most value in life. Next, describe how you actualize these values, or how or why you fail to actualize them. In doing this, you will begin to see how closely you are living your life according to your values.

Value	How actualized	How not actualized

71. In what way would you say you are a religious or spiritual person?
72. What is your religious background?
73. Has your religious or spiritual faith been of help to you during your life? _____ In what ways?
74. Do you meditate, pray, or perform a regular religious ritual?_____ What sort and how frequently?
75. Has your religious or spiritual practice been helpful during times of illness or difficulty? _____ In what ways?

SECTION VIII: CHANGE GOALS AND THE FUTURE

76. How many more years do you expect to live, and how do you expect to die?
77. Please write your own epitaph, about how you would like to be remembered.
78. Please write several reasons—things to accomplish, desires, interests, areas of life to explore, relationships, obligations—that you have to overcome or get relief from your current difficulties. Please do this carefully, and be specific.
79. What emotional feeling do you have when you imagine your future?
80. Please write the specific goals and achievements you expect to accomplish in your future.
81. What are some of the specific changes, things you will have to learn or give up, that you will have to make to achieve these goals?
82. How completely do you expect to overcome your current major and minor health, emotional, and life difficulties? (If experiencing any).
83. How long do you expect this process to take?

SECTION IX: INQUIRY INTO ILLNESS

This section is to be answered if you are currently experiencing an illness or if you want to explore an illness that you had previously.

84. Thinking back to the time of the first onset of the illness or symptoms you wish to explore, and your life situation at the time, write down several factors or reasons in your psychologic and family life that may have made you susceptible to that illness:
85. Before the initial symptoms or your decision to seek help, did you have any premonitions, dreams, thoughts, expectations, or worries that you might be, or become, ill? __________ Describe them.
86. List a few of the factors in your life today that might tend to maintain you in a state of illness or make it difficult to become well. These may be things that you do, things that you feel, fears of the future, benefits of being ill, feelings about yourself, or things that you can't do. These are the major obstacles to your getting well.
87. Draw a picture that represents to you, either literally or symbolically, your symptom or illness. Then look at your picture regularly, and become familiar with your feelings about it.
88. Draw a representation of the potential healing forces or powers within you that might have an effect or the power to heal your illness. You might draw the healing forces in action against your illness. Use this image as part of your healing meditation to depict your healing forces in action.

Fig. 14-8, cont'd. Personal Health Workbook.

interview significant patterns of maladaptive response to life stress and specific events and difficulties can be related to current symptoms. After this interview the client is asked to take the Personal Health Workbook home and spend some time each day reflecting on its questions.

The family is involved in this exploration because the condition of health or illness does not lie solely within the individual. Although symptoms may manifest physiologically within the person, the entire family system can have patterns that create and maintain symptoms. Minuchin and others[33] have demonstrated that a whole family can have a synchronized biopsychosocial system that leads to a breakdown in one member's body. The family, they suggest, has one body. When family patterns are altered to support greater flexibility and individual autonomy, then the symptoms disappear.[20]

Usually the spouse or the whole family will come in for one or more interviews to focus the health inquiry on the whole family. Illness can be a great disorganizer or transformer of family roles, creating potential health problems in others. One person's symptom makes demands and puts pressure on other family members, which might lead to guilt or resentment. It is often important for the whole family to air deep feelings so health can be maintained, enhanced, or regained in the various family members.

In one family, the husband was critically ill. The family conflict involved resentment at the husband, who had lost his job and did not attempt to get another. He perceived the others' criticism, and the family thought that this contributed to his breakdown. His illness enabled him to share his own fears and pain, which previously he was denying. In other families the core issues relating to the symptoms involve continual conflict in the couple or a pattern of avoidance or disengagement or overinvolvement. Either extreme can breed physical expression of the conflicts. For example, when an alcoholic husband reformed after 20 years, he developed a disabling heart attack that placed him once more as a dependent in his wife's care. Another woman become ill soon after she seriously considered leaving her husband.

Within a few sessions, the Personal Health Exploration helps clients make connections in their lives they have never seen before and explore issues they ignore or deny. The loose structure, which suggests areas of inquiry but allows the client to determine significance and focus, reinforces the client's autonomy. What is most interesting is how congruent the inquiry is with commonsense assumptions about illness. Thus, although the traditional biomedical model denies individual participation in the creation of symptoms or downplays its significance, individuals themselves spontaneously see these links. By guiding the individual and helping relieve guilt and find constructive outlets for difficult feelings, the process proceeds easily and leaves the client feeling much better and freer and healthier as a result.

Relaxation and Self-Regulation Training

The second phase consists of instruction in relaxation and self-regulation training. The goal is for each client to learn this basic skill of relaxation. Any of the approaches described previously may be used, and clients can practice them all before selecting the one that works best for them.

All clients must develop a change program, after careful consideration of how they individually experience stress and of the nature of their particular states of health. The health program usually involves some important changes in the following dimensions of life:

1. *Environmental change.* This includes changes in social involvements, work, living place, or anything else that surrounds us. The environment greatly influences how we feel and act.
2. *Behavioral change.* Behavior can be changed in relation to the family, the personal relationships, work, and everyday behavior. We often need to change our food or exercise behavior or the way we interact with those around us. Although it is difficult to change others, it is often most practical to change our own response to others, which in turn affects their response to us.
3. *Change in thinking patterns.* Worries are anticipated negative events or replays of past stressful events that activate our physical stress response even though they are simply thoughts. We often tell ourselves negative things about our potential, our expectations, or our abilities and in many other ways internally create messages and assumptions about our lives that help to create stress and pain. Beliefs, mental patterns, and negative thoughts can be modified using mental imagery, relaxation, self-hypnosis, and psychotherapy.
4. *Change in physical responses.* Our physical responses to life events can be modified by daily use and practice in psychophysiologic self-regulation. Using self-regulation can help overcome the negative effects of painful emotional states and overcome excessive stress when it occurs within the body. However constrained we are in other areas of our lives, we can always modify our physiologic responses to life events.

Development of a Personal Health Plan

After the personal inquiry and a period of relaxation training, the nurse and the client together develop a personal health plan, listing goals, resources available, skills needed, and concrete, specific steps to be taken to increase the client's health level. The client finishes the exploration with a sense of things that he needs to do to maintain, to regain, or usually to enhance his or her health.

As in all therapeutic relationships, the nurse, as a health resource guide, must be sensitive to the needs of the client and provide an atmosphere of openness, acceptance, and safety. Exploration is an intense experience and encourages clients to disclose very personal material. Encouraging clients to be responsible includes allowing them to decide what information will be disclosed and when. The task of the guide is to use *persuasion*, not force, in helping clients explore uncharted territory. The exploration does not have a time limit for completion. This is an active program to mobilize new coping skills to respond more effectively to the demands of life. At this stage, clients learn actively to modify negative habits, response patterns, or styles of life. For example, those who exhibit the time-dominated, hard-driving, easily frustrated type A behavior pattern will need to modify some of these qualities by changing the extent of their work schedules, learning to relax for short breaks during work, giving up control over projects to peers or subordinates, or practicing techniques of active listening. Clients who continually feel helpless and hopeless or who continually get anxious by expecting the worst will have to learn to modify these internal dialogues or assumptions about life, since they threaten future health.

The change program each client undertakes is different. Clients who are in life crisis often work through the effects of their life change or crisis emotionally, using conventional psychotherapeutic techniques, and sometimes find that their symptoms decrease or even vanish. Others, whose illness or symptoms grew up over time because of dysfunctional overreaction or misplaced reaction to stressful situations, learn to modify their responses and behavior.

To prevent illness, many clients commit themselves to making major changes in their responses to stress, the degree of conflict, anxiety, or emotional pain they regularly experience or to modifying a painful, stressful, or conflicting situation they have endured for years.

At this stage of the exploration process, a small group of people who think alike and are making changes in their lives can be very important. Self-help groups have a long history as adjuncts or alternatives to psychotherapy, helping people to cope with physical illness.[17,24] At the end of the Personal Health Exploration (see Fig. 14-8), the clients who wish to undertake modifying behavior, altering mental or psychophysiologic responses or changing relationships often join health self-help support groups, which continue for several weeks to a year or more.

HEALING THE HEALER

The holistic health perspective, as mentioned previously, looks at the health of the healer as well as the health of the client. The old adage, "Physician heal thyself," is reaffirmed. Nurses interested in promoting health in others need to be involved in improving and maintaining their own health status. Nurses would be wise to act as health resource guides for one another and monitor their own wellness levels. They need to be aware that their diet, exercise, self-care, and psychologic well-being all contribute to their overall health. This is especially important because nursing is a stressful profession, which increases the probability of nurses experiencing stress-related illnesses or burnout.

Burnout is a condition in which health professionals lose their concern and feelings for their clients and treat them in detached or even dehumanizing ways. Some cues that a nurse is suffering burnout include using derogatory language to discuss clients, minimizing involvement with clients, becoming very analytic, going strictly by the book, and joking about clients in a negative way.[32] Fortunately, nurses and other service-oriented professionals can learn specific health behaviors that will help prevent or alleviate burnout.[21,32]

Stress and the Nurse

Stressful situations are inherent in the practice of nursing. Difficult aspects of nursing include sensing that one's competence is on trial, feeling vulnerable to the same illnesses as the client, and constantly facing major issues, such as one's mortality. Other stresses result from the high visibility of nursing acts and the critical importance of never failing. A nurse might fear, for example, missing a high-risk factor in a client or feeling inadequate to work with a client who has difficulty understanding English.

Marshall,[31] describing major sources of stress among nurses, cites the job itself as the top stressor. Nursing involves heavy physical and mental work, and nurses must often work in understaffed conditions. Coping with clients' emotional states, such as anger, fear, and sadness, are a constant part of a nurse's work environment. Rotating shifts and inconsistent days off, other sources of stress, are both physically and socially disruptive and increase pressure. Other stresses include relatively low pay, lack of private areas for nurses to relax, and the frustration of not having enough time to teach clients necessary self-care activities.

Nursing is also stressful because there is often responsibility without concomitant authority. Often professional roles and responsibilities for various tasks are not clear-cut. If, for example, an adolescent female client at a community health center does not want a male physician to do her pelvic examination, the nurse may suggest that the client see a female nurse practitioner in another center who is a specialist in women's health care. This act may be interpreted as insubordination; when nurses go outside rigid established guidelines, often organizational support is lacking, and they may be reprimanded rather than rewarded for creative thinking.

Relationships with clients can also cause stress; the intimacy of client contact can be a pressure. Marshall[31] describes how the clients act as a mirror for nursing staff members and portray their own feelings before them. The more similar a client is to the nurse, the greater the impact. Caring for clients from different cultures and classes and personality differences also can be difficult; nurses deal with a large, ever-changing, and widely diverse population.

Struggle for Validation

Nurses often experience difficulty in trying to gain recognition and validation for the importance of their contribution to the medical team. They may encounter clashes with role definitions of other personnel or may not be highly respected within the institution or organization. Professional nurses have a relatively low status in the medical hierarchy, reflected in their low pay, yet there are high expectations of nurses who dedicate themselves to taking care of others, often at the expense of their own needs and wants.

The nurse-physician relationships can be a major source of tension. Physicians, who are given a high level of recognition and respect, do not always value the nursing role or the importance of health education and community work. Some physicians are uncomfortable with the natural dependence on nursing support and may act as though nurses are lower-class workers. Nurses may discover that interns who turned to them for help and direction become arrogant when they are residents.

Each nurse experiences these pressures differently. Variables include the nurse's level of experience, position in the organization, degree of specialization, the work setting, and differences in organizational structure. The climate of a facility, the attitudes of the staff, and the type of clients are additional factors. Personal characteristics and coping strategies also determine the stress experiences.

Preventing Burnout

Burnout refers to a generalized depletion of energy, lack of involvement, and inability to function well and achieve satisfaction. Burnout was first mentioned in reference to professionals working in human services. Those in the helping professions often have high expectations and emotional investment in their work. Frustration is inevitable due to conflicting demands, limitations of services, and bureaucratic obstacles. This can lead to burnout, causing the health professional to withdraw emotionally; become apathetic; and lose interest, energy, and dedication to their work. Fortunately, there are ways to deal with burnout.[21]

Certain strategies at both individual and organizational levels can help avoid burnout. Hartl[13] has described how developing an early warning system, performing reality testing, dealing with feelings and modifying attitudes, changing diet, increasing physical activities, using relaxation techniques, and finding emotional need fulfillment can increase a nurse's capacity to cope successfully with stressors and thereby avoid burnout.

The way a person perceives a stressor determines the amount of stress experienced. One of the first steps in modifying the degree of perceived threat is to separate the real from the imagined danger. Hartl talks of developing an inner *observer,* which evaluates the appropriateness of a stress response and can be used as an *early warning system.* By checking with the observer, the nurse can readily see that at times a real danger is present and the stress response is appropriate, whereas at other times it is unnecessary.

Hartl describes a four-step process in dealing with feelings:

1. Become aware of the feeling or sensation.
2. Label the feeling: anger, hurt, sadness, joy, excitement, and so on.
3. Decide the appropriateness of the feeling in the particular situation.
4. Express the feelings in a healthy way that will get what is wanted or needed and will not harm others.

Hartl believes that healthy expression of feelings prevents an unnecessary buildup of tension and that a good place to do this is in a support group.[13]

By modifying attitudes, the nurse can not only avoid unnecessary stress but also become more creative and fulfilled. One of the most important attitudes to nurture is a sense of unconditional acceptance of one's feelings, behaviors, and experiences. Self-forgiveness is another attitude that can eliminate the stress that comes from feeling guilty or ashamed. Mistakes should not be ignored but rather viewed neutrally; the nurse then can decide what to do differently in a similar situation.

Relaxation techniques, as described previously, are another important way to reduce stress and increase coping abilities. Nurses who practice therapeutic touch seem to avoid the occupational hazards of burnout.[43] Some other ways to reduce stress include having hobbies and having more spontaneity and play in life.

Interventions at the organizational level can also reduce stress and burnout among nurses. Studies have shown that professionals who actually express, analyze, and share their feelings with their colleagues have much lower burnout rates.[31] Providing shorter work shifts, lower client/staff ratios, and a variety of job tasks for each professional also seem to reduce job stress. Increasing sanctioned breaks, which include rest periods, the opportunity to do less stressful work occasionally, permission to go to the library or attend workshops or seminars as part of one's work, and an occasional mental health day off, help reduce job stress as well. Participation in a support group can assist nurses to understand the common sources of stress in their work and personal lives, to reexamine the reasons they became nurses, to explore their expectations, and to consider personal changes they may wish to make.

Nurses are a high-risk population for stress-related disease. Only through actively identifying sources of stress and instituting proper stress management strategies will the nurse avoid stress-related illnesses or burnout. No one is more qualified than nurses themselves to take charge of this. It is essential for nurses to be in charge of their own health and wellness.

SUMMARY

Nursing and the principles and practices of holistic health are very compatible. From the inception of the holistic health movement many nurses have been drawn to its focus on wellness. The possibilities for the use of holistic principles and practices are limitless. One nurse might be involved in teaching medical self-care classes; another might be a Touch for Health instructor teaching clients how to assess for allergies.

The more gentle forms of healing will increase in the future. Such activities as therapeutic touch, acupressure, relaxation techniques, and guided imagery will be basic nursing skills. When a nurse acts as a health resource guide, the client has the opportunity to explore the relationships and interdependencies among his body, emotions, mind, and spirit. Nurses will use many other techniques, such as autogenics, biofeedback, and hypnosis in their practice. The techniques themselves are not as important as the philosophy that underlies them. As the art of nursing develops, so will an active scientific investigation into holistic health and wellness. It is exciting to consider how nurses will integrate holistic health and wellness into their practice and lives.

References

1. Association for Holistic Health: Membership directory, San Diego, Calif, 1978.
2. Association for Holistic Health: Statement on holistic health practitions, San Diego, Calif, 1981.
3. Becker RO, Selden G: *The body electric: electromagnetism and the foundation of life,* New York, 1985, William Morrow.
4. Benson H: *The relaxation response,* New York, 1975, William Morrow.
5. Benson H, Stuart EM: *The wellness book,* Secaucus, NJ, 1992, Carol Publishing.
6. Brouse SH: Analysis of nurse theorists' definition of health for congruence with holism, *Holistic Nurs* 10(4):324, 1992.
7. Cousins N: *Head first,* New York, 1989, EP Dutton.
8. Dossey B, et al: *Holistic nursing, a handbook for practice,* Rockville, Md, 1988, Aspen.
9. Farquhar JW: *The American way of life need not be hazardous to your health,* Palo Alto, Calif, 1978, Stanford Alumni Association.
10. Ferguson T: *Medical self-care,* New York, 1980, Summit.
11. Flynn PR: *Holistic health: the art and science of care,* Bowie, Md, 1980, Robert J Brady.
12. Harris M: How to make it to 100, *New West,* 2(1):28, 1977.
13. Hartl D: Stress management and the nurse, *Adv Nurs Sci* 1(4):39, 1979.
14. Hill L, Smith N: *Self-care nursing,* Englewood Cliffs, NJ, 1985, Prentice Hall.
15. Holden C: Cancer and the mind-how are they connected?, *Science* 200:1361, 1979.
16. Holden-Lund C: Effects of relaxation with guided imagery on surgical stress and wound healing, *Res Nurs Health* 11:235, 1988.
17. Huvitz N: Origins of peer self-help psychotherapy movement, *J Appl Behav Anal* 12:3, 1976.
18. Ireton HR, Cassata D: A psychological systems review, *J Fam Pract* 3:2, 1976.
19. Jacobson F: *You must relax,* New York, 1962, McGraw-Hill.
20. Jaffe DT: The role of family therapy in treating illness, *Hosp Community Psychiatry* 29:3, 1978.
21. Jaffe DT, Scott CD: *From burnout to balance,* New York, 1984, McGraw-Hill.
22. Johnson MB: The holistic paradigm in nursing: the diffusion of an innovation, *Res Nurs Health* 13:129, 1990.
23. Karagulla S: *Breakthrough to creativity,* Santa Monica, Calif, 1969, De Vorss.
24. Katz A, Bender E, editors: *The strength in us: self-help groups and modern world,* New York, 1976, Viewpoints.
25. Knowles J, editor: *Doing better and feeling worse: health care in the United States,* New York, 1978, WW Norton.
26. Kreiger D: *Therapeutic touch,* Englewood Cliffs, NJ, 1979, Prentice Hall.
27. Kreiger D: Therapeutic touch: the imprimatur of nursing, *Am J Nurs* 75:784, 1975.
28. Kuhn TS: The structure of scientific revolution, ed 2, Chicago, 1970, University of Chicago.
29. Kulbok PA, Baldwin JH: From preventive health behavior to health promotion: advancing a positive construct of health, *Adv Nurs Sci* 14(4):50, 1992.
30. Macrae J: *Therapeutic touch, a practical guide,* New York, 1988, Alfred A. Knopf.
31. Cooper CI, Marshall J, editors: *White collar and professional stress,* New York, 1980, John Wiley & Sons.
32. Maslach C: *Burnout–the cost of caring,* Englewood Cliffs, NJ, 1982, Prentice Hall.
33. Minuchin S, et al: *Psychosomatic families,* Cambridge, Mass, 1978, Harvard University Press.
34. Narayan S, Joslin D: Crisis theory and interventions: a critique of the medical model and proposal of holistic nursing model, *Adv Nurs Sci* 2(4):27, 1980.
35. Nguyen TV: Mind, brain, and immunity: a critical view, *Holistic Nurs Pract* 5(4):1, 1991.
36. Progoff I: *At a journal workshop,* New York, 1976, dialogue House Associates.
37. Public Health Service: *Healthy people 2000: national health promotion and disease prevention objectives,* confer-

ence edition, summary, Washington, DC, 1990, US Government Printing Office.
38. Quinn JF: Building a body of knowledge: research on therapeutic touch, 1974-1986, *J Holistic Nurs* 6(1):37, 1988.
39. Quinn JF: Future directions for therapeutic touch research, *J Holistic Nurs* 7(1):19, 1989.
40. Randolph G: The yin and yang of clinical practice, *Topics Clin Nurs* 1(1):10, 1979.
41. Robbins LC, Hall J: *How to practice prospective medicine,* Indianapolis, 1970, Methodist Hospital of Indiana.
42. Rogers M: *The theoretical basis of nursing,* Philadelphia, 1970, FA Davis.
43. Sandroff R: A skeptic's guide to therapeutic touch, *RN* 20:13, 1980.
44. Schwartz G: *The brain as a health care system.* In Stone GC, et al, editors: *Health psychology,* San Francisco, 1979, Jossey-Bass.
45. Sehnert K: *How to be your own doctor (sometimes),* New York, 1975, Grosset & Dunlap.
46. Smuts JC: *Holism and evolution,* New York, 1926, Macmillan.
47. Thie JF: Applied kinesiology, *J Holistic Health* 30(2):31, 1975.
48. Thie JF: *Touch for health,* Santa Monica, Calif, 1973, De Vorss.
49. Travis J: Wellness education and holistic health–how they're related, *J Holistic Health* 1:25, 1981.
50. Travis J: *Wellness workbook,* Mill Valley, Calif, 1977, Wellness Resource Center.
51. US Department of Health, Education and Welfare: *Healthy people: the surgeon general's report on health promotion and disease prevention,* Pub No 79–55071, Washington, DC, 1979, US Government Printing Office.
52. Williams G: The lowest-tech medicine ever, *Longevity,* p 60, January 1992.
53. Wilson HS, Kneisl CR: *Psychiatric nursing,* Menlo Park, Calif, 1979, Addison-Wesley.
54. Wirth DP: The effect of non-contact therapeutic touch on the healing rate of full thickness dermal wound, *Subtle Energies* 1(1):1, 1990.

UNIT FOUR

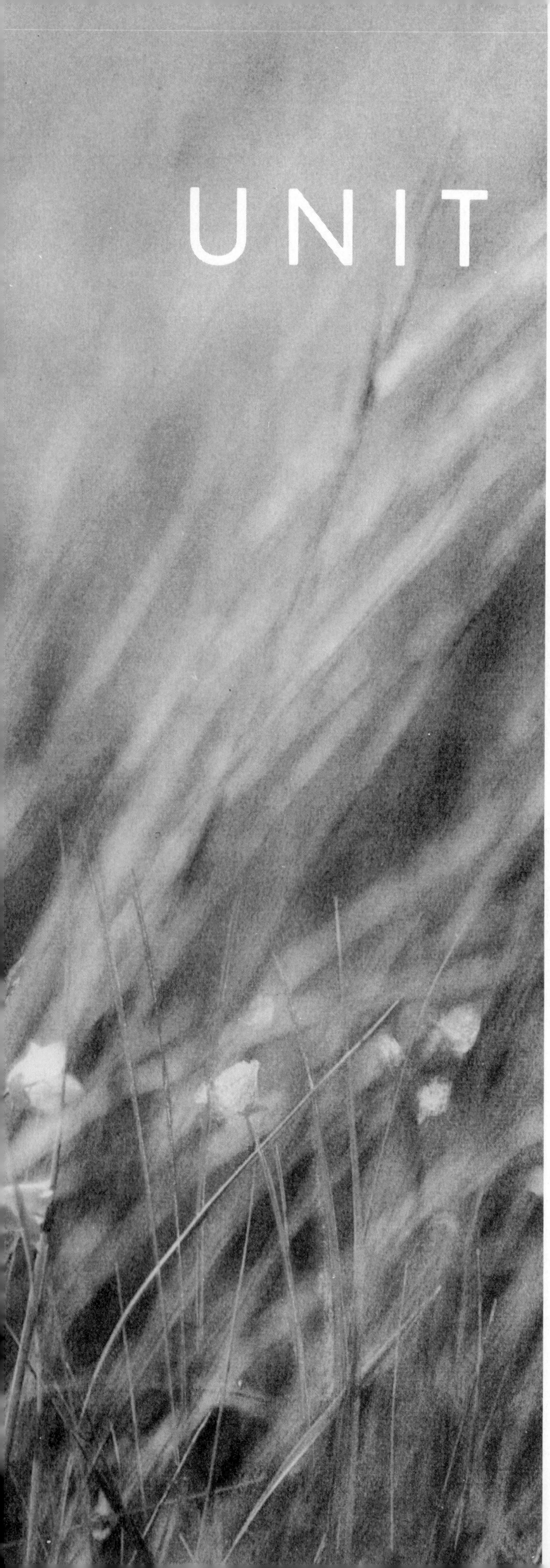

Application of Health Promotion

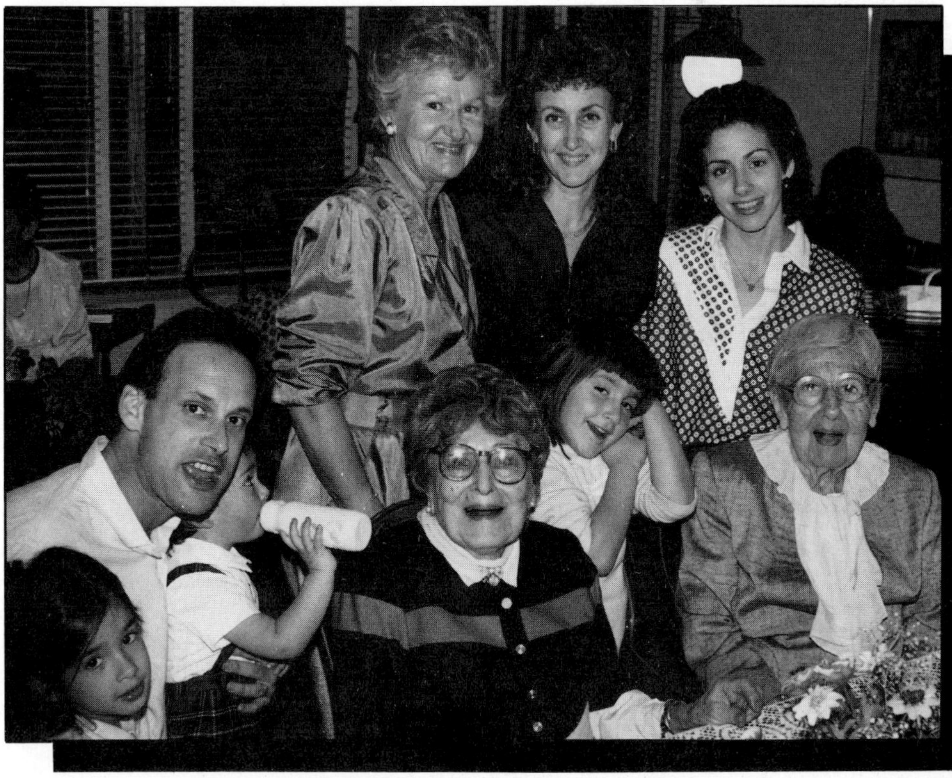

CHAPTER

15

Overview of Growth and Development Framework

Lois A. Hancock

Carol Lynn Mandle

Objectives

After completing this chapter, the nurse will be able to

- *Discuss the importance of development as a framework for assessing and promoting health.*
- *Contrast the terms* growth *and* development.
- *Discuss factors than can influence the rate and pattern of growth of an individual.*
- *Outline Erikson's theory of personality development.*
- *Outline the four stages of Piaget's theory of cognitive development.*
- *Outline the levels and stages of Kohlberg's theory of moral development.*

What causes persons to behave the way they do? Why do some eat a consistently balanced diet, whereas others overload on empty calories? How are individuals motivated to correctly brush and floss their teeth? Are some more prone to have accidents and crises? Are persons more receptive to health teaching at a certain age? When is a child old enough to be responsible for personal health practices?

These are the types of questions each nurse must consider while planning health assessment and promotion for clients. Multiple factors influence behavior: genetic potential, experience, development, and environment interact within persons to determine how each will respond to the many choices presented each day. Many of these choices influence an individual's health at present or at later life stages.

Unit Four focuses on development through the lifespan as a framework for health screening, education, and counseling. Assessment strategies must be appropriate and different for clients at each stage of development. The client may be an individual at some ages, such as the independent young adult, or may be a group or a family, as in the case of a young infant with inexperienced or anxious parents.

An understanding of human development can facilitate accurate assessment of health and health practices of clients at all ages. Health teaching is more appropriate when the nurse recognizes the client's developmental level. A mutually acceptable plan for health care and practices can be determined when the nurse understands the interplay between desire for compliance and the strength of social pressures at each age.

This chapter sets the stage for the study of health promotion at individual developmental levels by exploring basic concepts of growth and development and presenting an overview of three representative theories on development as applied to specific age groups. The following nine chapters each deal with a specific age level. Health assessment and promotion appropriate to each age are described based on the expected competencies for that age. The developmental periods described are prenatal; infancy; toddler; preschool age; school age; adolescent; and young, middle, and older adult.

DEVELOPMENTAL PERIODS

The *prenatal* period begins at conception and ends with birth. It is one of the most important developmental periods because of the extremely rapid rate at which development proceeds. The nurse involved with the care of the child will inevitably need to understand the influences of the prenatal period to obtain a meaningful history and to associate relevant factors from the prenatal period with the child's state of health at any current stage of development. This chapter includes the many changes that the expectant mother experiences and to some extent the adjustments of the father and other family members. The health-promotion needs of the expectant mother and the fetus are so intimately intertwined that they must be considered as a unit.

The period of *infancy* extends from the time of birth through the first 12 to 18 months of life or until the child begins walking alone and possesses the beginning speech sounds of language. The infant is totally dependent on others to meet basic needs.

The *toddler* period, from the time a child begins to walk and talk until about the age of 3, marks a significant time of physical and emotional development. Motor development progresses significantly, and the child achieves a degree of physical and emotional autonomy while maintaining the close identity with the primary family unit.

The *preschool* period, between about age 3 and the time the child enters the formal school setting at age 5 or 6, is distinguished by the child's increased interest and involvement with peers. Most children at this age have reached a level of physical and emotional ability to begin responding to their peers and having social interactions with many persons.

The *school-age* stage begins at age 5 or 6, which in Western culture is usually marked by entrance into school. At this point, children advance in cognitive abilities to a point that their interests turn away from the immediate family to the wider world of peers. They possess enough maturity to begin to relate to others as individuals in their own right and to practice advanced skills of socialization on their own.

The onset of puberty, usually between ages 11 and 14, marks the beginning of *adolescence*. In all societies, some significance is associated with this point in life. In the United States, adolescence is a period of transition, of adjustment, and of personal exploration and trial. In societies not technologically oriented, adolescence is more a time of entrance and acceptance into the adult world, and greater adult responsibilities are given to the adolescent at an earlier age. The end point of adolescence is reached when the individual demonstrates readiness to assume full adult responsibilities of financial, emotional, and social independence. Under usual circumstances in Western societies, this occurs between the ages of 18 and 21, but wide variations exist.[1]

Getting started in an occupation or career, finding and learning to live with a partner, starting and rearing a family, and beginning involvement in civic or community issues are the hallmarks of the *young adulthood* period.[3] Some of the decisions made at this time, such as choosing a mate and having and caring for children, may seem overwhelming to the young adult because of their long-term effects.

Middle adulthood has traditionally been a time of being established in a marriage, an occupation or career, and a community. In today's Western society, it may well be a time of continuing transitions. All persons at this stage must make adjustments to the physiologic changes of middle age.

Adjustments to decreased physical strength and health, retirement, reduced income, decreasing independence, and death of spouse, friends, and self are the traditional tasks of *older adulthood*.[3] As more individuals in our society live longer and maintain their good health, this becomes a time of continued involvement in work and active socializing. Some older adults find that their ability and desire to continue this active work and social life conflicts with cultural standards, such as mandatory retirement.

OVERVIEW OF GROWTH AND DEVELOPMENT

In today's world, the concepts of growth and development at times have expanded in proportion with advances in all fields of science. Increased ability to observe physical and biochemical events scientifically during intrauterine life has led to increased awareness and knowledge of the effects of fetal events on the individual's later life. The behavioral sciences have contributed to significant changes in the ways children of technologic societies are reared and taught. Discoveries in the physiologic and medical sciences have yielded the ability to alter the course of human life when deformity or debilitating disease occurs.

Research in the area of adult development has revealed that adults experience normative transitions that are as essential to their continuing development as the developmental landmarks are during childhood. Gerontology, the study of the aging process from maturity to old age, has shown that change and development continue through the later years.[3]

Concept of Growth

Growth refers to changes in structure or size. During childhood, the physical changes in weight, height, and body proportion are readily noticeable. During adulthood, continued, although more subtle, growth takes place in specific body parts. Metabolic and biochemical processes change as life progresses toward maturity; cells of the central nervous system change as maturity progresses.[5,6]

Growth Patterns

Expected patterns of growth exist for all persons. Growth is not steady throughout life. The two periods of very rapid growth–prenatal through infancy and the adolescence–are contrasted with the slower rate of growth during childhood and the almost imperceptible increases taking place after adolescence. These patterns can be seen in the height velocity grid in Fig. 15-1. The mean increase of 15 cm (6 inches) in height by age 1 and 9.25 cm (3½ inches) during the second year are in marked contrast to the mean of 5.4 or 5.5 cm (2¼ inches) per year from ages 8 to 10. The adolescent growth spurt, although not of the velocity of infancy, is a dramatic change from the preadolescent pattern. This type of growth grid is generally used when there is concern about velocity of growth.

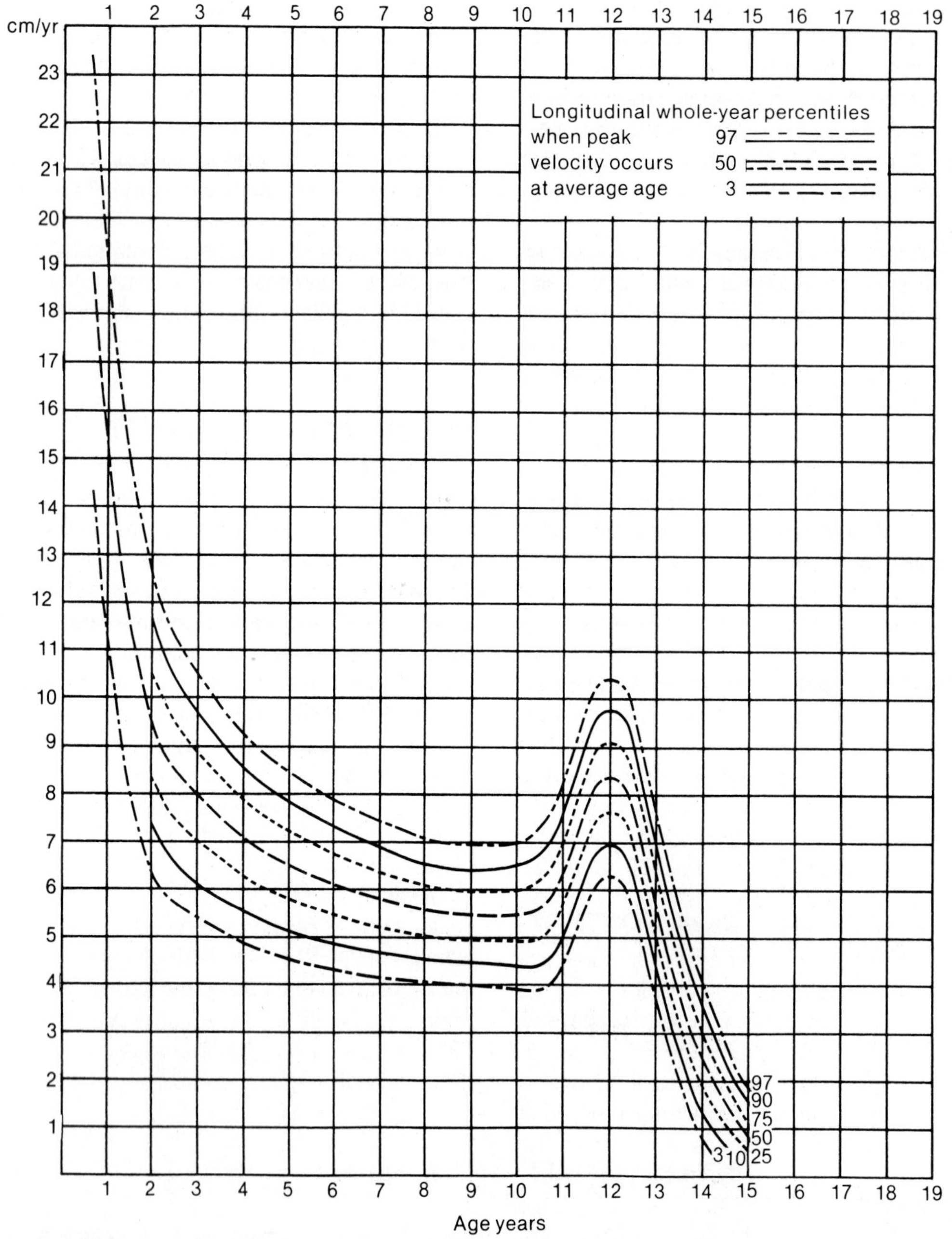

Fig. 15-1. Height velocity grid for girls. (Redrawn; courtesy J. Tanner and R. Whitehouse, University of London Institute for Child Health.)

Different parts of the body increase in size at different rates. For example, from conception to birth the head is the fastest-growing section; from age 1 to adolescence, the legs grow the fastest. The changes in proportion of body parts from infancy to adulthood are demonstrated in Fig. 15-2.

Standardized growth grids (see Figs. 17-4 and 17-5) give an indication of the expected flow of height and weight parameters for a given population. Although growth grids often indicate standards to age 18, they are less accurate once the adolescent growth spurt begins. The child's height (or length up to 36 months) and weight are plotted against age, and a percentile is obtained. For example, if a 9-year-old girl weighed 30.5 kg (67 pounds), she would be at the 50th percentile for weight. This tells us that approximately 50% of girls her age will weigh more and 50% will weigh less than she. Serial measurements plotted on a growth grid indicate a person's pattern of growth and are of greater value than an isolated measurement.

Any dramatic change in percentiles for a child should be investigated. The nurse gathers data on current diet, changes in diet, recent or chronic illnesses, and family stresses to evaluate any significant change in percentile.

Growth refers not only to the obvious changes in height and weight but also to the increases (and in old age the decreases) in size of individual organs and systems. Table 15-1 outlines the directions of growth changes that take place throughout the life cycle. The growth of some systems, such as the skeletal and muscular, is influenced by the sex of the individual, while the growth of other systems, such as the nervous and respiratory, are independent of sex.[5] Note especially the changes that take place in middle and old age. The nurse who has studied growth only from the perspective of children could be missing important differences among adult clients. The health history and physical assessment of a client should include all body systems but should also emphasize those systems undergoing the most change.

The rate and pattern of growth can be modified by intrinsic and extrinsic factors both before and after birth. Genetic endowment, maternal nutrition, disease, birth experience, and emotional factors can all influence an individual's potential for growth from conception through birth.[7]

Some postnatal environmental factors that influence an individual's potential for growth are nutrition, illness, and the opportunity for exercise. Other less obvious influences are the climate, air pollution, cultural practices, and child-rearing practices. Although the limits of growth are genetically determined, a person's growth may be hampered by illness or environmental deficits. A developing individual is most subject to the influence of these factors during periods of rapid growth. The timing of exposure to environmental hazards may determine to a great extent the amount and kind of effect of these influences. For example, if a mother in her first trimester of pregnancy is exposed to the rubella virus, an abnormality may occur because this period is critical for organ development in the fetus. If, on the other hand, the mother is exposed to the rubella virus during her last trimester of pregnancy, an abnormality is not likely to occur because this is not a time of rapid cell differentiation.

Concept of Development

Development refers to changes in skill and capacity to function. In contrast to growth, which is a quantitative or precisely measurable change, development is qualitative. Qualitative changes are more difficult to describe because they cannot be measured in precise units. Development evolves from maturation of physical and mental capacities and learning. The child cannot achieve maturity until physical growth is complete, and yet developmental maturity cannot be pinpointed at a particular point in life. Emotional maturity has many interpreta-

Text continued on p. 363.

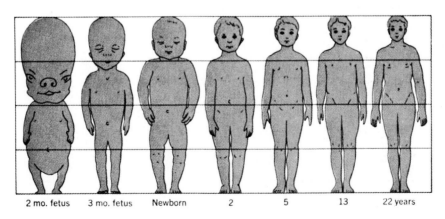

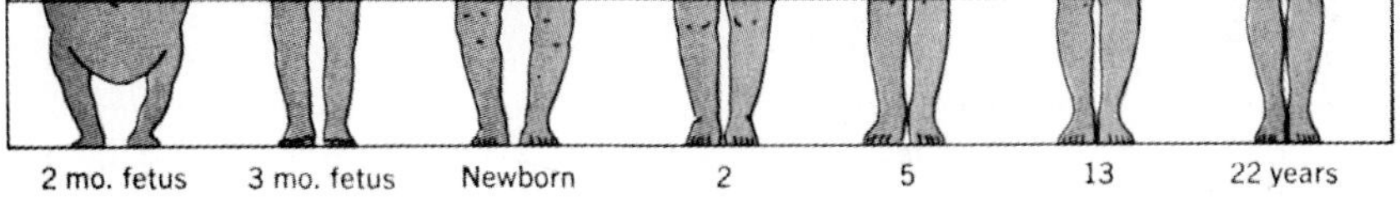

Fig. 15-2. Changes in body proportions from birth to adulthood. (From Crouch JE: *Human anatomy and physiology,* ed 4, New York, 1985, Lea & Febiger.)

Table 15-1. **Flow chart showing directions of growth changes throughout life cycle***

Overview of developmental changes	Prenatal→	Infancy→	Childhood→	Puberty and adolescence→	Adulthood→	Middle age→	Old age
Heart and circulatory system							
Action of heart and circulatory system is under control of autonomic nervous system. Throughout life cardiac rate is responsive to organ needs and emotional states (fear, anxiety, tension depression).	Heart formed and begins to beat about third week	Heart grows little more slowly than rest of body (weight doubled by 1 year, body weight tripled) Grows steadily during childhood With birth, considerable change in paths and relative volumes of blood flow, reflected in loss of certain fetal structures and changes in heart and major vessels		At puberty, heart takes part in rapid growth, reaching mature size with rest of body	Heart weight remains relatively constant after age 25 (only organ other than prostate that does not decrease in weight with age) Cardiac output decreases 30% to 40% between age 25 and 65 Cardiac power is less with age, whereas expenditure of energy is more than in youth. Capacity to increase rate and strength of beat during physical work is diminished		
	Heart rate high, approx. 150 beats/min	Heart rate falls steadily throughout childhood 130 beats/min	70-80 beats/min	60 beats/min in adolescence; rates differ from sexes	After maturity, women have slightly higher pulse rate than men, 65 beats/min (girls' temperature remains stationary, higher than boys'); men maintain same pulse rate in maturity (slightly lower body temperature than women)		
		Heart rate more variable during childhood–regular					
			Not until midchildhood does peripheral blood picture become same as adult				
Urinary system							
As a whole, parallels growth of body as a whole. Proportion of body water and solids follows pattern related to growth–tendency for human organism to dry out as life progresses. Function of kidneys, with other organ systems, is to help in regulation of internal environment of body.	Young fetus is about 90% water Urinary system begins in first month	Newborn is about 70% water Urinary system does not complete full development until end of first year All renal units immature at birth; thus, fluid and electrolyte imbalance occurs readily Kidney function adequate at birth if not subjected to undue stress	Composition of urine in healthy child (after age 2) changes very little as child matures; thus renal function and urinalysis can be used as monitor of well-being		Adult is about 58% water Glomerular filtration rate decreases about 47% from age 20 to 90		
						Renal mass decreases with age; renal flow decreases 53% (some researchers believe this is an adaptive change, compensating for declining cardiac output)	

Digestive system

As a whole grows as total body grows, although evidence suggests that various parts of gastrointestinal system undergo separate periods of growth, maturity, and senescence.

Before birth nutrients are supplied through placental circulation; digestion and absorption do not occur in the gastrointestinal (GI) tract

Stomach size increases rapidly first months, then grows steadily throughout childhood

Spurt of growth of puberty

Digestive apparatus immature at birth (food passes through rapidly, reverse peristalis common)

All actions of the GI tract (food intake, digestion, absorption, elimination) not only respond to physiologic needs but from birth to old age are sensitive to tensions and anxiety

Available data suggest generalized atrophy of entire GI tract with advancing age

Nutritional needs vary according to individual variation–decreasing metabolism→decreasing enzyme production→HCl→stomach volume–tone of large intestine may become impaired

Acidity of gastric juices varies over lifespan; low during infancy, rises in childhood; plateau about age 10, rise in puberty

Until decrease with senescence (also diminished taste)

Free gastric acid (HCl) more marked in boys

Salivary glands small at birth

Increase rapidly during first 3 mo; reach relative adult proportions by age 2

Special senses

Most are well developed at birth, although their association with higher centers comes about gradually during early life and diminishes with advancing age.

Begin very early in embryonic development–3 to 6 wk

Sense of touch is developed first, then hearing and vision

Vision: infant can perceive simple differences in shape but not complex patterns (greater proportion of total growth before birth); various dimensions of vision develop at various ages, eye muscles function at mature level 1st year, fusion begins 9 mo until 6 yr; refractive power changes over life cycle–hyperopia increases until eyeball reaches adult size (approx. 8 yr), then reverses trend toward emmetropia–postpubertal years–toward total myopia until 30–myopia decreases–hyperopia increases

---

Adapted from Sutterly D, Donneley G: *Perspectives in human development: nursing throughout the life cycle,* Philadelphia, 1973, JB Lippincott.

*This chart indicates only general trends and directions of growth and development; it is not all inclusive. No distinct ages, absolute values, or ranges of normal variations are intended in this flow chart.

Continued.

Table 15-1. **Flow chart showing directions of growth changes throughout life cycle—cont'd**

Overview of developmental changes	Prenatal→	Infancy→	Childhood→	Puberty and adolescence→	Adulthood→	Middle age→	Old age
Adipose tissue							
Although adipose tissue varies greatly from individual to individual, overall life time pattern exists. Fat accumulation varies greatly with body build and constitution. Relationship between caloric intake, amount of exercise, and utilization and/or accumulation of fat is not yet fully understood but is basis of much interrelated research today.	Accumulates rapidly before birth; peak at seventh prenatal month	Increases rapidly during first 6 mo	Decreases from first to seventh year in both sexes	Then begins to increase slowly to puberty		Typically both sexes tend to gain weight in 50s and 60s but do not maintain same body contours of earlier years at same weight (increase deposit on abdomen and hips)	Usually fat stores are lost after seventh decade in both sexes Sharpness in contours, increasingly prominent bony landmarks
	Premature infant may look wrinkled and scrawny because of lack of adipose tissue	(Gender differences are not noted in the body shape of prepubescent children)		Fat begins to accumulate slowly and continues uninterrupted in girls, producing feminine curves and accounts for much of weight gain	Some girls slim down after full maturation; many maintain about same amount of adipose as at puberty		
				Deposition of fat differs in body–amount decreases sharply at time of maximum growth spurt (increased weight caused by increase in muscle mass and bones)	After full maturation, fat accumulation begins→	(Continues→)	
Lymphoid tissue							
Lymphoid tissue is scattered widely throughout body and includes lymph nodes, tonsils, adenoids, thymus, spleen, and lymphocytes of the blood; follows unique pattern of growth, rapid in infancy and begins to atrophy at puberty.	Begins in last month of uterine life–immunoglobulins cross placenta at levels equal to mother's and continue for several months following delivery	Grows most rapidly during infancy and childhood, reaching maximum size a few years before puberty; parallels development of immunity		Then atrophies and is smaller in volume at full maturity than during childhood			Thymus so small that it is difficult to locate in older people
		Thus increased incidence of disease with increasing age of child					

Respiratory system

Growth parallels that of total body growth. Respiratory apparatus is a highly organized system of organs under nervous and hormonal regulation, which functions in coordination with rest of body. Sex difference in gaseous exchange becomes apparent during puberty.	Before birth, air sacs do not contain air; oxygen supplied through maternal circulation	When umbilical cord is cut, infant must use own breathing apparatus–breathing irregular at first both in rate and depth–fast in infancy–gradually slowing through childhood until full maturity is reached			No sex difference in respiratory rate at any time of life	Basal metabolism rate declines (rate higher in men than women)
		Respiratory exchange gradually becomes more efficient as life advances. Actual volume of air inhaled with each breath increases as lung size expands with general body growth. Vital capacity and maximum breathing capacity rise gradually in both sexes, increasing more in boys during puberty; adult men have more efficient respiratory exchange, are capable of greater feats of muscular exertion without exhaustion than women.				

Skeletal system

Bone growth passes through successive stages of development from connective tissue to cartilage to osseous tissue; completion of calcification indicates end of growing period and is thus useful measure of growth rate and physiologic maturity. Most growth ceases in adolescence.	Follows cephalocaudal law of development		Reserved during growth spurt		Maximum height in early 20s to 30s	Then gradual decline until onset of senescence
		After first year, legs fastest growing, 66% of total increase in height; longer puberty is delayed, greater the leg length				Thinning of vertebral disk beginning in middle years; most rapid in last decade
	70% of head growth before birth; bones of hands and wrist laid down in cartilage	Trunk fastest growing, 60% of total increase		Length of trunk and depth of chest reach peak growth speed last		
		At birth, shafts of metacarpals are ossified (and visible by radiograph); carpal bones begin to ossify	Growth of both sexes nearly even until onset of puberty in girls first (approx. 10½ yr) Boys begin approx. 2½ yr later, but markedly greater Peak in height comes before peak in weight			Spinal column shortens (osteoporosis) with thinning vertebrae–shortening of trunk with long extremities–reversal of growth proportions in infancy

Continued.

Table 15-1. Flow chart showing directions of growth changes throughout life cycle—cont'd

Overview of developmental changes	Prenatal→	Infancy→	Childhood→	Puberty and adolescence→	Adulthood→	Middle age→	Old age
Muscular system							
Number of striated muscle fibers is roughly same in all human beings. Tremendous difference in size, not only from fetus to adult but between adults, is caused by ability of individual muscle fibers to increase in size. Growth potential, however, is influenced by genes, hormones, nutrition, exercise, and possibly other unknown factors as well.	Muscle formation begins early assuming final shape by end of second month	Increases rapidly during infancy but slowly during childhood	Growth in both sexes is same in childhood	With onset of puberty, muscle strength is greater in boys (when muscle growth is stimulated by testosterone) Greatest increase begins in puberty; muscle size precedes muscle strength in boys	Muscle mass continues to increase gradually–maximum strength in early adulthood–then declines slightly–according to use and genetic constitution Will increase in bulk and strength as used		Until onset of senescence–atrophy and loss of muscle tone
			Increase in muscle size means increasing strength in children; increase in skill is more intimately related to maturation of nervous system				
Nervous system							
Growth and maturation of central nervous system (brain, cord, peripheral nerves, many sense organs) follow pattern reflected by changing size of the head.	Growth very rapid during intrauterine development; head increases at greater rate than rest of body	Has all the brain cells of first year, which will continue to increase in size; number and complexity of axons and dendrites will continue to increase			Function continues with use		Possible decrease in size and number of brain cells in senescence (?) (subject of study)
		All neural tissues grow rapidly during infancy and early childhood		(No neural growth spurt at puberty)			Decrease in myelin sheath, impulses decrease; slow down speed of action and reaction

		Brain grows rapidly after birth, reaching 90% of total size by age 2	By midchildhood, almost reaches adult size	Then slow increase to full maturity	Brain weight decreases with age	
	Segmented spinal nerves are mature, fully myelinated, and functioning at term (e.g., knee jerk), but acquisition of myelin in cortex, brainstem, and cord is closely correlated with observed behavior (myelinization of this tract follows cephalocaudal, proximodistal law)					Taste less acute, less discrimatory with advancing age Structural changes in CNS result in impaired perception
		Equipment for sense of taste and smell present at birth and perhaps most acute at that time)				
Reproductive system						
Organs of reproductive system show little increase during early life but rapid development just before and coincident with puberty. Maturation and fulfillment of reproductive functions of maturity (in female) are followed by involution in later years.	Genital organs form during uterine life; uterus undergoes growth spurt before birth (hormone stimulation from mother)	Female sex organs well formed but not functioning at birth (but have full quota of sensory nerves)	Quiescent during childhood→	Maturation at puberty (menstruation)→		Involution following menopause
		Uterus undergoes involution to half its birth weight	Regained size by age 10-11→	Adult size at puberty→	Maximum increase with pregnancy→	Begin to atrophy with advancing age
		In male–testes, as with ovary, remain dormant and small, not even growing in proportion to rest of body (with sensory nerves)	Until puberty, interslitial cells of Leydig reappear and secrete testosterone; so testes and penis continue increase in size (pubic hair appears)			
	Mammary glands develop in both sexes during fetal life	Enlargement of breasts at birth (both sexes)→	Nonsecretory during childhood until puberty→	Development rapid→	Enlarge during pregnancy, developing alveoli→	Atrophy with advanced age
	Sex hormones; until puberty girls and boys produce male hormones (androgens) and female hormones (chiefly estrogens) in small and roughly equal amounts					

Continued.

Table 15-1. **Flow chart showing directions of growth changes throughout life cycle—cont'd**

Overview of developmental changes	Prenatal→	Infancy→	Childhood→	Puberty and adolescence→	Adulthood→	Middle age→	Old age
Integumentary system							
Includes skin and its appendages and adnexa (nails, hair, sebaceous glands, eccrine and apocrine sweat glands). Although all skin is similar, this organ shows considerable	Hair, skin, and sebaceous glands fully formed in utero	Skin contains all its adult structures at birth but immature in function	Matures slowly until puberty (children prone to rashes)	Rapid spurt in maturation of skin and all its structures		Changes in skin most obvious sign of aging (exposure and environmental conditions)	
variability in different parts of body (and from individual to individual) and varies greatly during the lifespan.	Lanugo begins to decrease before birth and continues regression few weeks postnatally→		Replaced by body hair, less extensive distribution; marked difference in type and distribution of hair at puberty→			Decrease in regenerative and growth power decreases and skin loses elasticity	
	Activity of sebaceous decreases after birth→			Increases rapidly at puberty (more prone to acne)			
Endocrine system							
Consists of number of glandular structures scattered throughout the body. Although small in size, their hormones influence all growth and development of whole organism.	Immaturity of entire endocrine system puts infant at disadvantage if required to adjust to wide fluctuations in concentration of water, electrolytes, glucose, amino acids. All are interrelated, but each organ develops at own rate: Thyroid–increases from midfetal life to maturity; little larger in boys than girls; growth spurt at adolescence Adrenals–after birth decreases in size and continues throughout first year, increases again during childhood (but smaller than birth); spurts at puberty, reaching maturity with rest of body; greater increase in male gonads and testes and female ovaries–are endocrine glands as well as reproductive organs; follow genital type of growth pattern Hypophysis, or pituitary gland–produces or stimulates hormones that influence growth Parathyroids–produce hormones that maintain homeostasis of calcium and phosphorus Islets of Langerhans–dispersed through pancreas; produce insulin and glucagon						
						With age, decline occurs in all endocrine gland functions	

tions; it is difficult to describe completely the close interrelationships of all aspects of life. Physical, emotional, and social factors have made the exact study of human nature elusive and difficult. Philosophy and theology have long influenced the study of development and the thinking of those most earnestly seeking knowledge of the person. This is understandable, since children and adults are beings with the unique ability to think, feel, ponder, deliberate, and reason. The endless quest for understanding of development and life processes is enhanced through understanding of certain principles and characteristics that can describe but do not necessarily explain the developmental process.

Developmental Patterns

The pattern of development of physical and mental abilities shows certain common and predictable characteristics. All individuals follow a similar developmental pattern, with one stage leading to the next. Early development proceeds

1. From simple to complex, as demonstrated in the infant's ability to make basic "cooing" sounds before learning to refine those sounds into speech
2. From general to specific, as demonstrated by the infant's ability to use the whole hand before learning the finer control of the pincer grasp
3. From head to toe (cephalocaudal), as exemplified by the infant gaining neck and head control before controlling the movements of his extremities
4. From inner to outer (proximodistal), which is similar to the cephalocaudal principle in that the infant gains control of structures near his center before those farther away; the infant is able to coordinate the arms to reach for an object before being able to grasp it

Although developmental sequence is predictable, exact timing of the appearance of skills depends on the individual. Each follows a predictable pattern in a personal way and at a personal rate. For example, not all infants begin to crawl at the same time, but most crawl before walking.

Social expectations can influence developmental tasks; society expects an individual to make certain adjustments during each period of development. The ages at which the child is expected to master the developmental tasks are partly determined by the culture group. These tasks are similar to lessons that must be learned if the individual is to make a personal and social adjustment to the culture.

Development results from a combination of maturation and learning. Maturation refers to the emergence of the genetic potential an individual possesses. Learning is the process of gaining specific knowledge or skill as the result of experience, training, and behavioral changes. Maturation and learning are also interrelated; no learning occurs unless the individual is mature enough to be able to understand and change behavior.

Early accomplishments in development are crucial to successful later development, since the foundations laid in the early years often determine the individual's future adjustments to life. Early stages of development set the stage for the next steps in the sequence of expected development.[2]

Growth and development are complex, interrelated processes that are influenced by and in turn can affect the health of an individual. The nurse who understands these interrelationships is aware of the need for age-specific health screening, nursing history questions, and health teaching.

THEORIES OF DEVELOPMENT

Specific aspects of development of the person have been studied for centuries. Many theories of development are used in the study of individuals throughout the life cycle; the nurse may wish to refer to a text on developmental psychology to become familiar with some of these. Three widely used theories of psychosocial and cognitive development are used throughout this unit to gain a holistic view of the progression of individual development through the life cycle. These theories were developed by Erik Erikson, Jean Piaget, and Lawrence Kohlberg.

Personality Development: Erikson's Theory

Erikson described the development of identity of the self and the ego through successive stages that naturally unfold throughout the lifespan.[3,4] He studied with Freud and supported the psychosexual theory of development but based his theory on the need of each person to develop a sense of trust in self and others and a sense of personal worth. Erikson emphasized a healthy personality described in positive terms, not merely through the absence of pathology. Psychosocial adaptation is based on critical steps, with each requiring resolution of a conflict between two opposing qualities. The successful outcome of each stage results in specific lasting outcomes. Accomplishment of each successive task provides the foundation for a healthy self-identity. Each stage depends on the other and must be successfully accomplished for the person to proceed to successful accomplishment of the next. The influence of other persons and the environment is significant, but the motivation to achieve the challenges of identity arises from within.

Although each of the conflicts is predominant at a

certain stage in life, it is important to recognize that all the conflicts exist in each person to some extent at all times, and that a conflict, once resolved, may present again in appropriate situations.

These stages are summarized in Table 15-2. Each of these psychosocial stages is discussed more fully in the specific chapters on each developmental age.

Cognitive Development: Piaget's Theory

Another aspect of development is the progressive acquisition of higher levels of cognitive skills. Jean Piaget, a Swiss psychologist trained in zoology, viewed the child as a biologic organism acting on its environment. The child's main goal is to master the environment or, in other words, to establish harmony or equilibrium between self and the environment.

This cognitive theory is concerned primarily with structure rather than content, that is, with how the mind works rather than with what it does. It is concerned more with understanding than with prediction and control of behavior.[10] Piaget used the word *scheme* to describe a pattern of action or thought. A scheme is used to take in or assimilate new experiences or may be modified or accommodated by new experiences. Each person is striving to maintain a balance, or equilibrium, between assimilation and accommodation.[10,11]

Piaget described stages of cognitive development throughout the developmental years. Through a natural unfolding of ability, the child acquires sequentially predictable cognitive abilities. Given adequate environmental stimuli and an intact neurologic system, the child gradually matures toward full ability to conceptualize. Piaget's theory of cognitive development encompasses the time from birth to approximately 15 years of age. There are four distinct stages, and each is divided into a number of substages.[11-13] These stages are summarized in Table 15-3 and discussed more fully in specific chapters on each developmental age.

Piaget suggested that quantitative, but no further qualitative, changes in cognitive function take place after approximately age 15. This cognitive theory of development has far-reaching implications for the nurse in

***Table 15-2.* Erikson's eight stages of human development**

Stage (approximate)	Psychosocial stages	Lasting outcomes
1. Infancy	Basic trust versus basic mistrust	Drive and hope
2. Toddlerhood	Autonomy versus shame and doubt	Self-control and willpower
3. Preschool	Initiative versus guilt	Direction and purpose
4. Middle childhood (school age)	Industry versus inferiority	Method and competence
5. Adolescence	Identity versus role confusion	Devotion and fidelity
6. Young adulthood	Intimacy versus isolation	Affiliation and love
7. Middle adulthood	Generativity versus stagnation	Production and care
8. Older adulthood	Ego integrity versus despair	Renunciation and wisdom

Adapted from Erikson EH: *Childhood and society,* New York, 1993, WW Norton, with permission of WW Norton.

***Table 15-3.* Piaget's levels of cognitive development**

Stage	Age	Characteristics
Sensorimotor	0-2 years	Thought dominated by physical manipulation of objects and events
Substage 1	0-1 month	Pure reflex adaptations
Substage 2	1-4 months	Primary circular reactions
Substage 3	4-8 months	Secondary circular reactions
Substage 4	8-12 months	Coordination of secondary schemata
Substage 5	12-18 months	Tertiary circular reactions
Substage 6	18-24 months	Invention of new solutions through mental combinations
Preoperational	2-7 years	Functions symbolically using language as major tool
Preconceptual	2-4 years	Uses representational thought to recall past, represent present, and anticipate future
Intuitive	4-7 years	Increased symbolic functioning
Concrete operations	7-11 years	Mental reasoning processes assume logical approaches to solving concrete problems
Formal operations	11-15 years	True logical thought and manipulation of abstract concepts emerge

Adapted from Schuster C, Ashburn S: *The process of human development: a holistic lifespan approach,* Boston, 1992, Lippincott.

assessing health status and in teaching health promotion. Even the concept of health may not be understood by the child or adult who is unable to grasp abstract ideas.

Moral Development: Kohlberg's Theory

A specific aspect of cognitive development is the development of moral thinking and judgment. Kohlberg has postulated a theory of moral development based on interviews with young persons from school age through young adulthood. These interviews are focused on hypothetic moral dilemmas such as, Should a man steal an expensive drug that would save his dying wife?

The responses to these moral dilemmas indicate that there are distinct sequential stages of moral thinking. These stages depend greatly on cognitive development and always follow the same sequence. There are three levels of moral judgment, and each consists of two stages. These levels and stages are outlined in Table 15-4.[8,9]

In our society progression through the successive stages of moral development generally takes place during the school-age, adolescent, and young adult years. Not everyone progresses through all stages. In fact, only a minority of adults operate in stage 6 or even stage 5.[8] Beyond the very young adult years, a stabilization or increased consistency of thought and perhaps an increased correlation between moral judgment and moral action can occur.[8]

These theories of development provide the nurse with

***Table 15-4.* Kohlberg's stages of moral development**

Level and stage	What is right	Reasons for doing right
Level A: preconventional		
Stage 1: punishment and obedience	Avoiding breaking rules, to obey for obedience's sake, and to avoid doing physical damage to people and property	Avoiding punishment and the superior power of authorities
Stage 2: individual instrumental purpose and exchange	Following rules when it is in someone's immediate interest Using fairness, equal exchange, agreement	Serving one's own needs or interests in a world where one must recognize that other people have interests as well
Level B: conventional		
Stage 3: mutual interpersonal expectations, relationships, and conformity	Living up to what is expected by relatives and friends or what is generally expected in one's role as son, sister, friend, and so on "Being good" is important	Needing to be good in one's own eyes and those of others Following the "golden rule"
Stage 4: social system and conscience maintenance	Fulfilling actual duties to which one has agreed Upholding laws are to be upheld except if they conflict with other fixed social duties and rights Contributing to society, the group, or institution	Keeping institution going as a whole Using self-respect or conscience to meet one's defined obligations
Level B/C: transition		Basing reasons on emotions; conscience is arbitrary and relative
Level C: postconventional and principled		
Stage 5: prior rights and social contract or utility	Being aware that persons hold a variety of values and opinions, most of which are relative to one's group Realizing that some nonrelative values and rights, such as life and liberty, must be upheld in any society	Feeling obligated to obey the law because one has made a social contract to make and abide by laws for good of all; the greatest good for the greatest number
Stage 6: universal ethical principles	Acting in accordance with the principle when laws violate universal ethical principles Understanding the equality of human rights and respecting dignity of human beings as individuals	As a rational person, seeing validity of principles and becoming committed to them

Compiled from Kohlberg L: *The philosophy of moral development,* San Francisco, 1981, Harper & Row.

a framework for observations, interactions, and health care planning for individual clients and their family members. Each client and family exists in a larger community, and this community, whether on a local, state, or national level, can greatly influence the availability of health care and the climate of health promotion versus disease focus of care.

SUMMARY

Individuals make many choices that affect their health each day, and multiple factors may influence how these choices are made. The stage of motor, social, and cognitive development can greatly influence how the person perceives a situation and the choices arising from that situation. The nurse who has studied development has a clearer idea of how a person may respond to a given idea or situation at a specific age or stage of development. The basic outlines of Erikson's theory of psychosocial development, Piaget's theory of cognitive development, and Kohlberg's theory of moral development are explored in detail in the age-specific chapters as a framework for discussing health assessment and promotion.

References

1. Berger KS: *The developing person through childhood and adulthood,* ed 3, New York, 1991, Worth Publishers.
2. Berger KS: *The developing person through the lifespan,* ed 2, New York, 1988, Worth Publishers.
3. Erikson EH: *Childhood and society,* ed 35, New York, 1986, WW Norton.
4. Erikson EH: *Identity, youth and crisis,* New York, 1968, WW Norton.
5. Guyton AC: *Textbook of medical physiology,* ed 8, Philadelphia, 1991, WB Saunders.
6. Ham RS, Sloane PD: *Primary care geriatrics: a case-based approach,* ed 2, St Louis, 1992, Mosby.
7. Kenney RA: *Physiology of aging,* ed 2, Chicago, 1989, Mosby.
8. Kohlberg L: *The philosophy of moral development, vol 1,* San Francisco, 1981, Harper & Row.
9. Kohlberg L, Kramer R: Continuities and discontinuities in childhood and adult moral development, *Hum Dev* 12:93, 1969.
10. Phillips JR: *The origins of intellect: Piaget's theory,* San Francisco, 1969, WH Freeman.
11. Piaget J: *The child's conception of the world,* Totowa, NJ, 1929, Littlefield Adams.
12. Piaget J: *The grasp of consciousness, action and concept in the young child* (Translated by S Wedgwood), Cambridge, Mass, 1976, Harvard University Press.
13. Piaget J: *The psychology of intelligence,* London, 1950, Routledge & Kegan Paul.

CHAPTER

16

The Prenatal Period

Lois A. Hancock

Ellen F. Olshansky

Mary E. Abrums

Ann Marie McCarthy

Objectives

After completing this chapter, the nurse will be able to

- *Discuss development of a zygote into a fetus.*
- *Outline changes in the maternal reproductive, musculoskeletal, circulatory, urinary, and respiratory systems during pregnancy.*
- *Explain Apgar scores to a pregnant couple.*
- *Discuss some of the common "normal" discomforts of the pregnant woman and suggested relief measures.*
- *Interview a pregnant woman, focusing on the major developmental tasks of motherhood described by Rubin.*
- *Discuss change in the pregnant woman's self-concept and body image.*
- *Answer a couple's questions about sexuality during pregnancy.*
- *Discuss three viral infections known to have harmful effects on the fetus.*
- *Discuss the possible fetal problems caused by maternal drinking, smoking, and drug use during pregnancy.*
- *Answer a parent's questions about possible trauma to the infant during the birth process.*
- *Discuss the new father's reaction to his role of parent.*
- *Discuss with the pregnant woman her other children's possible responses to her pregnancy and the birth of the baby.*
- *Discuss the pros and cons and possible difficulties of working during pregnancy.*

The mystery of life before birth has fascinated scientists, philosophers, and theologians for centuries. When a child is conceived, many events occur that greatly affect the entire life of the developing individual. Some of these events are at present beyond human control; others only recently have been discovered and described. This new knowledge has led to speculation and experimentation with ways to protect and ensure a better life for the child and eventually for all human beings.

The process of conception, pregnancy, and birth involve the complex interaction of many factors, including the physiologic and psychologic change in the mother and the development of a conceptus into a viable newborn. The focus of this chapter is the mother and the developing fetus; it is impossible to discuss one without the other. The nurse must always keep both parts of this dyad view when seeking to promote a healthy pregnancy.

PHYSIOLOGIC PROCESSES

Age and Physical Changes

The physical changes during pregnancy discussed here include fertilization of the egg by the sperm, implantation of the fertilized egg into the uterus, embryonic and fetal growth and development, placental development and function, and maternal changes.

DURATION OF PREGNANCY

Pregnancy begins with the joining of a sperm and egg. Under normal, healthy circumstances a pregnancy ends approximately 9 months (10 lunar months) later with the birth of the infant. Because the last menstrual period (LMP) is a more certain date than the precise moment of conception, the weeks of pregnancy are counted beginning with the LMP. A pregnancy often is divided into three equal parts, or trimesters, when discussing the progression of fetal development and maternal changes. The estimated time of delivery (expected date of confinement, or EDC) is calculated by Nagele's rule: adding 7 days to the date of the first day of the LMP and subtracting 3 months. Thus, if a woman's LMP began on July 13, the EDC is determined by adding 7 days (July 20), subtracting 3 months, and arriving at April 20.

FERTILIZATION

The union between male and female sex cells and the beginning of life require several crucial factors, not all of which are fully understood. When the egg or ovum lies within the fallopian tube and is penetrated successfully by a sperm cell, a zygote is formed and division of cells begins. Both sex cells must be in a proper state of maturity before union can occur, and both sperm and ovum must be within the fallopian tube for about 5 hours for penetration to occur. The sperm must possess high motility and be able to secrete an enzyme or enzymes that aid in the dissolution of the membrane surrounding the ovum at the point of entry. Although the process of sperm formation, spermatogenesis, requires the slightly lower temperature maintained in the male testes, fertilization requires the basal temperature of the abdomen. The sperm must be uniform in size and shape and normally formed. The fallopian tube must be free from adhesions or obstructions to permit transport of the ovum and zygote. The period of fertility for the female is believed to be within 24 hours of ovulation. Since sperm are viable for up to 72 hours in the female reproductive tract, fertilization may take place if intercourse has occurred up to 3 days before ovulation.[7]

IMPLANTATION

Transport of the fertilized ovum into the uterine cavity usually requires about 3 days. The developing zygote appears to need this period because secretions from the glands lining the tube are important for the developing organism. When the uterine cavity is entered, the ovum remains unattached for an additional 4 or 5 days, receiving nutrition from secretions of the endometrium, the inner lining of the uterus. The cells that have formed around the developing zygote secrete enzymes that begin to digest and liquefy the endometrial lining and initiate conditions for attachment of the zygote, which begins placental development.

Fertilization triggers the production of greater amounts of progesterone.[16] This hormone already has stimulated the formation of endometrial cells rich in glycogen, proteins, lipids, and minerals, and the extra supply of progesterone stimulates further development of these nourishing cells, known as *decidua*. The decidua provides nutrition for the embryo for 8 to 12 weeks, but the placenta begins to function within a week after implantation and also helps nourish the developing organism.

FETAL GROWTH AND DEVELOPMENT

The stages of physical development throughout embryonic life are well delineated and described for each structural system of the body. Metabolic functions, particularly endocrine and neurologic, are less completely understood. The following description of embryonic development is that expected under normal conditions; development depends on these events occurring in a specified period and order. When cells do not develop adequately at the necessary point in time and sequence, abnormality in structure or function occurs, since development cannot proceed normally.

FIRST TRIMESTER

The first 3 months (trimester) of pregnancy are critical for the child's development and are characterized by extremely rapid cellular growth and differentiation of tissues into essential organs. By the time implantation occurs during the second week of gestation, tissues have begun to develop into distinct layers, differentiating according to types; these become the precursors of different body tissues. The rudiments of the central nervous system (CNS) have begun to develop, and within a few days of implantation blood cells that clearly belong to the developing organism have formed. By the end of the fourth week of gestation, the blood cells and rudimentary circulatory system have become fairly well formed in the trunk. The heart has assumed major anatomic characteristics and has begun to pulsate. The respiratory and gastrointestinal systems have developed in rudimentary stages, as have the skeletal and muscular systems of the trunk. The nervous system is in a critical stage of development; the groove that forms the spinal cord is accomplishing closure, and rudimentary structures for the major sensory organs of the eye and ear are developing. Limb buds are distinguishable by this point in gestation.

By the fifth week, the embryo has a marked C-shaped body, accentuated by a rudimentary tail and large head folded over a large, protuberant trunk. Fig. 16-1 illustrates the relative shape and size of the human embryo at about this stage of development in contrast to earlier and later stages. Each system now has been established in at least primordial form, and the umbilical cord organizes as a distinct unit. Five brain vesicles can be distinguished, and the nerve and ganglial tissues are more fully developed.

By the sixth week of gestation, the heart reaches a definitive human form with all septa intact, and the

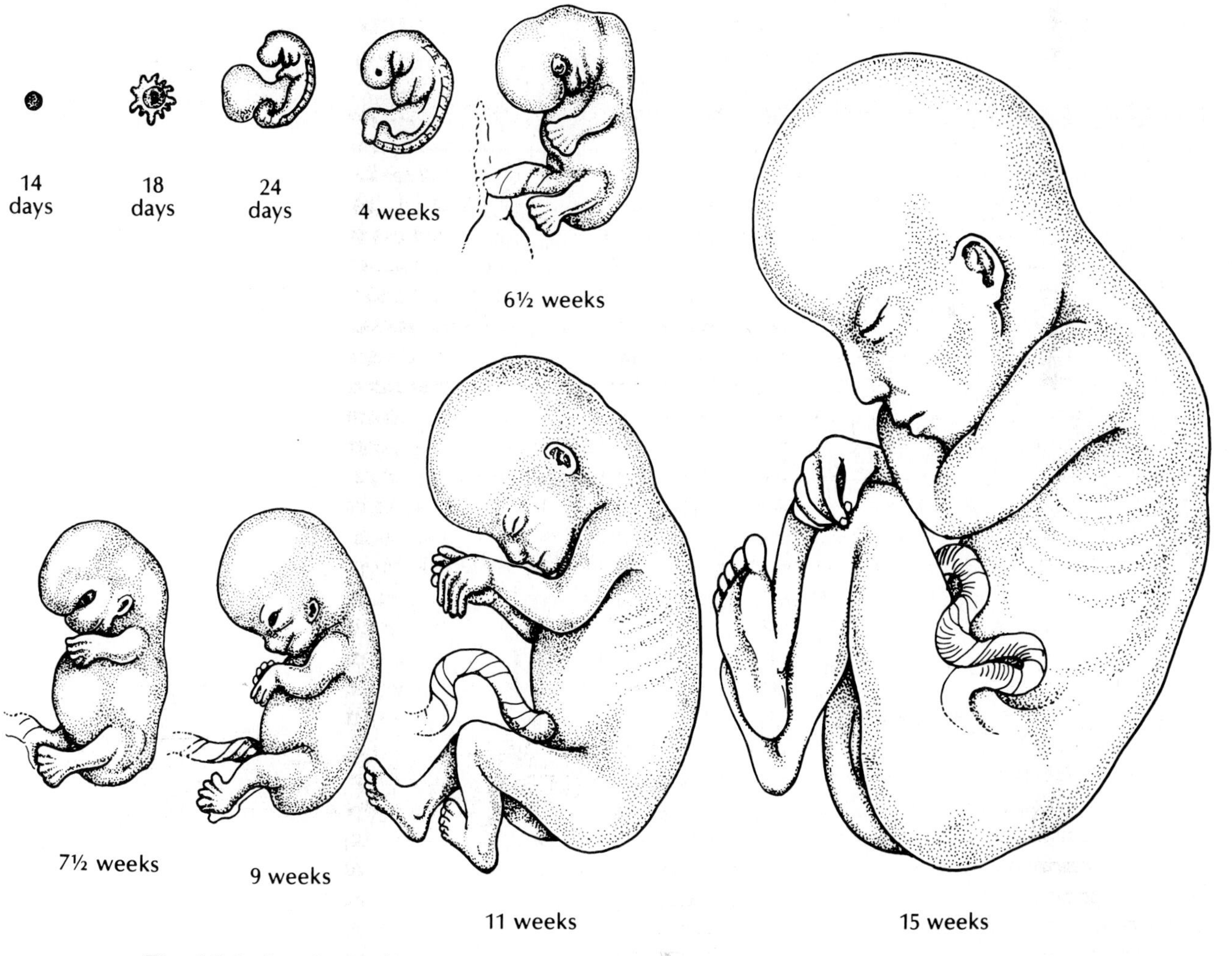

Fig. 16-1. Actual size of human embryos at early stages of development. Comparison of relative stages of external development also is indicated. (From Chinn PL: *Child health maintenance: concepts in family-centered care,* ed 2, St Louis, 1979, Mosby.)

circulatory pathway that characterizes fetal life is established. Limbs are now recognizable as arms and legs, although ossification of skeletal tissue has not yet occurred. The embryonic head and face are approaching a critical stage of development, since the ridges of the jaws and the tissues that form the tongue and palate are widely separated. The intestine begins to elongate and form loops, and the stomach begins to differentiate and assume the rotated position. the lungs now have formed the lobes, with the bronchi beginning to branch. The liver begins to produce blood cells. Although a gonad, which is the precursor to both male and female gonads, is distinguishable, it is impossible to determine the sex of the embryo because differentiation has not yet occured.[7]

Significant gastrointestinal and genitourinary tract changes occur during the seventh week of gestation; until approximately this point the rectum and the bladder-urethra are part of the same structure, with no external opening. During this period, the rectum separates from the bladder-urethra, and each forms into a separate tube; shortly thereafter, the urethral and anal openings form. Fetal circulation is established further with final formation of the inferior vena cava and differentiation of the cardiac valves. Eyelids begin to form over the lens of the eyes, and nerve fibers to the sensory areas of the head are developed more completely.[7]

At the end of the eighth week and before the end of the second month of gestation, the embryo reaches the fetal stage of development. The individual has not yet begun to assume a "human" appearance, but several external features are surprisingly advanced. The fingers and toes are well formed, and the fetus begins to assume a more nearly erect posture. The liver is very large, and the diaphragm is formed. The main blood vessel system is complete, and the lymphatic system has begun to form. Testes and ovaries are distinguishable, but external differentiation of sex is still impossible. Definitive muscles have formed for all parts of the body, and the fetus is capable of movement. The cerebral cortex has formed.

The tenth through twelfth weeks of development are particularly crucial for the development of the face and mouth, since the palate fuses completely, lips separate from the jaw, the cheeks become distinguishable as facial features, and the nasal septum forms the nasal passages. The kidney becomes functional, acquiring the ability to secrete urine, and the bladder expands into a sac. External genitalia become distinguishable as male or female, and internal sex organs begin definitive development for the appropriate sex. The lungs acquire definite shape. *Ossification* of the skeletal system begins, hair follicles begin to appear on the face, and the nail beds of the fingers and toes are apparent. The spinal cord reaches definitive internal structure, and the brain reaches the general structure of the human organ. Essential structures of the eye are formed and arranged in characteristic organization; the eyelids are fused.

By the end of the first trimester of pregnancy, the fetus is not yet capable of extrauterine life, but essential formation of the body structures is complete. Growth and maturation proceed throughout the remainder of gestational life, with many essential developmental events leading to the ability to sustain life.

SECOND TRIMESTER

Early in the second trimester, at about the sixteenth week of gestation, the fetus assumes a human appearance. The face has formed with the eyes close to the nasal bridge, the trunk and limbs have grown larger in proportion to the head, and hair begins to appear on the head. Metabolic function begins to develop with the acquisition of more mature glands; the pituitary, gonads, tonsils, and lymphatics acquire definite structure and begin to function. *Meconium* begins to accumulate in the intestine, indicating some activity of smooth as well as skeletal muscle. The lungs remain functionally immature throughout the second trimester, but their structure primarily is completed by the end of the sixteenth week. Blood formation becomes a function of the spleen. The bones of the entire skeletal system are apparent, and joint cavities begin to form. Muscular movements of the fetus are detectable by the mother early during the second trimester.

By the twentieth week of gestation, *lanugo* has developed over the entire body, and *vernix caseosa* begins to appear. Myelinization of the spinal cord begins and continues through infancy and toddlerhood. Enamel and dentin begin to form in the primary tooth buds. Growth and maturation of functional development proceed throughout the second trimester until, at about 28 to 32 weeks of gestation, the fetus theoretically is capable of sustaining extrauterine life.

THIRD TRIMESTER

The lungs, which are essential for viability, do not achieve adequate maturity until late in the third trimester. Pulmonary branching, formation of the alveoli, and the ability of the lungs to secrete surfactant remain grossly immature; at any point before 36 weeks of gestation, the fetus is in jeopardy of being unable to exchange gases adequately in the lungs and support extrauterine life. The analysis of amniotic fluid for the *lecithin/sphingomyelin ratio* is useful in assessing the ability of the lung to produce surfactant and for estimating gestational age.

During the third timester, the period of rapid growth and weight gain, the fetus collects fat in subcutaneous tissue, which changes fetal appearance from wrinkled and lean to rounded and smooth. The gonads achieve final structural form, and in the male the testes begin to descend into the scrotal sac late in the third trimester.

Cerebral fissures appear rapidly during the third trimester, and *myelinization* of the brain begins. All the sensory organs become functional, although at birth the sensory abilities of the infant are not fully mature. Reflexes begin to appear by the beginning of the third trimester, but only the Moro reflex usually is present during the early weeks of this period. The ability to suck begins to appear at about the thirtieth week, but the developing reflexes are immature and rapidly exhaustible. As the fortieth week (term) approaches, the reflexes and neuromuscular capacity of the fetus increase greatly, thus enhancing the chance for surviving in extrauterine life.

PLACENTAL DEVELOPMENT AND FUNCTION

Throughout embryonic and fetal life, the primary source of nourishment is the *placenta.* This essential organ begins to develop at implantation, when integration of the embryonic and decidual cells begins. The *chorionic and amniotic membranes,* which surround the fetus throughout gestation, also begin to form along with the placenta, as does the *amniotic fluid,* which provides a support medium for the developing infant and protection from injury.

The basic structure of the mature placenta (Fig. 16-2) allows interchanges between the mother and fetus in providing nourishment for the fetus and excreting fetal waste materials. Maternal blood flows through the intervillous spaces; the *chorionic villi* contain the fetal vessels. The unique structure of the tissues between the two circulatory systems permits exchange of certain molecules but prevents mixing of the two blood supplies.

We have long known that the placenta supplies the fetus with essential nutrients, provides for the excretion of wastes, and protects the fetus from harmful substances; however, these functions are not sufficiently understood to allow prediction of which substances will and will not cross the placenta. Molecular size was believed to control this, with the heavier molecules not passing the placenta. This may be a factor but is not the mechanism by which placental transfer occurs. Diffusion, facilitated diffusion, and active transport have been demonstrated to participate in the transfer mechanisms of the placenta. *Pinocytosis,* a form of active transport, transports larger lipid and protein molecules through the membranes.[7] Currently, a substance is presumed to be transferable to the infant unless substantial evidence indicates otherwise. This leads to increased concern regarding drug use during pregnancy and provides the safest guideline for maternal ingestion of potentially harmful materials.

Inspection of the placenta after birth reveals important clues to the adequacy of gestational life. The placenta contains 14 to 30 distinctive lobules, known as *cotyledons,* which are incompletely separated from one another by thin, septal partitions. The tissue of the placenta appears dark red, with the spongy maternal

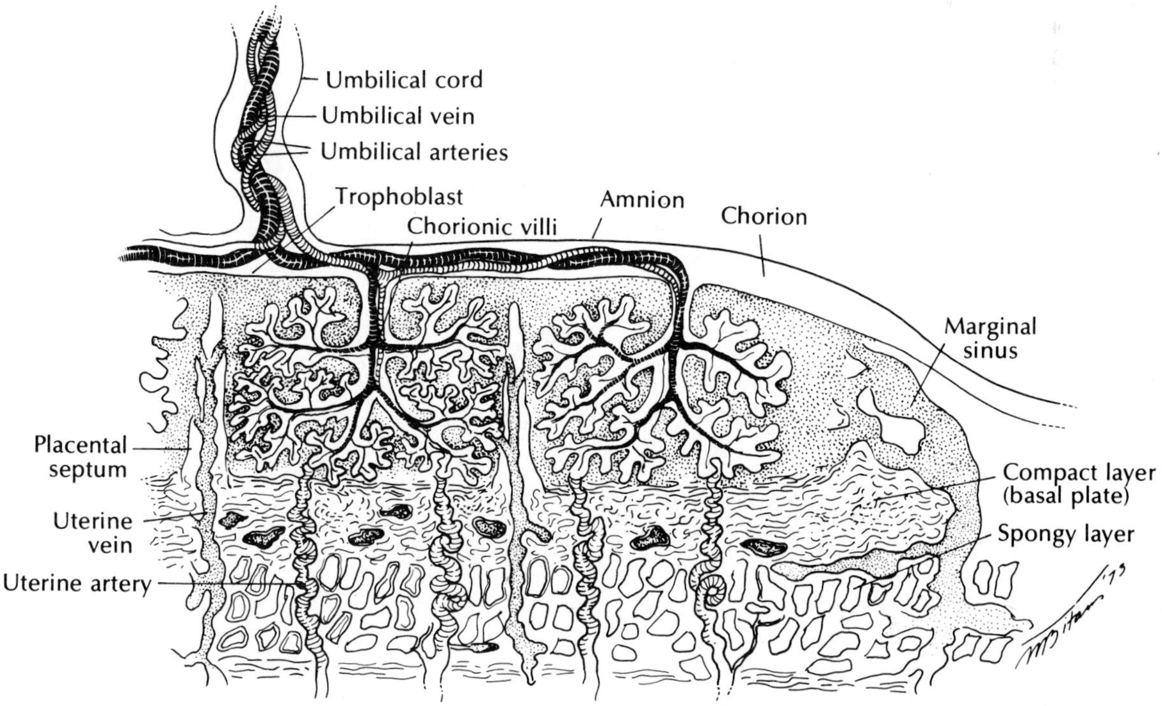

Fig. 16-2. Structure of mature placenta. (From Chinn PL: *Child health maintenance: concepts in family-centered care,* ed 2, St Louis, 1979, Mosby.)

side darker than the shiny fetal side, which is gray and glassy. The umbilical cord normally rises from near the center of the placenta, and the membranes rise smoothly from the rim. Abnormal insertion of the cord, necrotic areas of the placenta, abnormal insertion of the membranes, or two umbilical vessels rather than three are signals of possible problems that appeared during gestation but that may not be immediately apparent in the infant.

The fetus, who has continued to gain strength and maturity during the later weeks of gestation, generally assumes a position with the head resting in the lower maternal pelvis. Fig. 16-3 illustrates the relationship of the fully developed fetus to the placental and membranous structures. The membranes provide protection from infection for the fetus as well as a container for the amniotic fluid. As birth begins, the membranes rupture, causing the loss of amniotic fluid. When labor is imminent, this often stimulates strengthening of uterine contractions, but when rupture of the membranes is premature–more than 24 hours before delivery–risk to the infant from infection is great.

As gestation nears completion, the placenta decreases gradually in function, which is thought to be one possible stimulus for the onset of labor. When gestation proceeds beyond the point of fetal development, the infant's well-being is at considerable risk, since the source of nourishment and waste disposal is continually declining.

This discussion of fetal development gives only half of the story of the prenatal period. Maternal changes and the culmination of the prenatal period, labor, and birth are now addressed.

MATERNAL CHANGES

The physiologic changes that a woman undergoes during pregnancy are brought about by a combination of hormonal and mechanical changes. The hormonal influences tend to increase as the pregnancy progresses. The mechanical or hemodynamic changes reach a peak in the seventh or eighth month and then gradually decline.[7,9]

Signs of Pregnancy. The woman first begins to think she may be pregnant because she skipped a menstrual period, or experiences nausea and vomiting, breast changes, especially tingling and tenderness, followed by an increase in size, or urinary frequency. If any of these signs are present, the woman should seek a pregnancy test. A number of home pregnancy tests are now widely available without prescriptions. Women should be cautioned against relying on such tests, as false results can be caused by concurrent medication or substance use. Also, if the home pregnancy test is performed too early,

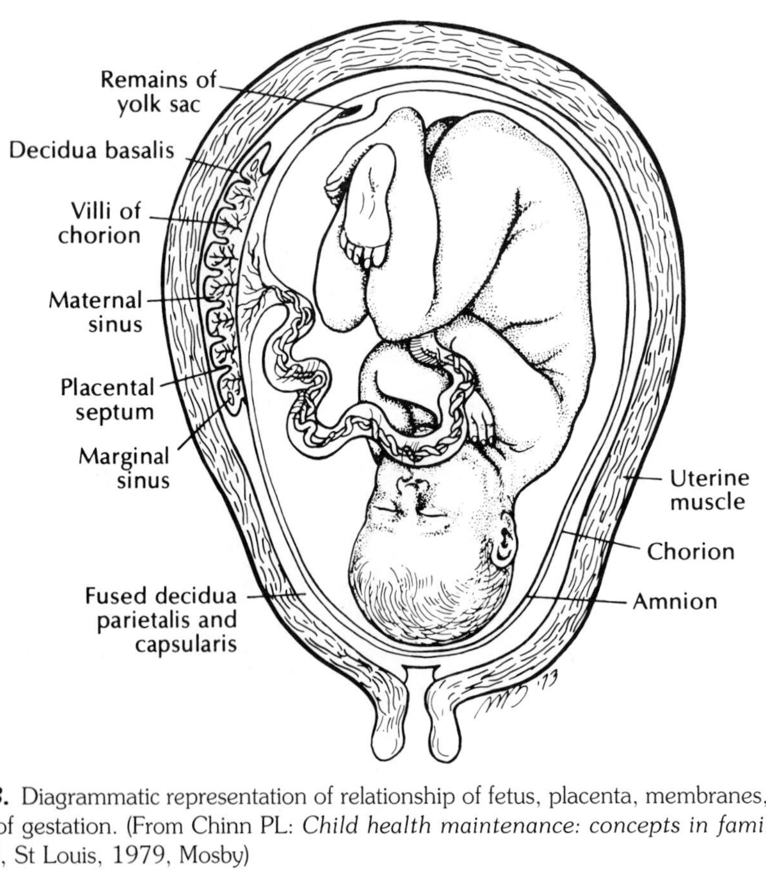

Fig. 16-3. Diagrammatic representation of relationship of fetus, placenta, membranes, and uterus near end of gestation. (From Chinn PL: *Child health maintenance: concepts in family-centered care,* ed 2, St Louis, 1979, Mosby)

a false negative outcome can result because the woman has not yet produced enough human chorionic gonadotropin (HCG) to be detected in her urine.

Probable signs of pregnancy–observable changes that carry a high degree of probability of pregnancy–can be observed by the health care provider. These probable signs have a degree of certainty that varies from 80% to 90% (see box below).

Until recently, the positive signs of pregnancy, which show that a fetus is present, usually did not occur until the second trimester (see box below). An ultrasound test made during the first trimester can demonstrate the presence of a fetus much earlier.

Adaptive Changes of Other Systems. Besides the obvious changes in the reproductive system, adaptive changes in many other systems occur during the three trimesters of pregnancy.

The urinary system undergoes dramatic changes that are reflected in a 50 increase in *glomerular filtration rate (GFR).* Starting in early pregnancy, the renal collecting structures become dilated, which is called the *physiologic hydronephrosis* of pregnancy. These changes are thought to result from effects of estrogen and progesterone.[7] The pregnancy hormones affect smooth muscle tone and glandular and mucosal secretions within the gastrointestinal tract. The results can be constipation, heartburn, and increased salivation. Although these symptoms do not result in serious problems, they can be very annoying for the pregnant woman.

Circulatory system changes begin early in pregnancy, as demonstrated by cardiac output increasing 30% to 40% by the end of the first trimester. An increase of 30% in total blood volume also takes place during pregnancy.[7,8]

Respiratory changes are manifested by a considerable increase in the volume of air breathed per minute resulting from the increased tidal volume. Increased alveolar ventilation leads to more efficient distribution and mixing of gas during late pregnancy.[7]

The musculoskeletal system undergoes an increase in elastic tissue and a softening of connective tissue, with a relaxation of the joints, especially the pelvic ones. This increased flexibility prepares the pelvic outlet for labor and delivery. Late in pregnancy the lumbar and dorsal curves of the spine are exaggerated, causing the characteristic gait of pregnancy. This also can be a source of low-back pain.

The metabolic and endocrine changes during pregnancy are dramatic. Increased thyroid activity is reflected in basal metabolic rate, radioactive iodine uptake, and thyroid size. Estrogen is the stimulus for the changes in thyroid function. Adrenal function is increased in pregnancy and is closely related to fetal adrenal function. More parathyroid hormone is produced by the parathyroid glands. The pituitary, especially the anterior lobe, which may double or triple in size, is very active throughout pregnancy.[7]

Reproductive System. Pregnancy changes in the reproductive system include uterine changes as well as changes in the breasts, vagina, vulva, and ovaries. The prepregnant uterus is about the size of a fist. The term uterus is large enough to enclose a 3.2- to 4.5-kg (7- to 10-pound) infant (sometimes even larger) and the placenta. As the uterus enlarges, the fundus can be felt higher in the abdomen. Fig. 16-4 illustrates the upper

❑ ❑ SIGNS OF PREGNANCY

Probable

Enlargement of the uterus
Softening of the uterine isthmus (Hegar's sign)
A bluish or cyanotic color to the cervix and upper vagina (Chadwick's sign)
Asymmetric, softened enlargement of the uterine corner caused by placental development (Piskacek's sign)
A positive test for human chorionic gonadotrophin (HCG) in the urine or serum

Positive

Detection of fetal heart tones by auscultation or use of a Doppler instrument
Palpation of fetal parts
Objective detection of fetal movements
Radiologic or ultrasonic demonstration of fetal parts

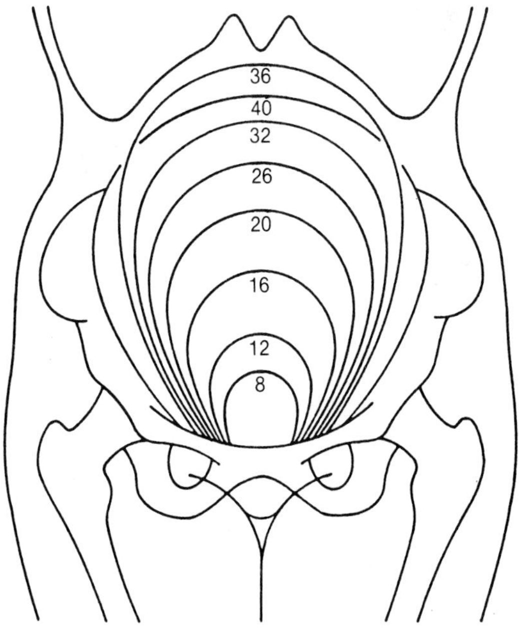

Fig. 16-4. Upper level of enlaring uterus at various weeks as pregnancy progresses. (From Smith D: *Mothering your unborn baby,* Philadelphia, 1979, WB Saunders.)

level of the uterus as the pregnancy progresses. The breasts begin enlarging early in the pregnancy and in late pregnancy may secrete small amounts of colostrum. The vagina and vulva receive a greater blood supply. Some women will notice an increase in vaginal secretions and a darkening of the vulva caused by the increased blood supply.

Many changes in the pregnant woman's body are stimulated by the hormones, *HCG* and *estrogen,* which are secreted by the placenta and the baby. Thus, the developing fetus contributes to the provision of an adequate environment for its growth and nourishment.

Normal Discomforts. The many changes in the woman's body can cause the "normal" discomforts experienced by some women at various times during the pregnancy. Table 16-1 lists these discomforts, the possible causes, and the teaching or suggestions that the nurse can offer. Often just knowing these symptoms are

***Table 16-1.* Normal discomforts experienced during pregnancy, probable cause, and nursing suggestions for relief**

Discomfort	Known or probable cause	Nursing suggestions for relief
Backache	Changes in posture, such as increased lumbar curve Excessive bending and lifting	Practice good posture Perform pelvic rocking Wear comfortable, low-heeled shoes Squat to lift Avoid prolonged sitting Sleep on firm mattress
Constipation	Pressure of enlarged uterus Slowed peristalsis caused by progesterone Side effect of iron supplement	Increase fluid intake, especially juices Eat high-fiber foods Exercise Drink warm liquids in morning Only if other methods fail, use mild laxative, stool softener, or glycerine suppository
Fatigue	Decreased metabolic rate in early pregnancy	Get full night's sleep Nap or rest during day Share work load when possible "Usually better after first trimester"
Hemorrhoids	Constipation Pressure of enlarged uterus	Relieve constipation with measures just listed Take sitz baths Use ice pack or witch hazel for local relief Reinsert hemorrhoid and do perineal tightening exercises Local preparation for analgesia
Leg cramps	Pressure of large uterus on blood vessels Fatigue or chilling Lack of calcium Sudden stretching or overextension of the foot Excessive phosphorus in diet	Take calcium supplement Practice gentle, steady stretch to relieve cramp Never massage cramping muscle Avoid toe-pointing when exercising
Leukorrhea (increased vaginal discharge)	Increased vascularity of cervix and vagina	Wear cotton crotch panties Wash genital area more frequently If infection develops, have physician treat Do not douche
Nausea and vomiting (may occur any time of day)	Increase in estrogen and progesterone levels Change (especially lowering) of blood glucose level	Eat small, frequent meals Eat dry cracker before getting up in morning Snack at bedtime Usually "stops after first trimester"
Urinary frequency (day and night)	Pressure of uterus on bladder in first and third trimesters Nocturia may result from increased venous return from extremities when lying down	(Explanation of why frequency is occurring) If interfering with sleep, reduce fluids in evening Rest during day
Varicosities	Increased vascularity of pelvic organs Venous return slowed by pressure of uterus Familial tendency Progesterone effect in smooth muscles	Avoid knee socks and tight elastic on underwear Elevate feet for 10 to 15 minutes several times a day Avoid long periods of standing Avoid crossing legs when sitting Wear support stockings

normal and expected increases the woman's sense of well-being and comfort. The nurse's role as educator is indispensable, especially for the woman in her first pregnancy.

Total Weight Gain. Total weight gain during pregnancy reflects not only growth of the baby and placenta but of the uterus, breasts, maternal fat storage, and increases in blood and other body fluids. Ideal weight gain is usually in the range of 24 to 32 pounds.[5,21]

Labor and Delivery. The culminating event of a pregnancy is labor and delivery. The woman's feelings, fears, and ideas about this momentous event are discussed with other psychologic factors in the next section. The events of a normal labor and delivery are discussed briefly as background for considering the physiologic changes in the mother and infant.

The precise cause of the onset of labor is not known, although several theories have offered explanations. Several factors probably interact, including distension of the uterus, mechanical irritation, progesterone deprivation, posterior pituitary action, and localized progesterone activity.[11] Labor usually begins at the end of 40 weeks, or the equivalent of 10 normal menstrual cycles. This suggests that some hormonal control, which participates in controlling menstrual cycles, also contributes to the onset of labor.

The placenta also may play an important factor in labor onset. Special hormones may be produced when the placenta has reached term and may be responsible for inducing labor. Placental aging, resulting in dropping of blood levels of estrogen and progesterone, also is believed to be an influential factor; this has a parallel in the menstrual cycles. With deterioration of the corpus luteum, blood levels of estrogen and progesterone drop, with menstruation beginning a few days later.

Labor may be conveniently divided into three distinct stages. The *first stage* is cervical dilation, beginning with the first true labor pain and ending with complete dilation. The presenting part of the fetus begins to press on the cervix and lower uterine segment as well as on the nerve endings around the cervix and vagina. The upper uterine segment is the active contractile portion, which becomes thicker as labor progresses and retracts the lower uterine segment and cervix, pushing the fetus downward. The lower uterine segment is the thin-walled, passive portion through which the infant descends.

Signs of true labor may be summarized as follows: (1) bloody show, or the escape of the plug of mucus that has corked the cervical canal mixed with a minimum amount of blood, (2) regular uterine contractions, (3) contractions increasing in intensity as time passes, (4) palpable hardening of the uterus during contractions, and (5) pain in both the back and the front of the abdomen. This last sign is not present for all women. Examination of the mother's cervix and vaginal canal reveals that the cervix has begun to dilate and that the presenting part of the fetus has begun descent into the birth canal but remains in a fixed position between contractions. Bulging or rupture of fetal membranes is a frequent result.[11]

The mechanisms of the first stage of labor accomplish two important changes in the cervix: effacement and dilation. *Effacement* refers to shortening of the cervical canal from a structure 1 to 2 cm in length to one in which the canal is replaced by a mere circular orifice with almost paper-thin edges. *Dilation* refers to the enlargement of the cervical opening from an orifice a few millimeters in size to an aperture large enough to permit passage of the baby. The primary forces that accomplish these changes are uterine contractions retracting the cervix and causing pressure of the membranes or the pressure of the presenting fetal part against the cervix and lower uterine segment. Effacement usually begins before the onset of the actual labor through the mechanism of *Braxton Hicks contractions,* which involve painless, irregular contractions of the uterus that occur throughout pregnancy.

During the *second stage,* the baby descends through the birth canal. The upper uterine segment greatly thickens, and abdominal muscles assist in the descent and expulsion.

At some point during the first or early second stage of labor the amniotic membranes rupture spontaneously, or they may be ruptured artificially. Once this occurs and the amniotic fluid escapes, the progression of labor tends to be an irreversible process. As descent of the fetus begins, the mother cannot resist contracting her abdominal walls and diaphragm and pushing downward during uterine contractions. This process is repeated at varying intervals and with ever-increasing force and strain. When the head is presenting, this force is applied directly to the fetal spinal column. The curve of the fetal spine tends to straighten, adding power to the push of the head downward. The fetal spine is usually parallel to the midline axis of the mother's abdomen or slightly to one side. The head accommodates to the mother's pelvis as it passes through the vaginal canal by turning first to one side then the other. Finally the head appears, with the diameter of the occiput visible at the level of the perineum; then the neck straightens, turning the head to one side in alignment with the position of the shoulders. When the shoulders pass through the pelvis and accommodate to the shape of the birth canal, the body continues to rotate. The posterior shoulder is usually born over the perineum first, and the anterior soon follows under the symphysis pubis. The body quickly follows, and the infant is born.

The *third stage* begins after the birth and lasts until placental expulsion is complete. Placental separation usually takes place within 5 to 30 minutes after completion of the second stage. Signs of placental detachment include (1) a rush of blood from the vagina, (2) lengthening of the umbilical cord outside the vulva, (3) rise of the uterine fundus and the abdomen as the placenta passes from the uterus into the vagina, and (4) the uterus becoming very firm and globular. It is essential to examine the placenta to determine if any parts are missing and remain in the uterus and to detect any abnormalities that may aid in determining the infant's condition and expectations for the transition to extrauterine life.

Many aspects of care are provided by professional members of the health team, but a woman's family or significant friends can be an important part of her care during labor and delivery. Many practitioners suggest that the way labor and delivery are experienced by the mother has a great effect on how she fills the mothering role for the infant. When significant others are available and willing to help her by support, encouragement, and physical care, nursing assistance often is needed to encourage their participation and sharing. The mother may be functioning at a disadvantaged level of ability during labor and delivery, with her dependence on others heightened considerably. When persons who have established a sharing, trusting relationship are present, the mother is better able to give to her infant in the mothering process. The most important aspects of health promotion during labor and delivery usually are accomplished in the months before delivery, as the nurse, through prenatal classes or individual teaching, prepares both the pregnant woman and her support person for the events.

Overview of Care. During the first stage of labor the mother must be encouraged to relax continually with contractions. Bearing down is avoided because it does not improve the progress of labor, and may cause cervical edema if the cervix is not yet fully dilated. During the second stage, however, when the cervix is fully dilated, bearing down becomes helpful in pushing the baby through the birth canal. Even when the laboring woman has had past experiences with delivery or when she is coping adequately with the demands of labor and using principles and techniques learned, she needs continuous reinforcement and reassurance regarding the progress of labor and the safety of her infant.[9]

When fetal monitoring is used, the nurse may assure the mother by explaining the purpose of the various leads and keeping her informed of the resulting information.

Physical care that promotes the mother's comfort and rest during labor is very important. Back rubs, frequent positional changes, assistance with elimination, provision of clean and dry linen, and assistance in keeping the skin dry and mucous membranes moist become progressively more significant to the mother as labor progresses. In many instances, such care given to the mother also affects the well-being of the fetus.

During labor and delivery, careful observation is essential. This includes

1. Any unusual fetal activity, described as precisely as possible
2. Presence of meconium when the membranes rupture or at any point thereafter
3. Fetal heart rate auscultation
4. Duration of any tachycardia or bradycardia continuing after a contraction

When observing an unusual sign, the nurse must report promptly to the physician or midwife with a complete description. Current fetal signs, as well as the former fetal patterns, are related to the following conditions:

1. Maternal physical condition
2. Medications administered; amount and time given
3. Frequency, type, and duration of uterine contractions
4. Intactness of the membranes and the presence or absence of meconium-stained fluid
5. Bleeding
6. Other significant changes in the mother's condition that occur at or near the time of altered fetal signs

CHANGES IN TRANSITION FROM FETUS TO NEWBORN

Birth of the infant signals new roles for the parents, and the mother's body starts returning to its prepregnant state. Birth also marks dramatic physical transitions within the newborn.

There is a relatively orderly continuum of adaption from fetal to extrauterine life. The events pass unnoticed and with relative ease in most cases. When difficulty occurs, however, care of the infant depends on understanding the normal events of adaptation during this period. Since normal transition depends on a fine balance of chemical, physiologic, and anatomic changes, stress is ultimately hazardous. Infants have demonstrated a relative resistance to the stress of *anoxia;* they can survive longer in an oxygen-free environment than can an adult. The search for a metabolic or biochemical basis for this relative tolerance has yielded no complete answer, and the long-term effects of mild oxygen deprivation are not known. Skillful detection of impending danger to the neonate from any stress can be a lifesaving and health-protecting measure.

Respiratory System. The most important and life-dependent change at the moment of birth is the establishment of respiration. The first inspiratory effort is mammoth. A negative pressure of up to 70 cm of water is required to move between 12 and 70 mm of air in to the lungs. The normal negative pressure of about 20 cm of water is sufficient to move air into the lungs once initial expansion is established. Obligatory respiratory effort greater than the normal pressure required continues to decline until a relatively stable, easy rhythm is established. Lung expansion greatly increases the capillary bed absorptive surface areas for gas exchange.

Circulatory System. Placental circulation ceases with the cutting of the cord or the complete detachment of the placenta. A rise in left atrial pressure and drop in inferior vena cava pressure occur, resulting in effective functional closure of the foramen ovale during the first 24 hours of life. Controversy still surrounds the exact mechanism of closure of the foramen ovale and the ductus arteriosus. Murmurs resulting from incomplete closure of these structures are not unusual in the neonatal period. The ductus arteriosus probably is not closed for several days; it either becomes functionally ineffective, or a normal reversal in flow continues before true closure occurs.

The sudden decrease in vascular pressure, which occurs with the expansion of the lungs at the moment of inspiration, causes the rush of blood flow through the capillary beds of the lungs for the first time. This vascularization of the lungs contributes to the dramatic changes in the blood flow through the greater vessels surrounding the heart and lungs.

A rise in plasma protein level and hemoglobin concentration occurs from a few minutes to 3 hours after birth. This is thought to result from a shift of plasma fluid from the vascular compartment and a loss of cellular water from the erythrocyte. This shift in turn may be the result of the redistribution of blood flow and capillary leakage. The altered pH and carbon dioxide and oxygen saturations (P_{CO_2} and P_{O_2}) at birth and their return to normal may account for the water lost from the erythrocyte. These factors also may be related to the edema of the neonatal period. In term infants, this usually is confined to the presenting parts; but in the premature infant it is more generalized.[7]

Gastrointestinal System. At birth the digestive and absorptive mechanisms necessary to handle the protein, fat, and complex sugars present in human milk are present. The neonate's source of energy for the first few hours is carbohydrate, with fat becoming important by the second day of life. Protein metabolism begins by the third day. Brain tissue continues to depend on carbohydrates as the energy source throughout life.

The liver is limited in its ability to function, especially in conjugating bilirubin and corticosteroid. Glycolysis occurs more rapidly in the first 12 hours of life than it does after 3 days. Lowered surrounding temperatures cause an increase in the metabolic rate, which in turn continues to contribute to metabolic acidosis or at least keeps the balance just on the acidotic side so that respiratory efforts to correct the imbalance remain relatively neutral. Increased metabolism is mediated further by adrenal medulla compounds (epinephrine, norepinephrine), which delay or disturb the adaptation of pulmonary circulation.

Renal System. The kidney of the newborn cannot concentrate urine as efficiently as the more mature kidneys of the older infant. The rate of fluid intake and excretion in the neonate is seven times as great in relation to weight as an adult. Thus, dehydration or overhydration are definite possibilities during this period.[7]

Nervous System. The nervous system of the neonate is incompletely integrated at birth but is fully functional in a life-sustaining sense. The autonomic nervous system, which is believed to be the most crucial system during transition, is the overall integrator and stimulator for maintenance of respiration, acidbase control, compensation of imbalance, and temperature control.

At first the infant is responding to the massive stimuli that occur during birth. Responses of the autonomic nervous system to the stimulation of the delivery process are demonstrated by the infant's behavior, as reflected in a massive wave of sympathetic system activity. Normal, healthy newborns will cry, look around with a wide-eyed expression, and move vigorously. Their heart and respiratory rates are elevated slightly, and they are likely to discharge urine and stool, and excrete mucus from the mouth. After this first reactive period, infants exhibit a reversal of these signs and enter a period of sleep and relative calm. With respiratory and heart rates decreasing, newborns exhibit very little spontaneous motion and are not likely to discharge mucus, urine, or stool. If an effort is made to stimulate them or to elicit neurologic responses, only minimum response will be obtained, and they will easily resume the appearance of deep sleep.

Usually, after 2 to 6 hours, infants spontaneously experience the second reactive period, which resembles closely the active, alert behavior exhibited immediately after birth. The intensity of the behavior is not as pronounced, but the same characteristics are again present. They then go through slowly declining periods, oscillating between rest and activity. At any point during the periods of stimulation, the newborn is at risk from the common hazards present immediately after birth, including respiratory, circulatory, and neurologic complications.

Nursing Interventions. The nursing implications of this adaptation process are great and involve specific protection of the infant and secondary prevention as the nurse observes and intervenes when necessary to assist in a safe, healthy transition from intrauterine life. First, the newborn should be allowed to pass through the normal physiologic stabilizing process with minimum disturbance and maximum observation. Bathing and feeding, for instance, should be delayed until behavior and physiologic mechanisms are stabilized, usually between 4 and 8 hours of age. The nurse's most reliable guideline, however, is individual behavior, not clock hours of life.

Mucus. Newborns tend to regurgitate during this period. Mucus is a normal product of intrauterine life and probably originates in the lung and gastrointestinal tissues. The amount of mucus produced varies greatly. Some controversy remains regarding the efficacy of gastric suctioning for alleviation or prevention of mucus being regurgitated into the upper esophageal tract, creating a danger for aspiration. When mucous production reaches a level at which aspiration becomes an obvious hazard, suctioning should be employed. If vomiting occurs, suctioning of mucus from the mouth with a simple bulb syringe may help, but the more effective approach is to remove material from the esophagus, then the stomach.

Apgar Score. Assessment of the newborn after the first few hours is essentially the same as assessment of the young infant (see Chapter 17). One technique, specific to the minutes just after birth, is the Apgar scoring system. Apgar scoring provides a simple and easily applied clinical measure for evaluation of the infant's general condition.[1] The score has been validated by many studies, and its usefulness in determining the condition of the infant as well as predicting future adaptation and neurologic development is well established. The scoring is made at 1 minute and 5 minutes of age and may be repeated until the infant's condition has stabilized. The total score is obtained by adding the values allotted to observations of heart rate, respiratory effort, muscle tone, reflex irritability, and color, as indicated in Table 16-2. The highest score possible is 10. A score of 8 to 10 indicates that the baby is adapting very well.

Gender

Gender differences also occur in fetal growth. Generally, males grow faster than females in the third trimester; and after 26 weeks, males are larger. At birth, males are slightly heavier and longer and have a larger head circumference than females.

There is also a gender difference in number of conceptions and births. More males are conceived, but more male embryos are spontaneously aborted as well. The exact cause of this greater loss of male embryos is not fully understood. More male embryos may succumb to X-linked recessive conditions during this time, or the female, having two X chromosomes, may have more protection from some of the hazards of early pregnancy. After birth, the male continues to have a lower survival rate than females; and by middle age, women are more numerous than men.

Race

Race can affect the fetus's health in several ways. The first is in rate of twinning. In the United States, nonwhites (mainly Blacks) have more twin pregnancies than Whites. Twin fetuses are at increased risk for a premature delivery and also place higher nutrition demands on the mother. Any premature baby is at higher risk because of less mature organs.

Race is also a factor in how often certain specific malformations occur. For example, *anencephaly* (absence of brain tissue) is more common in Whites than in Blacks, whereas *polydactyly* (extra fingers or toes) is more common in Blacks. Interestingly, the total number of malformations tends to be about the same across races that have been studied (white, black, Japanese).

Race may also affect fetal outcome because of its link to socioeconomic status. Pregnant women of minority races generally are less likely to have the economic resources to obtain a nutritious diet or early and ongoing quality prenatal care.

Genetics

Genetic influences during the prenatal period affect the survival or later well-being of the child through several known mechanisms. Abnormal chromosome number or structure, a mutant (abnormal) gene, and polygenetic inheritance are responsible for a significant percentage

***Table 16-2.* Apgar scoring**

	Score		
Sign	0	1	2
Heart rate	Absent	Slow (below 100)	Over 100
Respiratory effort	Absent	Weak cry, hypoventilation	Good strong cry
Muscle tone	Limp	Some flexion of extremities	Active motion, extremities well flexed
Reflex irritability	No response	Grimace	Cry
Color	Blue, pale	Body pink, extremities blue	Completely pink

From Chinn PL: *Child health maintenance: concepts in family-centered care,* ed 2, St Louis, 1979, Mosby.

of congenital malformations or defects.[18] *Down's syndrome* (trisomy 21) is the most well-known and most commonly occuring example of an extra chromosome. Extra chromosomes, deleted chromosomes, or translocations usually result in multiple malformations. Single malformations in an otherwise normal fetus, such as clubfoot, cleft palate, and neural tube defects, are thought to result from the combined effect of many genes.

More than 50% of spontaneous abortions have a chromosomal abnormality; thus, natural forces stop the development of many abnormal fetuses. Some genetic problems do not become apparent until later in life, but the basic defect was present from conception.

Not all malformations and multiple defect syndromes are genetically based. The environmental influences on the developing embryo and fetus are substantial. These influences, including infectious agents, drugs, radiation, chemicals, alcohol, and smoking, are discussed later in this chapter with the whole spectrum of environmental processes.

Modern techniques of amniocentesis, chorionic villi sampling (CVS), and chromosome analysis have expanded the possibilities for genetic counseling in the prenatal period. The nurse must know where these resources are available in the community and direct clients to these resources if any family history, previous pregnancy history, race, or maternal age indicates that a genetic defect or syndrome may be more likely for the fetus.

Nutritional and Metabolic Pattern

The large volume of evidence regarding the general effects of adequate nutrition on the viability, growth, and development of the unborn child conclusively indicates that this is one of the most important variables for satisfactory fetal health and well-being. Maternal malnutrition during pregnancy, which is usually a lifelong state of inadequacy, has been implicated as exerting a possible teratogenic effect on the fetus. The principal fetal system usually damaged is the central nervous system, leading to impaired intelligence performance later in life.[21] (See box on p. 380.)

The effects of poor nutrition are most severe for the young adolescent, who still has growth requirements, and for the mother with accumulated effects of several pregnancies, at which time prolonged poor nutrition more directly affects the fetus. Nutritional deficiencies of the mother during her own fetal, infancy, and childhood years contribute to the development of structural and physiologic disadvantages for supporting a growing fetus. Maternal stature and pelvic development, which evolve from the prior nutritional status as well as genetic endowment, may influence the difficulty of labor.[21]

Studies also suggest that improving the diet of pregnant women who have been poorly nourished throughout life does not always appreciably improve their ability to produce healthy offspring. Poor nutrition throughout life may be more significant than the inadequacy of the mother's diet during pregnancy. This superficially appears to conflict with the evidence supporting the proposition that the fetus derives most raw materials for development from the maternal diet and not, as formerly believed, from the mother's body structure and reserves. Maturity and development of all functional systems, such as essential enzyme systems, appear to depend heavily on a lifetime of adequate nurturance. Thus, utilizing dietary elements effectively may be impaired in the poorly nourished mother. Further study is required to understand fully these aspects of nutrition.

A major portion of families who eat poorly also suffer from socioeconomic limitations, and they may be strongly influenced by dietary practices of a subculture. These factors compound efforts to understand the influence of poor nutrition on fetal well-being. Although culturally based difference in food habits and beliefs are important, *poverty* keeps the diet inadequate in basic nutrients. It seems apparent that cultural differences in type of diet lose nutritional significance as adequate economic resources become available. Families of all cultural groups who are relatively affluent tend to choose and eat foods from each of the four basic food groups, although the manner of preparation and seasoning continues to vary according to cultural practices.

The additional dietary demands of the mother, which exceed those of the nonpregnant woman of comparable age, have been estimated in studies that have increased our understanding of normal physiologic adjustments made during pregnancy. Ideas on the demands of pregnancy have changed substantially as investigations have shown that the woman herself requires more metabolic energy and structural resources to support pregnancy adequately.[5,21]

Calorie requirements during pregnancy exceed those of the nonpregnant woman by about 200 kilocalories each day, resulting in a weight gain of about 25 pounds. If, at the end of 20 weeks' gestation, the woman has not gained at least 10 pounds, she should be considered a high-risk mother for delivering an ill infant. The former belief in the desirability to limit weight gain by limiting caloric intake during pregnancy was founded on the unsound notion that any fat or liquid weight gain was related to the development toxemia. Although the rate of gain and the total gain during pregnancy varies considerably among women, it is recognized now that avoiding weight gain by limiting caloric intake is seriously hazardous to fetal well-being. Low maternal weight gain, as well as being underweight at the onset of

HEALTHY PEOPLE 2000

SELECTED NATIONAL HEALTH PROMOTION AND DISEASE PREVENTION OBJECTIVES

THE PRENATAL PERIOD

- Reduce the infant mortality rate to no more than 7 per 1000 live births (Baseline: 10.1 per 1000 live births in 1987)

Special population targets

Infant mortality	1987 baseline	2000 target
Blacks	17.9	11
American Indians/Alaska Natives	12.5*	8.5
Puerto Ricans	12.9*	8

- Reduce the fetal death rate (20 or more weeks of gestation) to no more than 5 per 1000 live births plus fetal deaths (Baseline: 7.6 per 1000 live births plus fetal deaths in 1987)

Special population target

Fetal deaths	1987 baseline	2000 target
Blacks	12.8*	7.5*

- Reduce low birth weight to an incidence of no more than 5% of live births and very low birth weight to no more than 1% of live births (Baseline: 6.9% and 1.2%, respectively, in 1987)

Special population target

	1987 baseline	2000 target
Low birth weight		
Blacks	12.7%	9%
Very low birth weight		
Blacks	2.7%	2%

- Increase to at least 85% the proportion of mothers who achieve the minimum recommended weight gain during the pregnancies (Baseline: 67% of married women in 1980)
- Increase to at least 90% the proportion of women enrolled in prenatal care who are offered screening and counseling on prenatal detection of fetal abnormalities
- Increase abstinence from tobacco use by pregnant women to at least 90% and increase abstinence from alcohol, cocaine, and marijuana by pregnant women by at least 20% (Baseline: 75% of pregnant women abstained from tobacco use in 1985)
- Reduce the incidence of fetal alcohol syndrome to no more than 0.12 per 1000 live births (Baseline: 0.22 per 1000 live births in 1987)
- Increase to at least 90% the proportion of all pregnant women who receive prenatal care in the first trimester of pregnancy (Baseline: 76% of live births in 1987)
- Increase to at least 90% the proportion of pregnant women and infants who receive risk-appropriate care
- Increase to at least 60% the proportion of primary care providers who provide age-appropriate preconception care and counseling

*Per 1000 live births plus fetal deaths

pregnancy, is associated with infants who are underweight for gestational age and who risk the hazards of impaired neonatal adjustment that accompany low birth weight. The woman who is overweight at the time of conception also risks endangering the fetus if an attempt is made during pregnancy to lose her own body weight. The effects of *ketoacidosis,* which occurs as a result of caloric limitations, have been associated with neuropsychologic defects in infants.[11] Thus, with the exception of considering specific disease states, the nurse should advise the mother to eat a well-balanced diet according to appetite.[21]

The well-balanced diet needed by the pregnant woman is similar to the diet needed by all human beings, with specific increases of certain components, as recommended by the Food and Nutrition Board of the National Academy of Science.[5] The nurse should approach the diet of a pregnant woman in terms of the food offered to the entire family; asking a mother to feed herself differently from other family members is usually unrealistic and unacceptable. It may be tempting to recommend that limited resources be directed to upgrading nutrition for the mother and fetus, but such recommendations are futile if family needs are not considered.

Protein requirements during pregnancy are estimated to be about 1.2 grams per kilogram of body weight per day (g/kg/day), as opposed to the nonpregnant woman's requirement of about 1.0 g/kg/day. Animal protein should constitute the major source during pregnancy, since this contains the most complete supply of essential amino acids, but achieving this goal may be virtually impossible when resources are limited. Because the family's protein requirement is the most costly, the budget should consider this first; a larger proportion of nonanimal protein sources may be necessary.

The most important increase of intake during pregnancy besides calorie and protein is *minerals.* Increase in protein foods usually provides the extra essential minerals needed, particularly phosphorus and calcium. Calcium is deposited mainly in the fetus during the last month of gestation. The rapid deposition at this time requires that a good supply be stored from the early months of pregnancy to meet this demand and to minimize depletion of maternal calcium supplies. One quart of cow's milk each day supplies about 1 g of calcium; the requirement of the pregnant woman is estimated to be about 1.2 g daily. Other protein foods consumed in adequate amounts supply the extra amount.

Vitamin supplementation, a common practice among American physicians, is of unsubstantiated value. If the woman's diet is well balanced, the food sources of vitamins and minerals should be adequate to meet the needs of pregnancy, with the exception of *iron.* Supplementation with 30 to 60 mg of ferrous iron during the last 3 to 4 months of pregnancy can be beneficial in building and protecting maternal iron stores.[21] Some evidence points to the desirability of folic acid supplementation, particularly in the case of potential or real anemia or multiple pregnancy.

Fats and *carbohydrates* are needed in amounts that will supply the caloric requirements during pregnancy. Although some caloric increase is supplied by the extra protein, protein components are needed for the body-building requirements of pregnancy and fetal growth. Fats and carbohydrates remain the most important sources of energy, and they also supply essential vitamins and minerals. Supplementation with vitamins and minerals, although not known to cause harm to the mother or fetus if within reasonable limits, is usually a costly way to achieve nutritional improvement when compared with the cost of improving the dietary intake of the mother and family. The related benefits of increasing consumption of needed components that exist in the form of food may be more important than currently recognized.

The frequent practice of *pica,* or the eating of non-food substances, especially by economically deprived, pregnant black Americans, warrants special consideration. This phenomenon also occurs among small children, particularly when hunger and poor nutrition are common. This situation, combined with normal cravings for food or nonfood substances, can lead to a culturally acceptable practice of eating such materials as starch, mud, clay, soap, or plaster. Although this practice has been known to exist for centuries among many groups of people, the possible harm and the reasons for it occurring more commonly during pregnancy are not understood. The effect most reliably associated with pica is the presence of iron deficiency anemia, but whether this condition would occur in the absence of pica is not known.[21]

NURSING INTERVENTIONS

The best time to teach a woman about prenatal nutrition is before she is pregnant. Since most women do not seek prenatal care until they are pregnant, this information often is given later than is best for the developing fetus. Primary prevention intervention in this instance should begin with high-school health classes. Although women will not remember the details of the recommended prenatal diet for several years, they may remember that good nutrition is vitally important at this time and may seek further information when they are planning a pregnancy. Secondary prevention intervention occurs during the pregnancy through laboratory monitoring of iron levels and assessment of the woman's actual intake of essential nutrients, as well as her pattern of weight gain.

Elimination Pattern

FETUS

The fetus accomplishes all essential elimination functions through the placenta. Carbon dioxide, water, urea, and other waste products that pass through the placenta then are eliminated through the mother's body. By the end of the first trimester, the fetus is able to swallow, make respiratory movements, and urinate. These abilities, however, do not become functional as avenues to elimination until birth.[9]

PREGNANT WOMAN

The pregnant woman experiences changes in her elimination pattern because of hormone influences and mechanical forces caused by the enlarging uterus. These changes-urinary frequency in the first and third trimesters, constipation, and hemorrhoids-usually are experienced as normal, minor discomforts (see Table 16-1 on p. 374).

Activity and Exercise Pattern

FETUS

Early spontaneous movements of the fetus may be reflexive, stimulated by passive uterine movement, and may be present as early as 8 to 10 weeks. Ultrasound observation of fetal movement shows that repetitive movements occur by 12 to 16 weeks, "locomotive movements" of arms and legs by about 16 weeks, and hand-to-face movements by 24 to 26 weeks.[12,17] By the end of the second trimester fetal movement becomes more restricted because of lack of space in the uterus. Fetal movements are felt by the pregnant woman and have been shown to be a good indication of fetal well-being. A dramatic decrease in or absence of fetal movements for more that 8 hours may indicate fetal distress.

PREGNANT WOMAN

The weight gain and physical changes during pregnancy and the vigors of labor and delivery would seem to require that the pregnant woman be in the best physical condition of her lifespan. Historically, pregnancy has often been viewed as incapacitating or a sickness, and women were instructed to restrict their activities. Fortunately for today's woman, pregnancy is viewed as a normal, natural state, and she is encouraged to participate in any physical activity or sport that she enjoyed before pregnancy,[8,9] except for sports such as sky diving, which carries a risk of falling and thus trauma to the fetus, or high-altitude climbing, which carries a risk of low oxygen availability. A woman's choice of activities should be based on her interest; comfort and good judgment should determine how vigorously to pursue these activities. If a sport or activity causes undue exhaustion, muscle cramps, or joint pain, it obviously should be modified or discontinued. Because of normal change in the musculoskeletal system and the shift in her center of gravity as the uterus enlarges, the pregnant woman may want to choose different sports or exercises or a different level of participation later in the pregnancy.

The woman with a sedentary lifestyle before pregnancy should actually increase her activity level during pregnancy within moderate limits. A half-hour walk each day is a good introduction to a regular exercise program.

Specific exercises to prepare the woman for labor and delivery are needed. These are taught in prenatal classes and have been illustrated in popular books. For the self-motivated woman, a book of exercises may be enough of a stimulus to begin and maintain an adequate exercise program. For most women, a group situation may be a better method of regular exercise. The nurse needs to keep informed of exercise groups for pregnant women to relate these options to clients.

No scientific evidence suggests sexual activity should be restricted during a normal pregnancy, with the emphasis on "normal." Threatened abortion or history of abortion in the first trimester, early rupture of membranes, and some other complications of pregnancy do call for restriction of sexual intercourse or orgasm. The enlarging uterus will require some modifications in positions for intercourse. The couple's feelings about the woman's changing body may be the main barrier to their sexual relationship (see section on roles and role changes later in this chapter). The nurse's first step in primary prevention intervention in this area is to clearly state that sex is not a taboo subject but rather an accepted and essential topic for prenatal visits and classes.

Sleep and Rest Pattern

FETUS

Electroencephalogram studies have shown that the fetus has cyclic activity patterns. Four states of activity and alertness have been identified: awake, drowsy awakefulness, rapid eye movement (REM) sleep, and quiet sleep. Evidence suggests a diurnal (day/night) pattern is established during the fetal period.

PREGNANT WOMAN

Since the exact cause of fatigue during the first trimester is unknown, no preventive measure exists. The nurse can counsel a woman that this fatigue usually subsides by the fourth month. Rest breaks during the day and a full 8 hours of sleep can increase comfort during this time.

A full night's sleep is sometimes difficult to achieve because of the need to urinate several times throughout the night during the first and third trimesters and the positional discomfort some women experience during the third trimester (see Table 16-1 on p. 374 for ideas for relief). The pregnant woman who is fatigued and unable to get adequate rest may find that she has more negative than positive feelings about her pregnancy. The nurse should explore this and help the woman express her thoughts and feelings.

PSYCHOLOGIC PROCESSES

The dramatic physiologic changes during pregnancy are accompanied by many psychologic changes in the way the woman thinks about herself, her role, her body, her beliefs, and many other aspects of her life.

Cognitive and Perceptual Pattern

FETUS

Little is actually known about the cognitive and other psychologic processes of the fetus. There are anecdotal reports of persons "remembering" events that happened or music that was repeatedly played during their gestation, but these need further study before they can be accepted as evidence of prenatal learning and memory. More information is available about the *sensory* abilities of the fetus; it is known that all the sensory systems are functional or capable of functioning during the prenatal period. This includes vision, hearing, taste, smell, and touch, as well as proprioception and vestibular senses.[17]

Tactile, proprioception, and vestibular responses have been demonstrated in the first trimester. Hearing is functioning after 20 weeks, as shown by monitoring changes in fetal heart rate in response to pure-tone audiometry. After about 25 weeks, the fetus is startled by a loud, sudden noise; many pregnant women can attest to this. The fetus is capable of seeing by 28 to 32 weeks of age but has little opportunity to use this ability in utero.

Some women naturally offer sensory stimulation to the fetus as they sing to their unborn child or unconsciously or consciously rub or pat their abdomen. These actions may indicate a woman's desire to interact with her child; knowledge about her baby's sensory abilities may help her visualize and accept the fetus as a separate person. The nurse can include this kind of information in prenatal teaching sessions.

PREGNANT WOMAN

Physical and psychologic processes are closely intertwined as pregnancy progresses. Psychologic stresses and problems, as well as normal emotional growth, can affect the physical status of the pregnancy, the interactions of the family members, and the eventual relationship between mother and infant. When considering the emotional aspects of pregnancy, it is important to recognize that individual personality differences, the woman's environment, physical state, family, and sociocultural and spiritual background affect how the woman handles the psychologic changes.

Two major categories of psychologic influences are (1) the normal psychologic growth required of parents to prepare physically and emotionally for their new child and (2) the major internal or external stressors on the pregnant woman that can detract from her ability to provide the best environment for the developing infant. The pregnant woman undergoes many cognitive changes that ultimately result in psychologic readiness for motherhood.

Emotional Changes. The woman is assisted physically in this psychologic "work" by the hormonal changes occurring in her body. An increase in progesterone affects the woman's general mood, causing her to be more introverted, passive, and somewhat narcissistic. These mood changes are necessary for the woman to center her energy on the growing child and on her own growth and development as a person. In addition to the hormonal change, the actual presence, growth, and movements of the child developing within the woman become more and more a part of the woman's "experiential self." Rubin[16] states that as the woman's body grows and changes, she experiences a heightened "sensory perceptivity in the tactile and kinesthetic modalities." She receives immediate sensations of touch and motion and weight that she can share only partly with others, which results in a feeling of separateness and uniqueness. This awareness of the child also causes the woman to turn inwards. She frequently worries that the shift in energy away from the world toward herself and the child may cause her to lose contact, drift away from the valued relationships, and lose feelings of competence in areas of achievement.

As the woman is withdrawing, she also feels a sense of oneness with all life. At times the world seems to recede, and yet it encompasses the woman in new ways. Her introversion, as disconcerting as it sometimes may be to her, her family, and friends, allows her to prepare herself for the child. She spends her time "observing, interviewing, recalling in microscopic detail, sorting and classifying her findings and analyzing meaning . . . the interest, tolerance and patience for minute details is necessary preparation for rearing the very young child."[16] She constantly studies qualities of human relationships and is very intent on learning the meaning of behavior. This absorption in meaning causes an increase in sensitivity and perceptiveness; to others, she may seem overly sensitive and analytic.

The pregnant woman also may experience other emotional changes, such as wide mood swings, emotional lability, irritability, and changes in sexual desire. These experiences are caused partly by endocrine changes, physical discomforts, feelings about changing body image, the adjustments to work and in relationships, and demanding cognitive maturational processes.

The nurse must recognize that the "mood of pregnancy" can be different for different women and at varying times in the pregnancy. The shifting emotions reflect the great amount of physical and psychologic work needed for personal growth and development.

Factors Influencing Development. By drawing into herself, the woman works through the meanings of actions, studies relationships, experiences mood swings, daydreams, and fantasizes, thus accomplishing the developmental tasks of pregnancy. She then experiences a growing sense of adulthood, fulfillment, and integration–new maturity. This growth may coexist with her emotional disequilibrium.

These tasks may not all be accomplished during the pregnancy, but certain elements may need to be completed in the early postpartum period or even in the first few months of the baby's life. How a woman works at these developmental tasks will be strongly influenced by her age, her general feelings about the pregnancy, her life situation, her degree of stress, whether she has other children, and the influence of her loved ones.[9] A pregnant teenager who is still accomplishing the developmental tasks of adolescence may be searching for her own identity and may have difficulty incorporating the pregnant body or the role of mother into her self-image; cognitively she may still be in Piaget's stage of concrete operational thought and unable to think through new problems, such as making plans for the baby or even accepting the pregnancy until she feels the baby move. Table 16-3 outlines some difficulties adolescents may experience when the developmental tasks of pregnancy overlap with those of adolescence.

An older woman experiencing her first pregnancy may feel more isolated by her situation than does the pregnant woman in her twenties. More women are becoming pregnant at older ages today, however, and this sense of aloneness may be decreasing. Even the woman who greatly desires a pregnancy may feel ambivalence. Frequently she is well established in her career and family and needs to balance her growth and development in these valued areas with her new sense of changing self. Fears related to being at high risk because of age may increase her anxiety. She may worry about her ability to handle the physical demands of labor and delivery, the sleeplessness of motherhood, the fears of having an abnormal child, and the need to juggle conflicting responsibilities. Many times the older woman is hesitant to discuss her fears and conflicts with the nurse, since she feels that she should be mature enough to handle the pregnancy competently on her own.[9]

A woman with other children moves through the developmental tasks differently than the woman pregnant for the first time. She may worry about how to incorporate the new infant into all her ongoing relationships and whether she will have time to love the new baby or the older children as much as needed. She may have fears and anxieties about labor and delivery because of a previous negative experience. She may be much more aware of the problems involved with caring for a new infant and not be as effused with the excited "glow" of impending motherhood.[9] Developmentally she may have already worked through some of the tasks with her prior pregnancies but now must incorporate new dimensions into her role as mother.

Whether the pregnancy was desired and how supportive or welcoming the woman's family is are other aspects that will influence how rapidly and thoroughly the woman is able to understand and grow with her pregnancy. If the woman is under stress from finances, family, work problems and instabilities, or poor health, she may be inhibited from doing the work of pregnancy as she copes with day-to-day living.

Developmental Tasks. Rubin[14,16] describes four major developmental tasks that the woman seeks to accomplish in the process of learning to be a mother:

1. Ensuring safe passage through pregnancy and childbirth
2. Ensuring the acceptance of the child by significant persons in her family
3. Binding in to her unknown child
4. Learning to give herself

According to Rubin, "All four tasks are worked on concurrently and equally, somewhat as in weaving a tapestry, where one is developed to a point, then each of the other areas is brought forward, so that the whole piece is even."[16]

Each woman works through these tasks in her own style. Many manifestations of the psychologic work will be seen in the woman's fantasies and dreams, her interactions with others, her verbal comments, and her behavior. Each developmental task is described further in the following paragraphs.

Ensuring Safe Passage. The woman attempts to en-

***Table 16-3.* Developmental tasks of pregnant adolescent**

Developmental tasks	Actuality of pregnancy
Learn to accept and live comfortably with slowly changing body and associate sexual feelings and desires. Develop positive self-image.	Must deal with gross body changes, particularly huge abdomen and large breasts; skin is marred by chloasma and striae. Sexual feelings and desires may vary in intensity throughout pregnancy. Because of individual's own growth as well as needs of pregnancy, large amounts of food are needed; this is in conflict with the slimness so highly value in society.
Reorganize thought processes, with thinking becoming less egocentric.	Huge hormonal increases as well as the tasks of pregnancy lead to progressive introspection, dependency, and egocentric thinking and behavior.
Become independent of parents and gradually develop interdependence.	Psychologic dependency increases during pregnancy as young woman uses internal resources to cope with tasks of pregnancy. Since most adolescents are unable to support themselves, financial considerations increase dependency on parents; occasionally other extreme occurs–alienation from parents because of pregnancy.
Gain sense of identity through interaction, first with same-sex peers, then with heterosexual friends.	Being pregnant and thus different isolates adolescent from group. Firm foundation was established incompletely, if at all, with same-sex friends before physical relationship with opposite sex; thus, adolescent often is left without peers of either sex.
Take increasing responsibility for own activities.	Critical difference between adolescent and adult is ability to be responsible for oneself and one's activities; financial consequences associated with pregnancy alone can prevent young woman from taking responsibility. Lack of knowledge and maturity also affects ability to parent an infant, although society still tends to hold the teenager more responsible for the pregnancy.

Adapted from Bishop B: *The maternity cycle: one nurse's reflections,* Philadelphia, 1980, FA Davis.

sure safe passage for herself and her infant in many ways. She seeks out prenatal care in all forms: from health care professionals, books, movies, television, and advice from friends and family (see box on p. 386). The folklore of pregnancy becomes extremely important to some women, and they attempt to avoid activities they believe may be detrimental to the baby. Examples of such folklore are myths that the cord will strangle the infant if the mother raises her arms above her head or that viewing a handicapped person will cause the baby to be abnormal. Activities such as falling, experiencing a blow to the abdomen, or undertaking strenuous exercise involve new risks; normal everyday events can seem dangerous and threatening. In her growing protectiveness for herself and the fetus, the woman feels more and more vulnerable and avoids crowds, revolving doors, small spaces, and active children. She desires peace and serenity and yet hates to be alone. In her third trimester, she becomes exceedingly anxious about the delivery of her child. She is tired of being pregnant but fears the effect of delivery on her and her child's safety.[15,16]

Her dreams and fantasies echo her fears and desires. Frequently the pregnant woman needs to discuss her sleeping and waking thoughts, which may center on misfortune, especially in the third trimester.[14]

The woman who is able to discuss and work through these distressing thoughts can use the material for the growth process. She tries to avoid harmful places and behaviors; she attempts to prepare herself for delivery; and she seeks reassurance from friends and health professionals about the probability of having a normal child. However, nothing that the woman is able to do during her pregnancy will completely free her from these fears. Only the safe delivery of her normal child can fully accomplish this task.[15]

Ensuring Acceptance of the Child. The woman must feel that her child will be accepted into her family. The partner's receptivity to the child is particularly important; the woman may show new concern for the husband's acceptance of his role as father and for his dependability in all situations. Many fantasies about the sex of her child revolve around the partner's preference. The woman frequently judges the degree of receptivity to the infant by the amount of love and attention that

RESEARCH REVIEW PRENATAL

OBSTACLES TO PRENATAL CARE

Harvey SM, Faber KS: Obstacles to prenatal care following implementation of a community-based program to reduce financial barriers, *Family Plan Perspec* 25:32-36, 1993.

Purpose The purpose of this study is to identify obstacles to prenatal care among low-income women designed to reduce financial barriers.

Review Two hundred thirty-six women who received inadequate prenatal care (e.g., received no prenatal care, made fewer than five visits or initiated care in the third trimester) agreed to participate in the study. The most common reasons cited for inadequate prenatal care were financial obstacles. Among the most frequently cited by women included difficulty paying for prenatal care (70%), difficulty with medical insurance (55%), ambivalence or fear about pregnancy (46%), and transportation problems (42%). Logistic regression analysis was employed and identified six significant predictors of inadequate prenatal care. Implications are discussed which address the structural and personal barriers to good prenatal care. Such care is critical if the United States is to achieve its objective of no more than seven infant deaths per 1000 live births by the year 2000.

she herself receives during pregnancy. She accepts these inputs as messages that the child, as part of the woman, is welcomed.

Other information related to the importance of the family in enabling the woman to complete this developmental task is presented in the section on environmental processes.

Binding in to Her Unknown Child. The third developmental task is perhaps the most complex of the cognitive processes that the woman experiences. To accomplish it, the woman goes through two basic steps: first, incorporating and integrating the fetus as an integral part of herself, then growing in her perception to see the infant as a separate being. This task will not be completed until after the birth of the baby. The pregnant woman's fantasies clearly demonstrate her growing awareness of the child as a person. Many early fantasies are fleeting, highly changeable images. The woman may experience associative fantasies; when she eats an egg, she may think of the baby. Later fantasies in the second and third trimester are related more specifically to what the child will be like; the woman may eat a treat, for instance, and imagine that she is feeding the infant (seen as an older child) a favorite food. She frequently uses clothing to accomplish this imaginative work, seeing the baby in little girl or boy clothes. During the eighth month, she is ready to begin nesting activity. She thinks of the baby as an external reality and starts preparing the environment by readying the crib and the nursery. The process of binding is described further in Table 16-4.

Learning to Give of Herself. Although the actual mothering activity occurs after the birth, the learning process begins during pregnancy. The woman begins the task by examining what she will gain and lose by becoming a mother. She then explores the meanings of giving by examining how others give to her, how other mothers give to their children, and how she has given to others in the past.[16] If this is her first pregnancy, she may be concerned about this ability. If she has other children, she may fear she will not have enough to give or will give unequally. Outward manifestations of giving are important; the woman values gifts of companionship and concern and needs to have others give gifts to the baby. Gifts for herself and the baby are meaningful manifestations of her own and others' acceptance and ability to give to the child.[15]

The woman, according to Rubin,[16] has much ambivalence about the central task of giving birth. She prays for safe delivery and "for the true gifts of living–time, interest, companionship, concern and relief" during a time of anxiety and stress.

The pregnant woman's cognitive growth and development are extensive, with the intense drawing inward allowing her to focus on and accomplish the developmental tasks of pregnancy. The last two tasks of binding in and learning to give of herself demand that the woman change her self-concept to see herself first as pregnant and then as a mother, making pregnancy a kind of identity reformation.

Self-Perception and Self-Concept Pattern

To develop a maternal identity, the woman must first accept the pregnant body image. Early in the pregnancy the woman accepts the infant as part of herself, then

***Table 16-4.* Binding in to the unknown child**

Incorporation and integration of fetus as part of self	Perception of fetus as separate being
Goals	**Goals**
To ascertain and accept reality of pregnancy To incorporate fetus into body image and resolve changes in relationships to partner and own mother	To view fetus as an individual To take on personal mothering identity
Responses	**Responses**
1. Feels surprise at conception; asks questions of identity 2. Experiences ambivalence, a feeling of "not now" 3. Senses that thoughts turn inward; focuses on self 4. Seeks prenatal care as validating mechanisms 5. Feels special, as if having a secret; incorporates fetus into own body 6. Becomes more aware of self as person 7. Notices changes in body; may like these or show ambivalence 8. Buys maternity clothing 9. Manifests growing introspection 10. Accepts pregnancy 11. Reviews conflicts with own mother in role preparation 12. Reviews losses–what will be given up and the previous loss of family; may see the link between generations, with child representing lost family 13. Seeks new acquaintances who are pregnant or parents	1. Takes on maternal role by mimicry of mothering behavior, selecting behaviors that suit her personality 2. Begins to realize that fetus is separate being; conceptualizes fetus as having a personality 3. Searches for cues as to what baby will be like 4. Buys baby supplies 5. Attempts to involve others in feeling fetal movements, buying baby supplies, and so on 6. Takes active interest in children and what they do 7. Dreams and fantasizes about babies and sex of her baby 8. Feels body is "full of life" 9. May become more dependent on supportive nurturance of others 10. Makes plans for physical separation of delivery 11. Increases preparations for new family member 12. Lets go of former roles incompatible with mothering role 13. Has sense of waiting–too much time on her hands 14. Is increasingly protective of unborn baby; feels vulnerable 15. Feels sense of readiness coupled with anxiety for labor process, baby's normalcy, and her ability to mother

Data from Blair C, Salerno E: *The expanding family: childbearing,* Boston, 1976, Little, Brown; and Clark A, Affonso D: *Childbearing: a nursing perspective,* ed 2, Philadelphia, 1979, FA Davis.

gradually begins to see the baby as a separate individual, simultaneously taking on the new role of mother.

BODY IMAGE AND SELF-IMAGE

In the developmental task of binding in to the child, the woman first incorporates the infant into her self-image. The ambivalence seen in the first trimester is partly a result of the woman's need to make the pregnancy compatible with how she sees herself as a woman. For some women, alterations of the body are a traumatic part of pregnancy, whereas others feel a passive acceptance or love the pregnant body and enjoy showing it off.[8] In the second timester, the woman frequently begins to feel more positive about her changing womanly image. As she feels the baby move; as the increased estrogen and progesterone work to increase her sense of vitality, inner peace, and acceptance; and as her body begins to look pregnant and others respond positively to this change, the woman is frequently happier with herself and begins to love the baby as part of herself. Some women describe pregnancy as living in anticipation of joy. During the third trimester, however, the woman frequently becomes tired of the pregnancy; her sense of well-being is overcome by awkward movements, sleepless nights, the constant need to urinate, Braxton Hicks contractions, and other discomforts. Some women experience the infant's movements or mild contractions as pleasurable, sensual sensations, whereas others find them extremely uncomfortable. As the pregnancy nears its end, most women are very tired of the pregnant body, even those who have loved being pregnant. They yearn to have their former body boundaries back, to have the delivery behind them, to hold the baby in their arms, or to have someone else be able to carry the baby for awhile.

The nurse should realize that even though the woman gradually sees the infant more and more as a separate individual, her strong association of the baby being part of herself will continue even after bith, as seen in her bodily sensations postpartum. Some women experience phantom limb sensations and continue to feel the baby move inside; many cannot lie on their stomachs. Another manifestation of this continuing identification can be seen in the way the mother treats her baby. If she feels good about herself, she will feel loving toward the infant; if she feels ugly or unlovable, she may make uncomplimentary remarks about the infant's appearance.[16]

SEXUALITY

The pregnant woman's feelings about her sexuality are greatly influenced by her body image and whether the body image fits into her ideal of femininity. The reflections of others, particularly her partner, also influence such feelings. Many women develop a more positive sense of femininity during their pregnancy, which assists them in accepting their physical bodies. This may lead to a greater adjustment in their sexual interactions.

Women experience different feelings about their sexuality during pregnancy. Some women experience an increase in desire, whereas others experience a decreased need for sexual activity. Many women worry about the appropriateness of intercourse during pregnancy, fearing that it will cause miscarriage, infection, or early delivery or in some way may harm the baby. The couple can sometimes experience dissatisfaction because of restrictions in positions or movements, pain on penetration, an increase in vaginal discharge, breast tenderness, or the other physical discomforts of pregnancy, such as fatigue or heartburn.[8] Many women experience a decreased need for sexual intercourse but an increased desire for holding, touching, and other signs of physical affection.

MATERNAL ROLE

The pregnant woman's individual personality, level of maturation, and psychologic development will influence her readiness to assume the role of mother. How society and culture perceive motherhood and the role of women and how her views mesh with these perceptions will affect the ease of the transition. The family situation, availability of peer role models, and her relationship with her mother are also concerns. The internalization of the mother role occurs only after the birth, as the woman changes her behavior and interacts with the infant in a reciprocal relationship. The mother claims the infant in a social context instead of as a component of her self system. Only at this time can the woman fully understand herself and her behavior in relation to the child.[14]

NURSING INTERVENTIONS

The woman may feel overwhelmed by her feelings and thoughts during pregnancy. Although the physical changes are visible to and acknowledged by others, the psychologic changes are more hidden, especially if the woman feels guilty about her ambivalent or confused feelings. The nurse should include a discussion of cognitive changes and self-image in prenatal teaching. Whether in one-to-one sessions or in group classes, women and their partners should be encouraged to discuss their ideas and feelings. It is best to discuss these topics with both the pregnant woman and her partner, since the woman's self-image and thoughts and feelings about the pregnancy have a strong impact on this intimate relationship. The nurse must be open and nonjudgmental when the pregnant woman reveals ambivalent or negative feelings about her pregnancy. The nurse also should assess each woman's progress in taking on the mothering role as the pregnancy nears term. This information can be shared with the postpartum nursing staff so that they can continue to encourage discussion in this important area.

Coping and Stress-Tolerance Pattern

The amount of stress in the pregnant woman's life and her ability to cope with stress influences and is influenced by her physical and psychologic adaptations. Every pregnant woman experiences certain stresses as previously discussed. Many women also have one or more ongoing stresses they must continue to struggle with, such as poverty, marital difficulties, or unsatisfactory living or working conditions. Even the so-called normal discomforts of pregnancy, such as fatigue, nausea, or frequent urination, are stresses that call for modifications in the woman's routine.

Anxiety tends to be high in the first trimester as the woman makes her initial adaptations to her pregnancy and anticipated life changes. Feelings of anxiety related to the pregnancy itself tend to decrease during the second trimester and then increase during the eighth and ninth months as labor and delivery become imminent.[2,20]

A pregnant woman's anxieties may be represented in her dreams and fantasies. Many pregnant women report having dreams about their baby being deformed or dead, themselves dying, or a family member being injured. Other women may manifst their anxiety by increased reliance on smoking, drinking, or drug use, all of which can harm the fetus (see following sections on environmental processes). Other women demonstrate their anxieties through psychosomatic complaints and behaviors, such as nausea and vomiting after the first trimester, excessive eating, food cravings, sleeplessness, and fainting.[8]

The fetus definitely is affected by the mother's stress and her responses to this stress. Adrenocorticosteroids produced by the mother may cross the placenta to the fetus. Emotional disturbances and severe fatigue of the mother during the third trimester have been associated with increased motor activity in the fetus and increased irritability, higher heart rate, and gastrointestinal disorders in the newborn.[8] Excessive nausea and vomiting or food cravings for nonnutritious substances can result in insufficient fetal growth.

The pregnant woman may perceive a decrease in her ability to cope with not only the stresses specific to pregnancy but also with the everyday crises and stresses that she has managed in the past. She feels more vulnerable to risk and injury, especially in the third trimester. Her new feelings of ambivalence may make it difficult for her to even know what outcomes she wants from a given situation.

Some women use tension-relieving strategies that they have discovered themselves or they have seen others use, including listening to soft music, laughing it off, crying, sleeping, talking to a friend, meditating, exercising, swearing, and fantasizing. These are all safe for the fetus and can provide relief for many normal tensions and anxieties.

The nurse can play a key role in health promotion related to increasing the pregnant woman's coping abilities, whether in the office or clinic setting or during prenatal classes (see box to the right).

❑ ❑ NURSING INTERVENTIONS TO PROMOTE COPING DURING PREGNANCY

- Supply accurate information about pregnancy, labor, birth, and parenting. For many women this information will dispell some of their fears that are based on lack of understanding or misinformation. Some women may want to read extensively on these topics and should be given a list of resources. Others prefer a verbal method of learning and may need more extensive informational sessions with the nurse.
- Discuss the normalcy of anxiety, fear, and tension during pregnancy. Encourage each woman to express some of her own anxieties and discuss these in detail.
- Be nonjudgmental about a woman's negative thoughts and ideas.
- Support each woman in her self-initiated coping strategies unless they are harmful or potentially harmful to herself or the fetus.
- Monitor each woman's progress in recognizing and coping with the stress in her life.
- Refer the woman who is not developing adequate coping strategies for more extensive psychologic care.

Value and Belief Pattern

Among the many stresses of pregnancy is the shift in values and beliefs that the woman, and many times her partner, experiences. The major transition in role identity during and after pregnancy often necessitates transitions in priorities and values. The woman who has valued her career and economic security may find that she is questioning the importance of these goals. The woman who has had ongoing conflicts with her mother may find that her own ideas are moving closer to those her mother has always professed. She may call or visit her mother more often and find that, for the first time in years, she actually enjoys and respects her mother. The ambivalence of pregnancy is a manifestation of the questioning of goals and values.

Pregnancy has been described as the fulfillment of the deepest and most powerful wish of a woman, an expression of self-realization. Pregnancy also means giving up or delaying certain personal and professional goals and restructuring life to include the child. Her joy in the creative act of producing a child often is accompanied by fear stemming from her feelings of losing part of herself. She gives up some relationships and pleasures to take on other anticipated satisfactions. She may find that she values friendships with other mothers now, whereas in the past many of her friendships focused on work or school. She may find, much to her husband's confusion, that she values different qualities in him than she did before anticipating birth. Her husband is also likely to experience a shift in his values, as discussed later in this chapter.

Pregnant women and their partners also may experience changes in their spiritual values. Conception may be seen as a mystical event or miracle, which may lead to an increased faith in God or a favorite saint. Couples who have not attended church in years may begin talking about affiliating with a church or synagogue after the baby is born because they want religion to be a part of their child's life.

Religious beliefs may influence a woman's decision to undergo certain tests or procedures, such as amniocentesis and abortion. Some women can feel forced to have large families because their religion forbids contraception or encourages large families; each pregnancy may be seen as another unwanted but unavoidable burden.

The nurse can assist the pregnant woman in her exploration of goals and values through discussion during the prenatal period; as always, the nurse maintains a nonjudgmental attitude. If the nurse suspects that a woman's religious beliefs are a source of conflict during this time, she can refer the woman to an understanding minister, priest, rabbi, or elder. Sometimes the conflict has arisen because the woman has actually misunderstood her church's position.

Health Perception and Management Pattern

Women may view pregnancy as an illness, a completely natural healthy state, or a combination of the two. This perception influences her view of her changing body, the usual discomforts of pregnancy, such as fatigue or backache, and her choice of health- or illness-oriented care. The woman who sees herself as ill wants a care provider who will accept this view; the woman who sees herself as healthy and experiencing a normal part of life wants a care provider with a similar outlook. The pregnant woman who sees herself as healthy is likely to have a more positive view of the minor discomforts that can accompany pregnancy and to continue active participation in her family and job. The woman who sees her pregnancy as a time of illness may use this as an excuse to withdraw from her work and personal obligations.

A woman's acceptance of her pregnancy influences her health management practices. The woman who denies she is pregnant or has strong negative feelings about her pregnancy may fail to eat properly, to get enough rest, or to seek prenatal care. The woman who views her pregnancy as illness may refuse to participate in any physical exercise or demand medication for every discomfort. The nurse should be alert to these views and assist the woman to discuss her thoughts.

ENVIRONMENTAL PROCESSES

The drama of the development of a child from a few cells is matched by the all-pervasive changes occuring in the pregnant woman. Her self-concept, coping ability, and basic values and beliefs are changing at a rate she and her partner may find overwhelming. In addition to considering these changes, the nurse must be aware of the many environmental influences that can affect the mother and fetus.

Natural Processes

The outcome of most pregnancies is a whole and healthy infant. Certain genetic abnormalities and environmental hazards can influence the developing fetus, however, causing problems, such as spontaneous abortions and minor or serious congenital defects. Approximately 15% to 25% of all conceptions are spontaneously aborted; 6% to 7% of all live-born infants have congenital defects.[18] The infant also can be injured during the process and interventions of labor and delivery.

Harmful environmental agents, known as *teratogens,* also cause spontaneous abortions or congenital defects either by mutating genes or directly affecting the embryo or fetus. Also, these agents may not cause defects but may be toxic to the fetus. Unlike genetic abnormalities, which occur only at conception, environmental agents can affect the developing infant at any one point or over a period from conception to birth. The type of defect that potentially may occur in the infant depends on when during prenatal development the embryo or fetus is affected. Critical periods of development and the organ that may be affected if exposed to a harmful environmental agent are shown in Fig. 16-5. The first 14 days after conception are thought to be a period of "safety" from teratogenic agents. During this early period the embryo is more likely to be destroyed if it is affected by a potentially harmful agent.

Teratogens have been divided into six groups: (1) infections, (2) maternal disease or metabolic imbalance, (3) drugs, (4) substance abuse, (5) environmental chemicals, and (6) radiation. Each of these groups is discussed further, but first a review of some common prenatal tools used for diagnosing genetic abnormalities or fetal problems is presented.

PHYSICAL FACTORS AND DIAGNOSTIC TOOLS

A number of fetal problems now may be identified before birth through prenatal diagnostic tools, such as amniocentesis, ultrasound, CVS and alpha-fetoprotein (AFP) screening. Certain risk factors, such as family history or maternal age, are indications for their use. Problems that can be assessed include abnormal size or rate of growth of the fetus; chromosomal abnormalities, such as Down's syndrome; sex-linked disorders, such as Fabry's disease; inborn errors of metabolism, such as Tay-Sachs disease, and other disorders, such as neural tube defects and the maturity of fetal lungs. Many fetal problems cannot yet be diagnosed prenatally, however, including 85 to 90 of congenital abnormalities.[2,11]

Amniocentesis is the insertion of a needle into the amniotic sac, usually to withdraw amniotic fluid for diagnostic tests, most often to detect Down's syndrome, especially in the older mother. The test cannot be performed until the second trimester, when the uterus is larger, can be reached through the abdomen, and is filled with amniotic fluid. It is often done at about 16 weeks of gestation and is usually an outpatient procedure. To avoid damage, ultrasound usually precedes an amniocentesis and is also done during the amniocentesis to locate the fetus and placenta. To decrease the possibility of infection, strict sterile procedure is followed.

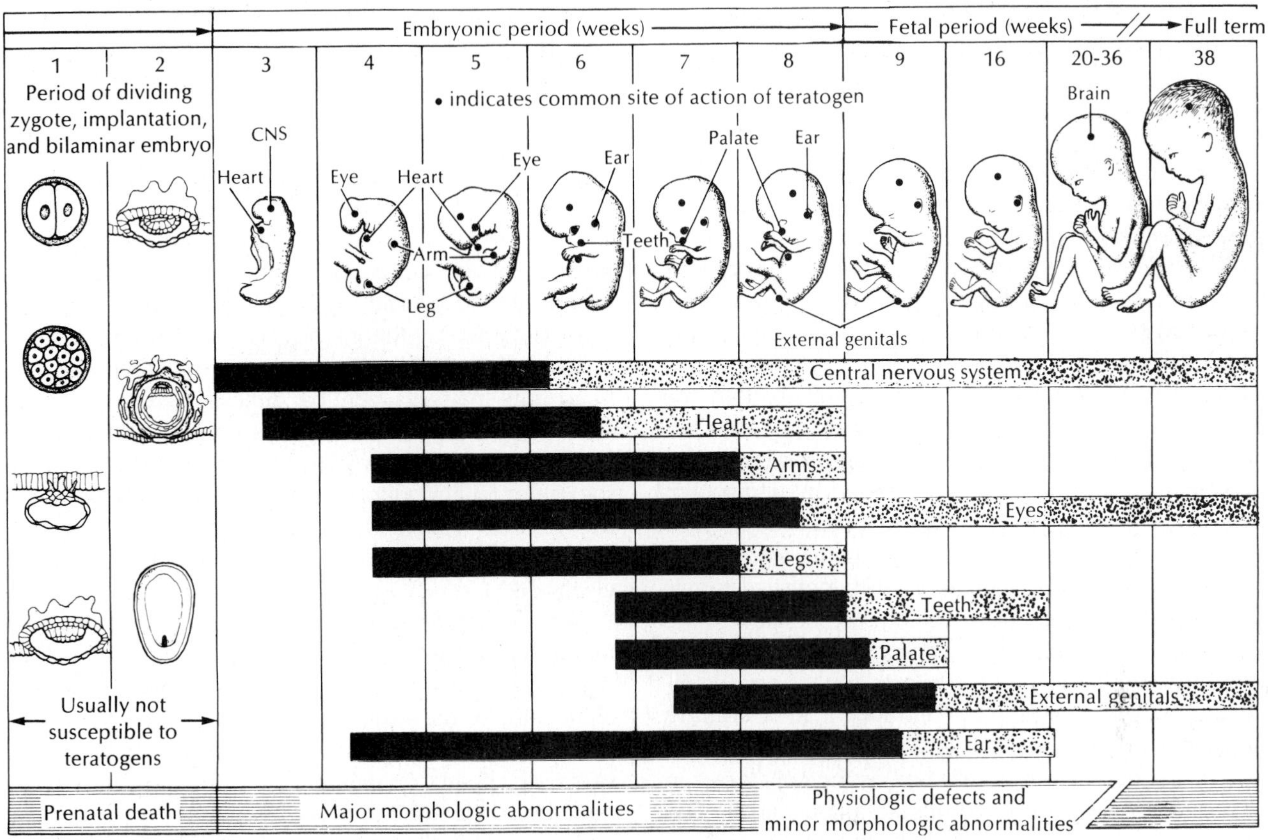

Fig. 16-5. Effects of teratogens on embryo and fetus. Dark areas indicate highly sensitive periods; stippled areas, less sensitive stages. (From Moore KL: *The developing human: clinically oriented embryology,* ed 3, Philadelphia, 1982, WB Saunders.)

Amniocentesis generally is considered safe; however, a 1% risk of a complication to either the mother or the fetus exists. Potential complications for the fetus include abortion, infection, hemorrhage, hematoma, premature labor, amniotic fluid leak, syncope, and fetomaternal blood mixture.

When informing parents of the procedure and receiving their consent, the nurse should be aware of the two areas of main concern: spontaneous abortion and puncturing the fetus. The rate of spontaneous abortion following the procedure is only 0.5% greater than the normal risk. Puncture wounds are also rare; if they occur at all, they tend to be minor.[11] Studies of children whose mothers had second-trimester amniocentesis have found their development and physical findings to be within the expected range.

Ultrasound uses high-frequency vibrational sound waves that pass through soft tissue, are reflected back by structures of different densities, and then are translated into an image of the various structures.[11] Ultrasound frequently is used in obstetrics as a diagnostic tool to confirm pregnancy (as early as five weeks); to localize the placenta before performing amniocentesis and when diagnosing bleeding; to identify multiple pregnancies; to estimate gestational age; to diagnose conditions such as hydatidiform mole, ectopic pregnancy, a few fetal anomalies, or polyhydramnios (large amounts of amniotic fluid) and fetal death; and to evaluate fetal position and presentation. Ultrasound can be done at any time during the pregnancy after 5 weeks of gestation, most frequently as an aid to amniocentesis and to estimate gestational age.

Ultrasound has been regarded as completely safe, noninvasive, and without the risks of radiologic tests. Recently, however, both consumers and health professionals have begun to question the possibility of both short- and long-term risks to the fetus; studies continue looking at the possible biologic effects on children over time. At present, it appears that exposure to diagnostic ultrasound has little or no risk to the mother or fetus.[2,11] The mother's ability to visualize the fetus via ultrasound may actually help maternal-infant attachment.[8]

CVS can detect disorders, such as Tay-Sachs disease, sickle-cell anemia, thalassemia, muscular distrophy, hemophilia, and cystic fibrosis but not neural tube defects. This test is performed between the ninth and twelfth weeks of pregnancy as an outpatient procedure. Chorionic villi are vascular projections from the blastocyst, which connects with the endometrium to form the placenta. A small sample of this tissue is aspirated with a catheter inserted into the uterus via the vagina. The amniotic sac is not punctured. Since this can be done much earlier than an amniocentesis, and requires only 5 to 10 days for a confirmed analysis of the tissue, parents can be informed much earlier in the pregnancy if there is a detectable fetal abnormality. (See box on p. 380.) There is some increased risk of bleeding, cramping, and spontaneous abortion after this procedure.[18]

AFP screening is a widely available method for detecting common congenital malformations of the central nervous system such as anencephaly, spina bifida, and encephalocele. AFP is synthesized in the fetal yolk sac and later in the fetal liver and is present in both the amniotic fluid and maternal blood serum. Maternal serum screening is done at 16 to 18 weeks. It is important to establish an accurate gestational age by ultrasound, since the levels of AFP change markedly during the pregnancy. Since 90% to 95% of infants with neural tube defects are born to parents with negative family and medical histories, this screening test should be done routinely to determine which pregnant women should have amniocentesis, specialized ultrasound, and determination of AFP levels in the amniotic fluid to confirm this diagnosis.[4] Serum AFP levels have a high rate of error and should never be relied on as the only factor in a decision to continue or terminate a pregnancy. The serum AFP is considered to be a screening test only.

The *stress test,* also known as the *oxytocin challenge test (OCT),* is used to evaluate the functioning of the placenta and fetus and to aid in assessing the fetus' ability to develop normally or to cope with the difficulties of labor and delivery. Contractions that are induced by oxytocin or occurring naturally are monitored on an external fetal monitor. Simultaneous tracings of both the contractions and the fetal heart rate are assessed to see how the fetus is coping. An OCT may be valuable in deciding fetal health and the best time for delivery in maternal illnesses or conditions, such as diabetes, pregnancy-induced hypertension (PIH), chronic hypertension, cyanotic heart disease, and chronic illness; in fetal conditions, such as postmaturity or intrauterine growth retardation; or when the mother has had a previous stillbirth.

An OCT may be done once or several times after about 34 weeks of gestation, often on a weekly basis. The risks of an OCT are the possibility of the oxytocin triggering labor and the difficulties that sometimes occur in interpretation.[2,11]

A *nonstress* test is similar to an OCT, but contractions are not induced; the fetal heart rate is monitored under normal circumstances. The indications for a nonstress test are the same as for an OCT; it also is used for the woman who needs assessment but cannot take the risks of an OCT, as in the case of threatened premature labor. The advantages of a nonstress test are its ease of administration and its lack of risks.

Fetal monitoring often is used during labor to assess how the fetus is coping with the contractions of labor. There are two types of monitors: external and internal. The external monitor is attached to the woman's abdomen, whereas the electrodes of the internal monitor are passed through the vagina and clipped to the cervix and the presenting part of the fetus, most often the head. Each of these types of monitors gives simultaneous tracings of the contractions and the fetal heart rate, which can be closely watched for indications of fetal distress caused by the intensity of the contractions.

Problems with monitoring can result because fetal heart rate patterns can be difficult to interpret, and problem patterns do not always correlate directly with fetal distress. Some parents may have concerns about the use of fetal monitoring during labor; both types limit the woman's ability to move freely. Others may be concerned about harming the fetus with the internal electrode.

Not all mothers need fetal monitoring during labor. Many are assessed successfully by auscultation; others may be monitored briefly with a fetal monitoring machine; and some require continuous fetal monitoring. Indications for fetal monitoring include fetal heart rate variations heard on auscultation, meconium staining, maternal conditions such as hypertension or diabetes, and fetal conditions such as postmaturity, abnormal presentations, and small size. Most are the same problems that were indications for OCT.[11]

The pregnant woman may be fearful and confused when the physician says that a diagnostic test is needed during pregnancy. The nurse can assist her by explaining the purpose of the test, describing the benefits and risks in terms of how it can help her and her baby, and supporting the woman during the test.

BIOLOGIC AGENTS

The biologic processes in the environment that can harm the fetus include infections and other health problems of the mother. The mother with a health problem, such as diabetes mellitus, usually is identified and appropriately treated; most persons are aware of the harm the fetus may undergo. The mother with an infection, however, especially a viral one, may not know she has it. If she is ill, she usually does not know the organism causing the illness. This often makes it difficult to identify if the fetus is at risk.

When discussing the effects of biologic processes on the fetus, the nurse must remember to correlate the time of infection or illness with prenatal fetal development to understand the possible congenital defects. Maternal infections occurring during the first trimester of pregnancy often result in severe defects. Infections later in pregnancy also can seriously affect the fetus, but defects of prenatal development are less likely. Fetal death and malformations are related conclusively to certain infections, particularly viral illness. Pregnancy appears to render many women more susceptible to viral illness. Most viruses are subject to placental transfer, and the rapidly developing tissue of the embryo seems to be more vulnerable to viral attack than at later periods of fetal life. Only the infections that tend to cause the most serious problems will be discussed.

Toxoplasmosis is a protozoa that infects persons through undercooked meat and the excretion of cats. The infected pregnant woman may not know she has toxoplasmosis or may have mild to severe upper respiratory symptoms. Most infected fetuses show no signs of the infection at birth. About one in seven infected fetuses will have a serious problem. Infants severely infected usually display such signs as rashes, hepatosplenomegaly, lymphadenopathy, myocarditis, pneumonia, jaundice, and severe central nervous system damage. Some infants show clinical symptoms months or years later, whereas others never have any clinical symptoms. Although this infection is rare, the sequelae to the infant can be so severe that pregnant women should avoid exposure and should be advised to avoid eating raw meat and unnecessarily handling cats or their excretions.

Syphilis is a sexually transmitted disease (STD) caused by the spirochete *Treponema pallidum,* which can be transferred to the fetus of an infected mother. Syphilis is well known as an infection of later pregnancy; although it is preventable and treatable, it still occurs during pregnancy and can remain undetected in the mother throughout the prenatal period. Syphilis affects about 4 in 1000 pregnancies. About 30% of all affected fetuses die, and the symptoms of those who survive vary widely. The infant may be born with localized mucocutaneous lesions, coryza, anemia, and generalized septicemia. Often, however, the infant appears healthy at birth, and symptoms appear during the second to sixth week of life. Occasionally a child survives without symptoms for 2 or more years, when widely varying manifestations of the disease appear. Relating the illness to congenital infection is difficult. The number of infants with congenital syphilis has been reduced by routinely checking for syphilis prenatally and by treating mothers found to have syphilis with penicillin or other antibiotics. Treating and curing the infected mother usually cures the fetus as well if intervention occurs in the first 18 weeks of the pregnancy.[11]

Rubella is a common virus of childhood, although about 20% of women reach their childbearing period without having had it. The symptoms of rubella infection are usually minor, and the mother may think she has a minor virus. However, infection in a pregnant mother in the first trimester can be devastating to the developing fetus, who also may become infected. The organ systems most often disrupted are the ears, eyes, and heart, with deafness the most common clinical manifestation in the infant. Once the fetus is infected, no treatment is available; however, rubella can be prevented. The current program in the United States has children immunized against rubella at 15 months of age and at approximately 10 years of age through the measles, mumps, and rubella (MMR) shot. Adult women who are not sure if they have immunity to rubella either from the immunization or the disease can have rubella titers done. Women with low titers then can be immunized. It is recommended that women not receive their immunization during pregnancy or within 3 months before becoming pregnant because of the chance that the immunization will harm the fetus in the same way the disease does. However, a study of 60 women mistakenly immunized against rubella during early pregnancy found no problems in the infants.[11]

Cytomegalovirus (CMV) is probably the most common infection that has possible serious complications for the fetus. An estimated 1% of all infants born in the United States are infected with CMV. Most mothers infected with CMV have very mild, often nonspecific symptoms. Approximately 10% of infants infected with CMV are born with cytomegalic inclusion disease (CID). The clinical manifestations of CID are very similar to those of toxoplasmosis, such as hepatosplenomegaly, cerebral calcifications, mental retardation, chorioretinitis, deafness, and microcephaly. Deafness has beeen found in as many as 10% of infants with CID. Unfortunately, at present no means exist to prevent or treat this viral infection. It is hoped that in the near future an immunization similar to the one for rubella will be developed.[11]

Herpes simplex virus infections are extremely common in today's society and are asymptomatic in about 90% of cases. However, this infection can be devastating to the newborn. Fetuses infected in utero often are aborted spontaneously or delivered with severe neurologic damage. Infants infected at birth may have localized or disseminated disease with clinical manifestations, including vesicular skin lesions, conjunctivitis, seizures, respiratory distress, gastrointestinal bleeding, and a fatal outcome. Most infants who become infected in the newborn period acquire the virus from the mother's infected birth canal. An infant delivered vaginally to a woman with active genital herpes has about a 40% to 60% chance of being infected. This problem can be greatly reduced by cesarean sections. The difficulty is often in identifying women with genital herpes.[2,11]

Chlamydia, gonococcus, group B streptococcus, and *Candida albicans* may be present in the woman's vagina or cervix and may infect the infant during a vaginal delivery. *Chlamydia,* which may be present in as many as 10% of women in lower socioeconomic groups, can cause conjunctivitis or pneumonia in the newborn. Gonococcus can infect the newborn's eyes and is commonly prevented by treating all newborns with either silver nitrate or erythromycin eye drops at birth. A group B streptococcus can cause septicemia or meningitis. *Candida albicans,* a common vaginal fungal infection, can cause the oral infection thrush in the newborn.[11]

Acquired immune deficiency syndrome (AIDS) is becoming more common among women and should be a focus for screening and counseling before and during pregnancy. Any woman in a high-risk group (i.e., an IV drug user, one who has bisexual partners or who has multiple sexual contacts) should be tested for antibodies to human immunodeficiency virus (HIV). For the woman who is HIV-positive or engaging in high-risk practices, counseling needs to begin before she considers becoming pregnant. Counseling should include both the impact of the virus on pregnancy and the effect of a pregnancy on HIV disease progression. There are many unknown factors regarding HIV and pregnancy. Some of the cautions are based on theoretic risks such as accelerated HIV disease progression during pregnancy because of the altered immune status that is known to occur during pregnancy. A number of risks have been documented. It is certainly possible that some of the early pregnancy discomforts, such as fatigue, anorexia, and weight loss, can mask the early symptoms of HIV infection and thus postpone definitive diagnosis. Also, the treatment of HIV-precipitated infections may be contraindicated during pregnancy and thus force a choice between treatment and continuation of the pregnancy.[10]

Infants born to HIV-positive women have an infection rate of 20% to 50%. Affected infants may not be seropositive for HIV for many months after birth, so it is difficult to determine if an infant has been spared from this syndrome.[10]

Because HIV is often a sexually transmitted disease, affected women should be screened for other STDs. Because of the alteration in immune response, that is, the hallmark of AIDS, the pregnant woman with AIDS or who is HIV-positive should be carefully monitored for the opportunistic infections that frequently occur. The pregnant woman with AIDS or HIV-positive serum should be closely followed by both an obstetrician and an infectious disease specialist. The nurse can be instrumental in assisting this woman to coordinate her many contacts with care providers, answering her questions, and working as a member of the team to provide optimal care for this mother and her child.

The nurse also needs to practice good preventive measures to minimize contact with affected body fluids such as blood, amniotic fluid, and vaginal secretions. Hospitals and birth centers have policies regarding the use of gloves, gowns, and so on, and the disposal of needles and other potentially contaminated equipment. These precautions should be used with all clients, not just those with known HIV disease.[10]

Pregnant women can have any of the infections of nonpregnant women. Since viruses usually can cross the placenta, one may suspect that fetuses are infected by many other viruses with varying results. To date, the viruses causing the common cold are not known to have the teratogenic effects of the infections discussed.[2]

A common symptom of many illnesses is fever. A high fever (*hyperthermia*) over a prolonged period in a pregnant woman can harm the fetus, especially in the first trimester. It must be determined whether the high fever or an underlying illness causing the fever has created the problem. Some reports have found a correlation between prolonged sauna bathing, hyperthermia, and resulting birth defects. The defects from hyperthermia primarily occur in the central nervous system, such as microcephaly, anencephaly, and hypotonia. Miscarriages, stillbirths, and premature deliveries also have been associated with high fever.[11] Until this issue is better understood, the nurse probably should advise pregnant women to avoid prolonged sauna use and high fevers. If a pregnant woman develops a high fever, she should be advised to contact her health care provider.

Immunizations are among the best preventive health care measures. Women may ask about immunizations when they are pregnant because they think they can protect their unborn child or they may need them for travel. Immunizations such as rubella and polio myelitis, however, generally are contraindicated because of the potential although not proved risk to the fetus. Vaccines from killed bacteria (cholera) or toxoids (tetanus and diphtheria) are probably safe, but since no conclusive data yet exist, these immunizations also are not usually given to the pregnant woman. Passive immunization with serum or gamma globulin is safe and not contraindicated if needed.

Pregnant mothers may have other health problems that can alter their own physiologic processes and cause harm to the developing fetus. Two relatively common problems are diabetes mellitus and cardiovascular disease.

Diabetes may be present before pregnancy or may develop during pregnancy, affecting both mother and fetus. Pregnancy increases the need for insulin. Complications from diabetes during pregnancy include polyhydramnios, acidosis, increased incidence of infection, vascular complications, and an increased chance of toxemia. Because of an increased incidence of intrauterine death after 36 weeks of gestation, these infants often are delivered by the cesarean method before 40 weeks. Neonatal complications include hypoglycemia, respiratory distress syndrome, hyperbilirubinemia, and hypocalcemia. These infants of diabetic mothers also have a higher incidence of congenital anomalies, usually one defect, such as a heart lesion or meningocele. Diabetes cannot be prevented, but the pregnant mother with diabetes needs close medical supervision and ongoing health teaching in an effort to control the diabetes as well as possible.[11]

Two major maternal cardiovascular problems that cause concern during pregnancy are heart disease and hypertension. *Rheumatic heart disease* is most common, and the major complications is the possibility that the increasing blood volume will result in congestive heart failure, threatening the mother's life. The fetus may be premature. *Chronic hypertension,* which is more frequent in mothers who become pregnant for the first time after age 30, increases the chance of stillbirths, premature delivery, and the development of preeclampsia, which increases the mortality rate for both mother and infant. Mothers with either of these problems must be monitored closely to prevent potential complications.[8,11]

Finally, maternal-fetal disorders sometimes occur and affect fetal development, such as *Rh-blood-group* incompatibility. The problem usually occurs when the mother has Rh-negative red blood cells and the fetus has Rh-positive blood cells. Maternal antibodies are developed against Rh-positive blood cells, or the major blood types cross the placental membranes and destroy the circulating fetal cells, with devastating effects on the fetus. The severity depends on the mother's isoimmunity and complex, inadequately understood factors, which seem to be best described as maternal idiosyncrasies.[11] The results include varying levels of hyperbilirubinemia and erythroblastosis fetalis.

This problem can be prevented by administering Rh_o (D antigen) immune globulin (RhoGAM), which avoids the mother's sensitization to fetal Rh-negative cells by inactivating fetal red blood cells in the mother before the mother can develop an antibody response. The ideal time to give this to the Rh-negative mother is (1) within 72 hours after delivery of her first Rh-positive infant or (2) after the first miscarriage or therapeutic abortion. The incompatibility does not occur during the first exposure but does later; RhoGAM prevents this from occurring in subsequent pregnancies.[11]

CHEMICAL AGENTS

Drugs ingested by the mother are the major chemicals potentially teratogenic to the fetus. The tragic experience with the tranquilizing drug *thalidomide* in the early 1960s has led to an extremely conservative approach in the administration of any drug for pregnant women. The fact remains, however, that during the most critical early weeks of fetal development, a woman usually is not aware that she is pregnant.

As illustrated by the thalidomide incident, drugs ingested during the first trimester can seriously interfere with normal fetal growth and development. The mechanisms for this is largely speculative. As the fetus matures during the second half of pregnancy, fetal response to drugs that cross the placental barrier seems to resemble more closely the neonate's response. The mechanisms of absorption, distribution, metabolism, and excretion of drug substances occur according to the ability of the fetal organs to perform these functions adequately. Differences in drug action at different fetal stages may depend on the maturity level of interdependent mechanisms developing at different rates during fetal life.[11] Drugs also may alter the placenta itself, or the placenta may react differently to this influence at various stages of pregnancy. The most common drugs that may cause congenital defects include those prescribed for the mother, over-the-counter (OTC) drugs, street drugs, nicotine from cigarettes, caffeine, and alcohol.

Women frequently become pregnant while on medication for other conditions or need to take medications during their pregnancy for health problems. Some of the more common drugs that have been studied for fetal effects include antibiotics, anticoagulants, and anticonvulsants.

Most antibiotics have not been found to harm the fetus. *Tetracycline* given to a pregnant mother between the fourth month of pregnancy and delivery, however, will cause abnormalities in tooth development, including brown spotting and unusual shape. Most teeth affected will be baby teeth, but if the antibiotic is given near the time of delivery, the permanent teeth can be damaged.

The oral anticoagulant *coumadin* has been found to cause defects in the developing fetus, including nasal hypoplasia, small size for gestational age, skeletal defects, retardation, and blindness. Although not normally used in the childbearing years, coumadin may be given to women who have had artificial heart valves or who have thrombophlebitis. A woman taking this drug who is pregnant or trying to become pregnant should discuss this with her physician.

The effects of *anticonvulsants* on the fetus have been well documented. Women with seizure disorders have conceived and carried to term infants while being treated with hydantoin, barbiturates, and other antiseizure medications. Infants born to mothers taking *hydantoin* (Dilantin) may have fetal hydantoin syndrome, with symptoms such as microcephaly, retardation, cleft lip and palate, and congenital heart disease. *Barbiturates,* such as phenobarbital, also are believed to cause retardation and other defects. *Trimethadione* (Tridione) causes spontaneous abortions, stillbirths, and a syndrome of typical malformations in 80% of pregnancies. The fetal trimethadione syndrome includes growth deficiency and mental retardation, with possible cleft lip and palate and heart defects. Women with seizure disorders should discuss their medication needs and other available drugs with their physicians before becoming pregnant and should be closely followed by both a neurologist and an obstetrician throughout their pregnancies.[6,11]

Pregnant women, as do virtually all Americans, frequently choose to treat their minor illnesses with OTC drugs. This is potentially dangerous, since these drugs may cause problems for the fetus. Research on both *acetylsalicylic acid* (aspirin) and *acetaminophen* (Tylenol) has not found these to be teratogenic, although toxic effects may occur. For example, aspirin alters platelet function and can cause maternal and newborn bleeding, and acetaminophen can be toxic to the liver. Certain ingredients in common cold remedies are associated with some birth defects. The antihistamine *chlorpheniramine* has been thought at times to cause polydactyly and gastrointestinal, eye, and ear defects. In general, since any drug has the potential for harming the fetus, all should be avoided during pregnancy.[11]

The nurse should include information on the known and probable effects of medications on the fetus in prenatal teaching. Most pregnant women who are aware of the risk to their baby will avoid medications not essential to their own welfare. (See box on p.380)

Drug abuse, including narcotics, tranquilizers, cocaine, amphetamines, marijuana, and others, is a serious health problem to both the mother and the unborn child. Again, all these drugs cross the placenta and can harm the fetus. The narcotics *heroin* and *methadone* cause problems, such as prematurity, intrauterine growth retardation, respiratory distress at birth, fetal addiction in utero, and neonatal withdrawal at birth. Signs of narcotic withdrawal in the newborn include tremors, irritability, hyperactivity, vomiting, diarrhea, sweating, poor feeding, and possibly convulsions. A neonatal syndrome similar to narcotic withdrawal has been reported in newborns whose mothers have taken tranquilizers, such as *diazepam* (Valium). No evidence suggests withdrawal in infants whose mothers took *cocaine* or *amphetamines,* although some animal experiments suggest that these drugs are teratogenic. *Marijuana* often is used during pregnancy, and studies have shown no fetal effects, although immunologic defects have been reported. To avoid these problems, nurses must recognize women who are drug abusers and help them seek appropriate help. This can be difficult, since drug abusers often try to hide this and are unable to change their lifestyle without extensive intervention.

Many women in today's society regularly drink *alcohol.* Alcohol crosses the placenta and reaches the same blood levels in the fetus as in the mother; it has been clearly shown to affect the developing fetus. Studies have divided maternal drinking into the following categories, with associated fetal risks:

1. "Regular" social drinking (two or more drinks daily)
   Intrauterine growth retardation
   Increased risk of anomalies
   Increased risk of stillbirth
   Decreased placental weight
   Behavioral decrements in newborn and infant
2. "Binge" drinking (five or more drinks on occasion)
   Structural brain abnormalities
3. Very heavy drinking
   Fetal alcohol syndrome

Fetal alcohol syndrome (FAS) (see box on p. 380) was described first in the literature in the early 1970s, although this has been mentioned throughout history. A typical facial appearance and retardation are common findings in the FAS child. Mothers-to-be frequently ask how much alcohol is safe; the answer is not yet known. Since alcohol is a teratogen, with devastating results at high levels of intake, most health professionals now believe women should avoid all alcohol during pregnancy. Since serious harm occurs during the first trimester and often earlier, women who are trying to conceive may choose to avoid alcohol even before they know they are pregnant.

Cigarette smoking by pregnant mothers has been shown since the 1940s to cause fetal problems. Today, the effects of maternal smoking are known to include an increase in rate of spontaneous abortions, low birth weight for age, preterm delivery, placenta previa, abruptio placenta, vaginal bleeding, congenital anomalies, and premature rupture of the membranes. All these can put the fetus at risk for illness or death. Long-term sequelae may include learning difficulties in the school years. Many women ask how much they can smoke when pregnant. The more the woman smokes, the more harm to the infant. Studies generally define "heavy smoking" as more than a pack of cigarettes a day. The best advice for pregnant mothers or women considering pregnancy is not to smoke at all, which can be very difficult to the woman who has smoked for a long period and has a serious habit. The nurse can play a major role in preventing potential problems to the fetus by supporting and helping a pregnant woman to stop smoking.[2,3] Some suggestions of the Florida and American Lung Association that the nurse can offer to help the woman decrease and ideally stop smoking include the following:

1. Extinguish each cigarette after the first puff, then relight.
2. Smoke cigarettes only halfway down.
3. Buy only packs, not cartons.
4. Buy one pack at a time.
5. Change brands each pack.
6. Refuse any cigarette offered, saying, "My baby and I don't smoke."
7. Never keep your cigarette in your hand; put it down after each puff.

8. Do not empty your ashtrays for a week.
9. Wrap your cigarette pack in paper and record on the paper each cigarette smoke, the time of day, and your activity at the time. This will increase your awareness of when and where you smoke.
10. When you have the urge to smoke, try an alternate activity (e.g., exercising, visiting or phoning a friend, or pursuing a hobby).

Caffeine is another common drug found in coffee, cocoa, tea, cola, or chocolate. Mutations have been found to occur in laboratory animals from moderate amounts of caffeine, but no mutations, congenital defects, or cancers have been discovered in human beings. Studies have implicated excess caffeine intake during pregnancy, however, with problems such as spontaneous abortions, stillbirths, and prematurity. Excess caffeine was defined in one study as more than 600 mg per day, or eight cups of coffee or more per day. Although more research is needed, in general moderate caffeine is allowed, whereas excess caffeine is discouraged.[2,11]

Most environmental chemicals that are potentially teratogenic to the fetus have only been tested in the laboratory on animals, so their teratogenicity may not be completely known. Some natural substances found to be teratogenic in animals but not necessarily in human beings include insect and bacterial toxins; insecticides; herbicides; and fungicides, including DDT (dichlorodiphenyltrichloroethane). Polychlorinated biphenyls (PCBs) were found to cause a brown staining in infants of Japanese mothers who mistakenly ingested it in cooking oil. Studies on metals have found arsenic, nickel, and cadmium to be teratogenic only in animals, but mercury and lead are teratogenic to human beings. After pregnant Japanese mothers ingested fish contaminated with methyl mercury, an epidemic of infants born with cerebral palsy and microcephaly occurred. Some studies have reported stillbirths, abortions, and mental retardation in fetuses exposed to lead. This area needs much more study. In general, nurses should advise mothers to avoid environmental chemicals. Unfortunately, the mother may not even know she has come in contact with anything unusual.[11]

The final time the fetus may encounter drugs through the mother is at delivery. Women are again delivering their infants with no drugs or with as few as possible. Since understanding of specific drug actions remains limited, only a few drugs are used during labor and with varying degrees of confidence. Drugs administered during labor affect the fetus primarily by exaggerating the degree of fetal asphyxia or by influencing the rate and quality of the infant's recovery, adaptation, and neurologic behavior. Studies of visual attentiveness, sucking behavior, and neurologic and electroencephalographic features suggest that depressant effects may last as long as 4 days after birth.[11]

One of the nurse's roles during labor and delivery is to monitor the effect of any drugs on the fetus. The nurse should be familiar with the drugs administered to the mother and should use knowledge of fetal effects to care for the infant after delivery; any therapeutic agent has a potential for adversely affecting the fetus and newborn. In addition, carefully documented observations of infants exposed to maternal drugs during labor contribute significantly to understanding long-term effects of drugs.

MECHANICAL FORCES

In general, mild to moderate trauma from minor injuries to the abdomen rarely injures the fetus, who is well protected by the amniotic fluid. Major trauma such as a severe car accident, however, may cause problems. The nurse should advise the woman to wear both a lap belt and shoulder harness when in a car.[2]

The uterus is another mechanical force that may affect the fetus. Near the end of pregnancy, the fetus outgrows the uterus and becomes molded by it. This may be more pronounced in a multiple pregnancy. Positional deformities, usually of the head or extremities, may result. Most deformities return to normal either naturally or with some repositioning. Some children have congenitally dislocated hips because of this type of positioning. Since there is no prevention, the neonate needs to be examined closely for positional effects and parents reassured about the infant's future appearance.[17]

A final mechanical force the fetus must cope with is labor and delivery–opening the cervix and passing through the narrow vagina. Actually, very few newborns are injured in this process, and those who are usually recover with no sequelae. Some of the more common injuries that occur from birth trauma are[2,8]

1. *Molding*–a change in the shape of the newborn's head to match the birth canal shape and allow its passage. This is possible because of incompletely fused sutures.
2. *Caput succedaneum*–edema of the scalp from the head pushing against and dilating the cervix.
3. *Cephalhematoma*–blood from ruptured vessels collected under the skull.
4. *Forceps marks*–abrasions caused by the pressure of either forceps or the bones of the mother's pelvis.
5. *Subconjunctival hemorrhages*–capillaries in the sclera of the eyes rupture from changes in the neonate's intracranial pressure during delivery.
6. *Fractures* may occur from the general trauma. Common sites are clavicle, humerus, femur, and skull.
7. *Paralysis* of areas from nerve damage can occur, including brachial plexus palsy; resulting in limited use of an arm, and facial paralysis, with one-sided decreased tone and movement. Both are temporary problems.

8. *Other injuries* that are less common include central nervous system damage, intracranial hemorrhage, and spinal cord injury.

These traumas are often difficult to predict and prevent. However, some infants at risk for trauma, such as those who are extremely large or those who require a forceps other than the low forceps for delivery, are now being identified. Cesarean section is considered a safer method of delivery.

RADIATION

It is generally thought that the pregnant woman should not be exposed to x-rays unless the information is critical to the health of the mother or child. The potential dangers from diagnostic radiation are chromosomal changes and malignancy. Studies suggest that the chance of chromosomal changes increases in children of mothers who have received significant amounts of radiation to the ovaries. A few studies have shown this relationship with Down's syndrome. Several reports have found that diagnostic radiation during pregnancy is absorbed by the fetus and that the children later in life have an increased chance of developing malignancies. One report found the incidence of leukemia in children of women exposed to x-rays during pregnancy was three times greater than in other children.[11]

The National Council on Radiation Protection and Measurements has made recommendations concerning the exposure of pregnant and potentially pregnant women to radiation, including when radiologic studies should be done, how they should be carried out, and what protection should be provided.

Social Processes

ROLE AND RELATIONSHIP PATTERN

The "pregnant family," as it sometimes is called, is in a state of change throughout the pregnancy and the postnatal period as each person explores the meaning of new roles. Role relationships are also in flux as each member explores the interaction of the new role with the changed roles of other family members.[2] A pregnant woman without a partner may feel quite isolated during her pregnancy. She may look to family members or friends to fill new roles as she adjusts to her new situation.

The partner or husband of the pregnant woman faces many new situations; his partner may seem very different to him because of her own emotional response to this pregnancy, her introspection, her fantasies, her need for more rest, and her change in sexual drive. He may feel a rivalry with the fetus and later the baby because of the woman's need and desire to divide her time. He may resent the attention his partner receives during the pregnancy and the additional demands she may make on his time. He may experience more financial pressure because of the anticipated needs of the baby and the partner's need to stop work on a short- or long-term basis. He may undergo pressure to assume a more "adult" manner of living by giving up favorite hobbies or activities that his society views as dangerous or frivolous. A major concern may be his ability to fulfill the "father" role, or he may be confused about exactly what this role entails. His role models for fathering may be limited because he lives away from extended family and associates mainly with other men his own age who are not fathers. He may never have even held a baby before and may worry that he may drop or harm his own child. If his wife is ill during the pregnancy or experiencing complications, he may feel guilty about having started the pregnancy. Table 16-5 gives a more complete list of both the father's and the mother's emotional responses to a first pregnancy. Adjustments during subsequent pregnancies probably are greatly influenced by adaptation to the first pregnancy and experiences as first-time parents.[20]

The father often thinks that he must hide his own apprehensions and fears about his new role because he is expected to be strong and supportive of his partner during this time. The nurse needs to encourage the woman and her partner to talk about their needs, their ideas about their changing roles, and their apprehensions. Some prenatal classes include this type of discussion as an essential part of the preparation for a successful pregnancy,[2] and it is as essential as discussing the physical changes during pregnancy.

Other children in the family also experience role change during and after the pregnancy. The very young child, while not having a concept of "new baby" until he or she arrives, may experience a change in interaction with the mother, who may have less time for playing or be more irritable because of her fatigue. Later in the pregnancy, the types of activity the child and mother enjoy together may change. The mother may limit or stop active play because of her increased awkwardness. Once the baby arrives, this child may be kept away from both baby and mother by well-meaning friends and relatives. When permitted to see the newborn, the child may be constantly admonished to "be careful," "don't touch the baby," and "be quiet." The child also quickly comes to realize that he or she must share his parents with this new arrival. It is thus understandable that he or she may not accept the baby with open arms. Sibling relationships are discussed more fully in Chapter 18.

The older child better understands the newborn's significance but still experiences apprehensions about the effects on him or her and the family. Since he must share his or her parents with one more person, the older child may wonder if his or her parents will have time for

***Table 16-5.* Possible responses to first pregnancy**

Phase of pregnancy	Fathers' responses	Mothers' responses
First trimester	Fear of losing wife or child Self-doubt as a future father	Loss of interest in coitus Less sexual affectiveness Sleepiness and chronic fatigue Nausea Increased dependence
Second trimester	Increased respect, awe as quickening comes Name for fetus coined	Solemnity, hilarity, playfulness about fetal movements Talk about and with fetus: "*We're* going shopping" Increased eroticism
Third trimester	Fear of coitus harming fetus Abstinence difficult Envy and/or pride at wife's creativity Worry over birth Keen awareness of male/female differences	Lessened sexual activity Continence (often recommended by physician) Sleepiness Backache Abdominal discomfort Sexual isolation Heightened sense of femininity
Postpartum	Eagerness to resume marital relations Concern over endangering wife's recovery Sense of triumph in becoming a father Tenderness toward mother and baby	Pain and fear of harm from too early coital resumption Low eroticism Concern about husband's continued abstinence, often suggested by physician for 6 weeks after baby's birth Sense of completion as a mother
Pregnancy as a whole	Increased romanticism Increased nurturance Increased participation in family life Anxiety about costs Concern about lack of skills in baby care	Increased romanticism Increased optimism Family roles replacing marital emphases Fear of miscarriage, malformations, and/or death of baby Pride in accomplishment

Adapted from Duvall E: *Marriage and family development,* ed 6, New York, 1990, Harper & Row.

him. The older child may have been told that he will be a "big brother" now: does this mean he must give up his toys and his room and share his friends? He also may wonder at the changes in his mother, who seems more tired, less available, and perhaps even "sick" at times. Her enlarging abdomen may appear frightening.

The pregnancy can be a difficult time for children in the family, or it can be an exciting time of learning and growing. What happens depends heavily on the parents. The nurse can help parents make this a positive experience for the siblings (see box to the right).

Although the extended family does not usually live together in American society, the expectant grandparents also experience changes during the pregnancy of their daughter or daughter-in-law. The maternal grandmother, seeing her daughter assume the mother role, may view her daughter as more of a rival now that they are both mothers. The grandparents may be reminded of their own aging, resenting when their advice about pregnancy and parenting is unheeded. A positive outcome of the pregnancy may be a new closeness between a woman and her mother if the daughter turns to her mother to seek advice and share feelings. The nurse can encourage expectant parents to realize that this is also a transition time for their own parents.

Each family member also begins to establish an emotional attachment to the fetus or the imagined new baby. Maternal attachment to the fetus has been studied more than that of other family members. Deep feelings of attachment to the fetus and adjustment to the pregnancy

❑ ❑ NURSING STRATEGIES TO HELP PARENTS PREPARE SIBLINGS FOR THE NEONATE

- Explain the pregnancy and birth in a way appropriate to the child's age.
- Answer the child's questions.
- Encourage discussion and questions by talking about the new baby at relaxed family times rather than at busy, rushed times.
- Have the child participate in decisions, such as names for the baby, clothes, and toys.
- If sibling classes are available as part of the childbirth education process, encourage the parents and child to attend.
- Suggest that the child go to clinic or office visits with his mother.
- Allow and discuss negative comments about the pregnancy or baby.

have been shown to correlate with the mother's attachment to the child in the postpartum period. Studies suggest that strong social support is a major factor in the woman's development of high levels of attachment to her fetus. In working with pregnant families, the nurse needs to assess[13]

1. The woman's feelings of support from her family
2. The impact of the pregnancy on the woman and her family
3. Conflicts the woman and family experience in regard to their new roles
4. Coping strategies of family members
5. Information the family needs to facilitate role transition and relationships

COMMUNITY AND WORK

The woman with an outside job must ask several questions when considering pregnancy:

1. Is her work strenuous and possibly dangerous to the fetus?
2. Does the job involve exposure to toxic substances that could be teratogenic to the fetus or stimulate premature termination?
3. Does she work double shifts or unusually long shifts that will interfere with needed rest?
4. Does her job involve exposure to viruses or other organisms that may be harmful to the fetus?

If the workplace is safe, does not involve exposure to hazardous substances or organisms, and provides adequate breaks, the pregnant woman can continue to work unless her health becomes impaired. Most women choose to continue working throughout most of their pregnancy. Some will encounter social pressure at the workplace to stop working or take a less visible position because their changing bodies cause embarrassment to supervisors or other employees. Some employers because of a bad experience with other pregnant women, may fear that their pregnant employee will overuse sick time or seek a reduced work load. The pregnant woman must deal with these specific situations by being factual and assertive about her ability to continue her work. If a woman believes she has been unfairly treated because of her pregnancy, she can pursue the issue through a local women's rights organization. If she thinks her work situation is hazardous to her pregnancy, she may negotiate for a different type of job within that organization or seek other employment. Changing places of employment during a pregnancy may mean giving up accrued leave time or taking a lower salary. The woman needs to weigh these against the hazards of her other job and make the best decision for herself and her child.

Workplaces vary greatly in allowing leave time during and after pregnancy. Ideally, a woman has explored this when she interviewed for this particular job, but many women do not consider this until they are already pregnant. A woman often needs written verification from her physician that she needs leave time. Although she may plan to return to work shortly after delivery so as not to lose seniority or for some other reason, the woman should be counseled to allow sufficient time to regain her strength and prepregnant sense of well-being. She may not realize the demands of infant care, especially the night awakenings. The nurse can help women make reasonable decisions related to working by pointing out potential hazards in the workplace and providing information about the demands of child care. The nurse also may give clients copies of the recommended standards for maternity care and employment of the U.S. Children's Bureau. These are recommendations and thus not binding on employers but may be helpful to the woman in negotiating safer conditions or leave time.

CULTURE AND ETHNICITY

Every cultural group has specific ideas and beliefs related to pregnancy, childbirth, and childrearing. The nurse and other health care providers must be aware of the beliefs of their client's particular group to provide appropriate, usable information. Childbearing concepts generally focus on four aspects of a cultural system:

1. *Moral and value system.* What are the duties and obligations of each person involved in this pregnancy, birth, and childrearing? Who monitors this system? What are the repercussions for deviating from expected norms?
2. *Kinship system.* What are each person's rights, duties, and obligations based on their relationships to each other?
3. *Knowledge and belief system.* How does this culture define and understand the process of conception, labor, and delivery?
4. *Ceremonial and ritual system.* Which rituals or ceremonies are seen as essential to the child's acceptance into the family and community? Who must perform these rituals? Do the requirements of a particular prenatal care setting or hospital interfere with these rituals?

Information and advice given to the pregnant couple should be based on their cultural background. The nurse has an obligation to seek out information on the cultures represented in the community through community ethnic organizations, individuals from the community, and culturally focused professional literature.[2,8] Above all, the nurse must be open to a variety of viewpoints, judging them not against personal beliefs but in relation to the general concept of health promotion. Before approaching the family, the nurse must consider the following questions on culturally determined behaviors specific to the pregnancy and birth:[2,8]

1. Who may have a child? How often?

2. Who may father a child?
3. Is birth control permitted?
4. Is sexual activity limited during pregnancy?
5. What is acceptable behavior during labor?
6. Who may be present during labor and delivery?
7. Are certain foods restricted during pregnancy?
8. Who cares for the child?

The nurse also must determine how engrossed the woman is in her culture. Does she think that some or most of the childbearing ideas of her culture are "old fashioned" but feel obligated to follow them, at least superficially, because of family pressure? Since this can be a very difficult situation, the nurse can sometimes be a confidant for the woman who needs to vent her frustrations about cultural restrictions.

LEGISLATION

Both legislative actions and societal movements influence childbearing. In some countries, the government decrees how many children a couple may have and imposes economic or social sanctions to enforce these restrictions; although this is not true in the United States, the general societal trend is to have smaller families, and specific groups lobby strongly for restriction of family size.

The U.S. federal government is concerned about the health of pregnant women and decreasing fetal and infant morbidity and mortality. Through Medicaid, Title V maternal and child health grant money is awarded to states or districts to upgrade services for pregnant women and children. The money available for a given year is determined by the current administration and varies greatly from one to another. Many community health centers depend totally on this federal money and are forced to close or drastically reduce services when less money is allocated at the federal level. Local health departments usually offer free or low-cost prenatal care; the extent of services offered depends on state government allocation of funds.

The nurse should keep informed and inform pregnant clients about pending legislative action on health care issues related to the childbearing family. A well-written letter from a nurse to the local representative can influence decisions on health care issues. Clients also should be encouraged to express their views and questions to their representatives.

ECONOMICS

When the pregnant woman begins prenatal care, personal financial resources can influence the kind of care she receives, whether she works during or after a pregnancy, her acceptance of a pregnancy, her nutritional status, and many other aspects. The expenses of the pregnancy itself may be the determining factor in putting the woman or her family in a financial crisis. If the pregnancy was planned, finances should have been considered in making the decision, but this is not always true.

The nurse should inquire about finances so that she can make appropriate suggestions to each family. The Title V maternal-child programs or the local health department may be a resource for families. Many low-income women qualify for the WIC program, the U.S. Department of Agriculture's supplemental feeding program for women, infants, and children. This program provides such essential foods as milk, cheese, and eggs to the pregnant and lactating woman. The nurse may be able to assist with planning a budget for food and other essential needs based on what the individual family members need for good health rather than what they are in the habit of eating. Cultural practices also must be considered. Local food banks and secondhand clothing and baby supply stores may provide needed items for these families.

Many women are hesitant to discuss financial need. The nurse must inquire in a caring, sensitive manner and offer suggestions as she would for other needs of the pregnant woman.

HEALTH CARE DELIVERY SYSTEM

Options for care during pregnancy range from medical-based care by an obstetrician or general practitioner to more health-focused care by a nurse or lay midwife. A few women will choose to have their child assisted only by an untrained family member or friend, but this is uncommon. A woman's choice of care can be influenced by geographic availability of options, finances, previous experience, partner's preference, cultural or social acceptability of certain options, and preexisting or newly recognized risk factors.

A woman can also choose where she will labor and deliver and how much intervention she desires. The movement toward home births that began in the early 1970s continues and is seen as a more family-oriented, natural, health-focused experience. Some couples consider home delivery but choose a hospital because of available emergency equipment and personnel in case of unexpected complications. Some insurance will only cover hospital deliveries. In-hospital delivery can be in the traditional delivery room or the more homelike birthing room. The woman also may choose to go home within a few hours after the birth or to stay for several days. Pros and cons exist for both hospital and home deliveries. The nurse can help pregnant couples become aware of care and delivery alternatives available to them so that they can make an informed choice.

Among the other options available to the pregnant woman is the actual style of laboring and delivery. She may choose natural childbirth or a method of analgesia or anesthesia, as based on the methods available in her community. The nurse can assist the pregnant woman and her partner to choose the most appropriate method by providing information about all options in the community and encouraging questions about each.

Prenatal classes that focus on individual styles of laboring and birthing are a valuable resource for many pregnant families. The International Childbirth Education Association and many local groups offer a variety of classes for the expectant family (see box below) generally including the following:

1. *Early pregnancy* classes involve one or two sessions in the first trimester and focus on fetal development, physical and emotional changes during pregnancy, and resources in the community.
2. *Childbirth* classes during the third trimester focus on preparation for and progress of labor and delivery. Specific techniques of Lamaze, Bradley, or others are taught.
3. *Cesarean birth* classes are similar to childbirth education but are geared to the woman anticipating this form of delivery.
4. *Sibling* classes focus on a specific age range and introduce the siblings to the pregnancy and birth experience.
5. *Postnatal* classes focus on the basics of infant care.

The nurse can assist a woman or couple to assess their needs and choose the appropriate care options for them. The well-informed woman or couple can plan a childbearing experience that satisfies their needs and desires and is a safe, healthy experience for them and their baby.

Nursing Interventions

Probably the most important aspect of nursing care during the prenatal period is appropriate teaching. The assumption that a mother who is experienced or well educated understands and knows all that she needs to know about her own care during pregnancy is fallacious and can be dangerous to the infant's well-being.

To provide appropriate teaching, the nurse must perform comprehensive *assessment*. This first step in the nursing process allows the nurse to determine maternal and fetal physical and psychologic risk factors and the woman's information or misinformation about pregnancy and birth.

Various guides for assessment of the pregnant woman are available; a comprehensive one is shown in the box on p. 403. This data can be gathered over several visits. Table 16-6 outlines risk factors that the nurse should look for in the assessment; the nursing actions or indications for referral should be adapted for each client.

After the assessment is complete, the nurse can arrange a *teaching plan* for the client. If the woman will be attending group prenatal classes, the nurse should coordinate her teaching with what is covered in the classes so that undue repetition does not occur. The nurse teaching prenatal classes should give a list of topics to students so they can share these with their own health care providers. A client may be very knowledgeable in some areas, but rather than deciding this woman does not need prenatal teaching, the nurse should develop a more individualized program for her. Topics covered in prenatal teaching sessions include[2,8]

1. Interpretation of physical findings and laboratory results
2. Value of keeping appointments
3. Danger signs that should be reported
4. Breast care
5. Breastfeeding versus bottlefeeding
6. Exercise and activity
7. Clothing
8. Fetal growth and development
9. Physical and psychologic changes during pregnancy
10. Discomforts of pregnancy and relief measures
11. Effects of smoking, drinking, and drugs on the fetus

RESEARCH REVIEW — PRENATAL

PRENATAL EDUCATION

Taren DL, Graven SN: The association of prenatal nutrition and educational services with low birth weight rates in a Florida program, *Public Health Rep* 106:426-436, 1991.

Purpose The purpose of this study was to determine the influence of prenatal care on a woman's risk of having a low birth weight (LBW) infant.

Review A total of 9014 prenatal charts were included in a retrospective chart review. Demographic data were recorded for age, race, marital status, and county of residence. Prenatal care program included education on early signs of preterm labor, blood test for hemoglobin, use of iron-vitamins-calcium supplements, record of dietary recall, and seeing the same clinician at least 75% of the prenatal visits. Education on early signs and symptoms of preterm labor and screening for anemia were highly associated with fewer LBW infants, after controlling for other factors. Such care is critical if the United States is to achieve its objective of no more than seven infant deaths per 1000 live births by the year 2000.

❑ ❑ PRENATAL ASSESSMENT GUIDE

Aspects of adaptation

Age
Initial response to pregnancy
Planned or unplanned pregnancy
Feelings about pregnancy
Desired family size
Perception of pregnancy affecting present activities and responsibilities
Perception of parenthood affecting future activities and plans
Current developmental task of pregnancy; coping mechanisms, fantasies about pregnancy, changes in mood and effect on others
Sexual functioning during pregnancy; changes, feelings, problems
Nature of verbal interest expressed about self and fetus
Preparations for prenatal classes (type, when completed), place of delivery, other children in mother's absence, and new sibling
Menstrual history: problems, last normal menstrual period, expected date of confinement
Height and prepregnancy weight
Past obstetric history: dates, course, outcomes
Present obstetric status: course, abdominal assessment, quickening fetal heart sound, blood pressure, urinalysis, weight and pattern of gain, signs of any major complications of pregnancy
Past medical history: illness, date, treatment, outcome, surgery; childhood diseases; current immunization status; allergies; venereal disease; emotional problems
Family medical history: illnesses, emotional problems, genetic defects (both sides of family)
Loss of significant other in past year
Food intolerances (lactose, nausea and vomiting), food cravings, and pica
Iron-vitamin-mineral dietary supplements used
Elimination patterns: changes, problems with remedies used
Pattern of rest, sleep: difficulties, remedies used

Aspects of personal belief system and lifestyle

Date first sought prenatal care this pregnancy and in prior pregnancies
Reasons for seeking and receiving prenatal care
Beliefs about pregnancy and childbirth; cultural beliefs about childbearing (antepartum, intrapartum, postpartum)
Racial, ethnic group
Beliefs about role of father during pregnancy and labor and in child care
Perception of needs of fetus
Perception of needs of infant and proposed methods to meet these needs
Contraceptive history: methods used, failures or problems, knowledge of alternate methods, willingness to use

Aspects of personal belief system and lifestyle–cont'd

Patterns of use of tobacco, alcohol, prescription and nonprescription drugs, illegal drugs; perception of effects on health of self and fetus
Patterns of nutrient intake: food dislikes, history and method of dieting
Planned method of infant feeding; why chosen
Occupation: present, former, how long, work requirements, hazards, amenities, plans regarding current occupation
Recreational activities: plans to continue, use of seat belt in car, pets in home
Community activities
Perception of and prior experiences with health care personnel and agencies
Date of last physical examination, including breast examination, Pap smear, chest x-ray films, dental checkup
Breast self-examination done regularly; if not, interested in learning about?

Aspects of support

Address: how long there, housing accommodations, phone, plans to move (when, where, why?)
Level of education and future plans regarding
Religious preference; normal or active involvement
Marital status; years married
Father of baby; age, occupation, educational level, racial and ethnic group, religious preference
Family composition: household members
Communication patterns with significant others
Communication patterns with health personnel
Perception of support system (mate, family, friends, community agencies) available and willingness to use
Perception of meaning of this pregnancy to significant others; mate's response to news of pregnancy
Type of prenatal service receiving and perception of its adequacy
Available transportation
Social service and community agencies involved with: how long and contact person
Self-concept and perceived ability to cope with life situations
Body-image concept: prepregnant and current; response to physiologic changes of pregnancy
Mate's response to body changes in pregnancy
Feelings about parenting woman received as a child; history of separation from mother
Prior experiences with infants; knowledge of infant care
Feelings about previous pregnancies, labor, puerperium, and mothering skills
Knowledge of reproduction, labor and delivery, and puerperium

Adapted from Becker C: Comprehensive assessment of healthy gravida, *Obstet Gynecol Nurs,* p 376, Nov/Dec 1982.

***Table 16-6.* Characteristics of high-risk families during pregnancy**

Possible high-risk emotional behaviors	Possible problem	Nursing role
Pregnant woman		
Nausea and vomiting continue beyond first trimester	Possible rejection of pregnancy; depending on severity, can become hyperemesis gravidarum	Observe and assess severity of symptoms Note any indications of rejection of pregnancy or other emotional stress; inform physician Assists clients with decreasing vomiting and stress When advanced, help maintain food and fluid needs
Number of abortions before current pregnancy	Habitual abortion, which may have some basis in severe rejection of pregnancy	Explore client's feelings toward this and previous pregnancies when appropriate; convey information to physician Assume supportive role indicated by psychiatric assessment
Physical signs of toxemia, increased blood pressure, increased weight, edema, dizziness, albuminuria, and so on	Combination of physical and mental stress resulting in toxemia (etiology unclear); can be enhanced by emotional stress	Explore family situation to detect possible areas of emotional stress, such as marital problems, financial stress, overwork, poverty, and so on Assist family in lessening stress and provide emotional as well as physical rest
Extreme anxiety over pregnant state, childbirth, and so on	Misconception, unconscious conflicts, and lack of information	Offer explanation of pregnancy and childbirth processes and assist mother and family in coping with anxiety Provide opportunity to attend classes, obtain literature, and explore feelings openly
Verbal indication of inability to relate to new baby or expression of severe emotional deprivation and harsh discipline as a child	Possibility of child battering or neglect or less-than-optimum relationship with new child	Observe family situation and relate information to physician and childbattering team if applicable Makes arrangements to explore further on postpartum unit and in early home situation
Expression of difficulty in accepting maternal role or no evidence of taking in or taking on this role	Difficulty in mothering	Explore client's view of pregnancy Help client find opportunity to work through her negative feelings Relate problems to obstetrician and psychiatrist if indicated List follow-up observations on the postpartum unit to determine status
Evidence of attempted abortion	Rejection of pregnancy and mothering	Maintain nonjudgmental attitude, listen to client, and assist in eliminating guilt Refer to obstetrician and psychiatrist for evaluation and possible therapy or therapeutic abortion
Sleeplessness, excess irritability, anxiety, excessive depression or excitement, suspiciousness, preoccupation with trivia, and tense agitation	Psychoses of pregnancy; usually occurs postpartally and is estimated to occur in 1 of every 400 to 1000 pregnancies	Relate symptoms to obstetrician and encourage pregnant woman to seek psychiatric help

***Table 16-6.* Characteristics of high-risk families during pregnancy–cont'd**

Possible high-risk emotional behaviors	Possible problem	Nursing role
Fetus		
Signs of fetal distress, such as extreme hyperactivity, failure to thrive, and increased heartbeat	Possible response to severe emotional stress in mother or family situation	Relay observations to obstetrician Explore with pregnant woman possible areas of stress Help reduce stress
Husband		
Extreme nonacceptance of mother's changes during pregnancy, with lack of support to mother and mother's increased stress because of this attitude	Misunderstanding, lack of maturity, or inability to be father figure	Explore problems and misconceptions and provide anticipatory guidance and support so father can support mother Encourage seeking help from obstetrician, psychiatrist, or family counselor as indicated
Indications of nonacceptance of role of father or background indicating possible child battering	Nonacceptance of father role; possible faulty relationship to child, resulting in battering or neglect	Explore problems and give support in minor situations; if possibility of severe situation, refer to childbattering team or psychiatrist
Children (expectant)		
Regressive behavior, change in behavior, emotional anxiety (assessed in regard to age and normal areas of stress)	Fear of replacement or change in environment because of room or bed change and/or parent's stress	Anticipatory guidance *before* occurrence Plan with parents considering age and individuality of child so as to decrease amount of stress child experiences

Adapted from Littlefield V: *Emotional considerations for the pregnant family.* In Clausen J, et al, editors: *Maternal nursing today,* New York, 1976, McGraw-Hill.

12. Nutrition
13. Rest
14. Work
15. Body mechanics
16. Personal hygiene
17. Sex during pregnancy
18. Specific preparation for labor and birth
19. Superstitions and old wives' tales
20. Signs of impending labor
21. Supplies and preparations for the baby
22. Husband's responses
23. Siblings' responses

Many of these general categories are discussed along with nursing interventions earlier in this chapter. It is often helpful to prepare basic handouts detailing such information as danger signals during pregnancy so that each woman can post these at home.

SUMMARY

Pregnancy is a time of dramatic change; a new life is forming and developing, and the "pregnant family"–mother, father, siblings, and other close members–are all experiencing major changes in their roles and relationships with each other. Although all fetal development, changes in pregnant women's bodies, and role transitions among family members share common elements, each pregnancy is a unique experience for that individual family. The client is the pregnant family, even though the nurse most often deals directly with the pregnant woman. The nurse provides valuable resources and information that the family can use to meet their specific needs. The nursing goal is to assist each family to have a healthy pregnancy.

References

1. Apgar V: Proposal for a new method of evaluation of the newborn infant, *Curr Res Anesthesiol Analg* 38:260, 1953.
2. Bobak I, Jensen M, Zalar M: *Maternity and gynecological care: the nurse and the family,* St Louis, 1989, Mosby.
3. Castiglia PT, Harbin RE: *Child health care: process and practice,* Philadelphia, 1992, JB Lippincott.
4. Cohen F: Neural tube defects: epidemiology, detection, and prevention, *J Obstet Gynecol Neonat Nurs* 16(2):105, 1987.
5. Committee on Nutritional Status During Pregnancy and Lactation: *Nutrition during pregnancy,* Washington, DC, 1990, National Academy Press.
6. Conley N, Olshansky E: Current controversies in pregnancy and epilepsy: a unique challenge to nursing, *J Obstet*

Gynecol Neonat Nurs 16(5):321, 1987.

7. Guyton AC: *Textbook of medical physiology,* ed 8, Philadelphia, 1991, WB Saunders.
8. May KA, Mahlmuster LR: *Comprehensive maternity nursing,* ed 2, St Louis, 1990, JB Lippincott.
9. Mercer R: *First time motherhood: experiences from teens to forties,* New York, 1986, Springer Publishing.
10. Minkoff H: Care of the pregnant woman infected with human immunodeficiency virus, *JAMA* 258(19):2714, 1987.
11. Pritchard JA, MacDonald PC, Gant N: *William's obstetrics,* ed 18, Norwalk, Conn, 1989, Appleton-Century-Crofts.
12. Rubin R: Attainment of the maternal role, part 1, processes, *Nurs Res* 16:237, 1963.
13. Rubin R: Attainment of the maternal role, part 2, models and referrants, *Nurs Res* 16:342, 1967.
14. Rubin R: Binding in the post-partum period, *Maternal-Child Nurs J* 6(2):67, 1977.
15. Rubin R: Fantasy and object constancy in maternal relationships, *Maternal-Child Nurs J* 1(2):101, 1972.
16. Rubin R: Maternal tasks in pregnancy, *Maternal-Child Nurs J* 4:143, 1975.
17. Schuster CS, Ashburn SS: *The process of human development: a holistic life span approach,* ed 3, New York, 1992, JB Lippincott.
18. Stringer M: Chorionic villi sampling: a nursing perspective, *J Obstet Gynecol Neonat Nurs* 17(1):19, 1988.
19. US Department of Health and Human Services, Public Health Service: *Healthy people 2000: National Health Objectives,* Washington, DC, 1991, US Government Printing Office.
20. Walken LO: *Parent-infant nursing science: paradigms, phenomena, methods,* Philadelphia, 1992, FA Davis.
21. Worthington-Roberts B, Vermeersch J, Williams S: *Nutrition in pregnancy and lactation,* ed 4, St Louis, 1989, Mosby.

CHAPTER

17

Infancy*

Susan Pennacchia

Objectives

After completing this chapter, the nurse will be able to

- *Define the infant's health status and give examples of basic growth and developmental principles.*
- *State the developmental tasks for the infant and the behavior that indicates these tasks are being met.*
- *Interpret the immunization schedule and other safety and health promotion measures to a parent.*
- *Discuss the nurse's role in promoting parental attachment and preventing child abuse.*
- *Identify common parental concerns regarding infants and describe a model for parent education to allay these concerns.*
- *Describe accidents that occur during infancy and appropriate counseling for accident prevention and safety.*
- *List several characteristics of the infant that may be risk factors and contribute to health problems.*
- *Specify ways in which nurses can be active in making major policies and influencing legislation concerning health.*
- *Compare and contrast the mortality statistics between white and nonwhite races and discuss reasons for the differences.*
- *Describe governmental strategies to meet goals of improving infant health.*

As this text's focus has shown, an increasing emphasis on providing nursing services to improve, maintain, and promote health has been a major change in health care delivery. The belief that health is the right of all people rather than a privilege granted to some has served as a catalyst to expand health care systems and begin to focus on health early in the life cycle.

This chapter focuses on the infant and family during the infant's developmental period of 1 to 18 months. Since the infant is totally dependent for a time, this chapter addresses the infant's parents and significant others in terms of health promotion activities. The relationship initiated at birth between parents and infant is the basis for the interdependence required for the proper psychologic and physical development of the infant. Thus health care professionals need to focus on parent education as a means of fostering healthy, satisfying relationships within the family unit and promoting the development of healthy future generations.

The principles of normal growth and development are

*Material in this chapter related to the prevention or treatment of cancer was contributed by Marilyn Frank-Stromberg and Rebecca Cohen.

HEALTHY PEOPLE 2000

SELECTED NATIONAL HEALTH PROMOTION AND DISEASE PREVENTION OBJECTIVES

INFANCY

- Reduce growth retardation among low-income children ages 5 and younger to less than 10%. (Baseline: up to 16% among low-income children in 1988, depending on age and race or ethnicity.) *Note:* Growth retardation is defined as height-for-age below the fifth percentile of children in the reference population of the National Center for Health Statistics.
- Reduce iron deficiency to less than 3% among children ages 1 through 4. (Baseline: 9% for children ages 1 through 2.) *Note:* Iron deficiency is defined as having abnormal results for 2 or more of the following tests: mean corpuscular volume, erythrocyte protoporphyrin, and transferrin saturation.
- Increase to at least 75% the proportion of parents and caregivers who use feeding practices that prevent baby bottle tooth decay.
- Reduce nonfatal poisoning to no more than 88 emergency department treatments per 100,000 people. (Baseline: among children ages 4 and younger 650 per 100,000 in 1986 to 520 per 100,000 in the year 2000.)
- Increase use of occupant protection systems, such as safety belts, inflatable safety restraints, and child safety seats, to at least 85% of motor vehicle occupants. (Baseline: children ages 4 and younger, 84% in 1988 to increase to 95% by the year 2000.)
- Reduce the prevalence of blood lead levels exceeding 15 μg/dl and 25 μg/dl among children ages 6 months through 5 years to no more than 500,000 and zero, respectively. (Baseline: an estimated 3 million children had levels exceeding 15 μg/dl, and 234,000 had levels exceeding 25 μg/dl in 1984.)
- Reduce the infant mortality rate to no more than 7 per 1000 live births by the year 2000. (Baseline: 10.1 per 1000 live births in 1987.)
- Increase to at least 90% the proportion of babies ages 18 months and younger who receive recommended primary care services at the appropriate intervals.
- Increase immunization levels as follows: basic immunization series among children under age 2, at least 90%. (Baseline: 70% to 80% estimated in 1989.)

used as a structural framework for this chapter. Understanding these principles assists the nurse to identify deviations from the norm and to institute appropriate preventive measures.

To promote and maintain health during infancy, a balance between the infant's internal and external environmental forces must exist; any disruption places the infant in jeopardy. Several processes that greatly influence this balance are identified, and appropriate nursing interventions are outlined to assist the nurse in promoting a healthy infant population. (See the box above.)

PHYSIOLOGIC PROCESSES

Age and Development

Human development begins when a single sperm penetrates a mature ovum. Even though this event of conception occurs without notice, the developmental changes that follow are undeniable and wondrous.

After conception, nothing can be added to or subtracted from the individual's hereditary endowment. The belief that a mother can make her unborn child brilliant by devoting her time to intellectual activities simply is not true. On the other hand, if she establishes a favorable prenatal environment for her unborn child through good physical health and healthy attitudes, the chances of a favorable development are greatly increased. The box shown on pp. 409 and 410 presents an overview of infant growth and development, with special recognition of expected landmarks.[46,67]

During this early period of growth and development the infant totally depends on others within the environment to meet all personal needs. The major resources to meet these needs are the parents. To assist the parents in their understanding of their infant's progress, the nurse must know what behaviors to expect at certain

❑ ❑ GROWTH AND DEVELOPMENT DURING INFANCY (LANDMARKS INDICATED BY ITALICS)

1 month

Follows and fixes on bright object with eyes when it moves within line of vision
Still has head lag when pulled into sitting position
Displays tonic neck, grasp, and Moro reflexes
Turns head when prone but unable to support
Displays sucking and rooting reflexes
Holds hands in fists
Makes small, throaty sounds
Gains 5 to 7 ounces weekly for 6 months
Gains 1 inch monthly for 6 months
Cries when hungry or uncomfortable
Lifts head momentarily when prone

2 months

Posterior fontanel closed
Listens actively to sounds
Lifts head almost 45 degress off table when prone
Follows moving object with eyes
Recongizes familiar face
Pays attention to speaking voice
Assumes less flexed position when prone
Vocalizes; distinct from crying
Turns from side to back
Social smile appears

3 months

Visually inspects objects and stares at own hand with apparent fascination when it appears in field of vision
Has longer periods of wakefulness without crying
Laughs aloud and shows pleasure in vocalization
Holds head erect and steady; raises chest, usually supported on forearms
Smiles in response to mother's face
Begins prelanguage vocalizations–coos, babbles, and chuckles
Carries hand or object to mouth at will
Actively holds rattle but will not reach for it
Turns eyes to object placed in field of vision

4 months

Begins drooling, indicating appearance of saliva; does not know how to swallow it
Holds head steady when in sitting position
Recognizes familiar objects
Shows almost no head lag when pulled to sitting position
Rolls from back to side and abdomen to back
Inspects and plays with hands; pulls clothing or blanket over face in play
Begins eye-hand coordination
Chews and bites
Enjoys social interaction
Demands attention by fussing
Reaches out to people
Aware and interested in new environment
Grasps objects with two hands
Squeals

5 months

Reaches persistently; grasps with whole hand
Plays with toes
Smiles at mirror image
Begins to postpone gratification
Shows signs of tooth eruption
Sleeps through night without food
Weight is twice the birth weight
Sits with slight support
Vocalizes displeasure when desired object taken away
Able to discriminate strangers from family
Makes cooing noises
Squeals with delight
Looks for object that has fallen
Rolls from back to stomach or vice versa

6 months

Gains about 3 to 5 ounces weekly during the second 6 months
Grows about ½ inch monthly for 6 months
Able to lift cup by handle
Begins to "hitch" in locomotion
Sits in highchair with straight back
Begins to imitate sounds
Vocalizes to toys and mirror image
Babbles with one-syllable sounds: "ma; mu; da; di"
Has definite likes and dislikes
Likes to be picked up
Plays peek-a-boo
Makes "guh, bah" sounds

7 month

Eruption of upper central incisors
Bears weight when held in standing position
Sits, leaning forward on both hands
Fixates one very small object
Produces vowel sounds: "baba; dada"
Shows fears of strangers
Displays emotional instability by easy and quick changes from crying to laughing
Repeats activities that are enjoyed
Bangs objects together
Approaches toy and grasps it with one hand
Imitates simple acts

8 months

Feeds self with finger foods
Sits well alone
Stretches out arms to be picked up
Greets strangers with bashful behavior
Begins to show regular patterns in bladder and bowel elimination
Responds to "no"
Makes consonant sounds: *t, d, w*
Dislikes dressing and diaper change
Releases objects at will
Shows nervousness with strangers
Pulls toy toward self

Continued.

❑ ❑ GROWTH AND DEVELOPMENT DURING INFANCY (LANDMARKS INDICATED BY ITALICS)—cont'd

9 months

Creeps and crawls (backward at first)
Shows good coordination and sits alone
Responds to adult anger; cries when scolded
Explores objects by sucking, chewing, and biting them
Responds to simple verbal requests
Drinks from cup or glass with assistance
Pulls self to standing position
Begins to show fears of going to bed and being left alone
Imitates waving "bye-bye"
Releases objects with flexed wrist
Repeats facial expressions of adults
Uses thumb and index finger in pincer grasp

10 months

Sits by falling down
Says "da-da," "ma-ma"
Understands "bye-bye"
Looks at and follows pictures in book
Crawls and cruises about well
Pays attention to own name
Picks up objects fairly well
Extends toy to another person without releasing
Pulls self to standing position and stands while holding onto solid object

11 months

Able to push toys and place several objects in container
Attempts to walk without assistance
Begins to hold spoon
Stands erect with help of person's hand
May have lower lateral incisors erupting
Holds crayon to mark on paper
Imitates definite speech sounds
Reacts to restrictions with frustration

12 months

Babinski's sign disappears
Hand dominance becomes evident
Weight is triple the birth weight
Head and chest equal in circumference
Walks with help
Knows own name

12 months–cont'd

Slow vocabulary growth because of increased interest in walking
Lumbar curve develops
Uses spoon in feeding but often puts it upside down in mouth
Drops objects deliberately for them to be picked up
Shakes head for "no"
Plays pat-a-cake
Recovers balance when falling over
Tries to follow when being read to
Does things to attract attention
Imitates vocalization head

15 months

Creeps up stairs
Uses "da-da" and "ma-ma" labels for correct parents
Tolerates some separation
Drinks from cup well but rotates spoon
Asks for objects by pointing
Plays interactive games such as peek-a-boo and pat-a-cake
Expresses emotions; has temper tantrums
Walks without help

18 months

Anterior fontanel closed
Trunk long, legs short and bowed, abdomen protruding
Walks up stairs with help
Turns pages of book
Has short attention span
Begins to test limits
Has bowel movements when placed on potty at appropriate time
Indicates wet pants
Gets into everything
Fills and handles spoon without rotating it but spills frequently
Runs clumsily and falls often
Is extremely curious
Places objects in holes or slots
Becomes communicative, social being
Imitates behavior of parents, such as mimicking household chores

age levels. These developmental landmarks serve as a basis for giving parents anticipatory guidance regarding their infant (Table 17-1). Parents must be aware of age-appropriate behavior so they can anticipate and help facilitate these developmental landmarks. This knowledge, along with the nurse's anticipatory guidance, can promote closer family relationships.

In addition to the growth and developmental aspects, the infant must achieve several developmental *tasks* to facilitate a healthy personality progression.

DEVELOPMENTAL TASKS

Everyone faces developmental tasks in the course of growth and development and must accomplish them individually. Different practices in various societies affect the perception and resolution of the tasks, but all must be faced.[33]

The infant's first and most basic task is survival, which includes the physical tasks of breathing, sucking, eating, digesting, eliminating, and sleeping. Since many of these tasks involve the infant's mouth, this stage of life is

Table 17-1. **Parenting tasks for developmental landmarks in infancy**

Age (months)	Landmark	Parenting task
1	Lifts head when prone	Place infant in prone position and dangle colorful object above head
2	Social smile	Promote by talking to infant and allowing opportunity to smile
4	Squeals	Encourage and praise for doing
5	Rolls from back to front	Place infant in protected area (crib, playpen) and encourage to move by placing toy out of reach
8-9	Uses pincer grasp to feed self cracker	Make finger foods available
10	Pulls self to standing position	Provide safe environment: place chair or object of appropriate height in reach
11-12	Initiates vocalization	Talk to infant frequently and include in family gatherings
12-15	Walks	Encourage and provide clutter-free, safe walkway; praise for attempts
15	Drinks from cup	Supply cup with appropriate drink; do not scold for clumsiness in handling cup or spills
18	Mimics household chores	Give rags to help with dusting, allow to fold clothes, and so on

often referred to as the *oral stage* of development, reflecting the primary importance of the mouth as the center of pleasure. Duvall[17] outlines several more developmental tasks that need to be accomplished in infancy:

1. Achieve physiologic equilibrium after birth.
2. Establish self as a dependent person but separate from others.
3. Become aware of the alive versus inanimate and familiar versus unfamiliar, and develop rudimentary social interaction.
4. Develop a feeling of and desire for affection and response from others.
5. Manage the changing body and learn new motor skills, develop equilibrium, begin eye-hand coordination, and establish rest-activity rhythm.
6. Learn to understand and control the physical world through exploration.
7. Develop a beginning symbol system, conceptual abilities, and preverbal communication.
8. Direct emotional expression to indicate needs and wishes.

To assist the infant's parents in encouraging achievement of these developmental tasks, the nurse should discuss the importance of stimulation and environmental interactions. Recent information indicates that genetic potential, in terms of the development of the anatomic structures of the brain, is not reached at birth; many such structures are far from complete.[41] To continue growing, the brain depends not only on internal, embryologic, and maturational forces, but also on the interaction of external stimulation with these forces. Such stimulation, as provided by the mother, is necessary for a child to develop fully. This external stimulation seems to influence the internal, anatomic, and maturational processes by at least three different mechanisms:[11]

1. Stimulation favors progressive complex aborization of dendrites (the connection between nerve cells).
2. Stimulation increases the degree of vascularization of certain anatomic structures of the brain, such as the centers associated with vision.
3. Stimulation increases the process of myelinization, which is closely related to the rate of development of a variety of functions. (Myelin coats the brain and nerve tissue, which then become activated.)[32]

When counseling parents, the nurse should stress the importance of a variety of stimuli within the infant's environment. Several auditory and visual stimuli should be available (colorful mobile, television, radio, spoken voice, toys) to assist the infant in achieving developmental tasks. The sense of touch is an extremely important stimulus, bringing the infant in tune with the external environment and thus making it a reality. These parenting tasks are vital to the infant's developmental progression.[25]

CONCEPTS OF INFANT DEVELOPMENT

The study of how a helpless infant grows and develops into a fully functioning, independent adult has fascinated many researchers, including Lawrence Kohlberg, Erik Erikson, and Jean Piaget. Their theories present human development as a series of overlapping stages that occur in somewhat predictable patterns in an individual's life.[10] Since these developmental theories are presented in previous chapters, only specific application to the infant is discussed here.

Kohlberg is a leading theorist in the area of *moral* development. He states that moral development is prefaced by the child's ability to reason and thus follows a sequence that corresponds with the development of intellect. Moral development is not a component of the infant's emotional-social development (see Chapters 18 and 19).

Psychosocial Development. Erikson's psychosocial developmental theory is primarily concerned with a series of tasks or crises that each individual must resolve before going on to the next one. The central task during infancy is the development of a sense of *trust versus mistrust*. Establishing this basic trust or mistrust determines how the infant approaches all future stages of growth. The infant first develops a sense of trust in the mother or caretaker and then other significant persons in the environment. The infant's future relationships will be characterized by this trust, allowing for deeper commitments and intimacy. The infant needs maximum gratification and minimum frustration to provide the balance between inner needs and outer satisfaction, which results in development of trust.

Prompt, skillful, and consistent response to the infant's needs help in fostering security and trust; the mother essentially is relieving the infant's tension. Part of developing trust depends on the infant's ability to predict what will happen within the environment. If no predictability and disorganized routines exist, the infant will develop fear, anger, and insecurity, which lead eventually to mistrust.

The infant can show wants by crying but depends on the sensitivity and willingness of others to provide them. If the most important persons fail to do this, the infant has little foundation on which to build faith in others or self when adulthood is attained.

Cognitive Developments. Piaget's *cognitive* developmental theory focuses on intellectual changes, which occur in a sequential manner as a result of continuous interaction between the infant and the environment.[56] Piaget's *sensorimotor period* (up to age 18 months) describes the infant involved in mastering simple coordination activities to interact with the environment. The infant solves problems using sensory systems and motor activity rather than the symbolic processes that develop later.

Research has shown that fetuses are able to distinguish light from dark and that sight is present at birth. The rod cells in the retina of the eyes, which are responsible for light perception, are functional at birth; the retina, the organ of visual perception, is not fully developed until about 4 months of age. The infant, however, can perceive color and shape. Since infants startle in response to loud noises and quiet down in response to soft voices, their sense of hearing also is functioning. This can be tested with audiologic equipment at birth. Babies cry when stuck with a diaper pin and fuss when too hot or too cold; thus the senses of pain and temperature are operative as well. Touching, stroking, and rocking typically soothe a fussing infant. Infants also will react to different odors and tastes.

In addition to perceiving stimulation, the newborn is capable of reflexive behavior. Reflexes are responses normally exhibited after a particular type of stimulation.[51] They are unlearned, since the response occurs the first time following the stimulus. Some infant reflexes have survival value, such as the rooting and sucking reflexes. The rooting reflex, activated by lightly stroking the angle of the lips or cheek, helps the infant locate the food source. The infant will turn toward the side that is stroked and open the lips to suck. The sucking reflex is initiated when an object is placed in the infant's mouth. Together these reflexes ensure that the infant can obtain food. Infants also have reflexes for grasping, yawning, hiccoughing, coughing, and sneezing.

Armed with these reflexes and sensory capabilities, the infant is ready to begin interacting with the environment–seeing, hearing, touching, tasting, and smelling to acquire valuable information.

The infant progresses in various ways between birth and age 18 months, with early capabilities changing and becoming more intentional. Piaget outlines five stages within the sensorimotor period that describe the infant's development from the early reflexive behavior to differentiation between self and environment (see Table 17-2).

***Table 17-2.* Piaget's five stages of infant development**

Stage	Description
Stage 1: birth to 1 month	Modification of reflexes: —infant practices and perfects reflexes present at birth —sucking reflex becomes more refined and voluntary
Stage 2: 1 to 4 months	Primary circular reactions: —infant repeats behavior that previously led to an interesting event —activities involve only the infant's own body
Stage 3: 4 to 10 months	Secondary circular reactions: —repetitions involve events or objects in the external world —infant seems to perform actions with purpose —beginning of hand-eye coordination
Stage 4: 10 to 12 months	Coordination of secondary reactions: —infant combines two or more previously acquired strategies to obtain a goal
Stage 5: 12 to 18 months	Tertiary circular reactions —infant uses active experimentation to achieve previously unattainable goals —purposely varies movements to observe results

The infant in the sensorimotor period uses behavioral strategies to manipulate objects, to learn some of their properties, and to obtain goals by combining several behaviors. The infant's behavior is tied to the concrete and the immediate; schemes can only be applied to objects that can be perceived directly.

Knowledge of the two child developmental theories is extremely valuable to the nurse who interacts with infants. Understanding the infant's level of cognitive thought and emotional and social development helps the nurse to decipher a child's communications more meaningfully and interpret behaviors and the processes that motivate them more accurately. This knowledge can be incorporated in the nurse's anticipatory guidance to the parents. The nurse should stress that a variety of sensory and motor stimuli will foster learning within the infant's environment.

DENVER DEVELOPMENTAL SCREENING TEST

This test (DDST) is a standardized tool that screens for developmental problems in children from birth to 6 years old. The original DDST underwent revision and restandardization and was released in 1990 as the Denver II. Three purposes have been identified for administering the Denver II:

1. Screening apparently healthy infants for developmental problems
2. Validating intuitive concerns about an infant's development with an objective test
3. Monitoring high-risk children for developmental problems[21]

Four areas of development are screened: personal-social, fine motor-adaptive, language, and gross motor. Unique features of the Denver II are its recent and sophisticated standardization and its inclusion of norms for various subgroups based on place of resident, ethnicity, and mother's education.

The Denver II includes four "test behavior" descriptors to rate the infant's behavior during the test. This rating reflects the screener's subjective impression of the infant's overall behavior. Behavior ratings are made for compliance with examiner's requests, alertness and interest in surroundings, fearfulness, and attention span.

Although administration of the DDST is not difficult, only nurses or other personnel trained specifically in its procedures and interpretation should attempt it. This precaution is necessary to ensure the validity of the developmental norms established for the test.

The mother should be told before the test that it is not an intelligence test but a test of the child's developmental level. By adding the number of accomplished and unaccomplished items on the test form (Fig. 17-1), the screener makes an estimate of the child's developmental level. The child is scored *P* (passed) or *F* (failed) on each item by referring to guidelines on the instruction sheet (Fig. 17-2). The DDST can be administered with minimal materials and time. Ideally it should be administered to an infant at about 3 or 4 months of age, again at 10 months, and again at 3 years.[47]

The infant's growth index is also important. Physical growth (height and weight) is a valid health-status indicator that should be measured at each routine office or clinic visit. During the first year of life growth is very rapid. An infant who is growing properly is at low risk of developing a chronic disease.[57]

The nurse should plot an infant's length and weight measurements against exact chronologic age on growth grids. In 1986 the National Center for Health Statistics (NCHS) published growth grids, that have been standardized (Figs. 17-3 and 17-4) to present growth charts for female and male infants from birth to 36 months.

An infant's growth index, as determined by length and weight, is only one factor in assessing health status. The nurse needs to have an overall understanding of growth development principles to counsel parents regarding their infant's progress (see Tables 17-3 and 17-4).

Sex

The infant's sex is usually determined at the moment of fertilization. The parents usually first ask, "Is it a girl or a boy?" The answer has far-reaching effects for many family units. The infant's sex is one of the many important factors that influence the parent's way of relating to the infant to create a healthy environment (Fig. 17-5).

Studies have revealed many biologic and behavioral differences between male and female infants. Males are on the average larger and have proportionately more muscle mass at birth. Female infants are generally smaller but physiologically more mature at birth than males and are less vulnerable to stress.[43] Males show more motor activity, whereas girls display a greater response to tactile stimulation and pain.[2] As the infant develops, further differences are noted. By 6 months, females respond to visual stimulation with longer attention spans and are more socially responsive than boys; they also tend to sit up, walk, and crawl earlier than boys. Female infants develop language earlier and respond better than boys to speech. Thus from an early age females learn to communicate with language, whereas males use their bodies.[51]

The sex of the infant, a major concern of expectant parents, may well influence parental relationships and expectations. The infant's sex may evoke disappointment; a woman may feel disappointed in a girl primarily because she knows that her husband wanted a son. Today the trend is to produce one or two children–one of each sex–and provide for them. Since the birth rate is down in comparison to the 1950s and inflation rates are up, families are having fewer children. One can see the importance and stress of producing the "right sex" infant. Being the "wrong sex" can combine with other

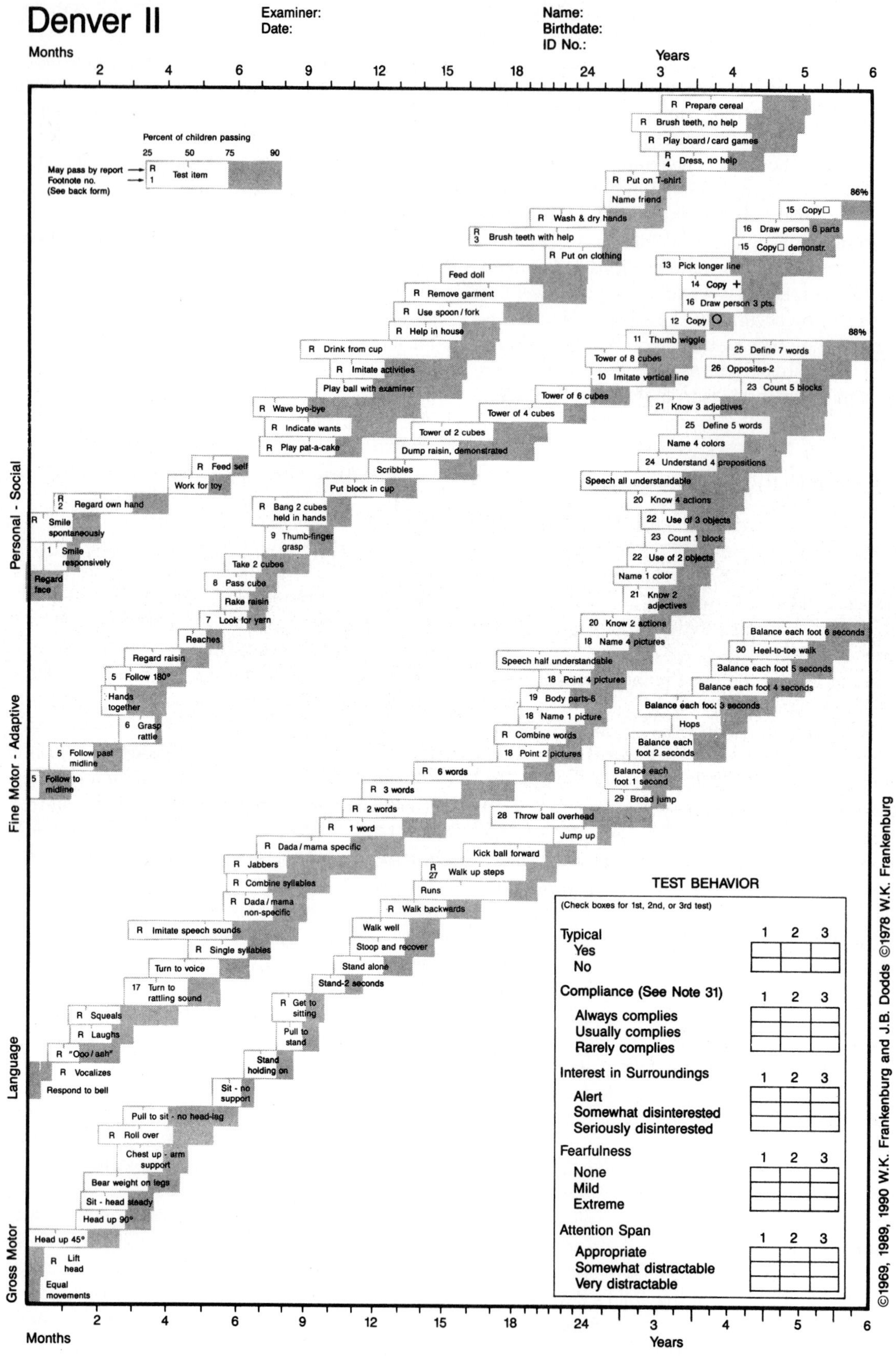

Fig. 17-1. The Denver II. (Courtesy WK Frankenburg, JB Dodds, University of Colorado Medical Center, Denver, 1990.)

1. Try to get child to smile by smiling, talking or waving to him. Do not touch him.
2. When child is playing with toy, pull it away from him. Pass if he resists.
3. Child does not have to be able to tie shoes or button in the back.
4. Move yarn slowly in an arc from one side to the other, about 6" above child's face. Pass if eyes follow 90° to midline. (Past midline; 180°)
5. Pass if child grasps rattle when it is touched to the backs or tips of fingers.
6. Pass if child continues to look where yarn disappeared or tries to see where it went. Yarn should be dropped quickly from sight from tester's hand without arm movement.
7. Pass if child picks up raisin with any part of thumb and a finger.
8. Pass if child picks up raisin with the ends of thumb and index finger using an over hand approach.

9. Pass any enclosed form. Fail continuous round motions.

10. Which line is longer? (Not bigger.) Turn paper upside down and repeat. (3/3 or 5/6)

11. Pass any crossing lines.

12. Have child copy first. If failed, demonstrate

When giving items 9, 11 and 12, do not name the forms. Do not demonstrate 9 and 11.

13. When scoring, each pair (2 arms, 2 legs, etc.) counts as one part.
14. Point to picture and have child name it. (No credit is given for sounds only.)

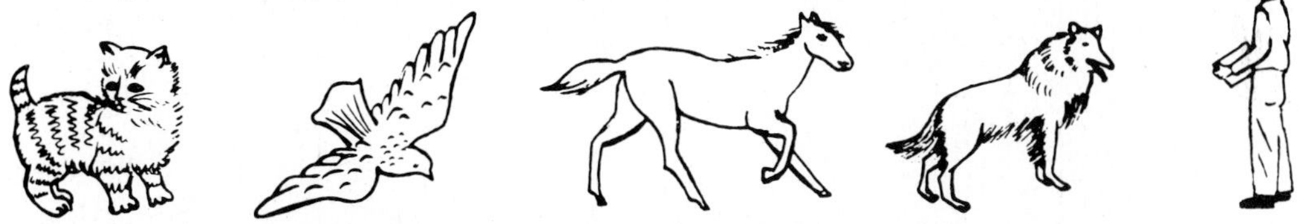

15. Tell child to: Give block to Mommie; put block on table; put block on floor. Pass 2 of 3. (Do not help child by pointing, moving head or eyes.)
16. Ask child: What do you do when you are cold? ..hungry? ..tired? Pass 2 of 3.
17. Tell child to: Put block <u>on</u> table; <u>under</u> table; <u>in front</u> of chair, <u>behind</u> chair. Pass 3 of 4. (Do not help child by pointing, moving head or eyes.)
18. Ask child: If fire is hot, ice is ?; Mother is a woman, Dad is a ?; a horse is big, a mouse is ?. Pass 2 of 3.
19. Ask child: What is a ball? ..lake? ..desk? ..house? ..banana? ..curtain? ..ceiling? ..hedge? ..pavement? Pass if defined in terms of use, shape, what it is made of or general category (such as banana is fruit, not just yellow). Pass 6 of 9.
20. Ask child: What is a spoon made of? ..a shoe made of? ..a door made of? (No other objects may be substituted.) Pass 3 of 3.
21. When placed on stomach, child lifts chest off table with support of forearms and/or hands.
22. When child is on back, grasp his hands and pull him to sitting. Pass if head does not hang back.
23. Child may use wall or rail only, not person. May not crawl.
24. Child must throw ball overhand 3 feet to within arm's reach of tester.
25. Child must perform standing broad jump over width of test sheet. (8-1/2 inches)
26. Tell child to walk forward, 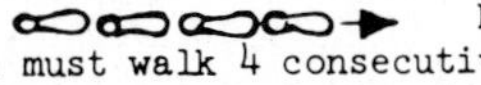 heel within 1 inch of toe. Tester may demonstrate. Child must walk 4 consecutive steps, 2 out of 3 trials.
27. Bounce ball to child who should stand 3 feet away from tester. Child must catch ball with hands, not arms, 2 out of 3 trials.
28. Tell child to walk backward, 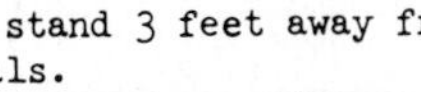 toe within 1 inch of heel. Tester may demonstrate. Child must walk 4 consecutive steps, 2 out of 3 trials.

<u>DATE AND BEHAVIORAL OBSERVATIONS</u> (how child feels at time of test, relation to tester, attention span, verbal behavior, self-confidence, etc,):

Fig. 17-2. Directions for administration of numbered items on the Denver II. (Courtesy WK Frankenburg, JB Dodds, University of Colorado Medical Center, Denver, 1990.)

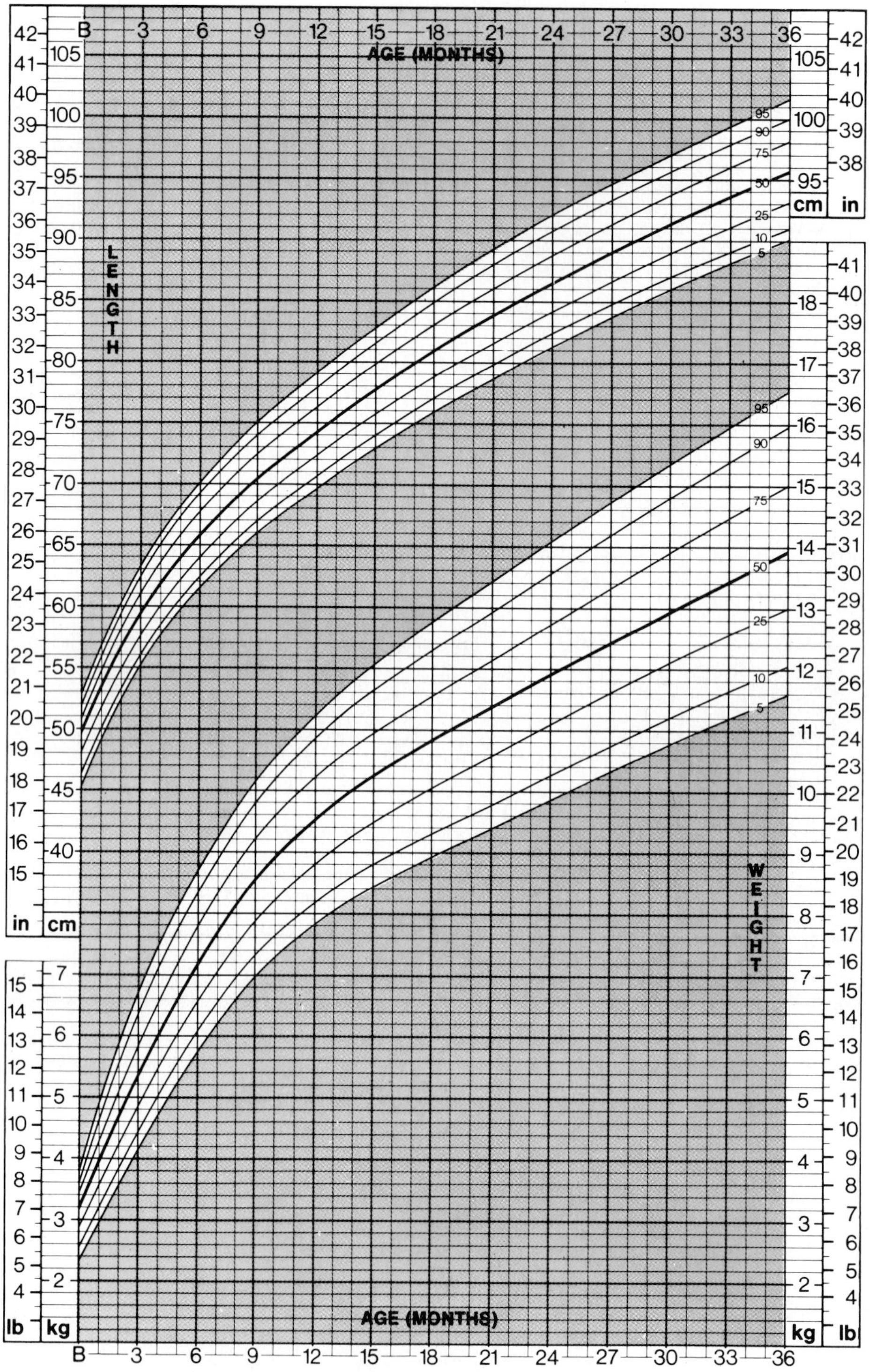

Fig. 17-3. Female infant growth charts.

factors to place the infant at potential risk for child abuse. The parents may find fault and place blame on the infant for not meeting expectations.[34]

Health intervention should focus on identification of high-risk families and promotion of a positive relationship between infant and parents. The nurse should enforce the good health, appearance, and potential developmental ability of the infant. Increasing the parent's feelings of adequacy and self-esteem will promote acceptance of the infant. Most important, follow-up care for these families should be a priority to ensure that adequate support and help are available.

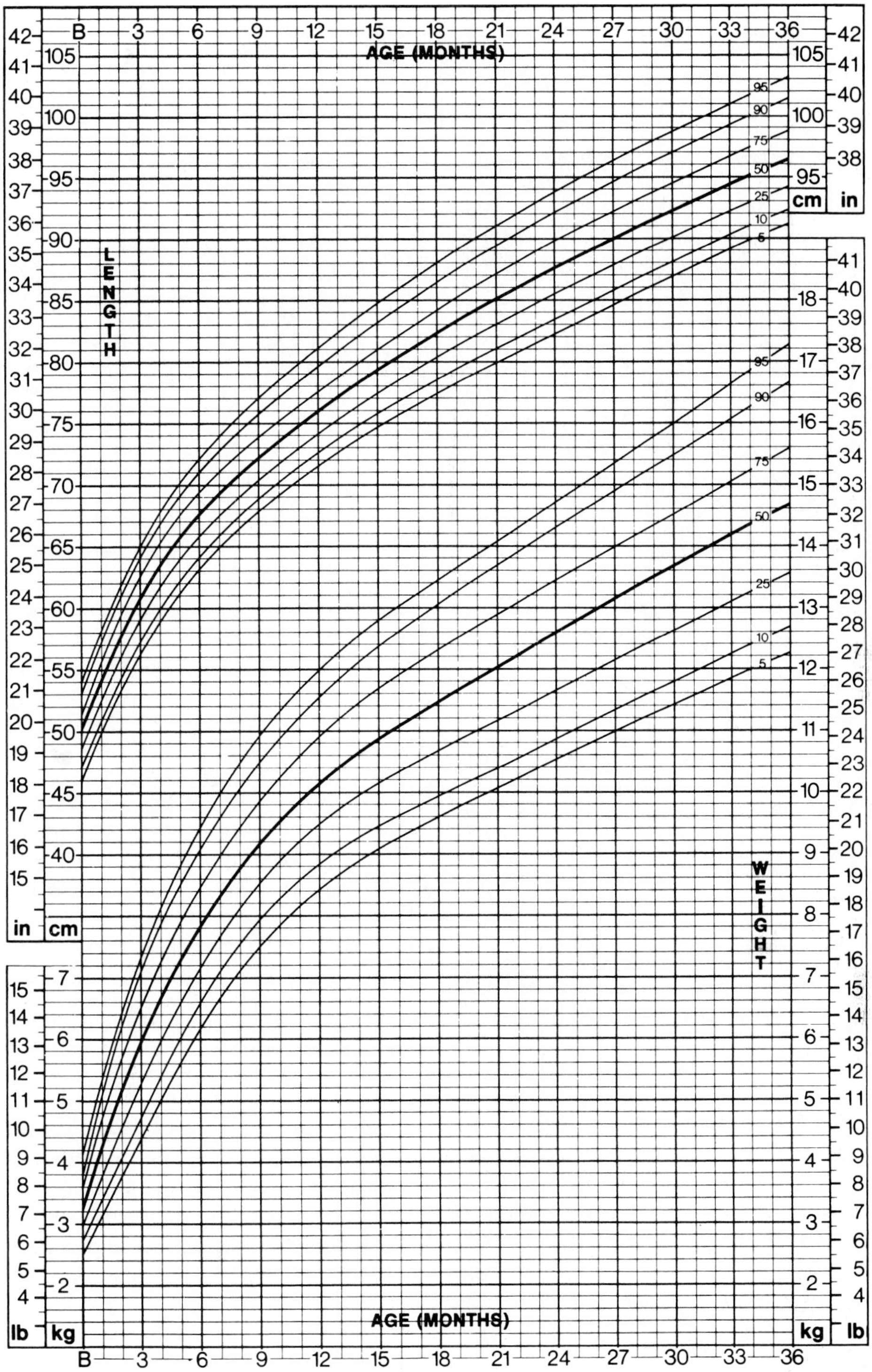

Fig. 17-4. Male infant growth charts.

Race

Race refers to the classification of human beings into groups based on particular physical characteristics, such as skin pigmentation, head form, and stature. Caucasoid, Mongoloid, and Negroid are the three racial types generally recognized.

There is a range of physical variation among people of different races with regard to growth rate, dentition, body structure, blood group, susceptibility to certain diseases, and a great many other variables.

In assessing an infant, the nurse not only collects data, but compares the data to the established norms–such as a standardized growth chart. If the norms chosen are not appropriate for the individual–if, for example, an

***Table 17-3.* Height and weight measurements for girls**

	Height by percentiles						Weight by percentiles					
	5		50		95		5		50		95	
Age*	cm	Inches	cm	Inches	cm	Inches	kg	lb	kg	lb	kg	lb
Birth	45.4	17¾	49.9	19¾	52.9	20¾	2.36	5¼	3.23	7	3.81	8½
3 months	55.4	21¾	59.5	23½	63.4	25	4.18	9¼	5.4	12	6.74	14¾
6 months	61.8	24¼	65.9	26	70.2	27¾	5.79	12¾	7.21	16	8.73	19¼
9 months	66.1	26	70.4	27¾	75.0	29½	7.0	15½	8.56	18¾	10.17	22½
1	69.8	27½	74.3	29¼	79.1	31¼	7.84	17¼	9.53	21	11.24	24¾
1½	76.0	30	80.9	31¾	86.1	34	8.92	19¾	10.82	23¾	12.76	28¼
2†	81.6	32¼	86.8	34¼	93.6	36¾	9.95	22	11.8	26	14.15	31¼
2½†	84.6	33¼	90.0	35½	96.6	38	10.8	23¾	13.03	28¾	15.76	34¾
3	88.3	34¾	94.1	37	100.6	39½	11.61	25½	14.1	31	17.22	38
3½	91.7	36	97.9	38½	104.5	41¼	12.37	27¼	15.07	33¼	18.59	41
4	95.0	37½	101.6	40	108.3	42¾	13.11	29	15.96	35¼	19.91	44
4½	98.1	38½	105.0	41¼	112.0	44	13.83	30½	16.81	37	21.24	46¾
5	101.1	39¾	108.4	42¾	115.6	45½	14.55	32	17.66	39	22.62	49¾
6	106.6	42	114.6	45	122.7	48¼	16.05	35½	19.52	43	25.75	56¾
7	111.8	44	120.6	47½	129.5	51	17.71	39	21.84	48¼	29.68	65½
8	116.9	46	126.4	49¾	136.2	53½	19.62	43¼	24.84	54¾	34.71	76½
9	122.1	48	132.2	52	142.9	56¼	21.82	48	28.46	62¾	40.64	89½
10	127.5	50¼	138.3	54½	149.5	58¾	24.36	53¾	32.55	71¾	47.17	104
11	133.5	52½	144.8	57	156.2	61½	27.24	60	36.95	81½	54.0	119
12	139.8	55	151.5	59¾	162.7	64	30.52	67¼	41.53	91½	60.81	134
13	145.2	57¼	157.1	61¾	168.1	66¼	34.14	75¼	46.1	101¾	67.3	148¼
14	148.7	58½	160.4	63¾	171.3	67½	37.76	83¼	50.28	110¾	73.08	161
15	150.5	59¼	161.8	63¾	172.8	68	40.99	90¼	53.68	118¼	77.78	171½
16	151.6	59¾	162.4	64	173.3	68¼	43.41	95¾	55.89	123¼	80.99	178½
17	152.7	60	163.1	64¼	173.5	68¼	44.74	98¾	56.69	125	82.46	181¾
18	153.6	60½	163.7	64½	173.6	68¼	45.26	99¾	56.62	124¾	82.47	181¾

Modified from National Center for Health Statistics (NCHS), Health Resources Adminstration, Department of Health, Education and Welfare, Hyattsville, Md. Conversion of metric data to approximate inches and pounds by Ross Laboratories, 1977.

*Years unless otherwise indicated.

†Height data include some recumbent length measurements, which make values slightly higher than if all measurements had been of stature (standing height).

Asian infant's growth is assessed on the basis of norms for Caucasian children–the comparison information will not be accurate.

The nurse working with families from a variety of racial groups needs to gain an understanding of each diverse background and how each relates to health and health care. In order to facilitate nursing care for a family from a different racial group than the health care provider's, it is essential that effective communication be established. Such communication will help to result in an understanding of the others' point of view and frame of reference. Each family member should be viewed as an individual, and there should be no stereotyping of all families within a racial group. Despite common language, color, or historical background, all members of a particular racial group are not alike. This diversity presents, without a doubt, considerable challenges for nurses working with families with young infants.[9] There are no universal norms by which to measure one's growth and skill capacity for all races. The nurse must recognize that there are differences and intervene appropriately. The orientation of health maintenance and disease prevention is basic to good health practices–regardless of anyone's racial group. This pervasive concept should be a major focus of all health care.

Genetics

The desired and expected outcome of any pregnancy is the birth of a healthy, "perfect" baby. Unfortunately, a small but significant number of parents experience disappointment when they discover that their baby has been born with a defect or genetic disease. A birth defect is an abnormality of structure, function, or metabolism. It is genetically determined or the result of environmental influences on the unborn child; often a combination of both may be the cause.[52] Many couples

***Table 17-4.* Height and weight measurments for boys**

	Height by percentiles						Weight by percentiles					
	5		50		95		5		50		95	
Age*	cm	Inches	cm	Inches	cm	Inches	kg	lb	kg	lb	kg	lb
Birth	46.4	18¼	50.5	20	54.4	21½	2.54	5½	3.27	7¼	4.15	9¼
3 months	56.7	22¼	61.1	24	65.4	25¾	4.43	9¾	5.98	13¼	7.37	16¼
6 months	63.4	25	67.8	26¾	72.3	28½	6.20	13¾	7.85	17¼	9.46	20¾
9 months	68.0	26¾	72.3	28½	77.1	30¼	7.52	16½	9.18	20¼	10.93	24
1	71.7	28¼	76.1	30	81.2	32	8.43	18½	10.15	22½	11.99	26½
1½	77.5	30½	82.4	32½	88.1	34¾	9.59	21¼	11.47	25¼	13.44	29½
2†	82.5	32½	86.8	34¼	94.4	37¼	10.49	23¼	12.34	27¼	15.50	34¼
2½†	85.4	33½	90.4	35½	97.8	38½	11.27	24¾	13.52	29¾	16.61	36½
3	89.0	35	94.9	37¼	102.0	40¼	12.05	26½	14.62	32¼	17.77	39¼
3½	92.5	36½	99.1	39	106.1	41¾	12.84	28¼	15.68	34½	18.98	41¾
4	95.8	37¾	102.9	40½	109.9	43¼	13.64	30	16.69	36¾	20.27	44¾
4½	98.9	39	106.6	42	113.5	44¾	14.45	31¾	17.69	39	21.63	47¾
5	102.0	40¼	109.9	43¼	117.0	46	15.27	33¾	18.67	41¼	23.09	51
6	107.7	42½	116.1	45¾	123.5	48½	16.93	37¼	20.69	45½	26.34	58
7	113.0	44½	121.7	48	129.7	51	18.64	41	22.85	50¼	30.12	66½
8	118.1	46½	127.0	50	135.7	53½	20.40	45	25.30	55¾	34.51	76
9	122.9	48½	132.2	52	141.8	55¾	22.25	49	28.13	62	39.58	87¼
10	127.7	50¼	137.5	54¼	148.1	58¼	24.33	53¾	31.44	69¼	45.27	99¾
11	132.6	52¼	143.3	56½	154.9	61	26.80	59	35.30	77¾	51.47	113½
12	137.6	54¼	149.7	59	162.3	64	29.85	65¾	39.78	87¾	58.09	128
13	142.9	56¼	156.5	61½	169.8	66¾	33.64	74¼	44.95	99	65.02	143¼
14	148.8	58½	163.1	64¼	176.7	69½	38.22	84¼	50.77	112	72.13	159
15	155.2	61	169.0	66½	181.9	71½	43.11	95	56.71	125	79.12	174½
16	161.1	63½	173.5	68¼	185.4	73	47.74	105¼	62.10	137	85.62	188¾
17	164.9	65	176.2	69¼	187.3	73¾	51.50	113½	66.31	146¼	91.31	201¼
18	165.7	65¼	176.8	69½	187.6	73¾	53.97	119	68.88	151¾	95.76	211

Modified from National Center for Health Statistics (NCHS), Health Resources Administration, Department of Health, Education and Welfare, Hyattsville, Md. Conversion of metric data to approximate inches and pounds by Ross Laboratories, 1977.

*Years unless otherwise indicated

†Height data include some recumbent length measurements, which make values slightly higher than if all measurements had been of stature (standing height).

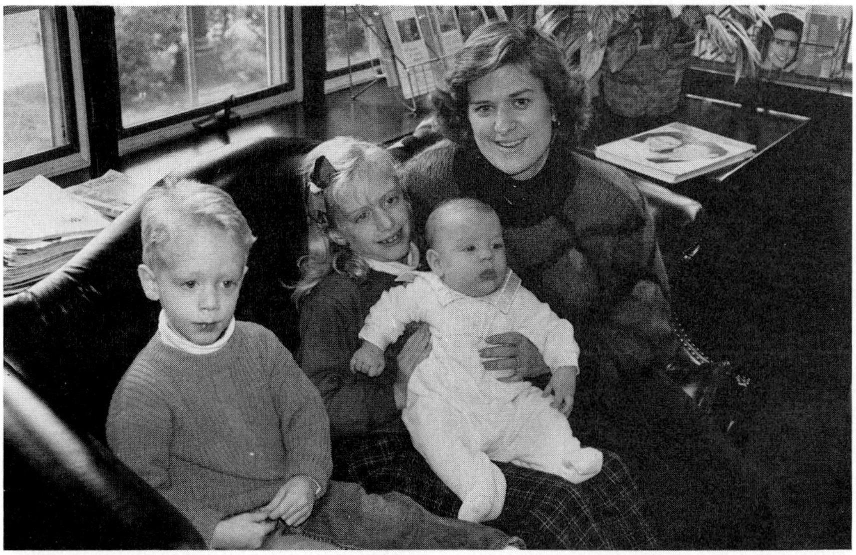

Fig. 17-5. A warm relationship between the parent and child creates the healthiest environment for the infant. (Photograph by Fredric J. Edelman.)

may refrain from having another child because they have had one with a serious birth defect and do not want to risk another. In these situations genetic counseling provides information that is needed to understand a hereditary disorder. Its major goal is to explain birth defects to affected families and to allow prospective parents to make informed decisions about childbearing.

Although specific birth defects may seem relatively uncommon, together they occur in about 7% of all births; the affected families number in the millions.[52]

Using the basic laws governing heredity and knowing the frequency of specific birth defects in the population, the genetic counselor can often predict the probability of recurrence of a given abnormality in the same family.[45] An important aspect of primary prevention is identifying families at increased risk and referring them for counseling. The aspects to be reviewed in the initial interview are[18]

1. *Maternal age.* The risk of having a child with Down's syndrome increases significantly for the mother over 35 years old. In this syndrome three chromosomes appear in the 21 chromosomal group (trisomy 21). Characteristic features include: upwardly slanting eyes; small, malformed ears; large, protruding tongue; broad hands and feet; and some degree of mental retardation.
2. *Ethnic background.* Several genetic disorders occur with higher frequency in certain groups. Eastern European Jews have a 10 times greater chance of carrying the Tay-Sachs gene than the general United States population. Tay-Sachs disease is characterized by abnormal deposits of lipids (fats) in the cells of the cerebral cortex, spleen, liver, and lymph nodes. It is transmitted by an autosomal recessive gene. Blacks have a much greater chance of carrying the sickle cell trait. Sickle cell anemia is an autosomal recessive condition occurring in 1:400 black births and causing severe hemolytic anemia crisis episodes.
3. *Family history.* Certain diseases, such as Huntington's chorea, hemophilia, or mental retardation, are often hereditary. Huntington's chorea, an autosomal dominant disease involving the brain, is characterized by deterioration of intellectual functions and involuntary movements of the limbs, face, and trunk. Once manifested, a steady deterioration leads to death after some years. Hemophilia is a sex-linked recessive coagulation disorder caused by a functional deficiency of a certain plasma clotting factor; bleeding is prolonged. Hemophilia is passed from an unaffected carrier mother to her male affected offspring and occurs in 1:10,000 births.
4. *Reproductive history.* Spontaneous abortions, stillborns, and previous liveborn children with birth defects or slow development may indicate an increased risk.
5. *Maternal disease.* Several maternal disorders are associated with higher frequency of birth defects, including diabetes mellitus, seizure disorder or mental retardation, and phenylketonuria.

Prenatal diagnosis offers the couple an alternative to having children affected with certain genetic disorders. For many this is not an acceptable option, since the only method of preventing genetic disease is to stop the birth from occurring. Chapter 16 discusses the various tests used for prenatal diagnosis.

The nurse's role throughout the genetic counseling process is to provide the vital link between the counseling team and the high-risk couple. The nurse should be involved in case finding, referral, and family education. The nurse must have a sound background in the principles of genetics to provide families with appropriate information as part of preventive health care guidance.

Nutritional and Metabolic Pattern

One of the most important aspects of health promotion in the infant is nutritional status. Many opinions have been expressed about the infant's nutritional needs. As research in this area continues, recommendations and opinions will change; however, some basic facts about nutrition remain fairly consistent. Infant nutritional requirements are based on what is considered necessary (1) to support life, (2) to provide for growth, and (3) to maintain health.

ESSENTIAL NUTRIENTS

Water, proteins, fats, carbohydrates, vitamins, and minerals are the essential nutrients needed in any diet. Since the first year of life is a period of rapid growth, nutritional needs during this period are especially important and always changing.

Water is vital to survival. Since the infant's body weight is approximately three-fourths water, the baby must consume large amounts of fluid to maintain water balance. Water requirements average 125 to 150 ml/kg body weight/day in the first 6 months of life to 120 to 135 ml/kg/day in the second 6 months.[31] The sources of water are fluids, primarily milk, and food; most strained foods are 75% to 85% water. Most infant diets meet the basic water requirement.

The infant also must consume sufficient high-quality *protein* to facilitate growth and development. Recommended protein requirements are 2.2 g/kg/day during the first 6 months to 2.0 g/kg/day in the second 6 months.[12]

Carbohydrates should supply 30% to 60% of the energy intake during infancy. About 37% of the calories in human milk and 40% to 50% of the calories in commercial formulas are derived from lactose or other carbohydrates.[44]

It is recommended that infants consume a minimum of 3.8 g/kcal and a maximum of 6 g/100 kcal of fat (30% to 54% of calories).[42] This quantity is present in human milk and all formulas prepared for infants. Significantly lower intakes, as in skim milk feedings, may result in an inadequate energy intake.

Vitamins are essential nutrients in the infant's diet that regulate metabolism and allow more efficient use of carbohydrates, fats, and proteins within the body. Breast milk or prepared fortified formula consumed in appropriate amounts generally meets the infant's needs.

Minerals are found in relatively small amounts in the infant's body but are vital elements in body structure and control of certain body functions. Mineral intake for infants appears to be adequate, except for iron and fluoride.

The full-term infant is born with adequate stores of iron to meet body needs for hemoglobin production up to approximately 4 to 6 months of age. After this time, body stores may need to be resupplied to ensure adequate levels. Although iron in human milk is highly bioavailable, both breast-fed and formula-fed infants should receive an additional source of iron by six months of age. Iron-fortified formula and cereals are the most commonly used food sources.

The commonly held belief that iron-fortified formula can cause constipation, loose stools, colic, and spitting up in some infants has not been documented in clinical studies.[48]

Fluoride, concentrated in the bones and teeth, helps reduce dental caries. The Committee on Nutrition of the Academy of Pediatrics has recommended that optimum fluoride for infants is 0.25 mg per day.[46] Supplementation is necessary when the diet does not contain sufficient fluoridated water.

A review of these requirements shows that milk, breast or formula, meets most of the infant's nutritional needs if consumed in adequate amounts. Thus no data support the theory that solid foods are needed to meet these nutritional needs, at least in the first 6 months of life. Despite this, many parents introduce semisolid foods to their infants as early as 2 weeks of age.

INTRODUCTION OF SOLID FOODS

No scientific evidence is available on the best time to introduce solid foods during infancy. Usually around 6 months of age, the infant is physiologically and developmentally ready to have solid foods, either commercial or home prepared. Some authorities feel that it decreases any tendency toward food allergies to wait until 6 months of age to introduce solid food. The timing for adding solid foods to the infant's diet depends on several readiness factors such as when the infant

- Has doubled his or her birthweight
- Consumes 8 ounces of formula and is hungry again in less than 4 hours
- Is 6 months old
- Consumes 32 ounces of formula a day and wants more

All infants develop according to their own schedules, and some are ready before others. The addition of foods should be governed by an infant's nutrient needs, readiness to handle different forms of foods, and the need to detect food allergies.[27] Traditionally, the sequence in which foods are introduced is (1) cereals, particularly rice because it is nonallergenic, (2) fruits such as peaches, pears, and applesauce, (3) vegetables, with yellow vegetables such as squash and carrots given before green vegetables like peas or beans, and (4) strained meats such as nonallergenic lamb or veal. A few tips to assist the parents in making the introduction of solid foods to their infant's diet a smooth process are as follows:

1. The infant's first solid foods should be very smooth and runny. Gradually the infant will be ready to accept a slightly rougher texture.
2. Pureed foods are used until the infant has teeth; chopped foods are used when the infant can chew.
3. Introduce only one new food at a time and in small amounts. If the new food is not tolerated or the infant is allergic to it, it can be identified quickly and discontinued.
4. The infant must learn how to handle solid foods. Because infants use sucking movements, part of the food is ejected from the mouth. With time and practice the infant learns how to take solid food from a spoon.
5. Do not mix solid foods together; the infant has to learn to appreciate different tastes and textures.
6. Do not add solid foods to the infant's formula bottle or make a larger hole to allow "drinking" of foods.
7. Do not start to reduce the milk supply until the infant is taking food successfully from the spoon.
8. Feed the solid food to the infant before the milk feeding.
9. Look at, smile at, and talk to the infant during feeding.
10. Involve the infant in the feeding experience. Potential introduction of foods is shown in Table 17-5.

WEANING

Weaning is a process. It is a gradual, caring process that introduces the infant to a cup from the bottle or breast. It should be started when the infant is ready,

Table 17-5. **First foods for the infant**

Age (months)	Addition
4-6	Iron-fortified rice cereal, followed by other cereal
5-7	Strained vegetables and fruits and their juices
6-8	Protein foods (cheese, meat, fish, chicken, yogurt)
9	Finely chopped meat, toast, teething crackers
10-12	Whole egg, whole milk (allergies less likely now)

usually by age 1 year. Many infants are ready for weaning at about 9 months. When the infant shows more interest in play and socializing than in the breast or the bottle or refuses to nurse, or nurses for shorter periods of time, it is time to wean. Developmentally the infant can usually approximate the rim of a cup by 5 to 6 months. The infant should be started at this age by periodically taking sips of water or juice. The infant may not be eager at first and needs to become accustomed to this new experience.

Some infants take to the cup readily; others are extremely reluctant to give up the bottle, especially the bedtime one. Allowing infants to sleep with propped bottles can lead to aspiration if the milk flows too rapidly or the infant becomes too sleepy to coordinate sucking and swallowing. Another potential problem that parents should be aware of is "baby bottle tooth decay": decay of all upper teeth and some of the lower posterior teeth from direct contact with sugar, syrup, honey-sweetened water, or fruit juice. Tooth decay occurs when the infant falls asleep and stops sucking on the bottle. The sugary solution pools around the infant's teeth and remains in contact with them all night. The carbohydrate of the solution is fermented to organic acids that demineralize the teeth until they decay. Parents can prevent this tragedy by not using the bottle as a pacifier. Some additional tips for counseling parents are as follows:

1. Keep a calm, relaxed attitude throughout the weaning process
2. Do not force an infant to use a cup; it is more detrimental to wean sooner than later
3. Introduce the cup for one feeding a day and progress from there until the breast or bottle is given up
4. Put only tap water into the bottle and give the infant juice and milk from a cup
5. Remember that infants like the accomplishment of using a cup; it is one of their first steps toward independence

ANTICIPATORY GUIDANCE

The infant progresses from a diet of milk to a diet of milk and solid foods within a short period. The nurse, in attempting to guide the parents to meet their infant's nutritional needs, must understand these needs, developmental capabilities, and family-infant relationships. The health promotion activity used in meeting infant nutrition focuses on parent education and positive reinforcement of their parenting abilities.

Elimination Pattern

The infant develops an elimination pattern by the second week of life, usually associated with the frequency and amount of feedings. Both breast-fed and bottle-fed infants progress to a pattern of fewer stools per day after the first few months of life.

A breast-fed infant's stools are orangish yellow and have a soft, even consistency, with a sourish but "clean" smell, unlike stools passed later in life. A bottle-fed infant's stools are harder and smellier and resemble those of an infant eating solid food. The breast-fed infant has many daily stools in the first month or two of life, progressing to one stool a day or even every 4 to 5 days in the later months before solid foods are introduced. The bottle-fed infant has two to four stools per day in the first month, tapering down to one or less daily at the end of infancy.[13]

For the first year of life an infant cannot control the bowels. Bowel evacuation remains under involuntary, reflexive control until myelination of the spinal cord is complete, usually by 14 to 18 months of age.[56] Overanxious parents should put toilet-training ideas aside until the infant is developmentally ready.

The stress in the United States culture for daily bowel movements makes many mothers concerned about their infant's elimination patterns. The breast-fed infant may go for several days without having a bowel movement, which is not usually a problem. If the infant's behavior and his feeding and sleeping patterns are normal, no elimination problem exists. A breast-fed infant rarely becomes constipated when consuming adequate amounts of breast milk. The nurse usually needs simply to reassure the parents and discuss normal elimination patterns.

Urination increases as fluid intake increases. An infant who voids six to twelve times a day in the first few months of life is usually healthy and well hydrated. Voiding is completely involuntary until sometime during the second year of life when bladder sensation develops. Irregular patterns of voiding describe the remaining period of infancy.

ANTICIPATORY GUIDANCE

Anticipatory guidance and health promotion concerning elimination patterns of the infant should consist of parental teaching and reassurance, with special emphasis on good hygienic practices. Reassuring the parents regarding the infant's inability to control elimination is important so that their expectations are not unrealistic. Despite what usually happens, the infant did not "save it up" until just after a clean diaper was put on.

Activity and Exercise Pattern

Physical activity and exercise contribute to development and coordination throughout the lifespan; infants receive their exercise through play. Initially infants engage in play with themselves–with hands or feet and sounds and by rolling and getting into various positions. By manipulating objects and achieving pleasurable sensations, infants learn about themselves and the objects in the environment.

ACTIVITY THROUGH PLAY

Although the word *play* suggests physical activity, the infant's first play is actually an exercise of his or her senses. The infant's first toys are visual ones. Through play, infants learn to hone their senses, to exercise their physical abilities, and to relate to other people. Most of the infant's play is solitary and repetitious. As each discovery is made, self-confidence and pride in the achievement are reinforced (as is the skill) through repetition.

As the infant enters the second half of the first year and becomes mobile, the family should provide the infant with increasing opportunities for spontaneous play and exploration. There must be a planned play period in an environment that is safe for the infant. The infant should have unrestrictive clothing so that movement can be free and unhampered. The caregiver should not interfere directly with the play but be attentive to the infant's needs.

A major nursing role in this area is assisting parents to promote play. The importance of providing opportunities for play appropriate for the infant's age should be stressed. The parents do not have to buy expensive toys; common household items (pots, pans, lids, spoons) provide excellent objects for play purposes.

ACTIVITY THROUGH STIMULATION

Parental stimulation of the infant is an important developmental technique, since the infant needs stimulation to learn about the world. This does not require expensive objects but instead involves experiences in sight, sound, and touch, which are free and can be provided by any parent. Examples of stimulating experiences for infants include

- Having lullabies sung to them
- Listening to tape recordings of heartbeat
- Seeing colorful mobiles in crib
- Being rocked in a rocking chair
- Having a familiar face smiling close by
- Having space to wander when developmentally ready
- Looking at themselves in mirrors
- Listening to music played in the household

ANTICIPATORY GUIDANCE

Knowledge of developmental landmarks allows the nurse to guide parents regarding proper play and stimulation for infants. Handing a 15-month-old boy a ball and placing him in the fenced-in backyard to "play" is not enough. These activities must provide interpersonal contact as well as activity and exercise. Activity and exercise, through stimulation and play, are extremely important for adequate and healthy development.

Sleep and Rest Pattern

The amount of sleep infants need is closely related to their rate of growth; at first infants sleep about 80% of the time, as demanded by their rapid growth. As growth begins to slow down toward the middle of the first year of life, less sleep is needed. The 12-month-old infant sleeps only 12 of 24 hours, a pattern that remains almost unchanged through the second year. To assist parents in understanding normal sleep and rest patterns, the nurse should stress that no set schedule exists (Table 17-6).

NURSING SUGGESTIONS

Health promotion activities also should help the parents to determine the individual needs of their infant. The nurse can stress that longer sleep patterns are signs of maturation in the infant and that sleep and rest are recognized as having a significant impact on the infant's growth and development. The nurse can offer the parents helpful comments for promoting infant sleep patterns, such as the following:

Table 17-6. **Normal sleep patterns for infants**

Age (months)	Hours in 24-hour period
2-3	Low: 10 Average: 16½ High: 23 (Two to four naps)
3-4	Low: 8-10 nightly High: 11-12 nightly (Two or three naps daily)
6-12	11-12 nightly (Two or three naps daily)
12-18	8-12 nightly (One or two naps daily)

1. Provide a quiet room for the infant that is separate from the parents' room.
2. Learn behavioral clues that signal the infant is going to sleep and not socially interacting.
3. Learn to become sensitive to sleep cycles and rest periods that the infant is establishing and base care accordingly.
4. Attempt to schedule feeding times during wakeful rather than drowsy periods.
5. Learn that certain cycles are intrinsic to infants and that each infant is unique.
6. Perform rituals for the infant (being rocked, having bedtime story read) to provide comfort and security and let the infant know the expected behavior.

If parents express a sleeping concern, the nurse must assess their reactions to consider their definition of the concern, to assess the sleeping environment, and to observe the infant's own unique sleep patterns. Only then can the nurse's health promotion approach be individualized to assist the family in caring for the infant.

SUDDEN INFANT DEATH SYNDROME

Recent studies of infant sleep have focused on abnormal patterns associated with sudden infant death syndrome (SIDS). Current research centers on sleep pathophysiology, particularly in relation to apneic spells lasting longer than 10 seconds. Physiologic variations in heart and respiratory rates during sleep are normally controlled by the carotid body network and brain stem reflexes. The mechanism of the relationship between apnea and SIDS is not well substantiated. It is thought that a sleeping infant can become hypoxic with positional narrowing of the airway and respiratory inflammation. For unexplained reasons, in SIDS these mechanisms probably fail to work during sleep and respirations cease.

Sudden infant death syndrome refers to the sudden and unexpected death of an infant who has been previously healthy, with the cause of death unexplained after a thorough postmortem examination (see box on this page). SIDS occurs in about 4 out of 1000 live births.[39] The sudden deaths of apparently healthy infants has been scaring people at least since Biblical times. Researchers point to the unexplained, tragic death of an infant in the book of Kings I as the first known reference to this phenomenon.[58] Much research, debate, and uncertainty surround this phenomenon. Its etiology remains a mystery.

Current research from abroad suggests that healthy infants should be put to sleep on their backs or sides. Those studies suggest that in certain countries, the number of SIDS cases dropped dramatically when parents stopped putting their children on their bellies.[57] After reviewing reams of research from abroad, the American Academy of Pediatrics concurred. The nation's leading pediatric group is reversing decades-old advice: Lay your infant down to sleep on its side or back–not its tummy. Experts who have studied sleep positions and the incidence of SIDS say the old recommendation of putting infants to sleep on their bellies was based on little more than conventional wisdom that infants are less likely to choke if they vomit during the night.[50]

❑ ❑ SIDS FACTS

1. Incidence is highest between 1 and 8 months of age.
2. Families of lower socioeconomic status with a history of heavy smoking or drug abuse are at greater risk.
3. Low-birth-weight infants are at greater risk of dying from SIDS than term infants.
4. SIDS most often occurs during the infant's sleep cycle.
5. Peak incidence is at 2 to 3 months of age.
6. Peak incidence is during the fall-winter season.
7. SIDS affects more male infants than female.
8. SIDS is a specific disease entity.
9. No evidence to date suggests hereditary or contagious causes.
10. SIDS is unexpected and unexplained.
11. No sign of distress, crying, or coughing is apparent at the time of death.
12. A mild upper respiratory infection may be present in some infants but not all.
13. Autopsy findings are remarkably similar, including pulmonary congestion, intrathoracic petechiae, edema, and inflammatory infiltrates in the upper airway.

From a preventive perspective, apneic monitors have been used in certain cases. Infants considered to be at high risk for SIDS include (1) survivors of SIDS, (2) subsequent siblings of SIDS victims, and (3) premature infants with recurrent apneic episodes during sleep. Controversy still exists over this type of respiratory monitoring at home, since parents face a heavy psychologic responsibility when left in charge of their young infant's life. Also, it increases their anxiety and protectiveness of the infant. As a prevention measure, however, it may save the infant's life.[15]

When an infant dies suddenly, unexpectedly, and for no apparent reason, a crisis occurs. The parents are devastated and totally unprepared for this shock, reacting with intense guilt, blaming themselves and each other, and agonizing over the part they may have played in the infant's death. Because so many unanswered questions remain, these feelings are universal. They feel there is something they could have done to prevent it. In the majority of cases, there isn't. The first sign that something was wrong is often death.

The nurse is in an excellent position to help the family through this crisis period. Helpful guidelines include the following:

1. Allow the parents and other family members to mourn in their own way.
2. Let them know that help is available when they need it.
3. Present the factual information available about SIDS to help alleviate their guilt.
4. Inform them that their reactions to the loss are not abnormal and many other parents have had similar experiences.
5. Review the autopsy findings with them to substantiate the definite cause of death and to reduce guilt.
6. Reassure them that accepting the reality of the loss takes time.
7. Stress that communication is important in the adjustment process following a crisis.
8. Give the parents and family the opportunity to *share* the experience of losing an infant to SIDS by being a good listener.

Dealing with the family's grief is not an easy task. Many families find strength in God to help them through this difficult time. Other family members and close friends can assist the family in their grieving process.

Many receive solace and support from talking to other parents who have lost an infant to SIDS. Several parent groups are available from local chapters of the SIDS Foundation; the nurse can refer them to the foundation in their area.

The nurse's major supportive role to families coping with SIDS is listening and offering compassionate guidance through the weeks and months to follow. The nurse should encourage and allow parents to talk about their infant. Too soon, family and friends expect the surviving family to be "over it." One is never "over it." It is only put in perspective and not so near the surface.

Nursing assessment of the infant at risk for SIDS includes observing the infant for apneic episodes. Usually, however, nursing assessment consists of observing for appropriate grief patterns in the survivors. Nursing diagnoses for sudden infant death might include the following:

- Spiritual distress related to coping with the possibility of death
- Ineffective family coping: compromised related to potential loss of an infant
- Dysfunctional grieving related to the parents' inability to cope

Nurses should also discuss with the family their feelings about caring for future children. Life may appear out of control, and parents may believe that they cannot care for another infant. The feelings need to be resolved before another pregnancy is contemplated.

When dealing with the families of SIDS victims, nurses may feel uncomfortable and helpless. As health professionals, they may speak in terms of easing the pain or alleviating the guilt of these families, but many times simple nonverbal human contact is sufficient to express concern and understanding.

PSYCHOLOGIC PROCESSES

Cognitive and Perceptual Pattern

Cognition is the process by which an individual recognizes, accumulates, and organizes the knowledge of the environment, beginning with the perception or recognition of an event within that environment.[16] Cognitive development is concurrent with biologic, adaptive, and psychosocial achievement. The infant's biologic and cognitive developmental patterns (Piaget's sensorimotor period) are discussed earlier in this chapter. The focus in this section is on the infant's sensory modalities and language development and the importance of infant stimulation to both developmental areas.

From birth infants possess sensory capabilities; all sensory organs are well developed and functioning. As the infant is cared for and handled, the special senses become organized neurologically into a pattern of behavior that will greatly influence subsequent development.

VISUAL PERCEPTION

The infant's initial visual impressions are unfocused, strange, unfamiliar, and without meaning. Since everything is new and only somewhat significant, visual stimuli must be moving, bright, or flashing to capture the infant's attention. The infant's eyes are well developed at birth, but the muscles that attach the eyes to their sockets are weak. This weakness may be stressful to parents, since the infant's eyes do not appear to function together. They can be assured that most infants coordinate their eye movements by 3 months and that by 6 months this function is mature. Table 17-7 summarizes visual developmental milestones for the infant.

AUDITORY PERCEPTION

After the amniotic fluid drains out of the middle ear several days after birth, the infant's hearing becomes acute. Hearing is one of the better developed senses in the infant; even the fetus can hear in utero and responds to loud sounds. The newborn can distinguish sound frequencies and turns toward a voice or other sound. The infant may be familiar with the mother's voice very early in life. Sounds gradually gain significance and meaning when they are associated with caregivers, food, and pleasure.

The ability to listen and to discriminate among sounds is an important task during infancy. The closer the infant is to the sound, the easier it can be discriminated.

***Table 17-7.* Visual developmental milestones during infancy**

Age (months)	Milestones
1-3	Stares at objects Follows light with eyes Looks toward sounds
3-5	Fixates on objects 3 feet away Accommodation begins to develop Follows moving objects well Looks at and grabs objects Visual acuity is 20/200
5-7	Developing hand-eye coordination Ultimate color of iris is established Eye movements coordinated and mature Searches for fallen objects
7-12	Depth perception begins to develop Demonstrates interest in small objects Reaches for unseen object Visual acuity is 20/100
12-18	Looks at pictures with interest Able to identify forms Convergence becomes well established Identifies forms

Adapted from Chinn PL: *Child health maintenance: concepts in family-centered care,* ed 4, St Louis, 1989, Mosby.

Groundwork for verbal ability begins to develop long before words appear, and many believe that infants whose mothers talk to them tend to speak earlier than infants not exposed to such sounds.[3] Table 17-8 summarizes the infant's auditory development.

***Table 17-8.* Progressive auditory development of infants during infancy**

Age (months)	Development
1-2	Startled by sounds (Moro's reflex) Quiets when hears voice Turns head toward familiar sound
3-5	Searches for sound in room Stops sucking to listen Locates sound below ear
6-8	Reacts to changes in music volume Recognizes familiar sounds
9-12	Listens to talking Responds to simple commands Begins to differentiate between words
12-18	Begins to show voluntary control over responses to sound Begins to develop gross discrimination by learning to distinguish between sounds

Adapted from Chinn PL: *Child health maintenance: concepts in family-centered care,* ed 4, St Louis, 1989, Mosby.

OLFACTORY PERCEPTION

The ability to smell is fully developed at birth. The infant has many receptors in the nose but lacks the cilia that line the inside of the adult's nose. As a result, the infant has a keen sense of smell, since odors reach the receptor cells easily. Within 2 weeks after birth, an infant can differentiate the odor of the mother's milk from others', an ability developed when the infant is held close.[55] At this time the infant begins associating the parents by detecting their body odors, a perception important to infant-parent bonding.

GUSTATORY PERCEPTION

The sense of taste is present at birth, and salivation begins at about 3 months of age. The four primary sensations generally agreed on are sour, salty, sweet, and bitter. The taste buds for sweet tastes are more abundant during early life than in later life, which may account for the preference for sweets characteristic of the infant and child.

TACTILE AND MOTION PERCEPTION

Tactile sensation is well developed at birth, particularly in the lips and tongue. Perceptions of motion and touch are perhaps the most important of all senses. Rocking and other motion are sensations of equilibrium picked up by the middle ear. Skin-to-skin touching should be performed regularly; it has been documented that touch helps relieve the unspent tensions infants develop and also accelerates neuromuscular development.[49] Infants respond with pleasure to rocking and other motion, as well as to tactile sensations of warmth, closeness, and cuddling.

LANGUAGE DEVELOPMENT

Language development, an important aspect of the infant's cognitive and perceptual pattern, is affected by intellectual development, maturation of the central nervous system, development of the organs of speech, and exposure to human verbalization.

As with other areas of development, the acquisition of language follows a definite sequence. During the first 2 months most of the infant's sounds are vowels and are made mostly in the front part of the mouth.[20] Crying is the means of communication during this period. Cooing sounds are heard at about 2 to 3 months, usually in response to an adult's voice. By 6 months babbling sounds are heard, and by 9 to 10 months the infant forms two-syllable sounds. By 12 months, words such as "mama," "bye-bye," and "dada" are emerging. From 15 to 18 months an expressive jargon with rhythmic intonations develops, but words are recognized only rarely. The infant uses jargon along with pointing to express wishes.

NURSING SUGGESTIONS

The nurse's knowledge and understanding of an infant's cognitive and perceptual behavior facilitates interaction with infants and serves as a guide in parental counseling. The major focus should center around *stimulation,* since each of the infant's senses is receptive to environmental stimulation. This activity helps the infant learn from the environment. When an infant is exposed to appropriate sensory stimulation, greater curiosity, improved mental capabilities, accelerated neuromuscular growth, enhanced gastrointestinal functioning, quicker weight gain, more rapid language development, and pleasing mother-infant interactions are likely to occur.[25]

Parents are the primary providers of pleasurable and stimulating experiences for the infant. The nurse can assist them by offering suggestions regarding suitable stimuli for each sensory modality.

Self-Perception and Self-Concept Pattern

Self-perception has a pervasive influence on all aspects of life. Self-concept consists of a set of attitudes regarding what each person thinks, believes, and feels about the self. These attitudes form a personal self-belief that is an abstraction referred to as "me." Many believe that the infant determines self-existence by first noting that actions such as crying or smiling have an effect on others, which depends on receiving feedback.[35]

Studies confirm that infants have the ability to identify themselves and therefore a self-concept. Infants at four months of age were found to be particularly fascinated with their images in mirrors and smiled more at themselves than at pictures of other infants.[63]

As the infant continues to grow and mature, many circumstances combine to influence self-concept. How others relate to the infant's body and the continuing messages the infant receives from the body lead to knowledge of a physical self. Abilities to use the body to influence others in the environment may lead the psychologic self to conclude that someone cares about the infant.[55]

The infant's development of body image is gradual. At birth the infant has diffuse feelings of hunger, pain, anger, and comfort, but no body image. At first all the infant knows is the self, regarding the external world as an extension of self. Only when infants begin to experience the environment through sensory modalities are they able to distinguish their bodies from animate and inanimate objects.

NURSING SUGGESTIONS

The nurse can play a vital role in assisting parents to foster the development of a positive self-concept and good body image in their infant. The nurse can first identify personal self-concept and how it influences clients.[28] The nurse should stress that the infant's self-concept is influenced by how the parents treat the infant in the environment. Basically infants and young children incorporate their parents' reflected interactions (good or bad) of them into their own view of self. Parents must understand that their infant's self-concept is an important, continuing event. What the infant knows and later believes about the self will affect all interactions with others, and by influencing what the infant will later attempt, the self-concept may have broad effects on the development of new skills.[30]

Coping and Stress-Tolerance Pattern

The term *stress* implies intense reaction to an experience and changes in usual behavior. Stress is a normal phenomenon that occurs throughout the life cycle when an individual experiences a developmental or situational crisis.

DEVELOPMENTAL CRISIS

Developmental crises are turning points or periods of great change. Most stressors the infant experiences are a necessary part of growth and development. For example, learning new skills creates stress. The infant who is not able to move forward while learning to creep experiences stress. The infant expresses this stress by crying for help. Other stressors are more psychosocial in nature, such as being left with a babysitter or in an unfamiliar place.

SITUATIONAL CRISIS

Situational crises are not anticipated easily and do not necessarily occur as part of the normal growth and development process. One major situational crisis during infancy is separation from the significant other. Three distinct phases are evident in the reaction to separation.[67]

1. *Protest.* Infant cries loudly, screams for mother, and refuses attention of substitute caregiver.
2. *Despair.* Infant stops crying and becomes less active, withdraws, and becomes apathetic.
3. *Withdrawal.* Infant takes an interest in surroundings but tends to ignore or reject mother if she returns because she did not meet the infant's needs.

Initially, with no time framework and no understanding of waiting, the infant has little ability to cope with

NURSING INTERVENTIONS TO ASSIST IN STRESSFUL SITUATIONS DURING INFANCY

- Attempt to meet the infant's needs promptly.
- Allow favorite toy or item of security to be present during stressful experiences.
- Allow familiar caregiver to be present to calm infant.
- Attempt to keep the number of strangers interacting with infant to a minimum.
- Attempt to provide a warm and accepting environment for the infant.
- Allow freedom of expression (crying) to reduce tension in the infant.
- Identify the infant's established daily routine and try to follow through.
- Reinforce the infant's need for expression.
- Establish a trust relationship with the infant.
- Provide opportunity for play so that the infant can "vent" fears.
- Provide emotional support for the parents so they may in turn give support to their infant.

stress. As the infant matures more and gains a feeling of security from the caregiver, he begins to wait a short time to have his needs met without protest. When the infant experiences stress, he reacts by crying, the main tool of communication. The infant gradually learns to tolerate greater stress as time progresses.

NURSING INTERVENTIONS

Nursing suggestions to assist the infant and family in stressful situations are listed in the box above. The nurse can facilitate coping behaviors in the infant by allaying anxiety in the infant's caregiver. The stressful situation and the problem-solving activities can be turned into growth-producing experiences for the family, with coping capacities strengthened for the future.

Value and Belief Pattern

A value is a standard or principle considered to be good or proper. When persons communicate, they send both the content message of the spoken words and the message of who they are and what they believe. Values are pervasive and important and give a focus to people within a particular culture. Since values are attitudes learned from significant others within the environment, value-belief patterns are not developed in the infant. The infant has not yet reached the cognitive level of incorporating the parents' values into the behavioral system. The parents, through parenting behaviors, serve as a model for their infant as he or she develops into a boy or girl.

NURSING INTERVENTIONS

By understanding and respecting the parents' value system, the nurse can work within their framework of values in the counseling situation. The nurse also communicates personal values to the family. To work successfully within a different value system, the nurse should incorporate the following attitudes concerning value and belief patterns into the nursing process:[29]

1. Believe in the ultimate worth of the infant and the family regardless of their behavior or situation.
2. Grant families the freedom to make their own informed choices and to experience the responsibilities and consequences of their decisions.
3. Use knowledge of the family's value system in specific ways to reward and reinforce positive health practices.
4. Value the growth potential inherent in developmental and situational crisis situations.
5. Recognize own value system and its influence on behavior.
6. Work with families without applying personal value system in judgment of their behavior.
7. Broaden value system by accepting lifestyles different from own.

The nurse also must influence the behavior of parents, who will have the greatest influence on developing their infant's value and belief patterns. The nurse can accomplish this by (1) modeling, by living congruently with professed values; (2) acting as a consultant by sharing pertinent information with parents; and (3) modifying his or her own values.[6]

Modeling can be a potent influence on another individual's behavior. In the counseling situation the family looks to the nurse for guidance and assistance in promoting healthy childrearing practices. How the nurse interacts with the infant, listens to the parents' concerns, and demonstrates respect for the family unit are all influencing factors on changing behavior. The following is an example of behavior modeling that can influence the family's health promotion practices.

The clinic nurse speaks to Mr. and Mrs. Gates regarding the importance of infant stimulation to promote normal growth and development patterns. While stressing this activity, the nurse avoids eye contact with their infant, rarely touches the baby, and offers no suggestions to the parents on how to carry out this stimulation. The nurse gives lip service to infant stimulation but fails to model the behavior that would be appropriate for the parents to incorporate in their activites.

Second, the nurse can act as *consultant* to influence values. Advice on childrearing practices is overwhelming to parents; everyone has opinions. The nurse often must listen before giving advice to determine whether parents will accept advice and to allow them to decide about its usefulness. Repeated attempts to convert parents to the nurse's value system may only make them defensive and resistant to the advice.

Third, the nurse can influence value and belief patterns by expressing values and attitudes but remaining *open* to other approaches. Parents should realize that they are free to change and are not bound to traditional values expressed by others outside their value system.[41]

The nurse using these communication skills can deal with families more effectively. The nurse's open attitude increases the likelihood that the parents will discuss their concerns and adhere to the health promotion guidelines the nurse has given them.

Health Perception and Health Management Pattern

Health promotion is aimed at assisting the infant and family toward changing behavior to produce greater physical and emotional health in adulthood. To provide this, the nurse encourages childrearing practices that promote normal growth and development, fosters attitudes and values compatible with health, and teaches appropriate use of health services.[37] The nurse promotes the infant's health through the parents, who determine the care practices for the dependent infant.

Health is largely a subjective judgment; each person's perception of health is related to physical and mental capabilities, self-concept, relationships with others and the environment, and personal goals and values in life.[45] Knowing this, the nurse should use every opportunity to convey confidence in the parents' health perception and management patterns and their ability to act to promote the infant's health. If parents learn and adopt behaviors that promote their own health, they are more likely to ensure that the health needs of their infant are met. Such parental modeling increases the chances of good health practices being retained throughout the child's life.

The goals of nursing practice with infants and their families are to promote individual motivation for health, to assist the family to identify health needs, and to develop problem-solving skills using the family's own resources. To meet these goals, the nurse needs to identify the family's perception of good or bad health practices, which greatly influences participation in health-promoting activities. Health perception is influenced by age, sex, educational level, cultural orientation, financial status, and occupation. When parents believe the infant is more susceptible to a health problem if promotional behavior is not enacted, they become more motivated to adopt the behavior.

The nurse's task is to help the parents recognize the infant's susceptibility and the potential consequences if healthy practices are not instituted. The nurse must work within the family's health perception framework to become acquainted with the characteristics that strongly influence the infant's health. Unless caregivers meet their own dependent needs, they will be unable to meet their infant's developmental needs.[33]

The nurse supports the parents, building up their parental confidence and self-esteem, providing information on meeting their infant's needs, and reinforcing their health perception and management patterns.

ENVIRONMENTAL PROCESSES

Natural Processes

PHYSICAL AGENTS

This area refers to various objects within the environment that could affect the infant's health status. The whole realm of accident prevention and safety promotion is applicable here.

Accidents are always unexpected and in retrospect usually could have been prevented. Adults take for granted living in a world designed by adults for adults. They need to remind themselves constantly that infants also live in this complex world and that, although they learn at a remarkable rate, infants are unaware of most environmental dangers. This renders them extremely vulnerable to accidents–a major problem and a challenging field for preventive measures.

Accidents occur in many situations: in the home, in the street, on the playground, and in automobiles. Regulation car seats prevent infant injury in some car accidents (Fig. 17-6). The majority of accidents, how-

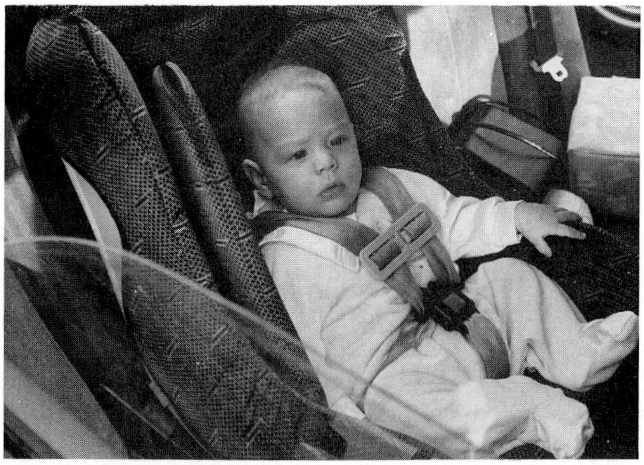

Fig. 17-6. Regulation car seats can prevent injury to infants in many accidents. (Photograph by Fredric J. Edelman.)

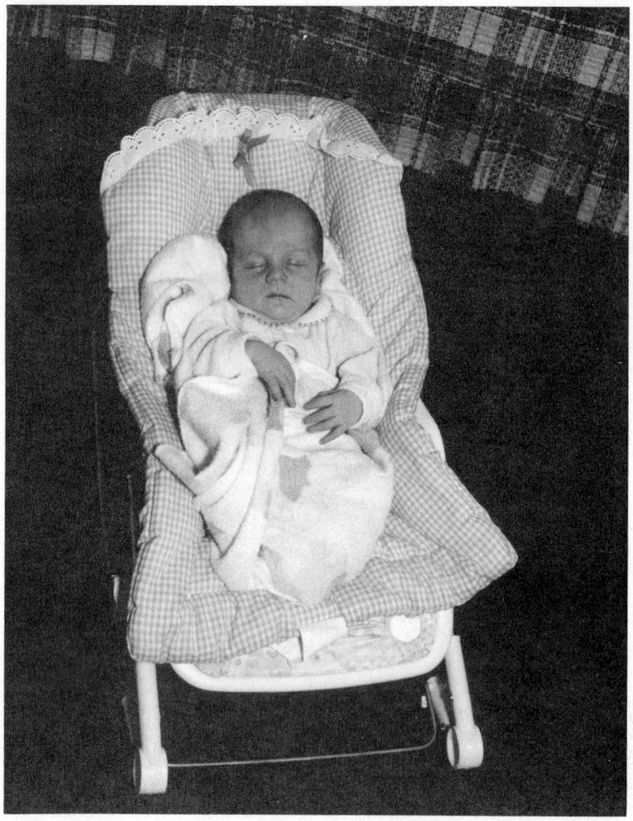

Fig. 17-7. When in doubt, the safest place for an infant is the floor.

ever, occur in the home environment. Their number and seriousness are closely linked to the infant's developmental stage. Accidents tend to increase with the mobility of the infant, but even a 2-month-old can wiggle or flip off a high place.

Nurses have the opportunity to help parents and caregivers anticipate and understand the common hazards of early life and to provide specific guidance for accident prevention.

Falls. Falls are most common after 4 months of age, when the infant has learned to roll over, but they can occur at any age. The best advice is never to place an infant unattended on a raised surface that has no type of guardrails. When in doubt, the safest place is the floor (Fig. 17-7).[28]

The following are some safety tips to assist parents in preventing falls:[54]

1. Keep the crib sides up and securely fastened whenever the infant is in it.
2. Place the infant seat in the playpen or on the floor; always strap the infant in securely.
3. Check highchairs, strollers, and carriages for safety, and restrain the infant if very active.
4. Lock windows if the infant is capable of climbing on the windowsill.
5. Clean up spills of food or liquids immediately from the floor.
6. Remember polished floors are hazardous, especially if throw rugs are present.
7. Close off stairways with doors, gates, or some other safety device as the infant becomes mobile.
8. Do not leave items in the crib that the infant could use to climb out.
9. To prevent falls, set the crib mattress at the lowest adjustment once the infant can pull to standing position.
10. Strap the infant into a shopping cart to prevent falls.

Burns. Burns are the most frequent and frightening of all accidents during infancy. Since nearly all burns are preventable, the attendant caregiver can experience severe guilt.

Burns may be caused by fire from matches or other sources, hot liquids, ultraviolet light from the sun, electricity or electric outlets, and heating elements such as radiators, registers, and floor furnaces. The following are safety tips to assist parents in preventing burns:

1. Keep the infant out of the sun when ultraviolet rays are strongest, generally 11 A.M. to 3 P.M.
2. Sunscreens, longer clothing, and a hat with a brim are essential if the infant is exposed to the sun.
3. Remember fireplaces can be a serious hazard. Fine-mesh screens attached to a frame are safer than free-standing ones. Be careful never to leave an infant alone in a room where a fire is burning; make sure the fire is out before going to bed.
4. Avoid bathing the infant in a sink or adult tub near hot water faucets. Test the bath water temperatures *before* putting the infant into it; keep one hand on the infant at all times during the bath.
5. Be sure all the infant's clothing is made of nonflammable materials.
6. Avoid handling hot liquids near the infant.
7. Turn the handles of cooking utensils toward the back of the stove.
8. Keep all electric cords short, especially those for coffee pots; keep cords out of the infant's sight as much as possible.
9. Cover electric outlets with protective plastic caps.
10. Place a barrier in front of any heat-producing element, especially floor heaters.
11. Keep all matches and lighters out of the infant's reach.
12. Teach the older infant the meaning of "hot."
13. Close oven doors when the oven is in use or is cooling.
14. Be attentive to keeping the heat of cigarettes or cigars away from the infant.

Aspiration of Foreign Objects. Any small object that an infant puts in the mouth has the potential to be aspirated. Parents should be advised that objects such as

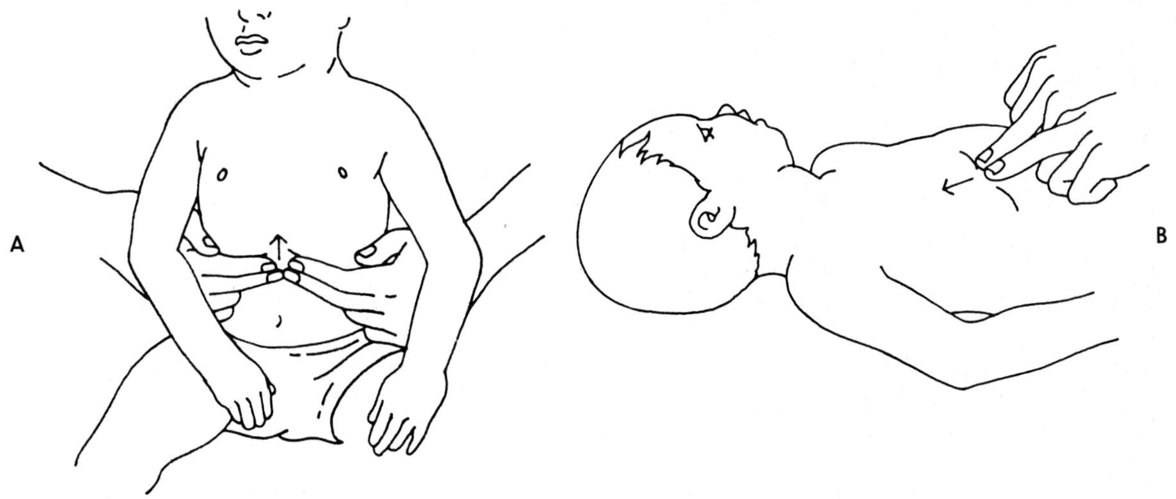

Fig. 17-8. The Heimlich maneuver for infants can be done two ways. **A,** Place infant in lap, reach around, and with index and middle fingers of both hands placed against abdomen, above navel, and below rib cage, give quick upward thrust. **B,** Position infant face upward on firm surface, face infant, and deliver upward thrust with same fingers. Repeat maneuver if necessary.

safety pins, peanuts, beads, coins, hot dogs, paper clips, nuts, corn, buttons, popcorn, chips, apple with peel, and parts off broken toys frequently are aspirated. Almost anything can fit into this category and also into the infant's mouth. Carelessness of the caregiver, relative, friend, babysitter, or toy manufacturer in leaving small objects available and within reach or giving toys unsuited to the infant's stage of development most often cause such accidents.

In one method employed when choking occurs, the infant should be placed across the adult's knees–face down in a prone position on an incline, with the head at the lower end–and thumped sharply between the shoulder blades.[47]

The nurse should give parents another basic method to prepare them for an incident of aspiration. The successful *Heimlich maneuver* should be learned and used in a life-threatening situation caused by aspiration of a foreign body (Fig. 17-8).[56]

Prevention of aspiration of foreign objects is a better treatment. Some safety measures for parents and caregivers of infants are listed in the box on this page.

The entire balance of safety for infants rests on allowing them plenty of opportunity to explore and play within the environment while at the same time protecting them from harmful physical agents. According to the American Academy of Pediatrics, the greatest threat to the health of infants is not illness but injuries, many of which can be prevented. As a nurse it is important to inform the infant's primary caregivers how to childproof their home. Tips for childproofing are summarized in the box on p. 432.

Biologic Agents. The fetus is protected from biologic agents by the placental barrier and the mother's defense system. After birth, however, the infant is thrust into an environment filled with infectious agents that cause disease. These bacterial or viral organisms can be found in food, crib, air, pets, parents, siblings–literally everywhere. Even the healthiest environment harbors disease-causing agents. Although the infant cannot escape exposure to these pathogens without being totally isolated, immunizations are given to assist the infant's defense against communicable diseases.

❑ ❑ NURSING INTERVENTIONS TO PREVENT ASPIRATION OF FOREIGN OBJECTS BY INFANTS

Keep all small objects out of an infant's reach.
Avoid propping bottles and making large holes in nipples to prevent aspiration of formulas into the infant's lungs.
Discourage the use of powder for infants to reduce risk of aspiration pneumonia from inhalation of zinc stearate.
Burp the infant well before placing into the crib; place on his or her side.
Older children should not give food to the infant, who may choke on it. An adult should be close by to supervise children around infants.
Adults should not set a bad example by putting pins or other objects in their mouths; older infants mimic them and may do likewise.
Inspect all toys for loose, removable parts that potentially could reach the infant's mouth.

❑ ❑ HOME CHILDPROOFING TIPS

1. Remove any heavy, sharp, or breakable objects from tables and low shelves.
2. Bolt bookcases to the wall and remove heavy books to prevent falls.
3. Test floor and table lamps to be sure they cannot be pulled over.
4. Disconnect unused appliances and wrap up cords. Close reachable outlets with safety covers. Secure all other cords so that radios, telephones, toasters, and the like cannot be tugged down.
5. Tie drapery and blind cords out of an infant's reach.
6. Choose stair gates with openings too small for an infant's head and child-resistant fasteners such as pressure bars. Avoid accordion or expandable gates with openings that can trap an infant's head.
7. Install smoke detectors and check the batteries at least once a month to make sure they are working. Use sturdy screens in front of fireplaces.
8. Place crib, play yard, and highchair well away from heaters, fans, and electrical outlets to prevent injuries.
9. Put childproof latches on drawers and cupboards. Store all cleaning compounds and detergents in a high, locked cupboard.
10. Buy all medicines in bottles with childproof lids and keep them in their original labeled containers for identification in case of accidental ingestion.
11. Put lids on garbage pails, and never leave any harmful materials in them, such as sharp can lids or spoiled food.
12. Regularly check floor for objects small enough to be swallowed.

AIDS. Acquired immunodeficiency syndrome (AIDS) is an acquired immunodeficiency spread by contact with the retrovirus HIV through blood and body secretions. The virus attacks the T lymphocytes, affecting formation of T4 (T-helper or T-inducer cells), the cells responsible for directing the immune response. The infant with HIV infection is unable to resist normal infection. Transmission of HIV from mother to infant is the most likely reason for childhood HIV. Transmission of the virus can occur during pregnancy, at delivery, and during breastfeeding.[4]

Because infants can retain maternal antibodies for HIV infection for as long as 15 months, diagnosis of HIV infection in an at-risk infant (one whose mother is infected) is extremely difficult. After the child is 15 months old, positive antibody test results are considered reliable, as is a positive HIV culture. Although signs and symptoms of illness can occur at any time, they usually begin in the first 2 years of life. In infants the behaviors of the disease include failure to thrive, oral candidiasis, recurrent bacterial infections, persistent pulmonary infiltrates, and chronic diarrhea.[5]

Nursing assessment centers on a careful and complete history of the infant and mother, signs and symptoms of the disease, growth and development history, and psychosocial concerns. Parents must be carefully assessed to determine their level of anxiety; knowledge of the disease process including prognosis, treatment, and transmission; and awareness of resources, support systems, coping strategies, and perception of the infant's needs.

No other disease in the past has seemed to cause so much public awareness and panic as AIDS. Part of this behavior is ignorance. Nurses play a major role in educating the public regarding the disease process, its mode of transmission, and most of all preventive measures. Preventive education should begin with the very young. Most school health programs include information on AIDS. School nurses can contribute to the success of these programs as can nurses working in prenatal clinics to spread the "prevention word." Nurses in all settings can engage in research related to AIDS to gather further clarification of this fatal disease.

Although the infant is not an active participant in the spread of HIV, it is very important that parents know how it is transmitted and not allow their infant to become a passive participant because of their high-risk behaviors.

The two types of immunizations are active and passive. In *active* immunizations a substance is introduced into the body that stimulates the production of antibodies to a specific antigen. This substance is generally a toxin of the disease organism; depending on the virulence and certain other characteristics of the organism, it is used in the vaccine in a live, killed, or attenuated form.[30] The attenuated form is alive, but its virulence has been reduced significantly by treatment with laboratory procedures that use, for example, heat or chemicals. Examples of active immunizations include diphtheria, tetanus, and pertussis (DTP); polio (OPV); and measles, mumps, and rubella (MMR). Active immunization affords lifelong immunity.

Passive immunization consists of the injection of already formed antibodies. After an individual has been exposed to a disease, a passive immunization is given to prevent contracting the disease. Passive immunizations provide a short immunity, usually 1 to 6 weeks. They will protect the person until the danger of contracting the disease from exposure is over. Passive immunization also helps to reduce the severity of the disease once contracted. Because of the short duration, active immunization is still needed to remain immune. Passive immunity occurs naturally in newborns by maternal anti-

Table 17-9. **Recommended immunization schedule for infants**

Age (months)	Immunization
Birth	HBV-1
1-2	HBV-2
2	DTP-1, OPV-1, HbPV-1
4	DTP-1, OPV-1, HbPV-2
6	DTP-3, HbPV-3
6-18	HBV, OPV-3
12-15	MMR, HbPV-4
15-18	DTP-4

Source: Modified from American Academy of Pediatrics: *Report of the committee on infectious diseases,* ed 23, Elk Grove Village, Ill, 1994, The Academy.

Key: DTP–diphtheria, tetanus, pertussis; OPV–oral polio vaccine; HbPV–hemophilus b polysaccharide vaccine; HBV–hepatitis B vaccine; MMR–measles, mumps, rubella.

bodies passed through the placenta or in breast milk.

The Committee on Infectious Diseases of the American Academy of Pediatrics recommends immunization schedules, which are revised periodically as new information arises. Table 17-9 gives the current recommendations for healthy infants.

Immunization provides one of the most cost-effective means of preventing infection in infants. Its importance is accentuated by the fact that viruses cannot be destroyed by currently available antibiotics; thus immunization offers the only means of control. Emphasis must be placed on educating parents about the importance of immunization. To motivate them to have their children immunized, the nurse can work toward (1) increasing health education to achieve greater health maintenance knowledge, (2) providing health services that make immunizations feasible and available, (3) developing a close relationship with the family, and (4) continuing surveillance of the immunization status of every infant in the health care system.

Nutrition Problems. These include undernutrition, in which infants do not receive an adequate supply of an essential nutrient, or overnutrition, in which they receive more of a certain nutrient than is needed for healthy growth and development.[63] For infants in the United States, both of these problems are present. Table 17-10 will help the nurse in counseling parents regarding nutrition problems in their infant.

Food Additives. In addition to their questionable nutritional value, additives in commercial baby food may negatively influence an infant's health status. The purposes of food additives vary, including (1) addition of nutritional value; (2) preservation or extension of shelf-life; (3) aid in processing preparation; and (4) improvement of flavor, color, and texture.[42]

Commercially prepared baby foods are generally safe, nutritious, and of high quality. In response to consumer demand, baby food manufacturers have removed much of the added salt and sugar their products once contained and have eliminated most food additives.

As an alternative to commercial baby food, a parent who wants the infant to have family foods can "blenderize" a small portion of the table food at each meal. This necessitates cooking without salt or sugar, though, as the baby food manufacturers do. Making baby food is easy and economical. Several written resources are available for the parents interested in more details about home baby food preparation.

Parents need to be encouraged to read baby food labels carefully. Nurses can obtain lists of baby foods and their ingredients from the manufacturers. The best overall recommendation nurses can make to parents is that they provide their infants a well-balanced diet and avoid excesses.

Drugs. Drugs today are important to many persons, but often caregivers are not alert to their potency in the hands of infants. A strange phenomenon occurs between drugs and infants: a parent can coax, bribe, or threaten in a vain attempt to get the infant to swallow prescribed medicines, only to find later the same infant stuffing that drug into the mouth.

Aspirin is the medicine most commonly ingested, with acetaminophen and vitamins close behind. Acetaminophen, the active ingredient in Tylenol and other aspirin substitutes, is becoming increasingly popular with parents as a good antipyretic. Vitamins themselves are usually harmless; however, many contain iron, making them potentially lethal. Infants are attracted to them because of appealing colors and flavors.

Recent changes in packaging and limits on the tablets dispensed in each bottle have reduced deaths resulting from overdose. Drug manufacturers are using childproof caps more and more frequently as a safety measure. Even though a concerted effort is being made by the manufacturers, childproof bottle caps vary in their effectiveness.[19] Frequently the safety caps are "adultproof," and children can readily open them.

All this seems to point to the dangers of medications, regardless of the dispensing bottle. *All* medications still need to be kept locked up when infants are in the home. Some additional guidance helps prevent accidents involving drugs:

1. Use a prescription drug only for the purpose for which it has been ordered. Do not "prescribe" it for a similar condition in the infant.
2. Discard unused drugs by flushing them down the toilet; many infants have been poisoned from eating tablets found in the trash.
3. Request safety tops on all prescription drugs.
4. Keep all medicines under lock and key.
5. Have the telephone number of the nearest poison control center readily available.

***Table 17-10.* Nutritional inadequacies during infancy**

Nutrient	Requirement	Excess	Deficiency	Sources
Water	Age 3 mo: 140-165 ml/kg 6 mo: 130-155 ml/kg 9 mo: 125-145/kg 12 mo: 115-135/kg	Abdominal pain, headache, water intoxication	Thirst, dehydration	Breast or formula milk
Protein	Age 6 mo: 2.2 g/kg 12 mo: 2 g/kg	Dehydration	Reduction in growth rates	Egg yolk, breast or formula milk
Fat	30%-50% of total calorie intake	Obesity, atherosclerosis, hyperlipidemia (lipemia) later in life	Dry, thickened skin; weight loss	Breast or formula milk
Carbohydrate	50-100 g/day	Obesity, dental caries, diarrhea	Ketosis, weight loss	Milk, prepared baby foods
Vitamins A (retinol)	5000 IU*/day	Anorexia, irritability	Impaired vision; dry, scaly skin; failure to thrive	Milk, yellow vegetables
D	400 IU/day	Anorexia, weight loss, calcification of soft tissue	Poor bone and teeth development	Milk, sunlight (30 min/day)
C (ascorbic acid)	35 mg/day	Unknown	Coagulation problems	Citrus fruits, vegetables
B_1 (thiamine)	0.5 mg/1000 kcal	Unknown	Fatigue, insomnia	Pork, liver, wheat germ, grain, cereals, milk
B_2 (riboflavin)	0.6 mg/1000 kcal	Unknown	Skin and visual problems	Leafy vegetables, dairy products
B_6 (pyridoxine)	0.3-0.6 mg/day	Unknown	Irritability, seizures, anemia	Bananas, brewers' yeast, liver
B_{12} (cobalamin)	0.3-1.0 mg/day	Unknown	Dyspepsia, sore tongue, fatigue	Lean meat, eggs, fish, milk
Niacin	8 mg/1000 kcal	Unknown	Pellagra, skin problems, diarrhea	Dairy products, meats, peanut butter
Minerals Calcium	360-800 mg/day	Unknown	Bone and teeth problems, growth retardation	Milk, dairy products
Iron	10-15 mg/day	Cardiovascular collapse	Anemia	Enriched cereals, liver, beef
Potassium	6mEq*/day	Heart block	Muscle weakness, fatigue	Meats, fish, whole-grain cereals
Sodium	6 mEq/day	Edema	Dehydration, muscle cramps, nausea and vomiting	Table salt, milk, cheese, preservatives

Data from Chow MP, et al: *Handbook of pediatric primary care,* New York, 1984, Wiley; and Pipes PL: *Nutrition in infancy and childhood,* ed 4, St Louis, 1989, Mosby.
*IU, international units; mEq, milliequivalents.

The major thrust in giving parents guidance in accident prevention should emphasize two approaches: (1) eliminating specific environmental hazards, such as drugs, from exploring infants and (2) supervising infants while they play and gradually replacing supervision with training for safety.[26]

Plants. House plants are another source of poisoning for infants. Most of us do not think of house plants along with foods when we think of poisoning because we do not think of eating them. But infants test almost everything by putting it in their mouths, and a number of plants can be deadly if eaten. As a result, plants are one of the leading poisoners of infants, and amateur foragers must learn the hard way that everything that looks good to eat is not.

Household plants are frequently placed on the floor where the leaves or flowers are attractive and easy to pull off and taste. The best treatment for plant poisoning is prevention, which in this case means prior knowledge. Table 17-11 identifies several common household and garden plants that are poisonous. It is essential that the nurse know which plants are harmful when ingested and to inform parents of the potential dangers to infants.

The National Clearinghouse for Poison Control Centers lists plants as the third most commonly ingested poison after aspirin and household cleaning agents.

Table 17-11. **Poisonous parts of common house and garden plants**

Plant	Toxic part	Symptoms
Apple	Seeds	Releases cyanide when ingested in large quantities; may be fatal
Azalia	All parts	Nausea, vomiting, dyspnea, paralysis; may be fatal
Buttercup	All parts	Inflammation around mouth, stomach pains, vomiting, diarrhea, convulsions
Castor Bean	Seeds	Burning of mouth and throat, excessive thirst, convulsions; one or two seeds are near the lethal dose for adults
Croton	Plant juice	Gastroenteritis
Daffodil	Bulb	Nausea, vomiting, diarrhea; may be fatal
Diffenbachia	All parts	Intensive burning and irritation of the mouth and tongue; death can occur if base of tongue swells enough to occlude air passages
English holly	Berries	Nausea, vomiting, diarrhea, central nervous system depression; may be fatal
English ivy	Leaves and berries	Dyspnea, vomiting, diarrhea, coma and death
Hyacinth	Bulb	Nausea, vomiting, diarrhea; may be fatal
Iris	Undergound stems	Digestive upset
Jasmine	All parts	Hallucinations, elevated temperature, tachycardia, paralysis
Lily of the valley	All parts	Arrhythmia, mental confusion, weakness, shock and death
Mistletoe	Berries	Acute stomach and intestinal irritations with diarrhea; may be fatal
Oak tree	Acorns	Kidney failure, gastritis
Oleander	All parts	Digestive upset, bloody diarrhea, respiratory depression, cardiac arrhythmia, blurred vision, coma and death
Philodendron	All parts	Burning of lips, mouth, and tongue; swelling of tongue; dyspnea; kidney failure and death
Poinsettia	Leaves	Severe irritation to mouth, throat, and stomach; may be fatal
Potato	All green parts	Cardiac depression; may be fatal
Tomato	Green parts	Cardiac depression; may be fatal
Violet	Seeds	Taken in quantity, cathartic effects can be serious to infant
Yew	Foliage, seeds, bark	Nausea, vomiting, diarrhea, dyspnea, dilated pupils; death is sudden

Safety education should be stressed at all well-baby conferences beginning in the first six months of life. Prevention of plant poisoning and other accidents depends on a reciprocal relationship between protection and education that must be related to age. Safe behavior is a learned behavior, gradually acquired in a progressive process with increasing age. The box on this page lists specific safety measures for parents to prevent plant poisoning during infancy.[32]

Toxins. Infants are at particular risk from toxic factors in the environment; as dependent, developing organisms, they are inherently vulnerable. In general, the exposure of infants to potential toxicants is quite different from that of adults because of differences in physical environment, activities, and diet. Daily activities of infants, such as proximity to the floor or carpet indoors and the lawn or soil outdoors, hand-to-mouth behaviors, and smaller body size and composition place them at great risk for environmental toxins. Studies suggest, for example, that the normal activity of infants may expose them to higher levels of lead or of pesticides applied indoors or to the lawn.[53]

Certain *pesticides* used to control insects that feed on cereal grains, fruits, and vegetables are notorious for their slow accumulation in human tissue. Over sufficient time, exposure to relatively small amounts may result in the build up of toxic doses.

Lead is another environmental toxin that has no known physiologic role in the human body. Although lead is essentially a contaminant, most persons take in a certain amount daily through air, food, and drink. Studies have revealed a very high lead content in dust, dirt, and soil. Lead in the air primarily comes from automobile emissions.[14] Absorption of lead is closely related to

❑ ❑ NURSING INTERVENTIONS TO PREVENT PLANT POISONING IN INFANTS

- Keep plants out of reach of infants and young children.
- Never eat any part of a plant except those parts grown or sold as food.
- Keep jewelry made from unknown seeds or beans away from exploring infants.
- Learn to identify poisonous plants around your house and garden.
- Do not use unknown plants as medicines or teas.
- Pay close attention to infants at play inside and outside.
- Seek help whenever anyone chews or swallows a poisonous plant.
- Be aware that infants are more susceptible than adults to the effects of poisonous plants.

particle size. Airborne lead of small particle size is readily absorbed through the lungs, whereas larger particles fall to the ground.

Infants are very vulnerable to lead exposure for several reasons. In proportion to their weight, infants breathe in more air and thus more lead than do adults. In addition, they breathe closer to the ground, where a higher concentration of lead is found. Their dust-raising play and habit of putting their hands in their mouths add to their consumption of lead. They also have a greater rate of gastrointestinal absorption of lead and other chemicals. Both exercise and blockage of the nasal passages increase mouth breathing, and the mouth is a far less capable filter than the nose. Thus mouth breathing, coupled with their greater frequency of respiratory tract infections, exposes infants to a greater amount of environmental toxins.[26]

Human potential and development clearly are important natural resources, and a growing body of evidence now links increased exposure to lead in the environment with an impaired intellectual performance and potential. Clinical lead poisoning affects many children, but it is a preventable disease; excess lead in the infant's environment is made by and should be prevented by human beings.

Infants do not necessarily escape noxious chemicals when they go indoors. The contaminants that cause *air pollution* are about the same indoors as out, with perhaps more carbon monoxide, nitrogen dioxide, and various hydrocarbons–from tobacco smoke, poorly vented heating and cooking equipment, and aerosol sprays. Many air pollution aftereffects may not be seen during infancy but may show up in problems affecting both physical and mental well-being over a lifetime.

Among the acute illnesses of infancy, respiratory disease is number one, representing between 50% and 75% of all pediatric disease.[54] Besides the inconvenience and incapacity induced by respiratory diseases, medical costs are high. Almost all respiratory problems are aggravated by dirty air, and some are caused by it. Infants with chronic respiratory disease may become adults with respiratory problems.

Water pollution affects the infant by causing gastrointestinal disturbances. Parents and medical authorities are quick to blame food, teething, or a virus for simple diarrhea, when the underlying cause may come from the kitchen sink. Numerous strong chemicals are used today to help purify drinking water. These chemicals can irritate the delicate lining and cause disturbances in the infant's gastrointestinal tract. Nurses can encourage parents to boil all water before they give it to their infant to help eliminate any potential problem. See Table 17-12 for major pollutants and their health effects.

MECHANICAL FORCES

This area refers to the effects of motion or action of forces on the infant; the focus here is on *motor vehicle accidents.*

Automobiles present a danger to persons of all ages, but especially to infants. Usually the problem is improper restraint of the infant inside the automobile. Many parents are misled by thinking it is better to be thrown clear of an accident than to be restrained. Many also think that is is safer to hold an infant on the lap in the front seat than have the infant restrained in the back seat. On the contrary, these practices tempt fate and increase the probability of a fatality. A free-moving child not only distracts the driver but also is in a more vulnerable position to be thrown.

Adult seat belts are unsuitable for infants or children under 4 years of age because their pelvic structure is small; the American Academy of Pediatrics recom-

Table 17-12. **Major pollutants and their health effects**

Pollutants	Major sources	Effects
Carbon monoxide	Vehicle exhaust	Replaces oxygen in RBC, causes dizziness, coma, or death
Lead	Antiknock agents in some gasoline; old paint chips, metal pieces, pottery, soil	Accumulates in the bones and soft tissues; affects blood-forming organs, kidneys, and CNS
Nitrogen dioxide	Industrial wastes, vehicle exhaust	Causes structural and chemical changes in lungs; lowers URI resistance
Ozone	Formed when hydrocarbons and nitrogen dioxide react	Produces smog; irritates mucous membranes, causing coughing, choking, impaired lung function; contributes to asthma and bronchitis
Sulfur dioxide	Burning coal and oil; industrial processes	Increase in colds, coughs, asthma, and contributes to acid rain
Passive smoking	Tobacco products	High incidence of URI, pneumonia and bronchitis, asthma, link to cancer

Source: Environmental Protection Agency, 1992.

mends that safety seats for infants be used.[64] A variety of car seats are available: for infants up to 20 pounds the recommended type is the rear-facing, molded plastic shell seat, which includes a shoulder restraint and employs the adult seat belt.[67] The shield-type car seat, for the child weighing 24 to 48 pounds, offers maximum protection for the older infant (see Fig. 17-6).

The nurse also can suggest the following to parents regarding automobile safety:[42]

1. Never leave a child alone in a car.
2. Never hold a child in the lap in the front seat.
3. Always use an infant car seat that is properly installed.
4. Keep all car doors locked.
5. Use safety restraints for all passengers and the driver.
6. Continue to use car seats until the child reaches 40 pounds, then use adult seat belts.

Much of automobile safety is common sense, but the nurse must cover all areas in anticipatory preventive teaching. The importance of automobile safety cannot be overemphasized.

RADIATION

Radiation, in its broadest sense, means the transfer of electromagnetic waves through space.[3] Radiation of all types presents a potential hazard within the infant's environment. The risk is proportional to the amount of radiation and the length of exposure, as well as to the particular tissues involved; the infant's rapidly growing and immature cells are especially vulnerable.

The infant is exposed to two basic categories of radiation: (1) natural background radiation, which comes from cosmic rays and radioactive material naturally existing in the soil, water, and air; and (2) man-made radiation, which includes x-rays and radiation from nuclear power plants, microwave ovens, and other electronic devices found in the home.[64]

CANCER

Ionizing radiation is a prime example of an environmental agent that can cause cancer. Studies have demonstrated that harmful effects occur in the body exposed to radiation. The incidence of leukemia and other childhood cancers has increased in infants who were irradiated in utero when their mothers underwent pelvic x-ray examination during pregnancy.[61]

Most persons think of cancer as a disease of adults. Cancer, however, is the leading cause of death from disease in children over 1 year of age. The most common cancers found from infancy to age 5 years are Wilms' tumor, retinoblastoma, acute lymphocytic leukemia, neuroblastoma, and rhabdomyosarcoma. Since most childhood cancers' peak incidences occur during other developmental age-groups (toddler, preschooler), only retinoblastoma and neuroblastoma are discussed here.

Retinoblastoma. This is a rare malignant tumor of the eye, with both sexes affected equally often. The majority of these tumors are diagnosed before the child is 2 years of age. The tumor may result from genetic transmission of a defective gene or from spontaneous cell mutation. Hereditary forms of the disease are caused by autosomal dominance. Retinoblastoma occurs most often as spontaneous development, not the inherited type. Infants with the inherited type tend to develop bilateral disease; those with the spontaneous type may or may not have the tumor in both eyes.

Perhaps because retinoblastoma is a rare tumor, many health professionals fail to recognize the ominous significance of early clues, usually first noticed by parents. The result is frequently a delay in diagnosis and treatment.

Nursing intervention to identify risk factors includes a careful history, which usually reveals a slow progression of symptoms–cat's eye reflex, strabismus, painful red eye, and blindness. The nurse should ask the following questions to identify risk factors:

Do tumors of the eyes run in your family?

If so, can you tell me which relatives had this and what was done for these tumors?

Have you noticed your child having any *eye problems–crossed or lazy eyes, difficulty seeing?*

Have you noticed any changes in your child's eyes?

Nurses with physical assessment skills can perform screening and ophthalmoscopic examinations on high-risk infants and children. These eye tests include checking for the following:

1. *Visual acuity,* which can be determined by the fixation test, used to screen vision in infants and children 6 months to 5½ years of age.
2. *Red reflex,* which appears whitish in the infant with retinoblastoma–the cat's eye reflex, the most common presenting sign of this cancer.
3. *Lid lag,* which is found in exophthalmos.
4. *Strabismus,* which is determined by giving the cover-uncover test.

Nursing assessment of infants with signs and symptoms of retinoblastoma warrant an immediate referral to an ophthalmologist for further evaluation. Nursing diagnosis for retinoblastoma might include the following:[23]

- Altered family processes related to the child's illness
- High risk for injury related to sensory deficit
- Pain related to possible pressure from a tumor
- Disturbance in self-concept related to loss of eye

Neuroblastoma. This is a malignant tumor arising from the sympathetic nervous system. It is primarily a disease of infancy and early childhood: approximately one third of all clients are under 1 year of age at the time of diagnosis; more than 80% are recognized by age 5

❑ ❑ NURSING INTERVENTIONS TO PREVENT CANCER IN INFANTS

Identify high-risk infants from family history, physical examination, screening programs, and so on.
Educate parents, caregivers, and day-care personnel regarding the warning signs that may indicate the presence of cancer.
Refer and provide follow-up care for high-risk infants.
Update own knowledge concerning cancer and its continuing effect on the environment.
Be aware of the benefits and risks of x-ray examinations to reduce unneccessary ones.
Promote parents' personal habits that are favorable to their own and their infant's health.

years. Unfortunately, two thirds have metastasis when first seen, and frequently the symptoms or signs arising from the secondary spread bring the infant to the attention of health professionals.[61]

Neuroblastoma is an embryonal childhood cancer that appears to follow both a hereditary and a nonhereditary pattern. The literature has identified a number of families with more than one affected sibling. There may be a relationship between neuroblastoma and some anomalies of neural crest origin (neurofibromatosis, aganglionosis coli).[44] It is important to note that survivors of neuroblastoma may develop subsequent tumors, thus necessitating continued medical surveillance. Some experts recommend monitoring the *offspring* of individuals with neuroblastoma and examining them carefully for evidence of neural crest abnormalities. Stromborg and Cohen also state. "The finding of increased urinary excretion of catecholamines in the siblings of children with neuroblastoma supports the contention that all members of a family in which this tumor is diagnosed should be investigated for similar abnormalities."[61] Neuroblastoma produces excessive amounts of neuroactive catecholamines, which are found in the urine of clients with this tumor. Thus, vanillylmandelic acid (VMA) in excessive amounts in the urine may indicate this tumor.

The box above lists nursing interventions to help detect and prevent these tumors during infancy.

Social Processes

ROLE AND RELATIONSHIP PATTERN

The literature has explored extensively the effect of early bonding between parents and their infants, emphasizing that this initial attraction prepares for later development of love and affiliation.[24] The bonding process also has many implications for that infant's future development.[35]

Attachment and Bonding. The parent-infant relationship does not begin with the birth of the infant; many aspects have been molded by the life experiences of the parents long before they reached parenthood. The earliest effects on the mother-infant relationship will be influenced by the kind of mothering she received as an infant and by the concept of "mother" she developed as she grew up. Her overall self-concept as a person will affect her ability to relate to her infant, as will her relationship with the infant's father.

The establishment of this emotional bond between the mother and her infant is known as *attachment.* This emotional bond is considered crucial for the optimum physical and emotional development of the infant. The process of attachment is demonstrated by such maternal behaviors as how the mother holds, feeds, and looks at the infant.[8]

Various theories have attempted to explain the basis for attachment behavior. Freudian psychoanalytic theory emphasizes that the bond between child and mother develops as a result of the mother's satisfying the infant's innate needs related to the human need to socialize with another and to the physical needs for survival. Social learning theory contributes the principles of reinforcement to the attachment process; as the mother meets the infant's needs, discomfort is reduced or removed. The infant associates a pleasurable feeling of being satisfied with the mother, who becomes a "significant other" in the infant's life.

The bonding process is the basis for the mother-infant relationship, which in turn forms the basis for the necessary interdependence required for the infant's psychologic and physical development (Fig. 17-9).[36]

The process of bonding is also important for fathers. Recently a process called *engrossment* has been used to describe the behavior pattern noted in fathers when they interact with their infants. The major characteristics of engrossment include: (1) visual awareness of the infant; (2) tactile awareness, often expressed in a desire to hold the infant; (3) awareness of distinct characteristics, with emphasis on those features that resemble the father; (4) perception of the infant as perfect; (5) development of a strong feeling of attraction to the infant that leads to intense focusing of attention; (6) experiencing a feeling of extreme elation; and (7) feeling a sense of deep self-esteem and satisfaction.[7]

Klaus and Kennell[35] have formulated seven crucial principles in the process of attachment:

1. There appears to be a sensitive period in the first minutes and hours after birth when it seems necessary for the mother and father to have close contact with their infant for later development to be optimum.

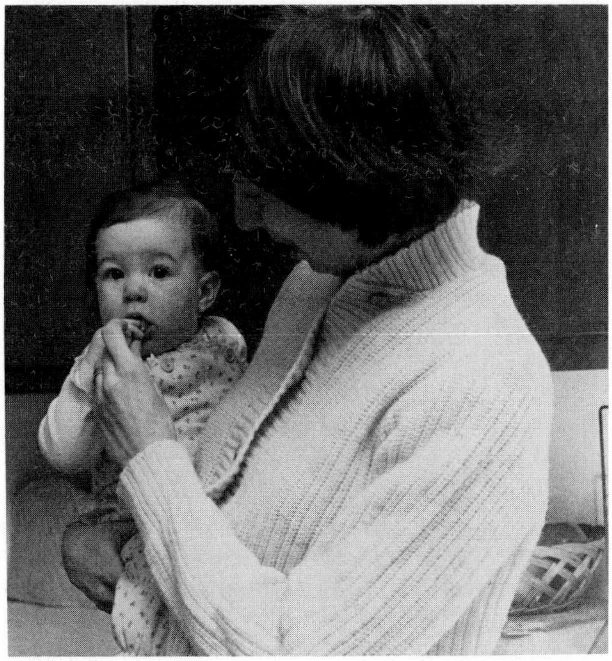

Fig. 17-9. The process of bonding is the basis for the relationship between the mother and child. (Photograph by Douglas Bloomquist.)

2. There appears to be species-specific responses to the infant in the human mother and father when the infant is first given to them.
3. The attachment process seems to be structured so that the parents become attached to only one infant at a time.
4. For attachment to occur appropriately, the infant must respond to the mother and father by some signal, such as body or eye movements. This principle has been called the "you can't love a dishrag" phenomenon.
5. Individuals who witness the birth process become strongly attached to the infant.
6. It is difficult for some adults to go through the processes of attachment and detachment simultaneously. Thus it is difficult for parents to attach to an infant while mourning the loss or threatened loss of another person.
7. Some early events may have long-lasting effects. For example, anxiety over an infant with a transient disorder in his or her early days may result in long-term concerns or behavior that will have implications for future development.

Just as the infant's behavior influences attachment, it continues to influence the evolving maternal-paternal-infant relationship as the infant develops. Studies have shown that if the process of attachment is interfered with, later problems are more likely to occur, such as child abuse, failure-to-thrive syndrome, and behavioral problems.[8]

Many factors are present when a relationship is being established and maintained. Most persons enter a relationship with unrealistic expectations; parents are no exception–they are going to be wise, patient, devoted, and nurture their infant. Because the parents' self-esteem is closely associated with their infant's interactions and accomplishments, disappointment, anger, and a disturbance in their infant's relationship may occur. In some instances this disturbed parent-infant relationship is short-lived, and nothing harmful develops from it. When a disturbed parent-infant relationship continues, however, the infant is at risk for abuse and failure-to-thrive syndrome.

Abuse. Infant and child abuse has always been a part of human history. Acceptable behavior toward infants is largely a learned phenomenon; the art of parenting is not as instinctively acquired as many believe. Abusing parents are seldom "monsters"; they are merely individuals attempting to cope with the demands of parenthood, often with little or no preparation for it.

The scope of the problem is extensive: estimates show that more than a million infants and children in the United States are victims of abuse.[10] Children under age 3 years are the most frequent victims. Studies have found that women are more frequent abusers than men because they are the primary caregivers. Men abuse more severely and often are involved in sexual abuse. Child abuse does not discriminate: it occurs in families of every race, creed, and socioeconomic class.

The child abuse syndrome is a clinical condition in infants who have suffered serious active or passive abuse at the hands of their parents or caregivers. Physical trauma is not the only facet, but it is the most overt indicator of a dysfunctioning family unit and a disturbed parent-infant relationship.[49]

Active abuse manifestations include

1. Brain injuries, subdural hematomas, and skull fractures;
2. Soft tissue injuries, such as bruises, lacerations, or burns; and
3. Fractures of the long bones and ribs; x-ray films frequently show multiple fractures in varying stages of healing.

Passive abuse manifestations include

1. Poor nutrition, failure to thrive, and severe malnutrition;
2. Poor physical condition: neglected safeguards against disease, poor skin condition, and lack of proper medical attention;
3. Emotional neglect–rejection, indifference, and deprivation of love; and
4. Moral neglect–allowing infant or child to remain in an immoral atmosphere.

Abusing parents often have common patterns of behavior. As children, they themselves may have been abused by their parents. In this way child abuse is recycled from generation to generation. The development of the maternal role that the infant depends on for health, progress, and survival begins in the early childhood of the mother herself. Unless she received love and mothering, she will have difficulty with a relationship that entails the complete dependency of another person. She may find the relationship with her own infant unrewarding, threatening, and frustrating. Feelings of inadequacy and guilt in the mother and father role compound the problems.

The parents are often socially isolated and have few persons to whom they can turn at times of crisis; they also cannot emotionally support each other. They may see the infant as the person who can provide the love, support, and nurturing lacking in their lives. When the infant does not fulfill their expectations, the risk of abuse becomes acute.[49]

The abused infant or child usually is singled out as someone who is different. This infant may be chronically ill, may have been premature, may be hyperactive, may have been the product of a difficult and complicated pregnancy, or may have an obvious birth anomaly. Early bonding disturbances–inadequacies in feeding, holding, and caring for the infant–are characteristic signals.

The long-term effects are profound. The victims lack basic trust, a major task of infancy, as well as confidence and self-worth. These deficits follow them into adulthood and parenthood, and the vicious cycle continues. One of the discouraging findings is that infants and children who were abused tend to grow up to be abusing parents themselves.[49]

Across the United States great interest has been generated in attempts to identify high-risk parents in the prenatal and perinatal period who have significant potential for later child abuse. Measures such as the following have been undertaken to help prevent child abuse:

1. Predictive questionnaires, given to mothers on postpartum units.
2. Recognition of mothers who appear to have difficulty relating to their infants through body language clues or verbalizations.
3. Closer hospital follow-up in the postpartum period by the public health nurse.
4. Crisis hot lines made available to parents in distress.

Before focusing on nursing interventions (see the box on this page), the nurse can make several observations using the following questions to assist in identifying a high-risk infant:

Does mother hold infant close and establish eye contact?

Does mother speak negatively about infant?

Does mother intensely dislike the duties of motherhood: diapering, feeding, and so on?

❑ ❑ NURSING INTERVENTIONS TO PREVENT ABUSE OF INFANTS

Promote and facilitate early parent-infant bonding.

Promote trusting nurse-client relationship.

Provide more frequent office visits and be available by phone.

Provide infant care instructions to enhance mothering ability.

Provide for community health person to make home visits.

Does mother expect too much of infant at a particular stage of development?

Does mother focus her attention on infant rather than husband?

Does mother have a good support system available?

Does mother act overly concerned about infant's sex?

Most communities are seeking ways to prevent child abuse through educational efforts, improved agency coordination, and development of new supportive efforts and services for parents and infants.[59] Laws for reporting abuse have been enacted in every state. It is mandatory that all cases of suspected abuse and neglect be reported. Everyone must assist in this endeavor to prevent continued abuse.

Failure to Thrive. Another problem that may stem from a disturbed parent-infant relationship is failure-to-thrive (FTT) syndrome. There is no unanimously agreed upon definition of FTT. The term is used to describe infants who fail to gain weight. It results from the failure to obtain or use necessary calories required to grow. A weight persistently below the percentile on a standard growth chart characterizes the FTT infant. Although failure to thrive may be due to an organic disease, it is most often the result of a disturbance in the relationship between the primary caregiver and the infant.

Five principal factors in the infant's growth and development are (1) adequate nutrition, (2) sleep and rest, (3) activity, (4) adequate secretion of hormones, and (5) a satisfactory relationship with a significant other who provides loving, human contact and stimulation. When this last factor is missing, the infant's growth is disturbed and development is delayed.[57]

The nurse must realize that the parent-infant relationship is reciprocal. The mother's failure to provide adequate emotional care and often adequate nutrition may result in an infant who fails to gain weight. This failure may be interpreted by the mother as a rejection of her mothering efforts, and this interpretation naturally reduces her self-confidence. This lack of self-confidence is reflected in her care; thus a negative pattern of interaction is established between mother and infant.[8]

The infant who is failing to thrive displays malnourishment and growth failure. The infant may have poor muscle tone, lethargy, an inability to cuddle, and delayed or absent speech patterns.[8]

The mothers of failure-to-thrive infants often show many of the following characteristics:[40]

1. Disrupted and disorganized home situations
2. Inability to assess her infant's needs
3. Inability to think about the future
4. Lack of nurturing when she was a child
5. Low self-esteem and feelings of inadequacy

The first nursing intervention is to assess the family relationships by asking questions and observing interactions.[45] The following guidelines may be helpful in the assessment process:

Do mother and infant have eye-to-eye contact frequently? How much body contact is present?

Does vocalization by mother evoke a smile from infant?

How much does infant cry? What is mother's reaction?

How does mother describe infant's feeding and sleeping patterns?

Does the mother describe her mothering tasks positively or negatively?

How does the mother perceive the problem? As infant's fault? Her fault?

Ask mother about her own health and impact on caring for infant.

Elicit family support systems present. Is mother isolated?

Have mother describe her home life and what changes have taken place within it.

The goals of nursing intervention after the assessment of family dynamics are listed in the box to the right.

NURSING INTERVENTIONS TO PREVENT FAILURE TO THRIVE IN INFANTS

Improve family interactions and relationships

Improve family's ability to cope with stress.

Increase parental self-esteem.

Discuss age-appropriate feeding techniques.

Praise positive parenting behaviors.

Review growth and developmental behaviors and encourage parents to foster them.

Provide adequate nutrition for the malnourished infant.

Teach parents their infant's nutritional requirements.

Demonstrate infant feeding position, formula preparation, and age-appropriate foods.

Help parents learn and interpret their infant's cues during interaction.

Promote adequate environmental stimulation

Demonstrate techniques of stimulation that will improve growth and development.

Teach reasons why stimulation is necessary for health promotion.

Improve family's awareness of and insight into problem area

Allow parents to vent their feelings toward infant.

Assist in identifying the infant's attributes and unique qualities.

Discuss stress within the family unit and assist the parents to use support system within the community: family, friends, clergy, social worker, nurse, and so on.

Continue counseling efforts at home through public health agency.

Refer to appropriate agency for financial, social, or other family needs.

Homelessness. Along with food, health, and personal safety, there is probably no greater basic need for human beings than shelter. The loss of these is detrimental to the health and well-being of all people. Homelessness in the United States is a national disgrace. Most estimates place the number of homeless at 3 million. One out of every four homeless persons is a child.[38]

It is not an exaggeration to say that the well-being of our next generation is being jeopardized by homelessness. It devastates every aspect of a child's life, doing damage with long-term implications that are still unknown. Homelessness endangers a child's health throughout childhood. Homeless infants are often exposed to unsafe and unsanitary conditions in shelters where infectious diseases thrive. Those dangers are combined with a lack of access to regular health care so that common childhood ailments like ear infections become very serious and sometimes life-threatening illnesses before they are treated.

Ear infections are among the most common problems encountered in pediatric practice. Usually, a 10-day course of antibiotics takes care of the situation. Rarely are long-term complications encountered. But for the homeless infant the story is different. Families are cut off from their regular clinics and providers. The struggle for basic life needs is intense. The poverty and isolation and disorientation of prolonged homelessness may be complicated by crack or alcohol abuse, provoked, at least in part, by situational despair. The very ability of a family to function is hampered or paralyzed.

So, for the homeless family, the fever caused by the infant's acute ear infection may not have the highest priority. Availability, accessibility, and affordability of medical care are serious questions. As a result, the infection is never treated, and the problem becomes prolonged. The infection evolves to a chronic state. Hearing and language development may be impaired.

Overall, these children simply do not receive routine, reliable health care. They remain at high risk for many health problems. Their medical problems remain undiagnosed and undertreated–if they receive medical attention at all. Medical complications and secondary problems abound. Furthermore, the conditions they live under–the squalor, the lack of safe food storage and preparation facilities, and the drug infested and physically dangerous environments, predispose children to a substantially increased rate of disease and injury.[65]

The pioneering work of Erik Erikson has defined the necessary stages of human development. Each level of maturation must be sequentially mastered, but it takes a secure environment, opportunities to succeed, and emotional support. The hidden tragedy for homeless children is the insult to their personal growth. These losses, as opposed to the loss of a home, may be irrevocable. Timing is critical in childhood to achieve critical developmental milestones.[66] Homelessness theoretically can be eliminated. The key factors must be increased affordable housing, increased income for low-income families, and strengthened service and support for families at risk of homelessness. Families at risk of homelessness for solely economic reasons can often be helped with short-term loans and grants. Community-based programs can help identify these families before they lose their homes.

Efforts should be made to link the homeless with all available programs and services, such as WIC, food stamps, Head Start, and housing subsidies. These programs should continue to provide assistance after the family is resettled in permanent housing. More comprehensive services will be needed by those families with special problems such as domestic violence, mental illness, or substance abuse. These programs need to be provided on an ongoing basis to help create stability for affected families.[66]

With a multitude of needs there must be a partnership in providing a multitude of resources. Nurses can take a leadership position in helping the homeless achieve a sense of security and adequate health care. Getting involved in community health care for the homeless and providing compassionate care gives the homeless a clear signal of hope and of concern about their plight. Bringing attention to this social problem by speaking to various community groups to get their help and support is another way that nurses can assist the homeless. Volunteering time in community shelters and organizing health care days through the local health department is still another way to address the problem. Nurses can become active in raising the nation's conscience and helping call attention to this national disgrace. It is imperative that housing and support services be provided to assist the homeless to regain a foothold in our society. With the right support services and health care, many of them can be stabilized and integrated back into the community. These families with infants are not "throw-aways," but people who have fallen on hard times and need someone to offer a helping hand. Through this help our nation's health can improve.

COMMUNITY

As infants grow and develop, their boundaries may extend beyond the home environment. Many mothers return to the work force while their infants are still very young and place them in community day-care centers.

Today, few young families can escape financial burdens. The two-income family is a way of life today, and the trend will continue. With more than half of all American mothers working outside the home, the need for day-care services is growing.

This is usually an emotional issue for families; the separation process can be traumatic for both infant and parent. The comforting realization in this dilemma is that most studies agree that the *quality* of time spent with an infant is important, not the quantity.[28]

The findings from social science research regarding the effects of day care on an infant's development and health can be summarized as follows: (1) little evidence suggests that day care permanently enhances or slows intellectual development; (2) day care can be used, even from earliest infancy, without damaging the mother-infant relationship; and (3) day care may lead to a slight increase in minor illnesses, but excluding ill infants from the center is not an effective means of reducing the spread.[62]

The question of how old their infant should be before starting in day care is a frequently asked question of health professionals. Many "experts" say a mother and infant should have 4 to 6 months together before the mother goes to or returns to work. Brazelton[7] makes a good case for the mother and infant going through 4 stages of attachment together before the mother goes to work. In the first stage, which takes 10 to 14 days, the infant learns to be attentive to the mother and the mother learns cues from the infant about being both ready and tired for attentiveness. The second stage, which lasts 8 weeks, is the stage of playful interaction when the mother learns how to recognize the infant's nonverbal cues and helps the infant maintain the alert state. The third stage, from the tenth week to the fourth month, is when the mother and infant learn to play games together. In the fourth stage, which occurs in the fourth month, infants rapidly learn about themselves and their world. Thus Brazelton suggests that a mother, when possible, spend the first 4 months with her new infant, but every mother must make her own decision.

A nationwide survey of family day care found that nearly half of all infants in day-care centers in the United States are cared for in one of three types of family arrangements:[7]

1. Private homes that provide informal day care to infants of relatives, friends, and neighbors
2. Regulated independent care licensed by state agencies
3. Regulated, sponsored care provided by licensed workers operating as part of home networks under umbrella agencies

The nurse has a viable role in assisting families with infants who need day care. Many factors must be reviewed when a family is looking for an appropriate day-care program; the nurse can counsel and guide the family in their search. Some nursing guidelines to help the family select a day-care center follow:

1. Promote awareness of the three types of day care available in their local communities.
2. Counsel parents on what to ask a prospective day-care facility.
   Licensed by the state?
   Open all year?
   Number of children present?
   Age range of children?
   Teacher-to-child ratio (for infants, 1:3 is recommended)?
   Describe day-care program.
   What meals are served?
   What is cost?
   Are there openings?
   Qualifications of caregivers?
   Are the caregivers happy and interacting with the infant?
   Are infants contented?
   Are parents welcome to drop in?
3. Assist parents to deal with separation behaviors manifested by their infant.
   Remain calm in situation.
   Attempt to reduce number of "strange" adults that interact with the infant and always introduce them.
   Encourage the parents to bring an infant's special cuddly toy from home to the day-care facility to promote security.
   Elicit the parent's understanding of the processes.
   Reassure parents that it takes time for the infant to make the transition from parent to another caregiver, and vice versa.
   Emphasize that at certain developmental levels "stranger anxiety" may heighten (8 months), and separation behaviors of crying and clinging may be repeated.
   Work toward promoting a good relationship between parent-infant-caregiver by providing opportunities for open discussions of concerns.

CULTURE AND ETHNICITY

The developing infant is subject to the influences of culture from the moment of conception. Partly because of the long dependency period, it is within the family environment that the infant experiences overall cultural attitudes. The parents' perceptions of illness, wellness, roles, patterns of childrearing, religious values, language, and health practices are all modeled for the infant. In short, culture helps to form the infant's view of the world.[9]

The family's ethnicity include ideas about health, illness, food preferences, moral codes, and family life that persist across generations and survive even the upheaval of coming to a new country. All multicultural groups confront repeated challenges as they transfer their families from familiar to unfamiliar surroundings. Infants are exposed to an appropriate mode of behavior that is in accordance with their family's cultural standards. They take cues for behavior from observing and imitating family members. These perceptions then are incorporated into their own self-concepts.[41]

To assess and plan appropriate interventions for multicultural families, nurses must be aware of their own cultural backgrounds. An important consideration is to look at all customs and values in relative terms, seeing none as altogether good or bad. Change is inevitable in family life, whether it is resisted or welcomed. An important function of the nurse is to help families monitor the rate of change acceptable to various members and reach a consensus. Key factors are listed in the box below.

The nurse must determine the power structure within a given cultural group. This knowledge may help dictate which family member to approach with the health teaching. Although the nurse might assume it would be

❑ ❑ FACTORS THAT FACILITATE MULTICULTURAL HEALTH CARE BY NURSES[41]

- Knowledge of the historical experience, recent and long term, of ethnic groups composing the community.
- Demographic data that include family size, socioeconomic status, and future expectations characteristic of diverse ethnic groups.
- Recognition of folk beliefs and cultural attitudes toward health and illness.
- Awareness of the nature of problems encountered by ethnic group members when they enter the health care system, including fear and distrust of health care professionals, language barriers, and discrimination by caregivers.

the infant's mother, this is not necessarily true. Among some American Indian tribes the grandmother, not the parents, has the authority over the grandchildren. In many Latin cultural groups, the infant's father, not the mother, makes decisions about the infant's welfare. The nurse also needs to know the cultural groups' practices and beliefs before planning interventions.

Approaches to infant care practices vary among cultural groups. In American culture the proportion of women choosing to breastfeed has steadily increased in recent years. Many factors are involved in the decision-making process–cultural beliefs about the role of women, female sexuality, mothering sense, family support or lack of it, and nurses' attitudes while working with the mother and infant. Nurses who deal with mothers need to be aware of the multiplicity of factors influencing feeding choice and should encourage and support parents in their decisions.

The family is the primary health care provider for the infant. It is the family that determines when an infant is ill and decides to seek help in managing an illness. Many cultural groups choose between components of traditional or folk beliefs that seem appropriate to them and Western medical treatment. The Vietnamese utilize both. For example, to decrease an infant's fever, a basil leaf is tied to the wrist with a piece of cheesecloth. For colic, a silver coin is dipped in wine and rubbed or scratched on the infant's back. Although the nurse may not feel that these practices are valuable, to pass judgment is wrong. Nurses must be cautious in imposing their own values, beliefs, and attitudes on clients. Rather than judging clients by the nurse's own cultural standards, the family should be viewed as a member of a different culture and the nurse should ascertain how this family's culture influences its health practices.

Nurses must actively work to reduce the experience of culture shock for families raising infants, remembering that American medical beliefs may seem strange to others. It is important for the nurse to remember that all behavior must be evaluated from within the context of the family's cultural background and experiences. Nurses who strive to foster health promoting attitudes and behaviors must begin at the most basic level: empathetic concern and respect for the individual. By incorporating the assessment of cultural beliefs and practices into the infant's plan of care, nurses can demonstrate respect, reduce alienation, and take a step toward developing culturally appropriate patterns of health promotion.

In addition to ethnic and cultural heritage, the nurse needs to incorporate the family's religious beliefs as well as communicate with understanding. Both are complex and multifaceted in form and function. Both have an impact on the family's sense of wellness and health practices. It is extremely important to respect another's language as well as his or her religion and work to achieve understanding and prevent barriers from forming.

Language. Language (and deafness) can create a barrier to health care and be a risk factor if it differs from that of the health care provider. Language is an important medium to understanding and working together. The nurse may avoid or tend to mumble a client's name when it is foreign; we all hesitate to express ourselves when the material is unfamiliar to us. The nurse must consider how the client, who speaks a different language, feels when he is unable to express himself or understand what is being said. Both parties may play the avoidance game.

The nurse must make provisions so that communication barriers are removed, including

1. Using a family member as interpreter to help in the communication process.
2. Using pictorial flash cards in the client's native language to assist in explaining instructions.
3. Sending a health care worker to school to learn the basics of the language to help in the interpreting process in the health care facility.

Even when the client speaks the nurse's language, it does not necessarily follow that understanding and comprehension of instructions will occur.

Religion. In our pluralistic and democratic society, Americans are being faced with the ethical and religious values impinging on health care services. Interestingly, some health providers act as if religion plays no role with clients in health care practices; thus they eschew the clients' religious or ethical concerns and deal mainly with the physical or psychologic problems at hand. The client's religious and ethical concerns are generally the major source for human values when evaluating health services.

Religious beliefs as risk factors focus mainly on decisions concerning treatment. An example may be the parents who refuse a needed blood transfusion, surgery, or other medically indicated treatment to save their infant's life. A court order is needed in many instances to treat these infants. This is the parents' decision based on their customs and beliefs and should be respected. It may be extremely hard not to intervene with an opinion regarding this, but usually it is unwanted. Religion is often a powerful force, and when the nurse causes conflict and interferes, a gap may be formed. This gap may force the parents to seek nonprofessional health care to help them with their health- and religious-related ideas about birth, death, stress, birth control, and other problems. The client's ethnic background should be investigated and understood thoroughly to work successfully with him.

Political Legislation. Health and well-being have become generally accepted rights of everyone, without regard to color, sex, age, economic or social status, or creed. The federal government has pledged to promote the general welfare of the United States in the belief that it belongs to everyone.

To fulfill this pledge, several goals were established to address areas of health concerns. One such concern was infant health. The goal, as described by the Department of Health and Human Services (HHS) states: "To continue to improve infant health, and, by 1990, to reduce infant mortality by at least 35 percent, to fewer than nine deaths per 1,000 live births."[64]

The infant mortality rate has been on a steady decline since the turn of the century, a result of better infant nutrition, improved housing, and improved prenatal, obstetric, and pediatric care.[64] To meet this goal of improving infant health, the major health problems in this age group must be reduced. The first and greatest hazard for infants is *low birth weight.* To address this problem, associated factors that increase the risk of low-birth-weight infants must be identified:

1. Maternal factors
   - Low socioeconomic status
   - No prenatal care
   - Preeclampsia and eclampsia
   - Hypertension
   - Chronic renal disease
   - Advanced diabetes
   - Malnutrition
   - Cigarette smoking (10/day or more)
   - Drug addiction
   - Maternal age (under 15 or over 35)
   - Alcohol abuse
   - Marital status
2. Fetal factors
   - Multiple gestation (twins)
   - Congenital malformation
   - Chromosomal abnormality
   - Chronic intrauterine infection
3. Placental insufficiency

Many of these factors can be prevented, or risks can be identified early and treated to prevent a low-birth-weight infant. The major focus for prevention is prenatal care for all women.

The second major threat to infant survival is *congenital disorders* such as malformations of the brain and spine (microcephaly and myelomeningocele), congenital heart defects (ventricular septal defects), and combinations of several malformations, such as Down's syndrome or Tay-Sachs disease.

Birth defects are responsible for one sixth of all infant deaths.[64] Many congenital abnormalities cannot be prevented, but many can be through prenatal screening and research to discover the "why" in the development of these birth defects.

Other factors identified by HHS that contribute to the high infant mortality rate are (1) injuries at birth, (2) sudden infant death syndrome, (3) accidents, (4) inadequate infant diets, and (5) inadequate parenting.[64]

The federal government's plans to attain the goal of healthy infants are to

1. Promote family planning services so that all pregnancies are planned and infants are wanted.
2. Provide pregnancy and infant care services through Maternity and Infant Care (MIC) projects to high-risk populations. Women, Infants, and Children (WIC) programs increase the nutritional status of both mother and infant.
3. Encourage educational efforts by schools, health providers, and the media to promote prenatal care.
4. Promote massive immunization efforts so that each infant is protected against communicable disease.

Nursing's Role. Roles for nurses are rapidly changing in response to a continually expanding knowledge base, consumer health care needs, and governmental legislation. The nurse can play a tremendous part in bringing about change in health care related policies by actively participating in groups involved with health planning.

The nurse's role in the development of health care policies takes on three stages: (1) identifying resources for the community to meet their specific need; (2) planning for resources not available to that community; and (3) coordinating the resources available to them to promote better use of them.

The nurse can become a member of a health planning council, a concerned citizen's group, or an advisory group to a local legislator or to a state health department grant task force. In this capacity the nurse's duty would be to inform the other committee members. Since nurses have first-hand experience with many community needs, they are in a good position to speak out on this issue and inform others of it.

The nurse within the local community also has several resources available to assist when a need is identified to promote the infant's health: (1) federal level–HHS; (2) state level–public health department; (3) local level–MIC clinics, well-baby clinics; and (4) community groups–parents anonymous, hot lines, LaLeche League, March of Dimes, SIDS groups.

Coordinating for resources, the nurse could actively participate in assessing the availability of services within the community and make recommendations to consolidate or expand existing ones. To make the public aware of community resources, their services, and existing needs is the basis of the nurse's role in developing policy.

Economics. Even in a society of considerable affluence, approximately 13% of the total population is below the poverty level.[60] These poor families tend to be characterized by having a lack of education, high unemployment rates, being large and headed by females, experiencing residential crowding, and having a lack of adequate bathroom facilities.[10] Virtually every major health problem is found more frequently in segments of the population with low income than in higher-income groups. The infant mortality rates in lower-income families remain significantly higher than rates of the higher-income family, despite an overall decrease in infant mortality rate nationally.[32]

Many studies have demonstrated that parents with low incomes are often unaware of their infant's developmental needs; they frequently are faced with many environmental and social stresses that demand their time, energy, and other resources.[13] Many parents have so many unfulfilled needs of their own that they cannot meet their infant's needs.

In many cases infants from poverty-level families have delayed language development. Their parents, with limited educational and life experiences, limit the amount of vocalization the infant will hear. Infants learn early language sounds from their parents, but their attempts at language must be reinforced.

Armed with this knowledge of how economics can affect the infant's growth, development, and health status, the nurse, before deciding interventions (see box to the right), needs to assess the family situation by

1. Establishing a relationship with the family to obtain pertinent information.
2. Evaluating home environment in which the infant interacts.
3. Eliciting parents' health perceptions regarding their own health as well as the infant's.
4. Completing a thorough physical examination on the infant to identify any problem areas.
5. Identifying community resources available to this low-income family.

NURSING INTERVENTIONS TO HELP ECONOMICALLY DEPRIVED FAMILIES AND INFANTS

Contact resource agencies, such as Aid for Families with Dependent Children (AFDC), WIC programs, MIC programs, and Medicaid to ascertain available services for the family.

Assume the role as an advocate for the poor family to assist members to interact with the array of health and social welfare agencies.

Participate in supporting legislation to reduce the social and economic stresses affecting poor families.

Use the knowledge of healthy infant-parent interactions to foster this within the family unit.

Be aware of a different value system when working with lower-income families, and do not let it interfere with developing a trusting relationship.

Offer the parents helpful hints on how they can facilitate their infant's development by using common household items: measuring spoons, plastic cups, and so on.

Emphasize need for protecting the infant's health by safety measures within the home environment and for receiving immunizations.

HEALTH CARE DELIVERY SYSTEMS

The U.S. health care delivery system is diverse and large; many different sectors emerge to provide infant care. The nurse within this huge, multidisciplined system must be a family advocate to facilitate its passage through the many facets of care. The box on p. 447 lists health care programs established for the infant and the family for the purpose of disease prevention and health promotion and maintenance.

The value of preventive health care has been validated; it is cost effective and is here to stay. As nurses' roles continue to expand within the various health care systems, their duty is to keep pace with the needs, concerns, and strategies available.[22] Since many conditions that cause morbidity or mortality in infants are preventable when health promotional practices are employed, nurses have the mission of working within the health care system to promote healthy infants.

NURSING INTERVENTIONS IN INFANCY

Health maintenance, promotion of wellness, and prevention of illness and injury are the goals emphasized throughout this chapter. The federal government has identified areas of concern and made recommendations to promote a healthy infant population. Table 17-13 lists a suggested schedule for health promotional infant care.

Nurses must become the "agents of prevention" within the health care system.[49] The increased opportunities for nurses to share in this major health care responsibility are exciting and challenging. If health maintenance/promotion and disease prevention are to become realities in the future of national health, nurses must take the initiative now to preserve the United States' most precious natural resource: its future generations (see box on p. 449).

❑ ❑ INFANT HEALTH CARE PROGRAMS

Government agencies

Department of Health and Human Services–office of Child Development (responsible for nationally funded health programs)
Food and Drug Administration (regulates any ingested substances)
United States Public Health Service (responsible for community's health)
State health departments (establish immunization requirements)

Voluntary agencies

National Foundation–March of Dimes (goal is to prevent birth defects)
Sudden Infant Death Syndrome Foundation (information, research, and education regarding SIDS)
Child Abuse Prevention Foundation (promote public awareness of problem)
Childbirth education associations (provide education to expectant parents)

International organizations

World Health Organization (WHO)
United Nations Children's Fund (UNICEF) (goal is to improve children's health worldwide)

Local agencies

Parenting education:
- College or school courses
- Hospital and clinic classes
- Cooperative extension services
- Social health department
- Childbirth education classes

Financial assistance–reduced fee health care:
- City or county health department
- WIC program
- Well-baby clinic
- Immunization clinic
- Prenatal clinic
- Family planning clinic

Ambulatory care:
- Pediatrician
- Family practice
- Pediatric nurse practitioner
- Public health nurse

SUMMARY

Society is changing, as are people's needs and ideas. Families today want more information and knowledge, and they are demanding that health care professionals be more responsive to their needs. Their demand has been a catalyst for the nurse's expanded health care role and responsibility for health maintenance.

Health maintenance and disease prevention practices applicable during infancy can be used in the nurse's expanded role. A three-pronged approach is stressed:

1. Giving anticipatory guidance to the family unit as the infant grows and develops.
2. Teaching and counseling to ensure the infant's optimum development.
3. Being a family advocate to ensure the safety and future development of the family unit.

Anticipating potential health problems during infancy and effectively intervening to avert them are nursing processes used to promote health. Many health problems, such as abuse, are avoided by early detection and reduction of risk factors. By anticipating problems and assisting families to avoid or minimize them, the nurse promotes health maintenance.

Using the infant's normal growth and development, psychosocial tasks, identified common health problems, and health maintenance strategies, the nurse can make an assessment of the infant, the family, and the infant's developmental status to provide anticipatory guidance.

In teaching, an essential component of the nursing process, the nurse transmits knowledge to families to ensure continuity of care and long-term health maintenance. In counseling, the nurse listens to the identified problem, assists the family to see the real issues, and allows the family to make its own decision regarding health care.

Since the infant is not in a position to advocate effectively, the nurse assumes this role to help ensure health maintenance. The ultimate goal of nursing intervention in maintaining the infant's health is future self-care. As the infant grows and matures, well-established family health maintenance habits can only enhance healthy future generations. The nurse is challenged to join this effort of investment in the future.

***Table 17-13.* Suggested schedule for health promotional infant care**

Age (months)	Promotional activity
1	Complete physical assessment Phenylketonuria (PKU) test Parent discussion includes: Basic infant needs–to be touched, held, fondled, rocked and talked to Appropriate toy–colorful mobile Nutrition–formula or breast
2	Complete physical assessment Immunizations: DTP and TOPV Parent discussion includes: Placing infant in prone position to allow lifting of head Need of infant to be exposed to variety of stimuli within environment Need of infant for change of scenery Discuss colic and other common problems
4	Complete physical assessment Immunizations: DTP and TOPV Parent discussion includes: Stimulation of infant Providing a mirror in which the infant may see reflection Being talked to and played with Appropriate toy–rattle
6	Complete physical assessment Immunizations: DTP Laboratory work: hematocrit levels Parent discussion includes: Accident prevention Teething and use of coal rings Allowing infant to crawl to explore environment Stranger anxiety
9	Complete physical assessment Parent discussion includes: Accident prevention Dental caries prevention–cleaning teeth with gauze daily Infant's need for space to crawl about Use of cup if weaning Use of finger foods Playing games with infant: Pat-a-cake Peek-a-boo Waving bye-bye Shaking hands Appropriate toys–blocks, stack toys, jack-in-the-box Fear of strangers
12	Complete physical assessment Immunizations: Tuberculin (TB) test Laboratory work: Complete blood count (CBC) Parent discussion includes: Accident prevention "Getting into things" Infant's need to touch and investigate environment under supervision Parent's need to read, show pictures, and repeat body parts to infant Infant's need for limited independence Sleeping patterns Appropriate toys–sets of measuring cups, nesting toys, pats and pans, wooden spoons
15	Complete physical assessment Immunizations: MMR Parent discussion includes: Negativism as normal aspect of development Age of curiosity in infant Toys appropriate for age–push-pull toys, balls Accident prevention Elimination patterns Discipline–stress positive aspects of behavior if possible
18	Complete physical assessment Immunizations: DTP and TOPV Parent discussion includes: Accident prevention Begin toilet training if child is ready Encourage vocalization Socialization with other small children Importance of reading to child Setting limits on behavior Coping mechanisms of parents

RESEARCH REVIEW

PRENATAL

INFANTS AT HIGH RISK

Cilenti D, Farel AM: Identifying infants at risk: North Carolina's high-priority infant program, *Public Health Nurs* 8:219-225, 1991.

Purpose The purpose of this study was to evaluate the implementation of a statewide program to meet the needs of infants at risk for developmental delay.

Review Data on infants enrolled in North Carolina's High-Priority Infant Program (HPIP) between July 1983 and June 1988 were examined. Information on the characteristics of the program, types and volume of its services, and follow-up findings at 1 year of age for infants at greatest risk were assessed to indicate whether the program was meeting its objectives. Total number of infants enrolled in the program steadily climbed from 1013 to 4868. Information about the infant's developmental status was collected according to a tracking protocol. The most common health indicators for tracking visits were very low birth weight, gestational age 34 weeks and below, and respiratory distress syndrome. Evaluation of the program emphasizes health promotion efforts early in life to maximize the child's emotional and physical growth and functional abilities.

INJURY PREVENTION

Jones NE: Injury prevention: a survey of clinical practice, *J Pediatr Health Care* 6:182-186, 1992.

Purpose The purpose of this study was to determine what education and training pediatric nurse practitioners receive about injury prevention and control and what kinds of clinical activities PNPs perform with regard to injury prevention.

Review Sixty-four members of the Greater New York Chapter of the National Association of Pediatric Nurse Associates and Practitioners were administered a questionnaire. Data on demographic, professional, practice characteristics, education, and clinical activities in injury prevention and control for infants and children were collected. Results indicated that advice about child car restraints and automobile seat belts was routinely given by less than 30% of practitioners, information about smoke detectors was given by about 15%, and advice about firearms in the home was given by 7% or less. Implications for PNP health promotion activities are discussed.

References

1. American Academy of Pediatrics: Report of the committee on infectious diseases, ed 22, Elk Grove Village, Ill, 1991, The Academy.
2. Bardwick JM: *Feminine personality & conflict,* New York, 1981, Harper & Row.
3. Bee H: *The developing child,* ed 5, New York, 1988, Harper & Row.
4. Bellack JP, Edlund BJ: *Nursing assessment and diagnosis,* ed 2, Boston, 1992, Jones & Bartlett.
5. Betz CL, Poster EC: *Pediatric nursing reference,* ed 2, St Louis, 1992, Mosby.
6. Bloom BS: *Human characteristics and school learning,* New York, 1982, McGraw-Hill.
7. Brazelton T: *Working and caring,* Reading, Mass, 1987, Addison-Wesley.
8. Brazelton T, Cramer B: *The earliest relationship: parents, infants and the drama of easy attachments,* New York, 1990, Delacorte.
9. Bukathko D, Daehler M: *Child psychology,* Boston, 1992, Houghton Mifflin.
10. Bureau of the Census: *Characteristics of the population below the poverty level: 1991,* series P-60, N 119, Washington, DC, 1991, US Government Printing Office.
11. Castiglia PT, Harbin RE: *Child health care,* Philadelphia, 1992, JB Lippincott.
12. Cataldo CB, et al: *Nutrition & diet therapy,* ed 3, St Paul, Minn, 1992, West Publishing.
13. Chinn PL: *Child health maintenance: concepts in family-centered care,* ed 4, St Louis, 1989, Mosby.
14. Davis JM, Grant LD: *The sensitivity of children to lead.* In *Similarities and differences between children and adults: implications for risk assessment,* Washington, DC, 1992, ILSI Press.
15. DeFrain J, et al: *Sudden infant death: enduring the loss,* New York, 1991, Free Press.
16. Dickason EJ, et al: *Maternal-infant nursing care,* St Louis, 1990, Mosby.
17. Duvall E, Miller B: *Marriage and family development,* ed 6, New York, 1984, Harper & Row.
18. Farrell CD: Genetic counseling: the emerging reality, *J Perinatology/Neonatology Nurs* 2:21, 1989.
19. Fields R: *Drugs and alcohol in perspective,* Dubuque, 1992, William C Brown.
20. Foster RL, et al: *Family-centered nursing care of children,* Philadelphia, 1989, WB Saunders.
21. Frankenburg WK, et al: The Denver II: a major revision and restandardization of the Denver developmental screening test, *Pediatrics* 89(1):91-97, 1992.
22. Gettrust KV, Brabec PD: *Nursing diagnosis in clinical practice,* New York, 1992, Delmar Publishers.

23. Gulanick M, et al: *Nursing care plans for newborns and children: acute and critical care,* St Louis, 1992, Mosby.
24. Gunzenhauser N: *Advances in touch,* New Brunswick, NJ, 1990, J & J Consumer Products.
25. Gunzenhauser N: *Infant stimulation: from whom, what kind, when, how much?,* New Brunswick, NJ, 1987, J & J Consumer Products.
26. Hall JA: *Don't just say NO! Safety book for children,* Detroit, 1991, Personal Products Group.
27. Hamilton EMN, et al: *Nutrition: concepts and controversies,* St Paul, Minn, 1991, West Publishing.
28. Heins M, Seiden AM: *Child care/parent care,* New York, 1987, Doubleday.
29. Helvie CO: *Community health nursing: theory and practice,* New York, 1991, Springer Publications.
30. Hoekelman R, et al: *Primary pediatric care,* ed 2, St Louis, 1991, Mosby.
31. Ingalls AJ: *Maternal and child health nursing,* St Louis, 1991, Mosby.
32. James SR, Mott SR: *Child health nursing: essential care of children and families,* Menlo Park, Calif, 1988, Addison-Wesley.
33. Janosik E, Green E: *Family life: process and practice,* Boston, 1992, Jones & Bartlett.
34. Jensen MD, Bobak IM: *Maternity and gynecologic care: the nurse and the family,* ed 4, St Louis, 1989, Mosby.
35. Klaus MH, Kennell JH: *Parent-infant bonding,* ed 2, St Louis, 1982, Mosby.
36. Korones SB, Lancaster J: *High-risk newborn infants: the basis for intensive care nursing,* ed 4, St Louis, 1986, Mosby.
37. Kozier B, et al: *Concepts and issues in nursing practice,* ed 2, Menlo Park, Calif, 1992, Addison-Wesley.
38. Kraljic MA: *The homeless problem,* New York, 1992, HW Wilson.
39. Kyle D, et al: Ethnic differences in incidence of SIDS, *Arch Diseases Childhood* 65:830, 1990.
40. Lancaster JB, et al: *Parenting across the life span: biosocial dimensions,* New York, 1987, Aldine de Gruyter.
41. Leninger M: *Transcultural nursing: concepts, theories and practices,* ed 2, New York, 1988, John Wiley & Sons.
42. Levy MR, et al: *Life and health: targeting wellness,* New York, 1992, McGraw-Hill.
43. Lewis M, Worobey J: *Infant stress and coping,* San Francisco, Calif, 1989, Jossey-Bass.
44. Mahan LK, Arlin MT: *Krause's food nutrition and diet therapy,* Philadelphia, 1992, WB Saunders.
45. Malasanos L, et al: *Health assessment,* ed 4, St Louis, 1989, Mosby.
46. Marlow DR, Redding BA: *Textbook of pediatric nursing,* ed 6, Philadelphia, 1988, WB Saunders.
47. Mott SR, et al: *Nursing care of children and families,* Redwood City, Calif, 1990, Addison-Wesley.
48. Nelson SE, et al: Lack of adverse reactions to iron-fortified formula, *Pediatrics* 81:360, 1989.
49. Olds SB, et al: *Maternal-newborn nursing: a family-centered approach,* Redwood City, Calif, 1992, Addison-Wesley.
50. Peri R: What's the best way for baby to sleep?, *Georgia Journal,* April 16, 1992.
51. Pillitteri A: *Maternal and child health nursing: care of the childbearing and childrearing family,* New York, 1992, JB Lippincott.
52. Rhodes AM: Minimizing the liability risks for genetic counseling, *Mat Child Nurs* 14:313, 1989.
53. Ross JH: *Experimental method to estimate indoor pesticide exposure to children.* In *Similarities and differences between children and adults: implications for risk assessment,* Washington, DC, 1992, ILSI Press.
54. Schmitt BD: *Your child's health: a pediatric guide for parents,* New York, 1991, Bantam Books.
55. Scipien GM, et al: *Pediatric nursing care,* St Louis, 1990, Mosby.
56. Servonsky J, Opas SR: *Nursing management of children,* Boston, 1987, Jones & Bartlett.
57. Smith MJ: *Child and family: concepts of nursing practice,* New York, 1991, Mosby.
58. Smith S, Crockett K: Moms break tradition for SIDS prevention, *Miami Herald,* Florida, April 19, 1992.
59. Soditus C, Mock D: Interrupting the cycle of child abuse, *Mat Child Nurs,* 13:25, 1988.
60. Statistical abstract of the United States, ed 111, US Bureau of the Census, Washington, DC, 1991.
61. Stromborg M, Cohen R: Cancer, the case for preventive strategies (draft chapter), 1981.
62. Taylor JR, Kling DR: *Day care guide for parents,* New York, 1990, Carekits.
63. Ulene A, Shelov JA: *Bringing out the best in your baby,* New York, 1988, Macmillan.
64. US Department of Health and Human Services, Public Health Service: *Healthy people 2000: national health promotion and disease prevention objectives,* Pub No 91-50212, Washington, DC, 1991, US Government Printing Office.
65. US Senate Hearing: *Homeless children: are we losing a generation?,* Washington, DC, 1989, US Government Printing Office.
66. US Senate Hearing: *Homelessness: an American tragedy,* Washington, DC, 1990, US Government Printing Office.
67. Whaley LF, Wong DL: *Essentials of pediatric nursing,* ed 4, St Louis, 1993, Mosby.

CHAPTER 18

Toddler*

Lois A. Hancock

Objectives

After completing this chapter, the nurse will be able to

- *Discuss the physical changes that occur during the toddler period and relate these changes to health hazards for this age.*
- *Discuss with a parent the common behavioral problems related to eating during the toddler period.*
- *Discuss with a parent an appropriate plan for toilet training a 30-month-old toddler.*
- *Develop a teaching plan for discussion of sleep disturbances during toddlerhood.*
- *Explain to a parent why temper tantrums are age-appropriate behavior for toddlers.*
- *Prepare a handout for parents of toddlers concerning accident prevention in the home.*
- *Answer a parent's questions about sibling rivalry in the toddler period.*
- *Outline the recommended schedule of preventive health visits for the toddler and appropriate subjects for the nurse to discuss with parents at each visit.*

The beginning of the toddler period is characterized by the child becoming secure in the ability to walk and run and achieving a language ability sufficient to express most needs and desires. During this time, the body structure continues to resemble that of the infant more than that of the adult, and the child primarily is involved in developing a separate sense of self.

The toddler may be quite isolated from traditional health care supervision–past the age of frequent immunizations and not yet in school, where periodic screening may be required. Parents may fall into a pattern of illness care rather than periodic preventive visits and health promotion for their toddler. The child from 18 months to 36 months is not yet old enough to be an active participant in personal health practices (see box on p. 452).

PHYSIOLOGIC PROCESSES

Age and Physical Changes

The 24-month-old toddler appears chubby, with relatively short legs and a large head. Over the next 18 months, a relative decrease in the growth of subcutaneous adipose tissue occurs, and the extremities grow more rapidly than the trunk.[21]

The toddler has a marked lumbar lordosis and a

*Sections of this chapter are adapted from Chinn PL: *Child health maintenance: concepts in family-centered care,* ed 2, St Louis, 1979, Mosby.

HEALTHY PEOPLE 2000

SELECTED NATIONAL HEALTH PROMOTION AND DISEASE PREVENTION OBJECTIVES

TODDLER

- Reduce iron deficiency to less than 3% among children aged 1 through 4
- Reduce drowning deaths among children aged 4 and younger to no more than 2.3 per 100,000 (1987 adjusted baseline: 4.2 per 100,000)
- Increase use of occupant protection systems such as safety belts, inflatable safety restraints, and child safety seats to at least 95% of children aged 4 and younger
- Reduce acute middle-ear infections among children aged 4 and younger, as measured by days of restricted activity or school absenteeism, to no more than 105 days per 100 children (1987 adjusted baseline: 131 days per 100 children)
- Reduce nonfatal poisoning among children aged 4 and younger to no more than 520 emergency department treatments per 100,000 (1986 baseline: 650 per 100,000)
- Reduce the prevalence of blood lead levels exceeding 15 mg/dl and 25 mg/dl among children aged 6 months through 5 years to no more than 500,000 (1984 baseline: an estimated 3 million children had levels exceeding 15 mg/dl and 234,000 had levels exceeding 25 mg/dl)
- Increase to at least 30 the number of states which at least 50% of children identified as neglected or physically or sexually abused receive physical and mental evaluation with appropriate follow-up or a means of breaking the intergenerational cycle of abuse

protuberant abdomen. The 24-month-old still has a wide stance and a slight outward rotation of the legs at the hip. By 36 months, the toddler may be "knockkneed," and the fat pad in the instep gives a flat-footed appearance. These are not pathologic conditions but rather normal characteristics at this age. Intervention is needed only if the child does not progress to a more straight-leg, toes-forward position by school age.[12]

Growth rate, which has slowed during later infancy, continues to decelerate until about age 24 months and then remains relatively steady throughout the third year and until school age. Average gains during the second year of life are 2.5 kg (5½ pounds) in weight, about 12 cm (4 ¾ inches) in length (or height), and less than 2.5 cm (1 inch) in head circumference. The anterior fontanel has usually closed by 18 months, and the skull becomes thicker. By 24 months, the head is four fifths of adult size, and height is approximately half of final adult height for the individual.[24]

The toddler's stature may be measured as length, as is the infant's, or as height, as is the older child's and adult's. The nurse must note which measurement was used in standardizing the growth grid and measure the child in a recumbent position for length or a standing position for height. The difference in measurements is small but can cause confusion in interpreting the child's pattern of growth.

The kidneys become well differentiated by the toddler years, and specific gravity and other urine findings are similar to those of adults.[11] The daily excretion of urine for the 2-year-old is 500 to 600 ml (15 to 18 ounces); for the 3-year-old, 600 to 750 ml (18 to 22½ ounces) in 24 hours.[11] The toddler empties the bladder less frequently than the infant and has more voluntary control of urination because of maturation of the neurologic pathways to the bladder and sphincter.

The toddler's gastrointestinal tract reaches functional maturity and can handle most adult foods. The organs of the gastrointestinal tract continue growing to adulthood. The toddler tends to need more frequent meals and snacks than the older child or adult. Many older toddlers have sufficient voluntary control of rectal sphincters to accomplish successful bowel training.

Basically no difference exists in lung topography or function after infancy. Lung capacity, however, continues to increase as the toddler grows, and respiratory rate decreases from a mean of 30 breaths/min at 1 year to 25 breaths/min at 3 years. The diameter of the toddler's upper respiratory tract is small compared to older child's or adult's. This small diameter, coupled with the toddler's lack of judgment in deciding what to place in the mouth, can result in airway obstruction, which demands emergency action.

The anatomy of the ear and the throat continues to

resemble that of the infant more closely than that of the adult, but gradual increases in the size of the structures lessen the probability of communicating infection from one area to another. The tonsils and adenoids remain large during the toddler years.[21]

With the exception of reproductive endocrine functions, most endocrine organs become functionally mature during the toddler and preschool years, although function continues at a minimum. The production of glucagon and insulin may be limited or labile, producing variations in blood sugar levels that may be demonstrated throughout early childhood. The production of cortisol, aldosterone, and deoxycorticosterone by the adrenal cortex probably remains somewhat limited but seems to function more effectively in protecting the young child against the hazards of fluid and electrolyte imbalance than during infancy. Secretions of epinephrine and norepinephrine from the adrenal medulla increase sufficiently to perform homeostatic functions of the autonomic nervous system and to mediate certain aspects of increased emotional components of behavior. Regulation of growth during early childhood remains one of the most important functions of the endocrine system. Growth hormone, thyroid, insulin, and corticoids probably are the most vital hormones for normal growth and development during this period.[6,11,22]

Permanent circulatory pathways are fully established when the child reaches later infancy or toddlerhood. Changes in the system's function, including decreases in heart rate, increases in blood pressure, and changes in vascular resistance of various body areas in response to growth in the size of the vessel lumen, continue gradually. Heart rate is variable throughout life, and the normal range is wide at all ages. The range for toddlers is 110 ± 40 (2 standard deviations); the mean blood pressure is 99 to 100/60 to 65.[20] Getting the toddler to sit still for a blood pressure reading may be difficult, but it is worth the effort to obtain several baseline readings for future reference.

The capillary beds gradually increase their capacity to respond to heat or cold in the environment and thus participate more effectively in thermoregulation. Autonomic control of this function becomes more fully integrated into the total functioning of the central nervous system so that the child can now begin to take voluntary measures to relieve the discomfort of heat or cold. For example, the older toddler can put on clothing or move to warmer or cooler areas and assist physiologic efforts to maintain a constant internal thermal environment.

The immune system of specific antibodies continues to become established. Some common organisms of the environment have been encountered, and immune responses have begun to function adequately. When toddlers enter the world of nurseries and day care, exposure to new and different organisms is greatly increased, and they may experience a period when they seem to succumb to many minor respiratory and gastrointestinal infections. As immunity begins to develop against the organisms of the new environment, their resistance likewise increases. Despite environmental exposure, however, increases in immunoglobulin levels have been demonstrated to follow a well-defined pattern during early childhood. Immunoglobulin G (IgG) continues to rise sharply; immunoglobulin M (IgM) reaches an adult level during later infancy or early childhood; and immunoglobulin A (IgA) demonstrates a gradual increase during these toddler years.[6]

Passive immunity to communicable disease acquired through transfer of maternal antibodies during fetal life has disappeared by this time, but active immunity to certain communicable diseases through initial immunization series is usually completed by 18 months. The next scheduled immunizations–booster diphtheria-tetanus-pertussis (DTP) and oral poliovirus vaccine (OPV)–are during the preschool period.[4]

During the second year of life, the last of the 20 primary or deciduous teeth erupt. The sequence is generally the mandibular cuspids at about 16 months, maxillary cuspids at about 18 months, mandibular second molars at 20 months, and the maxillary second molars at about 24-months. Timing of these eruptions for an individual child may vary widely, but a difference in sequence should alert the nurse to inquire about early trauma to the mouth or familial traits for out-of-sequence tooth eruption.

A mature swallowing pattern without a forward tongue thrust and permanent lip and tongue habits, which influence the occlusion and development of arch and jaw relationships, are formed during the second and third year.

As discussed in Chapter 17, fluoride is an important aspect of preventive dental care and should be continued throughout toddlerhood. Families who move to a new community as their child gets older may not know if the water in that new community is fluoridated, so the nurse should make this information available. Other important aspects of dental care at this age that the nurse should include in health teaching are listed in the box on p. 454.[13]

Ossification of the skeletal system gradually declines during the toddler years as this process becomes more advanced in many areas of the body, but it continues until full stature is reached.

Increases in the size and strength of muscle fibers also continue. During this period, as during infancy, use of muscle tissues is the primary stimulus for increased size and strength. Children who tend to develop a significant amount of muscle mass during toddlerhood are responding to a combination of genetic inheritance and stimulation through use. Boys demonstrate this pattern more often than girls, but this is not a true sex difference, since differential hormonal control of body growth and

❑ ❑ NURSING INTERVENTIONS TO PROMOTE DENTAL HEALTH CARE FOR TODDLERS

Brushing

- Use a soft-bristled brush. The gauze method used during infancy is no longer adequate because the many teeth are too close together to allow a finger wrapped in gauze to reach all surfaces.
- Introduce just a moist toothbrush. After the toddler has accepted the toothbrush, begin using toothpaste.
- Toothpaste should contain fluoride.
- Toddlers do not have the motor coordination to brush their *own* teeth. They may enjoy "imitating" parents and put the toothbrush in their mouths, but an adult needs to be responsible for actual brushing.
- Brush daily; for many toddlers, this becomes part of the bedtime routine. If the child seems too tired to cooperate in the evening, the parent should choose some other time of day when this important task will not be forgotten.
- It is probably easiest for the parent to sit down and place the toddler in the lap while brushing.

Foods

- Limit high-sugar foods.
- If the young toddler still has a bottle, it should only contain plain water and should be eliminated as soon as possible.

Visits to the dentist

- The first visit to the dentist should occur as soon as all 20 primary teeth have erupted–never later than age 3.
- Many dentists suggest an inspection-consultation type of visit when the child is about 18 months old. This provides an early, enjoyable introduction to the dental examination.

development is not operative during early childhood.[6]

Full development of voluntary motor movement during early childhood is not presently understood. Myelination of the corticospinal tract is functionally advanced enough to support most movement, but achievement of full control does not occur until much later in life.

Throughout early childhood, voluntary motor movement is often accompanied by involuntary movements on the other size of the body. This mirroring of action is more pronounced in children who suffer some damage of the central nervous system, but the mechanisms by which this occurs are unknown. The toddler generally does not show complete dominance of one-sided body function. Thus, the toddler may still switch hands when eating, throwing a ball, or engaging in other "handed" activities.

Gender

Throughout infancy and childhood, boys are more likely to show atypical development and be affected by some common childhood illnesses. For example, during the toddler years *otitis media* is a very common infection, affecting more than two thirds of children by age 3. Many studies have shown that boys are affected more often than girls.[12] Boys also are physically handicapped more often than girls, with a 5:4 ratio for hearing problems and 3:2 for speech deficits. The reason for this is not known precisely, but one hypothesis suggests that girls, because of the double-X chromosome, have some protection not only from recessively inherited diseases but also from commonly encountered organisms. Another possibility is that, because of cultural expectations for boys to be "strong," "brave," and so on, even at very young ages, they are exposed to more potential dangers and stresses earlier.[2]

Race

Some differences in the rate of physical growth between races occur during the toddler years, just as during infancy. During toddlerhood, these differences may be most noticeable in the earlier eruption of teeth of black and Asian children when compared to whites. Blacks continue to be slightly taller and demonstrate some motor tasks a little sooner than white toddlers.

The issue of race's effect on health is complex, as discussed in Chapter 15. Is race a major reason why certain toddlers have more illnesses, or is race a cumulative function of nutrition, living conditions, socioeconomic status, family structure, and availability of health care resources? More study needs to be undertaken in this area. The nurse should look at socioeconomic factors as well as race and adapt health teaching to the individual family's situation.

Genetics

Most genetic problems are noted and diagnosed during infancy. These problems may influence the health status of the toddler, but management has ideally been instituted during infancy. A few genetic problems may be detected during the toddler years. The most frequent is a mild *developmental delay,* which is partly or fully genetically determined. These delays often are not diagnosed in infancy because the subtle language, motor, or cognitive deficiencies do not interfere with expected performance and behavior. If the nurse detects subnormal performance in a standard age-appropriate developmental screening test during the toddler years, the child should be referred for diagnostic testing.

Other genetic problems occasionally recognized during the toddler years are some *hematologic conditions,* such as sickle cell disease, resulting from homozygous sickle genes, or *spherocytosis,* an autosomal dominant trait. These may be detected during routine screening or when the child becomes ill and diagnostic laboratory tests are ordered. The toddler who shows slowed growth or failure to thrive may have a growth hormone deficiency of genetic origin. The nurse may recognize this late onset of failure to thrive during routine screening of growth parameters.

Another genetic problem sometimes not manifested until after infancy is *cystic fibrosis,* an autosomal recessive trait. This might appear as a persistent or repeated respiratory or gastrointestinal disturbance. The nurse may teach about or conduct the *sweat chloride test,* which helps to identify these children.

All these conditions should be referred to a pediatrician or appropriate specialist for definitive diagnosis and medical management. The nurse will continue to care for these families by providing health teaching and screening for related problems and complications.

Nutritional and Metabolic Pattern

By the beginning of toddlerhood, weaning from breast or bottle usually has occurred, and milk intake has decreased in proportion to solid or table foods (see box on p. 452).

The primary dietary concern in American society is prevention of *iron-deficiency anemia,* and adequate iron intake must be ensured, particularly as the toddler changes from iron-fortified milk formula to whole milk.[18] Other food sources of iron, such as meat, may be avoided or rejected by the toddler, and the family's resources may limit its provision. Eggs, specifically the yolk, offer a valuable source of iron that can be incorporated easily into the toddler's diet, particularly if the family is aware of the child's need for this important nutrient.

From 18 to 24 months, the toddler may still be switching from infant to adult foods. The use of prepared toddler foods during the transition from infancy to early childhood presents a special concern, since these products may not provide optimum nutrition or the food range needed by the child. Helping parents understand the information labels of all prepared foods is valuable in conveying both principles of nutrition and sound marketing and consumer protection. Also, the parent may not realize the expense of such foods, and when convenience in preparation is not a major consideration, the child may be fed more economically and nutritionally with the regular family diet. Little extra preparation is needed by the time the child's first molar teeth appear.

Table 18-1. Food pattern for toddlers, ages 2 to 4

Food group	Examples	Number/size of servings
Bread	Bread, cereal, rice, spaghetti, noodles, muffin, pancakes	Six
Vegetable	Carrots, greens, tomatoes, broccoli	Two
Fruit	Orange, strawberries, peach, watermelon	Two
Milk	Milk, cheese, yogurt	Two to three
Meat	Fish, chicken, beef	5 oz.
Total fat		53 g
Total sugars		6 tsp.

As during other periods of life, the food guide pyramid should be used as a guide in estimating the adequacy of the toddler's intake of all essential nutrients, and the family should be counseled accordingly.

The decreased rate of growth during later infancy and toddlerhood results in a decrease in needed calories and thus a decreased appetite. Toddlers need approximately 102 calories per kilogram of body weight. Parents who express concern about their toddler's intake should be reminded of this. Table 18-1 lists the recommended food pattern for the toddler.

One difficulty in obtaining an adequate dietary assessment is the difference between what is offered and what is actually consumed. This is particularly true for toddlers, who may at times be more interested in playing with a particular food than eating it. A prospective record, such as the one in Fig. 18-1, yields a very accurate record. A 3- or 4-day record presents a good picture of a particular child's intake.[18]

The eating *behavior* and *habits* of the young child present one of the major barriers in providing adequate nutrition. The toddler often begins to use mealtime as an occasion to assert individuality, control of the environment, and for simple exploration of food textures and qualities. Definite food preferences and food fads emerge.

The nurse should use the basic lifestyle of the family as a basis for offering counseling and guidance related to feeding, for families vary greatly in their expectations for feeding behavior and mealtime routines. For example, if the adults in the family consistently eat a wide variety of foods and enjoy mealtime together, their expectations of the young child will differ greatly from those who eat meals individually or have a limited variety of foods.

The parents need to explore their fundamental expec-

Instructions

1. Record all foods and beverages immediately after they are consumed.
2. Measure the amounts of each food carefully with standard measuring cups and spoons. Record meat portions in ounces or as fractions of pounds: 8 ounces of milk, 1 medium egg, ¼ pound of hamburger, 1 slice of white bread, ½ small banana.
3. Indicate method of preparation: medium egg, fried; ½ cup baked beans with 2-inch slice of salt pork; 4 ounces of steak, broiled.
4. Be sure to record any condiments, gravies, salad dressings, butter, margarine, whipped cream, relishes: ¾ cup of mashed potatoes with 3 tbsp of brown gravy, ¼ cup of cottage cheese salad with 2 olives, ½ cup of cornflakes with 1 tsp of sugar and ⅓ cup of 2% milk.
5. Be sure to record all between-meal foods and drinks: coffee with 1 ounce of cream, 12 ounces of cola, 4 sugar cookies, 1 candy bar (indicate brand name).
6. If you eat away from home, please put an asterisk (*) in the food column beside the food listing.

Day 1

Date ______ Day of week ______ Weight ______

Time	Food	Amount	How prepared

Fig. 18-1. Food diary for children. (Adapted from Pipes PL: *Nutrition in infancy and childhood,* ed 4, St Louis, 1989, Mosby.)

tations of the toddler's mealtime behavior and determine which are appropriate at different developmental levels. If the parents want the child to learn to eat the foods served at mealtime, they may need assistance in anticipating the necessary adjustments for the toddler to acquire these feeding behaviors. If the parents find that the toddler is disruptive of other family interaction during mealtime, they may prefer to continue feeding the toddler separately except for one meal each day.

Within the limits of family resources, the parents should understand the need to provide sufficient variety of foods to ensure adequate nutrition. The family may need specific directions and assistance in selecting such a variety and in preparing these foods so that the toddler will accept and be able to chew and swallow them adequately.

The nurse can make the following recommendations to the toddler's parents:

1. Offer simple, single foods; toddlers often reject mixtures of foods.
2. Offer a variety of foods but repeat the same foods often enough that the toddler recognizes them.
3. Encourage use of utensils but accept that toddlers still often need to use fingers.
4. Do not offer snacks within an hour before a meal, since this dampens the appetite.
5. Mealtime should be a pleasant time, free of distractions and discussion of previous "bad" behavior.
6. Do not use food as rewards or punishment for behavior.
7. Schedule meals and sleep periods so that the child is awake and alert during mealtime.
8. Serve small portions and offer seconds after the first portion is consumed.
9. Do not offer raw carrots, celery, or other such foods that could be easily aspirated.

A very important point to discuss with parents is that the toddler may at times refuse a meal altogether. The reasons for this range from asserting independence to simple tiredness. Parents should not be concerned or punish the child for this behavior. If a major family crisis follows, the toddler may learn how easily the parents can be controlled by refusing food and may continue this behavior. The nurse can help to avert this by explaining that a well-nourished child who skips an occasional meal is not in danger of malnutrition.

Use of a prospective *food record* for several days may reveal a typical toddler pattern of a hearty breakfast, medium-sized lunch, and a small or no dinner. This is very common in this age group and is a problem only because it is the opposite pattern for most families. When the evening meal is thought of as "the main meal" and the toddler does not eat it, parents may think their child will be poorly nourished. The nurse needs to demonstrate the adequacy of the nutrients the toddler already is receiving during the first two meals of the day and help the parent work out a plan to offer more of the essential foods at these meals.

The family who uses a *vegetarian diet,* with no meat, poultry, or fish, may need some assistance in offering a diet adequate in protein to the toddler. Plant proteins must be offered in appropriate combinations and proportions so that the amino acids are complementary. The toddler may not accept sufficient plant foods nor the correct proportions to meet protein needs. If the nurse is not well informed enough to discuss the details of a vegetarian diet with parents, the parents should be referred to a nutritionist or written information sources. An excellent pamphlet, "Teddy Bears and Bean Sprouts" (1989), covers the key points about vegetarian diets for young children. It is available from Gerber Products Co., Fremont, MI, 49412. Vegetarian diets that include prudently chosen plant foods and a reasonable amount of dairy foods are adequate to support normal growth and development.[23]

Elimination Pattern

Toilet training is often a major family concern as the infant grows into toddlerhood. For the family who has never experienced this challenge before, it can be a major dilemma, and yet many families are reluctant to seek advice and assistance. The nurse should anticipate this developmental task toward the end of infancy and initiate discussion with the parents to determine their understanding of the child's developmental signs of readiness for toilet training and discuss their attitudes and plans well in advance of their early trials.

The child's ability regarding toilet training depends on sufficient neurologic and psychologic maturation, including (1) local conditioning of reflex sphincter control (about age 9 months), (2) completion of myelination of pyramidal tracts (12 to 18 months), and (3) the ability to cooperate voluntarily (12 to 15 months). Psychologic readiness and desire to control urination and defecation usually does not develop until between 18 and 30 months of age and is significantly affected by parental expectations and attitudes.

Often parents begin toilet training before their child is ready, resulting in months of frustration. The nurse should respond to this by discussing the usual periods of readiness and assist them in planning approaches to use if they are not successful. If the child responds favorably to the toilet-training plan, the parents should be encouraged to continue with the established routine. If the child does not respond as desired, the parents should stop efforts for a few weeks and resume toilet training later.

Findings from a 10-year-study that may reassure parents concerned about when their child will be trained are as follows:

1. The average age for completion of daytime training was 28½ months.
2. The majority of children achieved bowel and bladder training at the same time.
3. The average age for completion (day and night) of both bowel and bladder training was 33 months, 10 days.
4. About 80% of children were trained completely after 3 years.
5. Girls were trained completely an average of 2½ months earlier than boys.

The nurse can assist parents with toilet training by suggesting the sequence listed in the box on this page.

The parent who can approach toilet training with a relaxed attitude and accept some delays and frustrations will have a better chance of success and more positive feelings toward the toddler.

❑ ❑ NURSING SUGGESTIONS TO FACILITATE TOILETING PROGRAM FOR TODDLERS

- When the child shows an awareness of elimination, usually between age 12 and 18 months, casually and consistently use the word(s) chosen to describe the action. Thus the child begins to associate a word with the appropriate action.
- Around age 18 to 20 months check for the prerequisite skills for toileting: toddler able to (1) walk well, (2) stay dry for at least 2 hours during the day, and (3) communicate the need for assistance.
- If these prerequisites are present, introduce the child to the potty chair. The potty chair should provide secure seating with the child's feet touching the floor. The toddler can set on the potty chair with clothes on at first.
- About a week later remove diapers and have the child sit on the potty chair. Encourage the toddler to stay on the chair for 3 to 5 minutes and always explain what to do ("Go potty") rather than what not to do ("Don't wet your pants").
- Because of the gastrocolic reflex, defecation is more likely after a meal, so this is a good time to place the toddler on the potty. If a pattern of defecation or urination is noticed, use it as a guide for placing the child on the potty.
- Praise the child for desired behavior; do not withhold praise until urination or defecation occurs. This is the desired end, but positive steps, such as sitting on the potty, grunting, and so on, also should be acknowledged.
- Ignore undesired behavior and never punish the child by scolding, spanking, or other punitive measures.
- As the toddler achieves success, strive for more independence by dressing in easy-to-remove pants, keeping the path from usual play areas to the bathroom clear, and providing a secure step-up to handwashing supplies.

The toileting process, during which attention is focused on the genital area, may precipitate an increased interest in *masturbation* or curiosity about other's genitals. The nurse should include this in early teaching about toilet training, giving parents time to consider their feelings and decide on how they will deal with these behaviors. Some parents accept the child's curiosity, whereas others may feel obligated to introduce sexual values and taboos.

The nurse can assist parents to approach the issue reasonably by explaining that almost all toddlers engage in masturbation at times and that it is not harmful. Masturbation provides a means for the toddler to become better acquainted with the body. Parents should not punish their toddler for masturbation but can suggest or offer other activities as a distraction. The older toddler can grasp the concepts of privacy during elimination and special body parts.

Many parents are uncertain about which words to use for the sex organs and elimination; "cute" words unrelated to the correct anatomic name or function are sometimes invented to avoid "embarrassing" words. The nurse should alert the parents to the implications of avoiding correct terms as the child becomes older and aware of them. Toddlers can pronounce and use the correct words.

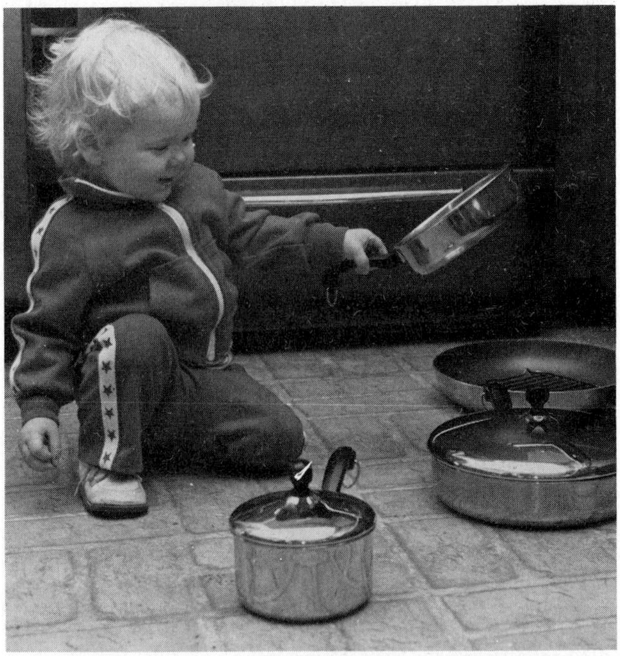

Fig. 18-2. Toddler's play may involve traditional toys or household objects. (Photograph by Douglas Bloomquist.)

Activity and Exercise Pattern

The toddler always seems busy: emptying wastebaskets, rearranging the contents of shelves and drawers, building towers, throwing and running after a ball, or removing and putting on clothes. Many activities are repeated time and time again, and many provide practice of newly realized motor skills.

The 18-month-old runs, pulls a toy, climbs, stacks three blocks, walks up steps, and "helps" around the house by running simple errands, dusting, or pushing a broom. This toddler uses a spoon with moderate to good success and scribbles, mainly off the paper.

The 24-month-old kicks a ball, throws a ball overhand, removes and may put on some clothing, and may enjoy some interactive games such as tag. This child is skilled in eating with a spoon, turns pages one at a time, and is able to keep the lines on the paper when scribbling.[18]

By the end of the toddler period, at 36 months, the child can pedal a tricycle, jump, stand on one foot briefly, wash and dry hands, and put on all clothing. This child copies a circle, uses a fork for some foods, and builds a tower of eight blocks.[18]

The toddler spends most waking hours playing, which encompasses a variety of activities, from exploring traditional toys and games to imitating "work" and repetition of motor activities (Fig. 18-2). Through imitation the older toddler can try out many roles and situations. This imitation, and fantasy play later on, becomes very prominent during the preschool years, as discussed in Chapter 19.

Toddlers delight in their own skills and love repeating actions for an appreciative adult. Verbal praise, smiles, or handclapping are effective reinforcers at this age. In their enthusiasm to try many activities, toddlers invariably take on tasks that are beyond their abilities. This results in frustration and sometimes the well-known temper tantrum. Tantrums and ways to deal with them are discussed under psychologic processes.

By 2 years of age, most toddlers are interested in other children, as manifested by looking at each other, exchanging toys, and saying "hi" or the equivalent. These social overtures are more common in those who spend more time with other children. Despite this interest in each other, play before age 3 is not really shared. It is described as *parallel play;* that is, toddlers may be doing a similar thing with the same toy, but each is working independently.[2]

When parents inquire about what toys and activities to provide for their toddler, the nurse can suggest the following:

1. Provide toys that challenge the child to develop new skills, that is, toys that require skills just above the child's present level but not so advanced that the child cannot achieve some success. For example, the toddler who has mastered pushing a hobby horse is ready for a tricycle.
2. Provide opportunities for new learning. This may be as basic as a book with pictures of new animals or a walk through the produce section of the grocery store to point out several fruits or vegetables.
3. Provide opportunities for social interaction but do not force "playing together." An hour in the park close to other toddlers provides many occasions for looking at other children or offering a toy.

4. Follow the child's lead. Let the toddler choose and explore new toys or objects–within safe limits.

A relatively recent phenomenon is some parents' desire to raise the smartest, best coordinated, or most musically talented child. These "superkids" receive intense instructions and practice in a subject or area chosen by their parents. This instruction, sometimes started before age 1, is almost always underway by the early toddler period. Some of these children have indeed shown the ability to learn at a younger age than was ever considered in the past. The main concern among child development specialists is that the time commitment and intensive drill may interfere with the child's need for self-structured play and exploration. Many unanswered questions remain about the long-term effects on these children.[7] The nurse can encourage parents who are considering this approach to consult with a child psychologist.

Sleep and Rest Pattern

SLEEP PATTERNS

The toddler requires less sleep time than the infant. Night sleep averages 8 to 12 hours at age 2, and naps become less frequent. Total nap time for the 2-year-old is about 30 minutes less than for that child at 1 year. Although the need for actual sleep has decreased, the toddler may need "quiet times," brief solo periods to unwind from a very busy or noisy activity. Sometimes the mother needs these rest breaks more than the toddler, and sitting together in a rocking chair for a soothing song or quiet music can be a calming experience.

The toddler may be very involved in an activity and not realize being tired. This is especially true when visitors are in the home or some interesting new toys have just been discovered. All parents know the overtired child who is exhausted but unable to relax enough to sleep. Parents can avoid this by scheduling nap and rest breaks even when there are house guests or holidays that may preempt the toddler's routine.

Many toddlers have a bedtime ritual. A typical pattern might be snack, bath, brush teeth, storytime, kiss parents, and light out. It is important to follow this ritual, since it seems to give the toddler a sense of security when ending the day. Changing this ritual can be very upsetting to the toddler. The nurse should encourage parents to follow the presleep ritual as closely as possible, even when visitors, family illness, or travel make this more difficult.

Many toddlers will try to delay sleep by calling for water, another story, another kiss, or other requests. Parents should be sure that the toddler has ample opportunity for interaction with them during the day, follow the usual bedtime ritual, and be very firm and consistent in resisting any requests for attention after the final goodnights have been said.

SLEEP DISTURBANCES

Some toddlers, from age 2 on, are fearful of the dark. A night light or a favorite toy can help to allay this fear.

Night terrors also may occur in the 2- to 4-year-old. These are unlike nightmares, which generally start around age 3, and result in the child wakening and being able to recall the frightening dream. The child experiencing night terrors does not waken completely but cries out, looks terrified, and cannot be aroused for several minutes. The child may believe animals or strange people are in the room or may be disoriented or not recognize the parents. After 5 to 30 minutes, the child falls back into a quiet sleep.[12]

Night terrors are rarer than nightmares. The parent needs to be assured that these episodes will stop spontaneously if not too much attention is focused on them. The parent should go and talk in a soothing voice but should not waken the child. If the child does waken, the parent should provide comfort and tuck the child back in bed.

Repeated requests for attention after bedtime, fear of the dark, and night terrors may precipitate the practice of bringing the child to the parents' bed. The toddler who is allowed to sleep with the parents after a frightening episode comes to expect to stay with them after any such incident. This can soon result in the youngster spending every night with the parents. Although parents may resent the loss of privacy and restricted sleep space, they may feel trapped in this situation by fear of doing harm by having the child sleep alone.

The nurse can help parents to avoid these difficult situations by counseling in late infancy, before these toddler-age problems arise. Important points to discuss with parents are as follows:[7]

1. These sleep disturbances result from the developmental level as the child begins to deal with ideas of separation and aggression.
2. Illness, a new sibling, moving, or frightening television shows or movies may be precipitating factors.
3. The toddler needs sufficient interaction with the parents each day to decrease the likelihood of demanding this attention after bedtime.
4. Parents need to be firm, fair, and consistent at bedtime and adhere to the expected ritual.
5. Excessive stimulation in the form of boisterous physical activity, arguments, or frightening stories should be avoided before bedtime.
6. A night light, favorite toy, or soft music may help the toddler fall asleep.

7. The toddler should not be moved from the bed after night terrors or nightmares but should be comforted and reassured that the parents are in the house.

Bedtime or nighttime disturbances can be very difficult to handle because they occur when parents are tired and probably less patient. They may need much reassurance that the child will outgrow these problems if they maintain a firm, caring attitude.

PSYCHOLOGIC PROCESSES

Cognitive and Perceptual Pattern

The toddler is intensely active and interested in the environment, poking, prodding, and sampling everything, even other human beings. The child thus gathers much data, which form a basis for beginning problem solving and symbolic thinking. In this discussion, it is important to remember that even though age ranges are stated, each toddler is an individual and may not precisely fit the description for the age. Also, as is true for all ages, the toddler may demonstrate certain cognitive skills in some situations but not in others. This is not totally understood but may relate to certain circumstances and stresses.

PIAGET'S DESCRIPTION

The young toddler, from 18 to 24 months, is in the last substage of the *sensorimotor period* in Piaget's description of cognitive development. As discussed in Chapter 17, the 12- to 18-month-old in substage 5 solves problems through a process of trial-and-error experimentation. The toddler in substage 6 has advanced to solving problems by mental rather than physical experimentation. Faced with a new object, this toddler does not immediately begin a series of physical manipulations to discover how this new thing works. The child may pause, look intently at the object, almost as if analyzing it, and then proceed to "solve the problem." Although not always succeeding on the first try and doing some analysis by physical manipulation, this child will do more and more problem solving on a mental level, manipulating images instead of real objects.

Object permanence is developed further during early toddlerhood. The older infant who fails to find a hidden object in the original hiding place will abandon the search. The child of 18 to 24 months who fails to find the object in the original hiding place will search in several possible hiding places. The toddler remembers that the object exists, that it has permanence, and knows that it can be made visible once again.

From about 24 months, until the early preschool years, the toddler enters the *preconceptual phase* of Piaget's preoperational period. This heralds the beginning of *symbolic thinking*, by which a word, gesture, or image (the *signifier*) stands for an object, person, or event (the *significate*).

The development of *language* plays a vital role in the cognitive development of symbolic representation. For Piaget, this type of symbolic act greatly enhances the act of *internalizing;* or mediating, the symbolic functions of the intellect.

Language does not fully represent the thought processes of human beings; it does not fully express the full richness or symbolic possibilities in thinking capacity. The ability to think about the relationships between the signifier and the significate exists before the ability to represent each in the form of language. The signifiers become internalized as images, and then a word is found that represents the meaning already acquired.

The toddler's language often reflects acquired meanings. For example, the word "mommy" may be used to represent a wide range of behaviors and actions in addition to its noun sense (mother). The context and differential vocalization inflection give it the intended meaning; "mommy" may mean "help me" on one occasion and "pick me up" on another. The continuing adaptive functions of assimilation and accommodation provide the child with the means to acquire internalized, differentiated, and more precise meanings between signifiers and significates gradually.

Between about 18 and 24 months, the toddler experiences a major transition in imitation and play. Piaget has labeled this stage the *invention of new means through mental combinations.* The child develops the capacity to imitate models that are not immediately present without using extensive trial and error. Imitation of nonhuman and nonliving objects occurs, which serves the important function of direct experience with object events in the world that are difficult for the toddler to understand. The relative absence of trial and error in imitation is indicative of the child having developed the ability to work out the pattern of experience before engaging in the activity. Play takes on increasingly symbolic functions and meanings. The toddler engages in repeating actions for fun and pleasure as previously, but now there is increasing symbolic meaning in the activity. An object such as a stone or a block of wood can now symbolize, in the child's mind, a person, animal, or any other object.

This make-believe form of play, or *ludic symbolism,* predominates throughout early childhood. Between ages 2 and 4 years, the toddler spends a significant portion of time acting out whole scenes of imagined events. Imaginary companions are frequently present, which serve the important function of mirroring the child's self or being a sympathetic audience for the child as the self is allowed full unrestrained expression and experimentation through play. During this period, the child uses play to act out what is forbidden in reality; this provides important trial experiences with taboo behaviors and offers an essential means of expressing socially unacceptable parts of the self that need some acceptable outlet. For example, the child may pretend to eat an infant sibling for dinner, expressing a dimension of ambivalent feelings toward the infant in a manner that is not punished and that provides a discharge of hostile or angry feelings.[17]

Toddlers are very *egocentric,* seeing everything through their own perspectives and not even realizing that other ways of viewing things may exist. This is reflected in language and activities. Although not purposely being selfish, toddlers have no concept that another child or adult may have different thoughts or perceptions from their own. The 2½-year-old may come running into a room and ask the parent, "Where is it?" The parent's response, "Where is what?" is very confusing to the toddler, who assumes the parent must be having the same thought.

This overview of Piaget's description shows that the toddler is becoming more proficient as a problem solver and is using some symbolic thinking. These skills enable the toddler to mentally manipulate reality and begin to contemplate the future and recall the near past.[2]

VISION

The toddler's sensory abilities develop from infantile levels to more adult ranges. From 18 to 24 months, visual acuity is 20/40 and accommodation is well developed. Depth perception is still immature, although better developed than in the infant. From 2 to 3 years of age, visual acuity is 20/30 and convergence is smooth. This older toddler is able to recall visual images, which contributes to an increasing skill in describing past events. The child is able to fixate on small objects or pictures for up to 30 seconds.

The possibility of development of *amblyopia* is greatest from infancy through the fourth year. Amblyopia is loss of vision or diminished vision caused by disuse of that eye. This disuse usually results from *strabismus,* a deviation of line of vision from the midline because of extraocular muscle weakness or imbalance. Marked and continuous strabismus usually is noticed early by the parents and health care provider and treated; the more subtle deviations often go unnoticed until the older toddler or preschool years.[15] Every toddler should be screened for strabismus as part of the routine eye examination done by the physician or nurse practitioner during well-child visits. Strabismus can be treated by patching the unaffected eye or by corrective surgery. Best results are obtained when the condition is diagnosed and treated during the infant or toddler years.

Other signs of possible visual problems the nurse may observe or parents may report in their toddler include the following:

1. Rubs eyes excessively
2. Shuts or covers one eye, tilts head, or thrusts head forward
3. Has difficulty reading or doing other work that requires close use of the eyes
4. Blinks more than usual or is irritable when doing close work
5. Holds books close to eyes
6. Is unable to see distant things clearly
7. Squints eyelids together or frowns
8. Has red-rimmed, encrusted, or swollen eyelids
9. Has inflamed or watery eyes
10. Develops recurring styes

HEARING

The development of hearing capacity, which is critical for the development of speech and language, reaches essential maturity by age 3 to 4 years. However, during this period the child begins the lifelong process of learning to listen and comprehend.

Studies estimate that all human beings listen to about 50% of what they hear and comprehend only about 25%. Parents will express concern that their older toddler or young preschooler "must have a hearing problem" because the child does not always respond to being called. This concern should be investigated, but often the nurse will conclude that this is "selective inattention" to parental requests, which is typical at this age.

Listening ability includes (1) attending to what is heard, (2) discriminating between the various qualities of sound, (3) making cognitive associations with previously learned experiences, and (4) remembering. The quantity and quality of language used in the home is thought to be more important for the development of listening ability and, therefore, receptive language than for the development of expressive language. Toddlers often seek repetition of auditory input, as seen in their seemingly endless repetition of sounds, words, or combinations of words. This repetition may be their way of organizing and practicing new language.

TASTE AND SMELL

The capacities to taste and smell, which have reached an optimum level of functioning during infancy, are influenced by voluntary control and associated with other sensory and motor areas. Thus, toddlers start to refuse tasting something that looks displeasing to them. They are able to react accurately to the sensation that a taste or smell arouses within them and begin to learn conditioned associations between certain smells and culturally acceptable values. The foods of the culture become palatable, and those unacceptable become displeasing. For example, children raised in a family that does not eat a certain meat will learn that this meat tastes bad, they even may be unable to develop a pleasurable association with such a taste later in life. Odors of body processes, such as sweating and elimination, become extremely offensive for children in some cultures, whereas in others they are not considered unpleasant.

LANGUAGE AND MEMORY

The toddler's cognitive abilities and increased sensory capabilities are demonstrated in language, memory, and decision-making abilities.

Both *receptive* and *expressive* language skills are developing rapidly during the toddler period. From 18 to 24 months, the transition from single words to short phrases occurs. These two- and three-word phrases most often are related to present events and describe an action ("daddy go"), a desire ("more cookie"), or possession ("my doggie"). Some landmarks of language for the child from 18 to 36 months are listed in Table 18-2. At all ages the ability to express words and ideas is not as advanced as the ability to understand language, the 30-month-old can understand up to 2400 words but uses only about 425 in speech.

By age 3, children have mastered the basics of language function, form, and content; these skills will continue to be refined throughout childhood and adolescence. Language development does not proceed at an even rate; plateaus, spurts, and hesitations occur in the toddler's progress. Parents are generally the most significant persons to the toddler and often provide much of the stimulation for language development.

Some suggestions the nurse can give to parents to facilitate their toddler's use of language are

1. Allow the child to make decisions about play.
2. Allow the child to initiate verbal interactions.
3. When the toddler says a sentence that is partly unintelligible, the parent can repeat the understood part as a question; they may help the toddler respond more clearly.
4. If the toddler does not seem to understand a question or direction, rephrase it.
5. Expand on the toddler's phrases: if the child says, "Daddy car," the parent can say, "Daddy gets into the car."
6. Do not criticize or make fun of the toddler's expressions.
7. Do not constantly correct the child's verbalizations; this may result in decreased verbalizations.

Memory in the toddler is demonstrated by recall of recent events or the need for exact repetition of rituals. Older toddlers can sing a simple song, but they generally do this by rote and may not be able to say the words by themselves. Visual and auditory images can be recalled and are important for language development.

The toddler is more skilled at *recognition* memory than recall memory; that is, the child can pick out objects shown earlier when they are put with new objects.

SCREENING

During the toddler years, routine assessment usually does not include testing of intelligence or specific cognitive skills. One of the most frequently used screening tools used during these years to assess overall developmental level is the *Denver Developmental Screening Test II (DDST II).*

The DDST II, discussed in Chapter 17, provides one means of screening for physical developmental problems.[8] This tool provides an estimate for the adequacy of motor skills that the child should be able to perform by a given age, but its usefulness decreases during the fourth and fifth years. Difficulties may arise when the tool is used with children who are bilingual or members of a minority subculture, since some items appear biased toward accepted U.S. culture. Insightful nursing judgment and further assessment may be needed to determine the accuracy of the test for a given child.

In using any developmental screening tool, the nurse needs to be fully prepared in the standardized techniques for administration, appropriate approaches to the child, and scoring and interpretation of results. The tool loses its effectiveness when inappropriate methods are used in administration, when the child's behavior is adversely affected by the approach of the nurse, or when the test is scored incorrectly. Anyone who anticipates using this tool for clinical practice must study the standardized methods, practice with supervision, and have initial scoring validated by an experienced user.[18]

Self-Perception and Self-Concept Pattern

The toddler's developing cognitive, language, and motor skills provide the means for the development of self-concept and self-esteem.

The toddler can separate from others by walking away and may no longer quietly cooperate when told to do something. Cognitive and language abilities have resulted in the ability to say "no" and to think of things to do on one's own. The desire to explore can take precedence over an adult's wish that the toddler go to bed. As the toddler becomes more aware of self, he or she tests this new concept over and over.

Table 18-2. **Landmarks of speech, language, and hearing ability during the toddler period**

Age (months)	Receptive language	Expressive language	Related hearing ability
18	Up to 50 words, recognizes between 6 and 12 objects by name, such as dog, cat, bottle, ball; identifies 3 body parts such as eyes, nose, mouth; understands the concept "now," and simple commands unaccompanied by gesture, such as give me the doll, open your mouth, stick out your tongue	Up to 20 words and 21 different phonemes; jargon and echolalia are present; uses names of familiar objects and one-word sentences such as go or eat; uses gestures, uses words such as no, mine, eat, good, bad, hot, cold, and expressions such as oh oh, what's that, all gone; use of words may be quite inconsistent, 25% of speech intelligible	Has begun to develop gross discrimination by learning to distinguish between highly dissimilar noises, such as doorbell and train, barking dog and auto horn, or mother's and father's voice
24	Up to 1200 words; in, on, under, identifies dog, ball, engine, bed, doll, scissors, hair, mouth, feet, nose, cup, spoon, car, key; distinguishes between one and many, and formulates a negative judgment–a knife is not a fork; understands the concept "soon," simple stories; follows simple directions; is beginning to make distinctions between you and me	Up to 270 words and 25 different phonemes; jargon and echolalia almost gone; averages 75 words per hour during free play; talks in words, phrases, and two- to three-word sentences; averages two words per response; first pronouns appear such as I, me, mine, it, who, that; adjectives and adverbs are just beginning to appear; names objects and common pictures; enjoys Mother Goose; refers to self by name, such as Bobby go bye-bye; uses phrases such as I want, go bye-bye, want cookie, ball all gone; 60% of speech intelligible	Refinement of gross discriminative skills
30	Up to 2400 words; identifies action in pictures and objects by use; carries out one- and two-part commands, such as pick up your shoe and give it to mommy; knows what we drink out of, what goes on our feet, what we can buy candy with; understands plurals, questions, difference between boy and girl, the concept "one," up, down, run, walk, throw, fast, more, my	Up to 425 words and 27 phonemes; jargon and echolalia no longer exist; averages 140 words per hour; names words such as chair, can, box, key, door; repeats two digits from memory; average sentence length is about two and a half words; uses more adjectives and adverbs; demands repetition from others, such as do it again; almost always announces intentions before action; begins to ask questions of adults; 75% of speech intelligible	
36	Up to 3600 words; understands both, two, not today, what we do when we are thirsty (hungry, sleepy), why we have stoves, wait, later, big, new, different, strong, today, another, and taking turns at play; carries out two- and some three-item commands, such as give me the ball, pick up the doll, and sit down; identifies several colors; is aware of past and future	Up to 900 words in simple sentences, averaging 3 to 4 words per sentence; averages 15,000 words per day and 170 words per hour; uses words such as when, time, today, not today, new, different, big, strong, surprise, secret; can repeat three digits, name one color, say name, give simple account of experiences, and tell stories that can be understood; begins to use more pronouns, adjectives, and adverbs; describes at least one element of a picture; is aware of past and future; uses commands, such as "you make it," and expressions, such as "I can't," "I don't want to"; verbalizes toilet needs; expresses desire to take turns; communication includes criticisms, commands, requests, threats, questions, answers; 85% of speech intelligible	Starts to distinguish dissimilar speech sounds such as the difference between "ee" and "er," although there may be some difficulty with the concepts of "same" and "different"

Adapted from Chinn PL: *Child health maintenance, concepts in family-centered care,* ed 2, St Louis, 1979, Mosby. In Weiss CE, Lilly White HS: *Communicative disorders,* St Louis, 1976, Mosby.

The toddler must explore the world, not just the physical aspects but the interpersonal aspects of relationships to other persons, to develop a true sense of independence. Exploring the physical world involves poking into, climbing onto, crawling under, tasting, smelling, and taking apart the objects encountered. The child explores relationships with others by searching for the limits of one's power: if a "no" or a temper tantrum allows one to control another person's behavior, he or she learns that his or her "self" is more powerful than the other person's "self." The toddler continually practices separateness as he or she develops a sense of autonomy.

This can be a trying and confusing time for parents. Their baby, who used to happily follow along, is suddenly saying "no" to requests and even offers of treats. The toddler may say a vehement "no" when offered a cookie and then scream and cry when the cookie is put away; the parent may wonder if the toddler wants the cookie or not. He or she probably does, but he or she also needs to express his or her autonomy by refusing it. Even the toddler must be confused by his or her conflicting desires.

The same toddler who displays such a strong need for independence may at times cuddle and even cling to the parent, realizing that independence can sometimes be frightening. The toddler must initiate this closeness; the parent must not force it.

The toddler's need for more autonomy may conflict with parental expectations, safety limits, or the rights of other children or adults. Any such conflict results in feelings of frustration. A typical toddler response to frustration is the well-known *temper tantrum*. Parents may feel totally unable to cope with these displays of frustration and give in to the child's desire, even if the desire is potentially unsafe or beyond the family budget. The toddler must practice independence but must not think that he or she can control the environment and other persons by tantrum behavior.

NURSING INTERVENTIONS

The nurse needs to assess each toddler-parent relationship to determine (1) how the toddler is expressing the need for independence, (2) how the parent perceives these actions, (3) how the parent responds to the toddler's independence, (4) what the toddler does when frustrated in exploring the environment or controlling personal and other's actions, (5) how the parent responds to the toddler's display of frustration, and (6) what provisions the parent is making to allow safe choices for the toddler. The nurse's teaching should focus on the aspects that are troublesome for an individual toddler-parent pair. Some general concepts to include are[2]

1. Fit the environment to the child's needs and abilities. Childproof the home so that the child can explore safely. Provide toys that the child can master. Give opportunities to play with more challenging toys, but do not make these the rule.
2. Give advance notice, about 5 minutes, of a change in activity, such as lunch time, nap time, and so on. Use simple games as a transition.
3. Make positive suggestions rather than giving commands.
4. Give two safe and acceptable choices when possible.
5. Let the toddler be "in charge" during play periods with the parent, choosing the book or game and deciding when to move on to another activity.
6. Allow "no's" in play situations and, when appropriate, in real situations.
7. When a command must be given, state it firmly and do not give in.
8. Set and enforce consistent limits so that the toddler will come to develop control within these limits.
9. If temper tantrums occur, glance to see that the child is safe, then ignore the child until behavior is acceptable. Give immediate attention when acceptable behavior is shown.
10. Praise the toddler's skills and abilities.

The toddler who is not allowed to develop a sense of autonomy experiences shame and doubt in self and abilities, missing an important step in the development of a positive self-concept.

Coping and Stress-Tolerance Pattern

As seen in Chapter 17, the infant copes mainly through motor activity. The toddler may continue to use some of these strategies, such as body rocking, change in position, restlessness, and turning away from a stimulus, but also is developing many new ways to respond to stress. The toddler begins to use basic problem solving as he or she deals with new situations, many of which result from environmental exploration. Other stresses may include a new sibling, new day-care arrangements, increased parental expectations related to toilet training, or changes in parental relationships, such as divorce or separation. Although older children and adults can recall past stressful situations and their responses, the toddler cannot draw from this store of memories or think of a wide range of possible responses.

Variables that influence a toddler's response to stress include (1) the child's state of health, (2) the nature and timing of information in preparation for the stressful experience, (3) the observed parental coping pattern, and (4) opportunities for autonomy and freedom of movement usually available to the child.[2]

The ill child does not have the same energy to deal with stresses as when he or she is healthy. The toddler should be prepared for stressful events shortly before they happen. The parent should not say to a 2-year-old, "You will get a shot tomorrow"; the toddler's understanding of tomorrow is vague, and his or her imagination has too long to deal with all the ramifications of "a shot." The parent should tell the toddler directly before this painful event occurs and then assist him through the experience by being close and reassuring. Avoiding the term *shot* altogether because of its association with guns and being injured or killed is probably best; *injection* can be used with the toddler. The child who is ill and requires a sequence of injections needs more ongoing preparation and opportunity to express fears and feelings. The child sees the parents' methods of dealing with stress and may adapt or imitate these.

Separation anxiety and regression are the two most characteristic toddler responses to stress. The child may also use denial, repression, and projection to direct the stress away from self.

Parents may need help in understanding and accepting their toddler's coping responses. A typical instance is the regression that is often a response to a new sibling in the family (see also role and relationship pattern later in this chapter.) *Regression,* or reverting temporarily to an earlier, previously abandoned developmental stage of behavior to retain or regain mastery of a stressful situation–in this case, the sudden appearance of a rival for his or her parents' time and attention–can be very beneficial to the toddler and very distressing to the parents. Toddler regression may take the form of losing toileting skills, crying more, wanting to be fed and dressed after mastering these skills, or reverting to "baby talk." The nurse can assist parents in recognizing this as a normal response of the toddler seeking to reaffirm a place in the family. This toddler needs verbal and physical demonstrations of the parents' love and the opportunity, through verbal play and motor activity, to work through these feelings.[5]

These early efforts at dealing with stress are essential steps to a more mature coping response as the child gets older.

Value and Belief Pattern

CONSCIENCE

Unlike the infant, whose behavior is largely unrestricted, the toddler is subjected to many limits, which are often put in the form of a moral dictum from an adult: "Good boy, you ate all your meat," or "No, don't hit your brother; that's bad." These limits sometimes are enforced through physical punishment, stern reprimands, or ignoring. Thus, the toddler is socialized into acting in accordance with adult wishes. The toddler develops some self-control through these efforts of parents and others, but this control continues to depend on their approval or disapproval. This is not an internally mediated conscience. *Conscience,* standards and prohibitions that have been adapted by the personality and that govern behavior from within, does not emerge until age 5 or 6, and it is rudimentary until age 9 or 10.[7] This does not mean that toddlers should not have limits set and enforced, but it does have implications for how these limits are set.

The young toddler may not have a good understanding of the word "no." Parents should still use "no," however, but should combine this with redirecting the child's attention to another activity that is acceptable. Thus, the toddler is helped to channel action and inquisitiveness into more socially acceptable occupations. Studies have shown that physical punishment and withdrawal of parental love do not lead to development of a conscience. The most effective conscience-building technique is an inductive explanation of the consequences of the toddler's action. Once the toddler has sufficient receptive language skills, the parent can give a brief, clear description of the outcome: "When you hit me, I hurt." Another effective technique is to explain rules and rights to the toddler: "You can play with the cars and trucks; you mustn't touch the TV." This helps the toddler develop acceptable moral feelings.[2]

Toddlers' moral behavior also is influenced by what others do. If they see others (family members, playmates, television characters) doing certain things, they assume that action is acceptable. This presents a problem when a toddler has been told, for example, "No, don't touch the stove, it will hurt you," but sees the parents and older siblings touching it all the time.

The toddler is more likely to "remember" rules and prohibitions when the parent or other adult is present; left alone, the child is more likely to try the forbidden act. Parents may need assistance to understand that their toddler is not purposely being "bad," but rather moral behavior, because of the child's level of cognitive and emotional development, tends to be influenced by situation, circumstance, and persons present. The ability to recite a rule does not mean the toddler has integrated it into a repertoire of actions.

SPIRITUAL VALUES

Toddlers from families with religious backgrounds often are taught prayers and songs with a spiritual theme, which sometimes are tied into "right" and "wrong" ideas. Toddlers certainly can learn the words to these simple prayers and songs, but parents may need to be cautioned that this does not mean that toddlers understand the full meaning of what is said. This early introduction into the family's religious beliefs is important as a socialization factor but should not be counted on to produce a "good" child.

An important aspect of teaching young children what is right and wrong was mentioned briefly but should be a major focus for the nurse working with parents. This is the technique of stating what is *acceptable* behavior and then reinforcing this behavior. Sometimes parents finds themselves constantly telling children what *not* to do. Could it be that children have been given so many prohibitions that they cannot think of any other alternatives? Another common mistake of parents is to "not disturb" toddlers when they are being "good." Thus, they receive no attention for acceptable behavior but probably are attended to when they misbehave. The nurse can teach parents the following points:[25]

1. State briefly and clearly the desired or acceptable action.
2. Praise desired behaviors.
3. Praise attempts at acceptable behavior, even if imperfect.
4. Vary the style of praise but always be enthusiastic and sincere.
5. Praise the child in front of others.

These techniques must be used repeatedly to produce the desired results: more frequent socially acceptable behavior.

Health Perception and Health Management Pattern

The toddler develops a sense of body image by seeing its parts, learning how to use it for locomotion, and exploring and observing others.

The toddler is exposed to concepts of health, illness, and related actions by the parents and others but may not develop any real understanding of these ideas. The child may come to know that being "sick" means feeling bad or not going to day care but has little if any understanding of the meaning of health. The toddler may perform or request some health promotion activities, such as brushing teeth, not because this will prevent caries, but because it is part of the evening ritual. Toddlers depend on their parents for health management.

ENVIRONMENTAL PROCESSES

Many environmental processes can affect persons at every age. Toddlers, because of their lack of judgment related to rudimentary problem-solving skills, level of physical coordination, lack of experience with many types of situations, and high level of curiosity about the environment, are at higher risk than at other ages.

Natural Processes

ACCIDENTS

Injuries are the most frequent cause of childhood disability and death. One out of every 10 toddlers is treated in an emergency room each year for trauma or poisoning. The number of accidents for females peaks in the toddler years, whereas for males two peaks occur: toddlerhood and adolescence. As is true for all ages, males have more accidents than females in the toddler period. Motor vehicle accidents are a major cause of injuries at all ages and are considered in a separate section that follows. Other agents that are discussed are related to structural elements or materials in buildings, fixtures, and furniture; toys; hazards from sports and recreational equipment or situations; drownings; and burns.

Structural Hazards. Houses and other buildings can be hazardous places for toddlers. Their desire to explore puts them in places where older children or adults would not think of going. The toddler will climb onto furniture or fixtures, out of windows, or into small spaces. One study estimated that there are 580 head injuries per 100,000 toddlers from furniture- or fixture-related accidents and 451 head injuries per 100,000 toddlers related to structural hazards. This number is only for head injuries; many more injuries affect other parts of the body from these causes.[12] The falls or injuries that result from these explorations can range from fatal head injuries to minor scrapes and bruises.

Preventive measures for these types of hazards include the following:

1. Have a locking gate or door on all stairs.
2. Carpet stairs to provide some padding in case the child does fall.
3. Use furniture with rounded edges.
4. Anchor or temporarily move bookcases, tables, or lamps that can be pulled over.
5. Keep chairs away from counters or tables to prevent providing "steps" for the toddler.
6. Have windows screened and made of safety glass.

Toys. Toys are another source of injury to toddlers. Hazardous elements of such objects include (1) toys or parts of toys that are small enough to be swallowed or aspirated, (2) flammable toys, (3) toys coated with poisonous paint, (4) stuffed animals with glass or button eyes or toxic stuffing, and (5) toys with sharp edges.

Parents need to inspect not only the toys that are in their own homes but also those given to the toddler outside the home by relatives, friends, baby-sitters, or day-care personnel. Many toys probably are safe for the older child in these settings but extremely hazardous for the toddler. This is one instance when "sharing" should be discouraged.

This discussion is part of the larger concept of "toddler proofing" the home or other settings where toddlers spend time. Ideally homes are "baby proofed" before the infant begins scooting and crawling. Baby or toddler proofing refers to the practice of removing all potential hazards from the child's environment. Hazards are related to motor and cognitive skills and change as the child matures. Thus, parents must reassess the safety of their home as their child gains new skills. Child proofing also includes removing or protecting those few irreplaceable or sentimental objects on display in the home. These objects may or may not be real safety hazards, but they do represent an emotional loss if accidentally destroyed by the exploring child.

Sports. Although sports and recreational equipment are recognized as a major source of accidents during childhood and adolescence, parents and health care personnel sometimes forget that these also can be hazards to toddlers. A primary danger is the improper storage of this equipment. Firearms that are left loaded and not locked up are an obvious hazard. Body-building weights and other heavy equipment look interesting to toddlers, who may pull these objects down on themselves. Unfenced playing fields close to toddlers' play areas present a hazard when the youngsters wander into a soccer or football game. Toddlers need to be supervised closely on swings and jungle gyms. They may be safe if playing alone, but when other youngsters are there, they can be hazardous to each other.

Drownings. Drownings are a major cause of death or serious sequelae in toddlers. For the child under 3 years of age bathtubs are a primary site of drownings. The toddler should never be left unattended in the tub nor be permitted to lean over the bathtub to play with water toys, since he could topple in, hit his head, and be unable to get out. Other water risks are swimming pools, natural bodies of water, and boats. All swimming pools should be fenced and have self-closing gates and latches. All children should wear a properly fitting life jacket when in a boat. Toddlers must be supervised constantly and competently whenever they are near any body of water. The American Academy of Pediatrics recommends that children under 3 years of age be accompanied by a parent at all times during any swimming lessons. The child should never be forced to put their face in the water (see box on p. 452).

Scalds. Burns, especially scalds, are another major cause of injury in this age group. A toddler or playmate may turn on a hot water tap and be unable to turn it off again. This hazard can be lessened by keeping hot water heater temperatures set below 130° F (54° C). In 1980, Florida was the first state to pass legislation limiting new water heaters to a preset temperature of 125° F (52° C). Other states have passed legislation that specifies a maximum water temperature in all rental units. Also, curiosity may case the toddler to overturn a pot of hot liquid on the stove. This can be avoided if family members put panhandles toward the back of the stove and do not leave cords from electric pots hanging within reach of the toddler. (See Chapters 17 and 19 for other types of burn injuries.)

Nursing Interventions. The specific intervention for the accidents discussed–teaching accident prevention–sometimes is not well received by parents. They may respond, "He has to learn sometime that water is hot (not to run into the soccer field, and so on)," or, "Well, now that he's been hurt once, he won't do that again." These statements indicate a lack of understanding of the toddler's cognitive level. In these cases the nurse needs to begin accident prevention teaching with a discussion of the toddler's developmental level. Written handouts may be a helpful way to make this information available to families and those involved in child care (see box on p. 452).

MOTOR VEHICLES

Motor vehicle injury is the leading cause of death in children from 1 to 4 years of age. Such accidents include passenger as well as pedestrian injury; for the toddler, passenger injury is more frequent. Many factors affect the risk of passenger injury: speed of the car, highway and road construction, type of vehicle, age of driver, alcohol intoxication of driver position in the car, and restraint (see box on p. 468).

Parents can definitely control some of these factors. Speed and alcohol use depend on the good judgment of the driver. Statistics indicate that cars with a wider wheel base provide greater protection for passengers in event of accident. Parents can take this into account when purchasing a new car. Rear seat position is safer than front seat; thus, children should always be in the back seat.

Probably the most effective preventive measure is the use of a crash-tested and approved toddler car seat. The nurse can provide a list of approved car seats and local retail outlets or agencies that lend or rent car seats. It is important to point out to parents that some infant seats are not appropriate for toddlers (see Chapter 17). The American Academy of Pediatrics has published a comprehensive pamphlet on choosing a car seat (1991 Family Shopping Guide to Car Seats, AAP Safe Ride Program, 141 Northwest Point Blvd., PO Box 927, Elk Grove, IL 60007-0927).

Unfortunately, not all families who own car seats use them consistently. Primary prevention must include the

RESEARCH REVIEW — TODDLER

SEAT BELTS AND SAFETY

Sharp GB, Carter MA: Use of restraint devices to prevent collision injuries and deaths among welfare-supported children, *Public Health Rep* 107:116-118, 1992.

Purpose The purpose of this study is to investigate mother's use of child passenger restraint devices (CPRDs) in a state which became the first to pass a child passenger law.

Review A total of 56 black women, receiving Medicaid and residing in inner-city Memphis, were interviewed about their use of restraints for children ages 0-3 years. About two thirds of the mothers said they rarely or never used CPRDs. Children ages 3 years were significantly less likely to be transported in child restraint devices than younger children. Consideration should be given to redesigning CPRDs to make them more acceptable to children and to building CPRDs into cars.

concept that car seats must be used *every* time the child is in the car to be effective. Most states have passed legislation requiring the use of approved child restraints. The nurse needs to be active in private and community action to get such legislation passed and enforced.[10]

BIOLOGIC AND BACTERIAL AGENTS

The toddler is susceptible to the same organisms as any other person but may succumb to common illnesses more frequently than an older child or adult, since the toddler has not built up specific resistance to many common organisms. A classic example of this is the annual number of upper respiratory infections (URI or common cold) in toddlers. Parents often become concerned because their toddler gets so many more URIs than anyone else in the family; it is not unusual for the toddler to have 6 to 10 episodes a year. This may be especially true for the toddler who is exposed to a variety of other young children in a group care setting or through older siblings.

The URI itself, although troublesome to the child and the caretakers, is not a major concern, but one of its common sequelae, mentioned earlier, *otitis media,* can produce long-term effects. The concern is decreased hearing acuity at a time when the youngster is acquiring many new language skills. Decreased hearing results from a buildup of secretions in the middle ear chamber when the eustachian tube is blocked by secretions or edema. The child with *acute* otitis media needs appropriate medical management. The child with *chronic serous* (fluid in the middle ear) otitis media needs careful monitoring of hearing status.[12] (See box on p. 452.)

This secondary prevention of complications of an existing condition is within the scope of the nurse's role. Hearing can be tested by use of pure-tone audiometry in the cooperative older toddler. For the younger toddler, more complex methods of conditioned response audiometry or brainstem-evoked response may be needed. These children should be referred to an audiologist. *Tympanometry* is a method of assessing the pressure in the middle ear chamber and provides valuable information about the progress of serious otitis media. Tympanometry is an easy technique to learn, and the equipment is relatively inexpensive and widely available.

CHEMICAL AGENTS

The toddler is exposed to the same pollutants in the air and water as any other person; these are discussed in detail in other chapters of this unit. Chemical agents of particular concern at this age are ingested poisons, such as household products, lead paint, drugs, cosmetics, pesticides, and plants (Fig. 18-3). The toddler, because of limited experience and cognitive level, does not know they are harmful. Many emergency room calls and visits are precipitated by a toddler's ingestion of a questionably or actually harmful substance. These acute ingestions are most likely to occur in the kitchen, bathroom, bedroom, or work area and are usually discovered by the parent or caretaker because of an open or empty container or a half-eaten leaf or other substance. (See box on p. 452.)

When parents or caregivers suspect that a toddler has ingested a poisonous substance, even if he or she appears perfectly healthy at the moment, they should call the poison control center. Each poison control center is part of a nationwide effort to provide immediate information regarding poisonings. It is very important that parents do not apply any first aid such as inducing vomiting without specific instructions. Vomiting could cause further harm if the child is drowsy, unconscious, or convulsing or if the substance ingested is a corrosive such as lye or a strong acid.[12] If vomiting is recommended by the poison control center, instructions are often given to use *ipecac syrup* to stimulate the

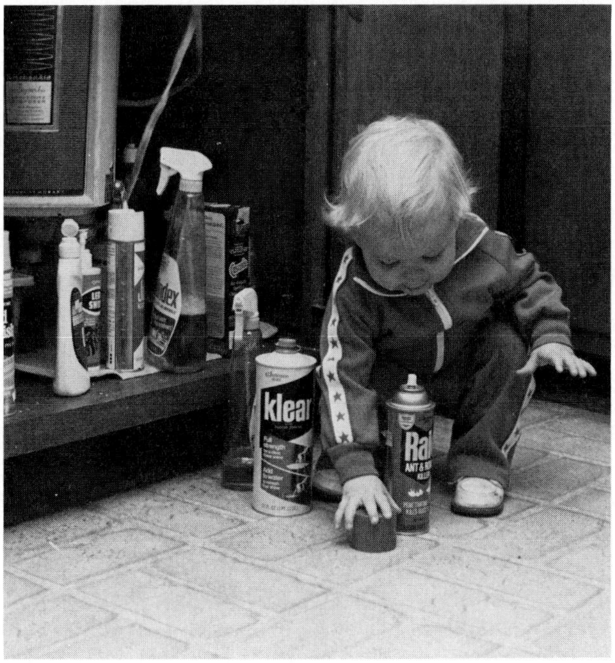

Fig. 18-3. Household cleaning supplies can be extremely dangerous. (Photograph by Douglas Bloomquist.)

❑ ❑ NURSING INTERVENTIONS TO PREVENT POISONING IN TODDLERS

- All household products (paints, drugs, cosmetics, garden products) should be in securely locked locations.
- A child should never be told that medicine is "candy."
- All products should be kept in their original containers for easy identification.
- No poisonous plants should be kept in the house. (A list is available through local poison control centers.)
- The child should not be left unattended in an outdoor setting where there are potential poisonous plants.
- The number of the poison control center should be posted next to every telephone.

vomiting rapidly. Parents must follow the administration instructions carefully, since ipecac in large doses can be harmful. This medication should be stored as carefully as any other medication or hazardous household product.

The nurse should discuss poisoning before the child begins to crawl or walk and then review this information when the child does begin to ambulate (see the box above).

Chronic poisonings, such as occur when a child sucks on an object coated with lead-based paint or eats lead-based paint chips, often are not detected until irreversible damage has occurred. Primary prevention involves teaching parents the dangers of lead-based paint; secondary prevention involves doing periodic screening of blood lead levels on all young children at risk. In certain settings, such as urban areas of older housing, all children should be screened. Consumer protection laws require that all toys and furniture manufactured for small children be free of lead-based paint products. However, many families paint their own furniture and play objects and may be unaware that the paint chosen has a lead base.[1] (See box on p. 452.)

The carcinogenic agents are basically the same for toddlers and preschoolers and are discussed in Chapter 19.

Social Processes

ROLE AND RELATIONSHIP PATTERN

By toddlerhood the child has learned who mother, father, and older siblings are and has established some kind of reciprocal relationship with each of them. The toddler may see one family member as the "fixer" of broken toys and bruised knees, another as the troublemaker who always takes away toys, and someone else as the peacemaker who smooths things out after fights. The child begins to establish a place in the line of family power by finding out who can be manipulated and who has the ability to set limits on behavior. The toddler's strongest motivator is the love and affection of parents. This may be difficult for parents to recognize when their toddler is in the midst of asserting independence.

Toddlers are more interested in the parents and siblings than they were as infants. They are curious about what these family members are doing and often imitate their actions. Toddlers are likely to prefer parents' or siblings' possessions to their own. Research has demonstrated that young toddlers are more responsive to playful social interaction initiated by the father. At age 2½ years, children were more cooperative, close, involved, excited, and interested in play with their fathers.[2]

Sibling Rivalry. A toddler often has to deal with a new member of the family–a tiny, sometimes loud creature who is unable to play, practically untouchable, and demanding of mother's time (Fig. 18-4). This new baby presents a dilemma for the toddler, who is very curious about this thing but frequently may be admonished to "don't hit," "don't poke," or "don't be so loud." Is it any wonder that love isn't the emotion foremost in the toddler's heart?

The regression that may occur in the toddler's skill

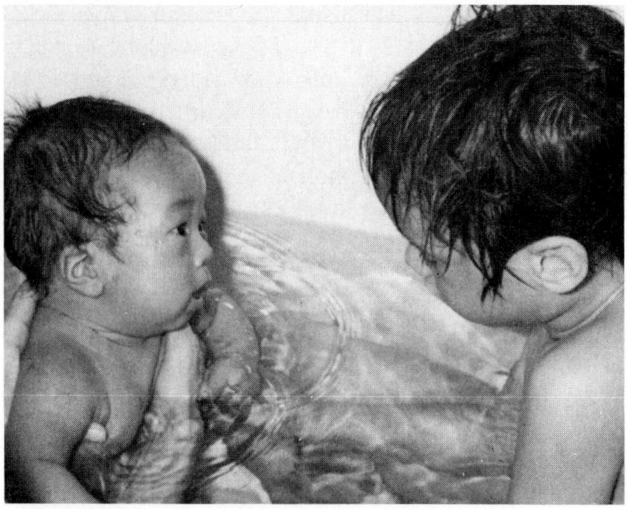

Fig. 18-4. Toddlers may have to learn to deal with new family member. (From Chinn PL: *Child health maintenance: concepts in family-centered care,* ed 2, St Louis, 1979, Mosby.)

level in response to a new sibling already has been mentioned. If parents are caring and understanding, the toddler will regain the former skill level within a short time. This not the end of sibling rivalry, however; it will continue but take other forms. All siblings feel competition from each other, and all siblings fight. Some competition is more subtle than others. Parents need to recognize sibling rivalry exists and may be most pronounced in the first 4 to 5 years of life. In these early years, siblings need adults to settle conflicts. Later, the adult can step back a little and help the siblings settle their conflicts among themselves.

Sometimes parents decide to treat siblings exactly the same to avoid any jealousy or rivalry. This does not solve the problem because the uniqueness of each child is unrecognized. Children, as with adults, have different likes and dislikes. It is important to a child's self-image to have particular likes and dislikes recognized and respected. This lets toddlers know that they are regarded as individuals.

Parents cannot stop sibling fighting by forbidding it, but it can be kept within reasonable limits. One way to tone down fighting is to remove the gain. Generally the desired effect in the toddler's mind is to see the self rewarded and the sibling punished. If parents do not reward or punish, or do not take sides, the gain is missing and fighting becomes less satisfactory. This does not mean that all fighting will stop, but the child will look for some other ways of getting approval.[25]

Parents and young children need to realize that not all family members are equal. Parents, because of their life experiences, should have more authority to make important decisions for the family and individual members. As children get older, they can share in this decision making, but it is ludicrous for parents to expect or allow toddlers to make important decisions.

The toddler, unlike the infant, demands some independence; this presents the first conflict in the parent-child relationship. Parents who have had experience with other toddlers or who have read about or discussed their behavior may be better able to deal with this new situation.

Sibling relationships and parent-child relationships can be difficult subjects for parents to discuss. They may think that any hint of discord indicates an unhealthy family. The nurse should include discussion of family relationships in her developmental teaching. Sibling rivalry and parent-child conflicts should be anticipated before they become major stresses. For example, sibling rivalry should be discussed before the new baby arrives, and the toddler's need for more independence should be discussed in late infancy.

Child Abuse. A major disruption in family relationships is child abuse. This tragic situation is not limited to one age and is more likely to occur with major change or turmoil in the family. The most frequent victims are males under age 3 years. The actual incidence of child abuse is unknown, since many cases go unreported (see box on p. 452).

Since young toddlers are unable to verbalize about abuse situations, health care providers must be alert to signs of abuse. Many of these may be difficult to differentiate from true accidents. The nurse should watch for (1) poor skin care; (2) malnutrition or failure to thrive; (3) minor bruises or abrasions; (4) soft tissue swelling, hematomas, or healed lesions; (5) injury to oral mucosa or frontal dental ridge; (6) bite marks; (7) retinal hemorrhage; and (8) discrepancy between history and physical findings.[14]

The nurse also should observe the child's attitude and behavior; children who have recently been abused may be hesitant to return home. Some children may withdraw from all adults or be excessively clinging for fear of complete rejection. Another way to assess potential abusive behavior is to differentiate behavior of parents according to typical reactions and attitudes versus reactions of battering or neglecting parents toward children's injuries.

In general, typical parental responses to childhood injuries include spontaneous reporting of the details of the illness or injury accompanied by concern, questions about progress and discharge, difficulty in leaving the child, and an attempt to identify with the child's feelings. These parents also may experience guilt for not protecting the child from the accident and may offer gifts to compensate for these feelings.

In contrast, neglecting or abusing parents often are hesitant to provide information about the illness or injury; they may seem evasive or even contradict themselves. In addition, they tend to be irritated at the inconvenience of being asked questions, seem angry with the child, or show little or no concern for the injury, prognosis, or discharge plans. Abusing parents tend to visit the child less and may even disappear during the examination. They may not exhibit guilt feelings and generally contend that the child was solely responsible for the injury. These parents do not mention good qualities about the child but rather are highly critical.

Although these signs of abusive potential certainly are not present in all abusing families and no one family exhibits all of these symptoms, their presence should alert the nurse to assess and observe further. The nurse also must remember that some of these signs may be found in nonabusing families; thus, their presence serves only as a cue to further assessment, not as a conclusive diagnosis.

COMMUNITY

The toddler's world may expand rapidly when he or she enters a day-care setting. The toddler years are when many parents decide that some experience in a group setting would be beneficial for their child. Counseling about day care should include the following areas of concern.

Feelings of Ambivalence or Guilt after Enrolling Toddler in Day-Care Settings. Regardless of the reasons for the family wanting or needing day care for the child, the traditional expectation of caring for the young child at home continues to influence the parents' concept of what they "should" do for their child. They need to be reassured that a day-care environment congruent with the family environment is not detrimental to the child, that they are not neglecting their parental duty, and that their choice or necessity arises out of achieving goals that ultimately will benefit the child. For example, if the parent must work to earn an income or needs to obtain job training or education or simply needs outside activity and stimulation for self-development, the child will benefit.[27]

Selection of Day-Care Setting. Several factors must be considered in selecting the day-care center. The economic factor is often the determining variable; but if possible, the family also needs to include such factors as convenience of location, range and flexibility of hours and services available, quality of the facility, and congruence of the center's philosophy of child care with that of the family. The parent may need assistance in determining the quality of day care and in estimating whether the day-care service follows their own philosophy. If a child has been placed in a setting that is detrimental to physical or emotional development, the parent may need assistance in selecting an alternate setting. Community action also must be taken to intervene at the setting to protect the health of all other children involved.[26] Parents can be directed to a local day-care referral agency or family day-care association for free pamphlets on how to choose a child care setting.

Ongoing Evaluation of Day-Care Setting. Changes in caregivers are hard on children, so parents need to make careful selections. However, making the initial choice of care settings is only the first step. Parents should be encouraged to reevaluate the care setting as their child matures. Some settings are wonderful for infants and young toddlers but cannot offer the range of activities and stimulation needed by the older toddler or preschooler.

Parents need to also monitor the ongoing safety and quality of their child's care setting. Parents should be concerned if they are not welcome to drop in and visit their child at any time, if the caregiver frequently seems overwhelmed, or if their child begins to exhibit unusual behaviors (i.e., anxious, withdrawn, tearful, always tired).

Anticipatory Provisions for Toddler's Care during Episodes of Illness. When toddlers first enter a day-care setting where other children are present, the frequency of episode illness usually increases dramatically until the child develops immunologic defenses against the infectious organisms encountered. The family needs to anticipate this probability and know what provisions will be made under such circumstances. Some large cities have one or more day cares that accept only children with short-term acute illnesses or common infectious diseases, such as chickenpox. Since this may place an additional financial burden on the family because of loss of income if the parent remains home from work to care for the child or makes alternate paid arrangements, planning for this added expense may ease the financial burden.[9]

Planning for Regulating and Controlling Parents' Physical and Emotional Resources. Often when parents work and then return home to the demands of caring for an active, dependent young child, their own physical and emotional capacity is rapidly depleted, and their ability to cope with the young child's demands wanes. The nurse should guide parents in recognizing their own limits of energy and help them identify ways in which they can conserve energy, obtain relief during difficult periods, and plan for their own restoration needs.

Anticipation of Separation Protest. An initial or transient reoccurring separation protest can be anticipated in the toddler period. The parent needs to understand that this is a normal reaction. They should plan firmly to leave the child soon after arriving at the day-care setting and clearly inform the child of this, saying they will return later in the day. The parent needs reassurance that the child will settle down soon and become involved in the day-care activities and that the early repeated episodes of protest will gradually decline.[16]

CULTURE AND ETHNICITY

The toddler continues to be shaped by the cultural values and beliefs of the parents and also begins to be introduced to the more ritualistic family practices. The way in which holidays, holy days, and birthdays are observed is very much culturally determined. The toddler is socialized into these rituals and comes to accept them.

Limit setting and discipline also are often culturally determined. Certain cultures expect even very young children to show unquestioning respect for adults. In the independent toddler, this expected "respect" for the parents rarely may be seen.

Health care practices also are culturally influenced. If the family views immunizations as dangerous or unnecessary, the child may go unprotected from these communicable diseases. If medication is not acceptable, the child may have to rely on the immune system for all diseases contracted.

Culture also influences what people think about the curiosity toddlers have about their bodies, especially genitals. If this sexual curiosity is considered "bad," toddlers may be punished for this developmentally normal action.

Unlike the older child, the toddler does not question the cultural practices of the family. The child may refuse to do certain expected things, but this is the need for independence, not a questioning of beliefs.

LEGISLATION

Local and state legislation specific to the toddler is directed mainly at safety. As mentioned earlier, some states have passed laws on approved car seats and limited temperature in hot water heaters.

A major legislative issue for this age group is the child abuse and neglect laws in each state. These laws generally state the purpose of the law: (1) to provide protection for a child or developmentally disabled adult, (2) to define abuse and neglect, (3) to require that a report be made to a designated agency in the case of actual or suspected abuse or neglect, and (4) to define the responsibility of the protecting agency. They also may provide for a central registry of reported cases of abuse. Nurses should be aware of the child abuse and neglect laws in their states and make this information available to others involved in child care.[12]

Another key legislative issue for the toddler is PL99-457, the Education of the Handicapped Act Amendment of 1986. This law creates a "discretionary program to assist states in planning, developing and implementing a statewide system" of programs for handicapped children from birth to 3 years of age. Nurses who work with young children with handicaps can investigate available programs in their state.

Other legislation pertinent to toddlers involves regulations concerning day-care settings. These rules usually pertain to size of facilities and fire prevention and may not deal with the qualifications of those actually caring for the children. Copies of these regulations can be obtained from the state licensing agency.

ECONOMIC FACTORS

Toddlers from low-income or unemployed families suffer the same effects of poverty as any child. The toddler definitely is not capable of contributing to the economic resources of the family. Economic resources may greatly limit parents' range of child care choices. Some services are available to this age group, such as public assistance; Aid for Dependent Children; and the Women, Infants, and Children (WIC) supplemental food program (see Chapter 7). The nurse can assist families to obtain these services for their toddler by making information about these services for their toddler available to families and directing them to appropriate personnel.

HEALTH CARE DELIVERY SYSTEM

As mentioned, the nationwide system of poison control centers is a health care resource available to and often used by families with toddlers.

Private physicians or nurse practitioners and public well-child clinics are the most frequently used resources for ongoing health maintenance or illness care for toddlers. Some public clinics may sponsor special immunization days for young children who do not receive routine health care.

Another program that serves the older toddler is *Early and Periodic Screening Diagnosis and Treatment (EPSDT).* This program usually is used more by the preschooler and is discussed in Chapter 19.

NURSING INTERVENTIONS FOR HEALTH PROMOTION

The toddler period presents one of the most interesting challenges in relation to approaching and relating to the child as an individual (see box on p. 473). Toddlers' reactions to health care workers often become conditioned as feelings of fear and apprehension and their limitations in experiences with persons outside their own family render them doubtful and uncertain of encounters with strangers. An effective approach to a child of this age requires knowledge of the developmental characteristics of the child and the incorporation of nursing behaviors that are personally comfortable and successful in establishing rapport.

Each of these factors influences the manner and order in which the nurse conducts the health assessment of

RESEARCH REVIEW

TODDLER

HEALTH PROMOTION ACTIVITIES

Richardson S: Child health promotion practices, *J Pediatr Health Care* 2:73-78, 1988.

Purpose The purpose of this study was to examine parents' child health promotion practices in several areas.

Review Parents of 605 children (ages 2-5) were enrolled in 33 day-care centers and responded to a self-administered questionnaire. In general, parents followed health-promoting practices in the following areas investigated: nutrition, safety, dental hygiene, immunization, personal hygiene, sleep and rest, and exercise. Highest scores were in immunization practices; 75% reported their child had all immunizations completed due to the requirement for enrollment in day-care centers. Parents reported low health practice associated with dental hygiene. Findings support that pediatric nurses can promote positive child health practices through parent education, focusing on benefits of daily health practices.

the toddler. The nurse should not follow a predetermined pattern; rather, each component must be approached according to readiness cues from the young child. Often developmental screening that involves play activities and motor movement is used initially to promote the child's familiarity with the environment and to help establish interaction with the nurse. Assessment procedures that require restraint or discomfort should be planned to be integrated into the assessment after the child is at ease and has established a sense of confidence. Activities that restore the child's comfort and sense of security should be planned to follow such procedures so that the toddler does not leave the encounter with a negative feeling of being manipulated into a frightening or uncomfortable situation.

The child's imaginative abilities may be used effectively when the nurse approaches the child with an age-appropriate toy, book, or game. Speaking in language that is appropriate, but not demeaning, helps in establishing contact. The overwhelming size difference between an adult and a young child may be overcome by kneeling and approaching the toddler at eye level. Colors in the nurse's clothing and pictures and toys in the setting all contribute to providing a sense of familiarity that may be missing from the white, polished environment of an office or clinic.

Toddlers need time to explore, to become familiar, and to "settle in" to a new environment. They may need time just to watch or stare at a new person. Having time to play with toys, listening to the mother interacting with those who are unfamiliar, and becoming accustomed to the smells and feels of the environment are very important to children. In addition, they need evidence of whether they can trust this new environment and those in it. When painful, discomforting, or threatening procedures must be done, time must be devoted to establishing a sense of trust and confidence. When children are warned immediately in advance of painful procedures, on the other hand, undue anxiety and fear are produced to the point that the safe and adequate administration of the procedure is hampered by the child's resistance.

Each protective health visit should include an interval history, measurement of growth parameters, physical assessment, developmental assessment, and discussion of age-appropriate developmental concerns. At the 18-month visit, the toddler receives his fourth DTP and third trivalent oral poliovalent (OPV) immunizations. If the fourth HbPV was not given at the 15-month visit, it should be given at the 18-month visit.[4]

At the 24-month visits, the toddler is screened for anemia and tuberculosis and has a urinalysis.[19] The nurse may take on the responsibility for a major portion of each of these visits, since the primary objective is health teaching and disease prevention. The health teaching and discussion of toddler development may be on an individual or group basis with parents. An advantage of the group approach is that parents may benefit from each other's experience with similar situations. Specific suggestions and information for many concerns of parents of toddlers already have been discussed.

The nurse also may contribute to the health of toddlers as a consultant to a day-care center, a leader of a toddler-parent discussion or play group through a community agency, or a speaker to a parents' organization. As always, the nurse must look beyond the needs of individual families and toddlers and become involved with community agencies and local and state legislative bodies charged with passing laws related to the health and welfare of these young children. This is the only way to ensure adequate health promotion opportunities for all children.

SUMMARY

The toddler period can be an exciting, challenging time for parents and their child to establish healthy and satisfying interactions and for the toddler to grow and develop into a more independent individual. The nurse promotes this healthy, satisfying outcome by screening for developmental delays and signs of disease and by providing ongoing information to parents about their toddler's needs and new skills.

References

1. Barker PO, Lewis DA: The management of lead exposure in pediatric populations, *Nurse Practitioner* 15(12):8-16, 1990.
2. Berger KS: *The developing person through childhood and adolescence,* ed 3, New York, 1991, Worth Publishers.
3. Briggs DC: *Your child's self esteem,* Garden City, NY, 1975, Doubleday.
4. Committee on Infectious Diseases, American Academy of Pediatrics: Haemophilus influenza type b conjugate vaccine, *Pediatrics* 81(6):908, 1988.
5. Dixon S, Stein M: *Encounters with children: pediatric behavior and development,* Chicago, 1987, Mosby.
6. Falkner F, Tanner J: *Human growth,* ed 2, New York, 1986, Plenum Press.
7. Fraiberg S: *The magic years,* New York, 1959, Charles Scribner's Sons.
8. Frankenburg WK, et al: *Denver screening manual,* Denver, 1990, Denver Materials.
9. Furman L: Infirmary style sick-child daycare: do we need more information?, *Pediatrics* 88(2):290-293, 1991.
10. Gallagher JJ, Trohanes PL, Clifford RM: *Policy implementation and PL 94-457,* Baltimore, 1989, Paul H Brookes Publishing.
11. Guyton AC: *Textbook of medical physiology,* ed 8, Philadelphia, 1991, WB Sanders.
12. Hoekelman R, et al: *Primary pediatric care,* ed 2, St Louis, 1992, Mosby.
13. Kronmiller J, Nirschel R: Preventive dentistry for children, *Pediatr Nurs* 11(6):11, 1985.
14. Krugman R: Recognition of sexual abuse in children, *Pediatr Rev* 8(1):25, 1986.
15. Magramm I: Amblyopia: etiology, detection and treatment, *Pediatr Rev* 13(1):7-15, 1992.
16. McCartney K, Galanapoulos A: Child care and attachments: a new frontier the second time around, *Am J Orthopsychiatry* 58(1):16-24, 1988.
17. Phillips JL Jr: *The origins of intellect, Piaget's theory,* San Francisco, 1969, WH Freeman.
18. Pipes P: *Nutrition in infancy and childhood,* ed 4, St Louis, 1984, Mosby.
19. Recommendations for preventive pediatric health care, committee on practice and ambulatory medicine, *Pediatrics* 81(3):466, 1988.
20. Scipien G, et al: *Comprehensive pediatric nursing,* ed 3, New York, 1986, McGraw-Hill.
21. Seidel H, et al: *Mosby's guide to physical examination,* ed 2, St Louis, 1991, Mosby.
22. Sinclair D: *Human growth after birth,* New York, 1985, Oxford University Press.
23. Trahms C: *Vegetarian diets for children.* In Pipes P: *Nutrition in infancy and childhood,* ed 4, St Louis, 1989, Mosby.
24. Vaugham VC: Assessment of growth and development during infancy and early childhood, *Pediatr Rev* 13(3):88-96, 1992.
25. Webster-Stratton C: *The incredible years: a trouble-shooting guide for parents of children aged 3-8,* Toronto, 1992, Umbrella Press.
26. Wong D: Helping parents select day-care centers, *Pediatr Nurs* 12(3):181, 1986.
27. Ziegler E, Hall N: Daycare and its effects on children: an overview for health professionals, *Dev Behav Ped* 9(1):38-46, 1988.

CHAPTER

19

Preschool Child

Lois A. Hancock

Objectives

After completing this chapter, the nurse will be able to

- *Discuss the physical changes that occur during the preschool years, and relate these changes to health needs.*
- *Discuss with a parent typical sleep disturbances of preschoolers and appropriate interventions.*
- *Relate the cognitive development of the preschooler to Piaget's theory.*
- *Discuss appropriate vision and hearing screening tools and approaches to use with the preschooler.*
- *Contrast the coping skills of the preschooler with those of a younger child.*
- *Outline the catch-up immunization schedule for preschoolers who were not immunized as infants.*
- *Discuss warning signs of cancer in the preschooler.*
- *Explain the concept of school readiness and the means to assess this readiness to a group of parents.*

The preschooler is characterized by a more mature body structure, an ability to control and use the body, and a facility with language that more closely resembles that of the adult. The major psychologic thrust of this period of development is mastery of the self as an independent human being, with willingness to extend experiences beyond that of the family. The end of early childhood is marked in most families of the Western world with entrance into formalized educational systems. (See box on page 476.)

PHYSIOLOGIC PROCESSES

Age and Physical Changes

The protruberant abdomen of the toddler disappears in the preschool years as the pelvis begins to straighten and abdominal muscles become better developed. The hips gradually rotate inward, replacing out-toeing with straight or slight in-toeing. Mild *in-toeing (metatarsus adductus)* is acceptable in the preschool years, but anything beyond a mild level should be investigated and treatment begun.[5]

Growth rate remains relatively steady between ages 3 to 6 years. The average preschooler gains about 2 kg (4½ pounds) of body weight and 7 cm (2¾ inches) of stature each year.[5] Head circumference increases less than 2 cm during the entire preschool period.

As early childhood progresses, the skin matures significantly in protecting from outer invasion and loss of fluids. The skin's ability to localize infection increases but remains less than mature. Secretion of sebum is negligible throughout early childhood, rendering the skin particularly dry. Changes occur in both color and curliness of the hair, which usually becomes darker and straighter than during infancy. The function of the

HEALTHY PEOPLE 2000

SELECTED NATIONAL HEALTH PROMOTION AND DISEASE PREVENTION OBJECTIVES

PRESCHOOL CHILD

- Increase to at least 80% of the proportion of providers of primary care for children who routinely refer or screen infants and children for impairments of vision, hearing, speech and language, and assess other developmental milestones as part of well-child care
- Achieve for all disadvantaged children and children with disabilities access to high-quality and developmentally appropriate preschool programs that help prepare children for school by improving their prospects with regard to school performance, problem behaviors, and mental and physical health (1990 baseline: 47% of eligible children age 4 were afforded the opportunity to enroll in Head Start)
- Reduce deaths among children age 14 and younger caused by motor vehicle crashes to no more than 5.5 per 100,000 (1987 baseline: 6.2 per 100,000)
- Increase to at least 80% the proportion of children ages 2 through 12 who have received, as a minimum within the appropriate interval, all of the screening and immunization services and at least one of the counseling services appropriate for their age and gender as recommended by the U.S. Preventive Services Task Force (Baseline data available in 1991)

eccrine sweat glands gradually increases, but the quantity of accrine sweat produced in response to heat or emotion remains minimal. Apocrine sweat glands remain nonsecretory during this period.

The kidneys have reached full adult maturity by the end of infancy and early toddlerhood. The only changes during the preschool years are in size. By the end of this period, daily excretion of urine is 650 to 1000 ml (19½ to 30 ounces). Under normal homeostatic conditions, the renal system is able to conserve water and concentrate urine on a level that approximates adult abilities. However, under conditions of stress this ability is still decreased, and the reaction of the renal system in the establishment of homeostatic balance probably is slower than that of the adult system.[18]

Growth of the various gastrointestinal organs continues through the preschool years, but no basic changes in function occur. Children who did not achieve full voluntary control of elimination during the toddler period generally do achieve this control by the end of the preschool period. *Acquired lactase deficiency,* an intolerance to milk manifested by diarrhea, may develop during the preschool years. This is more common in black and Oriental children and is managed by eliminating lactase from the diet.[11]

Lung capacity continues to increase, and respiratory rate decreases gradually. The preschooler can better judge what things are safe to put in the mouth, so generally fewer instances of choking and obstruction occur. As the ear gradually increases in size, the incidence of otiltis media decreases somewhat. The tonsils and adenoids remain relatively large.

The cardiovascular system enlarges in proportion to general body growth. Heart rate for the preschooler is 105 ± 35 (2 standard deviations). The mean blood pressure is 100/60.[5] Early *hypertension* may develop in the preschool years, thus monitoring blood pressure during this time is important. Hypertension is discussed in Chapter 20.

The preschool child is capable of maintaining adequate levels of hemoglobin if dietary intake of iron is sufficient. The bone marrow of the ribs, sternum, and vertebrae is fully established as the main site of formation of red blood cells, but the liver and spleen maintain the capacity to form erythrocytes and granulocytes during hematopoietic stress.[5,18]

The immune system continues a gradual development, as described in Chapter 18. The preschooler continues to build up immunity to common pathogens as exposure occurs. The child who joins a new preschool or play group may experience an increase in common contagious illnesses for a time.

All the primary teeth have erupted by late toddler or very early preschool years. The first permanent tooth may erupt at the very end of the preschool period. On the average girls tend to begin permanent tooth eruption about 6 months before boys.[5] Older preschoolers usually take responsibility for dental hygiene, although they may need gentle reminders to brush. Parents should continue to assist with and supervise flossing. Regular dental checkups are essential, since this is an age of caries formation (Fig. 19-1). The suggestions for promoting good oral hygiene in Chapter 20 also apply to the preschooler.

Musculoskeletal and neurologic system development has reached a level that allows for seemingly effortless walking, running, and climbing. Older preschoolers' ability to copy figures and draw recognizable pictures is an indication of their advancing fine motor abilities, and they are eager to demonstrate these skills to others. Practice, gains in muscle size, continuing associations between existing neural pathways, and the establishment of new pathways for already accomplished tasks are a few of the many complex factors that contribute to the advances in functioning observed during early childhood.[22]

Gender

As discussed in Chapter 18, boys are more likely to be affected by some of the common childhood illnesses. Preschoolers are more aware of their sexual identity and may imitate societal stereotypes more closely. Traditionally, boys were allowed or encouraged to take more risks and thus have been involved in more accidents than preschool girls, who may have been encouraged to choose more sedate activities. In today's society, boys and girls have a more equal opportunity to choose the same activities. It will be interesting to observe if accident statistics in future years reflect this change.

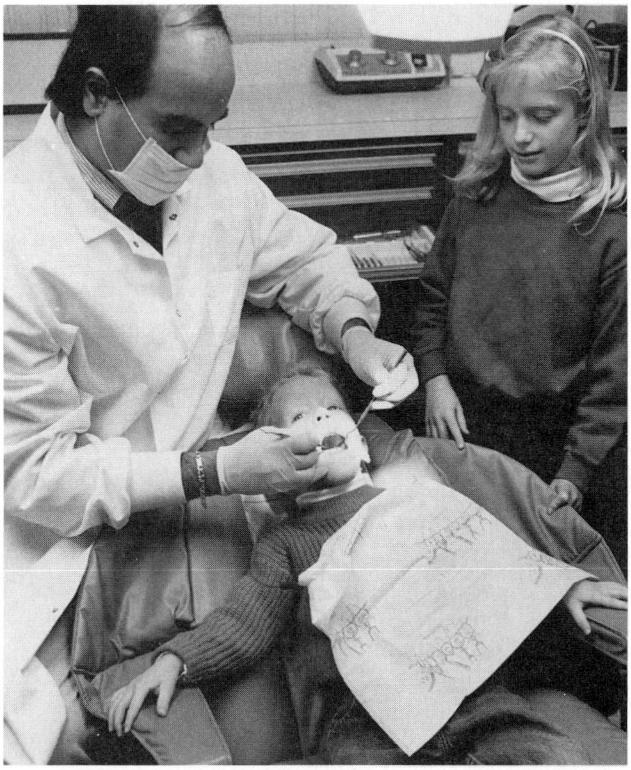

Fig. 19-1. Routine dental checkups should begin during the early preschool period. (Photograph by Fredric J. Edelman.)

Race

Race, with its related poverty or wealth, may influence health care practices at this age, as it does at all ages. Race also may influence dietary choices because of cultural preferences as well as economics.

Genetics

Few genetic problems do not manifest during infancy or toddler years, but these probably will be noted at adolescence. Although the preschooler's health may be influenced by genetic conditions diagnosed earlier in life, the nursing focus is mainly ongoing parent education and screening for complications of these conditions.

Nutritional and Metabolic Pattern

The average preschooler needs approximately 90 kcal/kg of body weight per day for health maintenance, activity, and growth. Table 19-1 shows a typical daily distribution of foods that will provide the essential calories and nutrients for the preschooler.

As early childhood progresses, intense expressions of food preferences emerge. This behavior is a natural outgrowth of the increased physical capacity to react to the taste and textures of foods and the realization that controlling the environment by expressing an opinion is possible. Preschoolers are more likely to reject cooked vegetables, mixed dishes, and liver. Older preschoolers are more likely to refuse to try new foods. Favorite foods for this age are meat, cereal grains, baked products, fruits, and sweets.[16]

Families vary in their tolerance of expressed individual food preferences, and children vary in their tendency to develop strong likes and dislikes. When a family and a child reach extreme differences over this matter, major conflict arises, and insightful counseling and support may be needed until some mutually satisfying solution is discovered. The nurse must (1) provide assessment of the nutritional adequacy of the foods liked and needed by the child, (2) help the family reach a comfortable approach in handling the situation, and (3) maintain a receptiveness to the wide range of possibilities that exist for all families in providing the essential nutrients needed for growth and development.

Many preschoolers eat at least one meal a day at the baby-sitter's, day-care, or school setting. Licensed day-

Table 19-1.* Food pattern for preschool children, ages 4 to 6

Food	Portion size	Number of recommended portions
Milk and dairy products		
Milk†	4 oz	Three to four
Cheese	½-¾ oz	May be substituted for one portion of liquid milk
Yogurt	¼-½ cup	May be substituted for one portion of liquid milk
Powdered skim milk	2 tbsp	May be substituted for one portion of liquid milk
Meat and meat equivalents		
Meat,‡ fish,§ poultry	1-2 oz	Two
Egg	1	One
Peanut butter	1-2 tbsp	
Legumes–dried peas and beans	¼-⅓ cup cooked	
Vegetables and fruits		
Vegetables‖		Four to five; to include one green leafy or yellow vegetable
Cooked	2-4 tbsp	
Raw	Few pieces	
Fruit		One citrus fruit or other vegetable or fruit rich in vitamin C
Canned	4-8 tbsp	
Raw	½-1 small	
Fruit juice	3-4 oz	
Bread and cereal grains		
Whole-grain or enriched white bread	½-1 slice	Three
Cooked cereal	¼-½ cup	May be substituted for one serving of bread
Ready-to-serve dry cereals	½-1 cup	
Spaghetti, macaroni, noodles, rice	¼-½ cup	
Crackers	2-3	
Fat		
Bacon	1 slice	
Butter or vitamin A–fortified margarine	1 tsp	Three to four
Desserts	¼-½ cup	
Sugars	½-1 tsp	Two

From Pipes PL: *Nutrition in infancy and childhood,* ed 4, St Louis, 1989, Mosby.
*Diets should be monitored for adequacy of iron and vitamin D intake.
†Approximately ⅔ cup can be incorporated easily in a child's food during cooking.
‡Liver once a week can be used as liver sausage or cooked liver.
§Should be served once or twice per week to substitute for meat.
‖If child's preferences are limited, use double portions of preferred vegetables until appetite for other vegetables develops.

care centers and preschools must serve an approved menu that provides a required percentage of the recommended daily allowances of basic nutrients. Parents should periodically inquire about what their child eats while away from home. Preschoolers in group settings may learn eating skills and food preferences from the teacher and other children.

The young preschooler is still struggling with the intricacies of using silverware. The older preschooler is skilled with a spoon, fairly proficient with a fork, and able to manage a knife for spreading soft foods on bread or crackers. The child may still need help cutting meat and pouring from a large, heavy container.

Preschoolers may enjoy helping to prepare family meals and are capable of making their sandwiches.

Elimination Pattern

By the end of the preschool period most children are capable of and responsible for independent toileting. They may still sometimes forget flushing or handwashing, a result of being in a hurry rather than lacking the skills. Preschoolers who have occasional "accidents" should not be teased or punished; they can be responsible for changing their clothes and gently reminded that they can do better next time. Enuresis and encopresis are discussed in Chapter 20.

Activity and Exercise Pattern

Play continues to be the main activity of this age group, as it is in the toddler years. The preschooler is an avid explorer; motor activities show more coordination and confidence. The child ventures farther from home than the toddler could. Many play activities involve other children.

The 4-year-old child separates easily from the parents, plays simple interactive games, dresses himself or herself, copies a number of basic geometric figures well, and draws a recognizable person. He or she enjoys using language skills in telling stories and asking questions. He or she can balance on one foot, jump, and run very well.[7] He or she loves an audience and enjoys practicing new skills and demonstrating mastered skills to others.

Play constitutes an important role in preschoolers' social and inner development. It is a vehicle for exploring and experimenting with the ways of the world, who they are, who they might become, and how they relate to others socially. The drama of play allows them to get outside of themselves and comprehend themselves momentarily from some other perspective. Play often reveals the child's inner reality and perception of the world.

Children "act out" the behavior of those familiar to them, rehearsing what has been demonstrated to them as appropriate behavior. Young children seldom assume the role of a younger child or infant in playing "house"; they more often assume mommy or daddy roles and use a doll for the younger child. Through play they learn to exert control over their own behavior; in voluntarily assuming an adultlike role, children consciously adopt a more mature form of behavior than is typical for their own age. Thus, children may be seen to practice expressing displeasure and anger in a play situation by vocalizing their distress, scolding the offending party, or using withdrawal of attention. If they were confronted with a similar but real anger-provoking situation, they would more likely respond with aggression, crying, or tantrum behavior. Observation of play reveals children's physical capacities in a more natural setting than that of the examination or testing environment and gives further evidence of their social and inner development.

Social competency can be estimated by observing a child's play in peer groups or through observing imitation play. The child who is a stranger in a peer group may be expected to stand back and simply observe other children for awhile and then approach and begin manipulating a toy object. During the preschool period, the child engages in more interactive play, particularly make-believe play. Two or more children may become involved in a make-believe plot, especially if toys and equipment are present that suggest a particular plot, such as toy kitchen equipment. Much of the preschooler's play involved fantasy. It is not uncommon for the 4- to 5-year-old child to invent an imaginary companion who plays, eats, and sleeps with her. The many aspects of fantasy and the preschooler are discussed in the section on cognitive and perceptual skills.

Most preschoolers are in a group setting for at least several sessions a week. At preschools and play schools generally some ground rules govern sharing of play materials, quiet times, and group activities. The preschooler is able to regulate activity better than the toddler and thus does not become frustrated by basic rules.

Although the preschooler's concept of time is not fully developed, he does have an idea of the passage of time, past and future. He may enjoy planning an activity with his parents. A trip to the zoo may be prefaced by getting library books about wild animals beforehand, selecting and helping to pack lunches the night before, and discussing what clothes to wear.

Many preschoolers spend long periods each day watching television. Although some excellent television shows are available for preschoolers, much more air time is devoted to adult themes and violence. A discussion of television viewing is presented in Chapter 20. Parents should keep in mind that preschoolers watching television

1. Do not have enough life experiences to interpret many of the issues presented in adult shows (violence, interpersonal relationships, moral decisions)
2. Could be missing opportunities for interacting with other children or adults
3. Cannot judge which shows are appropriate for them

Parents should choose which shows are appropriate for their child, and, if possible, should watch these shows with the child so there is an opportunity for discussion and for the child to ask questions.

Sleep and Rest Pattern

Most preschoolers sleep from 8 to 12 hours at night with wide variation from child to child. Many older preschoolers do not need a nap. The preschooler who does still nap usually requires only 30 to 60 minutes a day.[1] As with some toddlers, a "quiet time" in the afternoon may provide a welcome respite for the parent and a change for the active preschooler to relax before his afternoon activities.

BEDTIME RITUAL

Many preschoolers still need a ritual of activities at bedtime to help them make the transition from playing and being with others to being alone and trying to fall asleep. In a recent study of 109 preschoolers, 4- and 5-year-old children were more likely than toddlers to prolong the bedtime routine, insist on sleeping with the light on, take a treasured object to bed, request parental attention after being told good night, and experience delays in falling asleep.[1] The bedtime ritual may take 30 minutes or even longer. Vigorous resistance to bedtime may be more of a problem in the preschool than in the toddler period. This is especially true when such misbehavior was not effectively managed during the toddler years. Children who have learned to control the family by their bedtime behavior continue to use this power.

Nursing Interventions. When bedtime behavior has been a problem for a year or more or lasts for more than an hour, the nurse needs to gather a very comprehensive history, including (1) early episodes, (2) how they were handled and progression of events since first episodes, (3) current bedtime behaviors of the child and siblings, (4) responses of the parents and other family members, (5) feelings of the parents and child about each other and about the bedtime situation, (6) stressful events and changes that have occurred over the last several years, (7) behavior of the child at other times of the day, (8) parents' thoughts about why this has continued for so long, and (9) parents' ideas about how they can now deal with the situation.

The nurse then needs to observe interactions between the parents and child; an excellent way to do this is to go into the home when there is active interaction, such as at mealtime. In the office or clinic setting, the nurse can ask the parent to teach the child a task or give him or her directions. The nurse should be as unobtrusive as possible while observing the interaction. The firsthand observation of parent-child interaction, along with the detailed history, usually provides the nurse with adequate baseline information to decide if this situation can be dealt with in a primary care setting or should be referred to a child behavior specialist.

Reasonable bedtime rituals should be respected by parents. Repeated requests for attention after ritual is over should be handled firmly and consistently.

Discipline and management of misbehavior, which includes long-term bedtime resistance, is discussed under the role and relationship pattern later in this chapter.

SLEEP DISTURBANCES

Nighttime wakening is very common in the preschool years. In one study, this occurred at least once a week for 61% to 66% of preschoolers, and at least once every night for 19% to 33%. Just knowing how common this is may reassure many parents.

Night wakenings are of two types: night terrors and nightmares or anxiety dreams. As briefly discussed in Chapter 18, *night terrors* are frightening dreams that cause the child to sit up in bed, often scream, stare at an imaginary object, breathe heavily, perspire, and appear in obvious distress. The child is not fully awake and is unconsolable for 10 minutes or more, then relaxes and returns to a deep sleep. The child is unable to recall the dream and in the morning does not remember the attack. These night terrors may start about age 2, but are even more common during the preschool years. Night terrors are rarely seen in older children and adults and occur in only about 6% of preschool children. When they do occur, they can be very upsetting for the parent.

Nightmares and *anxiety dreams* are much more common causes of night wakening. Although infants and toddlers probably do have nightmares, their limited verbal skills make it difficult to document. From age 3 on, children have fairly frequent nightmares.[11] About one fifth of the night is spent dreaming; it is not surprising that many dreams are frightening for a child whose fantasy ideas and imagination are as active as the preschooler's. The child usually fully wakens and may feel fearful and helpless. He or she can usually vividly describe the dream at the time and often remembers it in the morning. A parent or baby-sitter should go to the child, listen to his or her description and fears, then reassure the child that he or she was only dreaming and encourage him or her to go back to sleep.

Use of the words "pretend" and "real" can be very helpful at this age. When the parent reads a story to the child or the child tells a make-believe tale, the parents can specify that these are "pretend" and did not really happen. The parent relating a true event can say, "This is real." As the child differentiates these two concepts, they can then be used in the future regarding nightmares and fears.

SUMMARY

Parents of a preschooler can benefit from knowing the following facts:

1. Bedtime rituals of 30 to 45 minutes are common for preschoolers. These rituals are very important to the child and should be respected within reasonable limits.
2. Night wakenings are very common in the preschool years. When the child wakens at night, he or she should be reassured and remain in his or her own bed.
3. Restricting frightening television shows and stories and discussing "real" versus "pretend" ideas and stories may help to lessen nightmares.

PSYCHOLOGIC PROCESSES

Cognitive and Perceptual Pattern

During the preschool years, the child makes great gains in conceptual and cognitive capacity. Concepts of time emerge, and the child gradually is able to differentiate today from yesterday and to think of tomorrow and the future. The child becomes more fully oriented in space and develops awareness of the location of home within the neighborhood. Structure and value order begin; the child begins to structure daily activities and value certain activities, objects, and people above others.

PIAGET'S THEORY

As discussed in Chapter 18, the older toddler enters the first substage of the *preoperational stage* described by Piaget.[15] The hallmark of this *preconceptual* substage was the ability to function symbolically using language. The preschool child demonstrates increased symbolic functioning during the *intuitive* substage, from age 4 to about 7 years. The cardinal rule of this and the following period is the *concreteness* of the thought processes in comparison with adult thinking. The preschooler, who is beginning to experience symbolic mental representations, simply runs through all the mental symbols as they would occur if he or she actually were participating in the event. An adult is capable of analyzing and synthesizing symbolic information, and mental connection with the real event is not necessary. The preschooler is not able to perform mental gymnastics, such as skipping from one part of an operation to another, reversing the operation mentally, or thinking of the whole in relation to the parts.

Concreteness is further characterized by the limitation of egocentrism. At this stage, children are unable to conceptualize another person's point of view. They can only think about meanings in relation to their own attached meanings and symbols and cannot understand why another person fails to follow these idiosyncratic communications.

Further, the child is unable to shift attention from one part of an object or event to another once attention is focused on a particular aspect. This is termed *centering* by Piaget and is illustrated by the child's inability to take into account more than one factor in solving a simple problem. For example, a child is given two identical cups containing equal amounts of water and is asked which cup contains the greater amount of water. During the preoperational period, the child responds that they contain the same amount of water The child is then asked to pour the water from each cup into two different containers: one flat and wide, and other tall and narrow. When asked which has more water, the child always identifies one, usually the taller, narrower container in which the water reaches a higher level. When the water is again transferred to the equal cups and the experiment repeated, the child continues to respond in exactly the same way as before.

This experiment also illustrates the trait of *irreversibility*. The child is not able to connect the reversible operation, the transfer of the water back into the original cup, and makes the logical conclusion that the differently shaped containers hold the same amount of water. The child cannot mentally associate that the transformation from one state to another is not a function of the amount of water but of the shape of the container.

Finally, Piaget describes the preoperative period of thinking as utilizing *transducive reasoning*. The child is not able to proceed from general to particular *(deduction)* or from particular to general *(induction);* rather, the child moves only from particular to particular in making associations and solving problems. For example, Piaget relates an association made by one of his children between being hunchbacked and being ill. When a hunchbacked neighbor could not visit one day because he had a communicable illness, the child was able to understand that the neighbor was ill. However, when the child was told later that the neighbor was better and that she could go to see him, her conclusion was that now his hunched back was straight and well. She was able to think in terms of being well or ill, but she placed the man in one or the other category and assumed he possessed all the attributes and meanings that she linked symbolically with either trait.[15]

The preschooler's cognitive development is reflected in his play as symbolic games become much more orderly and representative of reality. He or she begins to incorporate the reality of the world as it exists outside the self. The child increasingly seeks play objects that are models of authentic objects in the environment and increasingly imitates the social rules of society. Social interactive play becomes more predominant as the child develops a more secure sense of self.[15]

The preschooler may have one or more imaginary companions, who exist for varying periods. These fantasy companions may take the form of another child, animal, or other friendly or fearsome creature. The preschooler may save special chairs, insist that an extra place be set at the table and talk at length to this companion. Imaginary companions serve an important function in that they are totally controlled by the child and thus are not a threat to him or her. The preschooler can practice social interactions, control a fearsome beast, blame someone for naughty behavior, and so on without fear of scolding, shame, or attack, since the imaginary companion can do and say only what the child wills.

Sensory abilities contribute to the preschooler's skills in perceiving the world (see box on p. 476.)

VISION

Vision capabilities which are well developed by 2 years of age, continue to undergo refinement during the early childhood period; by about age 6 the child should approach a 20/20 visual acuity level. The possibility of development of *amblyopia* is highest from infancy through about the fourth year (see Chapter 18). Depth perception and color vision are fully established; the child is able to recognize subtle differences in color shading by the sixth year. Maximum visual capability usually is achieved by the end of the preschool years.

Changes in visual capacity throughout the rest of life are in the direction of deteriorating rather than increasing function. This phenomenon partly is caused by the refractive power of the lens and developmental changes that occur in the shape of the eyeball. In the normal sequence of growth the eyeball becomes increasingly more spheric, losing the short shape typical of infancy and progressing to the point where light converges accurately on the surface of the retina. This occurs at about 6 years of age. When this occurs before the sixth year, growth continues past the point of ideal light conversion, the eyeball lengthens, and the child may develop early myopic vision, which will progress with age. Glasses are always indicated for the child who develops *myopia* before about age 8.[11]

It is essential that the preschool child's vision be screened on a regular basis, usually by using the Denver Eye Screening Test or the Snellen Screening Test. The *Denver Eye Screening Test* is designed particularly for preschool children and includes detection of the commonly occurring visual problems, such as refractive errors, strabismus, and amblyopia.[11]

The *Snellen Screening Test,* when administered under standardized procedures, has the advantage of rendering a reliable estimate of the accrual visual acuity of the child. The child must be able to understand the test requirements of either pointing in the direction of the Es or naming the letters.[11]

The Snellen E chart usually is used for preschool children, and a version for testing by the parent at home is available from the National Society for Prevention of Blindness. Such home testing has been demonstrated to be very reliable and offers the advantage of obtaining an estimate for younger children who might not cooperate with such testing in a strange environment.

The pupillary light reflex provides a screening approach for *heterotropia,* a condition in which the child's eyes do not focus together to transmit good coordinated binocular vision. If the child has developed heterotropia, the light from a penlight held about 20 inches from the eyes reflects off the pupil slightly off center. Consistent and observable crossing of the eyes may be noted *(strabismus).* The cover test provides further evidence of a tendency for the child's eyes to cross *(heterophoria).* The child focuses on a spot first 14 inches away, then 20 feet away. While the child gazes at the designated spot, one eye is blocked completely for several seconds (the eye and eyelashes must not be touched) and then removed abruptly. If the covered eye moves from the line of vision of the uncovered eye, that eye has a tendency toward muscle imbalance and must be evaluated further.[17]

Color blindness presents a particular problem for younger children, particularly in relation to school, since many cues encountered there depend on the ability to distinguish colors. Early detection can result in the child receiving some assistance with learning to interpret visual perceptions so that the disadvantage is minimized. The nurse can screen for certain types of color discrimination difficulties by asking the child to respond to various colors in the environment; however, adequate testing for all color blindness types requires the use of a specialized test, such as *Ishihara's test,* which uses a series of cards with color-tinted letters and figures.[11]

The preschooler may be aware of some discomforts or limitations with vision. The nurse should gather history form the parents, including the questions listed in Chapter 18 about signs of eye problems. The preschooler should then be asked questions to elicit information about

1. Itching, burning or "scratchy" eyes
2. Poor vision
3. Dizziness, headaches, or nausea following close eye work
4. Blurred or double vision

HEARING

During the preschool period hearing develops to its optimal level, and listening, the ability to attend to and interpret what is heard, is more refined than in the toddler period. The 4-year-old begins to make fine discriminations among similar speech sounds, such as the difference between *f* and *th* or *f* and *s.*

The child's ability to hear is determined most accurately by audiometric methods. If an audiometer is not available, a rough estimate of hearing capacity can be made by whispering instructions when the child's back is turned and observing the ability to hear and respond accurately.

Most preschoolers enjoy demonstrating their abilities and cooperate easily with vision and hearing screening. The nurse can ensure that screening will be a positive experience by following certain points (see box on p. 483).

SENSORY PERCEPTION

Just as vision and hearing acuity reaches more mature levels during the preschool years, visual and hearing perception also becomes more mature. The preschool child may perceive visual stimuli in a diffuse, global manner and all in a detail-specific manner. The nature of the stimulus seems to be the main factor in determining which response will occur. The preschooler is very susceptible to visual illusions and has difficulty discriminating right-left mirror images, which explains the confusion with letters such as *b, d, p,* and *q.*

❑ ❑ NURSE'S INTERVENTIONS FOR SCREENING VISION AND HEARING OF PRESCHOOLERS

Being skilled in the use of the equipment.
Avoiding the term *test,* since even some preschoolers have come to associate test with anxiety and possibly failure.
Allowing the child to ask questions and examine the equipment.
Doing vision and hearing screening early in the visit before anything intrusive or painful.
Doing screening in a quiet, private area so the child is not distracted by people or noises.
Praising the child for cooperating.
If the child becomes distracted or tired, taking a brief break before beginning again.
Discussing the results of the screening with the child using simple, positive terms.

Auditory perception is at the level of accepting whole words or phrases without analyzing or selecting only certain sounds within the whole.

LANGUAGE

All theses cognitive and sensory abilities contribute to the preschooler's language development. By the time the child reaches the end of the preschool period, *expressive* language may be very similar to that of adults except for minor deficiencies in refinement, vocabulary, and structure. The degree to which a child fulfills this ability depends on the aptitude for language, the opportunity for using the language, the quality and quantity of language used at home, and the range of experiences to which the child is exposed outside the home. Regardless of the child's expressive capacity, the development of *receptive* language during the preschool years is believed to be vital, since this ability provides the foundation for later expressive ability. Throughout early childhood receptive capacity exceeds expressive capacity; the child comprehends the meaning of words and phrases that are not a part of the expressive vocabulary, and he or she can make associations between concepts even thought he or she cannot explain these concepts. Table 19-2 outlines the receptive and expressive language skills of the preschooler.

During the early childhood years the development of *rhythm* is an important dimension in the development of speech capacity. Between ages 3 and 5, the child begins to practice talking as an adult; this serves to develop neuromotor capacities for adult language and to stimulate verbal interaction, which develops vocabulary and a sense of grammatical structure. These attempts are characterized by hesitations, repetitions, and frequent revisions in speech, which may be labeled by adults as stuttering but actually represent normal speech immaturity. Many authorities believe that *stuttering* originates during this developmental period, arising not from an inadequacy in the child but from the response of adults to this normal broken pattern of speech. Such reactions are thought to include impatience in waiting to listen to the child's lengthy attempts to express her thoughts, which decreases the child's opportunities to use language, and the insistence that the child correct this pattern of speech before the capacity for fluent speech is developed.[9]

Suggestions that the nurse can make to parents to facilitate their preschool child's language development are listed in the box on p. 485.

MEMORY

Memory is an important component of language development as well as of learning in general. At the preschool level, the child may label pictures, group objects, or mimic others as ways to aid memory. The preschooler does not do these things with the precision of the school-age child. He or she can benefit from adult input about which stimuli or characteristics of an object or action should be used for grouping. Preschoolers may remember pictures better by saying the name of the picture, rather than just hearing the name of the picture when it is first shown.

Preschoolers do not use rehearsal or other *mnemonic strategies* (techniques for remembering things) spontaneously, but they use and benefit from rehearsal if it is suggested to them.[1] The nurse can test memory by asking the child to repeat an arbitrary sequence of numbers. By about age 5, children should be able to repeat four consecutively named numbers easily.

TESTING OF DEVELOPMENTAL LEVEL

Parents of preschoolers often ask how to tell if their child is ready for school or for a particular school program. School readiness can be thought of as the fit between the child's skill level, the child and family's psychosocial status, and the characteristics of the particular school program. Any questions about an individual child's readiness should only be answered after all of these components are addressed.[14] The developmental testing used during the toddler years is less accurate as the child approaches school age. Some appropriate tools can help to identify the child's skill level.

A widely used tool is the *PRESS,* or *Preschool Readiness Experimental Screening Scale* (see Fig. 19-2). Determinations of its validity indicate that it is reliable in assessing school readiness. The nurse can administer it easily during a health assessment. The

***Table 19-2.* Landmarks of speech, language, and hearing ability during the preschool period**

Age (months)	Receptive language	Expressive language	Related hearing ability
42	Up to 4200 words; knows words such as what, where, how, funny, we, surprise, secret, knows number concepts to 2, how to answer questions accurately, such as do you have a dog, which is the girl, what toys do you have.	Up to 1200 words in mostly complete sentences averaging four to five words per sentence; uses all 50 phonemes; 7% of sentences are compound or complex; averages 203 words per hour; rate of speech is faster; relates experiences and tells about activities in sequential order; uses words such as what, where, how, see, little, funny, they, we, he, she, several; can say a nursery rhyme; asks permission; 95% of speech is intelligible.	
48	Up to 5600 words; carries out three-item commands consistently; knows why we have houses, books, umbrella, key; knows nearly all colors, words such as somebody, anybody, even, almost, now, something, like, bigger, too, full name, one or two songs, number concepts to 4; understands most preschool stories; can complete opposite analogies, such as brother is a boy, sister is a ________; in daytime it is light, at night it is ________.	Up to 1500 words in sentences averaging five to six words per sentence; averages 400 words per hour; counts to 3, repeats four digits, names three objects, and repeats nine-word sentences from memory; names the primary colors, some coins; relates fanciful tales; enjoys rhyming nonsense words and using exaggerations; demands reasons why and how; questioning is at a peak, up to 500 a day; passes judgment on own activity; can recite a poem from memory or sing a song; uses words such as even, almost, something, like, but; typical expressions might include: I'm so tired, you almost hit me, now I'll make something else.	Begins to make the fine discriminations among similar speech sounds, such as the difference between *f* and *th* or *f* and *s*. Child has matured enough to be tested with an audiometer. At this age formal hearing testing usually can be carried out. Not only has hearing developed to its optimum level, but listening has also become considerably refined.
54	Up to 6500 words; knows what a house, window, chair, and dress are made of and what we do with our eyes and ears; understands differences in texture and composition, such as hard, soft, rough, smooth; begins to name or point to penny, nickel, dime; understands if, because, why, when.	Up to 1800 words in sentences averaging five to six words; now averages only 230 words per hour–is satisfied with less verbalization; does little commanding or demanding; likes surprises; about 1 in 10 sentences is compound or complex, and only 8% of sentences are incomplete; can define 10 common words and count to 20; common expressions are I don't know, I said, tiny, funny, because; asks questions for information, and learns to manipulate and control persons and situations with language.	

Adapted from Chinn PL: *Child health maintenance: concepts in family-centered care*, ed 2, St Louis, 1979, Mosby.

Table 19-2. **Landmarks of speech, language, and hearing ability during the preschool period–cont'd**

Age (months)	Receptive language	Expressive language	Related hearing ability
60	Up to 9600 words; knows number concepts to 5; knows and names colors; defines words in terms of use such as a horse is to ride; also defines wind, ball, hat, stove; understands words such as if, because, when; knows what the following are for: horse, fork, legs; begins to understand right and left.	Up to 2200 words in sentences averaging six words; can define ball, hat, stove, policeman, wind, horse, fork; can count five objects and repeat four or five digits; definitions are in terms of use; can single out a word and ask its meaning; makes serious inquiries–what is this for, how does this work, who made those, what does it mean; language is now essentially complete in structure and form; uses all types of sentences, clauses, and parts of speech; reads by way of pictures, and prints simple words.	

❑ ❑ NURSING SUGGESTIONS TO ENCOURAGE LANGUAGE DEVELOPMENT IN PRESCHOOLERS

Read to the child. Encourage the child to be an active listener by pausing at times during the story to ask such questions as, "What do you think will happen next?"; "Why do you think the boy said that?"; and "What would you do now?"

Praise the child's storytelling.

Always respond to the child's questions. At times a response must be delayed; for example, if the parent is driving in heavy traffic and the child asks a question that requires a complex answer, the parent might say, "That's a very good question, let's talk about that as soon as we get home." The parent should remind the child later of the question and respond if the child still is interested.

Never tease or criticize a child about his verbalizations. If the child is excited and talking so fast that he is fumbling over words, the parent might say, "I can't listen that fast. Slow down a little for me." This is much more encouraging than, "You talk too fast. No one can understand you."

Play games that are language focused, such as naming the colors of houses or kinds of flowers as parent and child walk to the store.

central concern is *not* measurement of intellectual level but rather screening for developmental lags or abnormalities that would interfere with the child's ability to succeed in the academic and social world of school. The tool was constructed for the average capabilities of 5-year-old children but may be useful in estimating readiness in children slightly older or younger.

When obtaining more specific scores of developmental age is necessary, the nurse may use one of the screening tools specific to the preschool child. Such screening tools provide only a rough estimate of ability but may be useful in identifying those children who need more extensive evaluation of intellectual capacity.

The *Bender Copy Forms* give an estimate of the child's visual-motor perception. Standard figures are presented and the child's attempts to reproduce the figures are timed and scored against normative data supplied with the test. This test does not depend on concepts or language peculiar to any cultural group; it is based on visual and motor perception of figures common to the experience of children in all cultural groups.[12]

The *Peabody Picture Vocabulary Test* is an easily administered test of verbal intelligence, but its use is limited to middlle-class children who have acquired standard English-speaking ability. The score obtained is a reliable estimate of verbal intelligence ability if the child fits into this cultural group. For children who have received insufficient language stimulation or who come from another cultural group, the score obtained is likely to be a false low score.

Draw-a-person and *draw-a-family* tests can be graded to give estimates of intelligence as well as interpreted in relation to emotional development; however, scoring of figure drawings requires administration under standardized conditions and evaluation by a qualified psychometrist. The nurse can obtain such drawings to assess general developmental expectations, fine motor control, and evidence of concept formation. The child's percep-

NAME ______________________ BIRTH DATE ______________

SCHOOL ______________________ DATE ______________

1. a. What color is grass? ______
   b. What color is the sky if there are no clouds? ______

2. a. Repeat four numbers (one success in two tries): 4-1-7-3 or 3-8-6-4 ______
   b. Recognize four tongue blades. ______

3. a. Does Christmas come in the winter or the summer? ______
   b. Where is your heel? ______

4. Draw a square (best success in two tries). ______

5. a. Comprehension and performance ______
   b. Personal-social maturity ______

TOTAL ______

Comments:

PRESS General Outline and Record Form. The children were asked to reproduce a standard 1-inch square.

Introduction

As the child is placed on the examining table and the records and equipment are organized, the nurse says:

1. "Mrs. Smith, as I examine Johnny I will be asking him a few question, so please don't talk to him for a few minutes." The nurse smiles and asks: "OK?"
2. "Johnny, I hear you're going to start kindergarten soon. Do you think you'll like that?"

Knowledge of colors

These questions are asked during the eye, ear, nose, throat (EENT) examination:

1. "I hear your teacher will want you to know colors. Do you know any colors yet?"
2. "If she asks you to color a house, what color should you make the grass?"
3. "And what color should you make the sky if there are no clouds?"

Knowledge of numbers

These questions are asked during the heart and lung examination:

1. "If the teacher tells you some numbers, could you remember them and repeat them back to her?"
2. "I'm going to tell you some numbers. Now you remember them and say the same number right back to me." (4-1-7-3 and 3-8-6-4)
3. "If the teacher asks you to count, could you do that?"
4. "Tell me, how many tongue blades are there?" At this point place four tongue blades on the table beside child.

General knowledge

These are asked as the abdomen, genitalia, and extremities are examined:

1. "I'm going to examine your tummy. You know where your tummy is, don't you?"
2. "Tell me, does Christmas come in the winter or summer?"
3. "Can you show me where your heel is?"

Fig. 19-2. Administration and scoring of the Preschool Readiness Experimental Screening Scale (PRESS). (From Rogers WB Jr, Rogers RA: *Clin Pediatr* 11:10, Oct 1972; and Rogers WB Jr, Rogers RA: *Clin Pediatr* 14:253, March 1975. In Chinn PL: *Child health maintenance: concepts in family-centered care,* ed 2, St Louis, 1979, Mosby.)

Drawing coordination

This is usually done at the end of the examination:

1. "If the teacher asked you to draw a square like this one (indicate the sample square), let's see you draw one just like it right beside mine. Take your time and make a good one."

General assessment: performance and maturity

These are best evaluated following the hearing and visual acuity tests when everything else is finished.

Scoring

COLORS. 1 point for knowing grass is green. 1 point for knowing the sky is blue. Any other answer, such as white, blue and white, or black gets no point.

NUMBERS. 1 point for repeating the four numbers in the same sequence. If the child misses the first set of numbers, try the second set. Score 1 point for *either* set of numbers repeated back correctly. 1 point for answering the correct number of tongue blades as four. If the child only counts "one, two, three, four," this is not given a point. You may then ask the child *one time only,* "Yes, but how many are there all together?" If the child does not answer four at this time, score 0.

GENERAL KNOWLEDGE. 1 point for answering *winter.* It is important to suggest winter first. Most children will give the second of two choices if they do not know the correct answer. 1 point for knowing the heel. The child must point to the heel or the Achilles tendon, not to the malleolus.

DRAWING COORDINATION. Allow the child to draw a second square if the first one is poorly done. Encourage the child to make the second more like the sample. Choosing the best square, score in the following manner:
2 points for drawing a good, readily recognizable square
1 point for drawing a fairly recognizable square
0 points for drawing a poor, unrecognizable square

COMPREHENSION AND PERFORMANCE. 1 point for those who reply promptly and follow instructions well (for example, during the hearing and visual acuity tests). 0 points for those who have to be coaxed, need frequent repetition of instructions, or need repeated clarification of what you ask.

PERSONAL-SOCIAL MATURITY. 1 point if the child seems reasonably mature and self-confident. 0 points for:
Excessive silliness or playing around
Overtalkative or hyperactive
Uncooperative, evasive, no interest
Unduly attached to mother
Generally immature compared with most 5-year-olds

It should be evident that the PRESS is not so much a standardized test with strict rules of administration as it is a set of standardized questions that can be blended into a physical examination. The nurse should note that it includes a few questions that are asked but not scored. These questions establish rapport and put the child at ease. They also serve as a lead-in to the test questions and serve indirectly in assessing the child's general maturity. Nurses may intersperse or substitute other lead-in questions if they think these would better express their method of dealing with children. It is important to ask the parent not to speak; an oversolicitious parent may interfere by offering help and encouragement.

Rating system

1. A score of 9 or 10 indicates high average to above average school readiness. A child in this score range should have no difficulty doing average or above average school work.
2. A score of 7 or 8 indicates average school readiness. A child in this score range should have little difficulty doing average school work.
3. A score of 6 indicates borderline school readiness. About half of the males and about a fourth of the females with this score may have difficulty in school. It is recommended that close liaison be maintained with teacher. If at any time the child is not functioning at class level, further study should be made at once.
4. A score of 5 or less indicates insufficient school readiness. Such children should be referred to a school psychologist or diagnostic center for further psychologic evaluation.

Fig. 19-2, cont'd. Administration and scoring of the Preschool Readiness Experimental Screening Scale.

tions of family relationships also can be assessed.

The 4-year-old child should be able to draw a person with at least six body parts that are placed in proximity to one another and in the appropriate locations. The child should be able to name the parts. The parts need not be accurate renditions but should resemble the actual body part and be rendered with strong, evenly flowing lines. The family drawing may or may not include all family members, and the drawing of each figure may not be as sophisticated as the child's actual figure-drawing capacity. The child should be able to name the family members shown and describe any of their unique characteristics from his point of view. He also should be able to identify which figures are big or little, as drawn on the sheet of paper.

The nurse provides a pencil and plain sheet of paper and asks the child to draw the best picture possible. The child is informed that the nurse will keep the picture but that another may be drawn to take home.

Self-Perception and Self-Concept Pattern

The preschooler starts with the basic concept of self that emerged out of his or her struggle for autonomy as a toddler. He or she continues to develop and refine this sense of self through both task-oriented and socially oriented experiences. Successful accomplishment of tasks builds self-esteem by reinforcing the preschooler's skills and capabilities. Social experiences of acceptance help this child feel successful in his role of son, brother, friend, and so on. The preschooler can try out other roles through a rich imagination. Pretend play of being the parents or baby allow the preschooler to imagine and act out the feelings of others–a safe way to experiment with new ideas.

ERIKSON'S THEORY

The preschooler develops a *sense of iniative* through his or her vigorous motor activity and active imagination. Erikson sees this as the central development in the emerging concept of self in the preschool years. Parents can promote the development of iniative by praising the preschooler's efforts to try new actions and ideas and by providing the opportunity for the child to see and try new things. This does not mean forcing or coercing the preschooler to do something new, but rather providing these options so that he or she may choose to experiment. The preschooler needs to have a feeling of mastery, which implies the need for repetition. When the preschooler achieves mastery over some actions, he or she is more confident about trying new ones.

Preschoolers who are ridiculed or told that their actions or ideas are bad or silly will develop feelings of guilt and inadequacy.

SEX ROLE

Another aspect of self-concept at this age is the sex role. The preschooler recognizes the two sexes and identifies himself or herself with the correct sex. Body image includes perception of sex organs as well. Preschoolers may be very curious about other persons' bodies and sexual function. Their questions should be answered simply and factually. Parents and others should not tease the preschooler about this interest or imply that such information is "dirty" or "bad." Positive self-esteem is based on positive feelings about all aspects of self, including the sex role.

NURSING INTERVENTIONS

Assessing self-concept can be difficult for the nurse dealing with the preschool child. The nurse cannot just ask how the child sees or feels about himself or herself. Various play approaches are useful in eliciting behavior indicative of the child's sense of self and self-esteem, future success or failure, sense of acceptance, and competence.

Doll or puppet play often is useful in observing a child's sense of self (Fig. 19-3). Dolls or puppets, including one that represents a young child of the same sex as the preschooler, should be the only toy objects available when this play is desired. If the child spontaneously begins to engage the dolls or puppets in make-believe activity, no further guidance should be given. If the child seems reluctant to begin play, the nurse begins a make-believe situation, such as going to the store, moving the dolls or puppets through the related activities and then involving the child. Often a preschooler continues the scenario for a time.

A related technique is *mutual storytelling.* The child is instructed that the nurse will begin a story and that the child will finish it. The nurse then begins with a standard line, such as, "Once upon a time there lived a (girl, boy, cow, monkey, etc.) who. . . ." The nurse then pauses to indicate that the child can pick up on the story. If the child is reluctant to participate, the nurse might continue the story for another sentence or two or ask the child what the figure in the story might be doing. As the child begins to supply details of the story, the nurse asks questions that encourage the child to fill in details or continue with the story, such as, "And then what happened?" or "How did the child feel?"

The child's story then is evaluated for several dimensions that indicate the child's inner nature. First, the emotional theme of the story should be noted and should be congruent with the child's tone and expres-

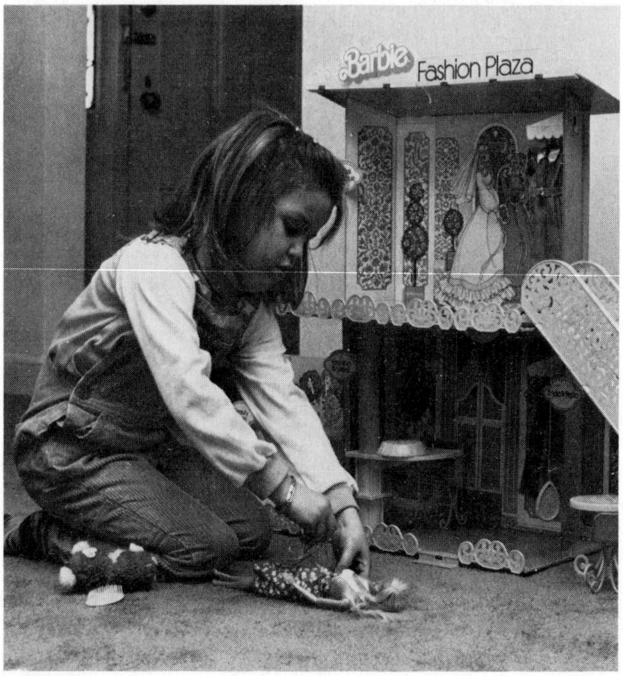

Fig. 19-3. Doll play often reflects child's sense of self. (Photograph by Douglas Bloomquist.)

sion. For example, if the child focuses on a theme of aggression and destruction but describes anger expressed by one of the characters in an emotionless monotone, incongruence of content and expression exists, which suggests that the child has difficulty in expressing feelings. Second, the possible meaning of the characters may be suggested by asking the child if he or she is like one of the characters at the conclusion of the story.

Interpretation of the child's behavior and responses in such play situations is highly speculative, and several encounters may be needed to determine possible themes or to estimate the child's self-esteem. In addition, it should be remembered that the nurse's personality and approach to the child has a significant effect on the child's ability to tell a story and on the spontaneity with which the child responds. The actual observed behavior and responses of the child should be recorded for future reference; interpretations must be avoided until validated by an experienced child health worker.

Coping and Stress-Tolerance Pattern

The preschooler uses the same types of coping mechanisms as the toddler: separation anxiety, regression, denial, repression, and projection. Protest behavior in the form of temper tantrums is usually not a common stress response for the older preschooler. If temper tantrums persist through the fifth year, the child may not have developed more mature coping responses because he or she found this to be a very successful method.

The preschooler has a larger range of experiences and memories from which to draw and thus may have more response options when a stressful event occurs. Some variables that determine positive coping resources in children are[1]

1. The range of gratification usually available to the child, which can help him or her accept substitute gratifications and find alternate solutions
2. The child's positive attitude toward life, including self-pride, resilience, and capacity to mobilize resources
3. The range and flexibility of the child's coping mechanisms and defenses
4. The capacity to regress and retreat to a level of function with less demands

Although the types of coping mechanisms are the same for toddlers and preschoolers, the preschooler should show more ability to verbalize frustration, less temper tantrum behavior, and more patience in trial-and-error experimentation to resolve a situation. The preschooler's problem-solving skills are more refined. Through *fantasy play* the preschooler may be able to look at and try out solutions or responses to stressful events.

Sometimes *projection* and fantasy in the preschooler lead parents to think that their child is lying. When faced with the question, "Did you break this dish?" the preschooler may respond, "No, Teddy did." He or she even may relate a detailed story of the toy bear's mishap. The child is projecting the blame away from himself or herself, and active fantasy thoughts help him or her tell the story. Parents should not accuse the preschooler of lying but rather should help him or her decide if the story is "pretend" or "real." These concepts of pretend and real can be very helpful in assisting the child to talk about nightmares, television shows, and stories, as well as in dealing with his or her own active imagination.[24]

The preschooler has a greater perceived ability to control and manage situations than the toddler. One way of controlling situations is by strict adherence to rituals or game rules. As already discussed, the preschooler has a longer and more rigid bedtime ritual than the toddler. The preschooler also dislikes "losing" and may control this situation by structuring the rules to assure winning. Older children and adults may be able to accept this structuring, but other preschoolers may become upset, since they also need to win.

Value and Belief Pattern

Preschoolers, as with toddlers, do not have a true conscience, but they are beginning to have some internal controls on their actions. These internal controls are not always consistent or effective but occasionally may be very strict, and the preschool child can feel overwhelming guilt. Fluctuations in behavior and the preschooler's feelings about those behavior depend very much on cognitive development.

Moral behaviors and moral feelings continue to be influenced greatly by modeling and inductive explanations. *Modeling* comes from many sources, not all of which are exactly what parents would want their child to do. Thus, parents may want to exert some control over what models are available to the child by screening television shows, carefully selecting day-care and baby-sitting situations, and monitoring play sessions. This does not mean the parent constantly is playing warden over the child, the parent is only verifying that the models for the child are acceptable. *Inductive explanations* can be more detailed than for the toddler but should be based on the individual child's cognitive level.

The preschooler's main motivation in controlling his or her behavior is the desire for parental love and approval. Disapproval from the parent does not mean that the preschooler is unloved, but it does mean that he or she feels a lessening of esteem in the parents' eyes. The fall in esteem is a motivator to change behavior. The resulting guilt from the perceived decrease in esteem is a step on the road to the preschooler developing a conscience.[6]

Moral actions for the preschooler may be linked to such simple actions as taking turns and sharing. These actions stem from the assumption that other persons have rights and desires that are equally important as those of the preschooler.

Preschoolers often express their values by stating who or what they like or what they want to be when they grow up. These values may change often, even within a few minutes. Preschoolers sometimes may use these statements of valuing as punishment for playmates or family members.

Preschoolers are famous for their "why" questions. When they direct these questions toward moral actions or feelings, they may be simply asking, "How does this work?" and not questioning the underlying parental value. This is also true when the child asks about the spiritual values the parent is trying to teach. This is an age when parents may enroll their child in Sunday school or other faith-oriented classes or activities. The preschool child generally enjoys the social aspects of these activities and receives some important modeling of values from the involved adults.

Health Perception and Health Management Pattern

Preschoolers have a fairly accurate perception of the outside of their own bodies based on what they can see and do; they may be very curious about the body of a member of the opposite sex. Their concept of what's on the inside of the body and how the internal functions of the body occur are vague and inaccurate. The internal body is seen as a hollow organ. Most preschoolers can name one or two things inside the body (blood, bones). Many of their questions about body function have to do with "having babies."[6]

By age 4 or 5, the child has amassed many beliefs about health from the family. He or she may begin to understand that he or she is partly responsible for his or her health. The preschooler often becomes very upset over minor injuries. Pain or illness may be seen as a punishment. The preschooler's declaration, "If you don't brush your teeth, your teeth will rot and fall out," is probably a statement of expected immediate and absolute cause and effect.

Although preschoolers are not completely responsible for their own health management, they certainly contribute by remembering to brush teeth, take medication, put on appropriate clothing for inclement weather, and perform other actions. Preschoolers' memory for such things may be sporadic, but they are at least beginning to be health care agents for themselves.

ENVIRONMENTAL PROCESSES

Natural Processes

The environmental processes that affect toddlers also affect preschoolers. Occurrence rates and outcomes differ in this age group most probably because of developmental differences. Preschoolers have more refined problem-solving skills, are more coordinated, and have more experience with a variety of situations. Although preschoolers can be expected to recognize and avoid some environmental hazards, they are still impulsive and immature in many ways and cannot be expected to recognize or avoid all dangers (Fig. 19-4).

ACCIDENTS

Preschoolers have fewer accidents than toddlers. Motor vehicle accidents, however, continue to be the major cause of fatalities for this age group.

Household furniture and fixtures also remain a hazard for preschoolers, as do structural features, such as stairs and windows. The occurrence rates for injuries in these categories remain almost the same in both ages. Nursery and toy injuries decrease during the preschool years. Sports and recreational injuries, however, increase markedly, from 8% to 21% during the preschool years.[11] This probably reflects preschoolers' increased involvement in group sports, riding bicycles, and using playground equipment. Parents should realize that pre-

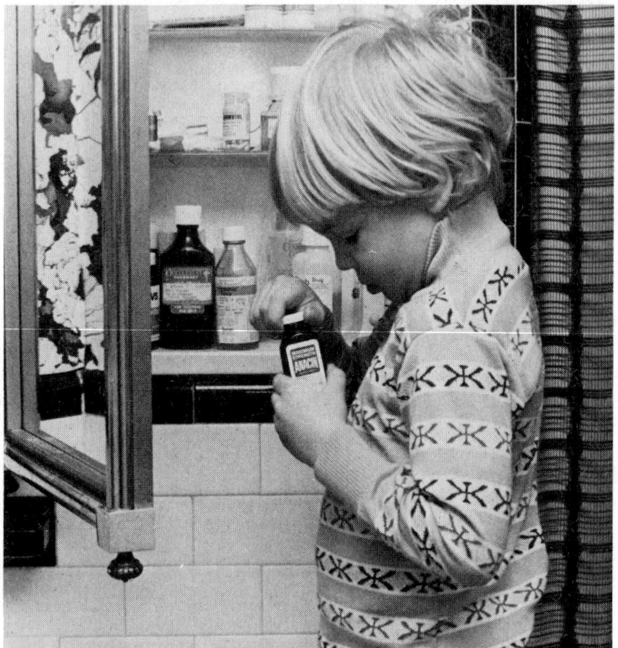

Fig. 19-4. Preschoolers are still impulsive and curious and cannot be expected to avoid all dangers. (Photograph by Douglas Bloomquist.)

schoolers need a broader range of play area and experiences, but providing age-appropriate limits and supervision remains essential.

Preschoolers do not have the skill or judgment to ride bicycles on the street; at this age, they need to learn about and deal with the hazards of sidewalk cycling. Preschoolers need instruction regarding safe use of playground equipment and require adult supervision. Group sports should be supervised by adults as well.

Preschoolers can begin to learn safe ways to handle basic tools, kitchen equipment, and cleaning supplies. They usually take pride in participating in house projects with a parent.

DROWNING

The child over 3 years of age is at lower risk for drowning in the bathtub but at greater risk for drowning in swimming pools or natural bodies of water. Preschoolers should receive instruction in water safety and swimming.

A preschooler is capable of learning the *Lanoue water survival technique,* a method of floating based on the principle that the body is naturally buoyant when the lungs are filled with air and that the natural floating position is face downward, beneath the surface of the water. He or she can and should learn this technique even before learning to swim. The preschooler should always wear a life jacket when on a boat, even if he or she knows how to swim. The preschooler should always be supervised when around water, even if it is shallow.

BURNS

Scalds and direct flame burns are major hazards for the preschooler. The measures discussed in Chapter 18 to reduce scald burns in the home apply to the preschool child as well. He or she should be taught about the dangers of matches, open flames, and hot objects.

MECHANICAL FORCES

As mentioned, bicycle accidents begin to be a greater source of injury in the preschool years. Many involve automobiles, and most of these result from the child's errors, such as going through a stop or yield sign. Parents need to set reasonable and age-appropriate limits about bicycle use. The transition from tricycle to bicycle is an excellent time to begin use of a bicycle helmet.

The preschooler as a passenger or pedestrian is at great risk for an auto-related accident. At this age, pedestrian injury is more likely than passenger injury. Preschoolers need to be taught proper street-crossing techniques and generally should be supervised when crossing streets. The preschooler who weighs more than 40 pounds (18 kg) can use an adult seat belt but should not use the shoulder harness. Preschoolers who weigh less than 40 pounds should continue using crash-tested and approved car seats or toddler restraints. The back seat is safer than the front, and all car doors should be locked. If the preschooler refuses to use the seat belt or appropriate restraint, parents must insist that the outing be postponed. Parents can give a good example by using their seat belt *every* time they are in the car. This example is the best safety teaching for the child and is especially effective with the preschooler who usually loves to imitate and please the parent. The child who has used a car seat from infancy on will generally accept the seat belt quite well.

BIOLOGIC AND BACTERIAL AGENTS

The preschooler may seem healthier to the parents because of fewer respiratory and gastrointestinal illness than as a toddler. The child has built up antibodies to many common organisms through exposure to them during the toddler years. Children who were not in group settings as toddlers and who begin preschool at age 3 or 4 usually experience an increase in these common illnesses, since they do not have immunity from previous exposure. This may be of great concern to parents and should be discussed by the nurse before the child begins attending a group setting.

Biologic agents important during this age include the recommended immunizations. For the child who was fully immunized as an infant, a booster dose of diphtheria-tetanus-pertussis (DTP) is given in the fourth year. Many states currently require that all children in a school setting be fully immunized or present a statement from their parent as to why they will not be immunized. Parents who have strong religious or other reasons for not accepting immunizations can continue to refuse for their child. However, many children have been protected only partly against these diseases because of parental forgetfulness or procrastination. Mandatory immunization is a good incentive for these parents.

Preschoolers who have received some of their immunizations do not need to repeat doses already given but simply continue from where they stopped as infants. Preschoolers who have received no immunizations follow the schedule in Table 19-3, as recommended by the American Academy of Pediatrics. The possible side effects of these immunizations are presented in Chapter 18. Parents should be fully informed about the potential side effects.[8,21]

Preschoolers with disabilities are often not sent to preschool because the parents wish to protect the child from inadvertent harm or even ridicule from the other children. Financially and socially disadvantaged children

Table 19-3. **Recommended immunization schedules for children in the United States not immunized in first year of life**

Recommended time/age	Immunization(s)[a,b]	Comments
		Younger than 7 years
First visit	DTP, Hib,[c] HBV, MMR, OPV	If indicated, tuberculin testing may be done at same visit. If child is 5 y of age or older, Hib is not indicated.
Interval after first visit		
1 mo	DTP, HBV	OPV may be given if accelerated poliomyelitis vaccination is necessary, such as for travelers to areas where polio is endemic.
2 mo	DTP, Hib, OPV	Second dose of Hib is indicated only in children whose first dose was received when younger than 15 mo.
≥ 8 mo	DTP or DTaP,[d] HBV, OPV	OPV is not given if the third dose was given earlier.
4-6 y (at or before school entry)	DTP or DTaP,[d] OPV	DTP or DTaP is not necessary if the fourth dose was given after the fourth birthday; OPV is not necessary if the third dose was given after the fourth birthday.
11-12 y	MMR	At entry to middle school or junior high school.
10 y later	Td	Repeat every 10 y throughout life.
		7 years and older
First visit	HBV,[g] OPV, MMR, Td	
Interval after first visit		
2 mo	HBV,[g] OPV, Td	OPV may also be given 1 mo after the first visit if accelerated poliomyelitis vaccination is necessary.
8-14 mo	HBV,[g] OPV, Td	OPV is not given if the third dose was given earlier.
11-12 yr	MMR	At entry to middle school or junior high.
10 y later	Td	Repeat every 10 y throughout life.

From American Academy of Pediatrics: In Peter G. ed. *1994 Red Book: Report of the Committee on Infectious Diseases,* ed. 23. Elk Grove Village, 1994, American Academy of Pediatrics.

If all needed vaccines cannot be administered simultaneously, priority should be given to protecting the child against those diseases that pose the greatest immediate risk. In the US, these diseases for children younger than 2 y usually are measles and *Haemophilus influenzae* type b infection; for children older than 7 y, they are measles, mumps, and rubella (MMR).

[b]DTP or DTaP, HBV, Hib, MMR, and OPV can be given simultaneously at separate sites if failure of the patient to return for future immunizations is a concern.

[d]DTaP is not currently licensed for use in children younger than 15 mo of age and is not recommended for primary immunization (ie, first 3 doses) at any age.

[e]If person is 18 y or older, routine poliovirus vaccination is not indicated in the US.

[f]Minimal interval between doses of MMR is 1 mo.

[g]Priority should be given to hepatitis B immunization of adolescents.

are sometimes kept out of preschool either because of lack of money or parents' lack of knowledge about the advantages of preschool as preparation for optimum school experiences. The nurse can help these families explore the pros and cons of preschool for their child and see that families obtain information about opportunities in their community and possible assistance with cost.

CHEMICAL AGENTS

The preschooler is exposed to the same environmental pollutants as any child or adult living in the same area. Specific chemical agents of concern during the toddler years continue to merit consideration, even though the preschooler can be expected to understand more clearly the concept of safe versus poisonous. Household products, drugs, pesticides, and poisonous plants should remain in adequately locked places or kept out of the house. Preschoolers should receive verbal explanations that something is poison or dangerous and why, but parents cannot rely on the child always to remember such cautions. The preschooler can identify certain warning symbols, such as "Mr. Yuk" stickers.

Cancer

From infancy to 5 years of age, the most common cancer is acute lymphocytic leukemia, which accounts for over one third of the cases of cancer in this age group. Other cancers commonly seen in this age group affect the eye (retinoblastoma), the kidney (Wilms' tumor), and the sympathetic nervous system (neuroblastoma). Cancer is the leading cause of death from disease in children over 1 year of age. Remarkable progress has been made in treatments which result in long-term survival of children with cancer. Early detection is the key to successful treatment.[23]

LEUKEMIA

Acute lymphoblastic leukemia (ALL) is the most common leukemia of childhood and accounts for about 70% of all cases. The incidence of ALL rises from the age 2 to a peak at age 5 and falls off through later childhood and adolescence. The risk factors for ALL are[13]

Sibling with leukemia
Identical twins of children with leukemia
Bloom's syndrome
Fanconi's anemia
Immune deficiency disease
Down's syndrome

It is believed that the risk of leukemia is increased at least 20-fold in Down's syndrome.[2,13]

Nursing Interventions. The dominant signs and symptoms of ALL are often sudden, but the child may have a prodromal period of weakness, malaise, anorexia, fever, and tachycardia. He or she frequently has pain in the bone, petechiae, and hemorrhages after minor procedures such as dental extractions. Another suspicious finding is an unexplained infection that does not respond to treatment. Early detection and treatment of ALL has resulted in a marked increase in 5-year survival rates.

Whenever leukemia is suspected, either because of the client's age, symptom, or known risk factors, the nurse should practice secondary prevention intervention by including the following in his or her assessment of the child:

1. Examination of the cervical and peripheral lymph nodes
2. Palpation and percussion of the liver and spleen
3. Inspection of the skin for systemic signs of leukemia such as pallor, purpura, petechiae, and chloroma
4. Inspection of the mouth for enlarged tonsils; hyperplasia of the gums; and red, friable gingivae
5. Palpation of the sternum, bones, and joints for tenderness and pain

Chloroma is a localized tumor mass that has a greenish appearance and may occur in the skin, orbit, or other tissues in granulocytic forms of leukemia.

School nurses and public health nurses working with Down's syndrome patients must be aware of the relationship between this genetic condition and increased risk for leukemia. Individuals with Down's syndrome should be followed closely for the early signs and symptoms of leukemia, as they have a 20-fold increased risk of leukemia.

WILMS' TUMOR

The majority of all cases of Wilms' tumor occur in children under 5 years of age. Girls are affected about twice as often as boys. A strong correlation exists between Wilms' tumor and several congenital malformations. The strongest association is with sporadic aniridia (congenital absence of the iris). One of every three children with this congenital malformation will develop Wilms' tumor. Other risk factors for Wilms' tumor are[13]

Family history of Wilms' tumor (autosomal dominant)
Children who have had Wilms' tumor
Children with trisomy defects (additional chromosome in an otherwise diploid cell)
Hemihypertrophy (muscular overgrowth of one half the body or face)
Genitourinary anomalies
- Hypospadias (uretra on underside of penis)
- Cryptorchism (undescended testes)

Nursing Interventions. A precise history is essential when attempting to identify the high-risk population associated with the development of Wilms' tumor. Children identified as high risk should be referred for continual evaluation and examined closely for any renal masses. Those nurses doing physical assessment should be aware that Wilms' tumor usually is found in one of the upper abdominal quadrants. The nurse or trained parent should obtain periodic abdominal girth measurements on high-risk children for monitoring early abdominal changes.

An excellent booklet designed to inform parents about the early warning symptoms and signs of childhood cancer is *Know the Warning Signs of Cancer in Children,* produced by the Cancer Association of Greater New Orleans. This booklet suggests making routine procedures, such as a bath, the time for parents to examine the child and outlines findings to discuss with the physician (see box on p. 494).

RETINOBLASTOMA

Although retinoblastoma is the most common intraocular tumor in younger children, it only occurs in 1 of 20,000 to 30,000 live births. It can occur either spontaneously or is *inherited* as a genetic mutation transmitted as an autosomal dominant characteristic. Familial retinoblastoma clients are especially at risk for secondary bone and soft tissue sarcomas.[19]

Nursing Interventions. The most important nursing action is to take a careful history, which usually reveals a slow progression of symptoms. Questions that help reveal risk factors are

Do tumors of the eyes run in your family?
If tumors of the eye run in your family, can you tell me which relatives were affected and how they were treated?
Have you noticed your child having *any* eye

❑ ❑ WARNING SIGNS THAT MAY INDICATE THE PRESENCE OF CHILDHOOD CANCER

Cancer is a leading cause of death in children less than 15 years old, second only to accidents. In this age group, one out of every five deaths is caused by cancer. In the United States each year 12.5 of 100,000 children develop cancer.

General

- Documented weight loss without explanation, failure to thrive
- Persistent poor appetite
- Easy tiring or lack of energy

Leukemia or lymphomas–"liquid tumors"

- (Cancer of the blood, blood-making system, lymph nodes)
- Persistent fever (more than 2 weeks)
- Bruising without injury and purple or red patches appearing on the skin
- Swollen glands (lymph nodes), unrelated to infection
- Persistent bone pain or limping
- Paleness of the lips, skin, nails, or lining of the eyes

Brain tumor

- Recurrent headaches, especially accompanied by vomiting particularly in the morning
- Reflection in the pupil of the eye (eye tumor)
- Unexplained, persistent changes in behavior

Kidney tumors

- Lump in the abdomen or enlargement of the abdomen
- Blood in the urine
- Bulging of the eyes
- Unexplained, persistent cough or chest pain
- A firm mass in the muscles

Make bath time examination time

- These complaints or physical findings should only be interpreted as a warning of possible serious disease. If present, you should consult your physician at once. Don't forget your children should be examined by a physician every year. The earlier cancer is detected, the better chances are for a cure. With current treatment methods of surgery, radiation therapy, and chemotherapy (administration of anticancer drugs), the survival rate of children with certain forms of cancer has been improved dramatically.

Adapted from the Cancer Association of Greater New Orleans, Inc., 211 Camp St., Room 600, New Orleans, LA 70130.

problems–crossed or lazy eyes, difficulty seeing? Have you noticed *any changes* in your child's eyes?

Nurses with physical assessment skills should perform screening eye examinations for high-risk children. These tests include checking for the following:

1. Visual acuity
2. Red reflex; in the child with retinoblastoma this appears whitish (cat's eye reflex). It is the most common presenting sign of this cancer
3. Ophthalmoscopic findings
4. Lid lag, which is found with exophthalmos
5. Strabismus, by doing the cover-uncover test

The cat's eye reflex and strabismus are the next most common presenting sign of retinoblastoma. If the nurse discovers any suspicious findings on the history or screening eye examination, the family should be referred for medical evaluation.

NEUROBLASTOMA

Neuroblastoma is a malignant tumor arising from the sympathetic nervous system. About 70% of these tumors begin in the abdomen, mainly in the adrenal gland. The other 30% originate in cervical, thoracic, or pelvic areas. Approximately one half of all clients are younger than 2 years at diagnosis; more than 90% are recognized by age 5. Unfortunately, two thirds of the children have metastases when first seen, and frequently the symptoms or signs arising from the secondary spread bring the child to the attention of health professionals.[13,19]

As many as 22% of all neuroblastomas are thought to follow a hereditary pattern. A number of families have been reported in the literature as having more than one sibling with neuroblastoma. Neuroblastoma may be related to some anomalies of neutral crest origin (neurofibromatosis, aganglionosis coli). It is important to note that survivors of neuroblastoma may develop subsequent tumors, thus necessitating continued medical surveillance. Because almost 25% of neuroblastomas appear to follow a hereditary pattern, some experts recommend monitoring the *offspring* of individuals with neuroblastoma and examining them carefully for evidence of neural crest abnormalities. Neuroblastoma produces excessive amounts of neuroactive catecholamines, which are found in the urine of clients with this tumor. Thus vanillylmandelic acid (VMA) in excessive amounts in the urine may indicate this tumor.

Nursing Interventions. Secondary prevention intervention includes the simple procedure of screening children at risk for catecholamines in the urine and for neurofibromatosis.

Social Processes

ROLE AND RELATIONSHIP PATTERN

Family members are very important to the preschooler, but peers become increasingly important as well. The preschooler gets ideas and information from his peers, which he introduces into family situations. The preschooler may question why rules or expectations are different at home than at a particular friend's house (Fig. 19-5).

Preschoolers are very much aware of sex differences related to expected jobs, activities, and competencies. They base their ideas of what is "girl's work" or "boy's work" on models in the home, at day-care or preschool centers, and on television. The preschooler tries out many roles through play, including family roles. As the mother or father in a play situation, the preschooler can set limits, punish, praise, and make outlandish demands on the "child" of the family.

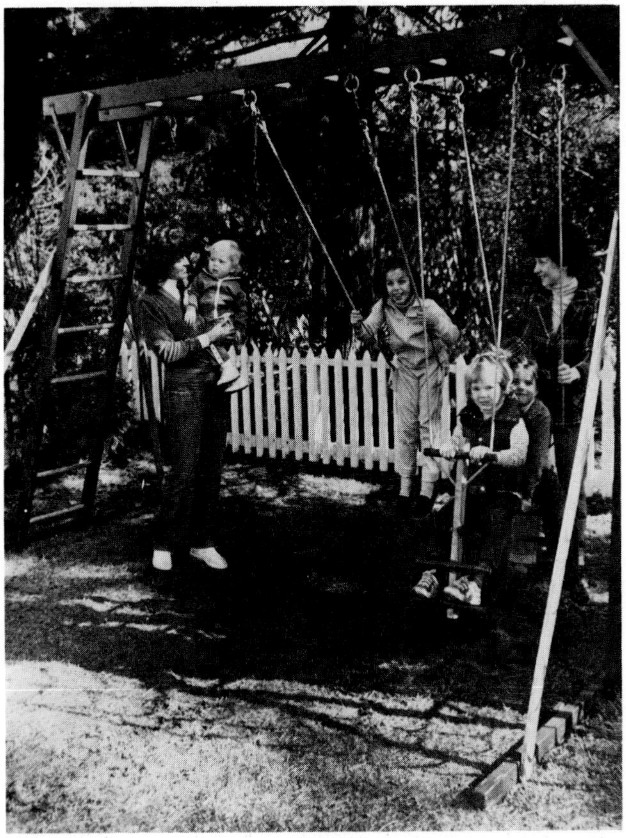

Fig. 19-5. Whereas toddlers stay close to their parents, preschoolers play more with other children. (Photograph by Douglas Bloomquist.)

Preschoolers are able to relate to older children in the family on a more equal basis. They still do not have the cognitive, motor, or language skills to keep up with these older siblings and their peers but are able to participate in some of their activities. One may admire an older sibling to the point of wanting to do everything exactly as the sibling does them. This may be flattering to the older child for a brief period but generally becomes frustrating if it persists.

The goal of social interaction during this period is school readiness. Through experience within the family and with peers and other adults the preschooler needs to attain readiness to interact in a group situation, follow directions, take turns, recognize others' rights, channel thoughts and actions to an assigned activity, and demonstrate increasing independence. School readiness assessment using a specific tool is discussed earlier in this chapter. The nurse who sees a preschooler over time, either in an office or clinic or at a group care or preschool setting, can assess the child's progress in development of social competencies. Comparison with the child's previous behavior is significant, and in most cases this outweighs comparison with other children of the same age, since the wide variations that normally occur among children tend to lead to undue concern for extreme behaviors that may be within normal limits. For example, a child who is temperamentally quiet, introverted, and subdued may appear more attached to his mother as school approaches in comparison to other children the same age. However, when comparing the child's social behavior with that of earlier years, the nurse may note progress toward independence. When mother is not available, the child makes sufficient adaptations to remain comfortable and secure.

Evidence of the preschool child's social competency can be obtained by discussion and evaluation of the child's drawing of her family. The nurse observes the drawing and responds to any comments or questions volunteered by the child. If the child asks for advice or assistance, the nurse encourages the child to proceed with the drawing just as he or she would like to do it. Positive encouragement and praise for the child's efforts may be made, particularly if the child becomes disinterested or is reluctant. After the drawing is completed, the nurse asks the child to identify the persons drawn and to describe individual characteristics. The names of each family member are written on the drawing, as well as any specific perceptions of the person that the child relates. Other questions such as, "What do you like best about your brother?" or "When do you get angry with your sister?" may be posed to encourage the child to describe the nature of family interactions. If an adult family member is present, the nurse explains the purposes of the drawing and interview and requests that the adult not participate until afterwards. Any areas of concern or questions need to be discussed, and the parent should be reassured of confidentiality. The child's perceptions may be verified with the adult at the conclusion of the interview, or further information can be sought to clarify them.

The *Vineland Social Maturity Scale* provides an objective, standardized estimate of social maturity. The tool provides a profile of the child's self-help skills, self-direction, locomotion, communication, and social relations. It is designed to measure the child's progression toward independence. Data are obtained by observing the child's behavior and interviewing the mother or primary caregiver. The tool may employ interview data alone if needed, but direct observation of the child's behavior is preferred.[4]

Divorce is a disruption in family relationships that may confront the preschooler. The child's response to this change in family circumstances primarily depends on his or her developmental stage and on the type of relationship he or she had with each family member before the divorce. The nurse must realize that a divorce is not an isolated incident but usually comes after a period of conflict, stress, changing relationships, and "hiding the problem from the kids." The preschooler definitely is aware of the stress in the home, although he or she cannot name this feeling or find its origin. The child may react to the changes in his or her parents in various ways, including regression, confusion, or irritability. He or she may express difficulty in comprehending what is happening by asking the same questions repeatedly, such as, "Is Daddy coming home for supper tonight?" or "Why doesn't Daddy stay here anymore?"

Parents in the midst of marital problems or divorce often do not have the psychologic energy or patience to deal with the preschooler's questions and altered behavior. Yet the child desperately needs closeness, patience, and consistent responses from his or her parents.

The nurse can serve as an advocate for the child by helping the parent (1) explore ways to deal with the child's regression and irritability, (2) develop skills in explaining the situation to the child, and (3) realize that the child, even if he of she is not currently manifesting problems in dealing with the family disruption, is deeply affected by it.[10]

COMMUNITY

Some preschoolers have had a variety of experiences outside of their family by age 3. This experience may be in group day-care settings, in church play groups, or through family involvement in other activities. Some 3- and 4-year-olds have had very limited experience outside the family, and a preschool setting is their introduction to a wider social arena. This is a time for parents to learn to "let go" in the sense of encouraging more independent activity in a safe, supervised setting. Preschoolers must test out their independence, interactive skills, and self-discipline as they learn to function in a group. Preschool provides a transition into kindergarten and first grade, where more group interaction skills are expected.

Selection of a preschool often is based on geographic closeness to the home or a friend's recommendation. This approach is practical and appropriate for many children.

CULTURE AND ETHNICITY

Preschoolers continue to be shaped by the cultural heritage of the family. Unlike the toddler, preschoolers may ask why certain practices are followed by the family; they also are likely to notice that not all people have the same practices. Their playmates may not celebrate the same holidays or have the same family rituals as their own family. As preschoolers have more experiences outside their own family, these differences become more obvious.

Preschoolers also are likely to notice ethnic differences in appearance and to decide that certain skin colors, eyes, and hairstyles, are "pretty" or "ugly." They are very likely to develop the same prejudices as their family or playmates.

Certain cultures put more pressure on the child to develop prosocial behaviors or take on more responsibility for younger siblings or household tasks as the school years approach. The preschooler may feel confused if the family's culture is different from that of most playmates. Confusion also can result when the child's parents have integrated their cultural background into the community standards, but the grandparents have maintained strict adherence to cultural practices, rituals, and perhaps childrearing ideas.

LEGISLATION

The preschooler is affected by the safety-focused legislation discussed in Chapter 18. The child also is beginning to be influenced by the school-focused issues discussed in Chapter 20.

ECONOMIC FACTORS

Poverty influences the preschooler as it does any child. Unlike the toddler, the preschooler may be more aware of the family's economic status. This is on the level of the family not having enough money to buy some toy rather than on a more comprehensive level of how limited economic resources influence the family's basic lifestyle.

Preschoolers realize that money or the special plastic

card the parent carries is necessary to get food, toys, and clothes, but they do not yet have a concept of economic values. The preschooler might trade an expensive item for a trinket that happens to look more interesting at the time. Preschoolers can be introduced to the concepts of earning money by completing chores around the house and of spending money by using their earnings to buy a treat for themselves.

HEALTH CARE DELIVERY SYSTEM

The preschooler has basically the same resources for health care as the toddler. As preschoolers enter a school setting, they are likely to be seen in a health care setting for physical and developmental screening as a requirement for admission to the school. For the child from a low-income family, this visit may come under the auspices of *Early and Periodic Screening, Diagnosis and Treatment (EPSDT)*, a Medicaid program. This screening is available to any child under age 21 who meets the economic criteria for Medicaid. Private offices, local health departments, and community clinics can provide an EPSDT examination. A preschool child can have one screening per year, which includes

1. Medical history
2. Assessment of physical growth, nutritional status, and mental development
3. Inspection of ears, nose, mouth, teeth, and throat
4. Vision screening
5. Auditory screening
6. Screening for cardiac abnormalities
7. Checking for anemia
8. Screening for sickle-cell trait
9. Urine sampling
10. Blood pressure reading
11. Assessment and updating of immunizations
12. Tuberculosis screening, if indicated
13. Referral to a dentist for diagnosis and treatment for children 3 years of age and older

Any health or developmental concerns identified at this screening are followed up by a participating physical. EPSDT is a comprehensive service that should be presented as a resource for eligible children. (See box on p. 476.)

RESEARCH REVIEW PRESCHOOL

HEALTH BEHAVIORS

Logsdon DA: Conceptions of health and health behaviors of preschool children, *J Pediatr Nurs* 6:396-406, 1992.

Purpose The purpose of this study was to examine preschool children's conceptions about health and their understanding of behaviors which are helpful and harmful to health.

Review Thirty preschool children were interviewed with data obtained through the use of a modified Preschool Health Picture Interview. It was a semistructured interview guide used in conjunction with a series of black-and-white photographs. Health conceptualized as a positive feeling state and the ability to participate in desired activities. Brushing teeth and eating were the highest ranked health promotion behaviors. Behaviors harmful to health were predominantly behavioral (e.g., standing on a chair reaching toward a kitchen cupboard; riding a bike on the street with a car directly in back of you). A t-test indicated the mean number of moral responses given by boys were significantly greater than the mean number given by girls.

PHYSICAL ACTIVITY AND HEALTHY DIET

Simons-Morton BG, et al: Promoting physical activity and a healthful diet among children: results of a school-based intervention study, *Am J Public Health* 81:986-991, 1991.

Purpose The purpose of this study was to influence the school environment in terms of effect on student diet and physical activity.

Review Two of the four elementary schools in one Texas school district were assigned an intervention and two to control conditions. Classroom interventions included health education, vigorous physical education, and lower fat and sodium school lunches. Nutrients and physical activity obtained during physical education were assessed as outcomes. Results indicated that students' posttest values were lower in the intervention schools (e.g., total fat, 15.5% to 10.4%; saturated fat, 31.7% to 18.8%). Physical activity increased in intervention schools. Efficacy of study demonstrates feasibility of modifying school lunches and activity to improve children's diet and physical activity.

NURSING INTERVENTIONS FOR HEALTH PROMOTION

Preschoolers are often very interested in the tools and procedures of a health screening examination. They may ask to see and try out the stethoscope, otoscope, and other diagnostic instruments. The nurse can explain the tests in age-appropriate terminology and expect the child to be cooperative for most of the visit. The preschooler may even show good self-control during injections but definitely needs a parent close by to offer support and encouragement. The nurse should include the preschooler in the history by directing questions to him or her about dietary intake and health practices, such as tooth brushing, favorite activities, friends, and so on. This is an optimum age for the child to begin to take some interest in health. (See box on p. 497 for research review of this age.)

The American Academy of Pediatrics' suggested schedule for preventive health care during the preschool years includes visits at 4 years and 5 years.[3] Each visit includes an ongoing history; growth, physical, and developmental assessment; and discussion of age-appropriate developmental concerns.

In addition to contact with preschoolers in an office or clinic, the nurse may be a consultant to a preschool or a nurse for a primary school and preschool. The school nurse's role in health promotion and prevention of illness is discussed in Chapter 20.

References

1. Berger KS: *The developing person through childhood and adolescence,* ed 3, New York, 1991, Worth Publishing.
2. Castoria H, Harris M: *Childhood leukemias.* In Hockenbery M, Coody D, editors: *Pediatric oncology and hematology,* St Louis, 1986, Mosby.
3. Committee on practice and ambulatory medicine, American Academy of Pediatrics: Recommendations for preventive pediatric health care, *Pediatrics* 81(3):466, 1988.
4. Doll LA: *Vineland social maturity scales,* Circle Pines, Minn, 1965, American Guidance Service.
5. Falkner F, Tanner J: *Human growth,* ed 2, New York, 1986, Plenum Press.
6. Fraiberg S: *The magic years,* New York, 1959, Charles Scribner's Sons.
7. Frankenburg W, et al: *Denver II screening,* Denver, 1990, Denver Materials.
8. Garber RM, Mortimer EA: Immunizations: beyond the basics, *Pediatr Rev* 13(3):98-106, 1992.
9. Guitar B: Stuttering and stammering, *Pediatr Rev* 7(6):163, 1985.
10. Hetherington EM, Arastik JD, editors: Impact of divorce, single parenting and step-parenting on children, Hillsdale, NJ, 1988, Laurence Erlbaum Associates.
11. Hockelman R, et al: *Primary pediatric care,* ed 2, St Louis, 1992, Mosby.
12. Koppitz EM: *The Bender Gestalt test for young children,* New York, 1971, Grune & Stratton.
13. Maul-Mellott S, Adams J: *Childhood cancer: a nursing overview,* Boston, 1987, Jones & Bartlett.
14. Palfrey J, Rappaport L: School placement, *Pediatr Rev* 8(9):261, 1987.
15. Phillips JL Jr: *The origins of intellect, Piaget's theory,* San Francisco, 1969, WH Freeman.
16. Pipes PL: *Nutrition in infancy and childhood,* ed 4, St Louis, 1989, Mosby.
17. Seidel H, et al: *Mosby's guide to physical examination,* ed 2, St Louis, 1991, Mosby.
18. Sinclair D: *Human growth after birth,* New York, 1985, Oxford University Press.
19. Stanfill P, Hayes F: *Neuroblastoma and related tumors.* In Hockenbery M, Coody D, editors: *Pediatric oncology and hematology,* St Louis, 1986, Mosby.
20. Stanfill P, Pratt C: *Retinoblastoma.* In Hockenbery M, Coody D: *Pediatric oncology and hematology,* St Louis, 1986, Mosby.
21. Task Force on Pediatric AIDS: Guidelines for human immunodeficiency virus (HIV)-inflicted children and their foster families, *Pediatrics* 89(4):681-683, 1992.
22. Vaughn VC: Assessment of growth and development during infancy and early childhood, *Pediatr Rev* 13(3):88-96, 1992.
23. Vietti TJ, et al: Progress against childhood cancer: the pediatric oncology group experience, *Pediatrics* 89(4):597-600, 1992.
24. Webster-Stratton C: *The incredible years: a trouble-shooting guide for parents of children aged 3-8,* Toronto, 1992, Umbrella Press.

CHAPTER

20

School-Age Child

Ann Marie McCarthy

Lois A. Hancock

Objectives

After completing this chapter, the nurse will be able to

- *Discuss the physical changes that occur in the child during the school years, including the wide range of normal values.*
- *Screen the school-age child for possible hypertension.*
- *Discuss with families some of the common sleep-related problems that occur in school-age children, specifically enuresis, sleepwalking, and sleeptalking.*
- *Describe the school-age child's cognitive stage of development and relate this to academic skills learned in school, such as mathematics and telling time.*
- *Discuss with parents ways they can enhance their child's self-concept.*
- *Discuss some possible coping behaviors for a school-age child undergoing stress.*
- *List the physical agents responsible for the most common accidents during the school years.*
- *Discuss the influence of peers on the school-age child.*
- *Explain to parents the school-age child's needs for social relationships, and relate this to the family's discipline practices.*
- *Discuss the possible influence poverty or affluence may have on a school-age child.*

The school-age years often are called the period of calm before the storm of adolescence. Changes do occur in this period, however, many of which are impressive when we compare the size and skills of a 6-year-old with those of a 12-year-old. Growth in height and weight is slower than it was in infancy and slower than it will be in adolescence but continues at a steady pace. The child develops new motor skills and perfects them through repeated practice. Mental abilities grow remarkably, with the child able to learn reading, writing, mathematics, and a variety of other subjects. As the child's motor and mental abilities expand, a sense of competence develops; this is influenced by the child's family, but now the influences of peers and others outside the family are becoming stronger.

For most persons the school-age years are the healthiest time of their lives. Their capacity to recover from injury or infection is rapid and relatively complete. Their energy level is high and may seem endless. (See box on pp. 500-501.)

HEALTHY PEOPLE 2000

SELECTED NATIONAL HEALTH PROMOTION AND DISEASE PREVENTION OBJECTIVES

SCHOOL AGE

- Reduce dental caries (cavities) so that the proportion of children with one or more caries (in permanent or primary teeth) is no more than 35% among children aged 6 through 8 and no more than 60% among adolescents aged 15. (Baseline: 53% of children aged 6 through 8 in 1986-1987; 78% of adolescents aged 15 in 1986-1987.)

Special population targets

Dental caries prevalance	1986-87 baseline	2000 target
Children aged 6-8 whose parents have less than high school education	70%	45%
American Indian or Alaska native children aged 6-8	92%*	45%
	52%†	
Black children aged 6-8	61%	40%
American Indian or Alaska native adolescents aged 15	93%†	70%

*In primary teeth in 1983-1984
†In permanent teeth in 1983-1984

- Reduce untreated dental caries so that the proportion of children with untreated caries (in permanent or primary teeth) is no more than 20% among children aged 6 through 8 and no more than 15% among adolescents aged 15. (Baseline: 27% of children aged 6-8 in 1986: 23% of adolescents aged 15 in 1986-1987.)

Special population targets

Untreated dental caries among children	1986-87 baseline	2000 target
Children aged 6-8 whose parents have less than high school education	43%	30%
American Indian or Alaska native children aged 6-8	64%*	35%
Black children aged 6-8	38%	25%
Hispanic children aged 6-8	36%†	25%

*1983-1984 baseline
†1982-1984 baseline

- Increase to at least 50% the proportion of children who have received protective sealants on the occlusal (chewing) surfaces of permanent molar teeth. (Baseline: 11% of children aged 8 and 8% of adolescents aged 14 in 1986-1987.)
- Increase to at least 50% the proportion of children and adolescents in 1st through 12th grade who participate in daily school physical education. (Baseline: 36% in 1984-1986.)
- Increase to at least 50% the proportion of school physical education class time that students spend being physically active, preferably engaged in lifetime physical activities. (Baseline: students spent an estimated 27% of class time being physically active in 1983.)

Continued.

HEALTHY PEOPLE 2000

- Reduce to no more than 15% the proportion of people aged 6 and older who engage in no leisure-time physical activity. (Baseline: 24% for people aged 18 and older in 1985.)
- Increase to at least 40% the proportion of people aged 6 and older who regularly perform physical activities that enhance and maintain muscular strength, muscular endurance, and flexibility.
- Increase to at least 75% the proportion of the nation's elementary and secondary schools that provide planned and sequential kindergarten through 12th-grade quality school health education.
- Reduce deaths caused by motor vehicle crashes to no more than 1.9 per 100 million vehicle miles traveled and 16.8 per 100,000 people. (Baseline: 2.4 per 100 million vehicle miles traveled (VMT) and 18.8 per 100,000 people [age adjusted] in 1987.)

Special population targets

Deaths caused by motor vehicle crashes (per 100,000)	**1987 baseline**	**2000 target**
Children aged 14 and younger	6.2	5.5

PROCESSES OF THE PERSON

Age and Physical Changes

Compared to the preschool child's body proportions, the school-age child has an overall slimmer shape, a result of changes in the amount and distribution of fat on the child's body and the longer legs relative to the rest of the body. The gradual decrease in fat stored from ages 1 to 6 years is followed by a reaccumulation and redistribution of fat from age 7 to puberty.[2]

During the school years growth is relatively steady, with the average gain of body weight about 3 kg (6½ pounds) per year and that of stature abut 6 cm (2¼ inches) per year. However, many children do have "spurts" of growth alternating with periods of minimum growth. During these years girls and boys are similar in size until puberty. At that time a preadolescent increase in growth tends to occur, in girls around age 10 and in boys around age 12.[10,28] This is the time when many girls tower over their male classmates. However, many variations still occur, with some late-maturing girls not beginning this growth spurt until ages 12 to 14, whereas early maturing boys may enter it at age 10. We can see why a classroom of 10- to 12-year-old children has a wide range of sizes for both sexes.[11]

The child's head continues to grow, but again at a much slower rate. After 5 years of age the head circumference grows only 1.27 cm (½ inch) per 5 years until full adult size at puberty. This is usually a change of measurement from about 51 cm (20 inches) to 53 or 54 cm (21 inches) and reflects the brain having now reached its adult size. The child's hair often darkens in color. Skin continues to mature and become less sensitive, approaching adult appearance and texture. Sebum and eccrine sweat production is minimal throughout childhood.

Most body systems reach an adult level of functioning during this age, if they have not already done so. The gastrointestinal system's maturity is seen in the child's ability to eat adult foods on a schedule close to an adult's, with fewer needs for the frequent snacks of the preschooler. By puberty all endocrine functions except those regulating reproduction approach adult capacity.

Differences in lung capacity occur during this period because of differences in size, but this variation is negligible. Respirations become slower, deeper, and more regular, changing from the 20 to 30 per minute of the preschool child to 17 to 25 per minute for the school-age child. The heart increases in size, whereas the heart rate slows down to the average adult heart rate of 70 to 100 beats per minute. Mean blood pressure is not as high in this age group as in adults.[12]

The long-term effects of *hypertension* in adults are well known. The realization that hypertension in adults may begin in childhood combined with elevated blood pressures in children possibly indicating other diseases have encouraged efforts to screen for elevated blood pressure in children. The Report of the Second Task Force on Blood Pressure Control in Children from the National Heart, Lung and Blood Institute presents percentile charts to use in defining normal ranges for children and in plotting children's blood pressures (Fig. 20-1). The report notes that children should have their blood pressure measured and plotted yearly, beginning at 3 years of age, and cautions that blood pressures can vary greatly. If an elevated blood pressure, defined as greater than the 95th percentile, is obtained in an otherwise normal child, the blood pressure should be repeated (usually twice) over time to try to see a pattern. Also, the child's height and weight should be noted. If a child is tall and lean or proportional for height, this BP reading may be normal.[31] Fig. 20-2 illustrates a rational sequence for evaluating the child with an elevated BP reading. Table 20-1 indicates the actual levels of significant and severe hypertension for children at various ages.[31]

Physical changes in this age group are notable in three areas: lymphoid tissues, teeth, and motor skills.

Throughout childhood the lymph tissue grows rapidly, reaching its maximum size before puberty, after which it begins to decrease in size, probably because of sex hormones. The lymphoid tissues of a 12-year-old are almost twice the size of an adult's. The larger lymphoid tissue in this age group can be seen in the size of many children's tonsils. What appears pathologically enlarged to a parent may be normal for that age.

The school child seems to be constantly losing or gaining a tooth. The first permanent teeth to appear are the 6-year molars, followed by the loss of the deciduous (baby) teeth, usually in the same order they erupted, and the appearance of the permanent teeth. Fig. 20-3 shows the 32 adult teeth and their average time of appearance. The child between ages 6 and 13 loses and gains about 4 teeth per year. A 13-year-old should have 28 teeth to replace the 20 deciduous teeth lost. When deciduous teeth come out, only the crown is lost; the root has been reabsorbed in the developing permanent tooth. As the child's mouth becomes filled with the larger, permanent teeth, the shape of the jaw and the child's facial appearance can change.

Dental problems, primarily caries, periodontal disease, and malocclusion, are among the most common

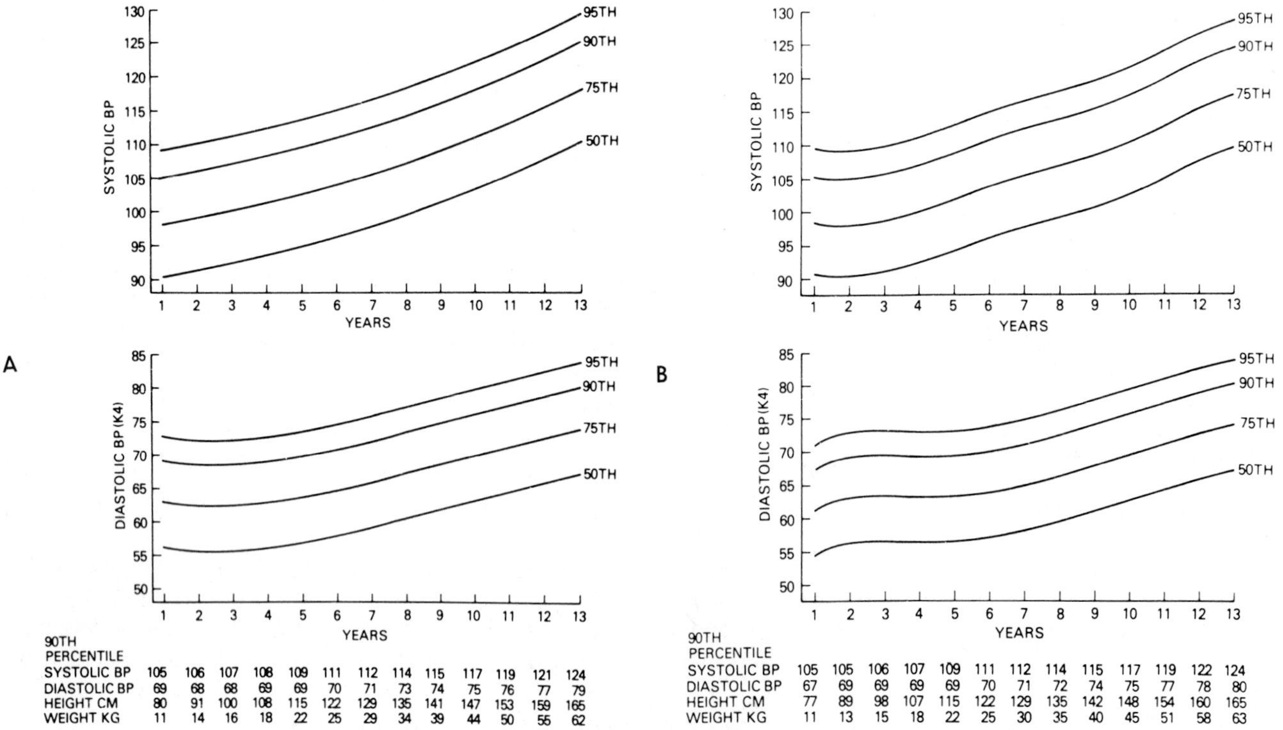

A — 90TH PERCENTILE

	1	2	3	4	5	6	7	8	9	10	11	12	13
SYSTOLIC BP	105	106	107	108	109	111	112	114	115	117	119	121	124
DIASTOLIC BP	69	68	68	69	69	70	71	73	74	75	76	77	79
HEIGHT CM	80	91	100	108	115	122	129	135	141	147	153	159	165
WEIGHT KG	11	14	16	18	22	25	29	34	39	44	50	55	62

B — 90TH PERCENTILE

	1	2	3	4	5	6	7	8	9	10	11	12	13
SYSTOLIC BP	105	105	106	107	109	111	112	114	115	117	119	122	124
DIASTOLIC BP	67	69	69	69	69	70	71	72	74	75	77	78	80
HEIGHT CM	77	89	98	107	115	122	129	135	142	148	154	160	165
WEIGHT KG	11	13	15	18	22	25	30	35	40	45	51	58	63

Fig. 20-1. Age-specific percentiles of BP measurements in **A,** boys, and **B,** girls–1 to 13 years of age; Korotkoff phase IV (K4) used for diastolic BP. (Reprinted with permission from the Report of the Second Task Force on Blood Pressure Control in Children–1987, *Pediatrics* 79[1], 1-25, 1987.)

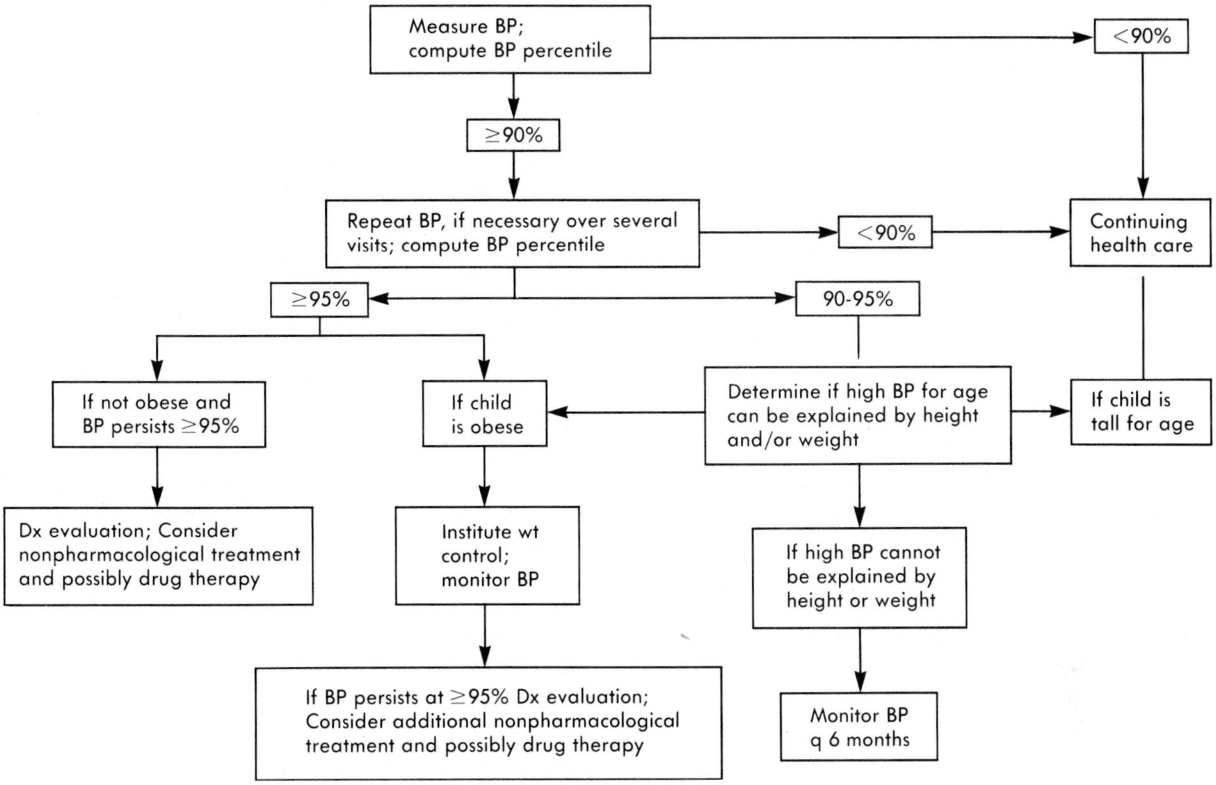

Fig. 20-2. Algorithm for identifying children with high BP. Note: Whenever BP measurement is stipulated, the average of at least two measurements should be used. (Reprinted with permission from the Report of the Second Task Force on Blood Pressure Control in Children–1987, *Pediatrics* 79[1], 1-25, 1987.)

Table 20-1. **Classification of hypertension by age group**

Age group	Significant hypertension (mm Hg)	Severe hypertension (mm Hg)
Newborn	Systolic BP ≥ 96	Systolic BP ≥ 106
7 days	Systolic BP ≥ 104	Systolic BP ≥ 110
8-30 days		
Infant (< 2 yr)	Systolic BP ≥ 112 Diastolic BP ≥ 74	Systolic BP ≥ 118 Diastolic BP ≥ 82
Children (3-5 yr)	Systolic BP ≥ 116 Diastolic BP ≥ 76	Systolic BP ≥ 124 Diastolic BP ≥ 84
Children (6-9 yr)	Systolic BP ≥ 122 Diastolic BP ≥ 78	Systolic BP ≥ 130 Diastolic BP ≥ 86
Children (10-12 yr)	Systolic BP ≥ 126 Diastolic BP ≥ 82	Systolic BP ≥ 134 Diastolic BP ≥ 90
Adolescents (13-15 yr)	Systolic BP ≥ 136 Diastolic BP ≥ 86	Systolic BP ≥ 144 Diastolic BP ≥ 92
Adolsecents (16-18 yr)	Systolic BP ≥ 142 Diastolic BP ≥ 92	Systolic BP ≥ 150 Diastolic BP ≥ 98

Reprinted with permission from the Report of the Second Task Force on Blood Pressure Control in Children–1987, *Pediatrics* 79(1):1-25, 1987.

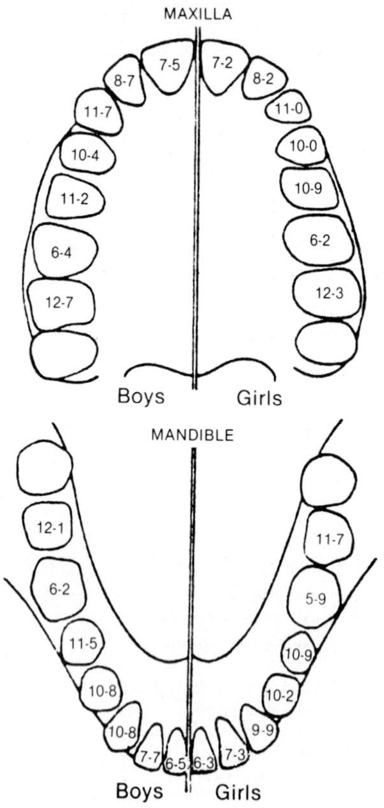

Fig. 20-3. Mean age in year and month (yr-mo) of emergence of permanent teeth for boys and girls. (From Sinclair D: *Human growth after birth,* London, 1978, Oxford University Press.)

health problems in school-age children today. The nurse can recommend the following measures to help the child and the family prevent some of these problems:[20]

1. Encourage children in this age group to be responsible for brushing and flossing their own teeth. Although thorough plaque removal once a day is usually sufficient, brushing more often may increase the probability of cleaning all tooth surfaces effectively. The American Dental Association (ADA) has several excellent pamphlets on appropriate brushing and flossing of teeth. These can be obtained from a local dentist or from a state dental association.
2. Continue to use fluoride; its role in preventing cavities and the various ways it can be administered are discussed in Chapter 17.
3. Change toothbrushes every 3 months.
4. Use a toothbrush with a straight handle, flat brushing surface, and soft, rounded bristles.
5. Purchase an electric toothbrush, if possible, since this may make brushing more fun and the child more willing.
6. Apply fluoridated toothpaste or rinses to the teeth daily.
7. Inspect the teeth frequently; children up to age 9 or 10 need parental supervision.
8. Use disclosing tablets occasionally to help assess adequacy of dental care.
9. Maintain an appropriate diet that is low in high-sugar food and frequent snacks.

With the rapid change in the number and type of teeth and the uneven growth in the child's jaw, this is the age when *malocclusion,* an unacceptable relationship of the teeth in one jaw to those in the other, first may be noted. A dentist should evaluate children with overbites, gaps in teeth, and other alignment problems. Some will grow out of their problems, but others may need orthodontic care to correct developing problems, to prevent potential problems, or to improve appearance.[20]

Neurologic, skeletal, and muscular changes combine to increase the child's overall *motor abilities.* In the nervous system myelinization becomes complete between 8 and 10 years of age, allowing the child more control over and more coordination with motor tasks.[2] The connection between the brain's two hemispheres, the corpus callosum, matures in both structure and function around 7 to 8 years, increasing brain function and integration. The child grows in height because of increases in the long bones; this growth continues into adolescence. Ossification, replacement of cartilage with bone, occurs throughout childhood.[29] The child's constant building of new bony tissue during the entire period of childhood accounts for the rapid repair of any fractures.

Muscle mass increases along with muscle strength. During the school-age years boys are slightly stronger than girls, but this difference is not really significant until adolescence.[29] With these changes the child now has the potential to perform more complex motor functions but must practice to perfect these skills. Children willingly carry out their newfound skills repeatedly and are rewarded when they see improvement in their skill level. They ride their bicycles, tie their shoes, throw the ball with their friends, and participate in a number of other activities requiring greater motor skills (Fig. 20-4). Table 20-2 shows a list of motor skills and when they tend to develop in school-age children.

Sex Differences

Girls tend to mature, enter puberty, and cease to grow earlier than boys. In general girls' physical growth is more regular, with fewer spurts and plateaus. Girls' teeth erupt sooner, and their bones ossify sooner. From birth girls have more fat, and after puberty they have a great percentage of body weight devoted to fat. Most physical differences between males and females become more pronounced after puberty. The earlier maturing process

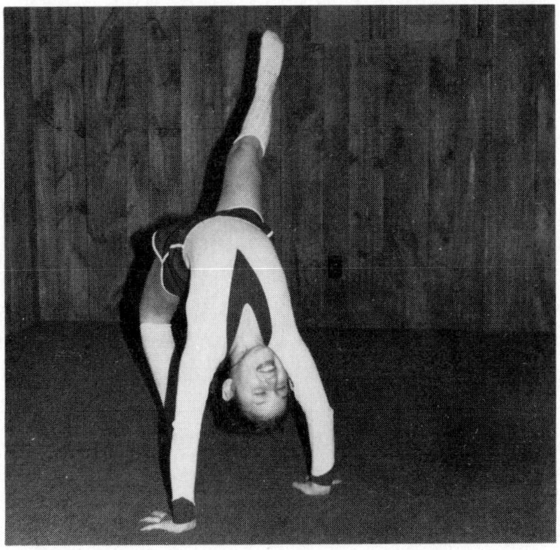

Fig. 20-4. Motor activities, such as gymnastics, become a challenge for children to master. (Photograph by Douglas Bloomquist.)

Table 20-2. **Motor development of the school-age child**

Age (years)	Gross motor	Fine motor
6-7	Balances on one foot for 10 seconds Can perform tandem gait Hops 25 times on one foot, 12 times on the other Pedals a bicycle	Spreads with a knife Holds pencil with fingertips Draws a person with three to six parts Cuts with a knife Aligns letters horizontally Ties a bow Draws a triangle Knows right from left
8-9	Has good body balance Enjoys vigorous activities Throws objects farther	When writing, spaces words and slants letters Draws a diamond Draws a three-dimensional geometric figure Good eye-hand coordination Bathes self Sews and builds models
10-12	Balances on one foot for 15 seconds Catches a fly ball Some awkwardness because of prepubertal growth spurt Possesses all basic motor skills	Similar to adult skills

of females occurs in many mammals and almost all primates.[3,29]

Two other areas of differences in the sexes are discussed in detail later in this chapter. First, girls tend to mature faster than boys in many psychologic and physical processes. This is understandable when one realizes that many psychologic processes, such as cognitive abilities and language skills, primarily depend on physical maturation of the nervous system. Second, boys tend to have some problems more frequently than girls, such as enuresis, encopresis, learning disabilities, and attentional deficit disorder.

Race

Black and Asian children mature at a faster rate than white children, including earlier dental development and menarche. Body proportions vary, especially sitting height compared to leg lengths. Blacks have the longest legs compared to sitting height, and Asians the shortest, which translates into blacks eventually being the tallest and Asians the shortest of the three racial groups. Blacks tend to have slimmer hips and more muscle and less fat in the limbs compared to fat in the trunk.[2,10]

As noted in previous chapters, in our society it is often difficult to separate race from socioeconomic conditions. Although statistics are based on differences in race, the major issue is one of *poverty*. Certainly not all black Americans are poor; but the number of poor blacks in proportion to the overall number of blacks is greater than the same ratio in whites.

Similar data are not as well documented for Asian children. However, we can surmise that, although many Asian Americans are economically not at poverty level, a number of new Asian refugee groups in the United States are poor and therefore may be exposed to accompanying malnutrition, overcrowded housing, school deficits, and health problems.

In looking at these differences, we see that it is not race, but poverty and the results of poverty that are the threats to the child's health.

Genetics

School-age children often are concerned about their rate of growth, time of menarche, and final height. The nurse cannot give exact answers to these questions, but knowledge of genetic influences helps in responding. Both parents contribute an equal amount to the end height of their children, but genes for being tall dominate over genes for being short. When assessing a child's height, even before looking at standardized growth charts, the nurse should look at the child's family. The child who plots on the third percentile for height compared to all the other children may have parents who are shorter than average, and therefore the child's shorter height may be expected.

Rate of growth also appears to be genetically influenced; the best example of this is *menarche.* An average difference of 2.8 months in the age menarche occurs in identical twins, 12.9 months for sisters, and 18.6 months for unrelated women.[2]

In general, most acute, life-threatening hereditary diseases have presented themselves before the school years. Some health problems that occur in the school years appear more frequently in certain families. These include obesity, learning problems, and enuresis. Each of these is discussed later in the chapter. (See the box below.)

Nutritional and Metabolic Pattern

School-age children, like all children, need a well-balanced diet. The average of 2400 calories per day required to meet growth needs is usually spread over three meals, and one to two snacks. As the child's size increases, the amount of food needed and eaten also increases.

Although some children in this age-group are willing to try new foods, many continue to dislike foods such as vegetables, casseroles, spicy foods, and liver and to like a small repertoire of foods. Some children who will not eat cooked fruits or vegetables will eat them raw. They may go through a period of wanting to eat just one food, such as peanut butter sandwiches, every day at lunch. This seldom hurts the child nutritionally and usually does not last long. Children frequently make their own after-school snacks and need supervision regarding the type.[26]

Families may eat only one meal a day together, most often dinner. This is an important social time for the family, and arguments about food should be discouraged. Parents and families play a role in shaping the child's food preferences and habits. A child's nutritional pattern usually reflects the parents' and family's patterns. Parents who skip breakfast may have trouble

RESEARCH REVIEW — SCHOOL AGE

HIGH BLOOD CHOLESTEROL

Davidson DM, et al: Family history fails to detect the majority of children with high capillary blood total cholesterol, *J Sch Health* 61:75-80, 1991.

Purpose The purpose of this study was to examine the predictive value of family history in detecting children with high blood cholesterol.

Review Finger-stick screening was done in 1118 children ages 9-10 whose parents provided parental and grandparental history of cardiovascular disease and risk factors. Mean blood cholesterol was 167.5 mg/dl with no significant sex or ethnic differences. Of 157 children with blood cholesterol over 200 mg/dl, 61 (39%) had a family history of myocardial infarction or hyperlipidemia; however, the prevalence of a positive family history varied from 2.8% in Vietnamese-Americans to 38.5% in Spanish students to 52.6% in all other children. Adherence to current policies recommending screening only children with a positive family history would result in failing to detect a majority of children from ethnic families.

CIGARETTE SMOKING

Flynn BS, et al: Prevention of cigarette smoking through mass intervention and school programs, *Am J Public Health* 82:827-834, 1992.

Purpose The purpose of this study was to test the ability of mass media interventions on cigarette smoking prevention programs.

Review A cohort of 5458 students received an educational intervention (via media) with specific objectives. Students were surveyed at baseline in grades 4, 5, and 6 with follow up annually for 4 years. Significant reductions were reported in smoking. For cigarettes per week, the reduction was 34%; and for smoking in the past week, the reduction was 35%. Results provide evidence that mass media interventions are effective in preventing cigarette smoking among high-risk youths.

convincing their children to eat breakfast. School children also are influenced by peers in their choice of food. The child whose friend is eating a candy bar usually prefers the same rather than an apple for a snack.[26]

School lunch programs exist in most school systems, ranging from those that receive federal support for milk only to programs in which children with financial need receive both breakfast and lunch. These meals must meet the guidelines established for a type A lunch under the National School Lunch Program, administered by the Department of Agriculture. The guidelines are based on the needs of a 10- to 12-year-old child and include the following requirements.[26]

1. Eight ounces of unflavored, fluid low-fat milk, skim milk, or buttermilk (Whole milk or flavored milk may be offered as a substitute, but a low-fat milk *must* be offered.)
2. Two ounces of protein-rich canned or cooked meat, fish or poultry, one egg, ½ cup cooked dry peas or beans, 4 tbsp peanut butter, or equivalent combinations of these foods
3. Two or more portions of vegetables and fruit to a total of ¾ cup
4. Bread or a bread substitute made with enriched flour

Television has a strong influence on children, and a large percentage of the advertisements during children's shows are devoted to sugary, nonnutritious junk food. Without parental guidance, school-aged children frequently make poor food choices. The nutrients that children tend to consume in quantities less than the recommended amounts are iron and vitamin C.[26] Although this age group is less and less willing to be guided by the parents, parents should discuss with their children what they want to eat, need to eat, and will eat.

OBESITY

The major nutrition problem in the United States is obesity.[15] There is some evidence that obesity in adulthood has its beginning in infancy or childhood.

Boys and girls with two slim parents tend to be slim, and boys and girls with two fat parents tend to be fat. This may be caused by a combination of genetic determinants and familial environmental patterns. For example, a child whose overweight parents constantly use food as a reward has a greater tendency to obesity than a child of thin parents who do not reward with food. More than 90% of obese children become fat because of excessive food intake. Obesity also tends to reinforce a pattern of decreased activity. The child who is obese is at greater risk for a number of physical problems, such as hypertension, carbohydrate intolerance, and coronary risk factors.[26]

The obese child is often ridiculed by peers in school and discriminated against by adults. This scapegoating, added to the child's frequently poor motor skills, reinforces an already low self-image. A cycle of isolation and poor performance may be set in motion.[26]

Helping the child who already is obese and has set lifestyle patterns requires intensive intervention. Treatment of obese children is often discouraging, with significant weight loss, especially maintained weight loss, a rare occurrence.[26] Programs of treatment have included caloric restriction, anorectic drugs, physical exercise, bypass surgery, and habit pattern changes, with varying degrees of success or failure. School-age children are a difficult group to work with because they are often not ready to admit their concerns about being overweight.

No matter how old the child is, any program instituted must involve the entire family. Family eating patterns or styles often need to be adjusted, and other family members must be willing to eat many of the same foods as the child. Unfortunately, even the best weight-reduction programs for children have poor long-term success. Prevention of obesity is much more desirable.[26] Some suggestions the nurse may give to parents interested in preventing obesity in their school-age children are listed in the box above.

❑ ❑ NURSING INTERVENTIONS TO PREVENT OBESITY DURING THE SCHOOL-AGE PERIOD

Parents need to evaluate their own nutritional values and patterns. Some use food as a reward or as an expression of caring and need help finding more appropriate behaviors.

Meal patterns may need to be assessed and altered. One family may eat only in front of the television, whereas another family may set up mealtime as a period of confrontation.

Family snacking habits can lead to poor snacking habits for the child, so the type of food available for snacking may need to be altered.

The child's snacking habits should be reviewed and changes made as needed.

Regular exercise is important to everyone and should be encouraged to the child.

Elimination Pattern

About 85% of children have full bowel and bladder control by 6 years of age. This includes undressing and dressing, wiping, flushing, and cleaning their hands. The child's elimination patterns are similar to the adult's, with urinating occurring 6 to 8 times a day and bowel movements averaging 1 or 2 times a day. For some school-age children, however, elimination continues to be a problem.

ENURESIS

The involuntary passing of urine at an age when control should be present is called enuresis. Primary enuretic children have never achieved bladder control, and secondary enuretic children have periods of dryness, usually for several months, and then display enuresis again. Enuresis should not be considered a disease but rather a variation of normal development.

Urinating at night, or bedwetting, is called nocturnal enuresis, and wetting during the day is called diurnal enuresis. Bedwetting occurs in 15% of 6-year-olds, 3% of 12-year-olds, and 1% of 18-year-olds and is more common in boys.

Nocturnal enuresis is involuntary wetting during sleep at least once a month. An organic cause is found in only 1% to 2% of such children, the most common being urinary tract infection. For the remainder, the etiology is probably a combination of factors including genetic predisposition; neurologic developmental delay, which includes both inhibition of the bladder contraction reflex and the child's slow waking response to a full bladder; reduced bladder capacity; and environmental factors, including family stress.

The school-age child with nocturnal enuresis faces a variety of problems. The child often is teased by classmates and siblings. A night away from home seems impossible because of fear of wetting. Parents may be angry at the constant bed changes and washes and try punishments, thinking the child should be able to control the problem. With all this stress it is not surprising that these children often have low self-esteem and poor self-confidence.[17]

Frustrated families frequently seek help with this problem. Once a physiologic problem, such as urinary tract infection, has been ruled out through a complete evaluation, treatment may be considered. The common treatments are wet alarm systems, drug therapy (Imiprimide), and hormonal therapy (desmopressin). Research has shown that the alarms are most effective.[17] Each method has advantages and disadvantages. Most take a commitment of consistency and time from the child and parents.

Because of the spontaneous cure rate with time, enuresis may be best treated by just explaining the problem to the family and waiting for time to cure it. No matter what treatment regimen or regimens are tried for a child, the nurse can include certain information when counseling the parents and child (see box on this page). The nurse can play a vital role in helping a family deal with nocturnal enuresis by providing information, support with treatment, and encouragement in dealing with feelings.

❑ ❑ NURSING COUNSELING FOR FAMILIES ABOUT NIGHTTIME ENURESIS

Enuresis is a common problem.

No serious physical problem is present, although the child may have a small or immature bladder.

It often is inherited; other family members may have had the same problem.

With time the child will be cured, usually by adolescence.

The child is not wetting the bed intentionally; it is not a conscious act.

The parents are not at fault.

If a treatment is tried, the child needs to be responsible for dealing with both the problem and the treatment.

Punishment when the child is wet should be replaced with praise when dry (positive reinforcement).

Some parents also wake the child to urinate before they go to bed.

A family plan for dealing with the wet bed and child can decrease family arguments. The plan may include who strips the bed, where sheets go, and so on. The child should play a major role in this process.

Diurnal enuresis is often called "daytime dribbling." This term accurately describes the pattern of urination for children who have it, most of whom are girls. They demonstrate "holding on" behaviors such as not voiding first thing in the morning, voiding only two to three times a day, and voiding exceptionally quickly. It is unclear why these children delay going to the bathroom and only partially empty their bladders, thus precipitating overflow incontinence. Evaluation of these children begins with a urine culture to rule out urinary tract infection. If symptoms persist after an infection is treated or if no infection is found, the "daytime dribbler" is treated by increasing fluids to prevent "holding" and establishment of a voiding routine. This routine includes voiding every 1½ hours and a conscious effort to empty the bladder completely. The nurse can be instrumental in helping the child and parents understand the problem and the treatment.[17]

ENCOPRESIS

Another elimination problem that can occur in children is encopresis. Encopresis may be defined as the persistent passing of stool into the child's underpants after age 4. A common time for this to occur is late afternoon. This incidence has been quoted at 1.5% in second-grade children. The vast majority of children with encopresis are boys of average or above average intelligence. These children retain stool at least part of the time. Many complain of recurrent abdominal pain, and a large percentage are also enuretic.

These children commonly have emotional difficulties, either before or resulting from the problem of encopresis. Nurses need to be aware of this childhood problem to identify the affected child, to refer the child for treatment, and to support the child and family during treatment. Treatment usually requires a specific bowel program coupled with counseling.[30]

Activity and Exercise Pattern

The school-age child usually is physically active. As discussed earlier, impressive changes in motor skills occur between ages 6 and 12. The child needs physical exercise or activities to enhance the development of strength, balance, and coordination. This occurs through group activities and organized sports such as Little League baseball; through activities of individual skill, such as gymnastics; and through unorganized play such as bike riding. (See box on pp. 500-501.)

The play and activities of this age-group incorporate other areas of the child's development, including social, personal, and cognitive aspects. The social aspects are of major importance. School-age children often prefer to interact with peers rather than family. This need is not completely satisfied in the school setting and carries over to their play and outside activities; many prefer to be with children of their own sex. Skill in motor tasks can both win the respect of other children and provide a feeling of self-accomplishment. Organized sports such as baseball teach team cooperation, competition, and other social skills. Organized activities, such as scouts and 4H clubs, teach children how to function in groups and what is involved in carrying out a task. This can prepare them for the discipline needed for a future job.

A child who performs well in these activities, especially when he receives prizes or trophies, feels good about himself, his competence, and his sense of industry. This feeling of self-accomplishment also is enhanced in the simple games played alone or with others, such as how far the child can hop or how many times she can jump rope.

New cognitive skills are incorporated into the child's activities. The abilities to count, sort, and group objects are seen in the pleasure children of this age receive from their collections of stamps, rocks, or other objects. Understanding the concepts of fair and consistent rules requires memory and logical reasoning. Many games, such as board games, integrate several intellectual skills. Reading can be used often in the child's daily life, reinforcing this new skill and bringing enjoyment to the child.

The nurse can help parents to promote healthy activities for children with some of the following suggestions:

1. Encourage reading. Parents can continue to read out loud with children, but now should include the child and possibly the whole family. Parents can also model reading as a routine leisure activity. Children can obtain library cards, providing both a variety of books and an added responsibility. Books in a series are particularly enjoyed by school-age children. Receiving their own magazines, such as *Electric Company* or *Highlights for Children* can be a special treat.
2. Monitor television use (discussed later in this chapter).
3. Support the child's outside interests. Some children prefer group, organized activities; others prefer individual pursuits.
4. Praise the child's success to encourage further development and a sense of self-worth.
5. Help children see both their strengths and weaknesses so they can learn to deal with both success and failure.
6. Encourage the child to participate in both group and individual activities to perfect a variety of skills.

Sleep and Rest Pattern

SLEEP PATTERNS

The majority of school-age children have no difficulties with sleep. Their sleep requirements and patterns are closer to the adult's than to the younger child's. Individual needs vary, but most children sleep between 8 and 12 hours a night without naps during the day. The difficulties often seen in earlier childhood with going to bed occur much less frequently. Most children and parents are able to agree on a bedtime, allow flexibility on nonschool nights, and keep to that agreement. If problems arise over the time set for going to bed, they may be a result of children testing parents who have not been clear and firm about their expectations or who have not been willing to discuss the arrangement with their children.

Children, like adults, experience rapid eye movement (REM) sleep alternating with non-REM sleep, with non-REM sleep consisting of four substages.

SLEEP DISTURBANCES

The most common sleep problems that occur in the preschool and school-age years are night terrors (see Chapter 19), sleepwalking, sleeptalking, and enuresis (discussed in the previous section). As a group, these have been called *disorders of arousal,* since they tend to occur between stages 3 and 4 of non-REM sleep, as the child is progressing toward waking up. They all have some similar characteristics: (1) they occur just before a switch to the REM state; (2) most occur 1 to 2 hours after going to sleep; (3) the same child may have more than one sleep problem; (4) a positive family history may accompany the problem; (5) boys have these more often than girls (4:1 ratio); and (6) the child does not recall the episodes. Stage 3 to 4 non-REM sleep may be affected by fatigue and stress, which are common in this age-group. Coupled with the normal CNS immaturity and the normal developmental changes in stage 3 to 4 non-REM organization, this may account for the increased occurrence of these sleep problems in children.

Approximately 15% of children between ages 5 and 12 have walked in their sleep at least once; only 1% to 6% have persistent sleepwalking. At times, it is associated with enuresis. Typically, 1 to 2 hours after going to sleep, the child sits up suddenly in bed and moves awkwardly. The type and amount of movement can vary from just sitting in bed to making repetitive finger and hand movements or to getting up and walking; usually the child stays in bed. If spoken to, the child may mumble. The episodes range from 15 seconds to 30 minutes. The child usually avoids hurting himself, although this is an area of concern and the child needs to be protected. Onset of the episodes is usually before age 10, and they stop by age 15. As with sleepwalking, sleeptalking is not purposeful. Usually the words are simple but difficult to understand, and the child quickly falls back to sleep. With CNS maturation both tend to be outgrown.[21]

Parents concerned about sleepwalking or sleeptalking can be reassured knowing that most children outgrow them. Parents need to watch the sleepwalking child and to protect him from hurting himself. Gates may be put at the top of stairs and sharp objects moved from the child's paths. Most parents find the easiest solution is directing the child back to the bed, where he will return to a normal sleep. Trying to wake the child is difficult and only seems to cause more confused behavior or loss of coordination in the child. If a child is having many episodes or if parents are particularly concerned, the child may need further evaluation and treatment.

Cognitive and Perceptual Pattern

The school-age child spends much time in settings that require mastering of new ideas and concepts–learning. Many elements make up the child's ability to learn; only a few are discussed here. The child needs to continue to develop cognitive skills; basic senses such as vision and hearing must be intact; language skills need to expand; and memory capabilities must increase. These elements, along with basic intelligence and the child's heredity and environment, encourage or discourage the child's learning. Unfortunately, many children in our society have difficulties in these and other areas that result in learning problems.

PIAGET'S THEORY

Piaget refers to the span from ages 7 to 11 years as the *period of concrete operations.* During this time the child is able to move from egocentric interactions to more cooperative interactions; to increase understanding of many concepts associated with objects, such as conservation; and to change reasoning from intuition to logic or rational operations, such as serial ordering, addition, subtraction, and other basic mathematic skills. The term *operation* refers to rule-governed actions carried out in the mind, such as ordering and relating. The operations of this period are termed *concrete* because the child's mental operations or actions still depend on the ability to perceive concretely what has happened. The ability to perform abstract thinking has not developed as yet. Children in this period are able to reverse these mental operations, which adds flexibility and control to their thinking (Fig. 20-5).

An interesting point to remember is that children are not deliberately taught the concepts and operations discussed here. They emerge; they are constructed by the environment and by experience, but they are not taught. This is a process; some aspects of the preoperational preschool child still occur in the school-age child. Younger school-age children still use magical thinking and are still egocentric.

The preschool child's egocentric thoughts, actions, and understandings in social and perceptual situations change in the school-age child, forming the groundwork

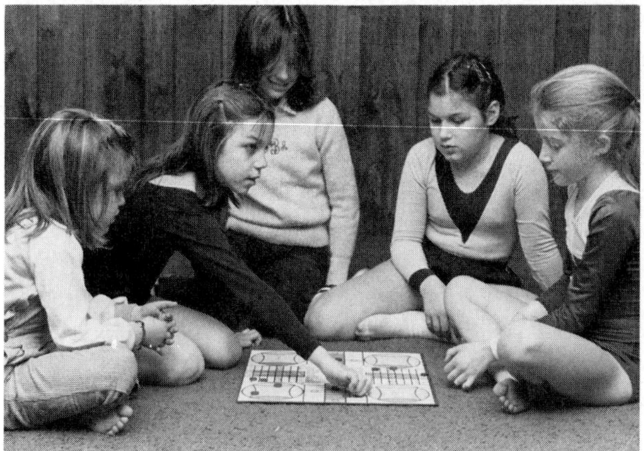

Fig. 20-5. The increasing cognitive skills of school-age children allow for cooperative interactions of progressive complexity, as this board game illustrates. (Photograph by Douglas Bloomquist.)

for the concepts and operations that develop. For example, the preschool or preoperational child, in talking with another child of similar age, engages in collective monologues. Each child pursues his or her private conversation regardless of what the other child says. During the concrete operations period, the child begins to be able to take into account the other child's point of view and to incorporate the partner's conversation into his or her own. Thus more meaningful intercommunication begins to emerge, and the children carry on a dialogue, each responding directly to what the other has just said. These traits do not emerge suddenly and completely; they tend to flow into one another, with the new skill being demonstrated in behavior only occasionally at first and then emerging with increasing frequency as the child's mental capacity and experience grow.[23,25,27]

The change away from egocentricity is seen in the child's perceptual abilities as well. An experiment in which the child is placed at a square table with three molded mountains of varying height on it illustrates this. Three empty chairs are placed at each side of the table. A doll is placed in each of the three chairs sequentially, and each time the child is asked what the doll sees when looking at the mountains from that side of the table. Before the concrete operations period the child cannot conceive of what the doll's view might be; the problem is often not sufficient to engage the child's interest. However, after about age 7 the child begins to show some interest in the problem and is able to represent erratically the doll's point of view. Toward the latter part of this period the child begins to accurately represent the doll's view from all sides of the table.[26]

The child in this period is able to understand a number of expanding concepts regarding objects. *Conservation* means that certain properties of an object remain the same in spite of changes in its other properties. A classic example is conservation of substance, mentioned in Chapter 19. Two identical glasses are filled with the same amount of liquid and shown to a child. Then the liquid from one of the glasses is poured into a third glass with a different shape. The child is asked if a difference exists in the amount of liquid in the two glasses. The preschool, preoperational child focuses on the different shapes and says yes. The concrete operational child realizes no change has occurred in substance despite the change in shape. Conservation of numbers, needed to understand basic mathematics, appears at about age 7, with some cultural variations. Conservations of quantity (substance, amount of space occupied by an object) also emerges at about age 7 or 8. Conservation of weight emerges at about age 9, whereas conservation of volume emerges close to the end of the concrete operational period.

The concept of *time* also develops during this period. Children begin to learn to tell time and to understand the passage of time during the early school years. By age 8 most children understand the difference between past and present; history becomes meaningful. The concept of human aging is more understandable, and the child can comprehend the difference between an 18-year-old and an 80-year-old person.[2]

Two major operations of the period are classifying and ordering. The child can now *classify* or group objects by their common element, understanding the relationship between groups or classes. For example, if given 12 wooden beads, some brown and some white, this child can understand that the beads can be grouped by their color and by their material. In contrast, the preschool child would only be able to focus on one property of the beads, such as the color. The newfound ability to classify is seen in the school-age child's interest in collections, such as stamps or coins.

Ordering things requires skill in seeing the relationships within a group or class. The child with a coin collection first groups all the quarters, nickels, and dimes together, then groups within these according to dates or other criteria. Children in school frequently are ordering their world: they line up in school according to height; they repeat numbers and letters in their classic order. These two operations are important in learning to read, in understanding the concepts of numbers, and in learning subjects based on relations, such as history (the relations of events in time) and geography (the relations of places in space).[2,24]

Thus during the concrete operations period the cognitive abilities needed to learn the basic concepts of mathematics, language, science, humanities, and social studies are developed. The child thinks differently than he did as a preschooler. The child considers others' views, can reverse thought processes, sees the relationships between objects and within a system, and can classify and order.

The child's *sensory abilities* also continue to develop.

VISION

Visual capacity should reach optimum function by the sixth or seventh year. The child's peripheral vision should be fully developed, and the ability to discriminate fine differences in shading of colors is fully developed. Acuity should be at maximum development or at least 20/30 in each eye, as measured by the Snellen chart. The child is able to coordinate eye movements, to see a single image, and to associate incoming visual stimuli with past and present mental images and functions. Throughout childhood further development of full visual potential occurs through use and practice.[12]

Physiologic changes occur in the eye during the school-age years. Eyes in the preschool years are normally hyperopic, with the image of an object falling behind the retina. However, unlike older individuals, preschool children do not need glasses, since they normally can accommodate their eyes to this by adjusting their own lenses. For most children, as the shape of the eye changes and grows in length and there is neurologic and behavioral maturation, their vision becomes normal (Fig. 20-6, *A*). However, 20% to 30% of school-age children do not have normal vision, and many of these deficits, as high as 75%, are not detected for a long period.[12]

Common *visual problems* in this age-group are myopia, hyperopia, and astigmatism. The most common, *myopia* or nearsightedness, which is often familial, is difficulty seeing distant objects because of an elongated eyeball that causes the image of an object to fall in front of the retina (Fig. 20-6, *B*). *Hyperopia,* farsightedness or difficulty seeing near objects, is no longer a developmental issue as it was for the preschooler (Fig. 20-6, *C*). *Astigmatism* is blurred vision caused by a poorly focused image on the retinas. All these usually can be corrected by glasses, but the problem may be in identifying the defects. For example, a child with myopia in the school-age years probably has never experienced maximum visual acuity and does not realize that the visual images being seen are not adequate. The delight and surprise when the world is first seen in full focus with glasses are long remembered.

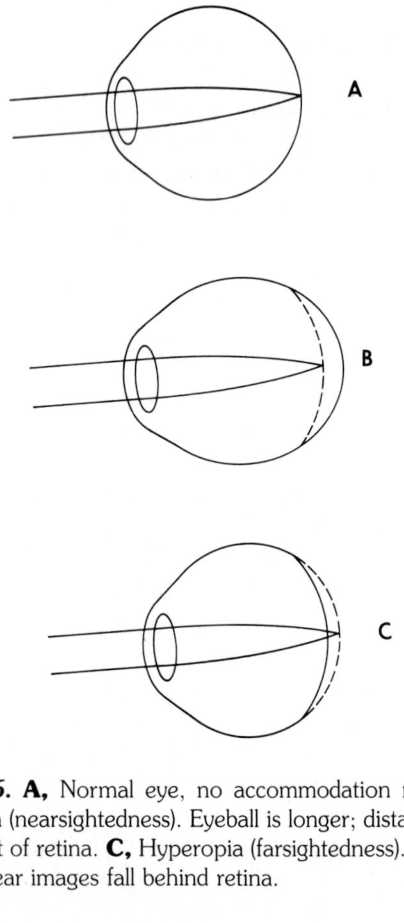

Fig. 20-6. **A,** Normal eye, no accommodation necessary. **B,** Myopia (nearsightedness). Eyeball is longer; distant images fall in front of retina. **C,** Hyperopia (farsightedness). Eyeball is shorter; near images fall behind retina.

HEARING

The child's hearing ability, or auditory acuity, is almost complete by 7 years of age, although some maturation continues into adolescence.[2] *Hearing deficits* are less common than visual deficits in childhood, but 3% to 5% of all school-age children have hearing deficits severe enough to interfere with school. *Chronic serous otitis media,* or fluid in the middle ear, is the most common cause of a hearing deficit in the early school years, as it was in the preschool years. All school-age children should have the periodic hearing evaluations that are normally done in schools. However, the nurse should be more suspicious of the child with a history of recurrent ear infections, which could cause persistent fluid in the middle ear. As discussed in Chapter 18, tympanograms are a valuable tool in detecting and monitoring this problem.[15]

PERCEPTUAL ABILITIES

Children often are taught through many senses at the same time: see a letter, hear the sound, and feel the shape. The child then has a number of ways to interpret and understand. For some children one of the ways is more effective than the others for learning, whereas other children learn easiest with many senses stimulated. By later childhood the child has begun to use these perceptions to form increasingly complex concepts and understandings of the world. Since no two children have exactly the same sensory acuity, sensitivity, or discrimination, all children build slightly different perceptions and conceptions of the world around them.

The area of perception most studied has been visual perception because of its role in learning to read. Studies have examined children's abilities to discriminate parts of a whole picture–to see a figure within a picture. Children usually progress from the preschool years, when they perceive visual stimuli more as a whole, to the school years, when they perceive the details more, and finally to the point where they perceive and integrate both. The role this plays in recognizing letters has been hypothesized. Children may first be able to differentiate between very different letters, such as *H* and *O,* but may have difficulty with letters similar in appearance, such as *b* and *d,* until they are better able to discriminate details.

LANGUAGE

Language develops remarkably during the school years. Most school-age children enter this period with the ability to understand and to speak a language but with just a beginning knowledge of reading and writing. By the end of this time most children have attained at least a functioning ability in both areas. Many skills are involved in the development of language, including visual perception for reading, auditory acuity and perception to understand spoken language, and fine motor skills for both articulation and handwriting.

Full capacity to imitate sounds linguistically develops during the childhood years. Between 6 and 7 years the child is able to produce properly the sounds *v, ch, l, sh, z, s, r,* and *th*. The sounds that children tend to have the most difficulty with are *s, l,* and *r*.[2] By 7½ years the child should be able to articulate all sounds.[2] The 6-year-old child usually has a spoken vocabulary of at least 2000 words, which then doubles by the sixth grade. The school-age child continues to develop in understanding the *syntax* (grammar) and *semantics* (meaning) of language. More complex sentences are used, and multiple meanings for the same word and the use of metaphors are increasingly understood.[2] The child should be able to recognize and correct spelling and grammar errors by the eighth or ninth year of life. The capacity to learn foreign languages is probably at an optimum level.

Reading and writing are the basic academic skills of a literate society. Much of the school-age child's time in school is devoted to learning these skills. Learning to read is a complex process, beginning with a recognition of letters and their sounds. Letters then are combined to form words that the child must learn to decode. Words then combine to form sentences, and so on. Few children learn to read by themselves. Most need help from teachers, parents, or older children. The best way for a child to learn to read is controversial. Some believe children learn best by sounding out the individual letters of a word (phonics), whereas others think learning the whole word as a chunk is better. There is value in both processes, and probably a combination of both is most effective. Considering the wide range of processes involved in reading–conceptual, perceptual, verbal, and motor–it is not surprising that many children have at least some difficulty in learning to read.[28]

Handwriting requires eye-hand coordination, motor control, and perceptual abilities. It is primarily a motor skill and is not necessarily reflective of intelligence. Many bright children and adults have poor handwriting, and vice versa. Boys tend to have more problems with legible handwriting than girls. Writing style does not approach adultlike maturity until the end of later childhood, but the child's writing should reflect the child's handedness, no reversal of letter forms should occur by the age 7 or 8, and the relative size of letters should be uniform. By the eighth or ninth year of life, letter strokes are firm, even, and flow with ease. For the individual who has difficulty with writing, learning to use a typewriter can be valuable.[28]

MEMORY

Memory abilities, both short-term and long-term, improve for the school-age child. Strategies that are used to remember information include organizing, classifying, and labeling information, strategies that the child in this stage of concrete operations has newly acquired. Rehearsal, repeating an item to be learned, is also a helpful memorization strategy. At age 5, children can use rehearsal if it is suggested or modeled; at age 10 they can rehearse spontaneously. Memory abilities can be improved through practice and rehearsal and by increasing the child's repertoire of strategies.[2]

INTELLIGENCE

The term *intelligence* has been used in a variety of ways and is often a confusing concept. Those who developed intelligence tests used intelligence to mean the quantity of information people possessed, their ability to think, and how that compared with others.

Scores on an intelligence test should measure the child's basic abilities and ideally should predict the child's future performance in school or society; however, this is not always true. Intelligence test scores tend to differ because each test, or each form of the same test, measures slightly different samples of abilities. Also, the nature of the tests tends to reflect the author's philosophy of the nature of intelligence. For example, the Stanford-Binet test places a heavy emphasis on abstract thinking; the Wechsler series emphasizes aggregate, or global knowledge; and the Peabody test emphasizes verbal skills. The younger the child, the less well developed these skills are, and the more difficult they are to measure. As language ability and mental functioning increase during later childhood, the measurement of intellectual capacity is more reliable and valid.

Children also take *achievement* tests, which measure the amount of information learned in a specific area. Although intelligence and achievement tests should measure different issues, basic ability versus learned achievement, their results correlate highly. Some believe this is because they both actually measure the same thing–achievement not ability.

The results of these tests are reported differently. Intelligence tests usually give an intelligence quotient (IQ): the ratio of the child's performance compared to others calculated by dividing maturational age (MA) by chronologic age (CA) and multiplying by 100 ($MA/CA \times 100 = IQ$). An IQ of 90 to 110 is average. Achievement tests compare the child's performance with other children and report scores as percentiles. A score of 50th percentile means the child is average in that skill, whereas a score of 20th percentile means the child is better than only 20% of other children his age in that skill, with 80% better than him.

Some of the tests used for this age-group to measure intelligence and development are listed in Table 20-3.

A discussion of intelligence must include mention of the controversy surrounding what role *heredity* and

***Table 20-3.* Common developmental and cognitive tests**

Test	Age (years)	Areas tested	Methods used to test	Comments
Alpern and Boll Developmental Profile	0-12	Five scales of development. 1. Physical age 2. Self-help age 3. Social age 4. Academic age 5. Communication age	Verbal responses from parents, teachers, others	
Bender-Gestalt (Bender Visual Motor Test)	3-4 to adult	Perceptual motor skills	Child copies geometric designs (nine in total), standard criteria for evaluating	
Goodenough-Harris Draw-a-Person	3-15	Gross mental age	Child asked to draw the best person he can; give points for body parts; score criteria used	Culture-free test
Peabody Picture Vocabulary Test (PPVT)	2½-18	Verbal intellectual capacity	Child told a word, then picks one picture out of four that corresponds	No reading necessary
Standford-Binet Intelligence Scale	2 to adult	Intelligence (global ability, not discrete areas of intellectual ability)	Series of standardized tasks	
Wechsler Intelligence Scale for Children (WISC)	5-15	Intelligence, two groups of tests, verbal and performance; gives verbal, performance, and full-scale IQ	Standardized tests	Very verbally oriented
Vineland Social Maturity Scale	1 to adult	Behavior, as related to ability to meet needs and responsibilities; categories include: 1. General self-help 2. Self-help in eating 3. Self-help in dressing 4. Self-direction 5. Occupation 6. Communication 7. Locomotion 8. Socialization	Direct observation; directed interview of child or caregiver	Gives social age quotient

environment play. At one point it was thought that basic intelligence is inherited and therefore fixed. However, it is now widely accepted that although some aspect of intelligence is inherited (to what extent is unclear), many environmental factors also influence it. Environmental opportunities for learning and the nature of these experiences greatly influence children's learning skills. Probably the greatest environmental influence is socioeconomic; children from poor families tend to have lower IQs by 10 to 20 points than children from middle-class families.[2] Why this difference exists is not clear and is probably caused by many subfactors, such as nutrition and parental stimulation. Society has tried to equalize some of these factors through nutrition programs, such as Women, Infants and Children (WIC), and preschool stimulation programs, such as Head Start. Others have suggested discontinuing the use of IQ tests, since they tend to label children early in life and influence, often negatively, their self-perception as well as their performance. The controversy of heredity and environment will continue for some time.

As previously stated, all these elements combine to allow the child to learn. With so many elements involved, however, it is not surprising that some children have problems learning. The reason for the learning problem may be a health problem, such as poor vision or hearing; an emotional problem, such as anxiety or depression; a cognitive problem, such as retardation or a learning disability; or a complex mixture of many issues. The child who comes to the health care system

❑ ❑ DIAGNOSTIC CRITERIA FOR ATTENTION-DEFICIT HYPERACTIVE DISORDER (ADHD)

Note: Consider a criterion met only if the behavior is considerably more frequent than that of most people of the same mental age.

A. A disturbance of at least six months during which at least 8 of the following are present:
   1. Often fidgets with hands or feet or squirms in seat (in adolescents, may be limited to subjective feelings of restlessness)
   2. Has difficulty remaining seated when required to do so
   3. Is easily distracted by extraneous stimuli
   4. Has difficulty awaiting turn in games or group situations
   5. Often blurts out answers to questions before they have been completed
   6. Has difficulty following through on instructions from others (not due to oppositional behavior or failure of comprehension), e.g., fails to finish chores
   7. Has difficulty sustaining attention in tasks or play activities
   8. Often shifts from one uncompleted activity to another
   9. Has difficulty playing quietly
   10. Often talks excessively
   11. Often interrupts or intrudes on others, e.g., butts into other children's games
   12. Often does not seem to listen to what is being said to him or her
   13. Often loses things necessary for tasks or activities at school or at home (e.g., toys, pencils, books, assignments)
   14. Often engages in physically dangerous activities without considering possible consequences (not for the purpose of thrill-seeking), e.g., runs into street without looking

B. Onset before the age of seven

C. Does not meet the criteria for a pervasive developmental disorder

Adapted from American Psychiatric Association: *Diagnostic and statistical manual of mental disorders,* ed 3, revised (DSM-III-R), Washington, DC, 1987, The Association.

with a learning problem needs a detailed, extensive evaluation.

LEARNING DISABILITIES

Some children with learning problems have learning disabilities. Many terms and definitions have been used to describe the impairments of these children who have normal or above normal intelligence and do not have visual, hearing, or motor handicaps or emotional problems.

The American Psychiatric Association classifies these as Specific Developmental Disorders. Examples are: developmental arithmetic disorder, developmental expressive writing disorder, developmental reading disorder, and developmental receptive language disorder. All of these specific developmental disorders are associated with impairment in academic functioning and are usually diagnosed after the child has experienced difficulty in the school setting. Some children have very minor difficulties that go practically unnoticed, while other children are so severely impaired that they may actually appear mentally retarded until appropriately diagnosed. It is certainly possible for an individual child to have more than one specific developmental disorder. It is also common for these children to develop behavioral problems as a complication of their inability to function well in the classroom.[28]

Another condition that causes difficulty in the child's adjustment to the school setting is Attention-Deficit Hyperactivity Disorder (ADHD). The essential features of ADHD are developmentally inappropriate degrees of inattention, impulsiveness, and hyperactivity.[28] This disorder has been given a wide variety of names in the past (Minimal Brain Dysfunction, Attention Deficit Disorder with and without hyperactivity) and is very difficult to assess since the child may manifest symptoms in varying degrees in different settings and with different people. The American Psychiatric Association has detailed the diagnostic criteria for ADHD (see the diagnostic criteria box above). Treatment of children with ADHD has been controversial and currently includes behavioral management, schooling alterations, and medications.

The nurse's role with the child who has a learning disability is varied. Detection of the problem, consultation during evaluations, and support and counseling for

❑ ❑ NURSING INTERVENTIONS TO PROMOTE COGNITIVE AND PERCEPTUAL HEALTH DURING THE SCHOOL-AGE PERIOD

Nurses need to help parents understand the child's level of cognitive ability to set realistic learning expectations. For example, the child who does not yet have an understanding of conservation of number is not ready for advanced mathematic skills.

School-age children are in the process of becoming less egocentric, but those working with them must remember this process is not yet complete.

Vision and hearing frequently are taken for granted. Parents and professionals need to remember that during the school years a child depends on these senses for learning but that this is also a time when many changes may be occurring. School-age children need frequent evaluations of their vision and hearing.

Language development and skills must be monitored. Often parents and family are so conditioned to a child's speech pattern that they do not recognize deviations from the norm. The child who has articulation problems beyond about age 6 or 7 should be evaluated.

Children in school undergo a variety of intelligence, achievement, and aptitude tests. Nurses working with these children should know the common tests used (see Table 20-3) and how to interpret results. This information will allow nurses to converse with other professionals about the child and to interpret information for parents and counsel them on their child's needs.

When assessing a child's cognitive abilities and learning potential, the nurse must do a thorough assessment of the child's family history and environment. Many problems associated with learning difficulties tend to recur in families, including myopia, delays in speech, and learning disabilities. Factors in the child's environment, such as divorce or poverty, may interfere with learning.

The first person to recognize or assess the child with a learning problem is often the nurse. In assessment, before jumping to the diagnosis of a learning disability, issues such as a vision or hearing deficit, a health problem, general immaturity, and environment deficit all should be considered and evaluated.

The child and family dealing with a learning disability need much support and counseling. They may need help in interpreting test results and educational plans, suggestions for dealing with behavioral problems such as increased activity, support in following appropriate medication or diet regimes, and counseling on how to cope with this usually hidden handicap.

---

the child and family are all possible nursing contributions. School nurses in particular play a vital role in the assessment and management of learning disabilities.

NURSING INTERVENTIONS

The nurse is often vital to the promotion of the child's overall cognitive and perceptual health and to prevention of problems in these areas. Some general considerations and suggestions are outlined in the box on this page.

Self-Perception and Self-Concept Pattern

Through each of the developmental processes of physiologic growth, cognitive development, learning capacity, and social development, children are engaged in an important process of self-discovery, of building and creating their own personalities, and of becoming exposed to a wider range of possibilities for their own behavior, attitudes, and values. Although a significant foundation for personality developed during infancy and early childhood, later childhood offers a valuable time during which children may begin to participate more actively in assuming specific traits and choosing values and attitudes.

ERIKSON'S THEORY

The stage of *personality development* described by Erikson for the school-age child is *industry versus inferiority*. The major task to be accomplished is full mastery of whatever the child is doing. The child's concerns tend to include both personal and social tasks. Erikson calls this a sense of industry; the primary hazard is the development of a sense of inferiority. Inferiority occurs with repeated failures at attempted tasks. The child can experience mastery through personal accomplishment and interaction with peers. Out of these dynamics the intense devotion and preoccupation with the peer group grow. The child is intense, interested, and involved and concentrates on developing knowledge and skills. As the child wields mastery of the tools of the culture in relationship to those of the peer group, a sense of worth and of understanding of the self is developed.[8,9]

SELF-CONCEPT

A child's self-concept develops over time and through a variety of experiences and relationships. The child's sense of self is influenced by how others see him, especially his peers. With increasing cognitive abilities, the child has a better understanding of what identifying factors–such as race, ethnicity, handicap, or sex–mean. Self-concept includes the child's self-esteem, sense of control, body concept, and sex role.

Self-esteem. Self-esteem has been defined as the extent to which the individual believes himself to be capable, significant, successful, and worthy. The younger school-age child has a limited self-concept, but this develops as the child successfully completes the tasks of this period–Erikson's sense of industry.

Although the child is increasingly moving his focus of interest out of the home, the base for a child to develop a high self-esteem is the family. Studies have shown that the parents of boys with high self-esteem were affectionate, supportive, and firm in setting behavior guidelines and that a strong parent-to-parent relationship existed.[2,32] For the child to fully appreciate and understand that he has succeeded, there must be approval and reinforcement by others as well as by self. Children need to know they have done a good job by parents verbalizing their pleasure. Other adults need to do the same, but often, as teachers or group leaders, they also reward the child who has succeeded in a task with badges, stars, or privileges.

The peer group's influence on the school-age child's self-esteem is unquestionable. Acceptance and a sense of belonging to a peer group adds to the child's feeling of self-worth. Competition with peers and its resulting success or failure helps develop the child's feelings of adequacy. Children are exposed to many situations through school, organized sports, and after-school activities. For some children there is little time for them to initiate their own interests.

The nurse must remember that a child needs to feel success at some task, and the completely structured activities for some children may not accomplish this. A child who succeeds in some things and is accepted by peers feels competent and worthwhile, is self-confident, and has a high self-esteem.[32]

Sense of Control. As the school-age child matures, a sense of control is developed over self and environment. The child begins to make choices and to feel in charge of herself. *Locus of control* refers to the source of the control, either within the child or outside in the environment. Children with an internal locus of control feel they are responsible for their behavior and accomplishments and tend to have higher levels of achievement than children who believe in an external locus of control. These children think that less reason exists for them to try hard at a task, since the results are determined not by them but by others or fate. Older children and girls tend to have a more internalized locus of control than do younger children and boys.[28]

Body Concept. The school-age child's concept of his body and its functioning also changes and adds to overall self-concept. By ages 8 to 11 children are aware that the parts of the body are a related whole.[2] The 11-year-old child can name twice the number of internal body structures as a 6-year-old. The most common structures named are parts of the cardiovascular (heart), musculoskeletal (bones), and nervous (brain) systems. Older children are more accurate in describing the location and function of the structures. For example, the 7-year-old knows the heart is important and that it beats, whereas the 13-year-old child knows that the heart pumps blood. Changes or differences in the body may be frightening to the school-age child. Loss of baby teeth might at first be upsetting until the child completely realizes this is a normal process and new ones will grow. Body differences, even as simple as freckles, may provoke ridicule and isolation. Children in this age-group often feel threatened by others with deformities.[2]

Sex Role. The preschool child learns his or her sex, that it is constant, and what general behaviors are expected. The child enters the school-age years with a strong identification with the parent of the same sex. The child then must learn the concepts and behavior of his or her sex role and incorporate them into self-concept.

Currently an increased awareness exists of the stereotypes regarding appropriate gender roles. Society has begun to narrow the dichotomy between sex roles and no longer encourages vast differences between men and women concerning occupation, interests, behavior, appearance, or personality traits. It will be interesting to see the effects on children with this change.

The school-age child's increasing awareness of the body and its functioning and a need for sexual identity combine to give the child a desire for knowledge about the biologic aspects of sexual function. Late in the school-age period, with the physical changes of puberty beginning, children often become increasingly concerned and curious about sexual issues. Children, especially between ages 9 and 12, are very attached to children of the same sex; it is not uncommon for them to explore each other's sexual organs. This is not true homosexual activity, although parents and children may have concerns that it is. The onset of changes varies for each child, so one girl may begin menses at 10 years and another at 13 years.

Children often are not sure whom to question, thus misinformation is passed throughout the peer group. Parents frequently are uncomfortable or unsure of what information to give to their children and when to give it.

Nurses play an important role in the area of sex education. When children are seen for routine health maintenance, the nurse should ask both child and parents questions regarding sexual development and concerns. The school is an ideal setting for group education programs. Some have incorporated these into the health curricula; others have special programs.

NURSING INTERVENTIONS

Ways in which the nurse can help children develop positive self-concepts are listed in the box to the right.

❑ ❑ NURSING INTERVENTIONS TO HELP DEVELOP A POSITIVE SELF-CONCEPT DURING THE SCHOOL-AGE PERIOD

Remind those working with school-age children that it is important for a child to succeed. All children need to believe they are good at something. Since not all children can succeed at all tasks, a variety of experiences should be provided so they can succeed at something. This helps them to deal better with failure and to try for more accomplishments and successes.

Parents need to learn the importance of giving positive feedback to their children, of setting realistic goals, and of helping the child attempt realistic tasks.

Children need to have some control over their lives and environment. School-age children should be allowed some choices to develop their sense of control and their decision-making skills. As children develop their concept of sex roles, if a goal is to develop a sense of equality of the sexes, then appropriate role models need to be provided.

The many questions children have about their bodily changes, including sexual changes, need to be acknowledged and discussed at home or at school. Families often have strong feelings on where these discussions should occur. However, some parents are unsure and benefit from the nurse's help in dealing with these issues. School nurses should play a vital role in developing sex education programs in the school.

Coping and Stress-Tolerance Pattern

An important aspect of development for the school-age child is learning how to cope with stress. Although many believe this child "has it made"–being cared for, going to school, and playing–he actually has many experiences in life that are stressful and need to be confronted. These include problems such as change, competition, frustration, and failures. Threats to the child's security, or stresses, cause feelings of helplessness and anxiety.

Many common coping strategies used by children are listed in Table 20-4. These mechanisms often are healthy, adaptive behaviors for the child, although he may become overwhelmed by his situation and not be able to move beyond his coping behaviors. Suggestions are given for ways the nurse can help the child use the strategies he chooses to deal with his problems, learn from them, and move on.

DIVORCE

A common stress in our society that school-age children must learn to cope with is divorce. At any one time 3 to 4 million children in the United States are undergoing the disruption of parental discord and separation.[14] The crisis aspect of divorce is time-limited, with much of the disorganization and readjustment occurring in the first 18 months. Children experience a feeling of loss, although they may hope that their parents will reunite at some point. This can delay their acceptance of the situation. Children's responses vary with their level of development. Their ability to cope with the divorce can be influenced by factors such as economic security, availability of both parents, and quality of parental interactions. Unfortunately, many parents are so involved in their own feelings that they are unable to support the children. Conflicts over custody, child support, and visitation rights add to the child's difficulty in coping.

Some children do not cope well with their parents' divorce and have emotional sequelae that can result in juvenile behavior problems or require long-term counseling.[14,32]

SOMATIZATION AND DEPRESSION

Children, like adults, use defense mechanisms to cope, with varying degrees of success. What works for some does not work for others; what is healthy in one situation may not be in another. Two mechanisms or

***Table 20-4.* The school-age child's coping strategies and nursing interventions for promoting coping**

Coping strategies	Nursing interventions
Use of defense mechanisms Regression Denial Repression Projection/displacement Sublimation Reaction formation	Accept child's use of defense mechanisms as temporary healthy coping responses, yet recognize and provide for child to move to more age-appropriate responses when ready. Help parents to understand and accept child's use of defense mechanisms as constructive way for child to deal with overwhelming threat until able to mobilize other coping resources.
Cognitive mastery (problem solving/ communication)	Ask child to tell you what he knows about his situation and encourage questions. Clarify misconceptions with honest, simple explanations; use diagrams, models, and equipment to supplement explanations. Encourage the child to verbalize her feelings about her situation and help her deal with them in a reality-oriented manner. Help child prepare ahead for stressful events by recalling what has helped him in past situations. Provide for self-expression, role reversal, and opportunities for controlling the situation. For the hospitalized child, try a personalized hospital memento book, body drawings, drawings of hospital situation, games, puppet play, and manipulation of hospital equipment; provide books such as Sarah Bonnett Stein's *About Handicaps;* have child continue schoolwork.
Controlling/holding behaviors	Encourage child to participate and make decisions. When appropriate, accept child's need to direct. Set consistent age-appropriate limits. Let child be responsible for self-care. Respond to signals for help.
Use of repetition	Use books and games to work through feelings again and again. Offer child opportunity to handle equipment as much as he desires.
Use of humor	Be a good listener; school-age children enjoy telling jokes and asking riddles. Be a good sport; school-age children enjoy playing jokes on others. Share anecdotes and cartoons that may relieve the child's tension.
Motor activity Aggression Protest behavior	Encourage optimum activity and action-oriented activities. Accept this behavior within reasonable limits. Do not take this behavior personally or respond with threats. Provide for aggression-release activities.
Withdrawal (resurgence of separation anxiety)	If child is separated from family, help parents understand that younger shool-age children may have resurgence of separation anxiety. Encourage parents to maintain contacts and keep child informed about home activities, siblings, and pets. Ask parents to bring child's games, collections, and favorite objects from home. Ask parents to request that child's teacher have his class send cards and letters.

Adapted from Vipperman JF, Rager PM: Childhood coping: how nurses can help, *Pediatr Nurs* 6(2):11-18, 1980. Reprinted with permission of the publisher.

strategies sometimes encountered in the school-age child are somatization and depression.

Some children, unable to cope with a situation and the resulting anxiety, transfer these feelings to a physical problem (somatization). The school-age child, unable to discuss or even admit his concerns, may complain of stomachaches or headaches, which are referred to as functional or psychogenic pain. Children may develop discrete, repetitive movement habits, called tics, which are usually a manifestation of anxiety or tension. The child with these problems often first needs to be evaluated to see if an underlying physiologic cause is present.[15] Then the child usually needs help in understanding his or her concerns and dealing with the behavior.

Depression does occur in children, although many persons, both professional and lay, have found this difficult to accept. The incidence has been hard to determine, but estimates ranging from 1.9% to 15% of school-age children with some depression have been quoted. In trying to define depression in children, most authors point out that they are not referring to the periodic sadness or disappointment that all children experience but to a more long-term syndrome in which the child's normal development and functioning are impaired. Factors that predispose a child to developing depression include emotional turmoil at home and loss of significant others. Factors that may place a child at risk for the development of childhood depression include[15]

Death of a parent
Divorce
Long-term hospitalization
Foster placement
Absence or chronic separation of parent and child
Parent(s) with psychopathology
Learning problems
Chronic illness or physical deformity
Rigid parents with uncompromising standards

The manifestations of childhood depression may be difficult to recognize. Behaviors that a depressed child might demonstrate include the following:[1]

Anorexia
Lethargy
Flat affect
Sad affect
Aggression
Weeping
Easily hurt
Hyperactivity
Irritability
Nonspecific somatic complaints
Fear of death of self or parents
Feelings of frustration
Feelings of sadness or hopelessness
Excessive self-criticism
Self-deprecatory feelings
Frequent daydreaming
Low self-esteem
Antisocial behavior
School refusal
Difficulty in school adjustment
Learning problems
Slow movements
Vacillating hostility toward parents and teachers
Loss of interest in previously pleasurable activities

However, nurses need to remember that many of these behaviors may be symptoms of other problems or may be normal for the child's level of development. Nurses can be instrumental in observing these behaviors and recognizing that a child may be depressed. Depending on the child, varying amounts of counseling will be needed. Nurses in schools and outpatient settings are often the ideal practitioners with the skill and time to help the child cope with a helpless feeling and its etiology. Often this counseling is done along with other psychologically oriented providers and includes methods of play therapy, family counseling, and individual guidance.

Value and Belief Pattern

Children make decisions everyday that involve moral and ethical issues. Should they tell the teacher which classmate broke the rule? Should they share their candy with a younger brother? Should they take the small toy that's just sitting on a friend's desk? For all these situations the child makes a decision based on his level of moral development.

Moral development includes moral behavior, feelings, and judgment. Behavior refers to the individual's actions; he may know he should not take a friend's toy, but will he? Feelings refers to how the individual feels if she does something she perceives is wrong; will she feel guilty if she takes her friend's toy? Both the child's behavior and how he feels are strongly influenced by environmental processes; the type of discipline the family uses, role models the child observes, with whom she identifies, and her rehearsal and practice. Judgment refers to the child's ability to figure out if something is right or wrong, a primarily cognitive, internal process.[2]

KOHLBERG'S THEORY

The stage of *moral judgment* in the school-age child is somewhat controversial. In general, most agree that the younger school-age child is at the preconventional level. Some children are in stage 1, punishment and obedience; but many are primarily in stage 2, individualism, instrumental purpose, and exchange. The child still does many things just to avoid getting in trouble (stage 1), but now he performs actions that will benefit him (stage 2). During later childhood most children progress to the next level, the conventional level, which includes stage 3, "good boy, bad boy," and stage 4, law and order. The age when the conventional level first occurs varies but usually occurs between ages 10 and 13. The conventional level or moral judgment shows a switch in focus, with the child looking to others for approval and to authority in society to define rules. This level coincides with Piaget's cognitive level of concrete operations and with the child's increased social involvement with those outside the home.[18,19,21]

The six aspects of moral development have been identified by Kohlberg as clearly developing during the school-age years in Western societies and are listed below:

1. The child enters this period judging behaviors in relation to real outcomes, or physical consequences. If children of this age are asked whether it is worse to break five cups while helping mother set the table or to break one cup while stealing a cookie, most would think breaking five cups is worse. As the school-age child progresses, the act begins to be judged in terms of the intention of the offender, and thus the stealing incident is considered the worse of the two acts.

2. Younger children view behaviors as totally right or totally wrong. Later they begin to be able to weigh several aspects of the situation and to use judgment in regard to the relative rightness or wrongness of the act.
3. Early in the middle years children state that an act is wrong because it brings punishment or displeasure from an adult. Later they develop the insight that an act is wrong because it breaks a rule, offends another person's rights, or harms another.
4. Reciprocity is used in terms of what will happen to the child when he or she offends or is offended. In other words, children are able to calculate that they would hit back when hit and that they would be hit if they were to hit someone else. By age 10 or 11, children can place themselves in another's position and begin to exercise the Golden Rule of "doing unto others as you would have them do unto you."
5. Younger children usually recommend severe punishment for the misdeeds of others. Later they begin to recommend a milder form of punishment and then an approach that would lead to the reform of the offender.
6. These children tend to view accidents or misfortunes as being punishments for wrongdoing. Later such naturally occurring misfortune is not confused with punishment.

MORAL BEHAVIORAL PROBLEMS

Some moral behavioral problems are common during the school-age years, such as lying, stealing, or cheating. Preschool and younger school-age children who lie frequently do so because of fantasy, exaggerations, or inaccurate understanding. As the child gets older, he may use the defense mechanism of denial to block upsetting situations. The resultant lie is then not a conscious act. Older children often lie because they are afraid of being punished or laughed at. Children may cheat because of a desire to win or do well in our competitive society; peer pressure can be an added stress that causes this. Children usually steal when they think they will not be caught and when they believe there is no other way to get what they want.[32] Although these actions can be quite upsetting for the child's parents, they are common developmental behaviors, and parents frequently need reassurance that the child is normal.

NURSING INTERVENTIONS

The development of morality in children often is not addressed by nurses, although it is frequently an area of concern for families. Nurses can help families in the area of moral development by the nursing interventions listed in the box on this page.

❑ ❑ NURSING INTERVENTIONS TO ENCOURAGE MORAL DEVELOPMENT DURING THE SCHOOL-AGE PERIOD

Help parents and those dealing with school-age children to recognize the normal level of moral development in this age-group, the importance of being accepted, and the rules of the group or society.

Support parents in developing fair rules and methods of discipline consistent with the child's moral expectations. Family meetings can be effective by the end of this period.

Counsel parents on how to deal with the minor behavioral problems of this age and on when to seek more in-depth counseling.

Support families in their personal choice of religion and religious education for their children.

Health Perception and Health Management Pattern

The school-age child understands what health is and what causes illness, but this is different than an adult's understanding. Some think that for younger school-age children the concept of health is too abstract.[2] But these children do have ideas about the symptoms and causes of illness. These ideas are a product of their cognitive level (concrete operations) and moral level (external rules and forces). One study has shown that children and their mother frequently see the same symptoms as signs of illness.

School-age children, when asked their ideas on what causes illness, usually state either the "germ theory," the "punishment theory," or the "external forces theory." Many children are able to state that germs played a role in their illness, but their understanding of germs is limited. Other children believe illness is caused by some action, with a resulting punishment. Closely tied to this is the belief that outside elements or persons cause illness, such as "the rain gives you colds." All these beliefs can make the child feel helpless, but they play a role in teaching these children health promotion concepts.[2]

Parents often spend much time teaching school-age children preventive health practices, such as personal hygiene, dental care, and good nutrition. Most children in this group still need some adult supervision in these areas. Many are probably unclear about the relationship between these "preventive measures" and how they prevent illness. Unfortunately, modeling their parents, children in our society are frequently passive health consumers, asking few questions and doing as they are told. This is partly caused by their need to obey authority figures and by the role model of most adults, who also are not assertive health care consumers.

An awareness of the school-age child's normal perceptions of health are important to the nurse counseling the child and his family on health promotion. Some suggestions to help the nurse in this area include:

1. When teaching children about preventing illness, begin by assessing their understanding of the cause or causes of illnesses.
2. Before teaching prevention, the nurse must first teach an understanding of the cause of illness.
3. Health promotion and prevention measures, properly understood, may give the child a better sense of control over health.
4. Children who believe they are being punished can be relieved by learning the true process of their illness.
5. Parents should be encouraged not to tell children, "If you're not good, you'll get sick," since this can add to their misconceptions.
6. Children can be taught to be appropriately assertive, questioning health care consumers through health education programs.

ENVIRONMENTAL PROCESSES

Natural Processes

School-age children, like all other age-groups, are exposed daily to agents or factors in the environment that have the potential of causing injury or illness. Many of these are harmless if used appropriately or if exposure is minimal. These include physical agents such as fires; mechanical agents, such as bicycles; biologic agents, such as bacteria; chemical agents, such as asbestos; and radiologic agents, such as x-rays.

PHYSICAL AGENTS

As previously discussed, accidents are the leading cause of death in children ages 1 to 14 years in the United States. In the school-age group accidental deaths represent 51% of all deaths.[15] However, most accidents do not result in death; about 17 million nonfatal childhood accidents occur each year and about 15,000 fatal ones. Although most nonfatal accidents are minor, some result in lifelong problems.

The agents, host, and environment can be considered in the accidents that occur in school-aged children. The type of accidents, or *agents,* have been found to vary with the child's age; the most frequent fatal accidents during the school-age period are motor vehicle accidents, followed by drownings, fires and burns, and firearms.[15] The most common nonfatal accidents tend to be caused by more simple agents and tend to produce simpler injuries. A study of emergency room visits showed that of the 498,000 visits made in one year by children ages 6 to 11 years, some of the major reasons for injuries were recreational equipment and activities, specifically bicycle, swing, and skateboard accidents.[15] Slightly older children had an increasing number of accidents from contact sports. Another study found that the most common types of accidents in children between ages 5 and 9 were cuts, falls, and burns. Both studies suggest a greater frequency of the minor accidents compared with the fatal ones.

Specific accident factors are associated with the *host,* in this case the school-age child. In general, accidents occur more frequently in school-age boys than girls.[15] The reason for this is not documented, although one can hypothesize that it is caused by differences in personalities, societal expectations, childrearing practices, and the activities of boys and girls. The agent varies with the sex of the host. For school-age boys, drowning is the most common fatal accident, and automobile accidents are second; for girls, automobile accidents are the most common, and drowning is fourth.[3]

The *physical environment* of the child can dictate the type or frequency of accidents, which occur in settings that include the home, neighborhood, and school. In 8- to 12-year-olds, only 30% of accidents occur indoors.[15] The majority occur outdoors, which means school-age children are at greater risk for automobile or bicycle accidents than for the poisoning or falls that occur indoors to the younger child.

The incidence of accidents is higher in the summer than the winter. This may be a result of children being outside more and the increase in accidents such as drownings and pedestrian motor vehicle accidents. The socioeconomic level may affect the child's physical environment, making him more likely to suffer from one type of accident than another. Space heaters may put poorer children at risk for burns, whereas a private swimming pool may put wealthier children at risk for drowning.

Social environment also can play a role in accidents; for the child this includes the family, school, and playmates. Many studies have shown that stress, both in the child and in the family, can increase the likelihood of an accident.[15] Often families have chronic stress, such as unemployment, with a sudden acute stress superimposed, such as the mother being ill, that results in an increased risk for accidents. Another vulnerable period for an increase in accidents is when parental supervision may be minimal, such as during holidays, a move to a new home, or family crises.

The more common agents or types of accidents for this age-group include drowning, burns, firearms, and recreational activities. Automobile accidents are discussed with other mechanical agents. Health providers

❑ ❑ WATER SAFETY PRACTICES

1. School-age and younger children should be taught to swim. Lessons can be incorporated into school gym classes or into outside recreational activities.
2. No one should swim alone, and children should swim only in areas where lifeguards are present.
3. School-age children should be taught basic lifesaving cardiopulmonary resuscitation (CPR) skills, through American Red Cross or school or community programs.
4. Backyard pools, when unsupervised, should be protected by high fences and locked gates.
5. Handrails and ladders in pools should be in good repair.
6. Areas around pools and diving boards need constant maintenance.
7. Children should be cautioned not to run or "fool around" along the edge of pools.
8. Swimming too soon after eating heavy meals should be avoided to decrease the possibility of cramps.
9. Children should be encouraged to know their own swimming abilities and not to be pushed by their peers beyond those abilities.
10. When on boats, children and adults should wear life jackets.

❑ ❑ FIRE PREVENTION PRACTICES

1. All homes should have smoke detectors and fire extinguishers.
2. All families should have planned escape routes from the home in case of a fire.
3. Family members should never smoke while in bed.
4. Appropriate fire escapes and plans should be provided for those sleeping on upper floors.
5. Children should be taught how to react in case of fire, including how to use the home extinguisher, call the fire department, and put out clothes fires.
6. Flame-retardant clothing should be used and cared for properly (read labels).
7. Night clothes that catch fire more quickly should be avoided, such as loose, flimsy nightgowns for girls.
8. Children should be cautioned not to use matches, cigarette lighters, and flammable liquids and materials. These materials should be stored safely.
9. Open fires such as fireplaces, need protective gratings.
10. Children should use stoves and other cooking facilities only with adult supervision.
11. Children should not be allowed to play with fireworks. Although each state regulates the use of fireworks, parents should monitor their children.
12. Children should be cautioned to never touch wires they may encounter, either on the ground or when climbing.

and families must always watch for these potentially harmful agents.

Drownings. Approximately 8000 drownings occur in the United States each year.[15] Water safety measures (see the box above) can help reduce this number, along with the many other injuries that occur around water, such as falls in slippery areas.

Burns. Each year more than 1 million Americans suffer burns.[15] Again, the majority of children who are burned live, often with physical and psychologic scars of varying severity. The two major types of accidental burns are scalds and flame burns. Scalds are more common in the infant, whereas flame burns are more common in the school-age child.

Children in this age-group receive their burns in various ways; many occur in residential fires, with 56% of fatal home fires associated with smoking. Other potential problem areas are playing with gasoline, firecrackers, matches, or chemistry sets; helping with barbecues or cooking; making candles; or just watching others do these activities. Electric burns occur in this group when children climb near high-tension wires and inadvertently grab one.

Several measures can be taken to prevent burns in children. One government intervention has been the *Flammable Fabrics Act,* which requires that fabrics used in children's sleepwear (sizes 0-14) be flame retardant–the material still can burn but at a slower rate. Children's sleepwear labels should be read to learn how to wash the garment appropriately. The nurse can offer suggestions (see the box above) to decrease the possibility of an accidental burn to the school-age child.

Firearms. These frequently cause fatal injury in the United States, including homicide, suicide, and accidents; approximately 20% of U.S. homes have a handgun.[15] Possibly the best means of preventing accidents with firearms is to ban them from private ownership. Experience with not allowing private handguns in England has shown a decrease in deaths and injuries. Families with firearms in the home should be encouraged to

❑ ❑ PLAYGROUND SAFETY PRACTICES

1. Playground equipment should meet the set standards. Sharp, protruding parts should be eliminated.
2. The area surrounding a playground should be cushioned adequately for falls.
3. Equipment should be located so as to avoid injury to other children.
4. Children should be trained to use any new equipment they obtain safely, such as a skateboard or a fishing pole.
5. Equipment should always be kept in good working order and securely fastened.
6. When involved in contact sports, appropriate protective equipment should be used.
7. During contact sports rules should be followed.

1. Store them safely in a locked area.
2. Store weapons and ammunition in separate areas.
3. Consider using nonlethal (wax) bullets.

Sports and Recreational Accidents. These are becoming more common during the school-age years. The types of injuries vary and include lacerations, contusions, hematomas, concussions, sprains, and fractures.[15] Children use a variety of equipment, including playground equipment, and increasingly are involved in contact sports such as football and hockey.

Injuries that occur during recreation periods can be prevented by several measures. The government's 1976 National Bureau of Standards has set standards for home playground equipment, regulating areas such as sharp edges, moving parts, and design of equipment. Nurses can help prevent accidents in this area through school education programs and by counseling families around a variety of issues (see the box above).[2]

Nursing Interventions. The advice nurse's can offer to parents may suggest that this type of *guidance* is usually successful in preventing childhood accidents. Unfortunately, studies in this area of health education have shown variable results, with some parents following the suggestions, but many, although they see the validity of the suggestions, not following through.[15] Some factors that have been found for why people do not follow through include a need for the action to be done frequently, the effort involved, a high cost, and discomfort in the use of the object. Most of these factors are perceived differently by different people. This type of education requires more study to learn the approaches that give the best results. However, since individual counseling is an integral part of health promotion and prevention, general strategies are suggested for the provider offering guidance on accident prevention (see the box on this page to the right). The box also lists community actions the nurse can support in this area.

❑ ❑ NURSING INTERVENTIONS TO PREVENT ACCIDENTS DURING THE SCHOOL-AGE PERIOD

Strategies for counseling

Discuss accident prevention at optimum times, such as the prenatal visit, the arrival of a new sibling, or after an accident.

Instead of all topics at once, discuss only the major concerns for the developmental level of the child at each well-child visit. For the school-age child this includes car, water, fire, and bicycle safety.

Repeat information at other visits to add to its importance.

Community actions

Use supplemental materials such as written pamphlets to reinforce the verbal information.

Support local and national legislation that sets standards for potentially harmful agents. Mandating standards has been one of the most successful accident preventives, as seen in the Poison Prevention Packaging Act and the Flammable Fabrics Act. Many nurses have been active in lobbying for bicycle helmet requirements in their states.

Consult with manufacturers on safe designs of materials used by children.

Report any objects that are potentially hazardous.

Participate in local activities that stress accident prevention, such as local offices of the National Safety Council.

Educate groups, such as school children and parent organizations.

MECHANICAL AGENTS

The two mechanical agents most often involved in accidents with the school-age child are cars and bicycles.

MOTOR VEHICLE ACCIDENTS

The leading cause of death in all groups of children from age 1 year to adulthood, these include children who are passengers in cars, pedestrians, and bicycle riders. In the United States, for children ages 3 to 12, deaths from pedestrian accidents outnumber deaths from passenger accidents. Accidents between automobile and bicycles account for one sixth of the injuries from motor vehicles in children between ages 5 and 14, but more than half of those killed in bicycle accidents are children.[13,15] Again, although not all motor vehicle accidents result in death, many children are left with long-term disabilities. (See box on pp. 500-501.)

Injuries to passengers in cars can be prevented or the

severity reduced by altering some aspects of the physical environment. Lower speed limits, not allowing driving after drinking alcohol, better automobile designs, and seat belts have all been shown to reduce the severity and number of accidents and injuries.

Studies have shown that car seats and belts used consistently and appropriately can decrease the likelihood of a child's death by 70% to 95% and decrease serious injury by 50% to 60%.[13] In spite of these impressive statistics, a large percentage of school-age children do not use seat belts. Educational programs directed at encouraging children to use their seat belts frequently have been ineffective. Reasons given for not using seat belts by parents and children included forgetting, difficulty reaching and fastening the belts, experiencing discomfort from the belt across their stomachs or necks, and driving short distances. One study found a strong correlation between parents' and children's use of seat belts; if parents role modeled the use of seat belts, children were more likely to use them. It has become clear that consistent use of seat belts by children will occur only if these and other safety devices are legally required and parents cooperate and provide role modeling.

For children less than 15 years of age living in an urban area, more than half of all the deaths from motor vehicle accidents are caused by pedestrian-automobile accidents. The injuries from these accidents tend to be more severe than passenger injuries, with a high percentage of head injuries. Many factors are involved in pedestrian accidents: Children often have difficulty interpreting traffic signs, judging how fast cars are going, and remembering to be careful crossing streets. Others have suggested that overcrowding, poverty, stress, and unsafe play areas may play a role. Supervision by adults decreases the likelihood of this type of accident, but effective preventive measures have not been clearly documented. Educational safety programs for children have not been successful in changing their pedestrian behaviors. Prevention lies in a better understanding of its causes and in a varied approach to the problem. However, most agree that children should be taught by their parents basic street safety principles of how to cross the street and how to obey traffic lights. Some potentially preventive measures are listed in the box on this page.

Bicycle Accidents. In 1980 approximately 60,000 injuries were related to bicycle (including tricycles)–motor vehicle accidents, with 26,300 occurring in the 5 to 14 age-group. The majority of accidents were minor, with only 410 deaths in this group. The following factors have been found to be risk factors associated with bicycle accidents:

1. Reckless riding and lack of control (riding double, trying stunts) are associated with 60% of accidents.
2. Mechanical or structural problems with bikes (brakes failing, chains slipping) account for 20% of children's accidents.

❑ ❑ STREET SAFETY PRINCIPLES

1. Older children and other adults can provide supervision as guards to help children cross streets.
2. Education programs for groups of children should involve the parents.
3. Streets in communities should be evaluated for areas at high risk for accidents, where stop signs or reduced speed signs may be needed.
4. Areas of greatest risk are often those with large numbers of children, such as playgrounds and schools. Children in these areas need adult monitoring and guidance, along with traffic controls such as reduced speed.

3. Bicycles that are not the right size of the child, primarily those too large, cause added risk.
4. Bicycles with elongated handle bars and low seats add to risk.
5. Hand brakes cause more problems than foot brakes.
6. In general, boys have more bike accidents involving cars than girls.

Bicycle accidents occur more frequently near the home and during the day, when the bicycle is being ridden for pleasure. Accidents increase when bicycles are used the most, in the summer and after Christmas. Children most often are hurt by the spokes of their bikes, frequently when they are riding on the back. The types of injuries include cuts, bruises, sprains, and fractures.

In helping to prevent bicycle accidents, teaching must encompass safety factors for both the bicycle and the rider. Parents should be cautioned to follow certain guidelines when obtaining a bicycle. The bike should be the right size for the child. When the child sits on the bike, his feet should be flat on the ground. When standing, at least an inch should be between the child and the center bar of a boy's bike. There should be easy access to the bike's brakes. Bikes with sharp, protruding parts or with slippery foot brakes should be avoided. As mentioned in Chapter 19, all children should wear helmets approved by the American National Standards Institute (ANSI) when biking. An ANSI approved helmet has these features:

- The outer shell is made of hard plastic or fiberglass
- The helmet liner is made from polystyrene foam and does not feel spongy when pressed
- The helmet is adjustable to the size and shape of the child's head, as the child gets older, the size can be adjusted by changing to narrower fitting pads
- The helmet does not limit hearing or vision
- When adjusted properly, the chin strap should hold the helmet securely on the child's head

Nurses should encourage parents to teach their children safe bicycling habits early in life. Suggestions for safe bicycling and safe bicycling in traffic, based on the American Academy of Pediatric's Child Safety Suggestions, are listed in the box on this page.

BIOLOGIC AGENTS

School-age children are constantly exposed to *bacterial, vital,* and other biologic agents that are potential threats to health. Compared to the preschool child, the school-age child has fewer illnesses.[15] The most frequent illness continues to be respiratory infections, most commonly upper respiratory infections (URIs). According to one study, in 1 year 61% of the days missed from school and 26% of visits to physicians were caused by respiratory problems. Most URIs have a viral etiology, but bacteria may play either a primary or secondary role. Two problems associated with URIs are streptococcal infection and otitis media.

Strep throat from group A beta-hemolytic streptococcus is a well-known problem, diagnosed by throat culture and treated with an antibiotic, most commonly penicillin. It can occur at any age but is most common in school-age children. A child with an infection from this strain of streptococcus may have a severe sore throat, fever, and malaise or may have only a minor sore throat.

The concern with group A beta-hemolytic streptococcal infections are the secondary complications and potential sequelae. More serious is the possible development of rheumatic fever or acute glomerulonephritis in a child following a streptococcal pharyngitis. Areas where close person-to-person contact occurs, such as schools, are prone to outbreaks. School nurses should be alert to children with possible strep infections for appropriate culture and treatment. Children being treated for strep throats with an antibiotic usually are considered to be noninfectious after 24 hours of treatment and then can return to school.[15] Children with throat infections caused by other strains of streptococcus, such as group B, do not usually need to be treated, since they are not associated with the same serious complications.

The frequency of *gastrointestinal infections* (influenza, gastroenteritis) decreases in the school-age years, although it is still the second most common acute condition of childhood after URIs. Most commonly caused by a virus, it results in vomiting and diarrhea. The older and larger school-age child is in less danger of rapid dehydration; he basically reacts to the illness the same as an adult and needs to be treated similarly. Gastroenteritis often affects several persons, so children in school again need to be monitored for outbreaks.

A skin disorder found commonly in this age-group is *infestation* with either scabies or lice *(pediculosis).* Both cause extreme itchiness, of either the body (scabies) or the hair (lice), and can spread to other children.

❑ ❑ BIKE SAFETY FOR SCHOOL-AGE CHILDREN*

Suggestions for safe bicycling

1. Parents should acquaint the child with a new bicycle, including braking, steering, and balancing.
2. The child should demonstrate to parents a basic ability in bike riding before being allowed to use it without supervision. This includes the ability to
   Stop the bicycle quickly by using the brakes.
   Start riding without wobbling a path 1 yard wide.
   Stop and dismount without falling, and
   Ride in a straight line close to the curb.
3. Parents should discuss where the child can ride. Safe areas for riding can be established and safe routes to and from school, friends' homes, and other locations can be mapped out.
4. Families should agree on some general rules for safe riding, such as not riding in the dark, barefoot, with someone else on the bike, in bad weather when brakes may not work, or with loose pants that could get tangled.
5. Bicycles should be inspected regularly to ensure they are in safe and good working condition, including properly inflated tires.
6. Children should wear ANSI approved helmets.

Suggestions for safe bicycling in traffic

1. Bicycle riders are subject to the same rules as automobiles. Traffic regulations, signs, and signals should be observed.
2. Local and state laws must be observed. This includes licensing, registration, and ordinances related to bicycle traffic.
3. If bike riding is done at night, the bicycle should have lights and reflectors, as required by local and state regulations.
4. Both hands should be on the handle bars at all times.
5. A basket or backpack should be used if objects need to be carried.
6. Children should ride on the side of the road traveling with traffic, keeping close to the side of the road; they should not ride two abreast.
7. Intersections should be approached with caution and may require walking the bike through on crosswalks.
8. Children should ride bicycles defensively, watching for cars, pedestrians, street dangers, and car doors opening.

Adapted from Betz CL: Bicycle safety: opportunities for family education, *Pediatr Nurs* 9(2):110, 1983. Reprinted with permission of the publisher.

*American Academy of Pediatrics Child Safety Suggestions, Copyright AAP, 1978.

School nurses especially need to be aware of these two conditions, since they can occur in epidemic proportions in schools. If these problems can be identified quickly, referral to a physician or nurse practitioner for appropriate treatment can be made and spread of the infection can be avoided.[7]

A biologic agent that today's school-age child is certainly aware of is the human immunodeficiency virus, the cause of AIDS. Of all ages, the young school-age child is at lowest risk for contracting AIDS, since perinatally acquired AIDS presents in infancy and toddlerhood, and most young school-age children are not taking IV drugs or engaging in high-risk sexual practices. The school-age child may well know a person with AIDS and has certainly heard something about AIDS from adults, older children, or the news. The school-age child needs to know basic facts about AIDS, how it is transmitted, and probably most important, that it cannot be transmitted through casual contact, such as being in the same classroom with a child with AIDS. Because of widespread misinformation and fear about AIDS, the surgeon general called for mandatory, explicit AIDS education beginning with 8-year-olds.[4]

Children with AIDS may attend school as long as their physician has determined that they are not in a period of heightened risk for contracting an illness from the other children. Thus during outbreaks of chicken pox, measles, or other illnesses, the child with AIDS should have home tutoring. The child with AIDS needs continual evaluation regarding the risks versus benefits of school attendance. Certainly, long periods of isolation from peers contributes to feelings of loneliness in the child with AIDS and may even appear to be a punishment for being ill.

The school nurse can be instrumental in providing age-appropriate educational materials to school-age children. Some resources for the nurse are listed in the box on this page.

By school age, most children have received their basic series of immunizations. Most states now require that the child's immunizations be up to date before entering kindergarten or the first grade (Table 20-5).

The child with only a few immunizations does not need to start from the beginning but can pick up where they were stopped. The child beyond age 6 should be given the adult vaccine, Td instead of DTP. Immunization to pertussis (whooping cough) is no longer needed, since the risk of the disease decreases with age, whereas the risk of immunization reaction may increase with age. The strength of the diphtheria antigen portion, "D" to "d," decreases, since reactions to this component of the immunization increase with age. Table 19-3 shows the recommended schedule by the American Academy of Pediatrics (AAP) for children not immunized in early infancy. The AAP recommends a booster MMR (measles, mumps, and rubella) just prior to entry into 5th grade. Research has shown that the immunity that develops after the toddler dose of MMR frequently does not last beyond 10 years. The 5th-grade dose ensures higher levels of immunity for these youngsters and provides coverage for young women as they enter their childbearing years.

❑ ❑ RESOURCES FOR AIDS EDUCATIONAL MATERIALS

American Academy of Pediatrics
Publications Department
PO Box 927
Elk Grove, IL 60009

American Red Cross
1-800-342-2437

Kidsrights
3700 Progress Blvd.
PO Box 851
Mt. Dora, FL 32757
1-800-892-5437

Network Publications
PO Box 1830
Santa Cruz, CA 95061-1830

San Francisco AIDS Foundation
333 Valencia St.
PO Box 6182
San Francisco, CA 94101-6182

***Table 20-5.* Guide to tetanus prophylaxis in wound management**

History of tetanus immunization (doses)	Clean, minor wounds*		All other wounds†	
	Td	TIG	Td	TIG
Uncertain or less than 3	Yes	No	Yes	Yes
3 or more‡	No§	No	No‖	No

From Report of the Committee on Infectious Diseases, ed 22 Evanston , Ill 1991. American Academy of Pediatrics. Copyright AAP, 1991.
*TD = adult-type tetanus and diphtheria toxoids. If the patient is younger than 7 years, DT or DTP is given (see text). TIG = tetanus immune globulin.
†Including but not limited to wounds contaminated with dirt, feces, soil, saliva, etc; puncture wounds, avulsions; and wounds resulting from missiles, crushing, burns, and frostbite.
‡If only three doses of fluid toxoid have been received, a fourth dose of toxoid, preferably an adsorbed toxoid, should be given.
§Yes, if more than 10 years since the last dose.
‖Yes, if more than 5 years since the last dose.

The school child who sustains an injury that puts him at risk for tetanus should receive prophylaxis according to the guidelines developed by the American Academy of Pediatrics (see Table 20-5).

CHEMICAL AGENTS

A number of potentially toxic chemical agents exist in our environment that the child is exposed to via inhalation, ingestion, or direct contact. As stated previously, children are thought to be particularly susceptible to chemical hazards. Two chemicals ingested by children on a regular basis are foods and drugs. Although normally safe, these can be harmful if used inappropriately. Other environmental hazards include exposures to pollution, heavy metals, and pesticides.

The nutritional needs of the school-age child are reviewed earlier in this chapter. As stated, children frequently eat foods with high sugar, salt, and fat quantities and with chemical additives. The effects of some of these additives have been questioned. On a short-term basis some are thought to cause allergic reactions; on a long-term basis some are implicated in the development of coronary disease and cancer. Nurses need to be aware that the child's diet may be a source of some health problems and should assess the child's intake and counsel the child and parents accordingly.

The incidence of *poisonings* decreases in the school-age years, since children are more aware of the appropriate uses of drugs and other agents around the home. However, drug concerns are still present. Older school-age children are increasingly exposed to recreational drugs, primarily through their peers and older children (see Chapter 21).

Pollution has become a fact of life. Air pollution irritates the eyes and the respiratory tract. Children with respiratory allergies, including asthma, can be particularly compromised when exposed to air pollution.

The *metals* that children may be exposed to include lead (see Chapter 17), cadmium, mercury, arsenic, and asbestos. Children exposed to these metals in toxic doses develop a variety of symptoms, both short and long term, with the type and severity varying with the metal. Mercury is particularly toxic to the developing central nervous system. Asbestos causes lung difficulties, but the response may be delayed for years. The child may be exposed to these through a variety of sources, including materials carried home from work on parents' clothes or in school buildings. The long-term effects of these metals on children still are not completely known.[15]

RADIOLOGIC AGENTS

The child is exposed to both naturally occurring radiation and man-made ionizing radiation. Radiation exposure occurs in varying degrees in the x-ray films taken for dental, bone, and other routine examinations; in radiation from nuclear plants and explosions; and in the radiation treatment for many childhood cancers. Children exposed to high levels of radiation have been found to be at risk for developing cancer in the future, with the risk greater to children compared to adults of developing leukemia, thyroid cancer, and breast cancer. Other problems documented following radiation exposure include mental deficiencies, psychiatric disorders, and compromised growth.[15]

Nurses and other health providers can and must play a role in the prevention of chemical and radiation hazards to children. This is an area where much work still needs to be done. Some beginning suggestions are included in the box on p. 529.

CANCER

The *cancers* most common in this age-group include leukemia (see Chapter 19), brain tumors and lymphomas, and central nervous system (CNS) tumors. Primary brain tumors represent 9% to 20% of cancers in this age; the second most common cancer after leukemia. These tumors occur slightly more often in boys, with a peak age at 5 to 10 years. The cause of CNS tumors is unknown. In children, unlike adults, most brain tumors are infratentorial (that is, brain stem, cerebellum). If the nurse suspects an intracranial lesion, the first step in assessment is a detailed history. Increased intracranial pressure is an early symptom in infratentorial tumors. The most common findings are vomiting, and disturbances of gait and balance. The lymphomas include Hodgkin's disease and non-Hodgkin's lymphoma. The incidence of Hodgkin's disease peaks from age 15 to 24 (see Chapter 21). Non-Hodgkin's lymphomas have a peak incidence in the school-age years. Boys are affected about three times more often than girls, and mortality rates in the United States tend to be higher in densely populated areas, particularly in higher education and income levels. The most common presenting symptom is abdominal pain. With appropriate treatment the 3-year survival rate is 50% to 80% for children with non-Hodgkin's lymphoma.[22]

Because of dramatic increases in life expectancy after treatment for some of the childhood cancers, an increasing number of school children return to school after successful treatment. These children present a challenge to the nurse, as they are in various stages of recovery or enjoying full health but feeling some threat of recurrence.

Social Processes

The daily life of the school-age child requires frequent interactions with other children and adults. These interactions occur within the family, at school, and in the

❑ ❑ NURSING INTERVENTIONS TO PREVENT CHEMICAL AND RADIATION HAZARDS DURING THE SCHOOL-AGE PERIOD

Become aware of the potential environmental chemical and radiation hazards in general and specifically for a local area. For example, rural areas may have insecticide spraying, factories may emit heavy leads, cities may have serious smog problems, and any area may have chemical waste dumps with potential leaks.

Know family member's occupations and living situations and their potential hazards.

Consider that some previously unexplained illnesses may be caused by these hazards.

Monitor the amount of radiation children are exposed to through x-ray films and the precautions taken, such as covering genitalia.

Work with community officials to locate potential hazards.

Know federal regulatory agencies as well as local ones and the roles they play in monitoring the environment:
- Environmental Protection Agency (EPA)
- Department of Labor–Occupational Safety and Health Administration (OSHA)
- Nuclear Regulatory Commission (NRC)
- Consumer Product Safety Commission
- Department of Transportation–National Highway Traffic Safety Administration
- Treasury Department–Bureau of Alcohol, Tobacco, and Firearms
- Department of Agriculture–Food Safety and Quality Service
- Department of Health and Human Services–Food and Drug Administration (FDA)
  - Centers for Disease Control (CDC)
  - National Institute for Occupational Safety and Health (NIOSH)
  - National Institute of Environmental Health Sciences (NIEHS)
  - National Cancer Institute (NCI)

community. Adequate social functioning is vital to the child's well-being during these years, since it often is the foundation for future relationships. The child is exposed to a variety of societal roles and interactions, the process of *socialization*. As socialization occurs, the child develops *social competence*, the ability and skills to participate effectively in the social interactions of society. This competence includes both the obvious social behaviors and an inner understanding of the appropriateness of behaviors.

Several elements play a role in the development of the child's social competence. The child's desire for a sense of industry encourages interactions, positive relationships, and accomplishments within society. Cognitive development is needed to understand relationships and to be able to problem solve. Moral judgment is needed for the child to understand consequences and fairness in relationships. Understanding and obeying authority is needed to maintain order in society. Social sensitivity is learned through social interactions and requires the child's ability to perceive the social cues of others, to understand the roles of others, and to communicate verbally with them. Social behaviors are also a part of social competence; these most often are learned through the imitation, role modeling, and reinforcement of others' behaviors. The interaction of all these elements produces a level of social competence in the child and simultaneously plays a role in the child's perception of himself; individuals frequently see themselves as others see them. Thus social competence and self-identify are closely related.[2]

ROLE AND RELATIONSHIP PATTERN

Families provide the child with a sense of security from the external environment. Within this safe setting the child begins to cope with the outside world. Families encourage the child's cognitive growth by exposing him to a variety of experiences and by instilling in him a desire to achieve.

Parents and children play many roles with each other and interact in a variety of ways; attachment, love, and companionship usually exist between them. Parents protect the dependent child and teach the learning child. The parent-child relationship is not completely equal, since parents are the authority figures who establish the rules needed for the functioning of the family and the safety and growth of the child. During the school-age years the child's increasing maturity, independence, and responsibility may begin to decrease the amount of parental authority.[32]

The school-age child begins to broaden her interests outside of the home, often encouraged by parents. Unfortunately, the child may become involved in so many activities that it becomes stressful for both child and parents. Intense relationships of earlier years must become less intense; family schedules and patterns are altered by the child's changing world. Studies have found that both mothers and fathers find this a difficult family period, with the lowest parental contentment with family life and with children occurring when the oldest child is between ages 6 and 13.

The relationships between *siblings* vary, depending on birth order, sex, and age differences. Sibling interactions have been studied in terms of outcomes such as intelligence and power. Siblings interact with each other in a number of roles, as playmates, teacher-learner, protector-dependent, and adversaries. The conflicts of

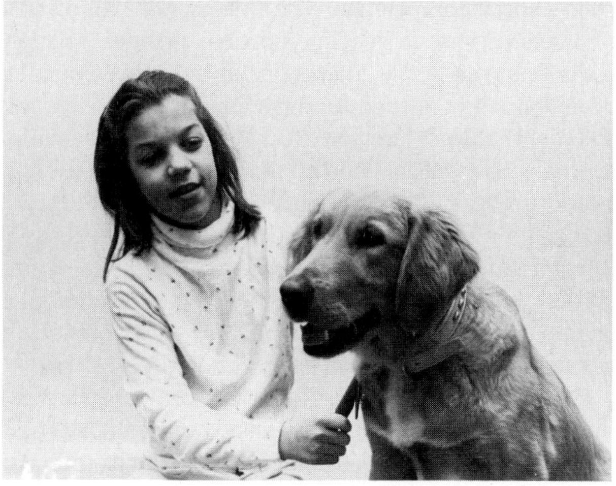

Fig. 20-7. As school-age children mature, they are able to take on more responsibilities, such as having pets. (Photograph by Douglas Bloomquist.)

siblings are expected, a result of feelings of jealousy and rivalry (see Chapter 18). School-age children can cope better with these feelings than preschool children, since they have outlets outside the family, including school and friends. Parents can minimize these conflicts by trying to understand each child's needs and level of maturity.[32]

As children mature, they take on more responsibilities within the family and the community. School-age children can learn responsibility for money, household chores, self-care, or pets (Fig. 20-7). This is the age when families often give allowances or children earn money through chores or small jobs such as paper routes.

The purpose of limit setting with children is to teach the child behaviors that are acceptable within society. Parents use many methods and philosophies of limit setting with varying degrees of effectiveness. However, some generally accepted concepts are applicable to the school-age child. Clear limits and expectations make it easier for the child to comply. Parents who express their feelings, explain why things happen, and listen to their children encourage the development of self-control. The child's self-esteem should be protected by constructive limit setting. Children model their behavior after the behavior of those they love: parents, friends, and other adults. Positive reinforcement, (such as rewarding the child for good behavior) is an effective form of limit setting. Punishment, a negative reinforcement, may stop an undesired behavior, but often only until the child can repeat the action and not be caught. Some families with school-age children find it helpful to have periodic family meetings where everyone discusses family issues, rules, and responsibilities. This cooperative effort results in increased understanding.[32]

Sexual Abuse. Unfortunately, relationships between children and adults, even their parents, are not always positive. Sexual abuse is a serious health problem that is becoming increasingly more apparent. The problem has been and frequently still is hidden, partly because (1) the child may be frightened or unable to talk about the situation, (2) families and society are reluctant to admit its existence, and (3) few agencies have handled these cases. This is changing, although slowly. Statistics on the number of American children assaulted are estimates only. Approximately 1 in 10 incidents are reported. The figure may be close to 750,000 children assaulted each year.

This type of abuse includes any sexual contact with a child; intercourse per se does not need to occur. The child is forced into the act by verbal threats, physical force, or offers of treats. Eighty percent of children know the person abusing them; one third of all cases involve the child's father; and many other abusers are relatives, family friends, baby-sitters, or others seen by the child as authority persons. The combination of the person's force and authority makes the child believe he has no power or choice. The child may think she must comply for a variety of reasons, such as to be good or to keep the family together. The feelings are complex and change as the child grows. Fear may give way to embarrassment and anger. Of the cases reported, 90% involve girls, although more boys may be abused than are reported. Cases of recurrent abuse often begin around age 6 years and continue until adolescence, when the child has more ability to either stop, change, or leave the situation. The long-term effects are usually serious. In adulthood these children often are depressed, unable to have trusting relationships, and likely to develop sexual and marital problems.

Nurses can help these children by recognizing those who are possibly experiencing abuse, and helping these children obtain assistance. A comprehensive list of characteristics that suggest sexual abuse (see the box on p. 531) can be used as an aid in identifying these families.

If a child is suspected of being sexually abused, an indepth interview and examination needs to be carried out by someone aware of how to approach the child and what to look for during the examination. Most authorities believe that children who describe sexual abuse are telling the truth, since the details are usually very specific and the trauma evident. Therefore a child's story should be believed until proved otherwise. This is an extremely complicated problem that is dealt with most effectively by a multidisciplinary team approach.[15]

COMMUNITY RELATIONSHIPS

The strongest relationships school-age children develop outside their families are with their *peers,* other children they encounter in their neighborhood and at

❑ ❑ SUGGESTIONS FOR IDENTIFYING SCHOOL-AGE VICTIMS OF SEXUAL ASSAULT

Family characteristics

Family secretive about many things
Antisocial behavior exhibited by family members
Poor impulse control shown by father
Signs of violence toward children
History of physical or sexual abuse of parents
Isolation of family in community; few friends
Denial of any trouble to the outside world; boundaries are rigid to outsiders but virtually nonexistent within the family

Characteristics of mother

Passive, easily manipulated
Dependent on daughter to assume maternal or marital role
Unable to contemplate severing relationship with man involved in the abuse for fear of losing the relationship, financial support, or sexual contact
Possesses poor self-image

Characteristics of father or other authority figure

Domineering and overpowering
Shows poor impulse control
Abuses alcohol
Was abused as a child
Denies that anything has happened
Tends to blame child or mother for what is happening

Behavioral signs in younger children

Fecal soiling
Regression in development milestones
Explicit knowledge of sexual acts
Excessive masturbation
Anxiety about being left alone with a particular person or about visiting a particular person
Open sexual behavior after age 6 or 7

Medical identification

Extreme distrust and fear of physicians or examinations
Somatic complaints (headache, stomachache)
Persistent sore throat resulting from gonorrhea
Sudden onset of bedwetting, day or night
Vaginal, rectal, or any genital discharge or irritation
Preoccupation with anatomy and an explicit knowledge of sexual behavior

School-associated identification

Depression or withdrawal
Hyperactivity and an inability to pay attention to school tasks; frequently labeled as "learning disabled"
Arrival at school very early
Afraid to go home; staying at school after everyone has gone
Poor self-image
Poor performance in school
Inability to get involved in any school activities because of inappropriate, heavy responsibilities at home

Adapted from Dennis LB, Hassol J: *Introduction to human development and health issues,* Philadelphia, 1983, WB Saunders.

school. Peers act as a new social system, becoming increasingly influential in the child's life. Children learn values, behaviors, and attitudes from their peer group, as they did from their families.[2] All children continue to be influenced significantly by their family, the culture of the family, and many other environmental factors, but the peer group now begins to influence lifestyle, habits, and speech patterns and formulates standards of behavior and performance. The standards of the peer group become vitally important, and all efforts are made to conform; it becomes more important to be accepted by the peer group than by anyone else. Conforming to the pressures of peers becomes an issue, especially when it interferes with the parents' expectations.

Children begin to face that their own goals, desires, and aspirations might be very different from those held by the peer group or the school, and they must find some way to cope and to perform according to the new standards if they are to succeed. Their success or failure may be judged more harshly among peers than they were previously among the family group. Whereas the devastation of failure with the group may be more severe than any they have experienced before, the feelings of success that come when they achieve group approval is a powerful and gratifying experience. The degree to which children are able to fit in socially, to make the adjustment, to learn to cope, and to receive satisfaction from the group is a powerful determinant of healthy socialization.

One type of relationship that develops between children is *friendship*. Three stages of friendship development have been described:

1. At the time the child enters school, friends are likely to be chosen based on specific acts or behaviors that the child identifies as pleasant or good. A single transgression perceived by the child can quickly change the child's feeling of friendship association, but in turn friendship can be readily reestablished by acts of good will between the children.
2. By about age 9 or 10, the child begins to sense the constant traits of trustworthiness in other children

and to identify as the basis for friendship those indications of a more consistent trustworthiness.

3. Toward the end of later childhood friends are selected because of a feeling of mutual understanding and willingness to assist with one another's innermost struggles.[2]

A child may have only one best friend or several important friends. Groups that form during this age are flexible and changing and may be goal directed, such as a sports team. These groups often have set rules or rituals that join the members. One notable aspect of the friendships and groups that develop during the school-age years is the tendency toward same-sex relationships. Certainly children have friends of the opposite sex, but the focus is clearly on friendships of the same sex. Later in the school-age years the development of heterosexual relationships begins with the first signs of dating and mixed parties.

School-age children become increasingly involved with adults outside the family, including teachers, coaches, and others, who become role models, influencing the child's view of the world and himself. Although this influence may not seem to be as significant as the child's peers, long-term ideas and beliefs often develop from these relationships. Children usually perceive some similarity between themselves and their models, who are often of the same sex with similar physical or behavioral traits. During these years children may or may not maintain a strong identification with the parent of the same sex, but they also tend to adopt other adult models with whom they can identify.[2]

CULTURE

The school-age child is more aware of the culture in which he or she lives than the younger child. Aspects of the American culture that the child must deal with include poverty and affluence, ethnic groups, working parents and day care, and the power of television.

Poverty. In the United States more than 17% (10.7 million) of children less than 18 years of age are in families whose incomes are below *poverty* level. Family conditions frequently associated with poverty include unemployment, inadequate housing, poor housing sanitation, poor nutrition, low educational levels, and difficult access to health and social services. The effects of this on children include higher mortality rates at all ages than those who are not poor and more days lost from school because of illnesses. Health care often is received sporadically without consistent coordination. For the school-age child poverty may influence all aspects of life, for example:

Physical Processes.

1. Poor nutrition, which can result in iron deficiency anemia, retarded growth, and other disorders
2. Poor dental care, which can result in caries and other diseases of the mouth
3. Poor health care, which can result in undetected or untreated problems, such as otitis media or strep throat.

Psychologic Processes.

1. School difficulties resulting from a variety of problems, such as poor health, sensory deficits not corrected, turmoil at home, or peer rejection
2. Poor coping strategies, such as depression or aggression from overwhelming stresses at home
3. Poor self-perception, resulting from lack of positive adult reinforcement or positive life experiences

Environmental Processes.

1. Accidents from unsafe home and neighborhood conditions
2. Other potential health hazards from environmental conditions, such as peeling paint and lead poisoning
3. Abuse and neglect from parents under stress who cannot cope

Nurses interacting with poor families and their children should know the many resources available to help them, as discussed in previous chapters. Signs of abuse, neglect, coping difficulties, and other health problems also need to be identified and appropriate measures taken. The nurse working with these children can intervene by helping these children in some way to succeed in something to give them a positive feeling for themselves. A relationship with a good adult role model or strong peer interactions can help accomplish this. Children from poor families who have strong family relationships that help them develop a positive self-image tend to do better socially over time.

Affluence. The social milieu opposite poverty, affluence, has not been examined or discussed with the same frequency as poverty. Children of the extremely rich are also potentially at risk for problems with development or health. Some aspects of great wealth that might have negative effects on the child include[3,16]

1. Frequent parental absences and subsequent weak family relationships; for the school-age child this may mean many years of boarding school separations
2. Frequent substitute caretakers of varying degrees of quality
3. Extremely high and often unrealistic parental expectations of the child to achieve in areas such as sports, academics, and social settings
4. Availability of many material possessions, with little awareness of choices or responsibilities involved
5. Often easy access to cars, drugs, and alcohol and their potential dangers

Nurses may have an opportunity to intervene with these families, but probably less frequently than with poor families; when possible, guidance to these parents should include

1. The importance and function of the role of parent, including love and support
2. The need to set realistic limits for appropriate behavior
3. The need to give their children clear values and responsibilities
4. Help in recognizing their individual child's abilities and needs and responding accordingly

There are two points to remember in discussing the children of poverty or affluence. First, many variables are involved for each child; all children are not influenced in the same way by their circumstances. Second, although the effects of both factors can be severe, the problems of affluence are probably easier to overcome than the all-pervasive problems of poverty.[21]

Ethnic Groups. Whereas preschool children notice racial and ethnic differences, school-age children are increasingly *aware* of these differences. This is a time when attitudes toward race develop, based on family and community attitudes. Studies of children 5 to 7 years of age show that the majority already identify with and prefer to play with those of their own race. Nurses must be aware of this identification and help develop it positively. Although prejudice exists, school-age children can be helped to see all groups more favorably, focusing on similar and positive aspects.[2]

Working Parents. Studies have shown that at least 50% of mothers with children between ages 6 and 17 work, and two thirds work full-time.

Many children return from school to a home without adult supervision. Many follow specific patterns, which may include beginning dinner in anticipation of their parents' return.

Parents and school-age children are often in conflict about how old is "old enough" to be home alone or with an older sibling. Although the school-age child may consider it a real marker of maturity to be home alone, recent research has raised some issues for consideration. Children who must look after themselves after school are significantly more isolated, reporting fewer opportunities to play outside or have friends visit. Children cared for by a sibling may be at risk for negative effects on self-esteem and social development.

Nurses can give guidance to families who must deal with the issue of after-school care for school-age children (see box on this page).

Television. Television is an integral part of and major influence in our culture. By the time the average child has finished high school, he has watched 15,000 hours of television, compared to 11,000 hours spent in school. Unfortunately, many TV programs and commercials can be harmful to children. In recent years consumer groups and health professionals have looked critically at TV's effect on children through various research studies. Areas of major concern have been the violence children see, commercials during children's programming, the unrealistic world depicted, and the passivity of TV viewing.

Violent acts are certainly a part of our society, but the statistics regarding TV violence are frightening. By the time the average child is 18 years old, he or she will have seen approximately 18,000 acts of TV violence, averaging 1 per minute in a typical cartoon. The violence during 1 hour of a children's program is on the average 6 times greater than in 1 hour of an adult program. Researchers have come to several conclusions:[16]

❑ ❑ SUGGESTIONS FOR AFTER-SCHOOL CARE OF SCHOOL-AGE CHILDREN

- Each child should be assessed to decide the appropriate after-school supervision. One 10-year-old might be able to be alone; another may not be ready. The child should play a role in this discussion, but the parents should make the decision.
- Alternatives may be considered: day-care homes, neighbors, other family members, older siblings, or after-school programs. Many public schools are beginning to develop day-care programs for older children before and after school.
- If the child is alone, a set schedule should be discussed with the child. This may include when the child should be home and whether or not a parent should be called.
- Specific guidelines should be discussed, such as after-school activities, use of television, whether or not playmates can enter the home, and where the child may or may not go.
- Emergency measures should be planned with the child; what to do if the child is sick, loses the key, or has a problem at home. Plans should include how to reach both a parent and another responsible adult.
- The child should be cautioned regarding strangers, including when he or she is coming home from school and when persons knock on the door or call on the phone.
- Time should be set aside for the parents and child to periodically discuss the arrangements to assess if they are appropriate for the child and the family.

1. All agree that watching TV violence results in increased aggressive behavior in children. One study suggested that school-age children are more affected in their aggressive actions than other age-groups.
2. Children learn new forms of violence from violent programs.
3. Because children are exposed to so much TV violence, they begin to show less emotional sensitivity when aggressive acts really occur in their lives.
4. Children become socialized, expecting and accepting aggressive behavior.

One positive note is that adults who discuss violence with children, pointing out that it goes against their own principles and results in pain, can help inhibit some aggression.[32]

The average child in our culture sees about 350,000 commercials by age 18 years. During 1 hour an average of 15 commercials, 5 program announcements, and 2 public service messages appear. The leading products advertised during children's shows are toys, cereals, candies, and fast-food restaurants. More than half of the commercials are for food, many of which are sugared foods potentially harmful to teeth and overall nutrition. Children, especially those under age 8, often cannot separate the program from the commercials and may believe they must buy what the TV people tell them to buy. Many families experience struggles and conflicts between children who want what they see and parents who must set limits. Authorities question the ethics of exposing children to any type of advertising. Interestingly, many of the earliest children's shows had no advertising; instead they were supported by the stations. This is an area in which our culture seems to have moved backwards.

The world presented on television does not reflect the real world accurately. In general three fourths of the characters seen on evening dramas are white, American males between ages 30 and 60. Others, including children, the elderly, women, and racial minorities, are underrepresented and stereotyped. Occupations tend to be oriented toward business, health, and law enforcement. Children identify their role models through play and fantasy with adults. Unfortunately, television presents many inappropriate role models in an unrealistic representation of our society.[32]

The hours children spend watching TV, as stated, is impressively high. Watching TV is a passive act. Many believe that children are taking time from either more active or more creative pursuits such as exercise and reading to sit in front of the television.

There are some positive aspects of TV viewing. A number of children's programs, such as *Mr. Rogers' Neighborhood* for younger children and *Call it Macaroni* for older children, are cognitively and developmentally appropriate for the children they want to reach. Unfortunately, these are still too few, and they are often only seen on public broadcasting stations.

❑ ❑ SUGGESTIONS FOR PROMOTING HEALTHY TELEVISION VIEWING IN CHILDREN

- Parents should be encouraged to watch TV shows with their children, explain and discuss them, reinforce what was learned, and discuss moral issues.
- Most children decide what they are going to watch; parents should play a more guiding role.
- Parents should evaluate programs: Are they age-appropriate, are the people and roles positive? Are the social issues at the child's level? Do they encourage values?
- The amount of time spent viewing television should be limited since other activities, including school, may suffer.

The fact is that television is here to stay, and our society must learn how to live with it. If used appropriately, television can be a valuable learning tool and a positive force for children.

Nurses and other health professionals need to consider assessment of TV consumption and promotion of good viewing habits as part of health care. The nurse can make suggestions to help promote better viewing habits and to teach more critical viewing (see the box above).

Nurses can play a broader role in TV programming for children through the groups that have been formed to monitor the presentation and development of such programs. The largest and one of the most active is

Action for Children's Television
46 Austin St.
Newtonville, MA 02160

LEGISLATION

Throughout this chapter laws beneficial to the health and well-being of the school-age child are discussed. These laws include safety measures such as product guidelines and flame-retardant clothes, and nutritional guidelines such as the school lunch programs. Another major law affecting school-age children is mandatory public education for handicapped children.

Public Law 94-142, put into practice in 1977, states that all handicapped children must receive appropriate public education. The ages of children served is 5 to 21 years, with many states beginning services at 3 years. Each child with special needs has the right to have an evaluation by school and/or health professionals, who then develop an individual educational plan (IEP) for that child. This law has done a great deal in responding to the educational needs of many children who were lost in the past.

Problems with P.L. 94-142 include (1) the cost to truly meet all the needs of all the children may be overwhelming; (2) too much paperwork is frequently involved; and (3) school systems may not have the appropriate qualified professionals or the money needed for the many support services. Other problems lie in defining "handicap" and an "appropriate education." Parents frequently are overwhelmed by the process involved in developing an IEP for their child. Others worry that the education of normal or gifted children will suffer because of the time and money committed to the handicapped. Nevertheless, the value of this law has made most involved believe strongly that the problems can be dealt with and that all children can benefit from it.[21]

Nurses involved with school-age children, primarily school nurses, have been active in the implementing of this law. The school nurse's role is discussed later in this chapter, but some suggestions for nurses specific to P.L. 94-142 are listed in the box below.

Many other laws to help the school-age child involve a variety of federal and local agencies; some are discussed in the following section.

NURSING INTERVENTIONS FOR HEALTH PROMOTION

The challenge for nurses working with school-age children is to maintain them in their normally healthy states and to prevent the development of illness, when possible. This is done through a variety of health promotion mechanisms, such as examination, guidance, education, and legislation. The school-age child is capable of playing an active role in personal health care and needs to be motivated to seek health and use various resources to attain, maintain, or regain optimum health. Aspects of the nursing process can be used effectively in various situations to maintain the child's health (assessing immunization status), promote health habits (teaching bicycle safety), and prevent illness (obtaining throat cultures for strep throat).

Nurses have many opportunities and settings in which to carry out their interventions; nurses and school-age children are able to interact during well-child evaluations and at school. Nurses in other roles, such as public health nurses and hospital nurses, also can play a role in health promotion, although these nurses often must focus more on helping the child and his family deal with an illness or crisis. Local and national groups affect the health of children through their activities and regulations and include organizations such as Boy and Girl Scouts, Big Brothers and Sisters, charities such as the Red Cross, and government agencies such as the Consumer Product Safety Commission. All these groups have a place for active nursing involvement, as a consultant, board member, or as child advocate.

❑ ❑ NURSING INTERVENTIONS TO PROMOTE P.L. 94-142

Know the process involved for the individual state.
Help identify children who require special educational services, especially preschool children.
Know the local school personnel work with special educational placements.
Be involved in assessing; taking histories, interviewing parents, and observing in the classroom.
Know the local support services available for referral.
Help parents understand the problems their child is having and the IEP for their child.
Become involved in local groups associated with children who have handicaps or learning problems.

Well-Child Care

The American Academy of Pediatrics recommends in their Standards of Child Health Care that children 6 years and older have a well-child examination at least every 2 years.[6] These examinations generally are done either by physicians or nurse practitioners. In the ideal situation the child has a primary health care provider, one person or practice where the child receives wellness care and the majority of illness care, and the remainder of his care is coordinated. Unfortunately, many American children still do not have this quality of care.

Table 20-6 gives an example of a possible health maintenance protocol for this age. Certainly not all areas are covered for each child at every visit. This type of protocol can be used by providers as a guide to the most important age-related issues about which information is obtained and guidance or education is given as needed for the individual child. The health history, physical examination, observations, general discussion, developmental tests, and laboratory tests done for all children can be added to discussions with others, such as a teacher or counselor, to obtain the information and data regarding the school-age child.

The nurse needs to encourage the school-age child to be an active member of the evaluation along with the parents. Children can give some of their own history, answer questions, and discuss their health concerns.

Table 20-6.* Health maintenance during the school-age period

Age (years)	Physiologic processes	Psychologic processes	Environment/social processes
6-9	Height, weight Blood pressure Dental–caries, bites, use of fluoride Diet–snacks Enuresis Exercise–motor skills, level of activity, attention Sleep patterns Vision and hearing screening	School level, adjustment, and progress Developmental level, including speech, cognitive level Stresses in child's life, coping patterns Self-care, hygiene Masturbation, homosexual play	Safety–use of seat belts, water safety, bicycles Immunizations reviewed and updated Responsibilities for household tasks, money, school work Relations with parents, siblings, peers, other adults Family activities Discipline After-school care Use of television Outside activities
9-12	Same as for ages 6-9 plus: Posture, scoliosis Menarche, stage of sexual development Acne	Same as for ages 6-9 plus: Habits such as drugs, alcohol, smoking Sexual activity	Same as for ages 6-9 plus: Time and place for privacy

*Includes areas for which information should be obtained through history, examination, observation, tests, and so on and guidance or education given.

During examinations the child's privacy should be respected. Some children in this age group want a parent present during their examination; others do not. If possible, spending at least some time alone with the child can be helpful. The examinations can also be a time for education of how the body works and how to keep it healthy. Information needs to be obtained on the child's school adjustment and performance, since this is a major portion of the child's life. School performance may reflect the child's cognitive and general development. If there are any concerns, the nurse will need to obtain more information through separate testing or discussion with school officials. Health education should be directed to both the child and parents for the best results. Activities that the child performs alone and together with the family can give a picture of relationships and adjustments.

School and the Nurse

As an integral part of the total community, the school system has specific responsibilities in health care and planning to provide a healthful school environment, an adequate school health service, and a comprehensive health education program. School systems vary greatly in the extent to which they fulfill these roles and agree that these are real functions of the school. Most schools take specific steps to ensure a level of safety and cleanliness in the environment, but an individual school may represent either extreme in providing a healthy physical and emotional environment. School health service in the United States and other countries also varies greatly. In some areas nurses, physicians, and other health care workers are integrally involved in the school health program, which includes health care and maintenance as well as education. In other areas the school health program considers educational aspects only. Programs range from an occasional mention of body care and the changes of puberty to a full program integrating physical and mental health principles into all aspects of the educational experience. (See Table 20-7.)

Although the ideal role of the school in providing health care remains a matter of debate, the school *does* influence and participate in children's health and well-being.[7] As they begin to spend an increasingly greater percentage of their waking hours in and around the school, this environment begins to exert an influence on their lives that at times may outweigh the current influence of the home. The attitudes that the school conveys in regard to health and well-being begin to influence children's attitudes, contributing to the shaping and formulation of the concept of health.

Comprehensive school health services require an interdisciplinary, coordinated effort between health care providers and educators. The nurse, either from the community or within the school, is often in a position to plan and direct comprehensive health care services for school-age children. These services should include

1. Planning direct health maintenance
2. Screening and health care for problems that interfere with the learning process
3. Providing nursing services for children with health problems

***Table 20-7.* Topics for health education during the school-age period**

Topic	Specific discussion areas
Nutrition education	Concept of basic four food groups Foods associated with dental caries Essential nutrients and their function Healthy snack foods
Body hygiene	Value of skin care, bathing, and grooming Care of minor skin injuries Hair care Dental care
Exercise and physical fitness	Physical fitness and sports programs Body mechanics, coordination Sleep and rest needs Prevention of injuries
Prevention of illness and accidents	Accident prevention with burns Water safety Life-saving instruction Bicycle and pedestrian safety Concepts of virus and bacterial illness Body defenses against disease Protection of vision; monitoring eye strain Protection of hearing; monitoring exposure to loud noises
Human sexuality	Community and parental awareness Consideration of sex role biases in society Preparation for the changes of puberty Ranges of normal changes that occur in puberty Life cycle changes Age appropriate information on AIDS
Prevention of drug abuse	Information about drugs, specifically tobacco, alcohol, street drugs Why people use drugs to cope or feel "grown up" General discussion about feelings and availability of drugs Healthy alternatives that can be used for coping

4. Coordinating referral services
5. Planning and implementing actions to ensure a healthy physical and emotional milieu for the school
6. Planning and participating in the health education curriculum

The role and responsibilities of each nurse depend on many factors in the particular setting, but some or all of these services are included.

Planning the *health maintenance* for the children of a school varies, depending on the type of health maintenance program. In one system the school nurses may try to ensure that each child has a primary source of health care, whereas in another system the school's nurse practitioners may be the primary providers. School nurses, for example, have monitored and updated the immunizations of children and identified children with potential health problems, such as scoliosis or strep throat. In either setting the school nurse needs to work collaboratively with the school's physician and the community physicians.

For many years school nurses have screened children for vision and hearing problems at regular intervals to detect children who were at a disadvantage in the classroom. With the passage of P.L. 94-142, nurses have expanded their role in identifying and caring for children with *learning problems.* Now school nurses frequently work closely with other school professionals in evaluating children whose school performance seems to indicate a problem, which is sometimes a physical one. The evaluating team often includes teachers, educational specialists, psychologists, physicians, and nurses. The role the nurse plays with the team in developing and implementing the child's IEP varies. Some school nurses have developed assessment tools that provide information to the team on the child's health, family interactions, and the family's perceptions of the problem. Interviews and home visits with the parents and child have been incorporated into these assessments.

Nurses in schools frequently see children with *minor illnesses.* Policies regarding the management of minor illnesses and accidents at school vary widely from state to state, community to community, and school to school. The nurse should be aware of all state and local laws and policies that affect the scope of nursing activity in the school and consider the legal implications of all such activities. Some systems allow only first-aid treatment and then referral to the child's physician. Other schools have developed standard protocols for the management of common problems. These protocols include guidelines on carrying out an adequate history and physical assessment, developing an acceptable plan of management, and consulting with the school physician. No matter what intervention the nurse takes, the child's parents need to be informed.

Not all health problems of children in school are minor. With the mainstreaming of children with handicapping conditions, nurses now may be involved in administering prescribed medications, watching for side effects, monitoring skin care, and performing various other nursing care acts.

Children with multiple health problems, as well as other children, often need the many services they receive *coordinated.* Since children spend much time in schools and often school professionals along with families recognize children's needs, the school nurse is an ideal person to make referrals and follow up on the recommendations. This process is most valuable when done with the parents, allowing them to take the primary responsibility while the nurse acts as a resource and advocate.

The school nurse can also play a role in developing a *healthy environment* for children at the school. A specific program for the prevention of accidents in and around the school should be planned by the school health care team. The school environment needs to be periodically evaluated for sources of health hazards. Potential health hazards include pedestrian and automobile traffic patterns, broken playground and classroom equipment, ice and snow, poorly maintained toilet facilities, and inappropriately prepared food. Fire prevention is usually mandatory by law and includes regular fire drills to acquaint teachers and students with the procedures used in the event of fire. Chemical hazards should be watched for as well.

The social milieu of the school is also important in providing a healthy environment. The social interactions of the children need to be watched and positive social relationships promoted. However, despite all efforts to provide for optimum social interactions, reinforcement from the group, and assistance with group interactions and coping with group stress, social problems continue to constitute a major concern for many children during this period. They may experience difficulty in making the initial transition away from the family and in establishing dependency and satisfaction from the group of peers. They may make the initial adjustment but then continue to interact with friends and adults in a relatively immature fashion, failing to form increasing mature social judgments and ways of interacting. When problems such as these arise, an evaluation of the underlying cause is needed. Nurses frequently find that these problems require the evaluation and support of a team of the school's health and educational professionals.

Encouragement of the school-age child's growing ability to serve as his or her own agent in health care provides the major thrust for *health education programs* in schools. The child needs adequate knowledge of all dimensions of health to make responsible choices to protect his or her health and to seek health care services when needed. Health education programs vary greatly, although all should be comprehensive, interesting, and age-appropriate. Whatever program is implemented in a school, the nurse should play an active role in developing, presenting, and evaluating the program. Areas frequently covered in the school-age levels are presented in Table 20-7.

SUMMARY

Many changes occur in children during the exciting period of the school-age years. The child's overall development progresses from the immaturity of the preschooler to the beginning of adolescence and eventual adulthood. The child's cognitive abilities increase dramatically, adding to the desire to master tasks and the ability to develop moral judgment. The child's world expands beyond the family unit as school and peers begin to exert a major influence. Opportunities for nurses to aid children during this period occur primarily in ambulatory settings, with the school nurse often the most effective and influential health care provider for this age group.

References

1. American Psychiatric Association: *Diagnostic and statistical manual of mental disorders,* ed 3, revised (DSM-III-R), Washington, DC, 1987, The Association.
2. Berger KS: *The developing person through childhood and adolescence,* ed 3, New York, 1991, Worth Publishing.
3. Berman BD, et al: After-school child care and self esteem in school age children, *Pediatrics* 89(4):654-659, 1992.
4. Berry R: Home care of the child with AIDS, *Pediatr Nurs* 14(4):341, 1988.
5. Committee on Infectious Diseases, American Academy of Pediatrics: Report of the commitee (Redbook), ed 22, Elk Grove, Ill, 1991, The Academy.
6. Committee on Practice and Ambulatory Medicine, American Academy of Pediatrics: Recommendations for preventive pediatric health care, *Pediatrics* 81(3):466, 1988.
7. Committee on School Health, American Academy of Pediatrics: *School health: a guide for health professionals,* 1987 ed, Elk Grove, Ill, 1987, The Academy.
8. Erikson EH: *Childhood and society,* ed 2, New York, 1986, WW Norton.
9. Erikson EH: *Identity, youth and crisis,* ed 35, New York, 1986, WW Norton.
10. Falkner F, Tanner J: *Human growth,* ed 2, New York, 1986, Plenum Press.
11. Graef JW: *Environmental toxins.* In Levine MD, et al: *Developmental-behavioral pediatrics,* Philadelphia, 1983, WB Saunders.
12. Guyton AC: *Textbook of medical physiology,* ed 8, Philadelphia, 1991, WB Saunders.
13. Hancock L: Safe biking–a bike helmet, *J Pediatr Health Care* 1(9):344, 1987.
14. Hetherington EM, Arasteh JD, eds: *Impact of divorce, single parenting and step-parenting on children,* Hillsdale, NJ, 1988, Lawrence Erlbaum.
15. Hockelman R, et al: *Primary pediatric care,* ed 2, St Louis, 1992, Mosby.
16. Reference deleted in proofs.
17. Hurley RM: Enuresis: the difference between night and day, *Pediatr Rev* 12(6):167-170, 1990.
18. Kohlberg L: *Development of moral character and moral ideology.* In Hoffman ML, Hoffman LW, eds: *Review of child development research, vol 1,* New York, 1964, Russell Sage Foundation.
19. Kohlberg, L: *The philosophy of moral develoment,* San Francisco, 1981, Harper & Row.
20. Kronmiller I, Nirschl R: Preventive dentistry for children, *Pediatr Nurs* 11(6):446, 1985.
21. Levine MD, et al: *Developmental-behavioral pediatrics,* Philadelphia, 1983, WB Saunders.
22. Maul-Mellott S, Adams J: *Childhood cancer, a nursing overview,* Boston, 1987, Jones & Bartlett.

23. Piaget J: *The language and the thought of the child,* New York, 1965, World Publishing.
24. Piaget J, Inhelder B: *The psychology of the child,* New York, 1969, Basic Books.
25. Piaget J: *The theory of stages in cognitive development,* New York, 1969, McGraw-Hill.
26. Pipes PL: *Nutrition in infancy and childhood,* ed 4, St Louis, 1989, Mosby.
27. Pulaski MA: *Understanding Piaget–an introduction to children's cognitive development,* New York, 1971, Harper & Row.
28. Silver AA, Hagen RA: *Disorders of learning in childhood,* New York, 1990, John Wiley & Sons.
29. Sinclair D: *Human growth after birth,* ed 4, New York, 1985, Oxford University Press.
30. Sprague-McRae JM: Encopresis: developmental, behavioral and physiological considerations for treatment, *Nurs Pract* 15(6):8-24, 1990.
31. Task force on blood pressure control in children, National Heart, Lung and Blood Pressure Institute: Report of the second task force on blood pressure control in children, *Pediatrics* 79(1):1, 1987.
32. Webster-Stratton C: *The incredible years: a trouble shooting guide for parents of children aged 3-8,* Toronto, 1992, Umbrella Press.

CHAPTER

21

Adolescent*

Jan Schurman

Lois A. Hancock

Gail Park Fast

Katherine E. Murphy

Objectives

After completing this chapter, the nurse will be able to

- *Explain to a group of young adolescents the expected body changes of puberty.*
- *Describe the stages in the development of secondary sexual characteristics of adolescents.*
- *Plan several nutritious menus for adolescents, taking into account their nutrient needs and food preferences.*
- *Discuss with a group of adolescents the course and treatment of acne.*
- *Contrast the cognitive abilities of the adolescent with those of the school-age child.*
- *Summarize Erikson's earlier stages of development, which are restaged as the adolescent establishes identity.*
- *Contrast the adaptive and maladaptive coping mechanisms commonly used by the adolescent.*
- *Contrast the various stages of moral development that could be represented in a group of 15-year-olds.*
- *Summarize the nurse's role in primary and secondary prevention of drug use and misuse by the adolescent.*
- *Discuss with a group of adolescents the pros and cons of sexual activity, pregnancy, and contraception.*
- *Discuss some current legislative issues that affect adolescents.*

*Material in this chapter related to the prevention or treatment of cancer was contributed by Marilyn Frank-Stromborg and Rebecca Cohen.

The period of adolescence, as with other developmental stages, is impossible to define in exact chronologic terms; it often is defined as beginning with the onset of puberty and ending with the achievement of a certain level of maturity. These landmarks are difficult to identify, however, and do not adequately describe the many complex factors that comprise adolescence in Western cultures. Adolescence may be conceptualized most appropriately as the period during which emancipation from the primary family unit is the central task of the individual.

The term *puberty* is used here to denote the period that involves the development and maturation of the reproductive, endocrine, and structural systems. *Adolescence,* on the other hand, refers to the period characterized by the psychologic, emotional, and social changes that result in the transition from child to adult. Adolescence usually begins just before puberty and lasts until adult roles and responsibilities are assumed. Cultural and social class variations are seen in the time of the end of adolescence. The college-bound adolescent generally holds moratorium on adulthood and has an extended adolescence while in school. The non–college-bound adolescent more quickly enters the adult world. The adolescent, who is in some ways a child and in other ways an adult, can present the greatest challenge to the nurse who is attempting to provide age-appropriate health care guidance and teaching (see box below).

HEALTHY PEOPLE 2000

SELECTED NATIONAL HEALTH PROMOTION AND DISEASE PREVENTION OBJECTIVES

ADOLESCENT

- Reduce dental caries (cavities) so that the proportion of children with one or more caries is no more than 60% among adolescents aged 15 (1986-1987 baseline: 78% of adolescents aged 15)
- Reduce untreated dental caries so that the proportion of children with untreated caries is no more than 15% among adolescents aged 15 (1986-1987 baseline: 23% of adolescents)
- Increase calcium intake so at least 50% of youth aged 12 through 24 and 50% of pregnant and lactating women consume three or more servings daily of food rich in calcium (1985-1986 baseline: 7% of women and 14% of men consumed three or more servings)
- Reduce overweight to a prevalence of no more than 15% among adolescents aged 12 through 19 (Baseline: 15% for adolescents aged 12 through 19 in 1976-1980)
- Reduce suicide among youth aged 15 through 19 to no more than 8.2 per 100,000 (1987 baseline: 10.3 per 100,000)
- Reduce by 15% the incidence of injurious suicide attempts among adolescents aged 14
- Reduce deaths among youth aged 15 through 24 caused by motor vehicle crashes to no more than 33 per 100,000 (1987 baseline: 36.9 per 100,000)
- Increase the proportion of high school seniors who associate risk of physical or psychologic harm with heavy use of alcohol, regular use of marijuana, and experimentation with cocaine

Alcohol 1989 baseline: 44%	2000 target: 70%
Marijuana 1989 baseline: 77.5%	2000 target: 90%

- Increase to at least 75% of the proportion of people aged 10 and older who have discussed issues related to nutrition, physical activity, sexual behavior, tobacco, alcohol, other drugs, and safety with family members on at least one occasion during the preceding month
- Increase to at least 90% the proportion of sexually active, unmarried people aged 19 and younger who use contraception that both effectively prevents pregnancy and provides a barrier against disease (Baseline: 78% at most recent intercourse and 63% at first intercourse; 2% used oral contraceptives and the condom at most recent intercourse [among young women aged 15 through 19 reporting in 1988])

PHYSIOLOGIC PROCESSES

Age and Physical Changes

In contrast to the slow, steady growth of the child, the adolescent experiences markedly accelerated growth. During this 2- to 3-year growth spurt, dramatic alterations in the adolescent's body size and proportions occur. The magnitude of these changes are second only to the growth rate from conception to birth and during infancy.

At this time sexual characteristics develop, and reproductive maturity is achieved. Physiologic functioning of adolescence occurs in a predictable sequence. The age of onset, magnitude, and duration of growth may vary greatly from individual to individual. Generally girls enter puberty earlier than boys–age 9 to 10 for girls, 10 to 11 for boys. The growth spurt for girls is generally early in puberty, whereas for boys it is a late pubertal event.

The physical changes experienced during adolescence are regulated by the *endocrine system;* the hypothalamic-pituitary-gonadal axis is particularly important. This system operates through a negative feedback mechanism. The *hypothalamus* responds to drops in circulating sex steroids by secreting gonadotropin-releasing factor (GnRF). This releasing factor stimulates the *anterior pituitary gland* to release *gonadotropins,* follicle-stimulating hormone (FSH), and luteinizing hormone (LH). The gonadotropins stimulate the male and female gonads, which in turn secrete sex steroids, estrogen and progesterone, from the ovaries and testosterone from the testes. This hormonal interaction is illustrated in Fig. 21-1.

During childhood this hormonal system remains dormant. The immature hypothalamus appears to be extremely sensitive to very low levels of circulating *sex steroids,* which inhibit the release of GnRF. The factors responsible for the changes in this system at puberty are not fully understood; just before puberty, the extreme sensitivity of the hypothalamus to sex hormones is believed to diminish. The hypothalamus initiates pituitary secretion of gonadotropins, which in turn stimulate maturation of the gonads.[17]

The sex steroids produced by the maturing gonads are primarily responsible for the biologic changes of puberty. Sex hormones replace growth hormone as the major regulators of adolescent growth. Recent evidence, however, suggests that growth hormone may play a synergistic role in the growth spurt with the sex steroids.[10]

Acceleration of growth during adolescence is first noted in the musculoskeletal system. During the growth spurt, the average female gains about 8 cm (3 inches) in height per year. The average male, in whom the growth spurt is more dramatic and lasts longer, grows at least 10 cm (4 inches) per year during this phase.

Changes in body proportion occur in a predictable pattern. The head, hands, and feet are the first struc-

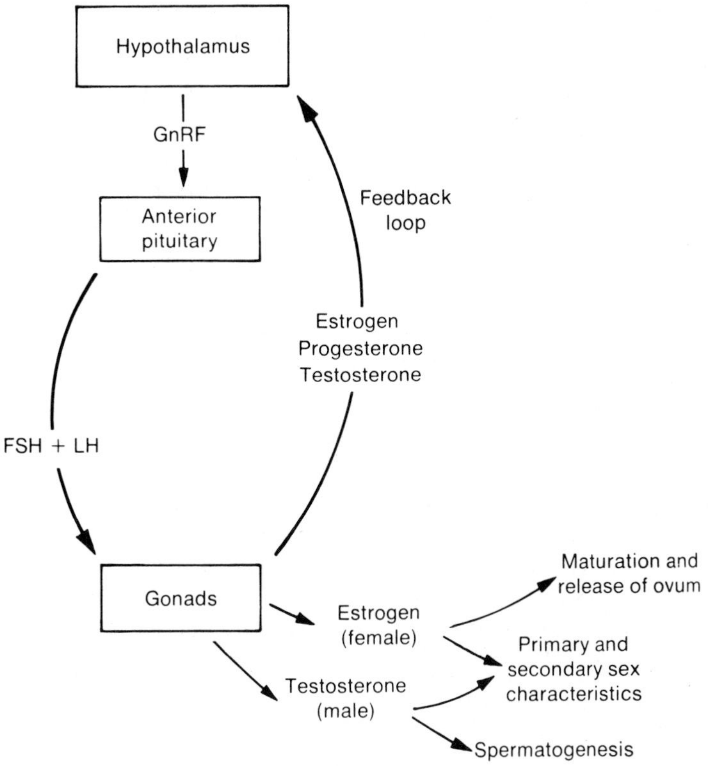

Fig. 21-1. Hormonal interaction between hypothalamus, pituitary, and gonads. (From Whaley LF, Wong DL: *Nursing care of infants and children,* ed 3, St Louis, 1987, Mosby.)

tures to reach adult status. Growth of the extremities precedes growth of the trunk, resulting in the leggy, awkward appearance characteristic of the young adolescent. Increases in shoulder, chest, and hip breadth follow.[10]

Although the size of the brain does not increase significantly during adolescence, the skull and facial bones undergo changes in proportion. Initially the forehead becomes more prominent. Later the maxilla and mandibula develop, and the jaw assumes its adult character. It is not uncommon for an adolescent's facial appearance to change dramatically within a few months.

Ossification of the skeletal system is not complete until late adolescence in boys. In girls, ossification is more advanced throughout childhood and is completed at an earlier age.

Both muscle mass and strength increase during the growth spurt. Muscle development is generally greater in males than females at similar stages of development.

A common skeletal deformity found in adolescents is *scoliosis,* a lateral S-shaped curvature of the spine. Scoliosis is a progressive disease stimulated by the adolescent growth spurt; the curve is usually convex to the right. Adolescent scoliosis is much more prevalent in girls than boys.[8] Some evidence suggests that it is a genetic disorder. Early intervention is important because untreated scoliosis can result in disfigurement, impaired mobility, and cardiopulmonary complications. The nurse should include scoliosis screening in the assessment of older school-age and adolescent clients. This secondary prevention intervention is accomplished by

1. Asking the adolescent to remove all clothing from the upper body. Adequate visualization of the entire back is essential.
2. Having the adolescent bend forward until the back is parallel with the floor. The feet should be together, legs straight, and both arms hanging freely. Inspect for any prominence of the ribs (rib hump) appearing on only one side. This elevation occurs on the convexity of a curve. Check also for hip or leg asymmetry.
3. Inspecting the back for any asymmetry, with the adolescent standing erect. Inspect and palpate for differences in shoulder or scapular height, a prominence of either scapula or hip, waist asymmetry, and malalignment of the spinous processes.

Referral for further orthopedic assessment should be made when any signs of scoliosis are detected.

Before the growth spurt, many children experience a temporary increase in body fat. During puberty, the proportion of total body weight comprised of fat declines, particularly in boys. At the end of the growth spurt, fat again begins to accumulate in both sexes. Following puberty, females have proportionately more body fat than males. This fat is distributed over the thighs, hips, breasts, and buttocks, contributing to their more rounded body contours. Research has shown that 18% to 20% adiposity is required in the adolescent female for menarche to occur.

Changes in the proportion of body fluids reflect general changes in the proportions of bone, muscle, and adipose tissue. The percentage of total body weight composed of fluid decreases throughout childhood. Boys and girls remain essentially similar in percentages until the changes in body composition occur. Then boys reach fluid composition of about 60% of total body weight, reflecting a greater percentage of muscle tissue, and girls reach an average of about 50% of total body weight in water, reflecting the larger percentage of body fat.

The basal metabolic rate (BMR) declines over childhood until reaching an adult level during adolescence. Throughout life, males have a slightly higher BMR, which is thought to be a result of androgenic hormones.[10]

During adolescence, the heart becomes larger and stronger. Blood volume and blood pressure increase, whereas the heart rate declines to adult levels. These cardiovascular changes occur earlier in females, consistent with overall growth patterns. Adolescent females generally have a higher pulse rate and slightly lower systolic blood pressure than males.

Blood pressure may fluctuate from time to time in an adolescent, but a systolic or diastolic pressure above the 95th percentile for age and sex should never be disregarded (see Fig. 20-1). Primary *hypertension,* discussed in Chapter 20, is being found even more frequently during adolescence than during the preschool and school years.[23]

Adult levels of all formed elements of the blood are found in adolescents. Hemoglobin levels are higher in postpubertal males (14 g/dl) than females (12 g/dl). These are minimum levels for each sex.

Respiratory rate decreases over childhood, reaching an average rate of 15 to 20 breaths/min during adolescence. Respiratory volume and vital capacity increase, particularly in males, because of their greater shoulder width and chest size. The laryngeal cartilage, larynx, and vocal cords grow, which produces the characteristic voice changes of puberty. Both male and female voices become deeper, with the effect more pronounced in boys.[10]

The liver, kidneys, spleen, and digestive tract enlarge during the growth spurt but do not change in function. They are already functionally mature by the early school years.

With the exception of the last four molars, which erupt between ages 17 and 21, a full set of permanent teeth is expected by age 12.[17] *Dental caries* are a significant problem during adolescence, particularly for those teenagers who have not had access to adequate dental care during childhood. Because of the changes in facial structure and proportions during the growth spurt, orthodontic bracing and repair is sometimes started in the adolescent years. As discussed Chapter 20, good dental hygiene, including daily brushing and flossing and a visit to the dentist twice a year, continues to be essential for maintaining dental health during the teenage years.[20] (See box on p. 542.)

The skin becomes thicker and tougher during puberty. Under the influence of androgens in both males and females, the *sebaceous glands* become active, particularly on the face, neck, shoulders, upper back, chest, and genitals. These sebaceous glands can become plugged and inflamed, leading to the common teenage condition of acne (see following discussion).

The eccrine and apocrine sweat glands become fully functional during puberty. The *eccrine glands,* which are found over most of the body, produce sweat, which helps eliminate body heat through evaporation. The eccrine glands located on the palms, soles, and axilla also produce sweat in response to emotional stimuli. The *apocrine glands* develop in relation to hair follicles and occur in the axillae, genital and anal areas, external auditory canals, around the umbilicus, and around the areola of the breasts. Apocrine sweat is produced continuously, stored, and released onto the skin in response to emotional stimuli only. The secretion is odorless when it reaches the skin surface but contains fats that are acted on by skin bacteria, producing characteristic odors.

The marked changes in body hair that occur during puberty are discussed in the next section on sex.

ACNE

Adolescents typically are concerned about their skin changes, which result from the hormonal changes of puberty. The sebaceous glands increase their production of sebum in response to a rise in circulating androgens. This increased sebum is a primary factor in the pathogenesis of *acne vulgaris.* The sebaceous follicles become plugged with sebum and debris, forming *comedones* (blackheads, whiteheads). Comedones are a productive environment for *Propionibacterium acnes,* which, when metabolized, releases fatty acids that irritate the wall of the sebaceous follicle. Inflammation occurs when a closed comedo ruptures, spilling its contents into the dermis.[20]

It is estimated that 80% of all teenagers suffer from acne; the degree may range from a few comedones to a severe inflammatory reaction. Its incidence within families suggests that hereditary factors are involved.

Since acne can have severe physical and emotional consequences, aggressive nursing intervention is required. Although the disease cannot be cured, it can be controlled. Thorough examination of the adolescent's skin and a discussion of the young person's perceptions of the problem are necessary to determine appropriate management strategies. Intervention should include teaching the client about the pathophysiology of acne. Knowledge allows the adolescent to become instrumental in its management and helps to dispel common myths about acne and its care.

The adolescent should know that washing with plain soap and water two or three times a day is the best way to remove dirt and oil. Vigorous scrubbing should be discouraged, since it can irritate the skin and lead to follicular rupture. The adolescent should not attempt to remove the pustules and papules that form. Squeezing the lesion may result in further irritation of the gland and permanent injury to the tissue.

Many nonprescription topical medications are available that contain benzoyl peroxide (Oxy-5, Epi-Clear, Persadox), which is also bacteriostatic and comedolytic. Unfortunately, these agents cause drying and peeling, so therapy is begun with application of a 5% strength once a day and after 2 weeks (if tolerated), increased to twice a day. The adolescent with inflamed lesions should be encouraged to seek medical attention; prescription medication may be necessary for more severe cases.

Adolescent girls need to be careful when selecting *makeup.* Most preparations if applied extensively over the face prevent adequate exposure to air and light, causing accumulation of dirt particles on the skin. Any cosmetic that has a grease or fat base should be avoided.

Sunlight may have a beneficial effect on acne; however, prolonged sunbathing should be avoided.

Stress may exacerbate acne in some adolescents. In such cases, stress-management techniques should be discussed.

The effect of *diet* on acne is a highly controversial issue. Current evidence indicates that dietary restrictions are not necessary.

The adolescent with acne needs support and understanding. The nurse can help the adolescent and their family understand that treatment does not result in immediate improvement. In fact, topical agents may initially make acne look worse, and improvement occurs slowly over several months.

The responsibility for management of the problems should clearly be assigned to the adolescent. The nurse should have periodic contact with the adolescent and the family to answer questions, reinforce teaching, and provide positive reinforcement.

Gender

Gender has a profound influence on the physical changes experienced by adolescents. The most obvious differences occur with maturation of the reproductive system. During puberty, both primary and secondary sex characteristics develop. *Primary* sex characteristics involve the organs necessary for reproduction, such as the penis and testes in the males and the vagina and uterus in females. *Secondary* sex characteristics are external features that differentiate male from female but are not essential for reproduction. Breast development, pubic hair growth, and lowering of the voice are examples of secondary sex characteristics (Table 21-1).

MALES

Sexual development in males begins with enlargement of the testes. As the testes grow, the scrotum also enlarges, and the scrotal skin becomes redder. Soon the penis grows larger, and longer and straight hair appears at its base. The development of pubic hair is often the first noticeable sign that puberty has begun. During this period, growth in height begins to accelerate.

As maturation proceeds, growth of the penis, testes, and scrotum continues. Pubic hair becomes thick and curly. Adult distribution of pubic hair describes extension of hair to the inner upper thigh.

Facial hair appears first at the corner of the lip. Body proportions change as the shoulder breadth increases. The voice begins to deepen. Some degree of bilateral or unilateral breast enlargement, called *gynecomastia,* may appear and frequently is discovered during peak growth rates. In the United States, this is most prevalent at 13 years of age. Gynecomastia is temporary and usually disappears by age 17.[6]

In males, *ejaculation* is widely considered to be the milestone of puberty. In the United States, boys experience their first ejaculation at an average age of 14. Ejaculation precedes fertility by several months.[10]

The primary and secondary sex characteristics continue to develop until late adolescence. In the average male the height spurt has decelerated, and sexual maturity has been achieved by age 18.

FEMALES

In females, development of the *breast bud* is usually the first sign that puberty has begun. The appearance of sparse, straight hair along the labia follows, although on some girls it may precede breast bud development. During this stage the height spurt begins, accompanied by the deposition of fat in the characteristic pattern described earlier. Over the next year pubic hair becomes more curly and abundant. Axillary hair appears, and the breasts continue to develop.

The internal reproductive organs grow throughout adolescence, reaching adult size between ages 18 and 20. The onset of menstruation, known as *menarche,* occurs about 2 years after the appearance of the breast bud. The average age of menarche in the United States is 12.8 years, with a normal range between ages 10 and 16.[10] Initially, menstrual periods are irregular and scanty and may not be accompanied by *ovulation.* A consistent pattern of ovulation is generally not established until 1 or 2 years after menarche.

Table 21-1 outlines the stages of development of the secondary sex characteristics in males and females. The relationship of these various changes is illustrated in

Table 21-1.* Developmental stages of secondary sex characteristics

Stage	Male genital development	Pubic hair development	Female breast development	Other changes
1	Prepuberty	Prepuberty; hair over pubic area similar to that on abdomen	Prepuberty; increased pigmentation of papilla only	
2	Initial enlargement of scrotum and testes; reddening and texture changes of scrotum	Sparse growth of long, straight, downy hair at base of penis or along labia	Enlargement of areolar diameter; small area of elevation around papillae	Usual time of peak height velocity for girls
3	Initial enlargement of penis; further growth of testes and scrotum	Hair becomes darker, more coarse, and curly; spreads sparsely over entire pubic area	Further elevation and enlargement of breasts and areolae, with no separation or contours	Usual point of onset of menstruation; facial hair begins to grow and voice deepens for boys
4	Further enlargement of penis and testes and scrotum; growth in breadth and development of glans	Further spread of hair distribution, not extending to thighs	Areolae and papillae project from breast to form secondary mound	Usual time of peak height velocity for boys; axillary hair begins to grow
5	Adult in size and contour	Adult in amount and type	Adult, with projection of papillae only; recession of areolas into general breast contour	

From Chinn PL: *Child health maintenance: concepts in family-centered care,* ed 2, St Louis, 1979, Mosby.
*As defined by Tanner JM: *Growth at adolescence,* ed 2, Oxford, 1962, Blackwell Scientific Publications.

Figs. 21-2 and 21-3. Familiarity with these relationships and stages can help the nurse accurately assess an adolescent's level of development.

NURSING INTERVENTIONS

The adolescent needs much support and information during the changes of puberty and the onset of reproductive function. Intellectual knowledge about the events of puberty should be obtained during later childhood. The nurse should never assume, however, that an adolescent has this information. In a tactful and unobtrusive manner, the nurse should estimate the teenager's knowledge of sexual functioning for both sexes and offer further explanation and clarification as appropriate. Males particularly need to be prepared for erections and nocturnal emissions. Many adolescent males are concerned about their height and the size of their genitals, linking these physical attributes to their attractiveness and virility. Early adolescence is an excellent time to begin to dispel cultural myths about male sexuality.

As with their male counterparts, adolescent females have many questions about the physical changes they experience during puberty. Menarche is perhaps the most significant event of female development; it signals the physical transition from "girl" to "woman." Menarche not only has physiologic ramifications but psychologic and social ones as well.

Preparation for menarche should begin in late childhood. Young women need to understand that the timing of menarche varies widely. *Amenorrhea,* the absence of an expected menstrual period, is not unusual in early adolescence. Stress, rigorous athletic training, or a very low proportion of body fat also can affect the menstrual cycle, causing missed periods.[24] The nurse can encourage the young woman to seek health care for these concerns. The sexually active young woman may experience much anxiety when she misses a period. The possibility of pregnancy needs to be considered along with the other causes of missed periods.

Dysmenorrhea is a common complaint of menstruating women. Characterized by a cramping, lower abdominal pain during menses often accompanied by nausea, vomiting, diarrhea, and headaches, it may last from a few hours up to 3 days. The onset of pain usually precedes or coincides with the onset of bleeding. In primary dysmenorrhea, no evidence of pelvic pathology exists; this disorder does not occur until cyclic ovulation has begun.[6]

Research has shown that women who experience discomfort during menstruation have excessive uterine muscle activity. Powerful uterine contractions cause ischemia, which in turn causes cramping pain. Evidence suggests that a relationship exists between prostaglandin levels and excessive myometrial activity. This hypothesis has led to the successful use of prostaglandin synthetase inhibitors such as ibuprofen (Motrin) and naproxen (Naprosyn) in the management of this problem.[6,20]

Dysmenorrhea is very prevalent among adolescents and is the leading cause of recurrent short-term absenteeism. Few adolescents who suffer from dysmenorrhea actually seek help for the problem. Communication with these young women about the causes and options for treatment of dysmenorrhea is important. The nurse,

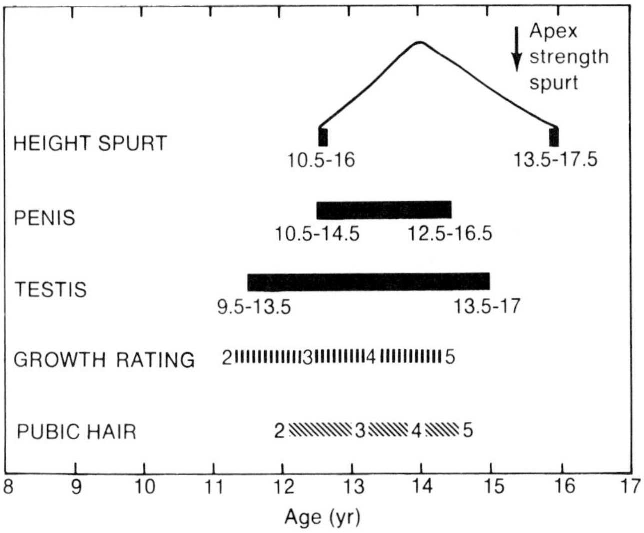

Fig. 21-2. Diagram of sequence of events at adolescence in boys. Single numbers *(2, 3, 4, 5)* indicate stages of development. Average boy is represented; range of ages when each event may begin and end is indicated by inclusive numbers below each event. (From Marshall WA, Tanner JM: *Arch Dis Child* 45:13, 1970. In Whaley LF, Wong DL: *Nursing care of infants and children,* ed 3, St Louis, 1987, Mosby.)

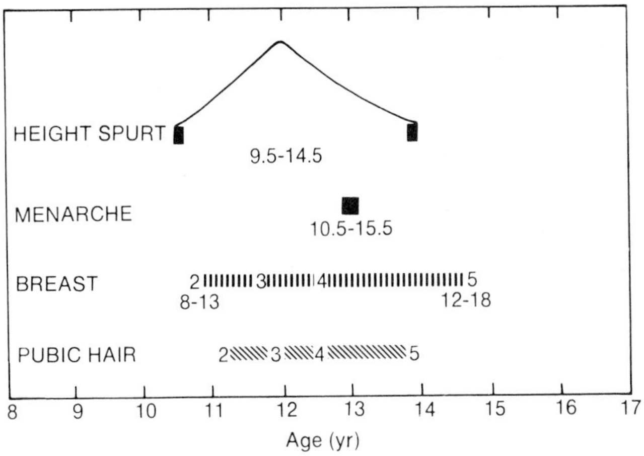

Fig. 21-3. Diagram of sequence of events at adolescence in girls. Single numbers *(2, 3, 4, 5)* indicate stages of development. Average girl is represented; range of ages when each event may begin and end is indicated by inclusive numbers below each event. (From Marshall WA, Tanner JM: *Arch Dis Child* 44:291, 1969. In Whaley LF, Wong DL: *Nursing care of infants and children,* ed 3, St Louis, 1987, Mosby.)

either in the school or in the primary care setting, is the logical health care professional to deal with this subject.

Race

Analyzing the relationship between race and the health of adolescents without considering environmental variables is impossible. Proper nutrition, economic stability, and access to health care services are examples of the many environmental resources necessary to ensure optimum development and health. Unfortunately, these resources are not equally distributed among the U.S. population. Racial minorities are more likely to grow up in impoverished environments.

Poverty, more than any racial or cultural factor, disturbs family functioning and health. The consequences of poverty among adolescent minorities contribute to increased homicide, violence, and incarceration rates; premature pregnancy; substance abuse; and drug trafficking. These psychologic and social problems lead to the increased morbidity and mortality found in this segment of our population.

There is a growing population of Indochinese refugees in the United States. A recent study of adolescent refugees from Southeast Asia showed that 52% had positive tuberculosis tests, 38% lacked some immunizations, and 10% were anemic. Many other physical and emotional problems were also identified.

Race cannot be isolated as the primary factor responsible for these different risk factors; however, nurses need to be aware that a relationship between race and certain health problems is likely to exist.

Genetics

Most genetic problems are discovered during infancy and early childhood. Some syndromes, however, may not be diagnosed until adolescence. These genetic disorders often are discovered during the assessment of a child with delayed pubertal development.

Turner's syndrome is caused by the absence of one of the X chromosomes in females. It is diagnosed most frequently during adolescence because of three outstanding features: (1) short stature, (2) sexual infantilism, and (3) amenorrhea. The incidence is estimated at 1 of 1500 to 1 of 10,000 live female births. Only a few girls with Turner's syndrome manifest all the possible features, which include a webbed neck; low-set ears; a shield-shaped chest with widely spaced, hypoplastic nipples; cardiac anomalies; learning disabilities; and ovarian hypoplasia. Treatment consists primarily of hormonal therapy and ongoing emotional support for the child and her family.[8]

Klinefelter's syndrome, also seldom diagnosed before puberty, is caused by the presence of one or more additional X chromosomes in males. This syndrome is the most common of all chromosomal abnormalities; the incidence is estimated to be 1 in 500 live male births. Characteristic features include a tall, eunuchoid figure; sparse facial and pubic hair; gynecomastia; firm, insensitive testes; a small penis; and sterility. Klinefelter's syndrome is associated with learning and/or behavior problems during childhood. As with Turner's syndrome, treatment usually involves hormonal therapy and counseling. If the nurse recognizes signs of either of these syndromes during routine screening, the child should be referred to a physician who is experienced in diagnosing and managing both the physical and the emotional aspects of these problems.

Most adolescents with delayed development do not have a genetic disorder; their pattern of growth merely falls at the far end of the normal curve.[14] Some cases of delayed growth result from inadequate nutrition. Whatever the cause, developmental delays can have a tremendous effect on the psychosocial development of the child. This is also true of children who mature earlier than their peers. These adolescents need ongoing assessment and support to promote development of a positive self-esteem.

Nutritional and Metabolic Pattern

A balanced diet is essential for optimum growth during adolescence; poor nutrition can retard growth and delay sexual maturation. The Food and Nutrition Board of the National Research Council[18] has recommended dietary allowances of the nutrients necessary to support adolescent growth (Table 21-2). These recommendations are considered to be the average daily requirements of males and females in a given age range.

Using age as a basis for determining the nutritional requirements of adolescents has limitations. Since wide variability exists in the timing of pubertal growth, the child's level of development should be considered when calculating specific nutritional requirements for each adolescent.[18]

The highest nutrient and energy demands occur at the peak velocity of growth. For example, a 13-year-old male in the middle of his growth spurt would have very different nutritional demands than another 13-year-old who had not yet experienced pubescent changes. Participation in sports or other forms of intense physical activity also increases nutrient and caloric requirements.[18]

In striving to become autonomous individuals, most adolescents spent increasing amounts of time involved in activities outside the home. Their lifestyles often

***Table 21-2.* Recommended dietary allowances of nutrients for adolescent male, female, and pregnant adolescents, ages 11 to 18**

		Males		Females		Pregnant females	
		11–14	15–18	11–14	15–18	11–14	15–18
Weight	(kg)	45	66	46	55	46	55
Energy	(kcal)	2700	2800	2200	2100	2500	2400
Protein	(g)	45	56	46	46	76	76
Vitamin A	(R.E.)	1000	1000	800	800	1000	1000
Vitamin A	(IU)	5000	5000	4000	4000	5000	5000
Vitamin D	(μg)	10	10	10	10	15	15
Vitamin D	(IU)	400	400	400	400	600	600
Vitamin E	(mg α T.E.)	8	10	8	8	10	10
Vitamin C	(mg)	50	60	50	60	70	80
Folacin	(μg)	400	400	400	400	800	800
Niacin	(mg)	18	18	15	14	17	16
Riboflavin	(mg)	1.6	1.7	1.3	1.3	1.6	1.6
Thiamine	(mg)	1.4	1.4	1.1	1.1	1.5	1.5
Vitamin B_6	(mg)	1.8	2.0	1.8	2.0	2.4	2.6
Vitamin B_{12}	(μg)	3.0	3.0	3.0	3.0	4.0	4.0
Calcium	(mg)	1200	1200	1200	1200	1600	1600
Phosphorus	(mg)	1200	1200	1200	1200	1600	1600
Iodine	(μg)	150	150	150	150	175	175
Iron	(mg)	18	18	18	18	18*	18*
Magnesium	(mg)	350	400	300	300	450	450
Zinc	(mg)	15	15	15	15	20	20

From Marina DD, King JC: *Pediatr Clin North Am* 27(1):125, 1981. Adapted from Food and Nutrition Board–National Research Council: *Recommended dietary allowances*, ed 9, Washington, DC, 1980, National Academy of Sciences.

include irregular eating habits, meal skipping, and snacking. Snacking can be a help or hindrance to good nutrition based on the nutrient content of the snack. The adolescent can be encouraged to select nutritious snacks such as fresh fruit and vegetables, juice, cheese, whole-grain crackers, and nuts. Eating at fast-food restaurants is popular in this age group. Fast foods tend to be high in calories, fat, and sodium and low in fiber, folic acid, and vitamins A and C.[18]

Adolescents often are dissatisfied with their appearance. Such dissatisfaction with body image is influenced by our predominant cultural ideals. Many adolescent females consider themselves to be too heavy and want to lose weight, whereas only 15% are actually obese. Many adolescent males think of themselves as being too thin and want to gain weight, although only about 25% are below average in weight (see box on p. 550).

The desire to be attractive and to fit in with one's peers may lead to unhealthy dietary manipulations. Fad diets are popular with teenagers. Rigid dietary practices, however, can result in malnutrition or other serious harm. In general, adolescent diets most frequently are deficient in calcium, iron, zinc, folic acid, and vitamins A and C.[18] Adolescent women, who diet more often than men, are most likely to ingest less than the required calories and calcium (see box on p. 542).

EATING DISORDERS

At one end of the spectrum is anorexia nervosa, which primarily affects adolescent females, although recent studies suggest that incidence among males may be higher than previously suspected.[20] This complex problem has underlying developmental and psychologic disturbances. The symptoms may include self-starving with significant weight loss, amenorrhea, compulsive physical activity, preoccupation with food, and a distorted body image. Typically the anorexic adolescent is described as a perfectionist or overachiever who always has performed well academically. This person's family also is achievement oriented, and often marital discord is present.[4]

The onset of the anorexic behavior generally is initiated in response to real or imagined obesity. With dieting, the adolescent begins to lose weight. Personal pride and positive reinforcement from others lead to continued dieting, which becomes the primary focus of the young woman's life.[4] Any feelings of hunger are denied rigidly. Eventually this adolescent becomes dangerously malnourished. Common complications of such a severely limited intake are fluid and electrolyte imbalances, hypotension, and constipation. Untreated, this disorder can progress to starvation and death. If the nurse suspects anorexia in any client, the young woman

RESEARCH REVIEW ADOLESCENCE

WEIGHT LOSS ACTIVITIES

Felts M, et al: Adolescents' perceptions of relative weight and self-reported weight loss activities, *J Sch Health* 62:372-375, 1992.

Purpose The purpose of this study was to examine perceptions of relative weight and the relationship of these perceptions to physical activity levels, time spent viewing television, and efforts to lose weight.

Review Data were collected as part of a larger study of health risk behaviors of North Carolina public school students using a modified version of the Youth Risk Survey (YRS). A total of 3437 9th through 12th graders responded. Of this sample, 25% perceived themselves as "too fat." Of that group, 68% were trying to lose weight. Females made up 75% of those reporting they were "too fat" and were trying to lose weight. White females were more likely to think of themselves as overweight than black females. Adolescents who reported themselves as "too fat" reported fewer days of strenuous activity, fewer hours of strenuous exercise in physical education classes, and more hours spent viewing television. Implications are raised which challenge schools and parents to provide more health-promoting activities for all adolescents.

should be referred to a specialist who is experienced with this complex problem. Recovery is a long process involving ongoing treatment of the entire family. Hospitalization is often necessary to prevent physical deterioration.

Another eating disorder is bulimia nervosa, a pattern of binge eating followed by forced vomiting and/or laxative use, a feeling of lack of control over eating, and body dissatisfaction. This is another complex situation and should be referred to a specialist for comprehensive evaluation and management.[4]

OBESITY

Obesity may be defined as weight that is 20% greater than ideal weight for a particular height. Although the etiology of this problem is undoubtedly complex, recent evidence suggests that a primary factor is inactivity. Fifteen percent of adolescents are obese. It is more common among girls than boys. The obese adolescent takes in too many calories for the amount of energy expended. Some may not be consuming excessive calories, but skipping breakfast and eating throughout the afternoon and evening is common.[18] (See box on p. 542.)

Obesity can be detrimental to the adolescent's self-esteem and social development. These teenagers often become trapped in a vicious cycle of social rejection, isolation, inactivity, and greater obesity. Unfortunately, obesity during adolescence has a poor prognosis; most obese adolescents become obese adults.[18]

Some methods for treating adolescent obesity are more successful than others. A holistic approach that addresses environmental, psychosocial, and physiologic factors is likely to be most successful. Dietary regimes which include rigid dietary restriction should be avoided to ensure that the nutritional demands of adolescent growth are met.[18]

Through periodic assessment of height and weight, nurses are often the first to identify obesity; their role in prevention is even more important. The suggestions for parents interested in preventing obesity in their children presented in Chapter 20 also are relevant for parents of adolescents, even though adolescents assume greater responsibility for their own eating and exercise patterns. Health classes in school are appropriate forums for discussion of nutrition and the related problems, such as obesity and anorexia.

Elimination Pattern

The renal and gastrointestinal systems are functionally mature during adolescence. Elimination patterns are consistent with those found in adults.

Activity and Exercise Pattern

During adolescence, the alterations in body composition and growth of lean muscle mass allows the teen to experience increased physical strength and endurance. For the first time, the young person has the ability to adapt to strain or stress equal to or in excess of that of the adult. This ability results from an increased capacity of the lungs and accompanying structures, which serves to restore oxygen to the tissues after intensive exertion and to facilitate recovery of normal function once the exercise is over. Heart rate, respiratory rate, reflexive shunting of blood from resting to working muscles, blood pressure, and electrolyte and fluid responses are among the many varied and complex reactions to exercise that reach their full capacity.

Many adolescents enjoy vigorous physical activity; participation in organized, competitive sports is popular. Activity levels vary greatly, however; whereas some adolescents lead very active lives, others are sedentary. Nurses who work with this age group need to assess their clients' patterns of activity periodically to determine appropriate strategies for health promotion and specific protection.

Adolescents who participate in athletic activities should be examined to ensure that they are physically able to cope with the demands of their sport.[24] Many schools require a yearly physical examination before participation in athletic programs is allowed. Stage of physical maturity is an important consideration in the evaluation of teenage athletes who will participate in competitive sports because increased strength accompanies sexual maturity. The Tanner scales, which characterizes sexual maturity into specific stages, is a useful tool for presports participation physical examinations. Athletes also need to be taught how to strengthen and condition themselves to prevent injuries.

Exercise affects the nutritional needs of the adolescent. Those who are physically active may have to increase their intake of both calories and nutrients to ensure optimum growth, whereas inactive teenagers may need to limit their caloric intake to prevent obesity. All young persons should be taught that good nutrition and regular exercise can improve their endurance, appearance, and general state of health and that these positive effects may extend into adulthood.

Sleep and Rest Pattern

During adolescence the amount of time spent each night in sleep declines. Although sleep patterns vary greatly among individuals, on the average adolescents sleep 8 hours each night. Working adolescents are most at risk for sleep deprivation and daytime sleepiness. The nurse can help employed adolescents problem solve regarding balancing work, school, responsibilities to their families, leisure time, and sleep.

PSYCHOLOGIC PROCESSES

The physical changes of puberty, as dramatic as they are, seem almost minor when compared to the psychologic and social changes that occur during adolescence. The young person moves from being a relatively dependent member of society to taking on full responsibility for self, actions, and sometimes another person, if parenthood occurs. By the end of adolescence, the young person is expected by society to assume a full adult role.

Cognitive and Perceptual Pattern

PIAGET'S THEORY

The early part of adolescence, ages 11 to 15, is the period when Piaget's *formal operations* begin. Thought processes develop into mature, adultlike patterns, with specific traits that allow for adult accomplishments in thinking. It is important to remember that not all individuals achieve this adult thinking capability at the same time. Piaget believes that development evolves as a result of the maturation of the cerebral structures. The main feature of this period of thought is that children can enter into the world of possibilities beyond the world of reality. They are able to think beyond the present and to consider things that do not exist but that *might* be. This type of thinking involves real logic and an organized, consistent approach to thinking. Piaget uses the term *formal* to represent the adolescent's focus on the "form" of thought, objects, and experiences rather than on the exact content. When they have attained the level of formal operations, adolescents think in a way that determines possibilities, ranks probabilities, problem solves, and makes decisions (Fig. 21-4). Still, they combine certain traits of cognition from earlier periods of life. They are capable of the fantastic flights from reality that are typical of the preoperational period and yet order their ideational material in a manner similar to organizational patterns used for sensory reality in the operational periods. Reality is recognized but becomes only a subset of many other possibilities.

As these patterns of thought emerge, adolescents are observed to be extremely idealistic, to constantly challenge the way things are, and to consider the way things could be or ought to be. They may totally discard what is. During the early part of the formal operations period, young persons demonstrate a kind of egocentrism in thinking. Their propositions and flights from reality allow them to see themselves as omnipotent and to bring reality in line with their own thinking. Although this trait may be irritating to others, it is a necessary stage before formal operational thinking. Once this has been mastered, adolescents can move on into more fully mature thought patterns that make use of the propositional, organized approach but that more fully account for the social and cosmic universe to which they are applied.

In solving a problem, adolescents in the formal opera-

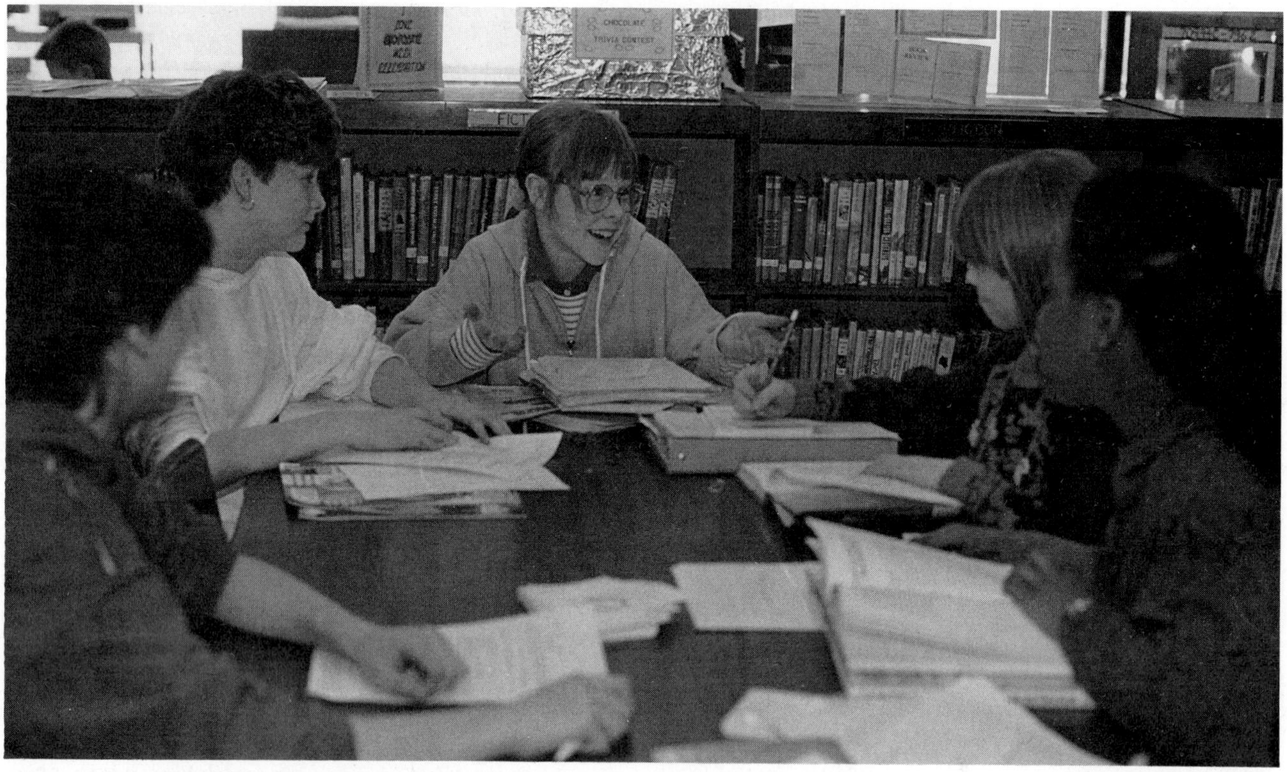

Fig. 21-4. The ability to think in abstract terms, a requirement for many high school courses, is developed during adolescence.

tions period can try out a variety of solutions in their minds without having to actually manipulate materials. They can operate solely through *symbolism.*[1] They can even hold several relevant variables constant while they systematically manipulate one and hypothesize about the outcome under each condition. This approach is the classic method of experimental science, but young persons rarely realize that they are using it with such sophistication.

These new cognitive abilities are reflected in the adolescent's behavior in several ways. The first change is that adolescents, because of their new ability to "think about their thinking," become very *introspective.* By middle adolescence, this introspection is quite marked, and the adolescent may assume that others are equally interested and almost or actually know what the adolescent is thinking. David Elkind points out that this gives rise to the adolescents' "imaginary audience." The imaginary audience provides the adolescent a means of evaluating, "How do others see me?" and leads to a sense of being the focus, special, unique, and exceptional. Being exceptional to the adolescent means being the exception, and this "fable of immunity" gives rise to the risk-taking behavior for which adolescents are so well known:

"I can get drunk on weekends and not develop a drinking problem."

"I can't get pregnant; after all I've had sex for 6 months and haven't gotten pregnant."

"I can take those hairpin turns at 50 miles per hour and not wreck."

Another behavioral manifestation of the adolescent's formal operations ability is an *intolerance* of things as they are. The adolescent can conceptualize things as they could be as opposed to how they are and also can think of elaborate means for achieving these changes. They can be vehement in trying to convince others of their viewpoint and untiring in the support of causes that seem to agree with their ideas. This idealism can also lead to rejection of family beliefs, religion, or social causes, which do not seem to be working fast enough to solve the problems of society. This often results in a major division between parent and adolescent.[19]

TIME ORIENTATION

Older adolescents look at time differently than they did as children. They realize that response to a problem can and often should be delayed to think through the possibilities for approaching the problem. They develop a future orientation and are able to delay immediate gratification to gain more satisfaction in the future.

SENSORY ABILITIES

The adolescent has a mature sensory repertoire. Touch, taste, smell, vision, hearing, and proprioception have reached full development by this period.

LANGUAGE

Advances in cognitive skills are reflected in an increased understanding of language. Formal operations and more abstract thought processes require expression in different words than did the more concrete thoughts of younger ages. Adolescents give more complex definitions, often including all possible meanings or uses. Interpretations of pictures or stories are more complex and abstract. Older teenagers are capable of using and understanding more complex sentence structure, although they, as with adults, may not use these routinely in their speech.

Both receptive and expressive vocabulary increase during adolescence. As at all ages, receptive vocabulary far exceeds expressive vocabulary. Vocabulary tests often are used to estimate intelligence quotient (IQ). The adolescent vocabulary often includes *argot,* that is, words devised and used by participants in a certain subculture. Parents often call this slang. This argot may be centered around such topics as drug use, popular dress, or activities or may be pervasive, in which case adults or "outsiders" may have difficulty following a conversation between two teenagers.

A more abstract thinking of the older adolescent is reflected in writing style. The younger adolescent is more likely to use a flamboyant, dramatic style, whereas the older adolescent's written expression is more objective and controlled (Fig. 21-5).

INTELLIGENCE

By the end of adolescence, adult IQ tests are used to evaluate level of cognition. IQ tests are based on thought processes and actual experience in the real world. Thus, for adolescents from a limited, restricted background, some of the situations presented or questions asked may seem very difficult because they are new. Also, adolescents of minority culture may perceive a situation or question from the perspective of their own culture and give an answer that seems in error but is actually true, based on their experiences. The nurse must consider differences in background in evaluating the intellectual capacity of the teenager.

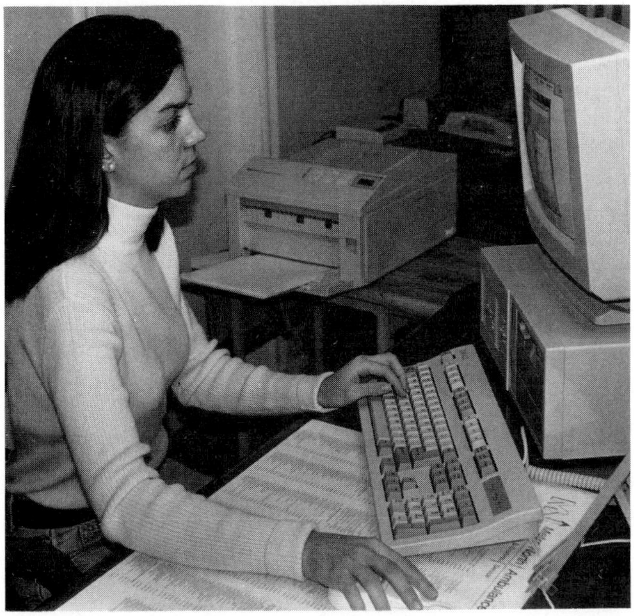

Fig. 21-5. Thinking in more abstract terms is reflected in older adolescents' writing style. (Photo by Fredric J. Edelman.)

Self-Perception and Self-Concept Pattern

ERIKSON'S THEORY

The central task of adolescence is the establishment of *identity,* with the primary risk being identity *confusion.* Erikson conceptualizes the youth culture that has developed in technologic societies as an attempt to establish identity formation. It may appear that the youth creating the culture are involved in a final rather than a transient or initial identity formation, but dedication to the adolescent culture provides a means of moving into and through the identity crisis of the period. Through the group, individuals find support and help with the many inner problems of developing a new body image, finding sexual identity, establishing intimacy with the opposite sex, and dealing with the many conflicting possibilities and choices of the present and future. Erikson views the adolescent clique as a means of testing one's ability to remain constant and loyal in the midst of inevitable conflicts of values.[7]

The adolescent identity crisis involves a restaging of each of the previous stages of development. The stage of infancy, with the development of trust in self and others, again is encountered as the adolescent looks intently for persons and ideals in which to have faith and prove oneself trustworthy. Groups of friends, cliques, or gangs can serve this function.

The stage of developing autonomy is reestablished in adolescents' search for avenues to express their right to will freely. At the same time, they must avoid the hazard of behaving in a manner that would expose them to self-doubt or to ridicule from their friends. They intensify their search for an occupational role through which they can express themselves in an autonomous, freely chosen direction. The accomplishment of this task and the avoidance of shame lead to an interesting paradox: adolescents would rather behave shamelessly in the eyes of their parents than be forced into behavior that would bring ridicule form their peers.

The third stage of life, when a sense of initiative develops, also is reenacted as young persons seek identity. Their unlimited imagination over what they might become is tempered only by a sense of guilt over the excessiveness of their ambition. Thus, they aspire to great accomplishment at one point, then loudly denounce themselves for exceeding the possible.

The school-age period of developing a sense of industry is carried into the adolescent period as teenagers begin to make a choice in occupation. The typical confusion and hesitation in making this choice arise from a fear of entering a career that will not afford them the chance to excel.

The extent to which the earlier tasks were completed or resolved successfully influences adolescents' success in finding an identity. Young persons who have experienced success are often very resourceful during adolescence in finding ways of making up a gap that might have been left in earlier stages of development. Erikson believes that when adolescents believe that society is depriving them of all forms of expression that permit them to integrate the various steps of their previous development, they resist violently and feel forced to defend their development of identity. When the threat of identity confusion is exceedingly great, delinquent behavior and potential alterations in mental health often occur. Such a threat is enhanced by conditions of poverty, racism, sexual orientation, dysfunctional family, chronic illness, and personal losses and grief. Erikson views society as posing special problems for our youth insisting on self-made identities that are characterized by strength, tolerance, readiness to take advantages of opportunity, and readiness to adjust to change. Society must present its adolescents with ideologies that can be shared by a very diverse young population and yet maintain the ideals of freedom of self-realization and choice.

The pursuit for something to be devoted to and the search for a meaningful ideology often create a puzzling combination of shifting devotion and sudden extremes in action. Erikson views this behavior as an attempt to try out various roles and to search for some stable principle that might last through the testing of extremes and into adulthood. Erikson devoted much of his work to finding interpretations of youth behavior related to the entire life history of the individual and thus to differentiating truly pathologic behavior during adolescence from that which is normal and useful in completing life's stages.[7]

BODY IMAGE

Self-image and self-esteem are very much tied to body image, and adolescents who perceive their bodies as being less ideal than their peers have less favorable feelings about themselves. As mentioned earlier, adolescent girls often view themselves as fat, and adolescent boys frequently view themselves as too thin. These young women want small hips, thighs, or waists; the young men want broader shoulders and more muscular arms (Fig. 21-6).

An important aspect of body image during adolescence is sexual characteristics. Young men are concerned with size of the penis and body and facial hair. A larger penis and more and early appearance of body and face hair is seen as desirable. Young women are concerned with breast size and onset of menstruation. Larger breasts most often are viewed as more feminine. The onset of menstruation is one rite of passage into adult femininity.

Because many sexual characteristics primarily are genetically determined, adolescents feel as if they are observing their bodies, waiting for the final result.

SEXUAL IDENTITY

The physical changes of sexual characteristics stimulate a change in the adolescent's concept of sexuality. Teenagers first fantasize about the pleasures of sex and then gradually experiment with dating, petting, and noncoital and coital contact.

Older adolescents who have had opportunities to work through their sexual role become comfortable with who they are and what their possible roles may be; they begin establishing intimacy with a partner or partners. This forms a groundwork for the long-term commitments of young adulthood. Sexual experimentation as a way of being accepted into a specific group or clique does not fall into the concept of true intimacy. As a final step in the acquisitions of sexual identity, however, intimacy often includes sexual activity. The outcomes and related responsibilities of sexual activity are discussed under social processes later in this chapter.

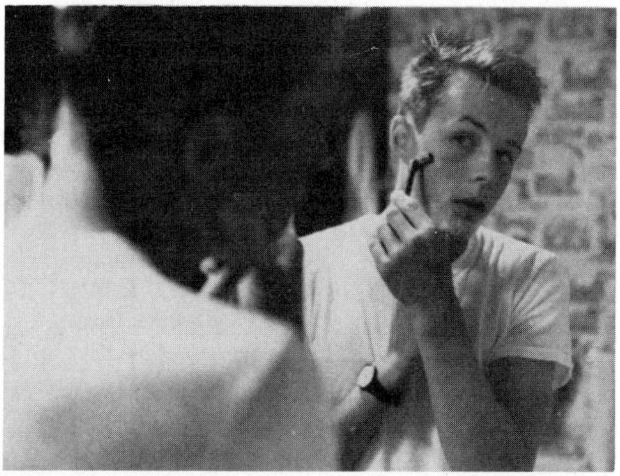

Fig. 21-6. Physical attractiveness is a great concern for adolescents. (From Wong DL: *Whaley and Wong's essentials of pediatric nursing,* ed 4, St Louis, 1987, Mosby.)

Coping and Stress-Tolerance Pattern

Each physical and psychologic change during adolescence produces some stress. When all these changes seem to be happening at the same time, the stress is compounded. Other stresses are competition, whether in sports, relationships, or school achievement; frustration involved in attempting new things and new ways of interacting; and the uncertainty of what lies ahead coupled with the need to make major life decisions about future education and relationships. Although parents are involved in some decisions and changes, the adolescent needs to separate from parents and may believe many choices must be made alone. Often the need to separate from parents and feel more independent is expressed as time spent away from home, alone in their bedroom, or absorbed in their music.

The adolescent may use egocentric behaviors as ways of dealing with the stresses of becoming more independent. The older adolescent is capable of using any defense mechanism that adults use. These forms of coping, if not used to excess, may be very adaptive. They allow the adolescent to move away from the stress briefly to reapproach the stressor with a fresh outlook and possibly turn the stressful situation into a constructive learning experience.[26]

Other coping mechanisms of adolescence and ways that the nurse can assist the teenager to use these in adaptive ways are listed in the box below.

DEPRESSION

All adolescents feel sad at times; depression is an all-pervasive sadness present much of the time. It is more common in adolescents than in school-age children. Nurses should ask adolescents if they are depressed as part of a routine history. Teenagers know what depression means and often welcome the opportunity to discuss this. The nurse should suspect depression if the teenager uses such words as low, blue, hopeless, worried, or discouraged and exhibits several of the following symptoms:

1. Change in weight or eating habits (more or less intake)
2. Insomnia or hypersomnia
3. Loss of energy; fatigue
4. Change in motor activity, such as inactivity to constant motion
5. Loss of interest in usual activities
6. Out-of-proportion feelings of self-reproach or guilt
7. Drop in school performance
8. Preoccupation with death

SUICIDE

A severe maladaptive coping behavior often related to depression is suicide. However, many adolescents who are suicidal do not have characteristics symptomatic of depression and could easily be overlooked when assessing suicidal risk. Between 1970 and 1980, almost 50,000 young people between the ages of 15 and 24 committed suicide. The suicide rate among adolescents increased 40% during the last decade, while the rates for other age groups remained stable. This dramatic rise was primarily among young men.[8]

These figures may not reflect the full scope of this problem. Many actual suicides probably are classified as accidental deaths. Suicide attempts are not included in

---

❑ ❑ COPING MECHANISMS OF ADOLESCENTS

Cognitive mastery. The teenager attempts to learn as much as possible about the situation or stressor. This is a common strategy for the adolescent with a chronic illness. The nurse can assist by clarifying any misinformation, sharing findings, and encouraging discussion of feelings along with facts.

Conformity. The teenager attempts to be a mirror image of peers; this includes dress, language, attitude, and actions. The nurse must respect this need for sameness and also can encourage discussion of feelings about differences between this teenager and peers.

Controlling behaviors. The adolescent needs to be in charge of some aspects of life and can no longer accept family and school rules without question as in the past. This need to control extends to health care. The nurse cannot just give directions or instructions but rather should present the possible options and allow the teenager to state preferences. Together they can work out an acceptable plan.

Fantasy. This may be used more by the younger adolescent. The nurse can encourage the teenager to use this fantasy thinking to develop creative plans to deal with the stressful situation.

Motor activity. Engaging in sports, dancing, running, or other high-energy activity can be a very effective tension-releasing strategy. The nurse can encourage safe activities and offer information about community resources for these motor activities.

these statistics, although estimates show that 50 to 200 attempts occur for every successfully completed suicide. (See box on p. 542.)

No one comprehensive theory adequately explains adolescent suicide. Because it is such a significant problem during middle and late adolescence, many believe the problem has developmental dimensions. Certainly adolescence is a period of considerable stress; if the adolescent's coping mechanisms and social supports are inadequate, suicide may be an outcome. Many suicidologists are convinced that suicide during adolescence is not an impulsive or spontaneous act and is selected only after other problem-solving methods have failed.

According to Teicher and Jacobs,[26] adolescents who attempt suicide have a characteristic presuicidal biography that indicates a gradual decline of the individual's ability to cope with stress, loss, and frustration. Problems begin in early childhood and frequently include one or more of the following:

1. One or both parents absent from the home because of separation, divorce, or death
2. Parent, relative, or close friend who attempted suicide
3. Extreme family conflict
4. Living with a person who is not a biologic parent
5. Frequent changes of residence
6. Parental alcoholism

These problems can cause the child great unhappiness and may lead to progressive isolation from satisfying social relationships.

During adolescence, the long-standing problems of childhood continue or worsen while the new problems of adolescence are added. Unable to resolve these escalating difficulties, the adolescent begins to feel helpless and hopeless. Before the suicide attempt, the adolescent perceives a rapid dissolution of any meaningful relationships. This may be precipitated by an event often mistaken as the reason for a suicide, such as a pregnancy, school failure, family fight, or terminated romance. The adolescent feels completely isolated and alone. Because previous attempts to resolve problems have failed, suicide is seen as the only option.

Fortunately, some adolescent suicides can be prevented. Distressed adolescents may give clues both verbally and nonverbally. Any one clue may mean nothing, but when several are noted, particularly in an adolescent facing difficult circumstances, they should be recognized as an important warning. Clues of suicidal risk can be classified into three groups: depressive equivalents, verbal clues, and behavioral clues (see box on this page).[2]

Identifying and treating these clues as serious forms of communication is essential. The nurse should not be fearful of asking adolescents if they have been contemplating suicide. If they have, they may be relieved to be able to talk about it; if not, asking them will not plant the idea. If the nurse suspects that an adolescent is suicidal, immediate referral should be made to someone trained in suicide intervention. A suicide threat should never be ignored. The adolescent in immediate danger of committing suicide should not be left alone.

A growing problem in some communities has been the phenomenon of "cluster" suicides. These can be suicides that occur within a limited time period and specific location or suicides in which victims share their thoughts together prior to the actual suicide. In response to the growing problem of youth suicide and fear of the cluster suicides, some schools have developed suicide-prevention programs. Nurses who work in junior and senior high schools can play an important role in development, implementation, and evaluation of such programs.

❑ ❑ CLUES OF SUICIDAL RISK IN ADOLESCENTS

Depressive equivalents are symptoms associated with depression: delinquency, aggressiveness, sexual promiscuity, running away, drug or alcohol use, headaches, abdominal pain, accident proneness, fatigue, slow speech, anorexia, sloppiness, and preoccupation with death.

Verbal clues are statements that indicate the adolescent is thinking of killing himself: "This world would be better off without me"; "I won't be around anymore."

Behavioral clues are actions that indicate the adolescent might be contemplating suicide; resigning from organizations, giving away cherished belongings, writing suicide notes, or exhibiting sudden changes in usual patterns of behavior (the good student who begins to fail, the quiet student who becomes aggressive).

DRUG USE

Other maladaptive coping behaviors are excessive use of drugs of any kind. Teenagers often see adults using drugs to relieve tension, so it is not surprising that they should adapt this socially sanctioned activity. Drug use and misuse is discussed later in this chapter.

❑ ❑ ❑

Exposure to stress and the resulting need to cope is a lifelong process. The teenager who learns adaptive ways to cope has a strong base to build on in the adult years.

Value and Belief Pattern

During adolescence, young persons acquire an intense sense of ideals, or a system of values evolved from what they project could be, not necessarily what is. They sometimes align their beliefs with a particular religion or intellectual school of thought or some other formal system that provides a basis for the formulation of the ideals. The teenager uses these ideals in weighing decisions between right or wrong, best or worst, important or not important. The ideal system may change drastically several times during adolescence, and this changing process provides the young person with different ranges of experience on which to later base lasting choices. Most adolescents assimilate the values and beliefs of their family systems; occasionally their values may be different from their family. When these new values conflict with parental ideas and beliefs about religion, social norms, and proper behavior, parents may demand certain behaviors, such as going to church, that the teenager believes are hypocritical. This creates much tension between adolescents and parents.

The ability to think abstractly allows adolescents to consider many moral issues that they did not think about or question in the past; it seems these issues never existed before. Teenagers struggle with such issues as: Is war justified? Is abortion moral? Is casual sex wrong? Is lying ever justified? Are the rich obligated to care for the poor? Some of these issues form the base of our political and societal standards. When teenagers question these and find they cannot justify society's stand, they may feel very alienated.

KOHLBERG'S THEORY

Kohlberg's research on the moral development of adolescents followed closely Piaget's work on cognitive development. Older children and young adolescents uphold a morality of law and order to determine right and wrong.[16]

As teenagers move into the *transitional level,* they begin questioning the status quo. Choice is based on emotions, and morality is arbitrary. At this point adolescents begin questioning societal standards and standing outside society while deliberating moral dilemmas, with no set principles for their choices and decisions.

Not all teenagers move through all successive stages of moral development, either during the adolescent or the young adult years. Even many adults operate at a conventional (law and order) stage of moral decision making. Adolescents pass through these stages at different rates and often find that they and their friends, who used to think alike about certain moral questions, now differ in their assessment of a situation.

The adolescent who advances to the *postconventional and principled level* of moral development finds moral decisions are based on rights, values, and principles that are agreeable to a given society. These rights and values may conflict with the stated laws and rules of the society. This person is able to understand and enter into contracts and agreements, recognizing the legal and moral points of view and seeing the conflict between the two. The teenager, for example, may engage in peaceful protest demonstrations.

In the final stage of the postconventional and principled level, *universal ethical principles,* the person bases right actions on the recognition of the validity of the universal principles underlying laws and social agreements. If laws violate these principles, the individual follows the principle, not the law.[16]

Adolescents are able to advance through these stages because of their ability to think abstractly about the human effects of certain values and because of their own growing experience with different ways of thinking. The school-age child does not have this wealth of experience nor the cognitive skills to view morality in this way.

Carol Gilligan[9] points out that Kohlberg's theory of moral development was based on research with an all-male population and does not reflect the development found in female adolescents. Young girls move from the generic platform of "good is rewarded" to the ability to define good as a relational attribute of caring for others. Young female adolescents acquire the ability for self-sacrifice, seeing good as caring for the many relationships in their lives. As her moral reasoning matures, she achieves a balance between what is good for herself and for others in her network of relationships.[9] Maturity in moral reasoning is situational and relational. Much research is currently being conducted on the topic of gender differences in adolescents' cognitive, emotional, and moral development. The nurse needs to be aware of new findings in these areas in order to work effectively with all teenagers.

The nurse can assist adolescents by being open to their way of thinking about moral issues and offering opportunities for dialogue between teenagers and adults and between teenagers themselves.

Moral thinking is not necessarily reflected in action. An adolescent may think something is wrong and be able to explain this feeling. Under pressure from peers or other stresses, however, the adolescent may act contrary to this expressed belief. This difference between knowledge and action is present throughout life.

Health Perception and Health Management Pattern

An important task during adolescence is to develop a stable, positive self-image. Young persons are very concerned about their physical development, appearance, and emotions. Does this egocentrism include an interest in health? If so, how do adolescents define their unique health care needs?

The needs of this age group largely have come from an analysis of morbidity and mortality rates. Using these measures, the health of adolescents appears to be very good. They have fewer acute illnesses than children, and the prevalence of chronic disease among teenagers is lower than that of adults. Adolescents are seen in physicians' offices less frequently than children or adults and are rarely hospitalized.

Many question, however, the validity of using these statistics as a measure of health. A more holistic perspective, which includes biologic, social, psychologic, and developmental factors, is necessary. A crucial component of an integrated understanding of adolescent health is consideration of the adolescent's own perceptions of health, illness, and health care services.[20]

Two studies in Minnesota organized high-school students into discussion groups to respond to questions about health and health care services. Data from these discussion groups were analyzed to identify recurrent themes. These adolescents saw health as more than the absence of disease. They viewed health as an optimum capability to pursue the activities of daily living with energy and involvement. Positive self-regard and psychologic well-being as well as a healthy, vigorous, and attractive appearance were seen as components of health.[14]

The adolescents in these studies indicated that major roadblocks to the attainment of good health were not only traditional medical problems but, more importantly, personal problems in relationships with others, particularly family, peers, and teachers. Other researchers also have noted that many health concerns of adolescents are related to psychosocial issues.

Even though adolescents are able to identify health problems that concern them most, they often are reluctant to seek health care. Some even deny signs and symptoms of an illness in an effort to maintain their activities of daily living, particularly contact with their peers. The following factors influence adolescents' health service utilization:

1. Severity of the illness
2. Duration of signs and symptoms
3. Restrictions on daily routine
4. Costs
5. Availability of a competent, sympathetic provider
6. Their awareness of a need for care

Proximity to health care is also an important variable for adolescents. Health clinics located within schools are emerging as a way to reach more teens. Both family and peers may serve as advisors in seeking health care, although peers become more important as the adolescent gets older.[14,20]

Adolescents are in the process of developing patterns of problem solving and health habits that are likely to last a lifetime. The cognitive and psychologic changes they experience may affect their adherence to preventive health care practices. Teenagers do not always consider the risks of their behavior and are unlikely to act differently from their peers. In striving for independence, they often will reject adult values and beliefs. A parent telling an adolescent to seek health or illness care may be met with great resistance. Nurses will be more successful in assisting the adolescent to manage health needs wisely if they treat him or her as a partner in planning care for which he or she will assume responsibility.[3,21]

ENVIRONMENTAL PROCESSES

Natural Processes

PHYSICAL AGENTS

Accidents continue to be the leading cause of death and injury in the teenage population, as for all children over 1 year of age. The types of accidents differ, with non-motor vehicle accidents decreasing and motor vehicle-related accidents increasing sharply. The non-motor vehicle accidents such as drowning, burns, and falls are discussed in previous chapters.

MECHANICAL AGENTS

Automobiles. Adolescents become increasingly mobile as they become progressively more independent. This increased mobility usually involves use of motorcycles and cars. Teenage drivers are overrepresented in fatal crashes, with the death rate for 18-year-old drivers greater than that of any other age group. Beginning at age 13, teenage passengers' death rates rise sharply and peak between ages 16 and 19. Nearly two thirds of these deaths occur in cars driven by a teenager and 45% to 60% of these accidents are alcohol related. Teenagers who drive need to be aware of traffic regulations and observe the speed limit. Knowledge of limits and regulations, however, does not prevent the teenager from giving in to peer pressure to try to set a record or perform other experimental maneuvers. The teenager may use driving as an outlet for stress or a way to assert independence.[5] (See box on p. 542.)

Driver education classes offered through the school can teach teenagers proper driving techniques and regulations. Unfortunately, the availability of such classes may encourage more adolescents to drive at a younger age than if they depended on family members or private driving classes. Communities that have eliminated high-school driver education programs have seen a sharp decline in teenage driver accidents. Each teenager should be considered on an individual basis regarding demonstrated level of responsibility, common sense, and ability to resist peer pressure. The teenager and parents should discuss these points and decide if the adolescent is responsible enough to drive. Age alone does not determine readiness for this increased level of independence.

Teenagers who have learned to drive still need some limits on automobile use. Parents and their teenager should negotiate these limits and periodically review and revise them based on the adolescent's safety record. Adolescents continually but *gradually* should assume more responsibility for their actions, especially when the consequences can be serious injury or death in an auto accident.

Motorcycles. Teenagers who ride motorcycles are also at risk for injury or death. Since head injury is a frequent outcome of motorcyle crashes, some states have passed strict laws requiring use of a protective helmet by any driver or passenger of a motorcycle. These helmets have been effective in reducing motorcycle injury and death but have met with much resistance. Unfortunately, because of public pressure, some states have repealed their mandatory helmet laws and have seen a sharp rise in fatalities among motorcyclists not wearing helmets.

Sports. Sports activities are extremely important during adolescence; they provide a means for social and personality development not afforded by any other activity. In addition to valuable exercise, sports provide experience in competition; team effort; and mature, acceptable conflict resolution and help develop self-esteem.

However, teenagers are particularly prone to sport injuries because their coordination skills are not fully developed, their judgment is often immature and inadequate, the epiphyses are not yet closed, and the extremities are poorly protected by stabilizing musculature. Also, school athletic programs often are underserved by health care workers, who can provide consultation in prevention of sports-related injuries and offer immediate care to injured players.

Sports-related injuries are likely to involve the head, spine, and extremities. Injuries to the head and brain are of special concern because of possible long-term neurologic damage or death. Spinal cord injuries also can result in long-term disability or death; cervical spine injuries are most common and are related to hyperflexion, hyperextension, or flexion compression of the vertebral column. Adolescents are prone to knee injuries because of the lack of strength and flexibility of the musculature and connective tissue surrounding the joint. Injuries tend to occur when the foot is locked to the ground or otherwise immobilized, and a lateral force causes the femur to adduct while the tibia rotates externally, with a medial hinging action between the femur and the tibia. Ankle injuries, particularly sprains, are also common. Foot injuries include puncture wounds, lacerations, and tendonitis.

The school nurse can practice primary prevention for sports injuries by advocating proper safety equipment and instruction, sports-focused physical examination for all participants, and strict regulations prohibiting an injured player from further participation until appropriate rehabilitation is completed.

BIOLOGIC AND BACTERIAL AGENTS

By adolescence a person has built up immunity to many organisms that cause the more common childhood illnesses. However, the sexually active teenager may come in contact with new groups of organisms: *sexually transmitted diseases (STDs),* including gonorrhea, syphilis, genital warts (condyloma acuminatum), genital herpesvirus type 2, chlamydial, *Trichomonas* and *Candida* infections, and AIDS.

Many adolescents over age 15 are at least occasionally sexually active. Young persons need to be aware of the prevalence of these infections and the means of prevention, detection, and diagnosis. Prevention is primarily through avoidance of sexual contact with an infected person; however, a partner's state of infection often is not recognizable. Many teenagers have heard of the more common STDs but may not realize that these diseases are practically epidemic in the young population.[13]

Viral STDs, like venereal warts (human papillomavirus [HPV]) and herpes simplex virus type 2 (HSV-2), have been recognized as serious and, to date, incurable infections that are associated with the occurrence and transmission of human immunodeficiency virus (HIV).[11] HPV is recognized as an oncogenic factor in the evolution of cervical dysplasia.[6,8]

CHEMICAL AGENTS

Drug abuse, or *substance abuse,* as it is sometimes called, does not start abruptly in adolescence and end before adulthood begins; but it is more widespread during the adolescent years. School-age children may try alcohol or tobacco or other easily available drugs; the use of such substances has been starting at younger ages in recent years.[5] Adults often use certain chemical substances to excess, but they are more likely to restrict their use to several agents rather than try a variety of drugs as teenagers are likely to do. There are four factors to consider when discussing the causes of substance abuse in teenagers. First, our society is oriented to using such chemicals as medications, alcohol, and tobacco to feel better, look better, look and act more social, have more energy, stay awake, go to sleep, be sexy, and so on. One evening of television viewing illustrates this very well. Some of the most famous music, theater, and sports stars have very openly modeled substance abuse for their fans.

Second, dysfunctional families (i.e., characterized by substance abuse, poor communication, rigidity, isolation, divorce, physical or sexual abuse) produce a higher percentage of teens who are substance abusers.[12]

Third, the individual teen may be predisposed because of depression, low self-esteem, pervasive anger, or excessive dependence.

Fourth, the peer group becomes very important in the middle teen years and may provide an overwhelming push toward drugs.[3]

Many adolescents use drugs once or on an infrequent basis; this is called experimental use. Others use drugs on a more regular, periodic basis, and a small percentage are compulsive users and are dependent on drug use.

The substances used and sometimes misused are classified according to their actions or availability. Some of these classifications are[8]

Depressants
- Alcohol
- Barbiturates
- Nonbarbiturate sedatives (especially methaqualone)
- Minor tranquilizers

Stimulants
- Amphetamines
- Cocaine
- Nicotine
- Caffeine

Hallucinogens/illusionogens
- Marijuana
- LSD
- Mescaline
- Dimethyltryptamine (DMT)
- PCP (phencyclidine)
- Psilocybin
- MDMA (methylenedioxymethamphetamine)

Opiates
- Heroin
- Morphine
- Codeine
- Meperidine
- Methadone

Volatile agents
- Toluene-based glues and paints
- Gasoline
- Alkyl nitrites
- Triethylene chloride (in typewriter correction fluid)

Some of these agents are easy for the teenager to obtain, whereas others required a major risk because of legal ramifications or places where the teenager must go to obtain them. Ethnic, geographic, and socioeconomic variables also influence choice of substance among teens. For example, white urban middle-class teens are more likely to choose alcohol and marijuana as "gateway" or initial substances. Rural and minority teens use inhalants more often as gateway substances.[25]

Although drugs usually are taken for the pleasurable or positive effects, they can also produce many negative effects.

Nurses must carefully assess their role in teenage drug use. If they believe their role is to prevent any use of drugs, the approach will be more rigid than if the goal is to prevent periodic drug use and dependence while accepting experimentation as a more acceptable form of experiencing this aspect of our culture (see box on p. 542).

Primary preventive intervention for chemical use should start in the school-age years. Establishing open dialogue between school-age children, their teachers, and the health care team is essential in providing openness and trust so that these school children can seek sound answers to their questions and discuss their concerns; of particular concern is the use that may be modeled in their homes. They need to discuss the underlying reasons why persons including their own parents may use drugs to cope with stress and fear, discuss healthy alternatives that can be used for coping, and experience the use of such alternate methods in the school setting. Young teens need to learn effective social skills to deal with peer pressure also and self-control skills. The use of alcohol and tobacco as a way of feeling "grown up" needs to be discussed, and the children should be encouraged to discuss and think about behavior that is more completely indicative of being "grown up."

During the adolescent years, the health education program should continue measures to inform teenagers of the hazards of drug misuse and abuse. Special attention should continue to be directed to the misuse of the socially sanctioned alcohol and tobacco products available to teenagers. The effects of health education on tobacco and alcohol use have not been confirmed as effective. Teenagers and children report, however, that drug education has influenced their decisions regarding use of drugs, alcohol, and tobacco, and the related health hazards are perceived accurately by those groups that have been surveyed. The young person tends to view the adverse health effects affecting the future and to indicate an intention to worry about that later. Primary prevention should be focused on providing information to help the young person make a responsible decision about drug use before experimentation. Age at first use is a critical risk factor for the development of substance abuse problems. The earlier the experimentation with drugs, the more likely that this teenager is dealing with a dysfunctional family or social environment.[15]

Secondary preventive intervention includes observing

for indications that a particular teenager may be using or abusing a drug, such as (1) a drop in school achievement; (2) personality change, such as more withdrawn, boisterous, or confused; (3) mood swings; (4) sleepiness or fatigue; and (5) behaviors noted for depression.

The nurse who suspects that a teenager is using or misusing drugs needs to approach the topic in a nonjudgmental way and attempt to find out the teenager's motivation as well as the extent of use. See Table 21-3 for common street names for drugs. These two factors will help the nurse make the best decision about referral for treatment or more information.

Because drug use is so common in the adolescent population, the nurse should routinely ask her school-age and adolescent clients about such use. The young person may choose to withhold such information, especially if this is the first encounter with the nurse. On the other hand, the adolescent may be relieved to know that the topic of drugs is acceptable in the health care setting and may have been wanting to discuss it with a knowledgeable adult.

CARCINOGENIC AGENTS

Radiation and temperature carcinogenic agents are discussed in previous chapters. Adolescents are affected by some of the same cancers as younger children, such as leukemia, osteogenic sarcoma lymphomas, and central nervous system tumors.

Adolescents begin to be at risk for some of the more typically adult-onset cancers because of tobacco use and exposure to carcinogens at a place of work. The nurse should always inquire about tobacco use habits, occupational history, and general respiratory environment at both the workplace and the home. "Smokeless" tobacco (i.e., snuff and chewing tobacco) is becoming more popular among young men. Surveys have shown from 8% to 30% of male high school students are regular users. Smokeless tobacco has been shown to cause oral-pharyngeal cancer.[8] Although the teenager may not have used tobacco for very long or have worked in an environment where there is asbestos or other respiratory carcinogens for more than a year or two, it is important to identify and inform the client of these risks.

Tobacco Use. The nurse's primary prevention focus should be on helping tobacco users to stop and keeping nonusers from starting.[6] Teenagers begin using tobacco for a variety of reasons: to seem older, to give in to peer pressure, or to imitate adult role models. Antitobacco discussions should start during the preadolescent years and continue through adolescence. One of the nurse's most important roles in helping teenagers to stop smoking is to serve as a role model. Nurses who smoke contradict all media coverage and scientific research pointing out the physical harm of smoking. Nurses cannot persuade a client to stop smoking if they have not. Research documents that fear tactics, nagging, preaching, and threats are not effective in convincing persons of any age to stop smoking. Because fear tactics have proved to be ineffective in changing smoking behaviors, serious efforts now are being made to create a social climate wherein smoking is not an acceptable behavior.

The nurse can assist teens to make rational decisions about tobacco use and occupational exposure to carcinogenic agents in several ways:

1. Conduct educational programs that unemotionally detail the known hazards of tobacco use.
2. Provide teenagers with educational material that further explains the health hazards of tobacco use or high-risk occupations.
3. Provide specific measures for those adolescents who desire to stop using tobacco or decrease occupational risk factors.

Many teenagers who want to stop tobacco use lack the information to help themselves stop. Nurses should be familiar with the antitobacco resources in their communities so that appropriate referrals may be made.[14]

Cancer. Older adolescents are entering the period of their lives when cancer of the reproductive and related organs is more common. For teenage women, focus is on cervical and breast cancer; for teenage men, on testicular cancer.

Peak incidence of *breast* and *cervical cancer* is during middle age and is actually quite rare in the teen years. Breast self-examination (BSE), which has been highly recommended for over 30 years, has recently been questioned as a routine practice for most young women. The extremely small number of breast cancers in teens weighted against the anxiety caused when a young woman finds a "normal" lump in her breast have caused some health care providers to deemphasize this practice for many teens. A genetic predisposition does exist for breast cancer, so the nurse should inquire into family history with the young woman. Certainly any young woman with a positive family history should be taught BSE.[20]

Following maturation of the breasts, young women can be taught how to examine them for early signs of cancer.

Regular examination of the breasts should follow each menstrual period. BSE can be taught during the physical assessment, but films and group discussions are helpful in reinforcing the importance and acceptability of this

Table 21-3.* Street names for drugs

Slang	Translation	Slang	Translation
A's	amphetamine	cokie	cocaine addict
Acapulco gold	high-grade marijuana	Coolie	PCP
acid	LSD, D-lysergic acid, diethylamide tartrate	copilots	amphetamines
angel dust	DMT or PCP sprinkled over parsley or tobacco	crank	methamphetamine hydrochloride
babo	Nalline Hydrochloride (brand of nalorphine)	crap	heroin
bag	packet of drugs	Cristina	methamphetamine hydrochloride
bagging	sniffing glue in a bag	crystal	methamphetamine hydrochloride, powdered or crystalline form
barbs	barbiturates	cubes	LSD
base	cocaine	DET	diethyltryptamine
Beast (The)	LSD	dexies	Dexedrine (brand of dextroamphetamine sulfate)
bennies	Benzedrine (brand of amphetamine sulfate)	DMT	dimethyltryptamine
Bernice	cocaine	dollies	Dolphine (brand of methadone hydrochloride) tablets
bhang	marijuana	DOM	dimethoxymethyamphetamine (see STP)
big chief	mescaline	downers	nonnarcotic central nervous system depressants
Big "D"	LSD	dusts	cocaine, PCP
black	LSD	dynamite	high-grade heroin
black beauty	methamphetamine	flake	cocaine
blow	cocaine	footballs	amphetamine tablets (oval shaped)
blue angels		gage	marijuana (term seldom used)
bluebirds		ganja	hashish
blue devils	amobarbital sodium	gee-head	paregoric user
blue heaven			
blues		geeze	injecting heroin
Blue Cheer	type of LSD	gold dust	cocaine
blues-and-reds	see rainbows	goof balls	barbiturates
blue velvet	paregoric in combination with amphetamine or antihistamine such as Pyribenzamine (brand of tripelennamine)	grass	marijuana (dried leaves, seeds, and stems of *Cannabis sativa*)
bombers	large marijuana cigarettes	H	heroin (diacetyl morphine)
bombido	injectable amphetamine	Harry	heroin (diacetyl morphine)
boo	marijuana	Harvey wallbanger	STP-LSD
booze	alcohol	hash	hashish (resin from *Cannabis*)
brown	heroin	hay	marijuana
brown dot	LSD	hearts	Dexedrine (brand of dextroamphetamine sulfate)
buds	marijuana	hog	PCP
bullets	Seconal (brand of secobarbital sodium)	honk	spray paint inhalation
bush	marijuana	horse	heroin (diacetyl morphine)
businessman's trip	DMT	hyke	Hycodan (hydrocodone)
buttons	dried tops of the *Lophophora* cactus (peyote)	ice	methyamphetamine (crystal)
cactus	mescaline	J	marijuana cigarette
candy	barbiturates	Jim Jones	marijuana cigarette laced with cocaine dipped in PCP
cap	capsules	joint	marijuana cigarette
cartwheel	white, round, double-scored amphetamine tablet	jug	ampoule of injectable drugs

From Neinstien LS: *Adolescent health care,* Baltimore, 1991, Williams & Wilkins.

*In treating adolescents for drug use, it is important for the practitioner to be familiar with drug slang. Drug slang constantly changes and no listing is ever up to date. Also, communities often have their own terms for drugs, and the translation may vary from locality to locality.

Table 21-3. Street names for drugs–cont'd

Slang	Translation	Slang	Translation
M	morphine sulfate	scag	heroin (diacetyl morphine)
magic mushroom	mushroom (*Psilocybe mexicana*) containing psilocybin	scat	heroin (diacetyl morphine)
mesc	mescaline	school boy	codeine
mese	mescaline (resin from *Lophophora* cactus–peyote)	sherms	PCP
meth	methamphetamine	shit	heroin or marijuana
Mexican brown	brown marijuana from Mexico	shrooms	hallucinogenic mushrooms
Mickey	combination of alcohol and chloral hydrate	Simple Simon	psylocybin (*Psilocybe mexicana*) from the Mexican mushroom
Miss Emma	morphine sulfate	smack	heroin (diacetyl morphine)
MJ	marijuana	snow	cocaine
mota	Mexican term for good marijuana	snowcap	cocaine sprinkled on a bowl of marijuana
nembies	pentobarbital sodium	spacebasing	rock or crack cocaine with PCP and tobacco
number	marijuana cigarette	speed	methamphetamine
orange	STP-LSD	speedball	heroin and cocaine injected
orange sunshine	form of LSD	splash	methamphetamine
Panama red	potent grade of marijuana from Panama	STP	dimethoxymethyamphetamine (see DOM) (serenity-tranquility-peace)
peace pill (PCP)	Sernylan (brand of phencyclidine), an anesthetic originally for dogs	stuff	heroin (diacetyl morphine)
peanuts	barbiturates	sugar	LSD
PG	paregoric	sunshine	LSD
piece of stuff	1 oz of heroin	tea	marijuana
pinks	secobarbital sodium	toot	cocaine
popper	amyl nitrate in ampoule form (generally sniffed)	trips	LSD
pot	marijuana	T's	talwin–pentazocine
powder	amphetamine sulfate in powder form	T's and Blues	pentazocine and tripelennamine
primo	marijuana cigarette laced with cocaine	T's and B's	pentazocine and tripelennamine
purple	STP-LSD	uppers	CNS stimulants
purple hearts	Dexamyl (brand of dextroamphetamine sulfate and amorbarbital sodium)	Water	PCP
rainbows	Tuinal (brand of amobarbital sodium and secobarbital sodium–red and blue capsules)	weed	marijuana
RDs	secobarbital	whacking	rock or crack cocaine with PCP and tobacco, smoked
red devils	secobarbital	Whites	amphetamines
reds	secobarbital	window panes	LSD in gelatin sheets
reds and blues	see rainbows	yellow jackets	pentobarbital sodium
roach	butt of marijuana cigarette	yellows	pentobarbital sodium
roaches	librium		
rope	hashish		
caviar	rock or crack cocaine with marijuana, smoked	juice	PCP
chalk	methamphetamine hydrochloride, powder form	junk	heroin (diacetyl morphine)
champagne	rock or crack cocaine with marijuana, smoked	junkie	heroin user
Charlie	cocaine	key	kilogram of marijuana
Chicano green	type of dark green marijuana	lid	1 oz of marijuana (approximate)
china white	heroine, fentanyl	Llesea	Mexican term for marijuana
chipping	periodic use of intravenously used drugs	locoweed	jimsonweed (*Datura stramonium*)
Christmas tree	Tuinal (brand of amobarbital sodium and secobarbital sodium)	ludes	methaqualone
coke	cocaine (extract of dried leaves of *Erythroxylon coca*)		

self-care responsibility. Detailed instructions on BSE are shown in Fig. 21-7. The nurse also should tell young women to make an appointment with their health care provider for a breast examination if they feel a breast mass.

Cervical cancer can be detected through a Pap smear, that is, obtaining and examining cells from the uterine cervical os, a procedure done during a pelvic examination. Sexually active teenage women should have a Pap test done yearly. The American College of Obstetricians and Gynecologists recommends annual examinations to begin by age 18, even if the young women is not sexually active. Teenage women are often reluctant to have these checkups. They fear pain, embarrassment and the public acknowledgment of being sexually active. The nurse should explain the purpose of the examination, the Pap test, and cultures to young women and strongly encourage them to comply with this preventive measure. The nurse can reassure the young woman that the exam will be performed gently and with sensitivity and that the sensation is one of pressure rather than pain. The nurse should also screen for high-risk factors for cervical cancer, such as[4]

1. Sexual intercourse before age 20

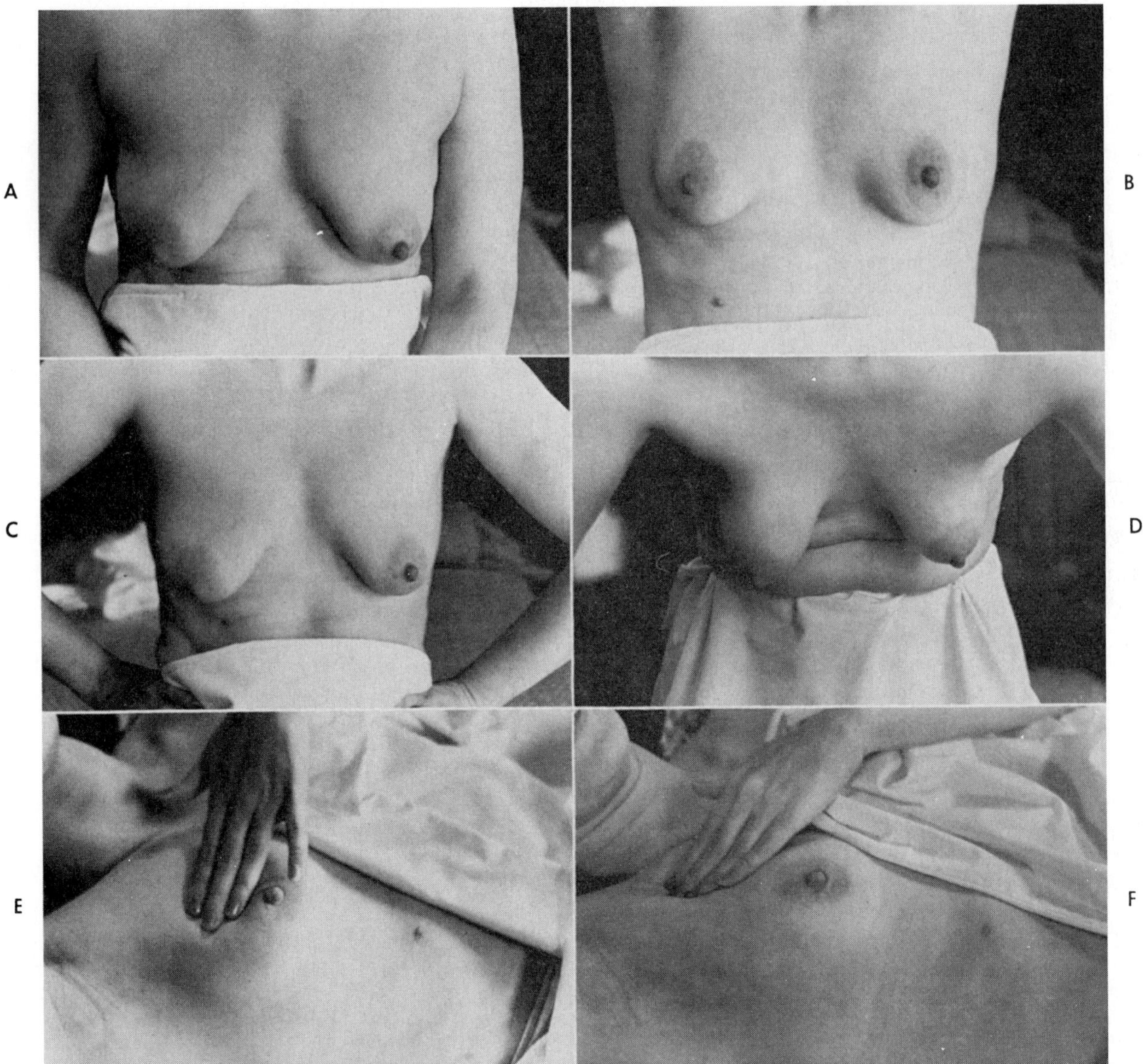

Fig. 21-7. Breast self-examination is accomplished as follows: **A,** Standing before mirror, woman visually inspects breasts for usual contour and appearance of visible excessive drooping, masses, or depressions. **B,** Same observations are made with arms raised over head. **C,** Arms then are placed on hips with pressure applied to hips, and breasts are checked for any unusual contour changes. **D,** Woman observes breasts for contour and symmetry as she leans forward. **E,** Lying on bed with pillow under shoulder, woman palpates breast near areola, **F,** toward neck and shoulder.

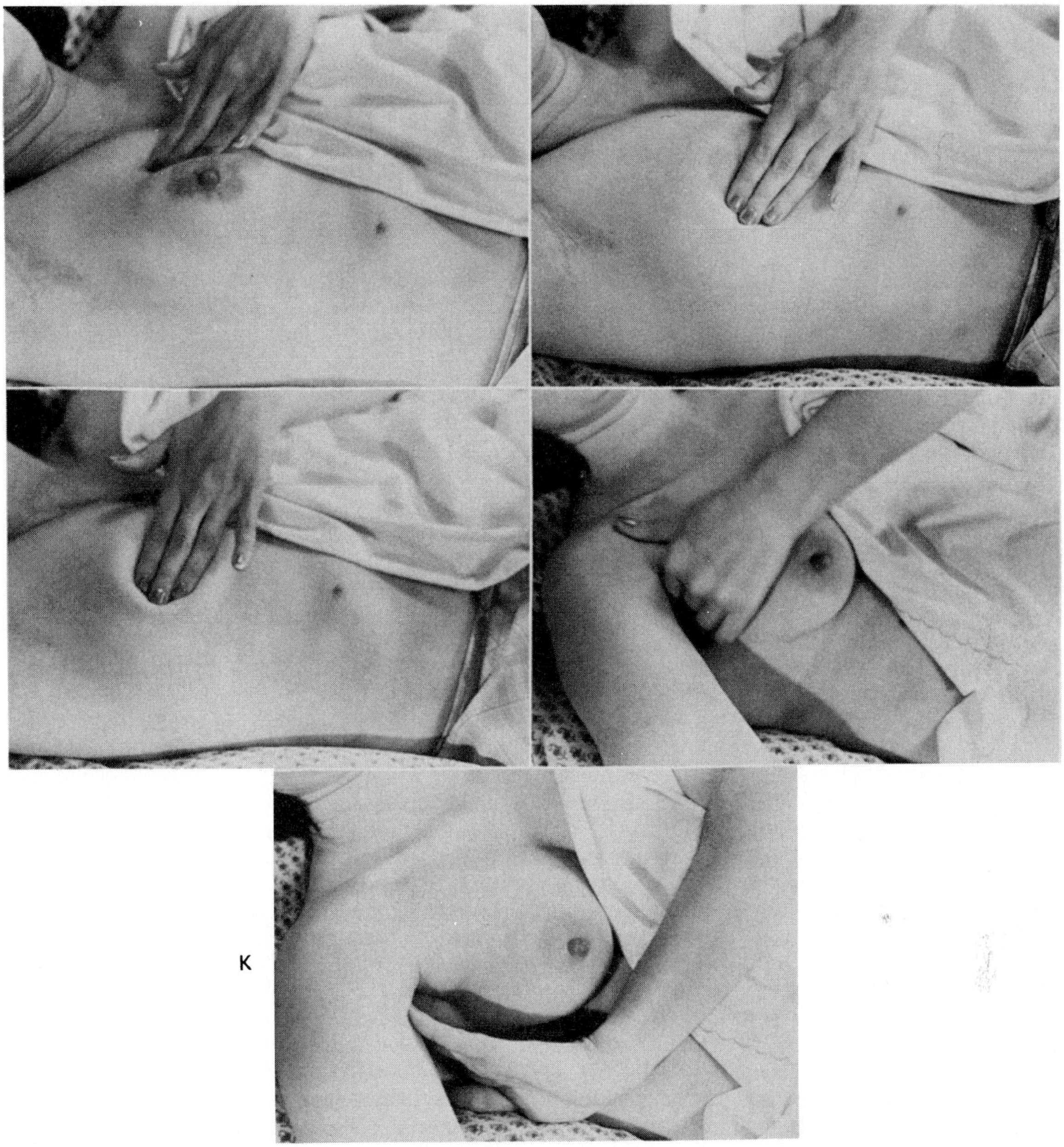

G H I J K

Fig. 21-7, cont'd. Lying on bed with pillow under shoulder, woman palpates breast **G,** toward sternum and, **H,** around and toward axilla. **I,** Woman palpates area beneath areola and nipple. Axilla is palpated over rib cage, **J,** and over arm, **K.** (From Chinn PL: *Child health maintenance: concepts in family-centered care,* ed 2, St Louis, 1979, Mosby.)

2. Multiple sexual partners
3. A sexual partner who has had many partners
4. Any history of sexually transmitted diseases
5. Any exposure to exogenous hormones (DES in utero or oral contraceptive user)
6. History of smoking or current smoker

Testicular cancer is one of the most common cancers in men between ages 20 and 35. Most testicular cancers are first discovered by the men themselves. If treated early, there is an excellent chance for total cure. Adolescent males should learn to do a testicular self-examination and continue this practice once a month for the rest of their lives.

The best time for self-examination of the testes is immediately after a bath or shower. While each testicle is rolled gently between thumb and fingers, any abnormal lumps should be noted. The epididymis, located at the back of each testicle, should be identified and not erroneously labeled an abnormal lump.

Although most teenagers do not like to think that they will ever have a cancerous lesion, the nurse needs to introduce this topic and teach the common methods of self-examination and the warning signs of cancer. This is an excellent time to begin a lifelong habit of self-examination.

Social Processes

ROLE AND RELATIONSHIP PATTERN

Until adolescence, the child depends very much on the parents. Striving for independence and self-identity, an adolescent pulls away from family. Parents feel their influence decrease as their teenager spends more and more time with peers, questions their basic beliefs and values, and becomes more mobile. This is a time of crisis for parents, and they may respond by setting unreasonably strict limits or asking intrusive questions about their teenager's activities, friends, and ideas. Another typical but more uncommon response is for parents to drop all rules and limits and assume that the adolescent can manage alone. Both these responses add further tension to the family.

The family with an adolescent also goes through a period of development. The adolescent is striving for a sense of identity and independence within society. The family is learning to let go; parents are focusing on their marital relationships, their aging parents, and their satisfaction with their work and goal attainment. The family may be described as in disequilibrium or in a normative developmental crisis.

Each member is temporarily unsure of their relationship with other family members. The family unit may undergo more stress than at any previous time.[6] Specific issues of conflict may center around

1. The adolescent moving psychologically or physically away from the family toward peers for support
2. The adolescent becoming more mobile
3. Power struggles developing over family rules, money, school performance, religion, privacy, choice of career, or school
4. New roles developing for other family members

Some families experience more negative outcomes than other families. Families whose parents maintain a willingness to listen and demonstrate an ongoing affection and acceptance of their adolescent have a more constructive, positive outcome during this adjustment period. This does not mean that parents do not disagree with their teenager's ideas or actions but rather that they are willing to hear what the adolescent has to say and to negotiate some limits.[21]

Parents may be very worried about substance abuse, early sexual experience, or other actions of their teenager but hesitate to verbalize such topics. Parents may need assistance determining the negotiable versus non-negotiable rules and how to voice their concerns in an honest, open way. Even if teenagers do not want to discuss these topics, at least they know why parents are concerned. (See box on p. 542.)

Siblings also experience changes in their relationship at this time. Older adolescent siblings may withdraw from the child just entering adolescence, adult siblings may empathize with the adolescent or assume a "parent" role, and younger siblings may emulate the older teenager. On the other hand, if there is prolonged, heated conflict between parents and adolescent, the younger sibling may regress in an attempt to escape the conflict.

The nurse can practice primary prevention of undue adolescent-parent and family conflict during this time by encouraging open communication between family members through family meetings, where each member is able to state views without criticism from others. The nurse also can provide information to both parents and teenagers about the conflicts at this time and the needs of family members during this transition. Secondary prevention for families who are experiencing unmanageable conflicts includes referral for family or individual counseling through an agency or practitioner experienced in dealing with adolescents and their families.

COMMUNITY: PEERS

Faced with the need to become autonomous, to achieve sexual function and identity, and to become economically self-sufficient and productive, the older adolescent turns from the family to peers and more intimate relationships.

Belonging to an informally organized clique, a crowd, a gang, or specific group is the primary means in Western societies for adolescents to make the transition from primary allegiance as a child in the family group to a colleague in the peer group. A sense of commonality develops within the group and follows no set rules or regulations but demands loyalty and group solidarity. This type of group membership requires that the individual lay aside personal goals and gain to achieve what is desired for the group as a whole. Identification with the group is proclaimed through conformity to standards of clothing, behavior, language, and values. This feature of the adolescent subculture persists despite the strong inclination in family and social structures toward greater levels of individuality. The adolescent group is a vehicle for movement out and away from the family unit, however, and as such it provides a means of achieving the goals of individuation.[27]

Teenagers talk a great deal with their peers. Whether on the phone or in person, they can discuss a 10-minute situation for hours on end. This sharing of thoughts and impressions is important for the adolescents to orient themselves to the norms of the group (Fig. 21-8). The telephone may provide a "safe" mechanism for the young teenager to converse with members of the opposite sex.

A same-sex best friend is very important, especially in the early adolescence. Best friends share their most intimate ideas and concerns and begin to experience a closeness and caring that will develop into the capacity

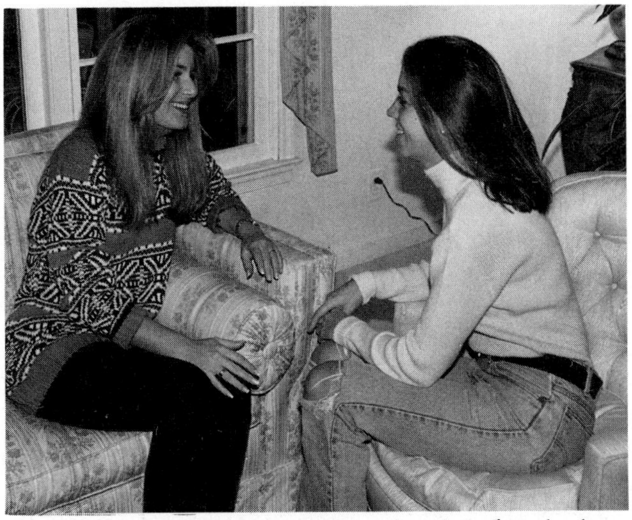

Fig. 21-8. Adolescence is a time when best friends share their ideas and talents. (Photo by Fredric J. Edelman.)

to form an intimate heterosexual relationship (Fig. 21-9).

Dating is a social custom developed by middle-class youth. Going steady means an exclusive dating situation. Some very young teenagers use the phrase "going steady" to indicate their relationship with a member of the opposite sex with whom they have never had a date but who may talk to them on the phone on a regular basis. Controversy surrounds young adolescents dating; certain churches disapprove of early dating, whereas some persons think early dating is a valuable educational experience in social skills and human relationships. Clearly, dating improves the adolescents' status among peers, while parents worry that it may lead to an early sexual relationship.

SEXUAL ACTIVITY

Teenagers become sexually active for a variety of reasons, which vary as the adolescent matures. Adolescents have sex for affection, because of peer pressure, as a symbol of maturity, spontaneous experimentation, to feel close, and because it feels good.

Adolescents 15 to 18 years old may take fewer risks and be more thoughtful about the reasons for having sex. Unfortunately, many of them may not use contraception or consider the possible outcomes of sexual activity any more than they did at younger ages. Older adolescents, ages 18 to 20, are more likely to plan for sexual intercourse by obtaining information about and using effective contraception.

Sexual activity is no longer the exception for teenagers; it has become almost a norm. Although gathering such data on younger teenagers is more difficult because of parental objections to surveys, several studies indicate that this younger group is also very sexually active. An indication of total numbers can be seen in the number of teenage pregnancies: among sexually experienced 15- to 19-year-olds, 32.5% have already had a premarital pregnancy.

The first step in primary prevention is involving parents and schools in the provision of accurate information and on sexuality, sexual decision making, contraception, and STD prevention.

Sensitivity to sexual preference is an important consideration in working with adolescents. Not all teens are heterosexual, and the nurse must have an open accepting approach in order to elicit an accurate sexual history and respond to the individual teen's needs appropriately.[22]

CONTRACEPTION

Adolescents need to become thoroughly acquainted with the available methods. Nurses must put aside moral judgments in counseling with individual teenagers and in recognizing a real health need. Both young men and young women should understand the methods of contraception, and they should know where to obtain help and advice when they need it. The community and the family of an individual teenager may have reservations or strong objections to the availability of such information, and the impact of these preferences should be understood and respected. The individual teenager, however, has the right and privilege to obtain information and to make a confidential choice that includes the consequences of the choice and the inherent responsibilities of the choice. Teenagers can be encouraged to know and understand the teachings of their culture, family, and religion regarding family planning and to make their own choice based on each aspect of the situation. The legal rights identified for minors in Ameri-

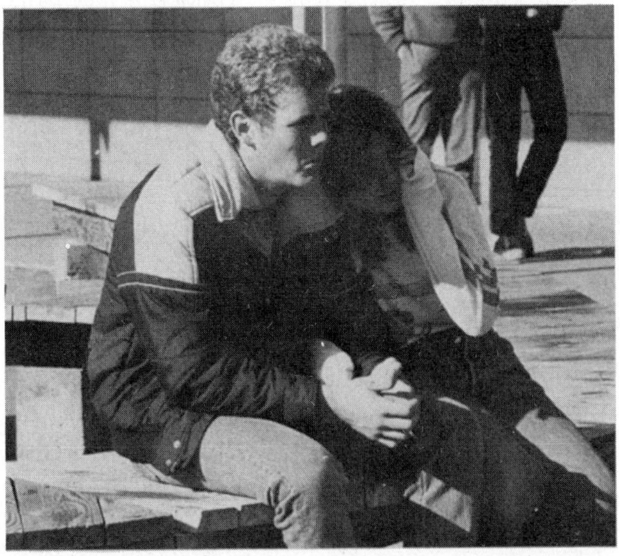

Fig. 21-9. Older adolescents are able to form and maintain a close relationship with a member of the opposite sex.

can society must be advocated if health care needs are to be met.[4]

The *rhythm method* of contraception involves determining the time of ovulation during the female cycle and abstinence from coitus during the normal lifespan of sperm before ovulation and for the lifespan of the ovum after ovulation. Ovulation usually occurs 14 days before the last day of a uterine cycle, but variation in timing of ovulation from cycle to cycle and from individual to individual makes exact prediction of this event difficult. To use the rhythm method, the woman's cycle must be fairly regular from month to month. As adolescents commonly experience irregular menstrual cycles, this is not a recommended method of contraception. However, many teens are unaware of ovulation patterns, fertile periods, and the lifespan of sperm, so clear discussion of these issues can increase the teen's reproductive knowledge base.

The *diaphragm* is a small, rubber dome molded onto a circular rim, which is fitted between the posterior farnix and the pubic bone to occlude the entry of sperm into the uterus. It is used in combination with a spermicidal cream or jelly and thus provides both a mechanical and a chemical barrier. The device must obtained from a health care agency and is not available in drugstores, as it must be fitted. Use of the diaphragm requires some amount of manipulation, which is troublesome and inconvenient for the adolescent. The overall failure rate is about 12%. The diaphragm has become increasingly popular, however, because of the relative safety of this method over all others in relation to the woman's own health.

The Food and Drug Administration (FDA) has recently approved a new barrier form of contraception, the *cervical cap*. This thimble-sized device is held in place over the cervix by suction.

The *condom* also is used to provide a mechanical barrier to the entry of sperm into the uterus. This method of contraception probably is attempted by most young teenage boys, and the peer-group sources of sex information usually include some description of the use of condoms. Condoms are recommended as a protection against STDs, but because only a portion of skin area is covered by the sheath, protection is limited. The sheaths are made of rubber or plastic and usually are supplied in a rolled form ready to be unrolled onto the erect penis. A small portion at the end of the sheath acts as a receptacle for the seminal fluid. The actual failure rate is about 10 per 100 woman years.

Chemical contraceptives also are readily available in drugstores without prescription. In the form of sponges, creams, jellies, and foams, their use is relatively simple and inexpensive. These preparations contain nonoxynol 9, which kills and immobilizes sperm and may provide some protection against STDS. However, they must be applied just before coitus and may be considered "messy" and involve touching the genital area. The actual effectiveness varies widely depending on use technique. When foam is used with a condom, the effectiveness is almost 100% and is as effective as oral contraceptives with the added benefit of reducing transmission of STDs.[6] (See box below for a research review on AIDS education.)

The female *oral contraceptive* prevents ovulation by chemically altering the usual endocrine cycle. Most forms contain estrogen, which raises the circulating level of this hormone early in the menstrual cycle. Since high levels of estrogen prevent the release of follicle-stimulating hormone (FSH) by the pituitary gland, ovarian follicles are not stimulated to mature, and ovulation is prevented. When progesterone is added to the estrogen preparation, the endometrium of the uterus is stimulated to develop as during a normal cycle, and withdrawal of the pill causes a menstrual period to occur that stimulates the normal ovulatory cycle.

The pill has certain bothersome side effects for many

RESEARCH REVIEW — ADOLESCENCE

AIDS EDUCATION

Ross MW, Caudle C, Taylor J: Relationship of AIDS education and knowledge to AIDS-related social skills in adolescents, *J Sch Health* 61:351-354, 1992.

Purpose The purpose of this study was to investigate the relationship between AIDS education, AIDS knowledge, and risk-related social skills.

Review Subjects (n = 490) were randomly selected from 10 high schools in urban and country areas. Questionnaires administered included the AIDS Social Assertive Scale (ASAS) and National AIDS Education Program AIDS Awareness Quiz for Young People developed as a standardized national measure for the federal government. Age, grade, hours of AIDS education, and sexual experience (condom use) were likewise ascertained. Results indicated that students at schools in the country and working-class areas had lower knowledge levels. Data confirmed a strong relationship between hours of AIDS education and AIDS knowledge.

women, including weight gain, nausea, breakthrough bleeding, and breast tenderness that simulate a pregnant state. Other side effects include headaches, regression of gum tissue around the teeth, eye complications, and increased blood pressure. Serious side effects that have been substantiated are the risks of thromboembolic disease, heart disease, hypertension, and cancer. Thus, the pill is never recommended for a woman who has had prior blood-clotting problems or who has a strong family history of these problems. The risk of serious illness or death from the use of the pill is less than that expected from normal pregnancy and childbirth; and the pill is still considered to be a safe, convenient, and reliable form of contraception. The woman who uses the pill enhances safety of use by having regular evaluations of her progress and her condition supervised by a health care professional. This often involves annual examination before the drug is renewed. Women who find remembering to take the pill daily difficult or impossible should use another form of contraception. The failure rate of the pill when it is used correctly is about 0.6%. Most instances of failure result from forgetting to take the pill regularly.

Progestin-only hormonal injections have been used worldwide for many years as a safe and effective method of contraception. Injections of medroxyprogesterone acetate (Depoprovera) inhibit ovulations and cause atrophy of the endometrium and thickening of the cervical mucus. The effectiveness is similar to over-the-counter products (OCPs) and it must be given every 90 days. This method provides long-acting contraception, amenorrhea or oligomenorrhea, and an alternative for poor pill takers or coitus-dependent methods.

Norplant is a silastic capsule which is placed subdermally in the medial aspect of the upper arm. It slowly releases lovonorgestrel into the bloodstream. This low-dose progestin provides contraception by thickening cervical mucus, reducing peristalsis of the fallopian tube, and causing the endometrium to be inhospitable for implantation. Ovarian follicles develop, and ovulation can occur. The actual failure rate is less than 1%; but of those pregnancies, 25% may be ectopic. Because ovarian estrogen is not suppressed, the endometrium will proliferate and shed unpredictably. Many adolescents find the unpredictable vaginal bleeding unacceptable. The capsules are relatively invisible and easy to place; removal can prove more challenging.[6] (See box on p. 542.)

PREGNANCY

When contraception fails or is not used and an unwanted pregnancy occurs, the problems for the adolescent are complex. Secondary prevention focuses on providing correct information regarding the options for continuing or terminating the pregnancy and referral to competent counselors or practitioners. Ideally the young woman, her family, and her partner should be involved in the decision of continuing or terminating a pregnancy; often it is the young woman alone who makes the decision. Her partner may have been a one-time or casual sexual encounter, and she may be afraid to confide in her family because she has never told them she is sexually active.

The adolescent of any age, but especially the very young adolescent who is pregnant, needs skilled counseling and support during this stressful time. She should be strongly encouraged but not forced to involve her parents. The adolescent who chooses to terminate the pregnancy should be referred to a clinic or private physician who is experienced with adolescents, and follow-up counseling should be arranged. The adolescent who chooses to continue the pregnancy should be referred to a practitioner who can provide not only the physical monitoring and care during pregnancy but also the emotional and developmental support that is essential for a positive experience with this pregnancy.

Table 16-3 outlines the developmental tasks of the pregnant adolescent. The nurse needs to be familiar with these developmental tasks and the possible range of their manifestations to interact with the pregnant adolescent. Many physical risks to the pregnant adolescent and her baby can be prevented or recognized and adequately treated through appropriate prenatal care.

SCHOOL

The school setting provides many important experiences for the adolescent: contact with peers, intellectual stimulation, and choices and restrictions of the community. It also can provide negative experiences, such as overwhelming competition, exposure to substance sellers and users, and peer pressure to rebel from parents and teachers.

Adolescents need to experience some degree of success in their academic life. Young adolescents are particularly vulnerable to slumps in relation to school achievement, since they are dealing with massive changes of their physical body, new social accomplishments, a new school situation, and the need to begin to establish new peer relationships. Their uncertainty regarding their ability in each of these areas and wavering in terms of their own identity are significant, whether these cause poor school performance or parallel events with no cause-effect relationship. Teenagers who are able to excel in school may find themselves in a particularly uncomfortable relationship with peers who envy their academic success. Thus, failure to achieve in school may result from the overwhelming need to experience group approval.

In addition, teenagers often experience conflicting messages about what is considered adequate achievement in school. The teachers in a junior high or middle school may define achievement in slightly different ways than what the child experienced in an elementary or primary school. Parents may begin to express increased concern as teenagers approach the stage when grades are important for potential college entry. Non–college-bound students must develop future life goals in a system which has not, in most instances, developed vocation and skill training alternatives.

Teachers and parents can contribute significantly to the nurse's understanding of the total situation of teenagers, and together they may be able to differentiate a serious problem from one that is within the range of normal adolescent behavior.

CULTURE

The family and ethnic influences that operated throughout childhood continue into adolescence. The adolescent may question or reject these influences more strongly than a younger counterpart, but the impact, especially when ethnically based, still exists because it can be seen by others. First- and second-generation adolescents of parents from the Pacific rim, Eastern Europe, or elsewhere must negotiate two cultures, languages, and expectations. These adolescents almost live a double life, resulting in increased stress that can pervade all aspects of their lives.

The "emancipated minor" provision of some laws recognizes that some adolescents do leave their family at an early age and assume adult responsibilities and independence. An emancipated minor is an adolescent who has not reached the standard legal age for certain privileges, such as consenting to marriage or seeking certain kinds of health or illness care but who is permitted to take on full responsibility for these decisions because he or she is economically and emotionally separate from his or her family.

Adolescents, as a separate segment of society, have a great deal of influence on the rest of society. Advertisers recognize the economic impact of this group and direct much of their strongest propaganda to them. The adolescent is mobile and often controls the money for his or her clothing and entertainment needs and desires. This control may result from working or being given an allowance, with very few guidelines about how to allocate it for needs versus desires. Adolescents are particularly vulnerable to advertising that stresses looking or acting similar to other teenagers or famous role models. As discussed earlier, adolescents are very peer-oriented and have an aversion to being different.

Adolescents from a minority group have a particular problem in relation to the culture of adolescence. They may desire strongly to "fit into" the predominant adolescent culture, which in our society is middle class, white, and Protestant. They may be able to fit one or perhaps two of these criteria but are unable to force fit into the other(s) because of economics, different appearance, or different education and experiences. Advertising does not feature the economically depressed or ethnic model, and their own peers are trying every means possible to look and act like the majority teenager. Further pressure comes from their own minority culture when they emulate the majority culture in ways the family sees as offensive to their ideas and beliefs.

The nurse needs to be aware of the current adolescent norms for behavior and to accept the teenager's real need to emulate the role models chosen. Some effective health promotion campaigns, such as cessation of smoking, have used famous role models. The nurse can use a similar strategy in promoting health care ideas to adolescent clients.

LEGISLATION

Many laws and regulations are aimed at the adolescent. Many deal with minimum age at which the adolescent may assume full adult privileges or responsibilities. The traditional rationales for these restrictions are that (1) youth do not have the experience, perspective, and judgment to recognize and avoid choices that could be detrimental to them, and (2) these youth require protection against exploitation by unscrupulous persons. A question often raised when considering minimum ages and the emancipated or "legally mature" minor is whether strict age criteria are appropriate for any adolescent, since development is variable and experiences are diverse.

Minimum age criteria to drive a motor vehicle and purchase firearms, alcohol, and cigarettes affect the health of adolescents not because these cause illness or death to every user but because there is higher risk of illness or accidents related to use and definitely to misuse of such agents. These restrictions are questioned periodically by groups of adolescents and adults but have not stirred the same emotional controversy as have the restrictions related to health care and information.

The restrictions recently questioned most strongly deal with issues related to sexual activity. The Supreme Court has affirmed the rights of all individuals to have equal access to contraceptive services, regardless of age or marital status, and the right of a minor to make decisions governing pregnancy termination. Despite these and other court rulings, the federal government, through certain members of Congress, has attempted to deny funding to agencies that provide family planning (contraceptive services, abortion) to any teenager under age 16 unless their parents are notified in writing by the agency. Advocates of this restrictive approach insist that teenagers are not capable of making these decisions by themselves. Opponents of this parental notification requirement insist that adolescents are not going to decrease their sexual activity if these resources are withheld but instead will seek this information and help from unsafe, irresponsible sources. The consequences could be increased unwanted pregnancies, with all the physical, emotional, and psychologic risks and increased illegal and probably improperly managed abortions. The teenager is trapped in the midst of these controversies.

The nurse also may feel trapped by the controversy and unsure how to deal with individual cases. An important point to remember is that the laws related to these sexual issues are in flux. Staffs in any health care setting who deal with adolescents must develop policies compatible with their knowledge of adolescent development, ideal and actual parental roles, and the range of community feelings toward and services available to teenagers.

ECONOMICS

The identification with peers, the essence of self-image during adolescence, includes dressing alike, having similar possessions, and going to the same activities or places. All these things require a fund of economic resources. Young adolescents and some older adolescents may be given an allowance by their parents that covers these desires. Many adolescents work to have money for these expenses and some, especially older adolescents, support themselves entirely. Money can be a major conflict between parents and their teenager. The parents may think that they should have the power to decide how a teenager spends money. Adolescents believe just as strongly that they know best how to allocate resources and how much money they need.

Teenagers vary greatly in their ability to manage money. Ideally, parents and adolescents should negotiate economic questions, with the parents becoming less controlling as the teenager gains more experience and expertise in these matters. Unfortunately, the emotional issue of holding on versus independence often interferes with economic discussions.

Some teenagers work not out of need for money but because they see work as a means of gaining experience and independence. Increased status among peers also may be related to work.

HEALTH CARE DELIVERY SYSTEM

Many health care resources theoretically are available to the adolescent. A basic problem in availability is that teenagers may not know about all their choices. They can continue to see their pediatrician or nurse practitioner in a pediatric center as they did as children, but this usually is rejected because of the young-child atmosphere at most of these settings.

School health programs often are available in junior high, high school, and college. Some of these programs are limited to mass screening for certain high-risk physical diseases and emergency care. Others offer a more comprehensive program of physical and mental health promotion.

Adolescent-focused clinics are available in many communities through both public and private agencies and, most recently, within schools. These clinics serve only adolescent clients, and staffs are oriented to the needs of this age group. Adolescents often feel more comfortable in these settings than in one where young children or adults also are served.

Adolescents can also make use of services such as family planning clinics. These settings may designate certain days and hours for younger clients, whereas others integrate them into the adult-oriented protocols. The pregnant adolescent most often finds prenatal care in a basically adult-focused setting, although more adolescent-specific programs are being developed. The basic physical needs of the pregnant adolescent may be the same as the pregnant adult, but the psychologic needs are very different and should be approached by a professional who has a comprehensive knowledge of adolescent development and responses to stress.

NURSING INTERVENTIONS FOR HEALTH PROMOTION

The adolescent is a rapidly changing individual. The nurse who works in an adolescent-focused practice needs to be well prepared in both pediatric and adult health promotion strategies, since these overlap in the adolescent years. The nurse also needs to have a thorough understanding of adolescent development and a recognition of the inherent dignity of each adolescent as a person.

The adolescent often is fearful about the procedures or possible diagnosis during a clinic or office visit, but at the same time needs to be in control of the situation. These conflicting feelings can be difficult to deal with together. The nurse can facilitate the adolescent's functioning in a health care setting by establishing that the adolescent is a partner with the health care provider(s) in promoting good health and screening for health risks.

The adolescent's questions should be answered fully and honestly. Since in many instances the adolescent is hesitant to voice concerns, information should be offered even if questions are not asked. A very effective approach to finding out about a particular teenager's concerns, especially about potentially embarrassing or stressful topics, is to say, "Many teenagers ask me about . . . Have you ever thought about this?" or "A lot of young people want to know about. . . ."

It is important to ask direct questions, even about sensitive topics: "Have you ever thought about suicide?"; "Are you depressed?"; "Are you sexually active?"; or "Do you use birth control?" Vague or circuitous questions imply a discomfort or lack of understanding and may cause the adolescent to be equally vague when responding.

Correct anatomic terms and descriptions of laboratory tests, disease processes, and possible outcomes are an essential component in treating the adolescent as an individual capable of being responsible for his or her own body. Nurses should avoid stereotyping adolescents because of their dress or behavior. Each is a unique individual despite striving to be like peers.

Adolescents should be encouraged but never forced to share their health care concerns with their parents. Nurses need to establish very clearly to themselves, the adolescent, and the parents that the adolescent is the client and that family members are seen as supportive to that client but not necessarily privy to all information exchanged between nurse and client.

SUMMARY

Adolescence is a period of dramatic change. These clients, who appear and act at times as children, at other times as adults, but most often in a category by themselves, can challenge the most experienced nurse. The many theories about adolescent development should form a background against which the nurse views each adolescent client as a unique, dynamic individual.

References

1. American Psychiatric Association: *Diagnostic and statistical manual of mental disorders,* ed 3, revised (DSM-III), Washington, DC, 1987, The Association.
2. Berger KS: *The developing person through childhood and adolescence,* ed 3, New York, 1991, Worth Publishers.
3. Capuzzi D, Gross DR: *Youth at risk: a resource for counselors, teachers and parents,* Alexandria, Va, 1989, American Association for Counseling and Development.
4. Comerci G: Eating disorders in adolescents, *Pediatr Rev* 10(2):37, 1988.
5. Committee on Adolescence, American Academy of Pediatrics: Alcohol use and abuse: a pediatric concern, *Pediatrics* 79(3):450, 1987.
6. Emans SJ, Goldsteen DP: *Pediatric and adolescent gynecology,* ed 3, Boston, 1990, Little, Brown.
7. Erikson E: *Identity, youth and crisis,* New York, 1968, WW Norton.
8. Friedman SB: *Comprehensive adolescent health care,* St Louis, 1991, Quality Medical Publishing.
9. Gilligan C, Lyons N, Hammer T: *Making connections: the relational worlds of adolescent girls at Emma Willard school,* Cambridge, 1990, Harvard University Press.
10. Guyton AC: *Textbook of medical physiology,* ed 8, Philadelphia, 1991, WB Saunders.
11. Helgerson S, et al: Acquired immunodeficiency syndrome and secondary school students: their knowledge is limited and they want to learn more, *Pediatrics* 81(3):350, 1988.
12. Hetherington EM, Arasteh JD: *Impact of divorce, single parenting and stepparenting on children,* Hillsdale, NJ, 1988, Lawrence Erlbaum Publishers.
13. Holmes KK, et al: *Sexually transmitted diseases,* ed 2, St Louis, 1990, McGraw-Hill.
14. Joffe A, Radius SM: Health counseling of adolescents, *Pediatr Rev* 12(11):344-351, 1991.
15. Kauffman JM: *Characteristics of behavior disorders of children and youth,* ed 4, Columbus, 1989, Merrill Publishing.
16. Kohlberg L: *The philosophy of moral development,* San Francisco, 1981, Harper & Row.
17. Lewis M, Volkman F: *Clinical aspects of child and adolescent development,* ed 3, Philaelphia, 1990, Lea & Febiger.
18. Lucas B: *Nutrition and the adolescent.* In Pipes PL: *Nutrition in infancy and childhood,* ed 4, St Louis, 1989, Mosby.
19. Muss RE: *Theories of adolescence,* ed 5, New York, 1988, Random House.
20. Neinstein S: *Adolescent health care: a practical guide,* ed 2, Baltimore, 1991, Urban & Schwarzenberg.
21. Patterson G, Forgatch M: *Parents and adolescents living together,* Eugene, Ore, 1987, Castalia Publishing.
22. Remafedi G, Blum R: Working with gay and lesbian adolescents, *Ped Annals* 15(11):773, 1986.
23. Report of the second task force on blood pressure control in children, *Pediatrics* 79(1):1, 1987.
24. Rice S: Clearing an athlete for sports participation, *J Musculoskeletal Med* 3(7):23, 1986.
25. Robinson D, Greene J: The adolelscent alcohol and drug problem: a practical approach, *Pediatr Nurs* 14(4):305, 1988.
26. Vaughan VC, Lett IE: *Child and adolescent development: clinical implications,* Philadelphia, 1990, WB Saunders.
27. Youness J, Haynie DL: Friendship in adolescence, *J Dev Behav Pediatr* 13(1):59-66, 1992.

CHAPTER

22

Young Adult

Elizabeth C. Kudzma

Johanne Quinn

Objectives

After completing this chapter, the nurse will be able to

- *Identify beliefs, attitudes, behaviors, and habits regulating the lifestyles of young adults.*
- *Identify developmental tasks congruent with adult maturity achieved during this period.*
- *Differentiate disease processes affecting the "younger" young adult and the "older" young adult.*
- *Identify physiologic, psychologic, and environmental factors that contribute to health problems for young adults.*
- *Describe specific health requirements for the young adult.*
- *Discuss the influence of genetic problems on healthy family functioning in young adulthood.*
- *Analyze cultural and ethnic risk factors affecting young adults.*
- *List occupational hazards that infringe on the young adult's welfare.*
- *Describe ways to reduce the incidence of sexually transmitted disease in young adults.*
- *State ways in which the nurse may help reduce risks associated with young adult behaviors of smoking, alcohol consumption, and drug use.*
- *Differentiate nursing roles in preventive intervention for healthy young adults in home and community environments.*
- *Delineate specific nursing interventions that may help ameliorate the effects of environmental factors on the young adult.*
- *Describe the nurse's role in family planning for the young adult.*

This chapter is the first of three chapters covering nursing assessment for health promotion and protection of healthy adults. Its focus is health promotion in the young adult, 18 to 35 years of age; the period ranges from the end of adolescence to the beginning of middle adulthood. The period before young adulthood can be described as preparation for assuming adult responsibilities and rights.

Interest has recently increased in phases of adult development. Popular books for the lay reader describing various crises and events in adult life have helped trigger this increased awareness.[68] Young adulthood comprises an extremely diverse group of people; it is a time of many physical and emotional changes and a period for learning by experience and experimentation. Health behaviors, safety practices, and attitudes about diet, exercise, sex, tobacco, and alcohol during this period often become lifelong habits. Preventable health concerns of young adults may be placed in two basic categories: (1) avoiding accidents, injuries, and violence that kill or disable[81] and (2) development of behaviors that promote a healthy lifestyle.[83]

Today approximately 26% of the population is composed of young people in the adult age group.[72] The cohort of young adults dropped by 9.7% from 1980 through 1986. The Census Bureau forecasts that this age group will continue to shrink. Also, the U.S. Bureau of the Census's *Current Population Report* indicates that the live birth rate per 1000 population for women between the ages of 20 and 34 was 2986 infants in 1988.[72] Nursing health promotion is particularly important for young adults because health education and protection directly influence the next generation.[38] (See box below.)

HEALTHY PEOPLE 2000

SELECTED NATIONAL HEALTH PROMOTION AND DISEASE PREVENTION OBJECTIVES

YOUNG ADULT

Specific Health Status and Risk-Reduction Objectives for young adults from *Healthy People 2000*[83] also discussed in this chapter:

1. Reduce the death rate for adolescents and young adults by 15% to no more than 85 per 100,000 people aged 15 through 24 (Baseline: 99.4 per 100,000 in 1987)
2. Reduce deaths among people aged 15 through 24 caused by alcohol-related motor vehicle crashes to no more than 18 per 100,000 (Baseline: 21.5 per 100,000 in 1987)
3. Reduce suicides among men aged 20 through 34 to no more than 21.4 per 100,000 (Baseline: 25.2 per 100,000 in 1987)
4. Reduce deaths among youth aged 15 through 24 caused by motor vehicle crashes to no more than 33 per 100,000 (Baseline: 36.9 per 100,000 in 1987)
5. Reduce overweight to a prevalence of no more than 20% among people aged 20 and older (Baseline: 26% for people aged 20 in 1976-1980, 24% for men and 27% for women)
6. Increase to at least 20% the proportion of people aged 18 and older who engage in vigorous physical activity that promotes the development and maintenance of cardiorespiratory fitness 3 or more days per week for 20 or more minutes per occasion (Baseline: 12% for people aged 18 and older in 1985)
7. Reduce the initiation of cigarette smoking by children and youth so that no more than 15% have become regular cigarette smokers by age 20 (Baseline: 30% of youth had become regular cigarette smokers by ages 20 through 24 in 1987)
8. Reduce the proportion of high school seniors and college students engaging in recent occasions of heavy drinking of alcoholic beverages to no more than 28% of high school seniors and 32% of college students (Baseline: 33% of high school seniors and 41.7% of college students in 1989)
9. Reduce alcohol consumption by people aged 14 and older to an annual average of no more than 2 gallons of ethanol per person (Baseline: 2.54 gallons of ethanol in 1987)
10. Increase the effectiveness with which family planning methods are used, as measured by a decrease to no more than 5% in the proportion of couples experiencing pregnancy despite use of a contraceptive method (Baseline: approximately 10% of women using reversible contraceptive methods experienced an unintended pregnancy in 1982)
11. Increase to at least 20% the proportion of people aged 18 and older who seek help in coping with personal and emotional problems (Baseline: 11.1% in 1985)
12. Increase to at least 50% the proportion of people who have received, as a minimum within the appropriate interval, all the screening and immunization services and at least one of the counseling services appropriate for their age and gender as recommended by the U.S. Preventive Services Task Force (Baseline data available in 1991)[83]

Young adulthood is usually the healthiest time of life (Fig. 22-1). Physical growth is complete by age 20; major concerns of biologic development are related to ensuring proper functioning of various body systems to provide optimal well-being.

The young adult's physical abilities are at peak efficiency, and body systems compensate optimally during illnesses so that health is maintained with minimum interruption. Nursing goals for individuals in the young adult group are oriented toward (1) prolonging the period of maximum physical energy and development of optimal mental, emotional, and social potential; and (2) anticipating and guarding against the onset of chronic disease through good health habits and early detection and treatment of disease when appropriate. Nurses should incorporate into their assessments both systemic and structural considerations.

Physical appearance is derived from genetic endowment; structural differences are evidence of unique familial genetic contributions. Height, strength, endurance, coordination, and speed of response are at maximum levels.[51] Full adult stature in men is reached around age 21; in women full growth usually occurs by about 17.

The peak of muscular strength usually occurs around age 25 to 30 years and then gradually declines by approximately 10% between ages 30 and 60. Most of this decline occurs in the muscles of the back and legs, with less occurring in the arms. Manual dexterity peaks in young adulthood and declines into the middle thirties.

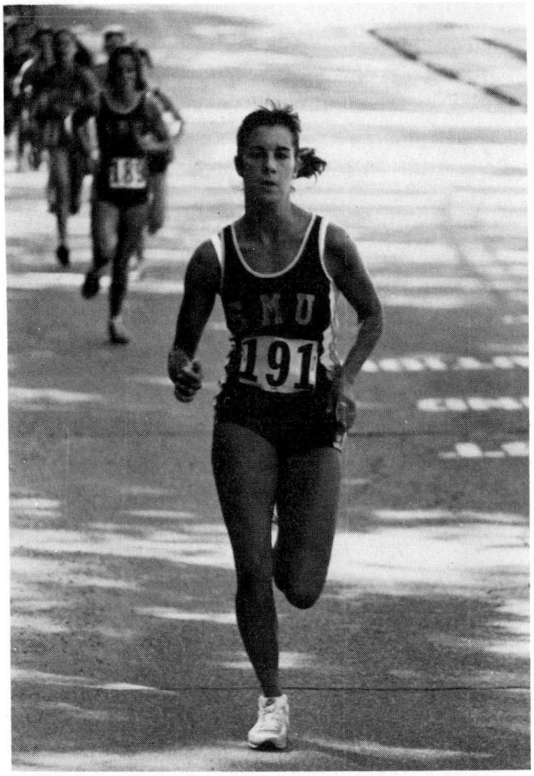

Fig. 22-1. Young adulthood is generally a healthy time of life. (From Arnheim DD: *Essentials of athletic training,* ed 2, St Louis, 1991, Mosby.)

HEALTH PERCEPTION AND HEALTH MANAGEMENT

Health and physical processes in the young adult are frequently taken for granted;[6] concern for health and well-being is lower among those in their twenties and starts to increase in the mid-thirties. Therefore health monitoring is both necessary and appropriate to detect health needs and incipient problems.[85] After the mid-thirties, there is an increased sense of the finiteness of life and the limitations imposed by work choices, well-being, money resources, and deterioration of physical abilities. For health care management, the young adult age span is split into two distinct age groups (18 to 24 and 25 to 35) according to the preventive services they require.

In the past 10 years, the assumption that all adults should have an annual physical exam has been replaced by more scientifically based information about health maintenance measures. Services offered in a health maintenance or screening program should meet certain criteria. A list of some of these criteria follows:

1. The condition for which screening is offered will have a serious effect on the quality or quantity of life.
2. Methods of treatment must be available and effective.
3. The condition must have a latency or asymptomatic period during which the disease may be detected with screening procedures, and treatment–if started promptly–will reduce morbidity or mortality.
4. Treatment during the asymptomatic period is likely to be much more effective than treatment started after symptoms emerge.
5. The cost of screening tests and programs must be acceptable and justified in terms of decreasing morbidity and mortality from the disease.
6. The prevalence of the condition must be common enough to warrant the cost of screening procedures and programs.[19]

Inability to satisfy each of these criteria means that a particular screening procedure or service is likely to be less effective. The rest of this section presents health maintenance procedures and screening with a significant core of agreement by experts regarding their effectiveness.[19]

Behavioral Health History

For young adults a behavioral history is important. In particular this should screen for risk factors of accidental death, a major cause of death and disability in this age group.[57] Also, the presence of such health risk factors as consumption of alcoholic beverages, drugs, and tobacco should be examined. After age 25, coronary risk factors should be explored; these include smoking, obesity, inadequate exercise patterns, and hypertension.

A behavioral health history that includes the behavioral and habitual aspects of health behavior and of problems for the young adult is most useful in examining and exploring these problems in an organized manner. The behavioral health history included here was developed for adults at the Health Cooperative of Puget Sound, Seattle (Fig. 22-2).[70] This history incorporates the Social Readjustment Scale, which rates life changes and occurrences for potential contribution to mental and physical disease.

Preventive Care

The basic goals of preventive care are (1) to maximize the period of optimum health status and (2) to detect incipient health problems at an early stage. At age 18 (around graduation from high school), a health appraisal is recommended. This clinic visit should include the taking of a family health history, past medical history, the behavioral health history just mentioned, and an exploration of life changes and stresses to which the individual has been exposed.

Table 22-1 illustrates preventive care important in the young adult period, along with the frequency of repeated screening services. As a general rule, the recommendation for most procedures is a repeat health history and visit at approximate 2-year intervals. Appropriate intervention in the young age group is directed toward correcting problems through history taking and counseling or avoiding them altogether. Subsequent counseling is directed more at rechecking and updating the earlier counseling given.

A physical examination includes a check of height, weight, and blood pressure, with an emphasis on the need to avoid obesity and (for women) education about the importance of breast self-examination (BSE), including the importance of repeating the technique monthly.

Social history

1. What organizations (community, church, lodge, social, professional, and so on) are you involved in? ______
2. List hobbies, skills, interests: ______
3. Do you live alone? ( ) Yes ( ) No
4. When did you last change residence? ______
5. (a) Marital status (circle one): single - married - divorced - widowed
   (b) Length of time ______
6. Were you ever in military service? ( ) Yes ( ) No
   (a) From ____ to ____ (b) Were you overseas during this time? ( ) Yes ( ) No
7. Has a close friend or an immediate member of the family died within the past 2 years? ( ) Yes ( ) No
8. List names and addresses of relatives or close friends in this area, indicating if friend or relative ______

Patient profile

1. Number years completed:
   Elementary school ____ High school ____ College__
2. Customary occupation ______ Employer ______
   For how long? ____ Is your work satisfying?
   ( ) No ( ) Yes

Habits:

3. Have you *ever* smoked cigarettes? ( ) No ( ) Yes
   a. How many? (check one) ( ) Less than ½ pack a day ( ) About one pack a day ( ) More than 1½ packs a day
   b. Do you smoke cigarettes now? ( ) No ( ) Yes
   c. For how long? (check one) ( ) Less than 5 years ( ) 5-10 years ( ) More than 10 years

Patient profile—cont'd

4. Have you *ever* smoked cigars or a pipe? ( ) No ( ) Yes
   a. If Yes, how long? ( ) Less than 5 years ( ) 5-10 years ( ) More than 10 years
   b. Do you smoke cigars or a pipe now? ( ) No ( ) Yes
5. Do you drink alcohol (wine, beer, whiskey)? ( ) No ( ) Yes
   If Yes, how much per day on the average?
6. Have you sometimes in the past year gotten drunk on work days? ( ) No ( ) Yes
7. Have you sometimes in the past year had alcoholic drinks (wine, beer, whiskey) in the mornings? ( ) No ( ) Yes
8. How much coffee, tea, or cola do you drink? (check one)
   ( ) None
   ( ) Less than 6 glasses or cups per day
   ( ) More than 6 glasses or cups per day
9. Do you use seat belts?
   ( ) Never ( ) Sometimes ( ) Always
10. How many miles do you drive per year? ______
11. Exercise: Describe type and amount per week ______
12. How much sleep do you *usually* get per night? (check one) ( ) 7 hours per night or more ( ) Less than 7 hours per night
13. Meals: Do you generally eat (check one) ( ) 3 regular meals per day? ( ) 2 meals per day? ( ) irregular meals?

FOR WOMEN; Do you examine your breasts each month for lumps? ( ) No ( ) Yes

Fig. 22-2. Sample behavioral health history form. (From Somers AR, et al: A whole-life plan for well patient care, *Patient Care* 11:83, 1979.)

***Table 22-1.* Developmental health monitoring**

Health problem	Ages 18-24 Procedure	Ages 18-24 Frequency (years)	Ages 25-35 Procedure	Ages 25-35 Frequency (years)
Smoking	History and counseling	At least once	History and counseling	Every 2
Obesity or poor eating habits	History and weight, counseling	Every 2-4	History and weight; counseling	Every 2-4
Problem drinking	History and counseling	At least once	History and counseling	Every 2-4
Accidental injury or death	History and counseling	At least once	History and counseling	Every 2
Unwanted pregnancy	Counseling	At least once	History and counseling	Every 2
Drug abuse	History and counseling	At least once	History and counseling	Every 2-4
Lack of exercise	History and counseling	At least once	History and counseling	Every 2-4
Hypertension	Blood pressure measurement	Every 2	Blood pressure measurement	Every 2
Breast or testicular cancer	BSE or TSE counseling	Every 1-2	BSE or TSE counseling	Every 1-2
Vision defects	Examination	Once	Examination	Every 4
Tetanus and diphtheria	Booster	Once if 10 since last one	Immunization	Every 10
Cervical cancer	Pap smear	Every 2-3	Pap smear	Every 2-3
Diabetes, proteinuira, bacteriuria	Urinalysis*	Once	Urinalysis*	Every 4
Birth defects	Rubella titer	Once in nonimmunized women		
Coronary artery disease	Serum cholesterol determination Triglyceride level	Once	Serum cholesterol determination*	Every 4
Anemia	Hematocrit or hemoglobin level*	Once	Hematocrit or hemoglobin level*	Every 4
Syphillis	Blood test*	Once	Blood test*	Every 4
Dental care	Dental examination and cleaning	Every 1-2	Dental examination and cleaning	Every 1-2
Tuberculosis	Skin test	Once	Skin test	Every 2-3

Adapted from Somers AR, et al: A whole-life plan for well patient care, *Patient Care* 11:83, 1979; and Frame PS: Health maintenance in clinical practice: strategies and barriers, *Am Fam Phys* 45(3):1192-1200, 1992.
*There is controversy whether this test should be done.

Testicular self-examination (TSE) should be taught to men, as well as what significant findings to report. Pelvic examinations of women generally are done, along with a Pap smear; the incidence of carcinoma in situ, thought to be a precursor of invasive cancer, is high in this group–1 in 1000 women. Increased screening is thought to be responsible for a decline in the incidence of this type of cancer. A rectal examination is not recommended unless symptomatology is present. Although after age 25, the emphasis is on modifying coronary risk factors, an electrocardiogram is not recommended in asymptomatic clients.[70]

Cardiac output and efficiency peak during the young adult years. Aging is responsible for degenerative changes in heart size and cardiac functioning;[61] but during the young adult years this decline amounts to less than 1% per year and causes little if any restriction.[36] Because cardiovascular disease is a primary cause of death in American adults, accounting for more than one third of all deaths annually, cardiovascular assessment of the young adult includes determining the presence of hyperlipidemia, hypertension, chest pain, or heart disease. A key risk-reduction objective for adults in *Healthy People 2000* is to reduce the mean serum cholesterol level among adults to no more than 200 mg/dl. (Baseline: 213 mg/dl among people aged 20 through 74 in 1976-1980, 211 mg/dl for men and 215 mg/dl for women.)[83] Parental hypertension is a risk factor for the development of hypertension in young adults; health history questions should elicit pertinent information about hypertension and coronary artery disease in parents and relatives.[23]

A predominant health problem for young black adults, especially males, is hypertension. This problem may result from a combination of factors–high-sodium diet, obesity, smoking, or high stress levels, as opposed to biologic inheritance–but many of the causes for higher hypertension incidence in this population are unknown. Hypertension frequently leads to severe complications; and more young black people than young Whites die as a result of chronic heart disease or cerebrovascular accidents.

The incidence of diabetes is also higher in Blacks.[80] Surveys show that the prevalence of diabetes is 15.8% in the black population, as compared to 7.0% in the white population.[17,80] These same surveys indicate that most diabetic persons under the age of 45 have insulin-dependent diabetes mellitus. Avoiding overweight and hypertension in young adults is critical, since estimates show that high blood pressure is a major cause of illness in this age group. U.S. statistics demonstrate that 13% to 17% of Whites and 26% to 28% of Blacks aged 20 and over have high blood pressure and weight problems.[17,83,84]

The frequency of coronary disease in young adults is greatly reduced when risk factors are at a minimum. The major risk factors for cardiac disease are smoking, drug abuse, hyperlipidemia, sedentary activity, poor dietary habits, emotional stress, genetic endowment, and physical illness, such as high blood pressure or diabetes.[33] The predisposition to develop coronary artery disease as an older adult is greatly reduced if coronary risk factors are minimized during young adulthood. A recent study reported that smoking over 25 cigarettes per day was associated with over five times the risk of fatal and nonfatal coronary events, and overall smoking alone accounted for approximately half those events.[90] In addition, young adult women who use oral contraceptives are at risk for cardiovascular disease–specifically blood clots, heart attacks, and strokes–especially if they are smokers.[26] It is sometimes difficult to convince individuals in this age group that someday they may be at risk for coronary artery disease and that modifying coronary risk factors such as obesity, lack of exercise, high blood pressure, and smoking is necessary during the young adult years.

Health Management, Decision Making, and Risk Taking

The decisions of young adults can affect their health and well-being. Their peak physical skills make young adults venturesome, daring, enterprising, and aggressive. Since at this time they often have had little close experience of death in significant others, they tend to take inordinate risks. A young adult is at greater risk for violent death from accident, suicide, or homicide.[83] Behaviors and practices related to violent death frequently illustrate the lack of a healthy sense of fear. Examples such as driving at high speed without a safety belt or driving after consuming drugs or alcoholic beverages are common.

During young adulthood personal interests multiply, and some can be hazardous. Sports like football, soccer, boxing, and others frequently involve personal contact and physical risk. Other young adults are interested in flying or scuba diving. A popular sport gaining interest among young adults is bungee jumping. Many of these activities make the individual susceptible to personal injuries and accidents; some may result in accidental death.

Health Management and Communicable Disease

Communicable diseases caused by many viruses affect young adults with varying degrees of severity. Influenza and *viral hepatitis* are difficult to control. They remain major health problems. Since 1983, viral hepatitis rates have gradually increased; hepatitis B infections continue to pose threats because the disease is carried by contaminated needles from illicit drug use.

Illnesses caused by infections with unidentified organisms can produce severe headaches, dizziness, fainting, and other unpleasant symptoms. Such organisms have caused large outbreaks of illness, such as Legionnaires' disease. Public health officials must use strict vigilance to monitor or retard disease transmission. Rubella in young adults is usually a minor disease; but if rubella is contracted during the first 12 weeks of pregnancy, the virus can cause severe malformations in the fetus. Clinically, prenatal infection or prematurity are the most common complications; however, more disastrous outcomes such as fetal abnormalities or intrauterine death are possible. Nurses should inform women of childbearing age before pregnancy (and preferably before childbearing age) that vaccination is available and is recommended in childhood. Many obstetricians routinely administer rubella vaccine to women following delivery. Rubella antibody titers, often done on women of childbearing age, should be done on unvaccinated clients who plan to become pregnant in the future. Women who chose vaccination should not become pregnant within 3 months of administration of the vaccine.

Public health authorities have reported outbreaks of rubella among teenagers and young adults who did not contract the disease as children and had not been immunized or had been vaccinated only before school age. Another vaccination at school age is recommended to preserve immunity through young adulthood. Nursing activities should be directed toward the identification of individuals who have lowered immunity to the disease. Vaccines should not be given to persons with known immunodeficiency or those on immunosuppressive therapy.

Other viral agents, such as genital herpes virus, human papovavirus (papillomavirus), may be spread through sexual contact. Genital herpes virus infections occur frequently in young adults with the onset of sexual activity. Of less consequence, yet still hazardous, is the

Epstein-Barr virus (a herpes virus), which causes infectious mononucleosis, a common viral infection afflicting young adults.

SEXUALITY AND REPRODUCTIVE PATTERN

Endocrine and Reproductive Functioning

In the female, the menstrual cycle should be well established by young adulthood. The usual duration of menses if 5 days, and the usual period between menses is 25 to 32 days. Menstrual irregularities include intermenstrual bleeding and prolonged heavy bleeding. Although the appearance of either is not always abnormal, these symptoms can indicate serious functional disorders and must be investigated.[69]

Cyclic hormonal functioning is responsible for regularities in the menstrual cycle and normal functioning of the ovaries and uterus. Increasingly research suggests that female hormonal functioning is indicative of a woman's feelings of well-being and cognitive effectiveness during phases of the menstrual cycle.[62] Problems typical of this age group include menstrually related alterations, such as premenstrual syndrome, dysmenorrhea, infertility, infections of the reproductive tract (in both the male and the female), and complications associated with contraceptive methods.

Common reproductive problems in the male include external conditions, mumps, orchitis, epididymitis, and occurrence of varicoceles and hydroceles. External conditions such as fungal infections, contract dermatitis, eczema, parasites like scabies and lice, and nonvenereal diseases like erysipelas, abscesses, or fistulas may occur in the scrotum. Mumps *orchitis* is a complication of mumps that occurs in 18% of cases in adult men; it can cause sterility and impotence. *Epididymitis* is a common infection caused by organisms that move from sites of established infection in the urine, urethra, prostate, or seminal vesicles. A *hydrocele* is swelling in the testicle caused by an abnormality in the lymphatic drainage; 90% occur after age 21. A *varicocele* is an abnormal dilation or twisting of the veins of the testicle that occurs most frequently up to age 25. Varicoceles can cause subfertility by affecting the number and mobility of sperm.

Male/Female Risk Ratios

Women have greater longevity than men at all ages.[67] On the average, women live seven years longer than men in the United States.[67] This may be partly because of female genetic composition or males' greater exposure to environmental hazards, such as accidents and dangerous industrial substances. Males also seek medical help less frequently than females and are lower users of health care services.[41]

Female/male illness and accident-risk ratios demonstrate considerable sex differences in the young adult years. Women are biologically stronger than men, outlive them, and naturally outnumber them; but a woman who neglects her health loses this edge. Males' shorter lifespans are related to attitudes involving risk-taking, competitiveness, dominance, and aggressiveness.[74] More deaths of men are caused by accidents, suicides, and homicides.[72,73] Other deaths result from drownings or are associated with activities of interest.[41]

Sex mortality differentials are higher for males among poorer populations. This may be attributed to higher rates of *homicide* rising from personal disagreements. Homicide is associated closely with alcohol abuse and frequently is related to robbery. Men are more likely to be both the offenders and the victims of homicide. Approximately 90% of all homicides occur between people of the same race, and many occur within families. The death rate from homicide among black males is slowly being reduced. The death rate among black males ages 15 to 24 was 72.5 per 100,000 in 1978. This figure had dropped to 66.8 per 100,000 by 1983.[72] Homicide also is correlated with easy access to firearms.

Suicide rates are higher in males: approximately four times as many men take their own lives. However, more women are known to suffer from depressive disorders and unsuccessfully attempt suicide.[88] Approximately 20% of all suicides occur in individuals under age 25.[74] In one study of 694 college freshmen ages 18 to 24, 54% reported having ever considered suicide, 26% had considered suicide during the last twelve months, and 10% reported having attempted suicide.[45] Suicide continues to be a major health problem, and some annual rates, especially for males and black females, continue to rise (Table 22-2).

Young adult women are more likely to contract *malignant neoplasms* at age 25 and over.[32,35,72] However, earlier detection of malignancies has decreased the mortality rates for females. Today more women have routine breast examination by a health care practitioner or regularly do breast self-examinations. It is recommended that women have routine Pap smears and mammograms.[35,65] A key health promotion objective included in *Healthy People 2000* for adults is to increase to at least 95% the proportion of women aged 18 who have ever had a Pap test and to at least 85% of those who have received a Pap test within the last 1 to 3 years.[83]

For the young adult woman, maternal mortality is decreasing. Health officials, however, are concerned that the maternal mortality rate targeted in the 1990

Table 22-2. **U.S. suicide rates for young adults by sex, race, and age, 1970-1988 (rates per 100,000 population)**

	Male						Female					
	White			Black			White			Black		
Age	1970	1980	1988	1970	1980	1988	1970	1980	1988	1970	1980	1988
All	18.0	19.9	21.7	8.0	10.3	11.5	7.1	5.9	5.5	2.6	2.2	2.4
15-19	9.4	15.0	19.6	4.7	5.6	9.7	2.9	3.3	4.8	2.9	1.6	2.2
20-24	19.3	27.8	27.0	18.7	20.0	19.8	5.7	5.9	4.4	4.9	3.1	2.9
25-34	19.9	25.6	25.7	19.2	21.8	22.1	9.0	7.5	6.1	5.7	4.1	3.8

Statistical Abstracts of the United States, Hyattsville, Md, 1991, National Center for Health Statistics 12.

Health Objectives for the Nation of 5 per 100,000 live births for the country or any ethnic group was not reached. Although maternal mortality had declined by 5% in 1983 (based on rates recorded 1979 to 1983), many factors continue to keep maternal mortality rates high in the United States in comparison to other developed countries. Universal access to prenatal care is a critical concern. High-risk groups like Hispanics and Blacks do not receive care appropriate to their needs. They lack proper insurance coverage, and our poorly developed health care systems lack formal referral mechanisms.[80]

Factors contributing to decreased incidence of maternal deaths include (1) compliance with prenatal care instructions; (2) more thorough knowledge and better management of prenatal complications, labor, and delivery; (3) more active participation of mothers because of prepared childbirth education; and (4) better management in the postpartum period, including the use of transfusions for control of hemorrhage or medications when indicated to prevent infections.[29]

Sex is a risk factor for morbidity and mortality related to cardiovascular disease. Young adult males have a higher incidence of cardiovascular disease. In 1988, 36% of all deaths of males occurred from heart disease; roughly 38% of these deaths were among males ages 15 to 44.[72] Studies also indicate that between 13% and 17% of Whites and 23% and 28% of Blacks have high blood pressure, with a majority more than 10% above ideal weight.[17,18,72]

Sexually Transmitted Disease

Sexually transmitted disease (STD) is a leading cause of bacterial infection and reproductive dysfunction in adults between ages 15 and 80.[5,17,39,66,81,82] Major reportable infections are herpes genitalis, chlamydia, genital warts, syphilis, and gonorrhea (Table 22-3). The most commonly reported infection is *gonorrhea,* which has reached epidemic levels in recent years; about 85% of reported cases occur in young adults. The incidence of gonorrhea is higher in Blacks and males. Racial differences in incidence are related to social factors rather than biological. Chlamydia and gonorrhea can be devastating for young adults. Contracting these diseases may result in severe complications that affect physical health and emotional well-being.

STDs cost millions of dollars for treatment and reporting.[81] Besides causing health problems for young adults, they impose tremendous demands on health care facilities. The incidence of STDs has increased worldwide in the past two decades; but the 1989 U.S. figures of reported cases show a slight decline. Reported gonococcal infections have decreased by approximately 22% since 1985 whereas veneral syphilis has increased since 1986.[5,72] Nevertheless, many cases go unreported because of emotional overtones of shame, silence, apathy, or ignorance.

The patient who seeks care for venereal disease typically presents symptoms of vaginal or urethral discharge associated with itching dysuria, the presence of a rash, or the appearance of ulcerated lesions. However, many STDs of lesser severity go unrecognized because of a lack of apparent symptoms. Consequently they are often responsible for chronic complications detected later. For instance, pelvic inflammatory disease (PID) is responsible for infertility in an estimated 75,000 women of childbearing age.[46] This occurs because women may be asymptomatic victims of gonorrhea and remain undiagnosed and untreated. PID is also responsible for more than 50,000 surgical procedures annually. In many of these cases, sterility occurs because of the necessity for total removal of the female reproductive organs. In other instances gonorrhea control is hampered because certain strains of the responsible organism have become resistant to penicillin and other antibiotics.[5,72]

Complications from STD in young adults are frequent. In addition to PID and its complications, young adult women have a greater incidence of ectopic pregnancy, abortions, stillbirths, and Bartholin's abscess.[4] Among males, gonorrheal complications also include disseminated gonococcal infection or epididymitis, prostatitis, and urethral stricture.

STD may affect the unborn or the young infant with complications such as fetal and infant deaths, birth defects, and mental retardation. In addition, chlamyda organisms are responsible for approximately 50,000 eye infections and 25,000 cases of pneumonia in infants annually.[5]

Nurses should be aware that STD and complications are reduced greatly with the proper use of condoms. Early diagnosis and treatment are essential, however, for intervention to be effective in cases where the disease has already been contracted. Nurses working with clients with STD must examine their attitudes toward this problem, as well as their attitudes toward sexuality and sexual behavior. Nurses must approach these clients with an open mind and in an objective manner; clients should be ensured that their lifestyles will be tolerated and their confidentiality respected.

The nurse's role in intervening in STD includes treatment and education. If a client has or is suspected of having STD, the nurse should obtain a complete history, including a sexual history, sexual contacts, previous treatment and test results, any signs or symptoms of a present infection, parental infections, the recent use of antibiotics, and any allergic reactions to antibiotics. If treatment is required, the nurse must be certain that the client understands the goals of treatment in an attempt to ensure cooperation and adherence to the planned treatment.

The nurse can serve as an educator, both of the individual client and of the general public. Health education regarding STD should include the modes of transmission, incubation periods, signs and symptoms, methods of treatment, complications from the lack of treatment, and repeated infections. Assessment of the client's knowledge will help to determine the understanding of what has been taught. It is hoped the nurse will promote the client's change of behavior and awareness of ways to prevent STD.

Another sexually transmitted disease is acquired immune deficiency syndrome (AIDS) which was identified as caused by human immunodeficiency virus (HIV) in 1983. Three routes of transmission have been demonstrated: (1) through innoculation with blood, (2) through sexual intercourse, and (3) through perinatal transmission. Routes other than these–having close personal contact or residing with an infected person, being a health care worker without exposure to blood, and suffering from insect bites–are not involved. Infectivity of the virus may be universal given exposure to a large enough amount of virus through an appropriate route. Since April 1985, blood products used in the United States have been screened for HIV, so the number of cases of HIV transmitted from blood products should be minimal. The incidence of HIV infection among homosexual men, the earliest recognized risk group, appears to be leveling. In the young adult, there is a growing concern about transmission through illicit intravenous drug use and heterosexual encounters.[21] There is some evidence that because of individual behaviors, social practices, and the period of time HIV first occurred in the population, its transmission in the United States will remain principally among homosexual and bisexual men and intravenous drug users, with less spread through heterosexual encounters than was the case in sub-Sahara Africa and Latin America.[44]

To date, there is no known cure for HIV disease or infection. Degrees of HIV disease are described. These are (1) demonstration of infection with the virus through antibody titer, but the patient is currently asymptomatic, and (2) clinical AIDS with severe immune deficiency and the inability to combat common environmental and opportunistic infections. Other signs are weight loss, loss of appetite, weakness, and a wasting syndrome that include an inability to function or work properly.[3] Definition of the clinical classification of HIV infection is continuously undergoing revision as new information and testing becomes available. For example, since January 1, 1993, the classification now includes CD4+T-lymphocyte count as a marker for immunosuppression.[11] One study of sexual risk reduction behaviors in young heterosexual adults demonstrated that higher levels of worry about contracting a sexually transmitted disease was a significant predictor of risk-reduction behavior implementation.[12]

Another, less serious reproductive condition is condylomata acuminata (genital warts), which is caused by the human papillomavirus and commonly seen in sexually active people. Untreated warts may grow into large masses and place the woman at increased risk of developing cervical cancer. In pregnancy, these warts become especially exuberant and may develop into sites of secondary infection. Infants born to mothers with vaginal warts often develop laryngeal warts.[5] Education is essential to prevent transmission and to make susceptible individuals aware of practices that increase exposure.[76]

VALUE AND BELIEF PATTERN

Developing values and beliefs is part of maturing into adult roles. Values–usually lifelong interests expressed in terms such as *good* or *bad*–are frequently reflected in behavior. Attitudes–frequently described as *likes* or *dislikes*–are changed most easily by influence. Beliefs–special attitudes based more on faith than on fact–are therefore usually part of background culture.

Young adults enter their 20s with habits, values, and beliefs acquired in childhood and adolescence. Unfortunately, many of these habits foster continuance of practices hazardous to health and well-being in later years. Irregular eating patterns, smoking, excessive use of alcohol, drug abuse, and reckless driving can result directly in obesity, hypertension, cardiovascular prob-

Table 22-3. **Summary of sexually transmitted diseases (STDs)**

Disease	Etiologic agent	Mode of spread	Incubation period	Clinical picture
Candida Albicans	Gram-positive fungus–*Candida ablicans*	Sexual contact; nonsexual; drugs, diabetes, pregnancy, oral contraceptives	Unknown	Male: itching, irritation discharge, plaque of cheesy material under foreskin Female: vaginal discharge; thick, white, cheesy, or curdlike material; vulva skin red and excoriated
Genital warts (Condylomata Acuminata)	Infectious papovarirus (papillomavirus)	Autoinoculations; sexual contact	Prolonged month or more	Digitating, papular, pedunculated lesions growing beneath or on prepuce, at external meatus or on glans and coronal sulcus. Lesions may be red or dirty gray and may remain singular and discrete; more often are in clusters.
Herpes genitalis	Herpesvirus type 2	Sexual contact	2-10 days maximum	Primary: large, discrete vesicles on erythematous base; painless inguinal adenopathy; vesicles rupture; lasts 4-6 weeks. Recurrent; clusters of small vesicles, more itchy than painful; lasts a few hours to 10 days; no adenopathy
Molluseum contagiosum	Pox virus group–DNA virus	Direct contact	14-50 days, average 30 days	Waxy globular papule, pinhead to pea-sized or larger; lesions elevated–shiny, translucent, and firm with no increase; pigmentation–center of lesions is small, dark-colored with umbilication from which curdlike substance may be expressed.
Nongonococcal Urethrin's (NGU)	*Chlamydia* group in half of cases	Sexual contact	1-3 weeks	Male: pain, frequency of urination, watery mucoid urethral discharge, symptoms milder than gonococcal urethritis, may coexist with gonorrhea Female: commonly a symptomatic carrier, vaginal discharge, dysuria, frequency of micturition

Adapted from US Department of Health and Human Services, Public Health Service, Centers for Disease Control: *Sexually transmitted disease summary,* Washington, DC, 1982, US Government Printing Office.

Laboratory test	Treatment	Contacts	Complications and sequelae	Nursing education message to emphasize
Wet smear	Nystatin (Mycostatin) vaginal tablets, miconazole (Monistat Vaginal Cream)		Relapse of problem, especially when pregnant; infection of newborn if mother not treated; superficial infection of skin and mucous membranes.	Arrange to return for other tests, arrange for test-of-cure in 14 days. Use good genital hygiene. Pantyhose serves as occlusive dressing, creating heat and moisture.
Microscopically	20% to 25% podophyllin in tincture of benzoin, desiccation, surgery	Examination of fingers, mouth, genitals of contact	Lesions may enlarge and produce tissue destruction. Giant condyloma, although histologically benign, may simulate carcinoma. In pregnancy, warts enlarge, are extremely vascular, and may obstruct the birth canal, necessitating cesarean section.	Return for weekly or biweekly treatment and follow-up until lesions have resolved. Partners should be examined for warts. Abstain from sex or use condoms during therapy.
Tzanck Test	No specific treatment; treat symptomatically	No specific follow-up	Males and females: neuralgia, meningitis, ascending myelitis, urethral strictures, and lymphatic suppuration may occur. Females: possibly an increased risk for cervical cancer and fetal wastage. Neonates: the virus from an active genital infection may be transmitted to the neonate during vaginal delivery.	Keep involved area clean and dry. Examine partner. Since both initial and recurrent lesions shed high concentrations of virus, patients should abstain from sex while symptomatic. Undetermined but presumably small risk of transmission also exists during asymptomatic intervals. Condoms may offer some protection. Annual Pap smears are recommended. Pregnant women should tell their obstetricians of any history of herpes.
Examination of crushed smear, wafer bodies	Desiccation and/or curretage of lesion	Examine contacts	Secondary infection, usually with staphylococci occur. Lesions rarely greater than 10 mm in diameter	Return for reexamination 1 month after treatment so that any new lesions can be removed. Partners should be examined.
Smears and cultures	Broad-spectrum antibiotics	Treat steady partner	Urethral strictures Prostatitis Epididymitis and infertility. Chlamydial NGU may be transmitted to female sexual partners, resulting in mucopurulent endocervictis and pelvic inflammatory disease, if pregnant, risk for spontaneous abortion stillbirth, and postpartum fever. Neonatal chlamydial infections such as ophthalmia or pneumonia may be acquired from infected endocervix during delivery.	Understand how to take any prescribed oral medication, if tetracycline prescribed, take 1 hour before or 2 hours after meals and avoid dairy products, antacids, iron, other mineral-containing preparations, and sunlight. Return for test of cure or evaluation 4-7 days after completion or therapy earlier if symptoms persist or recur. Refer sexual partners for examination and treatment. Avoid sex until patient and partners are cured. Use condoms to prevent future infections.

Continued.

Table 22-3. Summary of sexually transmitted diseases (STDs)–cont'd

Disease	Etiologic agent	Mode of spread	Incubation period	Clinical picture
Pediculosis pubis	*Pithirus pubis;* grayish ectoparasite 1-4 mm long with claws for clinging to hair	Sexual contact, occasionally from towels, clothing, toilet seats	Approximately 4 weeks	Intense itching, irritation of skin, pinhead-sized blood spots on underwear, nits attached to hair.
Scabies	*Sarcoptes scabiei;* female mite 0.3-0.4 mm, male somewhat smaller	Prolonged close contact with infected person	4-6 weeks	Severe itching worse at night, skin lesions papular and vesicular, burrows appear as grayish or black irregular lines.
Trichomonas vaginalis	Protozoan with undulating membrane and four flagella	Sexual contact	4-28 days	Male: slight itching, moisture on tip of penis, slight early-morning urethral discharge Female: itching and redness of vulva and skin inside thighs, strawberrylike appearance of cervix, vaginal discharge watery, copious, frothy
Gonorrhea	*Neisseria gonorrhoeae;* gram-negative diplococcus	Sexual contact	1 day 2 weeks, average 3-5 days	Male: frequency of urination, usually have dysuria, mucoid urethral discharges, purulent urethral discharge later Female: red, swollen cervix in 75% of females; symptomatic purulent vaginal discharge; frequency of urination; dysuria Anorectal and pharyngeal infections are common; may be symptomatic or asymptomatic.

Laboratory test	Treatment	Contacts	Complications and sequelae	Nursing education message to emphasize
Identification of organism on body	Kwell shampoo, lotion, creme	To be examined and treated	Secondary excoriations Lymphadenitis Pyoderma	Clothing and linen should be disinfected by washing them in hot water, by dry cleaning them, or by removing them from human exposure for 1-2 weeks. Avoid sexual or close physical contact until after treatment. Ensure examination of sexual partners as soon as possible. Return if problem is not cured or recurs.
Microscopic identification	Kwell shampoo, creme, lotion	Examine and treat all sexual contacts	Secondary bacteria infection occurs, particularly with nephrogenic strains of streptococci. Norwegian or crusted scabies (with up to 2 million adult mites in crusts) is risk for patients with neurologic defects and those immunologically incompetent.	Clothing and linen should be disinfected by washing them in hot water, by dry cleaning them, or by removing them from human exposure for 1-2 weeks. Avoid sexual or close physical contact until after treatment. Ensure examination of sexual partners as soon as possible. Return if problem is not cured or recurs.
Wet prep	Metronidazole (Flagyl)	Examine and treat steady partners	Secondary excoriations Recurrent infections common	Understand how to take or use any prescribed medications. Trichomoniasis or vaginitis; avoid alcohol until 3 days following completion of metronidazole therapy. Vaginitis: If tetracycline given, take 1 hour before or 2 hours after meals and avoid dairy products, iron, other mineral-containing preparations, and sunlight. Candidiasis: Wear sanitary pad to protect clothing. Store suppositories in a refrigerator. Continue taking medicine, even during menstural period. Refer sexual partners for evaluation. Return if problem is not cured or recurs. Use condoms to prevent future infections.
Female: culture from cervix Male: culture from urethra	Intramuscular penicillin	Examination and treatment of all contacts	10%-20% of women develop pelvic inflammatory disease and are at risk for its sequelae. Men are at risk for epididymitis, sterility, urethral stricture, and infertility. Newborns are at risk for ophthalmia, scalp abscess at the site of fetal monitors, rhinitis, pneumonia, or anorectal infection. All infected untreated persons are at risk for disseminated gonococcal infection (includes septicemia, arthritis, dermatitis, meningitis, endocarditis).	Understand how to take any prescribed oral medication, If tetracycline is prescribed take 1 hour before or 2 hours after meals and avoid daily products, antacids, iron, other mineral-containing preparations, and sunlight. Return for test of cure 4-7 days after completing therapy. Refer sexual partners for examination and treatment. Avoid sex until patient and partners are cured. Return early if symptoms persist or recur. Use condoms to prevent future infections.

Continued.

Table 22-3. **Summary of sexually transmitted diseases (STDs)–cont'd**

Disease	Etiologic agent	Mode of spread	Incubation period	Clinical picture
Syphilis	*Treponema pallidum:* spirochete with 6-14 regular spirals and characteristic motility	Sexual contact, prenatal syphillis, kissing, accidental inoculation	10-90 days	Primary: classic chancre is painless, indurated, and located at site of exposure. All genital lesions should be suspected to be syphilitic. Secondary: patients may have highly variable skin rash, mucous patches, condylomata lata, lymphadenopathy, or other signs. Latent: patients have no clinical signs.

lems, cancer, and accidental death.[74,83] Many may result from an inability to cope with life stress.

Whether these patterns of behavior are formed in earlier years or result directly from being a young adult, their long-range effects warrant prevention or early intervention in health management. Prevention can be directed toward changing value and belief patterns from those that encourage poor health practices to those that support optimum health behaviors. An understanding of the differentiation between values, attitudes, and beliefs is important so the nurse can distinguish one from the other and determine the relative difficulty of change; for example, attitudes can be changed more easily than values. Nursing interventions are more effective when the nurse can describe, discriminate, and identify value and belief patterns with practices known to maximize health.[50]

Values Involved in Parenting

Parenthood is anticipated by the majority of young adults; therefore, taking measures to ensure healthy offspring is a crucial goal. Genetic impairments are responsible for approximately one fourth of the serious malformations in newborns.[49] Two percent of all newborns are afflicted with congenital malformations. About 2000 genetic disorders are known; but very few are responsible for most genetic diseases in the United States today.[83]

Genetic factors influence biologic and personality development. If the individual with a genetic disease reaches adulthood, many problems occur, including fertility and transmission of the disease to offspring. Hereditary diseases, such as sickle cell disease and diabetes, can cause health problems for young adults when they are of childbearing age. For example, in sickle cell anemia the carrier state occurs in approximately 1 of every 12 black births. In addition, women diagnosed as having sickle cell disease have decreased fertility. If pregnancy does ensue, spontaneous abortion is a frequent complication, occurring in approximately 44% of cases.[9,88]

Values Regarding Prenatal Diagnosis and Genetic Impairments

For many genetic disorders, specific prenatal diagnoses have been available since the mid-1960s.[49] This has necessitated identification of high-risk pregnancies and requires the cooperation of the childbearing couple, who must provide accurate family medical and obstetric histories besides complying with suggested screening and follow-up care.[50] Decisions about reproduction and health care are based on current information on genetics and deleterious genetic factors. Some young adults now may be forced by this knowledge to think beyond their own reproductive ability to biologic destiny and reproductive issues of future generations.[88]

The finding of a malformed or genetically impaired fetus often results in the parents' decision to terminate the pregnancy. This decision, especially if it involves abortion, becomes a religious, ethical, and legal issue. Political debates and legislative mandates have greatly influenced the family control over many of these decisions.

Genetic counseling is an important nursing intervention during young adulthood. If a nurse suspects on the basis of a health assessment that an individual is at risk

Laboratory test	Treatment	Contacts	Complications and sequelae	Nursing education message to emphasize
Blood serology	Penicillin	Examine and treat all contacts	Both late syphilis and congenital syphilis are complications, since they are preventable with prompt diagnosis and treatment of early syphilis. Sequelae of late syphilis include neurosymphilis (general paresis, tabes dorsalis, focal neurologic signs), cardiovascular syphilis (thoracic aortic aneurysm, aortic insufficiency), and localized gamma formation.	Understand how to take any prescribed oral medications. If tetracycline is given, take 1 hour before or 2 hours after meals and avoid dairy products, antacids, iron, other mineral-containing preparations, and sunlight. Return for follow-up serologies 3, 6, 12, and 24 months after therapy. Refer sexual partners for evaluation and treatment. Avoid sexual activity until patient and partners are cured. Use condoms to prevent future infections.

for producing a child with a genetic defect, genetic screening should be discussed with the client. A genetic specialist gives technical explanations of genetic disorders; however, nurses have a supportive role in helping young adults to decide appropriately about whether or not to have children or to carry through a pregnancy that is at risk.

Ethnicity, Race, and Culture

Ethnicity and culture characterize a person's peculiarities and differences and place him or her within a particular race or subgroup of people. The young adult whose ethnic background separates him or her from the dominant culture is more likely to encounter prejudice, discrimination, or prejudgment. This can occur from specific differences of color or creed or of language, attitudes, values, preferences, and behaviors. The young adult is susceptible to these prejudices at work, at school, in health care delivery systems, and in the community. Since the young adult not only must meet personal needs but also frequently the needs of children or elders, it is crucial that nurses consider values specific to various cultures and ethnic backgrounds.

Race and ethnicity are important influencers of health for young adults. The longevity of nonwhite males and females has increased recently, a result of a decrease in birth-related fatalities and in deaths caused by chronic disability.[4] Blacks are still at risk for specific health problems, and the life expectancy of the average black person is shorter. Race and ethnicity may also influence the clinical response of an individual to drug therapy; unfortunately, many drug investigations underrepresent minority subjects in their study samples.[37]

Cultural Values about Fertility

Reactions to societal pressure have shifted the average age when both white and black women give birth. First births to white women aged 25 to 29 and 30 to 35 have increased substantially.[72]

Fertility rates per 1000 populations are proportionately higher among black women. This results from lifestyle preference or factors associated with approaches to sexual fulfillment. Studies have indicated, however, that noncompliance with or failure to use contraceptive measures properly has also led to higher birth rates among Blacks.[9] Studies also show that a smaller percentage of black women use contraceptive methods.[72]

Statistical reports in 1990 indicated approximately 57% of the births among black women were to unmarried women, compared to 17% of the births among white women. This was over 3 times greater the incidence for white women and 2½ times that of Hispanic women.[17,39] The abortion ratio in black women showed a slight increase from 1980 to 1987, rising from 642 to 648 per 1000 live births. The abortion ratio for white women showed a very slight decline in the same time period (376 to 338 per 1000 live births).[88]

Lifestyle and Culture

Race and ethnicity are closely related to educational and work-related decisions, which in turn affect choice of residence. Many Blacks must accept substandard housing or crowded living areas. This lifestyle, when compounded by insufficient economic resources, often affects health. Divorce can be an outgrowth of lifestyle patterns and socioeconomic conditions for black Americans. Divorce rates are proportionately higher for black females, and remarriage occurs less frequently than it does among white women in the same age range.[72] Poverty is seen more frequently in black families, and this often leads to inability to meet the basic needs of food, clothing, and housing and leads to decreased attention to health needs.

Culture, Values, and Minority Care

Obstacles and perceived barriers hinder entry into the health care system, especially for members of minority groups and recently arrived immigrants. In a study of 75 Vietnamese refugees (the Vietnamese are the largest group of Southeast Asians in the United States), newer arrivals were significantly more concerned about having a translator present in the health care facility, being understood by the health care provider, being able to understand oral and written instructions, and comprehending qualities related to the primary provider. These study subjects were also willing to be relocated to another clinic where a translator was available and to seek more frequent care if a translator could be present.[15]

NUTRITIONAL AND METABOLIC PATTERN

Good nutrition is essential to physical fitness, a state many young adults devote hours to attaining through desire, discipline, and determination. Because young Americans value slimness and athletic ability, healthy eating habits are a necessity, along with physical exercises.

An optimally functioning basal metabolic rate (BMR) in the young adult permits adequate oxygen uptake during normal activity and rest periods. Compensation for disturbances requires little disruption of normal functioning. Poor eating practices, however, can place the young adult at risk of being overweight or obese.[72]

The major principles governing energy and nutritional needs that may affect young adults are (1) size–heavier individuals require more nutrients than lighter people; (2) temperature–individuals in the tropics require less food than individuals in temperate zones; (3) growth–individuals who are still growing need more food, and usually more of each nutrient; (4) pregnancy–pregnant women require more nutrients to meet the needs of the developing fetus; and (5) activity–active individuals need more food energy.[57]

The young adult male needs about 1600 to 1800 calories per day to meet his body's basal metabolic needs; the young adult female requires only 1200 to 1450 calories a day to meet her needs. In addition to basal metabolic requirements, other calories are needed for digestion and activity; if the young adult consumes more calories than are utilized, overweight or obesity results. Since growth stops in the late teens, the BMR declines. If activity slows as well, more weight is gained.

Fig. 22-3 illustrates caloric intake by age, race, and sex. Note that increased caloric intake is high, particularly in males. Although white males tend to have higher caloric intake than black males, the caloric intake of white males levels off after age 15. For the black male

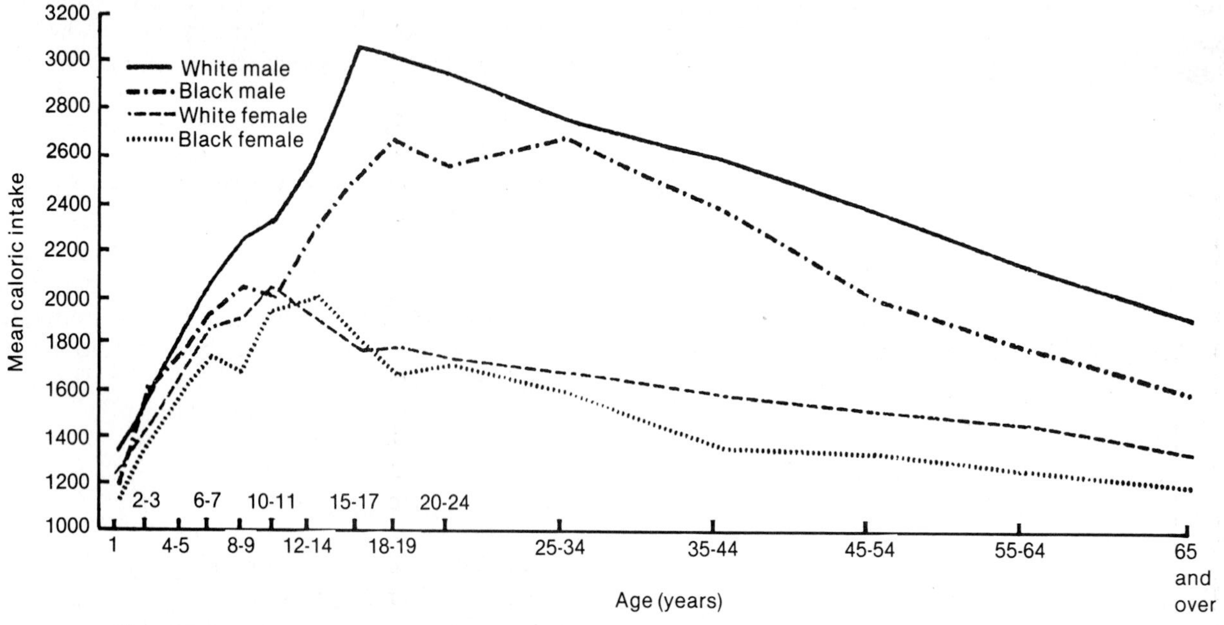

Fig. 22-3. Mean caloric intake of persons 1 to 74 years of age, according to race and sex: United States. Note especially intake during young adulthood. (From U.S. Department of Health and Human Services, Public Health Service.)

the increase in caloric intake continues through age 35.[87] Increased caloric intake without corresponding energy use may lead to obesity, a precursor to hypertension.

Good nutrition is especially important during pregnancy. Mothers-to-be should not only be concerned about food processing but also about using additives that could possibly be harmful to their unborn children or their other children. A recent concern has to do with pregnant women using newer essential trace minerals with unknown long-range effects. Iron-deficiency anemia is common in pregnancy, and iron supplementation is indicated for optimum growth of the fetus and supporting structures. Adequate maternal nutrition is necessary to avoid growth retardation in the fetus.[80,85]

Osteoporosis will be a significant health problem for elderly women who do not consume adequate amounts of calcium during the young adult years. One study indicated that three quarters of women aged 25 to 35 consumed less than 1250 mg of calcium daily and were therefore at risk for osteoporosis later in life.[10]

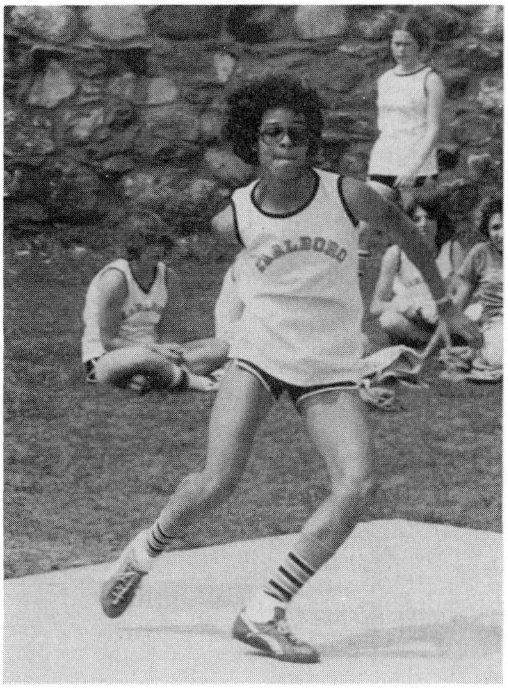

Fig. 22-4. Sports activities provide young adults with needed exercise. (Photograph courtesy Marlboro Newspaper.)

ELIMINATION PATTERN

In general, patterns of elimination are established by young adulthood. Health problems related to the gastrointestinal tract, including ulcers or colitis, can result from emotional stress. Although disorders of eating and purging usually start at an earlier stage of development, bulimia (vomiting), which may be associated with excessive use of laxatives, may continue during this period. The incidence of these disorders over the last 15 years appears to have increased rapidly.[8,64]

In pregnant women, disorders of elimination resulting from decreased bowel motility are common. Such disorders as constipation (often aggravated by iron supplementation) and hemorrhoids are usually treated conservatively by increasing fluids and roughage in the diet.

ACTIVITY AND EXERCISE PATTERN

Sufficient physical exercise is required to maintain physical fitness (Fig. 22-4). An individual who is physically fit has physical adaptability and ability to respond to increased activity, possesses energy needed to perform skills associated with daily living with sufficient reserve, and is able to live an active life with minimum risk of injury or disability. Inactivity is a predisposing factor to cardiovascular disease.[59]

Exercise to develop an optimally functioning cardiovascular-respiratory system is called aerobic exercise. Aerobic exercises depend on inspired air to continue expenditures of energy. They develop muscular fitness, endurance, power, and flexibility.[14] Inactivity leads to hypokinetic disease, which includes chronic fatigue, shortness of breath, obesity, ulcers, headache, backache, muscular weakness and atrophy, pain in the joints, high blood pressure, and accelerated degenerative processes.[57] To avoid these problems, young adults are encouraged to engage in fitness activities (Table 22-4 and box on p. 591), which increase the heart rate to approximately 150 beats/minute.[14] After 5 minutes of activity at this rate, the body is required to make adjustments in cardiovascular capacity by enlarging the lungs and capillaries in the lungs, muscles, and heart. Repeated aerobic exercises such as cycling, running, skipping rope, and walking (at least four times each week) produce physical fitness and decrease the likelihood of problems caused by inactivity.

Radiation and Sunbathing

Sunbathing is a popular social and recreational activity for young adults. Involvement in outdoor sports may also mean spending leisure hours in direct sunlight. Exposure to natural radiation from sunlight is linked directly to skin cancer, and approximately 400,000 cases of this type of cancer occur annually.[83]

Of increasing concern is the rise in popularity among young adults of tanning spas. The idea of maintaining a well-tanned body year round has gained appeal. Regrettably, this activity may lead to health problems similar to those encountered from natural radiation. The nurse

***Table 22-4.* Resources available to nurses assisting young adults to exercise**

Approaches	Purpose	Methodology	Resource example
Exercise	Control weight by combining diet and exercise Requires motivation Clients work to reach desired weight, then through behavior modification; goal is to stay at a certain weight	Motivation, exercise, diet (MED Method)	Exercise salons
Fitness	Bodybuilding to help increase muscle tone, strength, and muscle size Program is based on knowledge of how the body works and develops Objective is to vary resistance that the muscles work against during specific exercises using exercise technology	Muscle- and strength-building exercises	Fitness spas, Nautilus or Universal Gym
Movement exercise	Exercise with dance music to strengthen the body and trim pounds	Jazz dance to stretch, strengthen, and aid in loss of inches	Jazzercise
Total fitness workout	Exercise to music to improve cardiovascular capacity Clients learn how to achieve a "target heart rate" The energy needed is supplied by the oxygen inspired	Aerobic exercise done to music Begins with warm-up exercises and gradually increases exercises to strengthen the body and trim pounds.	Dancercise
Intense concentration exercise	To improve health while developing flexibility, strength, and coordination, along with regulation of breathing	Beginning level; learn to develop posture flexibility, strength balance, coordination, and stamina Advanced level; emphasis on inverted positions and seated postures	Yoga classes

should caution young adults regarding appropriate use of artificial tanning centers.

Although the goal of sunbathing is to achieve a fantastic tan, in reality individuals are exposing themselves to greater risks of cancer. Nursing activities should include education about excessive sun exposure and tanning, use of sunblocking creams and lotions, and knowledge about early recognition of skin symptoms that could indicate cancer. The use of sunblocking agents, such as paraaminobenzoic acid (PABA) is recommended, since these agents can be chosen on the basis of skin type and sensitivity to burning. Choices range from lotions or creams with double protection to those that totally block all burning radiation. The nurse should also advise young adults to avoid sunbathing during the two-hour period around noon, since two thirds of the day's ultraviolet light comes through the earth's atmosphere during that time.

Sports

The growing popularity of a variety of sports activities among young adults accounts for the recent increase of accidents in this age group (see Fig. 22-4). Bicycling and motorcycling were encouraged by environmentalists because they reduce pollution; however, the trend toward cycle riding was also stimulated by traffic congestion, the high cost of fuel, and an increased interest in healthful exercise. Cyclists are likely to be involved in accidents with automobiles. Older cyclists (15 and older) are responsible for a larger proportion of fatalities than they were a decade ago, when the highest rate of fatalities occurred among school-age riders. Nearly 80% of motorcycle accidents occur to individuals under age 30. More than 90% of these injuries occur among males, and most are a direct result of head injuries. In many instances, protective head gear was not used.

RESEARCH REVIEW YOUNG ADULT

EXERCISE

Bonheur B, Young SW: Exercise as a health-promoting lifestyle choice, *Applied Nurs Res* 4:2-6, 1991.

Purpose The purpose of this exploratory study was to examine differences between exercisers and nonexercisers in self-esteem, perceived benefits of exercise, and perceived barriers to exercise.

Review A sample of 108 university students completed 4 questionnaires (e.g., exercise self-report form, Borg Scale, Exercise Benefits/Barriers Scale, Coopersmith Self-Esteem Inventory). Using *t*-tests, a significant difference was found between exercisers and nonexercisers on self-esteem, perceived benefits of exercise, and perceived barriers to exercise. Exercisers demonstrated higher mean scores on self-esteem and perceived benefits. Exercisers participated at least 3 times per week for a duration of at least 20 minutes at moderate intensity and perceived fewer barriers to participation in exercise.

WORKSITE WELLNESS PROGRAM

Sherman JB, Clark L, McEwen MM: Evaluation of a worksite wellness program: impact on exercise, weight, smoking, and stress, *Pub Health Nurs* 6:114-119, 1989.

Purpose The purpose of this study was to evaluate the effects of a wellness program at the workplace in relation to its impact on exercise, weight, smoking, and stress of employee participants.

Review A quasi-experimental design was selected in which data were collected at specific intervals. Baseline data in the categories of exercise, weight, smoking, and stress were collected before program implementation, immediately (30 days) after its completion, and 3 months after its completion. The sample consisted of an experimental group and a control group. Individuals who participated in the wellness program constituted the experimental group. No significant differences were noted between the groups in the areas of exercise, weight, and smoking. Those who participated in the program decreased their level of stress on the job and increased their ability to express their feelings openly. Future research needs to focus on long-term evaluation of wellness programs.

Accidental death from drowning is unfortunately too common in young adults. Swimming, boating, and SCUBA diving, traditionally more popular with young males, are responsible for a high number of fatalities.

Amateur and professional sports activities generally pose few hazards to the participants when reasonable safety precautions are followed. Hang-gliding, parachuting, and flying home-built aircraft are responsible for a large proportion of air fatalities. Mountaineering, downhill ski racing, and bobsledding are other hazardous sports that can cause direct bodily injury. Relatively few fatalities are associated with professional contact sports like football, hockey, or boxing; but chronic injuries frequently cause discomfort. Chronic foot, ankle, and knee injuries are common in football and hockey; brain damage can result from repetitive head injuries in boxing.

The history of a young adult's recreational activities may attune the nurse to specific needs about safety education. The young adult should be encouraged to know and abide by the rules of the sport. Rules are constructed to ensure health and safety, to learn the sport well under appropriate instruction, and to promote good sportsmanship.

SLEEP AND REST PATTERN

Sleep usually follows fatigue, a feeling of tiredness, exhaustion, or need to rest. Young adults are subject to both mental and physical fatigue induced either by physical work or by inactivity and mental stress. Fatigue can be reduced in several ways. Mental stimulation can reduce fatigue by providing a new, challenging task; a change in activities can present new challenges. Changes in physical activity can also present different stimulation, such as learning new exercises or sports.[16,57]

Relaxation

Relaxation refers to a decrease in tension that reduces anxiety and fatigue. Relaxation relieves fatigue; assists in coping with anxiety; relieves stress, which contributes to high blood pressure, arteriosclerosis, heart attack, and stroke; aids in sleep; maintains alertness; and reduces the tendency to smoke or use drugs. Four techniques can be used to elicit the "relaxation response":

1. *Nonstimulating environment.* The ideal environment is free from noise and distractions. Quiet environments make repetitive thoughts and actions more effective.
2. *Mental stimulus.* A word or phrase can be used to shift the activity of the mind away from organized thought directed toward the external environment.
3. *Quiescent attitude.* Adopting an attitude of removal from external sources of stimulation and passivity toward the environment will induce relaxation.
4. *Posture.* Appropriate positioning, with a reduction in muscular tension, will induce relaxation.

Appropriate relaxation has been demonstrated to reduce systolic hypertension readings at least 10 mm Hg, lowering blood pressure levels from the borderline high blood pressure range to normal range.[7] This occurs because relaxation exercises counteract sympathetic nervous system activity, decreasing oxygen consumption, heart rate, respiratory rate, and blood pressure.

Nursing activities directed toward assisting clients in inducing relaxation consist of initial teaching, demonstrating the activity, and observing the client in a return demonstration (see the box on this page). Relaxation interventions may be helpful in assisting clients to cope with hospitalization or stress, and to reduce hypertension, thereby decreasing incidence of stroke (CVA) and heart attack.

Because young adults often keep erratic hours, they can be subject to sleep deprivation. One study found that young adults were sleepier than elderly subjects during the day as measured by onset of sleep during daytime naps. However, recovery from the effects of acute sleep loss after a night of total sleep deprivation was slower in the elderly than in the young adults.[58]

❑ ❑ NURSING SUGGESTIONS TO ASSIST THE YOUNG ADULT IN RELAXING

1. Find a quiet environment and a comfortable position.
2. Close eyes to block out extraneous stimulation.
3. Relax all muscles, starting with toes and feet and progressing toward head. Continue to keep them relaxed.
4. Become aware of breathing pattern. Breathe slowly in and out while counting slowly. Maintain this pattern for 10 to 20 minutes. Sit quietly after this is finished, first with eyes closed, later with them open, standing only at the conclusion.
5. Do not worry about success or failure of relaxation, maintain attitude of indifference toward environment and ignore distractions.

COGNITIVE AND PERCEPTUAL PATTERN

During young adulthood, the senses are most acutely developed. Visual acuity is best around age 20 and starts to decline at about age 40, when the development of farsightedness may indicate a need for prescription glasses. Hearing is also best at age 20; after this, higher tone sounds tend to be gradually lost. The other senses–taste, smell, touch, and awareness of temperature and pain–stay stable until age 45 to 50.

Intellectual maturity is requisite for adult decision making. The process of maturing requires that young adults acquire knowledge and develop skills and behaviors that improve the performance abilities gained as adolescents.[36,52] What is perceived as essential to acquire will depend on individual goals, values, attitudes, and practices as influenced by *intrinsic* (constitutional) and *extrinsic* (environmental) factors. Development of intellectual maturity also influences the selection of behaviors and attitudes that affect health and well-being.[48,63]

Piaget's Theory

Demonstration of mental capability is an important developmental goal for young adults.[36] Piaget's stage of *formal operational thought* evolves from concrete operational thought in adolescence and extends further into the reasoning process in young adulthood.[53] Formal operational thought was achieved by 67% of a sample of 60 college females.[77]

Achievement of formal operational thought allows the individual to analyze all combinations of relations and construct hypotheses capable of being tested. Young adult thought therefore is creative, astute, and insightful. Issues are usually approached objectively and realistically.[4] Young adults are energetic, contribute substantially to social and occupational decision making, and delight in productive dialogue.[47] Although they frequently take greater risks, using trial-and-error methodology, they demonstrate use of problem solving, reasoning, and analytic approaches.[36] The tendency to take greater risks can lead to health-related problems such as those already mentioned (accidents, homicide, suicide) and limit coping mechanisms available to manage situational problems (legal, financial, school, job-related) with which they have had little previous experience.

Intellectual Growth

Young adults use formal operational reasoning, assuming that the social environment and acquired experience provide sufficient cognitive and intellectual stimulation.[53] Organization of information influences memory and recall. Evidence shows that recall performance diminishes with age; at its peak in the twenties, it starts to diminish in the thirties. Improved strategies for organization of information may affect recall positively, however, and limitation of memory with increasing age probably is caused by retrieval mechanisms rather than storage mechanisms. Although the issue of adult intellectual growth is confusing, nurses cannot assume that full potential is realized early in young adulthood. Some growth is seen later; this may be related to stimulation afforded by the environment or influences of later education and experience.

Erikson's Theory

The major goal of young adulthood is to develop increased feelings of self-esteem, along with feelings of self-satisfaction.[16,47] In developing self-esteem, the individual learns to be truly open and capable of trust through the formation of intimate relationships, which are characteristic of this period. Erikson has described this stage of psychosocial development as *intimacy versus isolation and loneliness.*[16,31]

Passage of time is viewed as involving dynamic change in which the achievement of intimacy depends on the existence of a strong sense of self-accomplishment in the adolescent years. Erikson's concept of genuine intimacy extends beyond sexual intimacy to a broader view of mutual psychosocial intimacy with spouse, lover, parents, children, and friends.[13] Intimacy requires mutual trust and is characterized by reciprocal expression of affection. These interchanges are spontaneous for the young adult; relationships should be free and allow for self-disclosure. Young adults who are unsure of their identities may shy away from intimate contact or else embrace promiscuous intimacy lacking in true interrelatedness to others. This can result in a deep sense of isolation and consequent self-absorption. Healthy young adults search for continuity, sameness, or unity of relationships and regularities in life that provide meaning and avoid situations of little commitment.[16,28]

Moral Development

Young adults who have successfully mastered cognitive, social, and previous moral stages are usually able to use principled reasoning. Kohlberg has described this as the postconventional level of moral reasoning.[34,47] In this stage, the individual is able to differentiate self from the rules and expectations of others and to define right in terms of self-chosen principles. The individual at the postconventional level understands society's rules but goes beyond them. When society's rules or practices conflict, the person judges by principle. Therefore the interests of individuals can be weighed against the needs of society and the state, and violations of law can be justified when individual interests are in consonance with principles. Principled reasoning can provide a justification for social and political protest; during the Vietnam conflict, some students who participated in antiwar protests used principled reasoning to justify their actions. Gilligan studied the development of moral reasoning in women and girls; her findings indicate that women's moral judgments reflect less a rights perspective and more an emphasis on relationships as an alternative to seeing people as standing alone.[22]

The development of principled or high-level moral reasoning is possible in young adulthood; but it may not occur if cognitive and social factors stimulating increased moral reasoning are not present. Acts of personal violence representative of lower moral reasoning should not be present, but such acts are common in young adulthood, illustrating the need for addressing moral development concerns at earlier ages of education and socialization.

SELF-PERCEPTION AND SELF-CONCEPT PATTERN

During young adulthood, two emotional themes are evident. In their twenties young adults yearn to explore and experiment, keeping structures temporary and therefore reversible. These are individuals who move from job to job and relationship to relationship, remaining in a transient state. At the opposite extreme is the urge to prepare for the future by making firm commitments. Although young adults fear that the choices they make may be irrevocable, change is possible; and some adjustment to the original choice is to be expected.[48] During this period both men and women may question their value to society, the merit of their accomplishments, their success as sexual beings, and the probability of attaining their unfulfilled goals.[27,43]

Although the 1990s has seen an increase in unemployment rates, more women are working. Whereas women made up only 30% of the paid labor force by the 1950s, they accounted for more than 44% in 1988.[88] More than 65% of the women ages 25 to 35 are employed. Growing numbers of women with infants and children are employed. Employment, with all its benefits gained through wages, is a factor that can impinge on one's health and well-being. The gap in earnings, or pay equity issues between men and women, continues to grow. Access to insurance and pension benefits is not always available, especially to high-risk groups, such as minorities or persons receiving minimum wages. Even when there is access to health care, some types of employment expose individuals to occupational risks and hazards. As more mothers enter the labor force, the need for adequate child care has increased.

Many young adults are high achievers, and they seek opportunities to be challenged. Their goal is to acquire and demonstrate competence. An important component of their productivity is to be allowed *self-expression*. Unfortunately, the climate of many job settings restrains creativity. Stressful consequences of employment problems can be traumatic to the individual self-esteem and self-worth. The degree of stress can be compounded further by failure to receive a promotion or pay raise. Both a young adult and an older individual can be shattered at the loss of his or her first job, especially if it is the result of firing. Employment is more than a source of income; it provides self-esteem and social interaction.

One of the current issues affecting young adults is the inability to find jobs suited to their needs or particular goals. An even more stressful situation occurs among young adults who discover that their education or field of specialization has become obsolete or automated even before they have journeyed through the young adult lifespan.

Nurses need to be aware of problems arising from difficulties in the work world.[71] Since adjustment to the job market influences so many other aspects of daily living, young adults frequently require assistance in developing coping mechanisms to deal with this stress. Dealing with the initial stress often prevents further complications that might arise if the young adult turns to drugs, prescription medications, or alcohol to relieve anxiety and stress.

Young adult women share concerns and desires for success and job satisfaction with young men (Fig. 22-5). Many young women postpone childbearing until they have established careers; many are absent from the job only during a standard maternity leave. Young adult women who return to work when their children are very young often risk the emotional strain brought on by guilt feelings.[24]

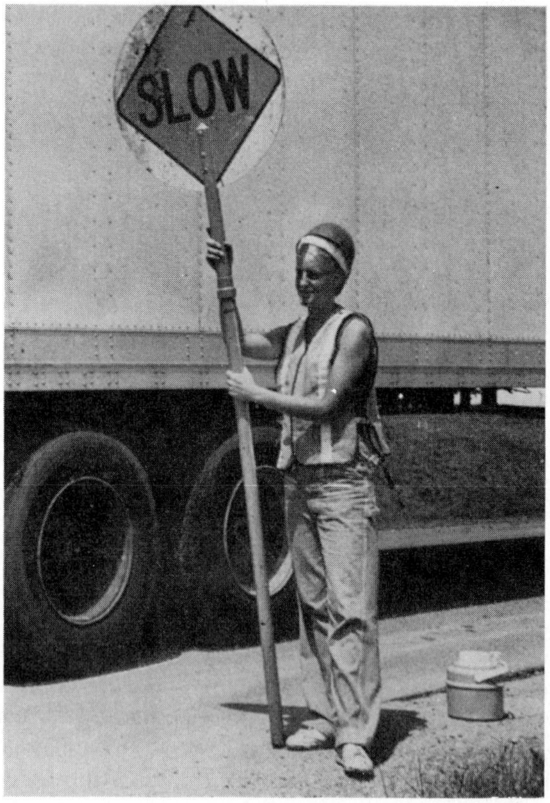

Fig. 22-5. Changing role of young adult women is evident in the workplace. (Photograph by David S. Strickler.)

Both working mothers and working fathers need to recognize that quality time with children is important. In addition to helping parents cope with the stress of being absent from their children, nurses can help them identify ways of providing quality supervision in their absence, through either private sitters, day-care programs, or friends and relatives.

Work can bring about happiness and fulfillment or lead to frustration and depersonalization. In addition, it is particularly significant to consider that dissatisfaction is a potential threat to well-being. For example, white-collar workers are reported to be more satisfied with career choices and work-related environments; they are professionally educated and usually afforded a higher percentage of job satisfaction with increasing age until later maturity. Women are more interested in extrinsic factors than men and less interested in relocating to obtain a promotion.[36,78]

The relationship of work to job satisfaction has been identified as a major cause of health hazards associated with stress-related illness. Job stress can lead to increased absenteeism, which is more common in young adults.[57,83] Nursing intervention in industrial settings can be directed toward improving both working conditions and employer-employee relationships.

COPING AND STRESS-TOLERANCE PATTERN

Assessment of Stress Levels

Because stress can play an integral part in the young adult's life, a health assessment should include questions to determine stress levels. Signs of increased anxiety, nervousness, depression, or somatic complaints may indicate a problem: divorce, loss of job, failure to be promoted, or financial difficulties. The nurse's role is that of a listener offering support and concern. The nurse may also believe that a referral to a therapist would be helpful; this might be suggested to the client. The nurse needs to recognize stress as a risk factor in the young adult to prevent further physical and psychologic problems.

Achievement Stress

Characteristic of young adult years is another potential risk to health–achievement-oriented stress. This differs from stress in situational crises in that the stress in an overachiever is brought about from internal pressures to succeed in relation to goals. Achievement stress often causes workaholic habits, including neglect to sleep and omission of meals. If this behavior becomes extreme, serious physical and emotional consequences can occur such as nutritional problems or burnout, which in turn lead to severe emotional and physical exhaustion. Workaholic behaviors may not be perceived by the individual and often go undetected until changes in body functions or behavior occur.

Health interventions aimed at helping the individual to identify and reduce stress factors are most effective.[60] Young adults are usually health conscious and willing to alter personal lifestyles and patterns of behavior according to their concept of health. Many have responded exceptionally well to the campaigns for physical fitness, exercise, and nutritional adjustment, which should increase their well-being and life expectancy.[83]

Accidents and Physical Injuries

Physical injury resulting in disability or death among young adults may be caused by misuse of firearms, poisoning by gases or vapors, ingestion of poisons from solids or liquids, or falls and accidents associated with drug and alcohol abuse. The largest pecentage of accidents occur before age 35, ages 18 to 21 being the peak years.

Auto accidents are a leading cause of death among young adults; they are responsible for more fatalities than all other causes of death combined.[83] Reducing speed limits has contributed to fewer fatalities, but traffic accidents continue to claim the lives of thousands of young adults annually. Mortality rates are higher in young adult males, but rates are increasing for females.[82,83] Reasons for continued high incidence in this age group include accessibility of cars to young adults and peer pressures to drive everywhere, often recklessly. Young adults often may be coerced into reckless driving–and alcohol or drug-related driving incidents.

This bleak outlook could be changed substantially by better awareness of safety needs. A majority of young licensed drivers today have participated in driver education courses to learn safe driving rules. Current campaigns encouraging and laws requiring use of safety belts are areas in which public education can be effective.

Accident prevention, although often considered appropriate for young children, should be included for the young adult. This includes helping the young adult understand the potentially fatal results of aggressive tendencies or thoughtless risk taking. If young adults are encouraged to reflect on the consequences of their actions, they may be more willing to control and change these behaviors.

Noise Pollution

Young adults are often exposed to high noise levels in occupational and recreational settings. Loud, high-pitched, and intermittent irritating sounds are becoming more frequent. Exposure to loud noise over time is directly related to impaired hearing and may also increased irritability and stress. Noisy conditions are very costly to industry in terms of mistakes, absenteeism, decreased efficiency, and lowered employee retention.[57,86] Young adults may be exposed in the work setting to noises from industrial machinery and equipment. Although this exposure cannot always be decreased, many young adults continue to expose themselves further by spending hours listening to stereo music at excessively high decibel levels. Dance clubs often provide social interaction within a very noisy environment.

Moderation in activities involving noise is to be encouraged. Ear protection may be necessary in some situations to prevent hearing disability. Recognition of noise hazards and appropriate education are early nursing strategies directed toward decreasing exposure.

Air Pollution

Young adults are often exposed to numerous pollutants in the environment. In industrial societies, waste is often added to the air faster than natural forces can remove it. Air is considered polluted when gases and particles are released in such amounts that health, safety, comfort, and outdoor employment are affected.

Motor vehicles are the largest source of air pollution; they release more than 90 million tons of particles and gases each year, most of which is either carbon monoxide or hydrocarbons.[57] Carbon monoxide can cause headaches, dizziness, and heart palpitations. In the sunlight, automobile exhausts become a photochemical smog containing ozone, which irritates the eyes and can cause respiratory irritation.

The second *Clear Air Act* (1970) requires each state to submit to the Environmental Protection Agency (EPA) a plan to achieve air quality standards. Pollution is heaviest in highly populated areas and heavy industrial sites. Industries have been slow to react to quality air legislation because the cost of removing pollutants must be passed on to the consumer. Air pollution can be controlled by better design of furnaces, smokestacks, engines, and other machinery where fuel is consumed. Some gasoline-powered machinery may be replaced eventually by electric, steam, or alternate engines. Particles can also be removed from the air using electrostatic cleaners after conventional burning of fuel.

No single method will reduce air pollution alone; in combination, however, these controls can reduce overall air pollution. Although air pollution is not a problem for young adults only, they frequently work in industrial settings and may be the group most affected.

Occupational Hazards and Stressors

Occupational hazards pose a threat of illness, injury, or death in all age groups. Occupational safety standards have contributed greatly to the reduction of work-related accidents. Legislation, including the *Occupational Safety and Health Act* (1970), resulted in improvement of work conditions along with the provision of health care facilities in many companies. But occupational hazards still are recognized as major contributing factors to poor health. For example, cancer rates are rising among industrial workers, and plastic workers exposed to vinyl chloride are more likely to develop liver cancer.[80]

Young adults should not be allowed to work in certain industrial settings without some vocational education or training to reduce hazards.[67] Even with the best precautions, however, young adults desire challenges, and they frequently accept hazardous employment; for example, working on offshore drilling rigs, on high bridges, or in nuclear plants. Regrettably, many young adults are unaware of their worksite hazards and risks to illness; many workdays are lost because of work-related injuries.

Because of their age, physical stamina, and quickness in response, young adults are the most likely candidates to be hired in positions requiring physical ability. A major objective to decrease hazards includes education about personal exposure risks, identification of work-related hazards, and the way in which severity of accidents often increases in combination with personal behaviors or habits. For example, young adults driving heavy equipment should avoid reckless behaviors or fast driving.

Other important objectives include routing physical evaluation and surveillance of the worksite by employers. Routine examination of workers in industries with known health consequences is important. Known conditions such as asbestosis, byssinosis, silicosis, and coal workers' pneumoconiosis have been greatly reduced because of better knowledge of disease processes and causative conditions. Working women who are pregnant also may expose their fetuses to industrial substances. Proper evaluation and temporary reassignment may be necessary.

Nurses in occupational settings, clinics, or private offices should explore with their patients their understanding of the dangers associated with the work setting. Objectives for preventive intervention require that known hazards and risks be identified early. The health history should include questions about the place of work, type of work, and young adults' understanding of the risks associated with their occupation. Occupational risk and mental health are closely related; stress associated with work, the use of alcohol or drugs, and a negative attitude toward work often result in occupational injuries. The nurse should counsel any troubled young adult about the potential for work injury.

Since so few jobs at industries have their own nurses or other health care providers, young adults need primary-care nurses to assist them. Frequently, work-related health issues arise that need attention, but job counseling aimed at changing other employment may be an appropriate referral for certain health problems. Employees in industrial settings should be seen on a periodic basis for health assessment, review of health history, and counseling.

Carcinogens

Exposure to environmental carcinogens is a potent stressor. Cancer is the second leading cause of death in adults. The 1988 statistics illustrate that cancer occurs as commonly in women as in men. Many deaths involve young adults.

Carcinogenicity in young adults is often associated with the work setting, smoking, and alcohol consumption. Environmental controls have limited the exposure to many hazardous chemicals; but the effects on health of many industrial chemicals is still unknown.[56] Altering behavior patterns to decrease the use of cigarettes and alcohol is increasingly meeting with success in young adults and should be the focus of nursing intervention.

Hodgkin's disease and breast cancer are among the leading causes of death from cancer in young adults. Fortunately, recent advances in the use of chemotherapy have drastically reduced the numbers of deaths. Breast cancer, a leading form of malignancy in women, has only recently been surpassed in incidence by lung cancer. Incidence rates for 1983 through 1987 and mortality rates for the United States in 1987 illustrate that 12% of all women will be given a diagnosis of breast cancer and 3.5% will die of the disease. An estimated 175,000 new cases were diagnosed in 1991.[25] The age-adjusted mortality rates have remained remarkably stable, but the upswing in incidence of breast cancer that began in the 1980s is mostly the result of an increase in detection of tumors measuring less than 2 cm in diameter. This is thought to reflect the wider use of screening mammography. Established risk factors related to breast cancer–a family history of breast cancer, early menarche, late age at first childbirth, late age at menopause, history of benign breast disease, and exposure to ionizing radiation–are related to weak or moderate elevations in risk of developing the disease. Alcohol consumption at a level of one drink or more per day is associated with a moderate increase in breast cancer risk in a number of studies. An increase in alcohol consumption by younger women may have contributed appreciably to the increased breast cancer incidence currently observed; in the Nurses' Health Study alcohol consumption at the age of 18 was three times higher among study participants born between 1960 and 1964 than among those born 40 years earlier.[25,37]

Lung and uterine cancer are of special concern to women. The recent high incidence of lung cancer and death is a consequence of women's delayed but relatively high smoking prevalence. Cervical cancer has decreased steadily over the years, probably because of the effective use of detection methods. Regrettably, uterine cancer continues to be found at higher rates among low-income groups.[37,72]

WAYS YOUNG ADULTS COPE WITH STRESS

Drugs

Misuse of drugs, a major threat for young adults, is associated with injuries, homicides, and suicides and is related to social problems–various criminal behaviors, as well as maladjustment to accepted norms. Drug abuse may be related closely to an inability to deal appropriately with adult responsibilities.

In 1988, 56.4% of young adults had some experience with marijuana; about 15% had tried strong drugs, such as cocaine (19.7%) or hallucinogens (13.8%). Among young adults ages 18 to 25, 15.5% currently were using marijuana.[72] This is an alarming problem, since fewer than 2% of the population, including young persons, had used drugs before 1962. The use of LSD, a popular drug in the 1960s, is on the rise again among young adults, with alarming reports of known usage among followers of rock bands. The increased use of illegal drugs among adolescents and young children also contributes to alarming statistical reports.

Medically prescribed drugs are another source for experimentation with chemicals in young adults. Used alone or together, barbiturates, amphetamines, or sedative-hypnotics reportedly bring about feelings of physical and psychologic well-being–feelings that may be desired by many troubled young adults. Continued use leads to physical and psychologic dependency. Barbiturates, consumed in combination with alcohol, are a leading cause of accidental death.

Use of anabolic steroids to improve muscle mass and athletic performance is increasing. Driven by the desire for an improved physique and increased strength, teenagers and young adults are turning to legal and illegal substances touted as physique boosters and performance enhancers. The risks of using steroids are enormous, and education should be aimed at modifying American sports and exercise values. Winning at sports does not justify endangering one's health; playing at one's highest level of ability is what is important. Would-be athletes should rely more on body building exercises than on gambling with their health as they strive to be bigger and stronger.[54]

Drug misuse is a cause of many health problems. As mentioned earlier, adverse social consequences of family maladjustment and crime increase; and resulting physical health problems account for more than 50% of the major acute and chronic problems of young adults.[83] Heroin users have higher mortality rates because of overdosage or chronic disability associated with hepatitis infections caused by contaminated equipment and with malnutrition.[83] Drug abuse in pregnant women directly affects fetal outcome. Use of prescription medications during pregnancy requires close medical supervision and strict compliance to the treatment regimen. Since most drugs cross the placenta, a developing fetus can be damaged by use of inappropriate drugs or treatment regimens. Gestational period is an important consideration when prescribing drugs. Fetal complications can also occur when drugs are self-prescribed and when they are taken before the woman is even aware that she is pregnant.

Nursing activities must include preventive strategies to curb the problem of drug misuse. Distribution of information about drugs, early treatment of complications, and drug treatment centers is part of the answer. Education must be directed toward reducing drug use and raising awareness of physical and psychologic complications of drug misuse. Nursing efforts aimed at increasing individual awareness and altering drug attitudes and behaviors are of critical importance.

Alcohol

Alcohol-related accidents among young adults ages 15 to 24 continue to be the leading cause of death; alcohol is a factor in more than 10% of all deaths in the United States, and 60% of all highway fatalities involving young adults are alcohol related.[85] Raising the legal drinking age to 21 reduces not only deaths and injuries related to motor vehicle accidents but also homicides and other violent deaths in general.[30]

Alcohol abuse is related directly to conditions affecting the adult, such as cirrhosis of the liver and various cancers. Recent reports have indicated that alcohol is a contributing factor in cancer of the esophagus, larynx, and oral cavity.[39] It is essential to modify or change the behavior patterns of alcohol consumption in young adults to decrease the frequency of chronic and disabling conditions.

Alcohol consumption has increased among young people and women. Alcohol is easily attainable, affordable, and more socially acceptable. Although young adults drink less regularly than older individuals, they tend to consume larger amounts of alcohol at one time. This causes quicker loss of control and increased potential for accidents. Dependency on alcohol is reported frequently among young adult drinkers.[32]

The increased numbers of women who work outside the home has increased opportunities for social drinking. Women who drink alcoholic beverages to excess are at additional risk for pregnancy complications, including *fetal alcohol syndrome,* noted by symptoms of central nervous system manifestations and gastrointestinal alterations in the baby. Nursing interventions include early identification of pregnant women who are heavy alcohol users. In addition, malnutrition may accompany heavy drinking; for pregnant women, this compromises their health status even more.

Smoking

Authorities agree that the greatest reduction in mortality from lung cancer can be achieved by cessation of cigarette smoking.[86] One of the nurse's most important roles in helping people to stop smoking is to serve as a role model; a nurse cannot persuade a young adult to stop smoking who does not demonstrate appropriate health behaviors.

The nurse must distribute information on the disease potential of smoking whenever possible. Individuals employed in high-risk occupations should be informed of the synergistic relationship between smoking and occupations related to asbestos and radiation exposure. Every assistance should be used to help those who want to stop smoking. Research indicates that fear tactics, nagging, preaching, and threats are ineffective in convincing people to stop smoking. Because fear tactics have proved ineffective, serious efforts are now being made to create a social climate where smoking is not acceptable. This approach reflects the concept of smoking as a social disease.

The most practical approach for nurses is

1. To conduct educational programs that unemotionally detail the known hazards of smoking
2. To provide clients with educational material that further explains the health hazards of smoking or high-risk occupations
3. To provide specific measures for those people who do desire to stop smoking or decrease occupational risk factors

The nurse needs to supply information on the "how to's" of smoking cessation. Many people think seriously about quitting but lack the information to help themselves stop. Nurses should be familiar with the antismoking resources in their communities so that appropriate referrals can be made.[75]

A three-goal unified approach is now recommended to decrease smokers in the United States:

1. Youth antismoking programs to prevent the acquisition of the smoking habit
2. Smoking-cessation programs to help current smokers quit
3. A less harmful cigarette for those who cannot or will not quit smoking

A nonjudgmental approach should be taken with individuals who refuse to stop smoking or are unable to do so. If appropriate, they should be urged to smoke cigarettes with tar yields of less than 10 mg, to smoke filtered cigarettes, and to smoke only half of each cigarette. The nurse should make it clear that switching brands only decreases the hazard at best (risk of lung cancer is dose and exposure related) and may not even do that for smokers who unconsciously increase the number of cigarettes smoked or alter their puffing patterns or put their fingers over the air holes of low-tar and nicotine cigarettes.

ROLE AND RELATIONSHIP PATTERN

Young adults interact with many people daily within their work, school, or community environments. By establishing relationships, they counteract social isolation. For many young adults, their most meaningful relationships occur in a variety of settings, including home, work, or community. Typically, young adults venture into their relationships with enthusiasm and passion; but they often are vulnerable to conflict or stress when relationships do not proceed in a smooth fashion. A shattered love affair with spouse or friend, a stressful work environment, or an unfriendly neighbor are situations capable of creating anxiety and maladaptation.

Adult friendships are more enduring than earlier relationships; but when these friendships become more intimate "love" relationships, they create a risk of disenchantment and disillusionment.[31] The focus of the relationship is the sharing of feelings or confidences; it involves a giving of self in an objective way to another. True relationships frequently are characteristic of a person who wants to give rather than to receive. Friendships are necessary in a constantly changing society; they provide a source of emotional support and a basis of stability for the development of the self-concept.[36]

Choosing friends and lovers is one of the most important occurrences of life. Establishing interpersonal relationships involves agreeable and purposeful interactions with others, not superficial but lasting and important contacts with another person.[36] Although interpersonal relationships can be created with persons of the same sex or the opposite sex, age is usually a less important factor than it was during adolescence. Friendships grow and mature in varying ways. The formation of intimate relationships develops within or outside a family context and sometimes in the work environment.

The young adult, in addition to achieving intimacy, must accomplish other developmental tasks for psychosocial maturation. These tasks focus on his or her ability to make decisions about career goals. Decision making about life and career directions is the task that heralds the transition from adolescence to adult status. Decisions usually entail establishing independence from the family of origin.[36] This often involves an actual physical move from the parents' home–going away to college, joining the military, getting an apartment–but movement away is not the sole indicator of independence (see Fig. 22-5). Frequently young adults remain in their parents' home for economic reasons, especially if life choices involve continued schooling or remaining unmarried. Gaining independence is secure when the young adult achieves an equal relationship with the parents and, if living at home, shares responsibilities for family maintenance. Under certain circumstances or in certain cultures, newly married young adults may share the home of one of their parents when they start their own family developmental roles.[1]

Exhibiting maturity by taking on adult roles and responsibilities is a developmental process. Most young men and women have the intellectual and emotional solidity to take on new social roles and venture into challenges with eagerness and a desire for mastery. Young adults feel more secure about themselves and the way they relate to others. They therefore begin to develop personal values, attitudes, and interests at work and in society.[36] They often speak out for causes that affect society; they remain committed to ideas and ideals until resolutions have been identified.

Young adults striving to accomplish psychosocial maturation are aware they have many common bonds and goals with peers. Similarities in view illustrate that all young adults experience the same conflicts, hopes, desires, disappointments, and urges in the process of change. Dissimilarity exists only in the timing and sequence of age-expected behaviors.[36] Accordingly, young adulthood is a time of transition and constant psychosocial growth.

Another important choice of this age group is the decision to start a family (Fig. 22-6). If procreation is the choice, a subsequent issue is the number and training of children. Additional thought must be given to considerations such as money, safety, family support, housing, the relationship to extended family members,

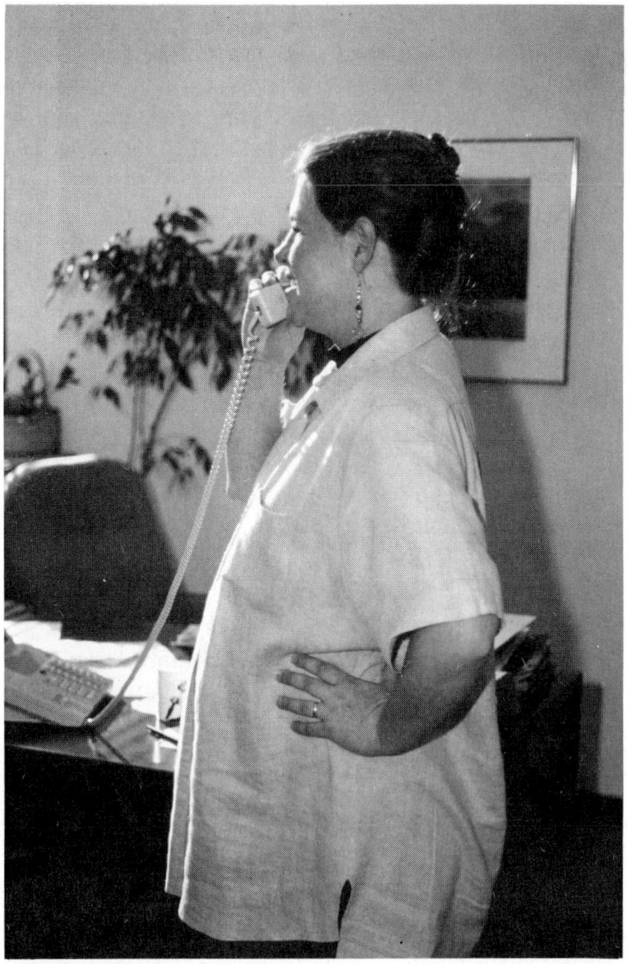

Fig. 22-6. Planning pregnancy and timing this event properly are critical decisions for many young adults.

and the roles and responsibilities of the nuclear family unit. Today it is important for young adults establishing a family to have open communication about self-development, which includes issues of dual careers, childbearing practices, and domestic duties within the home.[36]

Family development and harmony are major goals for many young male and female adults. Although family size and structure have undergone dramatic changes in the past several years, concerns about each individual member's health and safety continue as a prime focus within the family as a unit. Family life is influenced by the qualities of individual family members. Typically, the age of the individuals, job security, place in the community, and healthy patterns of living (good nutrition, personal cleanliness, physical fitness) are associated with healthy family adjustment. Therefore, the physical and mental health of one member affects all members. A young father of 35 recently diagnosed with cancer needs the support and cooperation of family members to cope during therapy and accept future adjustments.

Separation and Divorce

Divorce rates have been rising steadily in the last several decades, and rates are higher among young adults.[39] Although young black women have had higher rates, the rates among white women of varying socioeconomic standings are considerably higher than they were five years ago. Divorce makes more young women heads of households.

More women are entering the job market; this has been attributed in part to the increase in separation and divorce. Many stressors contribute to divorce. Socioeconomic factors often place unreasonable stress on marriages. Age at marriage is correlated with duration of marriage, and young adults whose parents have divorced also have a higher frequency of divorce.[39] In addition, society's willingness to protect the rights of women has encouraged more women to publicly make known intolerable situations they formerly were forced to accept.

Although dissatisfaction and unhappiness are frequent precursors to separation or divorce, the decision to dissolve a marriage is not easy. Considerable emotional strain exists for both partners, their children, and close family and friends. Divorce requires that young adults consider their basic values, individual personality and ego strength, future job potential, and socioeconomic factors that will ensure security and safety for themselves and their children. Consequently, divorced young adults often suffer severe emotional strain and depression. Some young adults are unable to adjust to role and status change and to threats to self-concept. For these reasons, support systems in the form of groups, individual counseling, or special social activities are critical.

As a result of divorce, many women and their young children are forced to find emergency shelter in publicly operated homes, including welfare hotels and congregate shelters. Looking at the statistics on homelessness, men tend to be the highest users of shelters for nighttime residence. Homeless women are more likely to be married than homeless men. Many homeless people hold jobs, on a sporadic basis, about 10% to 20% of the time. The percentage of homeless people with high school diplomas has increased over the past few years. Minorities are significantly overrepresented among the homeless in larger cities, reflecting the high proportion of minorities who live below poverty level.[20] Reporting on a survey conducted in 1990, the mayors of large cities cite an increase of approximately 24% in requests for emergency shelter, showing in some areas a 70% rise among single adults.[42,79]

The nurse working with young adults considering a separation or divorce must recognize the crisis that exists. They may need support from the nurse to help them work through this difficult time. Nurses should be aware of the fact that feelings of guilt, grief, and loss often are experienced by young adults going through a separation or divorce. Suggesting that young adults read articles or books on issues related to divorce is helpful, since it provides a reference point for their experiences. The nurse may also recommend marital counseling by a trained professional; this may be the most beneficial source of support for emotional well-being.

Unplanned Pregnancy

Unwanted or unplanned pregnancies are a constant source of stress to many young adults. Many children come before they are desired or are conceived when they are not wanted. The ability to control the timing of births is an important consideration for young adult women. Women often have goals for schooling or career that should take precedence over family development; interference in these goals often affects both future relationships and later mother-child relationships. Although some unplanned births are earlier than planned but are wanted later, 19% of unplanned births remain unwanted even after birth. These children have a greater potential for parental neglect and emotional deprivation.[82]

The timing of the first child forces individuals to alter their activities; these changes are age related and frequently occur in sequence. For example, according to the traditional ordering of events, schooling should precede marriage, and in turn marriage should occur before the birth of the first child.[42] For the young adult male, pregnancy can impose an increased financial burden on developing relationships long before schooling is complete or his first job is secured.

The unmarried couple undergoes similar experiences

with unplanned pregnancies; and such relationships often do not survive. This gives rise to problems concerning child custody and child support. On the other hand, conceiving premaritally often contributes to rushed early marriages.

Births to unmarried women increased during the 1980s, as more women chose to give birth but remain single. In 1988, half the infants of mothers under age 20 were born to unmarried mothers.[72,87] Although it is impossible to say how many of these parents did marry, studies have shown that when birth precedes marriage, a higher incidence of divorce clearly exists. This contributes to higher numbers of female-headed households throughout the young adult years.[39]

Factors such as family size, economic considerations, race, birth order, and disruption in family resulting from separation or divorce have been associated with unwanted pregnancy. Eliminating unwanted childbearing is a healthy goal, and for many young adults it involves making active decisions about pregnancy prevention.

Both married and unmarried young adults need information about contraceptives to decrease both the number of unwanted pregnancies and the need for abortions. The nurse's role in contraceptive counseling involves helping individuals to choose the methods appropriate to their needs. Patient education about the risks, side effects, and complications associated with a specific method and the effective use of such a method is vital. Several points should be considered by nurses who engage in contraceptive counseling:

1. Positive decision making and healthy family relationships are vital to emotional security.
2. When suggesting contraceptives, patient acceptability and skill must be considered to help the client make an appropriate decision.[26] Recent laws may restrict nurses and other health providers in some settings from engaging in abortion counseling.

Suicide

As mentioned previously in this chapter, suicide in the young adult population is a leading cause of death (see Table 22-2). Suicide occurs because many young adults are unable to cope with the pressures of adulthood. For some, pressure arises when dealing with interpersonal conflicts: marital problems, family discord, or the loss of a close relationship. For others, the precipitating event is one of personal resources, unemployment, or dissatisfaction with work or school. Many young adults try to solve their problems before the fatal incident but see no positive solutions; in many, a previous suicide attempt was their signal for help.

Nursing interventions should be directed toward identifying behaviors in the young adult who may be contemplating suicide. Some of the physical clues worthy of noting include: signs of self-neglect, depression, decreased muscle tone, slumped shoulders, slowed gait and speech, and drooped faces. Presuicidal individuals may also exhibit hypermobility, impaired reality testing, the expression of helplessness and hopelessness, impaired judgment and object relationships, decreased cooperativeness, anxiety and weight loss, an increased pain threshold, insomnia, and a radically changed affect.

The nurse should also be alert to other factors. Women may make more suicide attempts than men, but men succeed more often.[72] Suicide is more common among single or widowed individuals and most common among divorced persons.[39] Young adults are more likely to attempt suicide than older individuals, and professionals are more likely to attempt suicide than nonprofessionals.

The nurse working with the young adult should be aware of suicide as a potential problem. The nurse's contacts with young adults are preventive, since nurses assist in identifying young adults who may be contemplating suicide. In addition to identifying presuicidal behaviors, the nurse also should investigate the young adult's previous relationship patterns to determine which are complicated by feelings of worthlessness and defeat–danger signals suggesting close supervision and counseling. If the nurse identifies a young adult at risk for a suicide attempt, referrals to other professionals may be indicated.

ISSUES AFFECTING THE HEALTH OF YOUNG ADULTS

Neighborhood Resources

Community environment strongly influences the well-being of the young adult and sets the standard for the health of people and families living within a neighborhood. Neighbors can be a good source of support, which can be especially important to a young mother who does not have immediate family close by. Incompatible neighbors, however, can be a source of anxiety or stress. Nurses working in the community can facilitate the contact of individuals with common interests through community and religious activities and support groups.

Community resources for exercise and recreation are important to the young adult's physical health and emotional well-being. If such resources are available, the young adult can have the opportunity to exercise and release any stress or anxiety in a positive fashion. Schools within the community are a concern to young adults with school-age children. Parents dissatisfied with the public school system may feel additional pressure to provide private schooling. This may add additional financial burdens to a family who are already financially troubled.

Health Service Availability

The availability of health services within a community is also important for the young adult. Economic realities, however, are often responsible for inefficient or ineffective resources, especially for the young adult who is poor or belongs to a minority group. In some communities health services are lacking or, when available, do not consider the cultural customs and beliefs of the population they serve. In other communities the availability of public transportation may be a critical problem affecting the young adult's ability to make clinic visits.

The Impact of Homelessness

Homeless people were once mainly single men; today homeless families account for approximately one third of the estimated homeless population. Five factors have been shown to contribute to homelessness: the shortage of affordable housing, poverty, mental illness, alcoholism, and family disruption. Becoming homeless usually takes two phases: displacement from current housing and inability to relocate in substitute housing. In one study, women and their families stayed an average of two to eleven months in shelters before locating housing. Poverty was a key factor; welfare benefits were generally too low to cover high rents and there were long waits for public housing. Adequate housing might be located far from transportation and health care facilities, thus hindering access to health care.[20]

Culture and Ethnicity

The ethnic beliefs and health practices of young adults, especially young women of childbearing age, should be major nursing concerns. Young adult women and their unborn children sometimes practice inappropriate health behaviors because of beliefs and practices based on historic customs.

In the black American culture, little health care supervision occurs during pregnancy. Pregnancy is viewed as a state of wellness; therefore many women believe that prenatal care is not necessary.[71] Some women who do receive prenatal care fail to comply with instructions because they consider this type of care insignificant and passive, even though they and their children are prone to health deviations arising from socioeconomic factors, such as exposure to illness resulting from overcrowding and poor nutrition. Consequently, a high maternal and fetal mortality has developed over the past 20 years for the black population.[72] An estimated 60% of black women living in large, urban ghettos and rural areas fall into this high-risk category for maternal mortality.[9,83]

Health delivery methods in the United States are based on Western belief systems, which tend to be stereotypic and rigid in applications for specific clients. For example, women seeking birth control measures are expected to use the health clinics and keep their follow-up visits. Since health care providers have removed many traditional barriers once assumed to cause poor use of services (location, scheduling) by minority groups, nonattendance at scheduled clinic visits is often interpreted as noncompliance. However, a study recently indicated that utilization of preventive health services by Puerto Rican women was related directly to their cultural beliefs of modesty and their feelings of being male dominated.[17,18] In the American Indian culture, contraceptive education has gained little acceptance and fertility rates remain high–conception control is both culturally and religiously objectionable. Appropriate health strategies and interventions require that nurses identify cultural beliefs and health care practices that are harmful to their clients. Many cultural practices may be allowed because they do not affect appropriate health strategies. For example, food cravings are commonly seen in many pregnant women. In some cultures, excessive food cravings have been believed to cause birthmarks on the baby, supposedly corresponding in size and shape to the food that was craved.[9] In moderation, following dietary patterns directed by such cravings may not be harmful. When the craving leads to an unbalanced diet or to pica (eating unnatural substances), however, the pregnancy may be affected.[29]

Political Factors

Young adults are one of the major political constituencies in the United States. They support many causes and provide the time and energy to publicize issues related to the common good. Some of these issues have included nuclear power, war, pollution, and conservation. Relative to health, predominant issues have involved housing and health care in neighborhoods and rural areas and health, agriculture, and sanitation in foreign countries. Young adults have done and will do much to improve living conditions for future generations.

Demographic Considerations

To eliminate health problems for the population at all ages, nurses must concentrate on the whole societal environment influencing personal behavior and lifestyle. Thought and planning must be devoted to such variables as world population, food supplies, air, water, energy consumed, technologic advances, transportation, schools, housing, and health services. Resources should be protected for future generations, so that our lands will be kept esthetically acceptable and family life will continue to nurture the young. We must attempt both to alter past pollution mistakes and to consider today's environment. The future must be prepared by designing ways to preserve energy sources, control the economy, and ensure freedom as a peaceful nation. Many threats to our survival can be promoted and supervised most effectively by young adults.

Economic Factors

One of the young adult's tasks is to choose and develop a lifelong career pattern. This choice is related directly to economic factors; young adults want satisfying occupations that also yield adequate economic returns.

Economic issues may also affect other decisions. To deal with these issues and maintain a lifestyle in which personal needs can be met, young adults are electing to have fewer children. They are concerned about the desire for and timing of pregnancy. Many young adults consistently use some form of birth control. Although hazards associated with many contraceptive methods are greatly reduced, young adults may be concerned with the strain and constraints of pregnancy planning. Caring for aging parents can also cause economic stress.

Although goals vary greatly among young adult couples, they are generally concerned with acquiring material objects; the desire for house, car, furniture, or a vacation may necessitate that both work to meet financial obligations. This situation necessitates changes in roles and sharing of responsibilities, and open communication becomes a crucial component (Fig. 22-7).

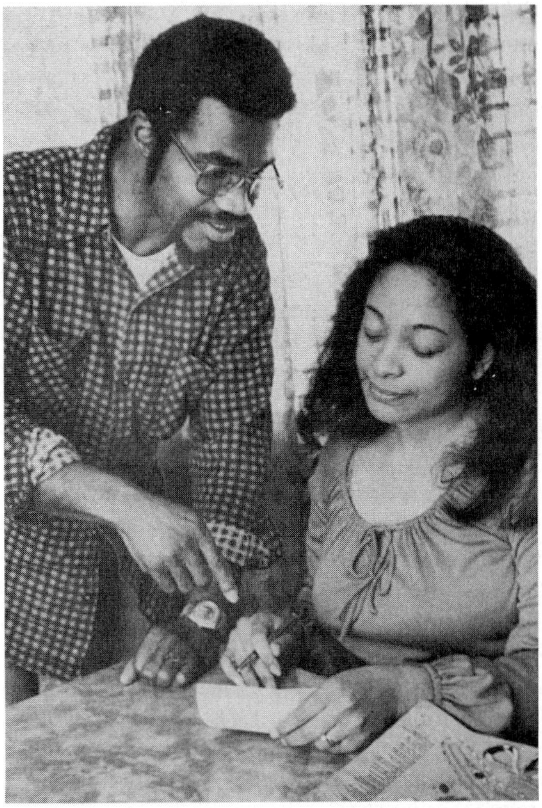

Fig. 22-7. Economic planning for family and future requires close cooperation. (Photograph by David S. Strickler.)

Dual Careers

For many young adults, dual careers place additional strains on their relationship because of different interests, separate friends, varying maturity levels, physical tiredness, and so forth. Such circumstances can provide a basis for domestic problems. Domestic quarreling may precede family disruption, leading to marital separation or divorce. In addition to the emotional strain placed on family members, domestic arguments may result in aggressive acts of abuse and personal injury. Young adults may also be faced with decisions about day-care facilities; the young woman may need support to resolve guilt feelings related to the separation from her child.

Some young adults who choose communal living are forced into this arrangement because of socioeconomic issues. Alternate lifestyles include living arrangements with individuals of the same sex or the opposite sex. Although these lifestyles are becoming more acceptable in today's society, they are still not viewed as appropriate for the development of young children. In many young adults unrealistic attitudes toward various lifestyles contribute pressures that lead to further stress and uncertainty.

Health Care Delivery System

For the young adult the principal settings for health care delivery are schools, worksites, and the community. In addition, traditional health care settings, such as hospitals and clinics, may have programs specifically designed to meet the needs of young adults.

The U.S. goals for "younger" young adults aim to improve health and health behaviors in this age group so that by the year 2000 mortality rates will be reduced by approximately 20%.[83] Specific goals are directed toward promoting healthy lifestyles, reducing fatal motor vehicle and other accidents, reducing alcohol and drug abuse that leads to death, and improving mental health status to reduce suicide and homicide.

SUMMARY

Nurses can promote health care measures and behaviors at all sites where young adults come into contact with the care delivery system. In community college, college, and university settings efforts can be directed toward health education curriculums with emphasis on positive health behaviors, establishment of peer counseling groups, and better utilization of sports and exercise facilities. Workshops on alcoholism, drugs, sports or dance and health, mental health and self-expression, relationships, and various aspects of gynecologic care have been effective in college populations. At the worksite, programs of employee counseling, blood pressure monitoring and treatment, exercise, smoking reduction, cafeteria nutrition management, and stress reduction have also been effective. Employee monitoring and commitment toward a safe and healthy work environment should be promoted. A health objective specific to worksites in *Healthy People 2000* is to "increase to at least 85 percent the proportion of work places with 50 or more employees that offer health promotion activities for their employees, preferably as part of a comprehensive employee health promotion program." (Baseline: 65% of worksites with 50 or more employees offered at least one health promotion activity in 1985).[83] Employee insurance programs should undergo continuous review to determine appropriate and comprehensive coverage for the insured group. Mental health, dental health, and maternity benefits should be analyzed and increased if necessary.

The nurse has an active role in the development of health care policy, which includes the following: (1) identification of resources, (2) planning for resources, and (3) coordination of resources. Since national objectives to promote health affect the lives of all young adults, available resources that provide services to meet these objectives must be identified. Accurate planning of services is essential–resources for health promotion and protection are limited.

Young adulthood is generally a healthy period, which challenges the nurse to be even more sensitive, insightful, and creative in implementing care for individuals within this age group. Important nursing interventions during young adulthood can include

1. Publicizing known health risk factors of this age group to young adults at schools, at worksites, and in the community
2. Providing specific techniques and methodologies to alter lifestyles, thus lowering or decreasing health risks
3. Knowing and identifying the signs and symptoms of health problems specific to this age group that merit further medical investigation
4. Finding opportunities for health promotion and protection in the many settings where young adults are found

References

1. Aamodt M: *Culture.* In Clark AL, editor: *Culture childbearing health professionals,* Philadelphia, 1981, FA Davis.
2. Alison L, Foster CD, Caldwell BB: *Homeless in America,* Wylie, Tex, 1990, Information Plus.
3. Allen J, Mellin G: The new epidemic: immune deficiency–opportunistic infections and Kaposi's sacoma, *Am J Nurs* 82(11):1718, 1982.
4. Amner C: *The new A to Z of women's health: a concise encyclopedia,* New York, 1989, Facts on File.
5. Benenson AS, editor: *Control of communicable disease in man,* ed 15, Washington, DC, 1990, American Public Health Association.
6. Benson ER, McDevitt JQ: *Community health and nursing practice,* ed 2, Englewood Cliffs, NJ, 1980, Prentice Hall.
7. Benson H, Proctor W: *Beyond the relaxation response,* New York, 1985, Berkley Publications.
8. Bruch H: *Conversations with anorexics,* 1989, Basic Books (edited by D Czyzewski, M Suhr).
9. Carrington BW: *The Afro-American.* In Clark AL, editor: *Culture childbearing health professionals,* Philadelphia, 1981, FA Davis.
10. Carter LW: Calcium intake in young adult women: implications for osteoporosis risk assessment, *JOGNN,* pp 301-308, 1987.
11. CDC revises AIDS definition, *Am Nurse* 25(3):20, 1993.
12. Cochran SD, Peplau LA: Sexual risk reduction behaviors among young heterosexual adults, *Soc Sci Med* 3(1):25-36, 1991.
13. Coles R: *Work and self-respect.* In Erikson E, editor: *Adulthood,* New York, 1978, WW Norton.
14. Cooper K: *Aerobics,* New York, 1992, Bantam Books.
15. D'Avanzo C: Barriers to health care for Vietnamese refugees, *J Prof Nurs* 8(4):245-253, 1992.
16. Erikson EH, editor: *Adulthood,* New York, 1978, WW Norton.
17. Foster CD, Landis A, Binsford SM: *Minorities,* Wylie, Tex, 1990, Information Plus.
18. Foster CD, Jacobs R, Siegal MA: *Growing up in America,* Wylie, Tex, 1989, Information Plus.
19. Frame PS: Health maintenance in clinical practice: strategies and barriers, *Am Fam Phys* 45(3):1192-1200, 1992.
20. Francis MB: Eight homeless mothers' tales, *Image* 24(2):111-114, 1992.
21. Friedland GH, Klein RS: Transmission of human immunodeficiency virus, *N Engl J Med* 317(19):1125, 1987.
22. Gilligan C: New maps of development: new visions of maturity, *Am J Orthopsychiatry* 52(2):199-212, 1982.
23. Hahn WK, Hite R: Blood pressure norms for healthy young adults: relation to sex, age and reported parental hypertension, *Res Nurs Health* 12:53-56, 1989.
24. Hamrick DD: *The working women.* In *Issues in health care of women,* New York, 1980, McGraw-Hill.
25. Harris JR, et al: Breast cancer, *N Engl J Med* 327(5):391-328, 1992.
26. Hatcher RA, et al: *Contraceptive technology: 1988-89,* ed 14, New York, 1988, Irvington Publishers.
27. Hogan DP: The transition to adulthood as a career contingency, *Am Sociol Rev* 44:261, 1980.
28. Hogan DP: The variable order of events in the life course, *Am Sociol Rev* 43:573, 1978.
29. Jensen MD, Benson RC, Bobak IM: *Maternity and gynecological care: the nurse and the family,* ed 4, St Louis, 1988, Mosby.
30. Jones NW, Piper CF, Robertson LS: The effect of legal drinking age on fatal injuries of adolescents and young adults, *Am J Public Health* 82(1):112-115, 1992.
31. Jordan WD: *Searching for adulthood in America.* In Erikson E, editor: *Adult-*

hood in America, New York, 1978, WW Norton.
32. Katchadourian HAP: *Medical perspectives on adulthood.* In Erikson E, editor: *Adulthood,* New York, 1978, WW Norton.
33. Keller KB, Lemberg L: Myocardial infarction in the young adult, *Heart & Lung* 20(1):95-97, 1991.
34. Kohlberg L, Lickons T: *The stages of ethical development: from childhood through old age,* San Francisco, 1986, Harper.
35. Koop, CE: *Early detection of breast cancer saves lives, surgeon general report,* US Public Health Service, Washington DC, March 1988, DHHS, US Government Printing Office.
36. Knox AB: *Helping adults learn: a guide to planning, implementing and conducting programs,* San Francisco, 1986, Josey-Bass.
37. Kudzma EC: Drug response: all bodies are not created equal, *Am J Nurs* 92(12):48-50, 1992.
38. Kulbok PA, Baldwin JH: From preventive health behavior to health promotion: advancing a positive construct of health, *Adv Nurs Science,* June 1992.
39. Lander A, Foster CD, Jones NH: *Women's changing roles,* Wylie, Tex, 1992, Information Plus.
40. Larson DE: *Mayo clinic family health book,* New York, 1990, William Morrow.
41. Lehman BA: Health sense: where the boys aren't, *Boston Globe,* p 29, Aug 15, 1988.
42. Levinson D, et al: *Periods in the adult development of men: ages 18 to 45.* In Schlossberg NK, Entine AD, editors: *Counseling adults,* Melbourne, Fla, 1986, Krieger.
43. Lowenthal MF, et al: *Four stages of life: a comparative study of women and men facing transitions,* San Francisco, 1975, Josey-Bass.
44. Mann JM, Chin J: AIDS: a global perspective, *New Engl J Med* 319(5):302, 1988.
45. Meehan PJ, et al: Attempted suicide among young adults: progress toward a meaningful estimate of prevalence, *Am J Psych* 149(1):41-44, 1992.
46. Menning BE: *Infertility: a guide for the childless couple,* Englewood Cliffs, NJ, 1988, Prentice Hall.
47. Murray RB, Zentner JP: *Nursing assessment: health promotion through the life span,* ed 4, Norwalk, Conn, 1989, Appleton & Lange.
48. Neugarten BL: *Adaptation and the life cycle.* In Schlossberg NK, Entine AD, editors: *Counseling adults,* Melbourne, Fla, 1986, Krieger.
49. Nhyan WL, Sakati NO: *Diagnostic recognition of genetic disease,* 1987, Lea & Febiger.
50. Niswander KR: *Manual of obstetrics, diagnoses and therapy,* ed 3, 1987, Little, Brown.
51. Papalia DE, Olds SW: *Human development,* ed 4, New York, 1989, McGraw-Hill.
52. Paul CR: *Psychosocial development of the young adult.* In Schuster CS, Ashburn SS, editors: *The process of human development: a holistic approach,* ed 2, Boston, 1986, Little, Brown.
53. Piaget J: Intellectual evolution from adolescence to adulthood, *Hum Dev* 15:1, 1972.
54. Pumping Up With Steroids, *US News & World Report,* 112(21):26-34, 1992.
55. Quinn TC: Screening for HIV infection, *N Engl J Med* 327(7):486-488, 1992.
56. Rao KS, Schwetz BA: Protecting the unborn: Dow's experience, *Occup Health Safety,* 1981.
57. Reed-Flora R, Lang TA: *Health behaviors,* St Paul, Minn, 1982, West Publishing.
58. Reynolds CF, et al: Daytime sleepiness in the healthy "old old": a comparison with young adults, *J Am Geriatric Soc* 39(10):957-962, 1991.
59. Rose KJ: *The body in time,* New York, 1989, John Wiley & Sons.
60. Schlossberg NK, Troll LE, Leibowitz A: *Perspectives on counseling adults: issues and skills,* Melbourne, Fla, 1986, Krieger.
61. Schroeder SA, Tierney LM, McPhee SJ, et al: *Current medical diagnosis and treatment,* 1992, Appleton & Lange.
62. Schulz DA: *Human sexuality,* ed 3, Englewood Cliffs, NJ, 1988, Prentice Hall.
63. Schuster CS, Ashburn SS, editors: *The process of human development: a holistic approach,* ed 2, Boston, 1986, Little, Brown.
64. Search for health, a report from the National Institutes of Health: *Anorexia nervosa,* Pub No 65-CHD-10/83, Bethesda, Md, 1983, US Government Printing Office.
65. Search for health, a report from the National Institutes of Health: *Find cancer early and save your life,* Pub No 15-NCI-4/88, Bethesda, Md, 1988, US Government Printing Office.
66. Search for health, a report form the National Institutes of Health: *Pelvic inflammatory disease,* Pub No 1-AID-1/88, Bethesda, Md, 1988, US Government Printing Office.
67. Search for health, a report from the National Institutes of Health: *Why do women live longer than men?* Pub No 51-NIA-11/87, Bethesda, Md, 1987, US Government Printing Office.
68. Sheehy G: *Pathfinders,* New York, 1981, Bantam Books.
69. Sloane E: *Biology of women,* ed 2, New York, 1985, Delmar.
70. Somers AR, et al: A whole-life plan for well patient care, *Patient Care* 11:83, 1979.
71. Spector RE: *Cultural diversity in health and illness,* ed 3, New York, 1991, Appleton-Century-Crofts.
72. Statistical abstracts of the United States, ed 111, National data book and guide to sources, US Department of Commerce, Bureau of Census, 1991, US Government Printing Office.
73. Stein GM, Mathein JD: Encouraging a balanced style of living, *Occup Health Safety* 21:36, 1981.
74. Stevenson JS: *Issues and crises during middlescence,* New York, 1977, Appleton-Century-Crofts.
75. Stromborg M: *Nursing's contribution to case finding and early detection of cancer.* In Manno L, editor: *Cancer nursing,* St Louis, 1981, Mosby.
76. Tkac D: *Everyday health tips 2000: practical hints for better health and happiness,* Emmaus, Pa, 1988, Rodale Press.
77. Tomlinson-Keasey C: Formal operations in females from eleven to fifty-four years of age, *Dev Psychol* 6:364,1972.
78. Troll LE: *Early and middle adulthood,* ed 2, Monterey, Calif, 1985, Brooks/Cole Publishing.
79. US Conference of Mayors: A status report on homeless families in America's cities, Washington, DC, 1990, US Government Printing Office.
80. US Department of Health and Human Services, Department of Agriculture: Nutrition monitoring in the United States, Pub No (PHS)86-1255, Hyattsville, Md, 1986, US Government Printing Office.
81. US Department of Health and Human Services, Public Health Center for Disease Control: *Sexually transmitted disease, summary,* Washington, DC, 1982, US Government Printing Office.
82. US Department of Health and Human Services, Public Health Service: *Health: United States, 1980, with prevention profile,* DHHS Pub No (PHS)81-1232, Hyattsville, Md, 1980, National Center for Health Statistics.
83. US Department of Health and Human Services, Public Health Service: *Healthy people 2000: national health promotion and disease prevention objectives,* DHHS Pub No (PHS)91-5012, Washington, DC, 1990.
84. US Department of Health and Human Services, Public Health Service: The 1990 health objectives for the nation: a mid-course review, Washington, DC, 1986, Office of Disease Prevention and

Health Promotion.

85. US Department of Health and Human Services, Public Health Service: *Prevention '82,* DHHS Pub No (PHS)82-50157, Washington, DC, 1982, US Government Printing Office.
86. US Department of Health and Human Services, Public Health Service: Proceedings of prospects for a healthier America, achieving the nation's health promotion objectives, Washington, DC, 1984.
87. US Department of Health and Human Services, Public Health Service: *Trends in teenage childbearing: United States, 1970-81,* Hyattsville, Md, 1984, National Center for Health Statistics.
88. US Department of Health and Human Services, Public Health Service: *Women's health: a report of the public health service task force on women's health services, vol 2,* DHHS Pub No (PHS)85-50206, Washington, DC, 1985, US Government Printing Office.
89. US Department of Health, Education and Welfare, Public Health Service: *The United States, 1968, 1969 and 1972 national fatality surveys,* Hyattsville, Md, 1978, National Center for Health Statistics.
90. Willett WC, et al: Relative and absolute excess risk among women who smoke cigarettes, *N Engl J Med* 322:130, 1987.

CHAPTER

23

Middle Adult

Donna Behler

Terry Tippett

Carol Lynn Mandle

Objectives

After completing this chapter, the nurse will be able to

- *Name three psychosocial changes that occur during the client's middle years.*
- *List two normal biologic changes that occur as a result of the aging process.*
- *Identify the major causes of mortality in the middle-aged adult.*
- *Complete a statement regarding the habits of middle-aged clients that alter their health status.*
- *Discuss the unique health problems related to the occupation of the adult between ages 35 and 65.*
- *Discuss the impact of psychosocial stressors on the middle-aged client and how these are affected by the client's culture and occupation.*

Middle adulthood is considered to include the years between ages 35 to 40 and 65. In this dynamic time, the adult experiences social, psychologic, and biologic changes.[94] The middle years represent a stage of maturation set within major economic productivity and family responsibility. A significant group of society, middle-age adults represent almost half of the population of the United States.

INDIVIDUAL PROCESSES

Age and Physical Changes

Although their onset is insidious, biologic changes come to the forefront during the middle years and affect most body systems.[19,56,81,89,93] The hair of the adult begins to thin and turn gray. The skin's moisture and turgor are decreased, and with the loss of subcutaneous fat, wrinkling occurs. This is even more pronounced if there has been much sun exposure through the years. The result can be a coarseness of the facial features.[10]

Fat deposition increases during these years with increases in weight gain. The body contour changes as "love handles" and "saddlebags" appear. These changes are caused largely by the more sedentary lifestyles, with no changes in dietary habits. The inactive lifestyle is compromised further by a decrease in energy; "I'm not as young as I used to be" is a common retort. This proclamation is legitimate, since the capacity for physical work decreases. The functional aerobic capacity is decreased, with a resulting decrease in cardiac output.[64,71]

In the musculoskeletal system, bone density and mass

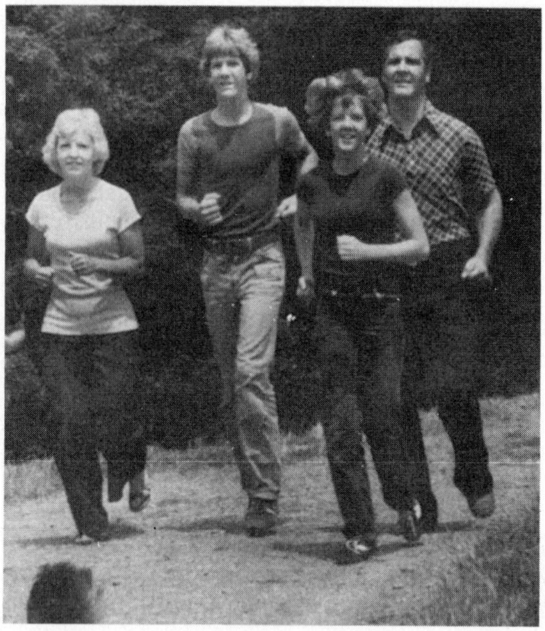

Fig. 23-1. Middle-aged adults should remain active but realize that their physical agility is decreasing as the aging process progresses. (Photograph by David S. Strickler.)

progressively decrease. It is true when 55-year-old adults say they were an inch taller when they were 18.[61] A 1- to 4-inch (2.5- to 10-cm) loss in height occurs as a person ages; thinning of the intervertebral disks accounts for about an inch. However, dramatic losses in height (as much as 4 inches) can occur with thoracic *kyphosis*. The wear and tear on joints predispose the adult to *degenerative joint disease,* with more frequent annoying backaches. The general decrease in muscle tone is categorized by many as "flab"[24] and reduces physical agility (Fig. 23-1).

In general, the functional capacity of all organ systems decreases. For example, in the gastrointestinal tract the following chain of events occurs: decreased metabolism leads to less enzyme production, resulting in lower hydrochloric acid levels and thus decreasing tone in the large intestine. As a result, the middle-age adult may complain of acid indigestion with increased belching.[24,71]

If the adult also leads a sedentary lifestyle, the effects of the diminished motility through the gastrointestinal tract can be more pronounced. It is well known that Americans eat more refined foods (foods that are low in bulk) compared to third-world nations. A low-bulk diet can contribute to the problem of constipation. In addition, many think a low-bulk diet is a main cause of the increased incidence of colon cancer in the United States.

Between ages 25 and 85, there is about a 35% loss of nephron units. The remaining nephrons increase in size and undergo degenerative changes. The entire weight of the kidneys decreases. Since blood supply is also diminished, the glomerular filtration rate is decreased by nearly one half.

Significant changes occur in the cardiovascular system as the blood vessels lose elasticity and become thicker. This predisposes middle-aged adults to coronary artery disease, hypertension, myocardial infarctions, and strokes.[21] Heart disease is the leading cause of death in the adult during the middle years.[35,72,96]

Menopause usually occurs between ages 45 and 55. There is much to learn about what exactly causes many of the symptoms that women frequently report. During this time, production of ovarian estrogen and progestrone ceases; the remaining estrogen is produced by the adrenal glands. As a result of the diminished estrogen level, a woman's secondary sex characteristics regress (loss of pubic hair, decrease in breast size). The female reproductive organs shrink in size, and vaginal secretions decrease. It is important to point out that no decline in libido occurs.[14]

The male experiences changes in his sexual response cycle as testosterone levels plateau, then decrease, as he approaches the end of the middle years. The testes undergo degenerative changes, the viable spermatozoa diminish, and volume and viscosity of semen decreases. In men, sexual energy gradually declines; it takes longer to achieve an erection, but it is sustained longer.[26]

Mortality Rates

The leading causes of death in middle adulthood are heart diseases, lung cancer, cerebrovascular disease, breast cancer, colorectal cancer, and obstructive lung disease. Reducing disabilities and deaths from these chronic conditions are national health promotion and disease prevention objectives.[96] (See box on p. 609.)

Many of these diseases are preventable, wholly or in part through behavior changes. Middle adults can influence their own health, as well as their children's, through a healthier lifestyle.

Gender

Male mortality rates have always been higher than female rates for the leading causes of death, with the exception of diabetes. The death rates of the middle-aged male from cardiovascular diseases plays a major part in this disparity. The incidence of lung cancer continues to slowly decrease for men (81.9 per 100,000) and increase for women (36.4 per 100,000) primarily due to the changing smoking and work patterns of women. Mortality rates also vary with sex

HEALTHY PEOPLE 2000

SELECTED NATIONAL HEALTH PROMOTION AND DISEASE PREVENTION OBJECTIVES

MIDDLE ADULT

- Reduce the death rate for adults by 20% to be no more than 340 per 100,000 people aged 25 through 64 (1987 baseline: 423 per 100,000 people)
- Increase years of healthy life to at least 65 years (1980 baseline: 62 years)
- Reduce coronary heart disease deaths to no more than 100 per 100,000 people (1987 age-adjusted baseline: 135 per 100,000 people)
- Reduce stroke deaths to no more than 20 per 100,000 people (1987 age-adjusted baseline: 30.3 per 100,000 people)
- Reverse the rise in cancer deaths to a rate of no more than 130 per 100,000 people (1987 age adjusted baseline: 133 per 100,000 people)
- Reduce overweight to a prevalence of no more than 20% among people aged 20 or older (1976-1980 age-adjusted baseline: 26% for people [24% for men and 27% for women])
- Reduce dietary fat intake to an average of 30% of calories or lean and saturated fat to less than 10% of calories (1985 baseline: 36% of calories from total fat and 13% from saturated fat)
- Increase complex carbohydrates and fiber-containing foods to five or more daily servings of fruits and vegetables and six or more daily servings of grain products
- Increase calcium intake to two or more servings daily
- Decrease salt and sodium intake
- Reduce iron deficiency in women aged 20 through 44 years
- Increase the proportion of people who use food labels to make nutritious food selections
- Increase to at least 75% the proportion of mothers who breastfeed their babies
- Increase to at least 30% the proportion of people who engage regularly, preferably, daily, in light to moderate exercise for at least 30 minutes per day (1985 baseline: 12%)
- Reduce to less than 35% the proportion of people aged 18 and older who experience adverse health effects from stress (1985 baseline: 42.6%)
- Reduce physical abuse directed at women by male partners to no more than 27 per 1000 couples (1985 baseline: 30 per 1000 couples)
- Reduce assault injuries to no more than 10 per 1000 people (1986 baseline: 11.1 per 1000 people)
- Reduce deaths from work-related injuries to no more than 4 per 100,000 full-time workers (1983-1987 baseline average: 6 per 100,000 workers)
- Reduce work-related injuries resulting in treatment, lost time from work, or restricted work activity to no more than 6 cases per 100 full-time workers (1987 baseline: 7.7 per 100 workers)
- Reduce destructive periodontal disease to a prevalence of no more than 15% among people aged 35 to 44 years (1985-1986 baseline: 24%)
- Reduce the incidence of HIV infection, gonorrhea, syphilis, chlamydia trachomatous, genital herpes, and hepatitis B
- Reduce cigarette smoking to a prevalence of no more than 15% (1987 baseline: 32% for men and 27% for women)
- Reduce alcohol consumption to no more than 2 gallons of ethyl alcohol per person (1987 baseline: 2.54 gallons)
- Reduce unintended pregnancies to no more than 30% of all pregnancies (1983-1988 baseline: 56%)
- Reduce infertility to no more than 6.5% (1988 baseline: 7.9%)
- Reduce the prevalence of mental disorders of adults living in the community to less than 10.7% (1984 baseline: 12.6%)

RESEARCH MIDDLE ADULT REVIEW

HEALTH PROMOTION IN MIDLIFE WOMEN

Duffy ME: Determinants of health promotion in midlife women, *Nurs Res* 37:358-362, 1988.

Purpose The purpose of this study was to investigate the relationship among perceived health locus of control, self-esteem, and perceived health status and the degree to which they explain midlife women's current practice of health-promoting lifestyle activities.

Review The sample for this study was obtained from a large southwestern public university. Of the 232 women who responded, most were married (61%), white (93.5%), and a mean age of 45.5 years (range 35 to 65 years old). Women who scored high on self-esteem, internal health locus of control, and low on chance health locus of control and reported their current health as high (good) were those who had high scores on self-actualization, nutrition, exercise, and interpersonal support subscales. In contrast, women who were older in age, had high health worry/concern scores, reported lower past health status (poor), and had low-chance health locus of control scores were the ones who scored high on health responsibility, nutrition, and stress-management health promotion subscales.

groups. Male deaths are lowest in married adults and highest in those who are divorced. Single, widowed, and divorced middle-aged adults generally have higher mortality than those who are married.

Chronic and degenerative diseases are less pronounced in females. The primary cause of death for both sexes over age 44 is heart disease. Women are more likely to have arthritis, colitis, and gallbladder disease (see box above). Men, on the other hand, are more likely to develop ulcers, hernias, and emphysema. Injuries also are more common in the male.[72,82]

Race

African Americans are the largest minority (14%) in the nation. Many risk factors are increased in black adults. Black adults between ages 25 and 64, for instance, have a cerebrovascular accident (CVA), or stroke, rate almost 2.5 times that of a white adult.[96] Race also is considered to be one of the risk factors in hypertension.[35] Blacks have an increased incidence and mortality rate in cancers of the lung, colon and rectum, prostate, and esophagus. The differences between the cancer rates in Blacks and Whites have been related partly to Blacks residing in lower socioeconomic areas, which may increase their exposure to industrial carcinogens. The educational opportunities available to Blacks in urban areas also may be limited. This could limit their knowledge of risk factors, significant signs and symptoms of disease, preventive self-care, and the location of health care resources.[101]

In looking at the 10 major causes of death in the adult, the three leading causes in both white and black

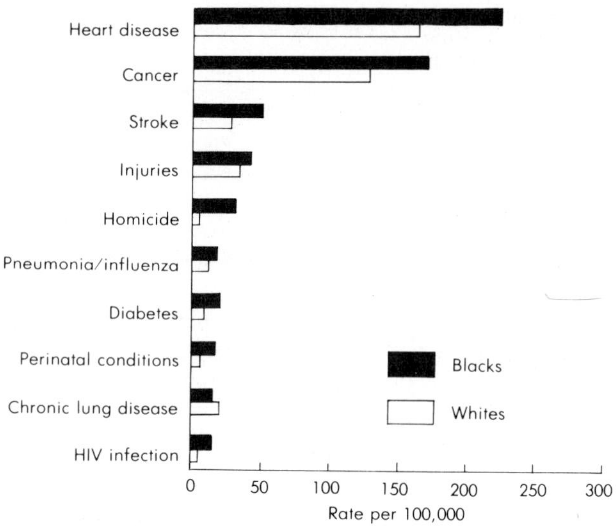

Fig. 23-2. Ten major causes of death in adults in the United States according to frequency of occurrence.

populations are the same: heart disease, cancer, and CVA. Homicide rates fourth in Blacks but seventh to eighth in Whites (Fig. 23-2).

Although the primary cause of death for both sexes over age 44 continues to be heart disease, the death rate is declining. The decrease has been similar for white males and black and white females but lower for black males (20%).[59,87]

Black men have the highest rate of stroke among all population groups, with a death rate about twice that of white men aged 25 to 65.

Similarly, since 1975 the age-adjusted incidence rates for lung cancer are higher for both black men and women than for white women. Colorectal cancer rates have fallen among white men and women, remained the

AMERICAN CANCER SOCIETY'S RECOMMENDATIONS FOR BREAST ASSESSMENTS OF WOMEN WHO HAVE NO BREAST SYMPTOMS AND NO FAMILY HISTORY

Less than 40 years old

Examine breasts monthly
Have a breast exam by a clinician at least every 3 years
Have a baseline mammogram between the ages of 35 and 39

Between 40 and 49 years old

Examine breasts monthly
Have a breast exam by a clinician every year
Have a mammogram every 1 to 2 years

Age 50 and older

Examine breasts monthly
Have a breast exam by a clinician every year
Have a mammogram every year

From American Cancer Society: *Special touch*, New York, 1987, The Society; and *Cancer manual*, ed 5, New York, 1990, The Society.

same for black women, and increased markedly for black men. Black women continue to have three times the cervical cancer death rate of white women.[96]

Breast cancer continues to be the leading site for cancer among women. Five-year survival rates for breast cancer are about 20% higher for white females than for black females (75% versus 63%).[65] As discussed in Chapter 21 on adolescence, since breast cancer is a major cause of illness and death among American women, all women should examine their breasts once a month;[20,75] and a clinical breast exam should be performed as part of regular (at least annual) health checkups.[28] The box above gives the current recommendations about breast assessments for different age groups for women who have no breast symptoms.[32]

The 5-year survival rate for all cancer sites combined is 50% for white patients and 37% for black patients.[96]

Genetics

The middle-aged adult may be at greater risk than the young adult for diseases known to be associated with genetics, or familial characteristics, including diabetes, hypertension, Huntington's chorea, arteriosclerosis, gout, obesity, heart disease, and alcoholism.

Some malignancies tend to run in families; for example, women with a personal or family history of breast cancer are at greater risk. Also, individuals with a family history of colorectal cancer, rectal or colon polyps, or ulcerative colitis are at greater risk for colorectal cancer.[2] In addition, the use of diethylstilbestrol (DES) has been linked with the development of cervical cancer and reproductive abnormalities in both male and female children of women who took DES while pregnant.[82]

HEALTH PATTERNS

Nutritional and Metabolic Pattern

Dietary factors are correlated with 5 out of the 10 leading causes of death in the United States: coronary heart disease, some cancers, stroke, noninsulin-dependent diabetes mellitus, and atherosclerosis.[96] The 1988 Surgeon General's Report on Nutrition and Health states that for the 2 out of 3 Americans who neither smoke nor drink, choices of eating patterns may determine their long-term health more than any other activity.

Physical activities and nutritional patterns are often correlated.[60] The middle-aged adult often leads a more sedentary lifestyle than the young adult, often because of the many convenience devices that infiltrate homes and workplaces and inadequate time. Unfortunately, this less active adult frequently does not alter any dietary habits. Consequently, one of the major health problems of the middle years is obesity.

OBESITY

The National Health Promotion and Disease Prevention Objectives for the Year 2000 include reducing overweight to a prevalence of no more than 20% of people (a 23% decrease) and reducing dietary fat intake to an average of 30% of calories (a 16% decrease) and saturated fat to less than 10% of calories (3% decrease). (See box on p. 609.)

Obesity is a contributing factor in many diseases, such as cardiovascular problems, stroke, and diabetes. Obesity is influenced by age, sex, race, socioeconomic status, and possibly genetics, with women generally having more body fat than men. Unfortunately, weight tends to increase with age. For men, this increase stops at about age 60; for women it continues. However, most adult-onset obesity begins during the middle years partly because of the more sedentary lifestyle.[91]

The prevention of obesity is the goal of weight management in the middle years. If the adult is obese, a clear-cut history of the onset is imperative. A lifelong history of obesity is much more arduous to alter than adult-onset obesity. A decrease in calories should be accompanied by at least 30 minutes of exercise three to five times a week. When calories are reduced and exercise is increased, weight loss is achieved and maintained.[71]

The weight-management resources available to the adult are plentiful. Weight-management programs using behavior modification may be found in varied settings, such as universities and worksites, Weight Watchers, Overeaters Anonymous, and TOPS (Take Off Pounds Sensibly).

If the nurse identifies a need for weight management and no program is available, a self-help group may be initiated. Input should be solicited from concerned clients as to time and place of meetings. A suggested list of topics generated by the clients could be assembled. A discussion of basic nutrition with appropriate handouts is a good place to start. Having adults write down their individual goals and keep a 1-week diet log is nonthreatening and helpful for future planning and also gives them some responsibility in the program.

HIGH-SODIUM DIET

High-sodium diets play a role in *hypertension,* especially when consumed over many years. The result may be an increase in total body fluids, which increases peripheral vascular resistance.[47] Salt contains about 40% sodium and is a contributing factor in 10% to 20% of Americans who are at risk for hypertension. On the average, Americans consume at least 4 to 5 g of sodium a day. The National Research Council of the National Academy of Sciences reports that between 1.1 and 3.3 g are adequate and safe.[47] A major contributor of dietary sodium is the salt found in processed foods.

HIGH-SATURATED FAT DIET

Lipid levels and ratios also have significant impact on cardiovascular morbidity and mortality. The National Heart, Lung, and Blood Institute regards a blood cholesterol level below 200 mg/dl as desirable. Yet the mean cholesterol level for Americans is 213 mg/dl, and about 60 million adults in this country are estimated to have blood cholesterol levels that place them at high risk for coronary heart disease. The Coronary Primary Prevention Trial showed that men at high risk were able to reduce coronary heart disease by about 2% for every 1% lower blood cholesterol level. Most people can lower their high blood cholesterol by reducing their intake of saturated fat, total fat, and dietary cholesterol and by normalizing their weight and increasing physical activity. Medications are available for those whose blood cholesterol levels remain significantly elevated despite diet modification.[84,96]

Gingivitis is common among adults who do not regularly brush their teeth and use dental floss. There is redness and swelling around the teeth which become more apparent. Bleeding of the gums while toothbrushing is an early sign. The gums may or may not be tender. If this inflammation is not adequately treated and controlled, periodontitis, involving bone destruction, may develop as well as tooth loss.

Regular oral hygiene and care are major factors in maintaining oral health. However, less than half of Americans receive regular oral health care. Middle adults not only have responsibility for their own care but that of their children. Low income is a risk factor. Untreated dental decay and tooth loss is higher in African Americans, Hispanics, American Indians, and Alaska natives than for the total American adult population.[96] Oral cancer is also a major problem not detected in the absence of good dental care.

Elimination Pattern

Aging brings a gradual decrease of tone in the large intestine. As mentioned, this change, accompanied by a sedentary lifestyle and lack of bulk in the diet, predisposes the adult to *constipation.* The mass media strongly encourage the population to rely on external controls instead of exercise and dietary means to solve this problem. Consequently, many adults are dependent on laxatives for normal bowel function.

As previously discussed, the degenerative changes in the nephron units occur during the middle years. Usually, however, the adult does not have any appreciable kidney malfunction.

If a woman has had multiple births and little exercise, she may begin experiencing stress incontinence during this time, which can be socially embarrassing.

Activity-Exercise Pattern

Regular physical activity increases life expectancy and quality of life. Regular physical activity can help to prevent and manage coronary heart disease, hypertension, diabetes, osteoporosis, and depression. It has been correlated with lower rates of back injury, stroke, and colon cancer and effective weight loss programs.[38,95,96,98]

Despite these benefits, few American adults engage in regular physical activity lasting 30 minutes three to four times a week. Nearly 25% of adults report no leisure time physical activity, and the prevalence of sedentary behavior increases with age.[96] Continuous, rhythmic exercise maintained for a period long enough to stress the cardiac system is desirable. Some suggested activities include brisk walking, jogging, swimming, bicycling, and skipping rope. Activities that focus on skill and coordination should be attempted by the adult over age 40 rather than those necessitating speed and strength. Moderation is the key, along with increased caution as the adult approaches age 65. Overexertion, evidenced by symptoms of dizziness, tightness in the chest, and unresolving breathlessness, should be avoided.

The nurse can initiate an exercise program with the middle-aged adult by asking the client what activities have been enjoyed in the past. If these are realistic today, the nurse should encourage the individual to rediscover them. If they do not appear realistic, new options can be explored with the client. Also, activities should be selected with consideration of potential for injury. Anyone at risk for heart disease (heavy smoking, high blood pressure, family history, diabetes, or prolonged lack of exercise) should have a complete history and physical examination before developing a rigorous activity program. For some of these individuals, an exercise test may be recommended. Proper equipment, including supportive shoes and thermally appropriate clothing, is also important.

To be health promoting, physical exercise should involve as many muscles as possible and be performed on a regular basis, preferably three to four times a week for a minimum of 30 minutes each time. The appropriate level of performance for aerobic exercise is determined by achieving a pulse rate that is established for each individual by taking the number 220, subtracting the person's age, and then computing 75% of that number. A 50-year-old person, for example, should not exceed a pulse rate of 128 (220 − 50 = 170 and 75% of 170 = 128).

Despite all of these considerations, the choice of activities and style should be an individual choice and approached as something done for oneself and for fun, not as another chore or responsibility of middle age.[37]

Sleep and Rest Pattern

Rest is a frequently omitted consideration for middle-aged adults, who spend less time in deep sleep and need less sleep overall. This change may be interpreted as insomnia, so the client may need reassurance that this is common. Regularly scheduled, quality sleep and occasional napping, when fatigued, are healthful guidelines.

Cognitive and Perceptual Pattern

It is a myth that at age 21 you reach your intellectual peak and it is all downhill after that. Continued learning is found throughout adulthood in such areas as reasoning, vocabulary, and spatial perception. Decreases may be seen, however, in reaction time and cognitive flexibility.[21]

INTELLECTUAL ABILITY

"Learning" intelligence accumulates through education and life experiences and continues to increase throughout life, as evidenced by those scholars and artists who are more productive in their middle years than as young adults.[21]

The theories of Havighurst, Piaget, and Bloom are relevant to the middle-age adult. Havighurst and Orr[39] see the adult in the middle years as the *learner-performer.* They conclude that the prime time to be in the learner role is when the developmental task for that role is to be accomplished. For example, to balance the responsibilities of caring for children and parents and work, the adult may explore new career options or creative endeavors.

Havighurst defines developmental tasks as the basic tasks of living to be achieved if the adult is to live successfully. They are dictated by the expectations of one's society, the physiologic changes of the body throughout life, and one's own value system and goals. Although initially described in the 1950s, Havighurst's developmental tasks of middle age are timely:[39]

1. Assisting children to become responsible, happy adults
2. Rediscovering or developing new satisfaction in the relationship with one's spouse. For the single adult this could mean a relationship with a sibling or significant other
3. Developing an affectionate but independent relationship with aging parents
4. Reaching the peak in one's career
5. Achieving mature social and civic responsibility
6. Accepting and adapting to biologic changes
7. Maintaining or developing friendships
8. Developing leisure-time activities

If career goals have been previously identified, reaching them can be very rewarding psychologically as well as financially. Along with career activities, the mature adult also has an increased social awareness and assumes more civic responsibility.

In Piaget's theory of cognitive development, *formal operations* is the final period. This begins at about age 12 and continues throughout life. He describes the thoughts of adults as being both flexible and effective. The adult can deal efficiently with complex problems of reasoning to include hypothesis testing.[34]

Bloom[9] has developed a hierarchy of cognitive levels in the adult learner.[77] *Knowledge* is the simplest cognitive level; the adult learner understands and can recall specifics. For example, the client defines "high blood pressure" in lay terminology.

Comprehension is the second level, as indicated by the learner grasping the meaning of the communicated message to relate it to other material. For example, the client gives one way that obesity influences high blood pressure.

The third level is *application.* Here the learner applies knowledge in the form of abstractions and ideas to concrete situations. For example, the hypertensive client begins a weight reduction and exercise program. In *analysis,* the fourth level, the adult breaks down material into its constituent parts while noting their relationship. For example, the client identifies values and life goals in determining actions to be taken for meeting health care needs.

The final levels, *synthesis* and *evaluation,* are at times difficult to achieve. The client is able to put together various elements to form a plan and then judge the extent to which the ideas, materials, and so on satisfy the established criteria. For example, clients may develop plans to improve their health care and increase their self-care responsibilities. In turn, they may validate their ongoing health care programs in relation to the expected outcomes they had formulated.

Perceptual Changes

Presbyopia, or farsightedness, is very common in middle-aged adults, even in individuals who have not previously had any vision problems. This condition is easily corrected by eyeglasses, which may only be needed for reading or close work. Other visual conditions that may not allow for ready correction include decreased peripheral vision and decreased visual sensitivity in the dark. Both conditions are due to the cornea becoming less transparent and are slow and subtle in development. Because all of these conditions are not readily detected by the individual, middle adults should establish a routine professional eye exam every year.

Another common perceptual change in middle age is presbycusis, or impaired auditory acuity. The first sounds to be lost are high sound frequencies, such as a woman's voice. Since this process is also subtle but important to the work environment and social interaction, middle age is also a time for auditory evaluations to be a part of routine examinations.

Beginning in the middle years, the sense of taste also diminishes. There is a progressive loss of taste buds, first affecting those located more anteriorly, which detect sweet and salt, and leaving the posterior ones, which detect bitter and sour. Consequently, this can alter a person's food preferences as well as present problems for those persons who insist on adding salt to make up for the deficit. Nurses can suggest using herbs and spices to add taste.

Self-Perception and Self-Concept Pattern

LEVINSON'S THEORY

In Levinson's research on men, a theory on "individual life structures" is posed. Levinson describes age-associated "seasons" or "eras." The midlife transition, beginning around age 40, appears to include reappraising one's life, integrating the polarities, and modifying one's life structure toward being who one wants to be.[58]

ERIKSON'S THEORY

In Erikson's eight stages of the life cycle, the last three are related to adulthood. Stage 7, *generativity versus stagnation or self-absorption,* most frequently is associated with the middle-age years.[22]

Erikson identifies the major task during this stage as generativity, which includes a feeling of productivity and creativity, as evidenced by reaching one's previously established goals. Generativity also encompasses a desire to care for others and is the opposite of what Erikson calls stagnation. Lack of accomplishment of middle age's developmental tasks results in stagnation or a tendency to direct most of one's interest and attention to self, thereby excluding others.[28,53]

Middle age is a time of critical self-review, and some persons are sad and disappointed in themselves and their accomplishments. Both women and men question their value to society, the merit of their accomplishments, their success as sexual beings, and the probability of attaining unfilled life goals. Women generally make this life assessment between ages 35 and 50, whereas men usually do not begin until about age 40. Since the male life assessment tends to come later, there is a potential problem for couples of approximately the same age. Women begin looking at changes they may want to make in their lives, whereas husbands still are content with the status quo. Such self-evaluation and lack of effective communication of personal needs to the spouse is a prime irritant to marriage stability.[13,28,97]

PHYSIOLOGIC CHANGES

The effect of physiologic changes on mental health is almost as critical during middle age as in adolescence. Some of the most obvious changes that influence self-esteem are graying hair, wrinkles, decreased visual and auditory acuity, and changes in body shape. How well these changes are tolerated to a great extent depends on the person's level of self-satisfaction and acceptance. Some try to hold onto youth by dressing like more youthful counterparts, whereas others adapt their attire to their age and position in life.[23,28,53]

It is controversial, but some researchers believe that hormonal changes during middle age lead to behaviors in both women and men that represent menopause, discussed earlier. In women decreased supplies of estrogen begin in the thirties; the loss of estrogen is thought to be responsible for the "hot flashes" and the mood changes that often occur. The concomitant emotional aspect of menopause seems to be related to the personality of the individual. Women who have a positive self-concept and who have coped effectively in the past are less prone to experience the full range of psychologic symptoms often associated with menopause. The most common changes include emotional lability, nervousness and anxiety, insomnia, fatigue, and depression.

Likewise, men often experience physical and psychologic reactions to middle age. The hormonal changes in males are more gradual and typically begin between ages 40 and 55. The symptoms are similar to those experienced by women, with the emotional effects related to other life events, past coping patterns, and general feelings of self-esteem.[23,38,53]

Coping and Stress-Tolerance Pattern

In a study of 100 women, aged 43 to 53, from working- and middle-class backgrounds, more than half identified the death of a husband, cancer, and the implications of getting older as their greatest concerns.[62] The significance of menopause was minimized, and many felt their health improved after menopause. Long-held myths about women during and after menopause were also dispelled in a 5-year study of 2500 middle-aged Massachusetts women. The following percentages of these women reported stress from children away from home (8.5%); children living at home (20.3%); children recently returned home (23.6%); husbands away from home (3.6%); husbands living at home (6.3%); parents/in-laws: receiving no care (13%), cared for outside the woman's home (49.1%), and cared for in the woman's home (52.7%). This study also found that stress was reduced by half if the woman had someone close who provided emotional support and practical help.[63]

Holmes and Rahe developed the Social Readjustment Rating Scale following much research, which indicated that a significant relationship exists between stressful life events and various physical illnesses.[30,31,42,43] An informative publication of the American Hospital Association entitled *Stress!* includes a variation of this scale that can be scored by the client.[4]

In a 45-year longitudinal prospective study of 173 men, Valliant and Valliant found that the extent of tranquilizer use before age 50 was the most powerful negative predictor of both mental and physical health outcomes at age 65. Another important predictor for health outcomes was the maturity of defenses against stress (sublimation, anticipation, altruism, and humor).[97]

STRESS AND HEART DISEASE

As reiterated throughout this chapter, heart disease is the number-one cause of death in the middle-aged adult. Haynes and others[40] studied the relationship of psychosocial factors to coronary heart disease using the 1965 to 1967 Framingham Study; 24 measures of psychosocial stress (PSS) were used (see box at right). In the male, aging worries were significantly correlated with systolic and diastolic blood pressures. Marital disagreement and personal worries were significantly correlated with diastolic blood pressure. Both diastolic and systolic pressures were significantly correlated with few lines of work changes (employed women between ages 45 and 64) and anxiety symptoms. Anger held in, anger discussed, tension, and anger symptoms were significantly correlated with diastolic blood pressure in this age group.

❑ ❑ PSYCHOSOCIAL FACTORS CORRELATED WITH CORONARY HEART DISEASE

Framingham type A
Emotional lability
Ambitiousness
Non-easygoing
No support from boss
Work overload
Marital disagreement
Marital dissatisfaction
Aging worries
Personal worries
Job changes in past 10 years
Line of work changes in past 10 years
Times promoted in past 10 years
Education mobility
Occupational mobility
Social class incongruity
Anger-in
Anger-out
Anger-discuss
Daily stress
Tension
Anxiety symptoms
Anger symptoms
Previous hospitalization for emotional disease

From Haynes SG, et al: The relationship of psychosocial factors to coronary heart disease in the Framingham study, *Am J Epidemiol* 107(5):372, 1978.

The worker between ages 45 and 65 was examined. Among male white-collar workers, the Framingham type A and ambitiousness scales also were significantly correlated with diastolic blood pressure. The correlation of anger symptoms and anger discussed with diastolic pressures was significant for white-collar women between ages 45 and 64.

The nurse who can identify the current stressful life events experienced by adults is better prepared to assist them to cope effectively and prevent additional stressors that can precipitate a decrease in physical or mental health.

Role-Relationship Pattern

Craig[21] notes that middle age is frequently a time of reassessment, turmoil, and change. This "painful stage" has been labeled as "midlife transition," "midcareer crisis," and "middle-age slump."[57] This turning point occurs for several reasons. Middle-aged adults recognize that their physical agility is decreasing; the inevitability of their own death is recognized, perhaps for the first time. Lifestyle choices have been made and are less flexible than at age 25. The adult identifies mistakes made in the past.

FAMILY

Duvall[26] delineates eight stages of the family life cycle, with stages 5, 6, and 7 in the middle years:

Stage 5–families with children, with the oldest child between ages 13 and 20; lasts about 7 years

Stage 6–families launching young adults, from the first leaving until the last; lasts about 8 years

Stage 7–families from empty nest to retirement; lasts about 15 years

The developmental tasks identified for the families in stages 6 and 7 approximate those of Havighurst; they focus on changes from a nuclear family to a marital couple. For example, in stage 6 the parents who are assisting their children to become independent may also be caring for their aging parents.[31] In addition, middle-aged adults fulfill multiple complex responsibilities within a variety of career, social, and civic positions.

Families with adults in the middle years have been described as both "postparental" and "launching" families. The children are leaving their homes of origin, creating their own family units, and pursuing their own careers. By supporting their children's efforts, parents can increase the self-esteem of their children and at the same time be effective role models. The parent assumes less of a parent-child relationship, interacting more on an adult-adult level. As the children are "launched," the parents may have uninterrupted time alone and time in which to share activities.

Family life may also be threatened by older children living at home or opposition to a child's partner and inability to establish satisfactory relationships with potential or actual partners or sons- and daughters-in-law.[8] Children leaving home may be anticipated with relief that the heavy care responsibilities of parenting are over or with dread over how to fill the void of time and inactivity. The empty nest syndrome may be complicated if the husband and wife have never learned to talk together and enjoy each other's company without the children.

At the other end of the family spectrum, aging parents can place demands on the adult child, since the elderly are frequently beset with health problems. A caring relationship is needed in which the need of the aged parent for independence is recognized.[4,5,13,27]

With our society's emphasis on youth, the adult must associate feelings of self-worth with personal integrity rather than body appearance or physical prowess. Friends of both sexes can be invaluable support systems. With the newly found free time after children have left home, the middle-aged adult can share favorite activities and learn new ones. Middle-aged adults should remind themselves how much and how well they are doing, especially considering the complexity of the demands placed upon them. Never before in history have families pursued such varied and individual-oriented goals as they do today.

Although for many Americans the concept of family is still of major importance, this concept is different from perceptions held by past generations. Parents and children in most families are involved in numerous activities, as evidenced by a "let's hurry or we'll be late" orientation. Even younger children often have schedules that must be met if they are to get to their dance, drama, play, or enrichment classes. None of these activities necessarily has a negative effect, but the cumulative influence places heavy demands on all family members. Also, many activities in which both children and adults are involved have a certain degree of competitiveness. For example, parents often get so emotionally involved in the athletic activities of their children that the failure of a 6-year-old to play a winning softball game causes a great deal of parental anguish. One has only to listen to the cheering of parents at a Little League game to note whose self-esteem is at stake. Shouts of "Kill her," "Grab the third baseman," and so on do not tend to engender feelings of team spirit or a notion of playing for the sake of having a good time.[28]

The effect of life events on mental health depends on personal strength of the individual, available supports, and the nature and number of events and their significance for the person. Three common examples of life events with potential disruptive effects are divorce, increasing number of two-career families, and caring for aging parents.[39] Their negative effects may be alleviated if assistance is provided early in the process of that change.

TWO-CAREER FAMILY–FAMILY AND WORK RESPONSIBILITIES

More and more women are in the work force.[59] Many feel the necessity for financial gain, especially with the increased cost of living and college expenses. Other women who are postmenopausal and have been separated from their last child have a newfound freedom and begin or rediscover a career. The husband may be a support person in this venture or on the other hand may feel threatened by his wife's new pursuit. These role changes can be stressors to the family.[65]

The relationship between marital status, with or without children at home, and employment status determines the psychologic status of the woman in her middle years. The educated woman who is married, has children at home, and has not worked since her marriage is at greater risk for psychologic disturbances.[63]

Love, hate, ambivalence, self-esteem, and the availability of support systems have been listed as intangible agents.[44] The anticipation of the last child departing from home includes many of these agents. Women who have lived vicariously through their children will be more affected, with depression a chief symptom.

Historically, there have been few prototypes for the two-career family. Women typically helped their husbands with farming or with the family business, but only since World War II have women made up a significant portion of the work force. In addition, women are becoming highly educated and motivated to pursue careers that often demand their time, attention, and energy. Both men and women are increasingly taking jobs that do not end at 5:00 P.M. The problems and challenges of the workplace are felt at home as adults carry projects and problems home with them.[53,63]

Also, job-related travel has increased in the last few years for both men and women. Travel by either partner means additional responsibilities for the parent who remains at home. Also, if one spouse travels far more than the other, feelings of resentment may develop, or the common ground for discussion of work events may be altered. The one who stays at home may feel "put upon" when the spouse is perceived as having so much fun. In contrast, travel is tiring and often hectic and is not usually as exciting as it seems to observers. Thus, the traveling spouse may come home tired and irritable and desire peace and quiet, which may conflict with the expectations of other family members.[53]

Men may feel threatened by highly successful and visible women. The traditional family prototype has been for husbands to gain recognition for their achievements outside the home and for wives to be supportive of the husband's career and provide a family environment that enriches the entire family. As women gain recognition and acclaim for their career accomplishments, even the most enlightened men may feel twinges of envy and discomfort. Men have few role models to turn to in learning how to be a participant in a successful two-career family. Thus, men may need as much, if not more, support than women in adapting to contemporary family styles. Opportunities to discuss what it is like to be a man in today's society can be helpful, such as in support groups by using volunteer professionals who provide services to various agencies and community resources.

In addition to the changes in women and the effect on families of two-career adults, the nature of the parental work environment is critical to family coping ability. Work that is emotionally draining, especially when it is filled with conflict, poses special threats to family stability. When one or both parents come home tired, angry, or frustrated from their experiences at work, they probably have limited emotional support to share with other family members.[46] Essentially, when persons gain self-esteem from their jobs and generally enjoy going to work, they tend to feel less frustration and dissatisfaction with themselves and their positions. They then are able to give more of themselves to other members of the family.[53]

Caring for Aging Parents. The needs of aging parents and of their own children may place additional demands on the adult in the middle years.[24] According to LeShan, the middle adult sometimes feels "caught between one's children and one's parents."[25] Both children and elderly parents may present unrealistic, excessive demands and be difficult to please.

Middle-aged adults may be faced with having frail and ill parents live within their own family unit or placing them into a nursing home. These dilemmas are complicated by the reality that their parents are growing older and may not have long to live. The recognition of their parents' impending death heightens the middle-aged adult's awareness of their own aging and mortality.[25]

Difficulties in caring for elderly parents can be somewhat lessened if potential situations are discussed before a crisis arises. This is particularly true if all members of the middle-adult family are working, space in their home is limited, and the community has few resources for the well and ill elderly. Although undesirable to many families, care of ill, elderly parents may eventually require placement in an institution. By anticipating these potential needs and dealing with them, middle-aged children and their elderly parents can further develop meaningful relationships with each other.[25,27,49]

Divorce. Divorce is a potential cause of mental health disruption. As the divorce rate has risen in recent years, individuals and families have been faced with new and often multiple problems. One study estimated that 20 million children under age 18 live with only one parent.[96,99] When a divorce occurs, each family member must confront the necessity to examine and often modify an accustomed style of living and adapting. In a 5-year study of 60 families, with a total of 131 children ranging from ages 3 to 18, Kelly and Wallerstein[99] found the first year after a divorce to be the most difficult; money constituted a major source of disruption. They also found that divorce is essentially a time-limited crisis for all involved that taxes the usual coping mechanisms such that adults have diminished abilities to parent effectively during the acute stage of adjustment.

Death. Like divorce, death of a spouse may result in grieving for the loss of companionship and the lost "planned-for" future–freer from the responsibilities of work and children. The surviving spouse may find oneself unprepared to be "single again" and live alone. The loneliness may be exacerbated by ill or dying peers and parents. Middle-aged adults become increasingly aware of the finiteness of life, thinking not only of the number of years since birth but also the number of years left to live. The midlife review is a common outcome of this recognition.

Middle age is important when looking at the career clock. Issues that need to be considered include midcareer changes in occupations as well as preretirement planning. Retirement is a major turning point; to many it is the transition from middle age to old age and the period of work to the period of leisure.[50]

Adults are working to the age of retirement, and many are entering new careers later in life. As adults progress through the middle years, they become increasingly aware of the time remaining until retirement: "Can I readjust my goals?" "Is there disparity between where I am in my career and where I would like to be?" Consider the 60-year-old veteran nightclub singer whose goal to cut a solo album has not yet been achieved. The heightened awareness of age and the decreased likelihood of finding another suitable job can precipitate increased anxiety or depression in this singer.[50]

WORK

Perhaps the most common role that middle-aged adults share is being workers. Much of their pride and sense of satisfaction is derived from their work (Fig. 23-3). In middle-aged working-class adults, work is equated with being "grown up"; one can easily recall the "What do you want to be when you grow up?" questioning of youth. Success and achievement are evaluated in terms of their jobs and family life. The work ethic still persists, especially with individuals born during the depression. Much of their conversation evolves from what they do: "My name is Leslie Smith. I am a real-estate agent." To be mature is to be a responsible, hard-working individual.[28,86]

Middle-aged adults make up most of the work force of 110 million people. Vocations play a major role in their levels of wellness. Approximately 10 million injuries occur every year: 3 million are severe, including 3400 to 11,000 deaths and 1.8 million total disabling injuries.[96]

More than 20% of fatal occupational injuries involve highway vehicles, while others include falls, nonvehicular injuries, blows, and electrocutions.

Although the number of fatal occupations appears to be decreasing, work-related illness and injuries appear to be increasing.[96]

Workers in mining, agriculture, fire fighting, and construction are at greater risk to die from a work-related injury (Fig. 23-4). Poor housekeeping and poor design predispose the worker to falls and other illnesses.[96]

Accidents are twice as high among smokers. Possible explanations include the loss of attention, the use of one hand for smoking, and irritation of the eyes.[35]

In addition, thousands of middle-aged adults die each year in car accidents that occur less than 11 miles from their homes.

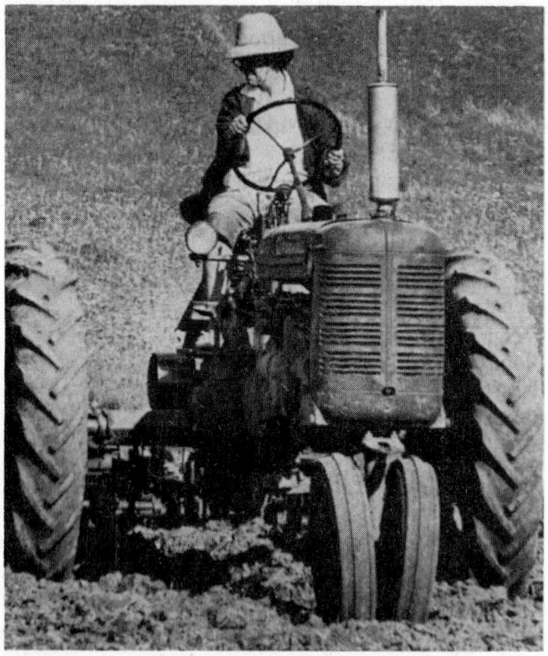

Fig. 23-3. Adults derive much of their pride pride and sense of satisfaction from work. (Photograph by David S. Strickler.)

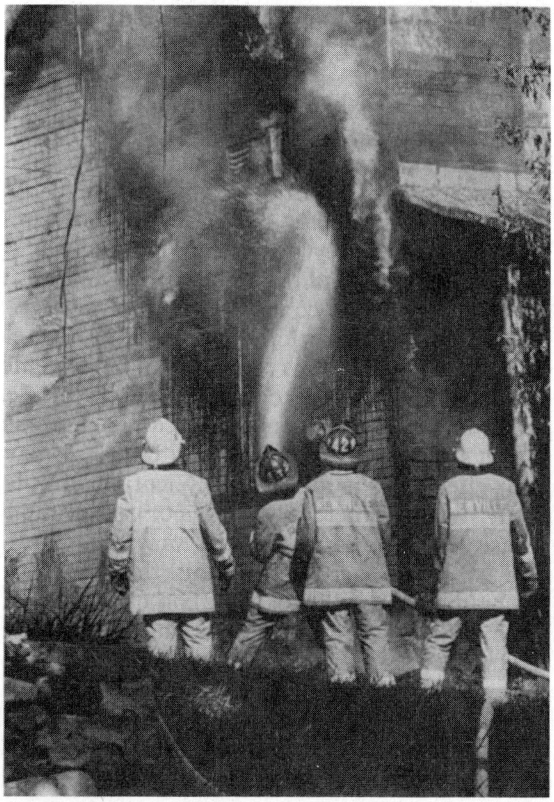

Fig. 23-4. Workers in mining, agriculture, construction, or fire fighting are at greater risk for work-related injury or death. (Photograph by David S. Strickler.)

Many accidents that contribute significantly to the morbidity and mortality of adults can be prevented. Fixing faulty steps, repairing faulty electric wires, securing carpets, and using rubber mats in the bathtub are just a few of the many preventive measures. Other work-related problems include lung diseases, musculoskeletal injuries, and occupational cancers.

Sexuality-Reproductive Pattern

More women in their 30s and 40s are continuing–or even beginning–to have children,[36,78] as well as to continue in satisfactory pattern of sexual functioning throughout the middle and older adult years. The fertility rate among women 35 to 39 years of age increased throughout the 1980s to the present level of 22.8 live births per 1000 women.

Abnormal genital bleeding and secondary amenorrhea are common gynecologic complaints that are indicate serious physical problems. Abnormal genital bleeding is the most common reason for gynecologic office visits by adult women. Although pregnancy and menopause are the most common causes of secondary, amenorrhea, other conditions related to abnormal pregnancy, functional disorders, physiologic changes, or pathology must be considered.[66]

After menopause many women enjoy sex more, when no risk of pregnancy exists. On the other hand, menopause may bring many challenges to a woman. Although changing, American culture still values women in part for their youth, beauty, and childbearing ability. Middle-aged women may confront their own aging for the first time and may be perplexed as to what their special roles should be.[8,64,100] Although men and women frequently enjoy very satisfactory sexual relationships throughout the middle adult years, men in their middle age are more vulnerable to sexual dysfunction than women. Middle-aged men often first experience problems with premature ejaculation, impotency, and retrograde ejaculation between ages 40 and 50.[24,44,80]

As with adolescents and young adults, sexually transmitted diseases continue to be major public health problems in the middle-aged adult. Women and children bear an inordinate share of sexually transmitted diseases' burden: sterility, ectopic pregnancy, fetal and infant deaths, birth defects, and mental retardation. Cancer of the cervix may be linked to sexually transmitted herpes II virus.[33] As with many other health behaviors and diseases, the full impact of this disease on the life of an individual and family may not be realized until middle age. Counseling about sexually transmitted diseases needs to continue throughout the adult years. Adults need accurate information about the causes, preventions, and treatment of sexually transmitted diseases to promote responsible sexual behaviors.[30,90]

Value and Belief Pattern

When adults make decisions affecting their lives, it is usually the result of a very personal, complex pattern of values and beliefs. Much of what people value or believe to be true is formed early in life and can be the most difficult to alter. Normally people do not spend much conscious thought at abstract explanations of the meaning of life and why certain things are valued. During times of an illness or crisis, however, persons frequently take time to review their value system and seek meaning as to what is important.[48,92]

A crisis at any age can be a turning point when both increased vulnerability and increased potential are present. If the crisis is successfully managed, a *virtue* or strength will evolve. Erikson names "caring" as the middle-aged adult's strength.

Committed responsibilities for the care and welfare of others promotes moral development. If lived with generativity, middle age has many opportunities to live life with higher principles. The middle adult can differentiate between personal wants and needs, duties demanded by society, and principles by which to live.[38] Kohlberg's work on moral development delineated these phases as Conventional and Post-Conventional. His studies of men described State 3 as an interpersonal definition of morality, whereas Stage 4 is a societal definition, based on law and order. Kohlberg concluded that most American adults were in these phases of moral development. In contrast, Stage 5 is the concern and willingness to sacrifice for the well-being of others.[52] Subsequent studies on moral development in women, as well as men, by Gilligan demonstrated gender differences in describing high morality. Women discussed issues of selfishness versus responsibility, of exercising care with and avoiding hurting. Men described terms of justice, fairness, and rights of individuals. Gilligan concluded that there is a different process of moral development in women in our society.[32,33] This model is summarized in Table 23-1.

***Table 23-1.* Gilligan's model of moral development in women**

Level	Characteristics
1. Individual survival	What is practical and best for self, realizing connection to others
—transition from selfishness to responsibility—	
2. Goodness as self-sacrifice	Sacrifices wants and needs to fulfill others' wants and needs
—transition from goodness to truth—	
3. Nonviolence	Moral equality between self and others

Valuing others, having relationships, and being responsible to others enables women to make the transitions of moral development. Women do this through raising children, developing more junior employees, and community service. Such commitments increasingly treat others as equals and gradually develop a sensitivity to and desire to change barriers to human worth and equality, such as racial prejudice, homelessness, inadequate access to health care, and weapon stockpiles.

Health Perception and Health Management Pattern

To promote health in the middle-aged adult, the nurse performs a health assessment that includes the person's values and beliefs, lifestyle patterns, general perceptions of health, and health practices.[81]

HABITS

The self-destructive habits of the middle-aged adult that have been practiced for years–cigarette smoking, alcohol, and overeating–begin to have visible side effects. As pressures increase, it is tempting for adults to turn to substances such as these as a crutch for coping with multiple stressors. Prevention is extremely important, since withdrawal from any of these substances is a difficult process. (See environmental processes later in this chapter.)

RISK FACTORS

The nurse needs to keep in mind that the major risk factors for adults in the middle years, as seen in chronic disease, are environmental and behavioral; thus, they can be changed.[96] Helping adults to take care of themselves and to change, if indicated, can be accomplished on an individual or group basis. Whether the nurse-client interaction is one-to-one or in a group depends largely on the setting and when the needs are identified.

A few of the health promotion needs of the middle-aged adult are acceptance of aging, exercise, and weight control. Decreasing or stopping cigarette smoking and alcohol intake also may be identified needs. Preventive health screening is vital. The adult should have input into and control of as many of these behaviors as possible. (See box below.)[54]

To help adults identify their specific risk factors, a *Health Hazard Appraisal questionnaire** has been developed. Suggested changes in living habits appear in order of priority on a computer printout or can be tabulated by hand. Clients are able to compare their risks with others in their age, sex, and racial group. How changing their lifestyle or habits will reduce these risks

*Prepared by John W. Travis, MD, the Society of Prospective Medicine and Interhealth, Inc., 1983. Updated with US Department of Health and Human Services: *Healthy people 2000: national health promotion and disease prevention objectives,* Washington, DC, 1990, US Government Printing Office; and American Cancer Society: *Cancer manual,* ed 8, Boston, 1992, American Cancer Society, Massachusetts Division, Inc.

RESEARCH REVIEW — MIDDLE ADULT

RECRUITMENT AND RETENTION IN HEALTH PROMOTION PROGRAM

Brill PA, et al: *Am J Health Promot* 5: 215-221, 1991. The relationship between sociodemographic characteristics and recruitment, retention, and health improvements in a worksite health promotion program.

Purpose The purpose of this study is to explore the relationship among sociodemographic variables, recruitment, retention, and health improvements.

Review Employees in the Dallas, Texas School District (n = 11,830) were given a health screen consisting of health habit assessment, measurement of clinical variables, physical fitness testing, and a medical examination. Thirty-three percent of employees were successfully recruited into the program. Recruitment rates were almost identical for men and women (32% versus 33%, respectively) but varied across ethnic and education groups. Blacks, younger employees, and noncollege graduates were less likely to be recruited. Sixty-nine percent were retained in the program, as defined by participation in the second screen. Women were more likely to be retained than men (71% versus 64%, respectively). Overall, participants showed an improvement in physical fitness and general well-being, lost weight, and decreased smoking. Changes were consistent across various demographic groups.

❑ ❑ SCREENING EXAMINATION: AGES 35 TO 65

Database

Health history–initial update with nurse or physician examination (PE)
Health hazard appraisal–initial screening
Social Readjustment Rating Scale (SRRS)–initial, then every 3 years

Physical examination (every 3 to 5 years until age 40, then annually) emphasizing

Weight
Blood pressure, pulse
Breast
Pelvic
Prostate
Testicular
Visual
Mouth
Skin

Laboratory procedures

Tuberculin skin test
Pap smear with gonoccal culture
Hemoccult–three stools for hemoccults with PE after age 50
Colonoscopy/Sigmoidoscopy–every 3 to 5 years after age 50 as indicated
Mammography–screening at 35 every 2 years, then yearly after age 50

Laboratory procedures–cont'd

Urinalysis–examined by provider at time of PE
Serum cholesterol
Renal plasma flow (RPR)–initial screening
Chest x-ray film–with PE if heavy smoker
TD booster–every 10 years
PPD (purified protein derivative of tuberculin)–every 2 years if negative
Influenza vaccine–follow current recommendations
Counseling and testing for HIV as indicated

Self-care education and counseling (with physical examination; individualized according to client's risk factors)

Injury prevention
Stress reduction
Exercise
Diet–cholestrol, fat, sodium, fiber
Breast self-examination
Testicular self-examination
Dental care
Mouth care
Sexually transmitted diseases
Contraception
Skin protection from ultraviolet light
Alcohol and other drug abuse
Smoking cessation

From American Cancer Society: *Cancer manual,* ed 8, Boston, 1992, American Cancer Society, Massachusetts Division, Inc.; US Department of Health and Human Services: *Healthy people 2000: national health promotion and disease prevention objectives,* Washington, DC, 1990, US Government Printing Office; and *Guide to clinical preventive services: an assessment of the effectiveness of 169 interventions.* Report of the US Preventive Services Task Force, Baltimore, 1989, Williams & Wilkins.

also is considered. The Health Hazard Appraisal should be completed so that self-care education and counseling can be planned more effectively.

Total health risks of middle-aged adults are composed of group risks (age, sex, race) and personality.[39] Precritical secondary prevention includes periodic selective screening for the detection of disease before it becomes clinically apparent, such as using breast self-examination.[59] A suggested screening examination appears in the box above.

Chronic conditions are defined as those that last for more than 3 months. Approximately 13% of the population report limitations caused by chronic conditions. A significant increase is seen between the ages of 45 and 64, with 25% to 30% of the population symptomatic. The percentage is slightly higher in the male.[55]

Chronic conditions found in the middle-aged adult include heart conditions, arthritis, impairments of the back and spine, chronic obstructive lung disease, mental and nervous conditions, and dental disease.[50]

Diseases[16-18] and behaviors for which screening is recommended in the middle-aged adult include the following:*

1. *Smoking history.* Heavy smoking increases the risk of carcinoma, chronia obstructive lung disease, arteriosclerosis, and coronary artery disease. Smoking cessation markedly decreases morbidity and mortality from these diseases.
2. *Alcohol screening.* Alcoholism is found most frequently in men over age 30. A positive family

*Prepared by John W. Travis, MD, the Society of Prospective Medicine and Interhealth, Inc., 1983. Updated with US Department of Health and Human Services: *Healthy people 2000: national health promotion and disease prevention objectives,* Washington, DC, 1990, US Government Printing Office; and American Cancer Society: *Cancer manual,* ed 8, Boston, 1992, American Cancer Society, Massachusetts Division, Inc.

history is a key risk factor. Approximately 70% of deaths from cirrhosis of the liver is related to heavy alcohol use.

3. *Obesity.* Adults who are 20% or more over their ideal weights have a 50% greater mortality rate, primarily from cardiovascular disease and diabetes.
4. *Heart disease and stroke.* Despite dramatic declines in mortality from heart disease and stroke in the past two decades, about 7 million Americans are affected by coronary artery disease, and cardiovascular diseases still cause more deaths in the United States than all other diseases combined. Reductions in major risk factors–high blood pressure, high blood cholesterol, and smoking–are having a significant impact on cardiovascular mortality.[6,47,96]
5. *Lipid profile.* A baseline blood test is indicated. Studies have shown that a correlation exists between hyperlipidemia and myocardial infarction in men between ages 30 and 59.

   Approximately 30% of adults in the United States have high blood pressure. People with uncontrolled high blood pressure are at three to four times the risk of developing coronary heart disease and as much as seven times the risk of developing a stroke as do those with normal blood pressures. Overall, Blacks have a higher prevalence of high blood pressure than Whites (38% versus 29%). Although surveys indicate that most adults with high blood pressure are aware of their condition, only about 25% to 33% have their blood pressure under control.[96] This remains a problem despite the fact that many can reduce their blood pressure to normal through programs of physical activity and weight loss, reduced sodium and alcohol intake, and stress management; and medications are available for those who cannot.[87]
6. *Breast cancer.* Breast cancer is a leading cause of cancer deaths (150,900 newly diagnosed cases and 44,300 deaths in 1990), involving approximately one out of ever nine women in the United States. Risk factors include female sex, family history, and age over 50. In the United States the incidence of breast cancer rapidly increases from 20 per 100,000 at age 30 to 180 per 100,000 at age 50. A family history of premenopausally diagnosed breast cancer in a first-degree relative (e.g., mother or sister) is a risk factor of about two to three times that of the average women in the general population. Other risk factors include history of benign breast disease, first pregnancy after age 30, menarche before age 12, menopause after age 50, obesity, high socioeconomic status, and a history of ovarian or endometrial cancer.[19,68,96]

   Early detection is critical, because the 5-year survival for localized breast cancer is 90%. The recommended screening tests for breast cancer are breast self-examination, nurse or physician examination, and mammography.[2,35,70,96]
7. *Ovarian cancer.* There were approximately 20,500 new cases and 12,400 deaths from ovarian cancer in 1990. Risk factors include being over age 60, nulliparity, late first pregnancy, late menopause, and family history. Women who have endometrial or breast cancer have twice the risk of developing ovarian cancer. Jewish women have higher rates.[2,35,96]

   The overall 5-year survival rate is only about 30% because symptoms usually do not manifest until the tumor presses on other structures. Women over age 40 with an enlarged abdomen or unexplained digestive symptoms (distention, discomfort, gas) need to be examined. There are no official recommendations to screen for ovarian cancer in asymptomatic women.[1]
8. *Uterine cancer.* There were 46,500 new cases and 10,000 deaths due to uterine cancer in 1990. Endometrial cancer primarily affects women between ages 50 and 64. Risk factors include a history of infertility; estrogen therapy; late menopause; and a combination of diabetes, hypertension, and obesity. (The postmenopausal woman should be strongly encouraged to report any vaginal bleeding.)[66]
9. *Testicular cancer.* The white male entering the middle years is at higher risk, although this tumor can occur at any age. Early detection and treatment, including testicular self-examination, decrease mortality rates appreciably.
10. *Colorectal cancer.* Ninety-five percent of colon cancers are found in adults over age 45.[1,65] A positive family history is significant. Dietary patterns should be assessed, since some evidence indicates that diets high in beef and/or low in fiber may be contributing factors. Fecal occult blood testing every 1 to 2 years and sigmoidoscopy as indicated are important in the early diagnosis of colorectal cancer.[2,35,96]
11. *Oral cancer.* This is most common in men over age 40; smoking is a primary risk factor. The client should report any mouth pain, sores, or lumps and have regular dental care.
12. *Tuberculosis.* Tuberculosis (TB) is a highly contagious disease. The incident of tuberculosis is increasing in the United States after experiencing a steady decrease from 1963 to 1985. More than 22,000 cases of TB were reported in 1987. About one third of these cases occurred in black Americans, 14% in Hispanics, and 11% in Asians and Pacific Islanders who have immigrated to the United States. Tuberculosis is 150 to 300 times more common in the homeless than in the general

population. Compromised immunity due to infection with the HIV virus is greatly contributing to the increased incidence of TB.

Tuberculin skin testing with the Mantoux test is the primary means of identifying TB in asymptomatic persons. Early detection is important because of the efficacy of isoniazid (INH).[2,35,96]

13. *Syphilis, gonorrhea, and HIV.* Sexually active middle-aged adults in urban low-income groups are especially at risk. (See Chapters 21 and 22 for discussion.)
14. *Glaucoma.* The adult over age 40 is at greater risk, especially with a positive family history. Controversy, however, surrounds the cost-effectiveness of routine tonometry. (See Chapter 24 for discussion.)

ENVIRONMENTAL PROCESSES

Natural Processes

PHYSICAL AGENTS

Ionizing radiation is a prime example of a physical agent that can cause cancer. Among the best known examples of cancer potentially caused by medical procedures using x-ray films and radiation are (1) bone cancers in clients treated with radium used for the treatment of tuberculosis; (2) thyroid carcinomas from radiation treatment for enlarged thymus glands; and (3) breast cancer from mammographic techniques, which may increase the incidence and, therefore, should be used with great caution.

Water pollution has become another major concern; several industrial and agricultural wastes have been recovered in rivers and lakes from which drinking water is obtained. Such waste includes benzene and chlordane.

Air pollution from auto exhausts, burning fuels, and industrialization have warranted smog alerts and air pollution indexes. These are especially important to the individual with chronic obstructive lung disease (COLD).[96]

In looking at occupational injuries, the nurse needs to explore the particular work environment; agriculture (forestry, fisheries); mining (anthracite, bituminous coals, oil and gas extraction); food production (meat packing, dairy products, bakeries).[45] Safety boards should establish standards in conjunction with recommendation from the Occupational Safety and Health Administration (OSHA).

Noise pollution in industry is a potential problem for the middle-aged adult worker. Hearing loss can be prevented if federal guidelines are followed with regard to noise exposure levels. Hearing-conservation programs should be enforced.[102]

Occupational exposures to excessive noise, radiation, sunlight, and vibration can produce such problems as COLD, cancer, and degenerative diseases in the middle-aged adult. Of approximately 50,000 chemicals in the workplace, more than 2000 have been reported to be potential human carcinogens.

BIOLOGIC AND BACTERIAL AGENTS

As noted throughout this text, the occurrence of health or disease is influenced by the interaction between the agent, host, and environment. Agent factors can be biologic, physical, chemical, or psychologic. Many of these agents are transmitted through the air or come in contact with certain vehicles, such as water or food. They enter through the respiratory or gastrointestinal tracts. The size of the agent is important; if it is very small, the portal of entry is the respiratory tract. Several of the categories merit special discussion in relation to middle adulthood.

Viruses. *Hepatitis A* is caused by virus infection, with transmission occurring primarily through the fecal-oral route. This host-agent interaction usually occurs in the middle-aged adult living in an environment with poor sanitation and having close contact with an infected person. The person also may be exposed through contaminated food and water. *Hepatitis B* is transmitted primarily in the blood or plasma of the infected persons. This is particularly significant in the adult employed in health care settings. Routes of exposure include (1) inoculation by contaminated needle (hospital employees, drug abusers), (2) minute skin cuts or abrasions (laboratory workers), (3) mucosal surfaces such as in the mouth and eyes, (4) sexual contact (virus is carried in saliva and semen), and (5) indirect transfer via vectors or inanimate environmental surfaces.[35]

Hepatitis B is an occupational hazard of medical and dental personnel, with surgeons, oral surgeons, and pathologists at highest risk, six times more than the general population.

Occupational Hazards. The biologic causes of occasional disease include bacteria, viruses, *Rickettsia,* fungi, parasites, and food poisoning. Because these are often limited to identifiable occupations, they can be more easily diagnosed, treated, and prevented (Table 23-2).

CHEMICAL AGENTS

As agents, nutrients include a wide variety of substances that increase the risk of morbidity and mortality in the middle-aged adult. These include assorted chemicals and drugs.

Since approximately 100 million workers are in the United States, occupational hazards are a serious threat to national health. Exposures to toxic chemicals, asbestos, coal dust, cotton fiber, ionizing radiation, physical

***Table 23-2.* Occupational biologic hazards**

Disease	Target organ	Occupational source	Exposed occupations	Preventive measures
Fever (*Rickettsia*)	Systemic	Placental tissue, excreta from infected cattle, sheep	Laboratory workers, farmers, slaughterhouse workers	Hygiene, immunization
Histoplasmosis (fungal)	Lung	Fowl droppings	Farmers, poultry workers, demolition workers	Dust control, environmental sanitation
Hookworm (parasite)	Small intestine	Larvae in human feces penetrate skin	Farmers, sewer workers, recreation workers	Environmental sanitation; use of shoes, boots, gloves
Tetanus (bacteria)	Nervous system	Soil	Construction workers, farmers	Immunization
Rabies (virus)	Central nervous system	Wild animals Cows	Laboratory workers, veterinarians, hunters	Immunization of human contact with dogs, cats, skunks, foxes, bats, raccoons

Adapted from Cohen R: Occupational biologic hazards, *Occup Health Nurs* 28(8):34, 1990.

hazards, noise, and stress can precipitate numerous health problems. For the middle-aged worker, these include cancers, lung and heart diseases, decreased hearing, bodily injuries, and mental health problems.[96]

If the home of the middle-aged adult is located near an industry, there is the risk of exposure to toxic chemicals that may pollute the air. Contaminants also may be carried home on the clothing from the workplace.

The National Institute for Occupational Safety and Health (NOISH) estimates that 100,000 Americans die each year from occupational illnesses.[96] Skin diseases represent the largest category of occupational illness (43%), followed by repeated trauma (14%).

Workers at increased risk are coal miners, wood handlers, and asbestos and coke workers. *Pneumoconiosis* is found in about 15% of coal miners, with *black lung disease* implicated in thousands of deaths per year. Wood handlers and asbestos workers have increased risk of certain cancers. In addition, the asbestos worker has an increased risk of death from *mesothelioma* and *asbestosis*. Approximately 2 million workers each year have been exposed to benzene and vinyl chloride, which may be carcinogens.[96]

Nine out of 10 American industrial workers may be inadquately protected from exposure to at least 10 of the 163 most common hazardous chemicals. More than 2000 of the 50,000 chemicals found in the workplace are suspected human carcinogens.[96]

Tobacco. Many 50-year-old adults have a 30-plus-year history of cigarette smoking. Cigarette smokers have nearly twice the heart disease death rates of nonsmokers, with the risk being proportional to the amount of smoke inhaled and the number of cigarettes smoked.[47] Smokers are at higher risks for colds, chronic bronchitis, emphysema, and cancers of the mouth, lungs, esophagus, pancreas, and bladder.[2] More blue-collar workers smoke (51%) than white-collar workers (37%).[73] A study of 2092 urban adults found that knowledge about smoking's health effects was generally lower among women, older adults, Blacks, those of lower education levels, and current smokers.[12]

Few smokers realize that cigarettes contain 2000 known chemicals, including tar, nicotine, hydrogen cyanide, formaldehyde, and ammonia. Cigarette smoking is for most smokers an addiction to *nicotine*, which is absorbed into the bloodstream. It acts in the two divisions of the nervous system to affect the central part of the brain and the spinal cord as well as the peripheral portion that controls the arms and legs. Effects of nicotine stimulation can be seen in both electroencephalograph changes as well as in hand tremors. In addition, nicotine acts to stimulate the heart, leading to an increased pulse and elevated blood pressure. Although smokers often believe that cigarettes have a calming effect, this is misleading. Nicotine stimulates the body, whereas increasing levels of carbon monoxide cause lethargy. Thus, smokers may feel calm, although they are actually having their sensations dulled by the elevated level of carbon monoxide.[47]

Additive effects can lower midexpiratory flow values, as from chlorine, cotton dust, and beta radiation. Profound effects can also be seen with asbestos interaction. In a 4-year study of 370 asbestos insulation worker, 24 of the 283 cigarette smokers died of bronchogenic carcinoma. None of the 87 nonsmokers died. Workers who smoke have eight times the risk of lung cancer, as compared to all other smokers. Those workers exposed to asbestos have *92 times* the risk of nonsmokers.[35]

Food Additives. Much controversy recently has surrounded food additives and their relationship to disease,

the nurse. These can be categorized as official, voluntary, and service agencies. Councils of community services often publish a directory of services that is most helpful. Official agencies include those that are state and federally funded, such public health departments and drug treatment centers. Voluntary agencies include the American Cancer Society, the American Lung Association, and Alcoholics Anonymous. Many educational and self-help programs are sponsored by these organizations. The American Lung Association sponsors a "Stop Smoking" program, which can be conducted on a group basis in a work or community setting (see box below).

❑ ❑ COMMUNITY RESOURCES FOR HEALTH PROMOTION DURING MIDDLE ADULTHOOD

Advocacy

Family and children's services
Legal services
SAGA

Adult education, community centers

American Red Cross
Community centers
Public Schools
YWCA
YMCA

Alcohol/drug abuse treatment and rehabilitation

Alcoholics Anonymous
Mental health centers
Hospital alcohol and drug abuse programs
Local council on alcohol and drugs
Narcotics Anonymous
State departments of mental health–alcohol and drug division
Veterans' hospitals–mental health unit

Clinics and health centers

Community clinics
Health departments
Planned Parenthood clinics
United Neighborhood Health Service

Community planning, organization, and development

Chambers of commerce
Councils of community
Metro development and housing agencies
Metro planning commissions
Metro social service departments
Urban leagues
State commissions on the status of women
State law enforcement planning agencies

Consumer affairs

Better Business Bureaus
State Division of Consumer Affairs

Counseling

American Red Cross
Family services

Counseling–cont'd

Rape and sexual abuse centers
Social service departments
YWCA

Crisis intervention services

Crisis call hotlines
Rape and sexual abuse centers

Employment counseling, training, and placement

Career counseling centers
Employment security offices
YWCA Displaced Homemakers Program

Environmental protection

State health departments
State departments of conservation
State departments of public health
State environmental councils

Health education and promotion

American Red Cross
Arthritis Association
American Cancer Society
American Lung Association
Dietetic Association
Diabetes Association
Heart Association
Kidney Foundation
Academy of Medicine
Council on Alcohol and Drugs
Tel-Med (recorded messages)
State dental associations

Spouse abuse

Crisis intervention centers
Legal services
YWCA

Women's organizations

Homemakers Back to Work
Junior League
League of Women Voters
National Council of Jewish Women
YWCA Women's Resource Center

Other agencies include professional organizations, such state nurses' associations the American Medical Association (sponsor Tel-Med program), bar associations, YMCAs, hospice programs, and the Women's Occupational Health Resource Center.*

NURSING INTERVENTIONS FOR HEALTH PROMOTION

The nurse in the community and industry has the responsibility to assess the health status of the adult client. The nurse first must understand the hazards to which the individual is exposed by listening to the client, conferring with other individuals in the same environment, and reviewing available health and safety data.

As a health educator, the nurse can initiate programs that emphasize helping clients to accept more responsibility for their own health. This can be on a one-to-one basis or in a seminar fashion. For example, with the goal of "early detection of high blood pressure," the nurse in the community or industry could (1) increase consumers' knowledge of hypertension, (2) screen clients who have sought health care for any reason, (3) set up mechanisms to screen clients outside of the health care system, and (4) refer and follow up on all clients with blood pressure elevations.[47,79,85]

The target groups identified by the nurse should have common needs, such as those exposed to a particular chemical, smokers, women just entering the workplace, men nearing retirement, and substance abusers. In a work environment, the occupational health nurse (OHN) also can assess absenteeism rates for any trends. In gathering data, this nurse can initiate research projects with multidisciplinary input.[74]

The preemployment physical examination not only provides the employer with information about proper placement but also provides a baseline health assessment.[61] This frequently is the only assessment that the individual has had in years.

The OSHA mandates that the employee have *a healthy and safe work environment.* Therefore, it is essential that the adult's health history be completed. History of hypertension, arthritis, cancer, hernia? Any significant family history? Smoker? How many packs per day? Taking any medications? Medical limitations must be addressed, such as decreased visual acuity means no driving or dermatitis means no oils, chemicals, or solvents. Removing a worker from a particular job may be indicated if the worker would endanger coworkers, had a disease condition that would be aggravated by the job, or was taking prescribed medications with potentially harmful side effects.[8]

*National Clearinghouse for Women Workers, Policy Makers and Others, 320 East 43rd St., New York, NY 10017.

The nurse in the community and in industry needs to reiterate some key safety issues to the adult, such as wearing seat belts and observing speed limits. With a decrease in visual acuity, driving at night becomes more hazardous. The middle-aged adult's reaction time is also decreasing, which reinforces the need to enforce recommendations by the National Highway Traffic Safety Administration for specific interval retesting.

With an increase in leisure time, the middle-aged adult is at greater risk for recreational accidents. As noted, moderation should be stressed. Alcohol is a depressant and should be avoided in activities that require attentiveness.

Protection from burns is essential; 56% of fatal residential fires are cigarette-related, such as smoking in bed. Falls can occur at any age, and safety measures should be considered for the entire family, with preparatory planning for aging parents A few suggestions to the adult would be to avoid highly waxed floors, poor lighting, high beds, and bathtubs without nonslip bottoms.

Handgun availability is controversial at best; however, about 20% of American households have them. If the client feels strongly about having a gun, safety measures to avoid accidental injury should be discussed, such as security locks and proper storage.

The Occupational Safety and Health Act of 1970 was designed to ensure that workers were employed under safe and healthful working conditions. The act is applicable to every employer who is engaged in a business affecting commerce. The employer must ascertain that the workplace is free from recognized hazards and must comply with the act. OSHA has offices in most major cities and can provide recommended standards for occupational agents.

Nurses can actively participate in the safety committee of the industry in which they are employed. If no such committee exists, many protection measures will fall on the nurse. Pope[74] suggests the following:

1. Tour the facilities on a regular basis. Be familiar with resource books, laws, and available codes.
2. Develop a toxicology chart with symptoms of overexposure and current treatment. Update this frequently.
3. Be a role model in safety issues; wear safety glasses, protective footwear, and gloves, and do not smoke.
4. Discuss the preemployment physical with the employee, with emphasis on risk factors. Monitor health problems and exposure levels in the work setting.

It is essential that the worker know the protective clothing that should be worn, sanitation measures for the work environment, general hygiene measures, and proper immunization. The food handler, for instance, should have an annual TB skin test, wear clean clothing and appropriate hair protection, and use good handwashing technique. The nurse should not assume that workers know how to protect themselves and others.

A major challenge to the nurse is to encourage workers to assume responsibility for protecting their own health. Nurses cannot evaluate workers' complaints, however, unless they have a knowledge of their specific working conditions as well as the organization and community as a whole.

Increasingly, organizations are interested in promoting the health of their employees for many reasons, including to enhance their recruiting efforts and to minimize lateness, absenteeism, turnover, physical and emotional inabilities to work, disability, costs, and health and life insurance costs. Health promotion programs are increasingly recognized for their vital contributions to the financial viability of organizations.[1,41,69,76,101]

Health promotion programs within an organizational setting can be categorized in one of three levels: (1) awareness, (2) lifestyle change, and (3) supportive environment. The goal of a health program at the level of awareness is to increase the individual's awareness or interest in a particular health issue (e.g. smoking cessation). Examples of awareness programs include special events, flyers, lunch seminars, meetings, and newsletters. Changing health behaviors or status are not the goals of awareness programs but are goals of lifestyle change programs.

Lifestyle change programs last at least 8 to 12 weeks and include assessment, education, and evaluation components to help individuals implement long-term changes in health behavior and status.

To maintain these long-term changes in health behavior and status and develop a healthy lifestyle, a supportive organizational environment is needed. Such an environment includes health promoting physical settings, corporate policies and culture, ongoing programs, and employee ownership of programs.[52]

Five models of nurse-managed primary health care delivery at the worksite have recently been proposed as part of the American Nurses' Association's program for reform of this nations health care system, "Nursing's Agenda for Health Care Reform." Each model is developed to enable employers to fulfill the goal of providing accessible, quality, and affordable care at locations familiar and convenient for employees. These designs assist employers in introducing or expanding health care services at the worksite, controlling health care costs, and meeting the health care needs of their employees.

SUMMARY

Nurses are in a position to help the middle-aged client improve the quality of life, both for the present and the future, through the identification of risk factors, health promotion, and appropriate nursing interventions. Nurses work in a variety of health care settings available to healthy middle-aged adult clients: outpatient clinics, occupational health clinics, and private practice.

Health promotion and protection are aimed at the personal habits and lifestyle of adult clients to improve their biologic and psychosocial development. Strategies to help an adult client achieve a higher level of health include individual or group counseling based on identified risk factors, providing self-help information that is most relevant to the middle-aged adult, and describing available resources.

Through these strategies, the nurse is better able to motivate middle-aged adults to assume more responsibility for their health behaviors. Changes may be effected after years of poor health practices, thus decreasing the adult's risk of disability from chronic disease–heart disease, cerebrovascular accident, and cancer.

References

1. Alexy B: Workplace health promotion and the blue collar worker, *AAOHN J*, 38:12-16, 1990.
2. American Cancer Society: *Cancer manual*, ed 8, Boston, 1992, American Cancer Society, Massachusetts Division, Inc.
3. Reference deleted in proofs.
4. American Hospital Association: *Stress!*, AHA catalog no P010, Chicago, 1989, The Association.
5. Archibald PG: Impact of parent caring on middle-aged offspring, *J Gerontol Nurs* 6(2):78, 1980.
6. Avis NE, Smith KW, McKinlay JB: Accuracy of perceptions of heart attack risk: what influences perceptions and can they be changed?, *Am J Public Health* 79:1608-1612, 1989.
7. Reference deleted in proofs.
8. Bischof L: *Adult psychology*, New York, 1989, Harper & Row.
9. Bloom BS: *Taxonomy of educational objectives. Handbook I. Cognitive domain*, New York, 1984, Longman.
10. Brincat R: A study of the decrease of skin collagen content, skin thickness and bone mass in postmenopausal women, *Obstet Gynecol* 70:840-845, 1988.
11. Reference deleted in proofs.
12. Brownson RC: Demographic and socioeconomic differences in beliefs about the health effects of smoking, *Am J Public Health* 82:99-103, 1992.
13. Burgel BJ: *Innovation at the work site: delivery of nurse-managed primary health care services*, Washington, DC, 1993, American Nurses Publishing.
14. Burnett R: *Menopause*, Chicago, 1987, Contemporary Books.
15. Reference deleted in proofs.
16. Centers for Disease Control: *MMWR* 41:(20):1, 1992.
17. Centers for Disease Control: *MMWR* 41(26):463, 1992.
18. Centers for Disease Control: *MMWR* 41(30):548, 1992.
19. *Cigarette smoking facts about your lung*, New York, 1989, American Lung Association.
20. Cope DG: Self-esteem and the practice of breast self-examination, *Western J Nurs Res* 14:618-631, 1992.
21. Craig CJ: *Human development*, ed 5, Englewood Cliffs, NJ, 1989, Prentice Hall.
22. Darling-Fischer C, Leidy NK: Measuring Eriksonian development in the adult. The modified Erikson psychological stage inventory, *Psych Rep* 62:747-754, 1988.
23. Davis G, Jones A: *Personality development: stages of growth*. In Lancaster J,

editor: *Adult psychiatric nursing,* New York, 1980, Medical Examination Publishing.
24. Dickelmann N: *Primary health care of the well adult,* New York, 1977, McGraw-Hill.
25. Duffy ME: Determinants of health promotion in midlife women, *Nurs Res* 37:358-362, 1988.
26. Duvall EM, Miller B: *Marriage and family development,* ed 6, New York, 1984, HarperCollins.
27. Edinberg MA: *Talking with your aging parent,* Boston, 1988, Shambhala Publishing.
28. Erikson EH: *Childhood and society,* anniv ed 35, New York, 1986, WW Norton.
29. Fedlman E: *Nutrition in the middle and later years,* New York, 1986, Warner.
30. Flaskerud JH, Calvillo ER: Beliefs about AIDS, health and illness among low income Latino women, *Res Nurs Health* 14:431-438, 1991.
31. Friedman MM: *Family nursing theory and assessment,* ed 2, New York, 1986, Appleton-Lange.
32. Gilligan C: *In a different voice: psychological theory and women's development,* Cambridge, 1982, Harvard University Press.
33. Gilligan, C: *Mapping the moral domain,* Cambridge, 1990, Harvard University Press.
34. Ginsburg H, Opper S: *Piaget's theory of intellectual development,* ed 2, Englewood Cliffs, NJ, 1979, Prentice Hall.
35. *Guide to clinical preventive services: an assessment of the effectiveness of 169 interventions.* Report of the US Preventive Services Task Force, Baltimore, 1989, Williams & Wilkins.
36. Hansen JP: Older maternal age and pregnancy outcomes: a review of the literature, *Ibstefriend Gynecol Survey* 41:726-742, 1986.
37. Harris SS, Casperson CJ, Defriese GH, Estes EH: Physical activity counseling for health adults as a primary preventive intervention in the clinical setting, *JAMA* 261:3590-3598, 1989.
38. Hatziandreu EI, et al: The cost effectiveness analysis of exercise as a health promotion activity, *Am J Public Health* 78:1417-1421, 1988.
39. Havighurst RI, Orr B: *Adult education and adult needs,* Chicago, 1956, Center for Study of Liberal Education for Adults.
40. Haynes SG, et al: The relationship of psychosocial factors to coronary heart disease in the Framingham study, *Am J Epidemiol* 107(5):362, 1978.
41. Hellings P: Using nursing research: instructor's manual: critiques of research on health promotion and primary care nursing, NLN Pub #15, 2297, 1989, National League for Nursing.
42. Holmes T, David E: *Life change events research 1966-1978, an annotated bibliography of the periodical literature,* Chicago, 1984, Greenwood.
43. Holmes T, David E: *Life change, life events and illness: selected papers,* Chicago, 1989, Greenwood.
44. Hymovich DP, Barnard MV: *Family health care, vol 1, General perspectives,* ed 2, New York, 1979, McGraw-Hill.
45. Hymovich DP, Barnard MV: *Family health care, vol 2, Developmental and situational crises,* ed 2, New York, 1979, McGraw-Hill.
46. Johnston RL: The holistic experience of stress, opportunity for growth or illness, *Occup Health Nurs* 28(12):15, 1980.
47. Joint National Commission on Detection, Evaluation and Treatment of High Blood Pressure: The 1984 report of the Joint National Commission on Detection, Evaluation and Treatment of High Blood Pressure, *Arch Intern Med* 114:1047, 1984.
48. Kerr MJ, Ritchey DA: Health promoting lifestyles of English-speaking and Spanish-speaking Mexican-American migrant farm workers, *Public Health Nurs* 7:80-87, 1990.
49. Killeen M: Health promotion practices of family caregivers, *Health Values: Achieving High Level Wellness* 13:3-10, 1989.
50. Kimmell DC: *Adulthood and aging and interdisciplinary, developmental view,* ed 3, New York, 1989, John Wiley & Sons.
51. Reference deleted in proofs.
52. Kohlberg L, Lickona T: *The stages of ethical development: from childhood through old age,* New York, 1986, HarperCollins.
53. Lancaster JB, King BJ: *An evolutionary perspective. In her prime: a new view of middle-aged women,* South Hadley, Mass, 1985, Bergin & Garvey.
54. Leavell HP, Clark EG: *Preventive medicine for the doctor in his community: an epidemiologic approach,* ed 3, New York, 1965, McGraw-Hill.
55. Lee PR, Estes C: *The nation's health,* ed 3, Boston, 1990, Jones & Bartlett.
56. Leitch CI, Tinker RV: *Primary care,* 1978, Philaelphia, FA Davis.
57. LeShan E: *The wonderful crisis of middle age,* New York, 1973, David McKay.
58. Levinson D: *The seasons of a man's life,* New York, 1986, Ballantine.
59. Lindberg SC: Periodic preventive health screening schedule for adult women and men, *Nurse Prac* 5(5):9, 1980.
60. Linder MM, Motley CP, Crump WJ, Pierce PJ: Health maintenance for adults, exercise and nutrition: practical applications of the USPSTF recommendations, *Consultant* 32:37-50, 1991.
61. Lindsay R: Prevention of osteoporosis, *Clin Orth Rel Res* 222:44-59, 1989.
62. Loevinger J: *Ego development,* San Francisco, 1976, Jossey-Bass.
63. McKinlay J, McKinlay S: Massachusetts women's health study. 9th annual scientific sessions, The Society of Behavioral Medicine, Boston, April 1988.
64. Miller J: *Toward a new psychology of women,* ed 2, Boston, 1986, Beacon Press.
65. Miller JR, Janosik EH: *Family-focused care,* New York, 1980, McGraw-Hill.
66. Murata JM: Abnormal genital bleeding and secondary amenorrhea: common gynecological problem *J Obstet Gynecol Neonat Nurs* 19:26-36, 1990.
67. Reference deleted in proofs.
68. Nemeck MA: Factors influencing black women's breast self-examination practice, *Cancer Nurs* 12:339-343, 1989.
69. O'Donnell MP: Design of workplace health promotion programs, *Am J Health Promot,* Royal Oak, Mich, 1986 (monograph).
70. Olson RL, Mitchell ES: Self-confidence as a critical factor in breast self-examination, *J Obstet Gynecol Neonat Nurs* 18:476-481, 1989.
71. Overfield T: Obesity: prevention is easier than cure, *Nurse Prac* 5(5):25, 33, 62, 1980.
72. Philosophe R, Serbel MM: Menopause and cardiovascular disease, *NAACOG Clin Iss Perinat Women's Health Nurs* 2:441-451, 1991.
73. Pierce JP, et al: Trends in cigarette smoking in the United States: projections to the year 2000, *JAMA* 261:61-65, 1989.
74. Pope R: Control and prevention in occupational health: the nurse's role, *Occup Health Nurs* 29(1):12, 1981.
75. Price JH: Urban black women's perception of breast cancer and mammography, *J Comm Health* 17:191-204, 1992.
76. Pruitt RH: Effectiveness and cost efficiency of interventions in health promotion, *J Adv Nurs* 17:926-932, 1992.
77. Ray OS: *Drugs, society, and human behavior,* ed 3, St Louis, 1982, Mosby.
78. Redwine F: Pregnancy in women over 35, *Female Patient* 13:30, 1988.
79. Reilly D, Oermann M: *Behavioral objectives: evaluation in nursing,* New York, 1990, National League for Nursing.
80. Rew L: Correlates of health promoting lifestyles and sexual satisfaction in a group of men, *Iss Mental Health Nurs* 11:283-295, 1990.

81. Samuels M, Samuels N: *The well adult,* New York, 1988, Summit.
82. Sandelowski M: *Women, health, and choice,* Englewood Cliffs, NJ, 1981, Prentice Hall.
83. Reference deleted in proofs.
84. Sempos C, et al: the prevalence of high blood cholesterol levels among adults in the United States, *JAMA* 262:45-52, 1989.
85. Simmons JJ, et al: A health promotion program: staying healthy after 50, *Health Educ Q,* 16:461-472, 1989.
86. Smelser NJ, Erikson EH: *Themes of work and load in adulthood,* Cambridge, 1980, Harvard University Press.
87. Smith ED: The role of black churches in supporting compliance with antihypertension regimens, *Public Health Nurs* 6:212-217, 1989.
88. Spector RE: *Cultural diversity in health and illness,* ed 3, East Norwalk, Conn, 1991, Appleton-Lange.
89. Spence A: *Biology of human aging,* Englewood Cliffs, NJ, 1989, Prentice Hall.
90. Strader MK, Beaman ML: Theoretical components of STD counselors' messages to promote clients' use of condoms, *Public Health Nurs* 9:109-117, 1992.
91. Strasser AK: Pre-placement screening: an exercise in preventive medicine, *Occup Health Safety* 28(5):23, 1979.
92. Stuart E, Deckro J, Mandle CL: Spirituality in health and healing: a clinical program, *Holistic Nursing Prac* 3:35-46, 1989.
93. Sutterly DC, Donnelly GF: *Perspectives in human development,* Philadelphia, 1978, JB Lippincott.
94. Troll L: *Early and middle adulthood,* ed 2, Monterey, Calif, 1985, Brooks/Cole.
95. Tucker LA, Bagwell M: The relation between aerobic fitness and serum cholesterol levels in a large employed population, *Am J Health Promot* 6:17-23, 1990.
96. US Department of Health and Human Services: *Healthy people 2000: national health promotion and disease prevention objectives,* DHHS Pub No (PHS)91-50213, Washington, DC, 1990, US Government Printing Office.
97. Valliant G, Valliant C: Natural history of male psychological health. XII. A 45 year study of predictors of successful aging at age 65, *Am J Psych* 147(1):31-37, 1990.
98. Volden C, Langemo D, Adamson M, Oechsle L: The relationship of age, gender and exercise practice to measures of health, lifestyle, and self esteem, *Appl Nurs Res* 3:20-26, 1990.
99. Wallerstein JS, Kelly JB: Divorce counseling: a community service for families in the midst of divorce, *Am J Orthopsychiatry* 47:4, 1977.
100. Watson GL: *Feminism and women's issues: 1974-1986: an annotated bibliography and research guide,* Hamden, Conn, 1989, Garland.
101. Weitzel MH, Waller PR: Predictive factors for health promotion behaviors in White, Hispanic and blue-collar workers, *Family Comm Health* 13:23-24, 1990.
102. Wright M: Education: the key to preventing hearing loss, *Occup Health Safety* 49(1):38, 1981.

CHAPTER

24

Older Adult

Anne Griswold Peirce

Terry T. Fulmer

Carole Lium Edelman

Objectives

After completing this chapter, the nurse will be able to

- *Identify normal aging changes in the older adult.*
- *Evaluate morbidity data according to age, sex, and race.*
- *Discuss nutritional factors that affect the health promotion of the older adult.*
- *Analyze environmental factors that have impact on older adults.*
- *Recognize risk factors that occur with activities of daily living in later adulthood.*
- *Enumerate the five most prevalent conditions and the five leading causes of mortality among older persons.*
- *Discuss environmental, biologic, physical, and mechanical agents that contribute to disability, morbidity, and mortality in later maturity.*
- *Analyze political and social issues that influence the well-being of the elderly.*
- *List the leading causes of accidents among older adults and suggest preventive measures.*
- *Identify major resources available for health teaching for elderly.*

Gerontologic nursing is a dynamic specialty area that has rapidly moved to the forefront of curricular, research, and practice agendas in recent years. This new emphasis is largely a result of what some have called the "demographic imperative." In 1900 only 4% of the population lived to the age of 65. Today it is expected that most people will live to be at least 65 years of age, a stunning indicator of how dramatically things have changed during the 20th century (see box on p. 633).

Gerontology, the study of normal aging, includes all sciences that contribute to the nurse's understanding of age-related changes in human function. Clearly, by the year 2000, the term *lifespan* will take on dimensions heretofore unknown (see box on p. 634). One major factor is the group of elderly individuals who are over the age of 85. This old-old group is the most rapidly growing subgroup of elderly. In fact, U.S. Census projections estimate that the population over 85 will nearly triple by the year 2020.[49] This observation has major implications for service delivery systems as we now know them.

RESEARCH REVIEW OLDER ADULT

HEALTH PROMOTION AMONG OLDER ADULTS

Duffy ME: Determinants of health-promoting lifestyles in older persons, *Image: J Nurs Scholarship* 25:23-28, 1993.

Purpose The purpose of this study was to determine the degree to which selected components derived from Pender's Health Promotion Model (1982) explained engaging in health promotion practices in a sample of persons 65 years old and older.

Review Data on 447 persons 65 years old and older were obtained by contacts with staff who managed retirement and senior citizen centers. A 2-hour interview was conducted by a trained interviewer. The research hypothesis was tested using canonical correlation analysis. Three significant canonical variates were demonstrated, explaining 88.7% of variance. Healthy older persons with high self-esteem and internal locus of control reported practicing five of the six health promotion strategies (e.g., self-actualization, health responsibility, nutrition, exercise, and stress management). Men with higher income and self-esteem but poorer health less often exercised or ate well. Older married subjects with higher incomes who were internally controlled were more likely to engage in exercise, health responsibility, and stress management.

INCENTIVE–HEALTH PROMOTION SCALE

Pascussi MA: Measuring incentives to health promotion in older adults: understanding neglected health promotion in older adults, *J Geron Nurs* 18:16-23, 1992.

Purpose The purpose of this study is to report the development and preliminary testing of the Incentive–Health Promotion Scale based on a concept analysis and two theoretical frameworks.

Review Pilot testing of the Incentive–Health Promotion Scale was done on two samples of older adults at senior citizen centers in a Midwestern city. In phase I, content validity and reliability were established. In phase II, 30 older adults were randomly selected to respond to several statements based on Likert Scale (1 to 6, Strongly Disagree to Strongly Agree). Incentives for health promotion among older adults include fitness and health, appearance, medical advice, socialization, independence, pressure, fun, feel good, and belong. Tools to measure healthy lifestyle are currently available and are continually being refined.

PHYSIOLOGIC PROCESSES

Age and Physical Changes

By 1984, the number of Americans 65 years old or older was approximately 28 million, roughly 12% of the population. By the year 2030, that percentage is projected to increase to just over 18% of the population. In fact, the fastest growing age group in the country is that of adults age 75 and older; the number of people in this age group is expected to increase by approximately 70% by the year 2000.[75]

Aging results in physiologic changes, have a cumulative effect in the continuum of biologic, psychologic, social, and environmental processes.[15] Goldman indicates four characteristics of physiologic aging: it is universal, progressive, decremental, and intrinsic. The physiologic changes that occur are normal for all people, but they take place at different rates and depend on different individuals' lifestyles and the environments in which they live.[23]

Normal aging may be viewed as those inevitable and irreversible changes that occur with time. Although generalizations are dangerous, especially since variability increases with age, most age-related biologic changes show growth and development peaking in the thirties, with subsequent linear decline until death. Specific normal age-related changes in their relationship to problems typical of the older adults are show in Table 24-1.

Although most normal aging changes are intrinsic by nature, older adults undergo some changes that are extrinsic and depend on their lifestyles. Thus, despite the misconceptions that abound, health promotion is as important in later adulthood as it is earlier in life (see the

HEALTHY PEOPLE 2000

SELECTED NATIONAL HEALTH PROMOTION AND DISEASE PREVENTION OBJECTIVES

OLDER ADULT

- Reduce coronary heart disease deaths to no more than 100 per 100,000 people (a 26% decrease)
- Reduce stroke deaths to no more than 20 per 100,000 people (a 34% decrease)
- Reduce disability from chronic conditions to no more than 8% of people (a 15% decrease)
- Increase to at least 80% of receipt of home food services by people aged 65 and older who have difficulty in preparing their own meals
- Increase to at least 60 percent the proportion of providers of primary care for older adults who routinely evaluate people aged 65 and older for urinary incontinence and impairment of vision, hearing cognition, and functional status
- Reduce significant visual impairment among people aged 65 and older to a prevalence of no more than 70 per 1000
- Reduce epidemic-related pneumonia and influenza deaths to no more that 7.3 per 100,000 people aged 65 and older (a 20% decrease)
- Reduce deaths among people aged 65 to 84 from falls and fall-related injuries to no more than 105 per 100,000
- Reduce edentulism to no more than 20% in people aged 65 and older (a 44% decrease)
- Reduce to no more than 90 per 1000 people the proportion of all people aged 65 and older who have difficulty in performing two or more personal care activities

Table 24-1. **Basic changes accompanying aging and their possible extrapolation to illnesses, symptoms, signs, and problems typical of the elderly**

Organ or system	Basic "normal" aging change	Disease(s) or problems
Arteries	Increased peripheral resistance; diminished aortic elasticity	Abdominal pulsation, bruits, and aneurysms
	Increased systolic and diastolic blood pressure	Positive correlation between blood pressure and morbidity: unclear if this is cause and effect or simply a correlation related to a third factor; possible protective effect on brain of moderately elevated blood pressure
	Arteriosclerotic and artherosclerotic changes in blood vessels	Occlusion of arteries leading to ischemia
Gastrointestinal tract	Diminished hydrochloric acid secretion (probable)	Association with increased iron deficiency anemia as well as possible association with gastric carcinoma and/or other absorption difficulties
	Diminished large bowel motility	Diminished frequency of bowel movements
	Diminished hepatic synthesis	Diminished serum albumin
	Decreased sensitivity to thirst	Constipation; dehydration
	Decreased absorption of calcium	Malabsorption; osteoporosis
Renal	Decrease in size of urinary bladder	Incontinence and frequency
	Decrease in size of kidneys and number of glomeruli; diminished renal blood flow, glomerular filtration rate, and tubular function	Drug toxicities when kidney is a major route of excretion; greater tendency toward at least transient, if not permanent, renal insufficiency in the presence of dehydration, diuretics, hypotension, or fever

***Table 24-1.* Basic changes accompanying aging and their possible extrapolation to illnesses, symptoms, signs, and problems typical of the elderly–cont'd**

Organ or system	Basic "normal" aging change	Disease(s) or problems
Genital tract	Enlarged prostate gland	Prostatic obstruction
	Weakening of the pelvic floor	Stress incontinence as well as cystocele and urethrocele
	Diminished vaginal and cervical secretions	Pruritus; dyspareunia
	Some, though not total, decrease in sexual function	Fear of impotence; embarrassment at sexual desires
Musculoskeletal system	Decreased synthesis and increased degradation of bone	Osteoporosis and/or fracture
	Diminshed muscle size and strength	Fatigue
Eye	Decreased accommodation to light; decreased ability to distinguish between various intensities of light	Accidents
	Increased density of lens	Cataracts
	Loss of elasticity of lens	Presbyopia
	Change in aequeous kinetics	Glaucoma
Mouth and teeth	Resorption of gum and bony tissue surrounding teeth and bone of mandible	Loss of teeth and periodontal disease
	Decreased saliva flow	Malnutrition; disturbing symptom of "burning tongue" (Glossopyrosis)
	Decreased number of taste buds	Weight loss
Ears	Anatomical change in inner ear as well as cochlea	Diminished hearing of high-pitched sounds (presbycusis)
Heart	Decreased cardiac muscle and catecholamine level	Diminished cardiac output (50% decrease by age 65); increased congestive heart failure
	Increased calcification of valves	Murmurs from aortic and mitral area and/or endocarditis; valve stenosis and/or insufficiency
	Calcification of the skeleton of the heart	Conduction defects; irritability of the cardiac muscle may result in alterations in rhythm
	Sclerosis of the conduction system	Most cases of complete heart block are of unknown origin
Lungs	Decreased elasticity and increased size of alveoli	Changes in lung mechanics, such as decreased vital capacity, maximal voluntary ventilation (MVV), and increased closing volume
	Decreased diffusion and surface area across the alveolar-capillary membrane	Diminished Po_2
	Diminished activity of cilia and decreased cough reflex	Impaired bronchoelimination and increased incidence of pneumonia
Immunologic status	Decreased T cell function	Increased negativity in skin tests such as PPD possible relationship to increased prevalence for malignancies
	Maintenance of secondary immune response (B cell antibody)	
Psychologic status	Role changes	Retirement
	Losses	
	Physical	Correlation with increased death rate within year of loss of spouse
	Psychologic	Depression
	Social	Loss of significant others, family, and friends
Hormones	Decreased metabolic clearance rate and plasma concentration of aldosterone	Decreased sodium reabsorption
	Decreased estrogen; diminished ovarian function	Postmenopausal decrease of secondary sex characteristics
	Decreased insulin response and peripheral effectiveness	Hyperglycemia
	Increased ADH response to hyperosmolarity	Inappropriate ADH with hyponatremia
	Insensitivity of pituitary gland to TRH in older healthy men	Men less likely to develop hyperthyroidism

Continued.

***Table 24-1.* Basic changes accompanying aging and their possible extrapolation to illnesses, symptoms, signs, and problems typical of the elderly–cont'd**

Organ or system	Basic "normal" aging change	Disease(s) or problems
Brain	Probable decrease in brain weight and/or number of cells in specific areas	Memory loss and/or senile dementia
	Alteration in sleep patterns; older persons tend to dream less and have increased periods of wakefulness	Increased complaints of insomnia
	Increased atherosclerosis of cerebral vessels	Multi-infarct dementia
	Increased activity of monoamine oxidase enzyme	Mental depression
	Decreased reaction time	Decrease in IQ scores when speed of response is a factor; some aspects of IQ (verbal and vocabulary skills) increase in late life
Skin	Decreased response to pain sensation and temperature changes	Accidents
	Decreased response to temperature and vibration; increased pain threshold	Burns
	Decreased subcutaneous fat; loss of fat padding over bony prominences	Decubitus ulcers
	Atrophy of sweat glands	Difficulty in body temperature regulation
	Decreased ability of body to rid itself of heat by evaporation	Heat stroke

Adapted from Libow L, Sherman F: *The care of geriatric medicine,* St Louis, 1981, Mosby. Prepared with the assistance of Rein Tidenksaar, P.A.-C., Jewish Institute for Geriatric Care, New Hyde Park, NY, and Assistant Professor of Allied Health, Health Sciences Center, State University of New York at Stony Brook, Stony Brook, NY.

❑ ❑ MISCONCEPTIONS ABOUT THE NEED FOR HEALTH CARE IN THE ELDERLY

- Disease is unavoidable in the elderly
- The results of poor health habits are irreversible
- Elders are unwilling to change
- There is no point in promoting health in the elderly

Source: Walker SN: *Am J Health Promotion* 3(4):47-52, 1989. Used with permission.

box above.) Extrinsic factors can affect intrinsic factors; they are discussed under environmental processes in this chapter.

Demographics

LIFE EXPECTANCY

Life expectancy is the number of years an individual can expect to live based upon statistical probability. A baby born in 1900 had a life expectancy of 46.3 years for males and 48.3 years for females. However, a baby born in 1982 has a life expectancy of 70.8 years for males and 77 years for females.[49] It is apparent that women tend to live longer than men and that the proportion of females to males does not remain constant with advanced age. The probability that an older woman will become a widow is relatively high. In 1989 half of all women over the age of 65 were widows.[7] Many women do and will continue to face the prospect of living their final years without the companionship, social support, and friendship of husbands. When giving consideration to members of the 75 and older age group, differences between percentages of widowed males and females becomes even more dramatic. Older men are twice as likely to be married as older women.[75]

MORTALITY RATES

Between 1950 and 1987, there was an 18% drop in the age-adjusted mortality rate for older adults.[49] The current standard of living, nutrition, prevention and treatment of infectious diseases, and progress in medical care have all sharply increased the survival rate for persons born in the United States. Once these individuals reach adulthood, they are very likely to survive to old age.

The leading causes of death for those over 65 are seen in the upper box on p. 637. These are then broken down by sex in Table 24-2. The death rate for heart disease, the leading cause of death, continued to decline in 1992. Over the last 15 years, the death rate for

❑ ❑ **LEADING CAUSES OF DEATH OF THOSE 65 YEARS OF AGE OR OLDER**

- Heart disease
- Cancer
- Cerebrovascular accident
- Chronic obstructive pulmonary disease
- Pneumonia
- Influenza
- Injury

Source: US Department of Health and Human Services: *Healthy people 2000: national health promotion and disease prevention objectives,* Boston, 1992, Jones & Bartlett. Used with permission.

***Table 24-2.* Five leading causes of death by sex**

Male	Female
Heart disease	Heart disease
Cancers	Cancers
Accidents	Cerebrovascular disease
Cerebrovascular disease	Diabetes
Chronic obstructive pulmonary disease	Accidents

Source: US Department of Health and Human Services: *Health United States 1991 and prevention profile,* May 1992.

❑ ❑ **CORONARY HEART DISEASE RATES PER 100,000, BY RACE**

Black	
Men	208
Women	129
White	
Men	185
Women	90
Native American	
Both sexes	110

Source: National Center for Health Statistics: *Health: United States,* DHHS Pub No 90-1232, Public Health Service, Washington, DC, 1990, US Government Printing Office.

coronary heart disease has declined by 40%.[71] The decrease (28%) was similar for white males and both white and black females, but lower (20%) for black males (see the lower box on this page and the box on p. 634).

The age-adjusted rate for stroke (see box on p. 634), the third leading cause of death in women and fourth in men, declined by 50% between 1970 and 1987.[49] High blood pressure has been implicated in cardiovascular disease. According to *Healthy People 2000,* high blood pressure increases the risk of heart disease 3 to 4 times and of stroke 7 times.[71] High blood pressure increase with age and also with race. Eighty-three percent of black females 65 to 74 have elevated blood pressure. In all, 38% of Blacks have high blood pressure, compared to 29% of Whites.[71]

Five-year survival rates for breast cancer, the leading cancer among women, are about 20% higher for white females than for black females.[49] Survival rates for breast cancer in women have not changed significantly between 1977 and today.

MORBIDITY

In general, health deteriorates with aging through an accumulation of chronic disorders and disabilities. Thirty million Americans have some dysfunction attributable to chronic disease, and 33% of these individuals are over 65 years old. This is the case even though the elderly account for only 11% of the population.[9] Table 24-3 lists the top 10 chronic disorders (1989) in this country. The proportion of medical events caused by selected conditions for persons over age 65 is shown in Fig. 24-3 (p. 641). In 1988, 29% of those over 65 said their health was fair or poor, compared to 7% of those under 65.[76] While life expectancy has increased, elderly people average 12 years of life with a chronic disease or condition (see box on p. 634).[49]

Race

Although women have longer lifespans among both Whites and Blacks, Whites have up to 7 years greater life expectancy at 60 years than do Blacks (Table 24-4). The table shows that Blacks have shorter lifespans than

***Table 24-3.* Age and chronic health problems**

Chronic conditions	Number of conditions per 1000 population: Under 45 years	65 and over
Arthritis	30.2	480.4
High blood pressure	42.1	394.4
Hearing impairment	39.6	295.6
Heart disease	32.5	276.6
Orthopedic impairment	93.8	172.7
Chronic sinusitis	130.2	169.4
Diabetes	6.3	98.3
Visual impairment	22.3	95.0

From Hampton FR: *The encyclopedia of aging and the elderly,* Copyright © 1992 F. Roy Hampton. Reprinted with permission by Facts on File, Inc., New York.

***Table 24-4.* Death rates, all causes, by sex, race, and age, per 100,000 resident population, 1987**

Age	Race	Sex	1987
65-74	Black	Male	4737.6
		Female	2874.5
	White	Male	3548.4
		Female	2001.8
75-84	Black	Male	9240.7
		Female	6145.7
	White	Male	8212.2
		Female	5075.2
85+	Black	Male	15,226.1
		Female	12,313.2
	White	Male	18,434.9
		Female	14,486.9

Source: National Center for Health Statistics: *Health: United States,* DHHS Pub No 90-1232, Public Health Service, Washington, DC, 1990, US Government Printing Office.

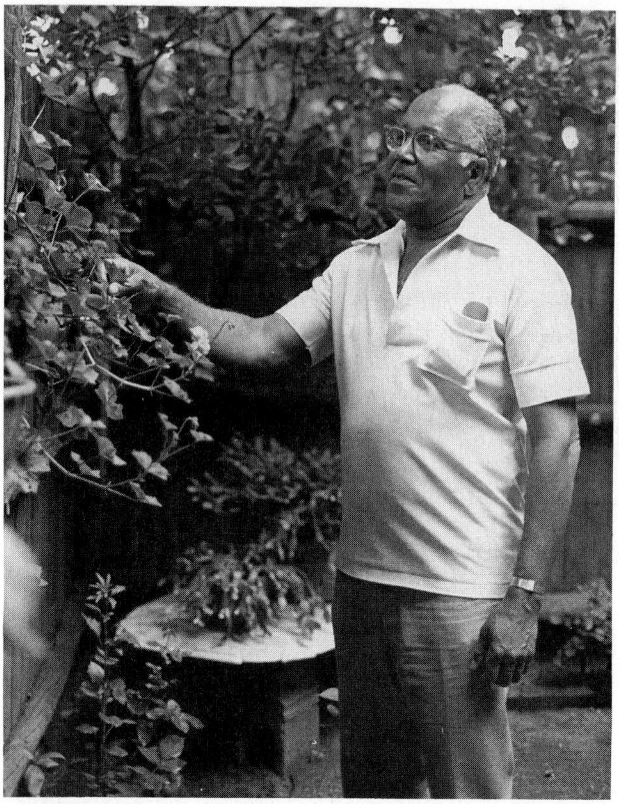

Fig. 24-1. Black adults over the age of 84 are likely to outlive their white cohorts. (Photograph by David Strickland.)

Whites. Older Blacks also rate their health as fair or poor at a higher rate (48%) than older Whites (29%).[75] However, the table also demonstrates the hardiness of very old Blacks. Those who live past age 84 are likely to outlive their white cohorts (Fig. 24-1). The total number of elderly Blacks has also increased, now representing 8.3% of all those over the age of 65.[75]

Genetics

Genetics and heredity, once thought to have great influence on lifespan, are not considered to be as important today. Although an individual from a family of long-lived relatives may live a very long life, these hereditary factors are but one part of successful aging.[31,69]

The attainment of longevity can no longer be attributed to any single factor. Physical, psychologic, social, and environmental features are interwoven to influence the lifespan.

Nutritional and Metabolic Pattern

Aging and longevity are affected by the nutritional intake of the older adult. A multiplicity of factors makes assessment of the older adult's nutritional status complex. Each assessment involves taking into account the interactions among social, cultural, economic, and physiologic factors. Lifelong eating habits continue through the older adult years. The aged are no different from other age groups in succumbing to food fads or advertisements that profess to partially or completely cure various ailments or to make them look and feel younger.

Many aged individuals live alone. When one eats alone, the outcome is often either overindulgence or lack of interest in food. Meals on Wheels is a program that encourages both the attainment of good nutrition and human contact for older adults who cannot prepare their meals. Other community feeding programs operate under Title VII of the Older Americans Act. Nutrition sites are strategically located in outreach centers and senior centers, where their purpose is to provide at least one nutritionally sound meal daily and to facilitate congregate dining to foster social contact and relationships. *Healthy People 2000* proposes to increase to 80%, the delivery of home food services to those in need (see box on p. 634).[71]

Lower incomes and inflation constantly erode the purchasing power of older adults. Therefore, they often rely on foods that satiate hunger but provide empty calories. Programs like Food Stamps have the potential to increase the purchasing power of older adults who qualify. But many older adults are hampered by limited transportation from acquiring the food stamps at designated sites.

According to Timiras, research seems to indicate that while digestion and motility change little with increasing age, the absorption of nutrients may decrease.[69] Older persons may be at risk for malnutrition as a result of physiologic change.[1] Sensory changes, dental problems, and gastrointestinal changes can create problems for older adults trying to main adequate daily nutrition. RDAs (Recommended Dietary Allowances) for caloric

❑ ❑ GUIDELINES FOR IMPROVED EATING HABITS IN OLDER ADULTS

- Caloric consumption that encourages weight control
- Program of regular exercise
- Increased consumption of complex carbohydrates
- Elimination of refined sugars
- Overall reduction of fat

intake, protein, carbohydrates, fat, vitamins, and minerals have been established by the National Academy of Sciences and the National Research Council for the young and middle-aged; but there are no RDAs for specific nutrient intake for those over 65 although there is an RDA for total caloric intake in this age group. The RDA identifies 2000 to 2800 calories for men aged 51 to 75 and 1650 to 2450 calories for those 76 years of age and older. The range for women 51 to 75 years of age is between 1400 and 2200 calories and for those 76 years of age and older 1200 to 2000 calories. Williams has stated that the caloric requirements of older adults are highly individual according to their activity level.[76]

The American Geriatrics Society has noted that there are many causes of failure to eat adequately, including depression, illness, and finances. The box gives some recommendations for improving eating habits (see the box above).

Elimination Pattern

Bowel and bladder functions in the older adult are normally only slightly altered by physiologic changes of age, but they can develop into problems severe enough to interfere with the ability to continue independent living.[1,32,69] Deviations from taught behaviors relating to bowel and bladder functioning can lead to ridicule, chastisement, and social withdrawal.

In the older adult the bladder retains its tonus, but its volume capacity decreases. Because of this situation, many healthy persons over the age of 65 are annoyed and troubled by the increasing frequency and urgency of their need to urinate. Urinary incontinence is a common and frequently debilitating problem. Although approximately 15% of older adults residing in the community have this problem, it has been estimated that as many as 25% to 35% of hospitalized and 40% to 60% of institutionalized elderly are affected.[53] Principal causes of urinary incontinence are listed in the right box on this page.

❑ ❑ CAUSES OF URINARY INCONTINENCE IN OLDER ADULTS

- Fecal impaction
- Hypercalcemia
- Hyperglycemia
- Medications, such as dieuretics, sedatives, and others
- Coffee, tea, and alcohol
- Pseudodementias
- Attention-seeking behavior
- Environment, such as poor access to bathrooms
- Urinary-tract infections
- Age-related vaginal changes
- Pelvic floor incompetency
- Neurogenic bladder
- Bladder outlet obstruction

It is not uncommon for older adults to avoid social activities because of problems with incontinence. Regular toileting and fluid restrictions before rest periods may reduce problems. Also, bladder retaining can be started as a means to help with incontinence.

In a grounded research study, Dowd found that seven women, aged 58 to 79, reported that incontinence was a threat to their self-esteem.[13] The women who felt "normal" were those who had effective continence systems. The sample reported that it was important to them to feel that they were in charge by having continence systems, by being prepared, and by organizing their lives to accommodate their systems. It was also important to the women's self-esteem to accept the incontinence as a manageable problem and to feel it an acceptable part of their lives (see box on p. 634).

Older adults may express concern, with bowel function, and they frequently discuss these problems with the nurse. Bowel problems that the nurse will encounter among this age group are constipation, fecal impaction, and bowel incontinence. Constipation may present as a serious problem to the elderly who use more laxatives, exercise less, take in decreased amounts of dietary bulk, use drugs that slow intestinal motility, and have inadequate fluid intake. Diet plays a significant role in problems with intestinal motility and constipation. Dietary modifications, such as the addition of fiber, can stimulate the colon and resolve constipation. Bran–6 to 15 g/day–has shown itself to be the most effective dietary additive in reducing the number of constipated days.[1] In a random mail survey of elderly Australians, 35% of men and 46% of women reported frequent use of dietary supplements such as bran. Similar findings have been reported in the United States.[30]

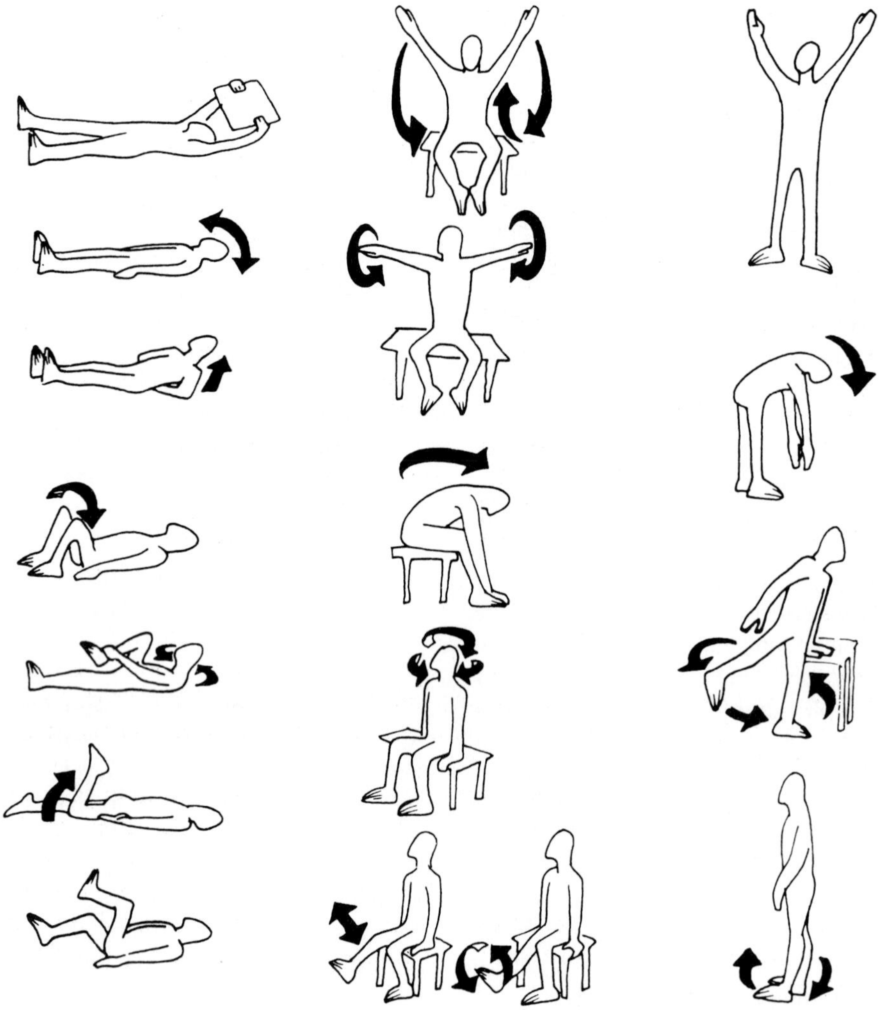

Fig. 24-2. Bed-lying, sitting, and standing exercies. (From Ebersole P, Hess P: *Toward healthy aging, human needs and nursing responses,* ed 3, St Louis, 1990, Mosby.)

Activity and Exercise

For optimal health maintenance of both psychologic and physical well-being in the older adult, physical activity is necessary. Nagler reported that although 30% of hip mobility is lost by age 40, exercise can increase the range of motion of any aged person.[47] He notes that joint stiffness and muscle shortening and weakening are more related to lifestyle than to aging. Regardless of chronological age, physical immobility hastens the aging process. In the older adult exercise is designed to maximize the rhythmic activity of large muscles and minimize the high activity of small muscles. Exercise like swimming, walking, and running maximize large-muscle usage.[16] Yet it is estimated that fewer than 30% of elders exercise regularly.[1] Before any exercise program is begun, the older person's physician should be consulted. Once it is started, activity levels should be increased gradually, and exercise should be perceived as a way of life rather than a short-term commitment. (See Fig. 24-2 for bed-lying, sitting, and standing exercises.) *Healthy People 2000* recommends that as much as possible all elders participate in light to moderate exercise that involves sustained rhythmic muscular movements such as those found in walking.[71]

The physiologic benefits of exercise include overall body toning, improved muscle support for good blood flow to and from the heart and the digestive system, favorable bowel function, appetite control, deeper respirations for better gaseous exchange, and a natural inducement for sleep. Activity should be paced for the older person's tolerance and should occur regularly. As with any new or vigorous activity, sufficient intermittent rest periods should be provided.

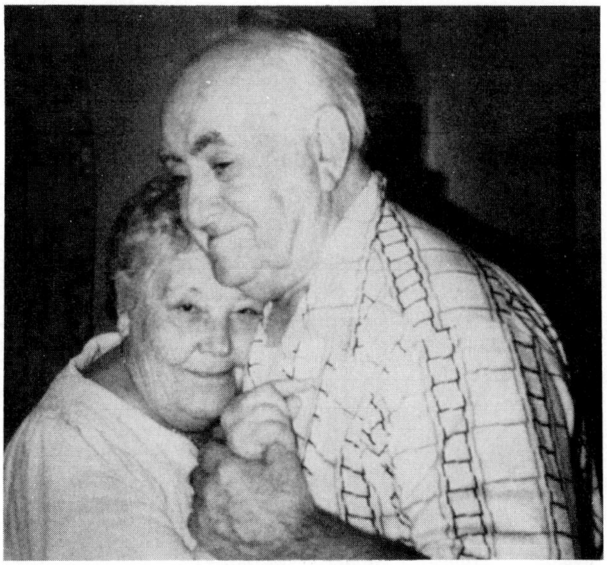

Fig. 24-3. Sexual feelings in the older adult include compan ionship, touching, and intimate communication. (From Ebersole P, Hess P: *Toward healthy aging: human needs and nursing responses,* ed 3, St Louis, 1990, Mosby.)

❑ ❑ GENERALIZATIONS ABOUT SEXUAL ACTIVITY IN OLDER ADULTS

- Sexual capacity is not lost
- Sexual activity decreases in frequency
- Differences in sexual activity are seen between men and women
- The sequential pattern of response doesn't change
- Illness often limits sexual activity
- There is a strong relationship between marital status and sexual activities
- Earlier established sexual patterns tend to continue
- Sexual performance wanes
- The stereotype of sexlessness is false
- Individual variations in sexual performance may be great

Sexual Activity

Sexuality is important to the older adult. Sexual feelings in this group shift form procreation to an emphasis on companionship, sharing, touching, and intimate communication, not just the physical act of coitus (Fig. 24-3). But older adults may be confronted with barriers to the expression of their sexuality by societal and cultural attitudes, poor health, and past trends. Nurses can assist older adults in many ways to feel comfortable with their sexuality. It is the nurses' responsibility to assist older adults in maintaining their sexual health by whatever criteria give them satisfaction.

The box on this page lists generalizations concerning sexual activity in old age. These are accepted statements and convey an appropriate picture of the older adult and sexual activity.

Sleep and Rest Pattern

The older adult needs rest and sleep to preserve energy, prevent fatigue, provide body relaxation, and relieve stress. Sleep is an extension of rest; rest is dependent on physical and mental relaxation. The older adult experiences more frequent and longer nocturnal awakenings and sleeps less than his or her younger counterpart. Both rapid eye movement and stage 4 slow wave sleep are decreased.[69] The quality of sleep generally deteriorates with age. Many older adults who fall asleep without difficulty have problems staying asleep.

A nursing assessment of the older adult's daily habits may show frequent napping during the daytime hours, as well as decreased physical activity leading to reduced sleeping during the night. A suggestion for increasing exercise and daytime activities and decreasing the number of daytime naps may be the best solution for reestablishing normal sleep patterns.

The "sundowning syndrome" is seen in some old adults who have mild to moderate organic brain syndrome. The symptoms of this syndrome present as disorientation, unusual behavior, and hallucinations seen at night. This syndrome can be treated with medication or with behavioral interventions.[20]

PSYCHOLOGIC PROCESSES

Cognitive

The cognitive processes in old age have been the subject of intensive study over the past few decades. While it is debatable what constitutes normal aging and what is disease in old age, it is clear that there are certain predictable changes in the cognitive processes with advanced age. These changes are manifested in individuals in varying ways because of the heterogeneity of the elderly, and therefore there are no age-specific normal patterns. Rather, there are predictable changes over time.[66]

Cognition, the act or process of knowing, takes in a wide array of factors, including those that are physiologic, psychologic, and sociologic in nature. Ebersole and Hess state that "the loss of cognitive capacity is the most feared of all human conditions."[15] The myth of senility in old age is one that is widely subscribed to in our culture, and it is important to clarify what is known and what is still in need of more research. Fig. 24-4 presents a histogram of reported memory changes for different age groups.

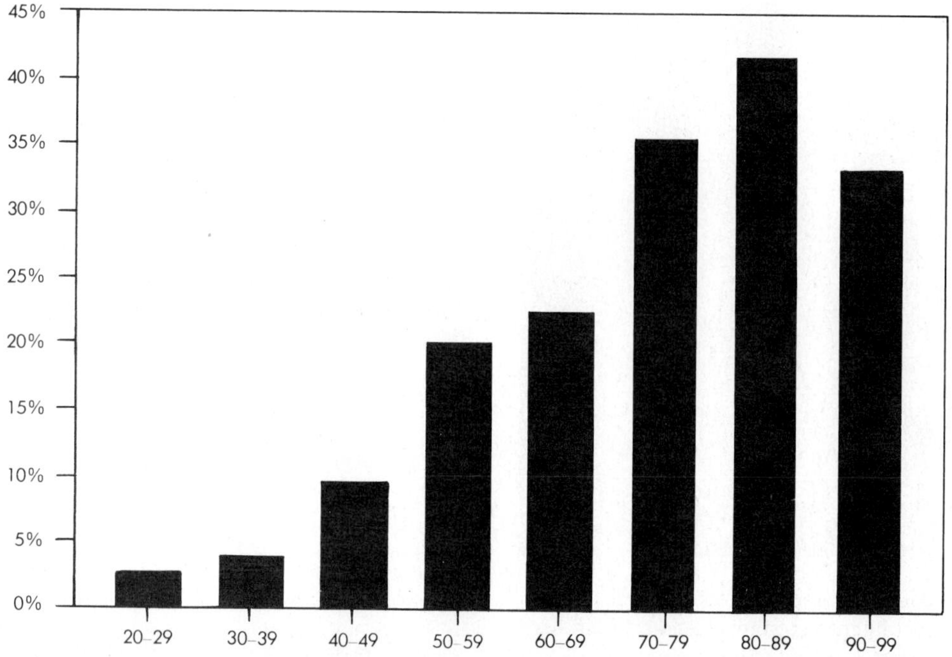

Fig. 24-4. Percentage of persons in one study reporting memory changes. (From Brocklehurst JC, Tallis RC, Fillet HM, editors: *Textbook of geriatric medicine and gerontology,* Edinburgh, Scotland, 1992, Churchill Livingstone.)

Physiologic Factors

With aging, brain weight decreases, and there is a shift in the proportion of gray matter to white matter.[14] The multiplicity of biologic changes in the brain is complex, and there is no consensus about how these changes translate into human behavior. Schaie describes old stereotypes that advanced the notion that old people are less capable of learning and lose their intellectual capacity. His work suggests that variables such as speed, performance versus potential, and pathology versus normal aging have major consequences related to data interpretation. He concludes that "reliable decrements until very old age (late 80s) cannot be found for all abilities or for all individuals"[64] In terms of pathophysiology, many diseases and disorders can affect cognition in old age. Alzheimer's disease, benign senescent forgetfulness, dementia, delirium, and depression are but a few of them. Their impact can affect judgment, problem-solving skills, and recall ability. Therefore it is important not only to clearly delineate the aging process from disease processes but also to be specific about the nature of the cognitive change and its progress over time. Certain medications have a dramatic impact on cognitive processes, and the pharmacokinetics of aged individuals produce variable outcomes.[63]

Cognitive processes have important and far-reaching implications, since the integrity of cognition has such a profound influence on an older person's ability to continue with self-care activities and remain safe. Further, cognition is what integrates the elder into the social sphere of life, providing a sense of love and belonging.

Sensory Factors

It may be that declining sensory function is responsible for cognitive changes, and it is important to evaluate the sensory sphere carefully. Elderly individuals have age-related changes in the five senses (Fig. 24-5). Visual acuity decreases because of a variety of structural changes. There is an increase in absolute light threshold, the lense becomes yellow, color discrimination becomes less acute, pupil size and its ability to constrict decreases, and peripheral vision diminishes. Cataracts–the opacification of the lens–are common in old age, as are the glaucomas, a group of eye disorders characterized by increased intraocular pressure. Broad-spectrum fluorescent lighting was preferred by elders in a research study done by Kolanowski.[33] That type of light may make it easier for the elder to discriminate colors and so improve visual perception. A summary of physiological and functional changes of the eye is presented in Table 24-5. (See also the box on p. 634.)

Hearing deficits are also common in old age, resulting from inner ear atrophy or sclerosis of the tympanic membrane. The inner ear can also undergo a number of changes, including those that are cell degenerative and nerve related. Sound threshold changes, with a concomitant difficulty in understanding what others are

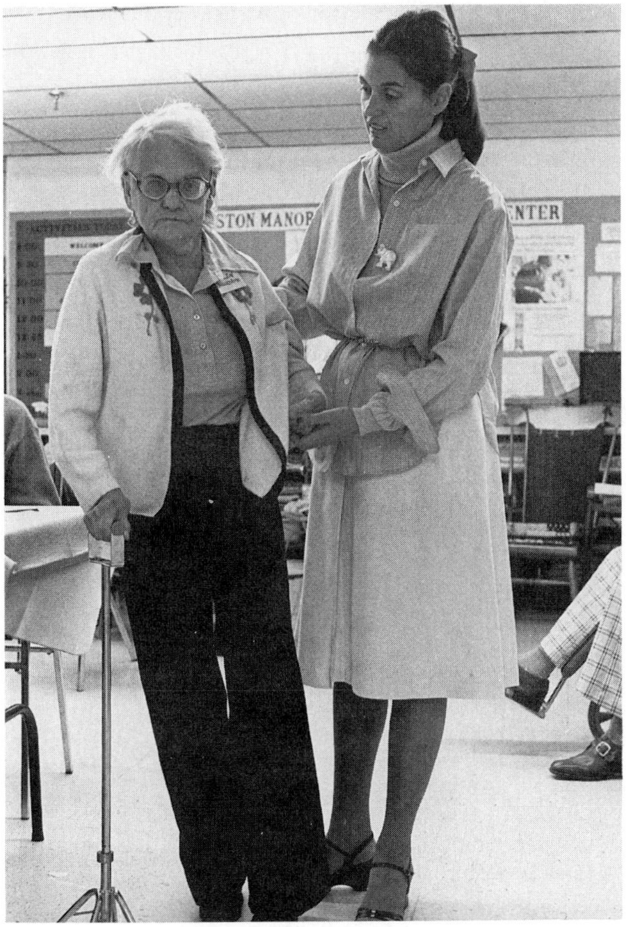

Fig. 24-5. Decreased sensory acuity and impaired balance further diminish the older adult's ability to interpret the environment. (Photograph by Douglas Bloomquist.)

Table 24-5. **Physiologic and functional changes of the eye**

Functional change	Physiologic change
Visual acuity	Morphologic changes in choroid, pigment epithelium, or retina Decreased function of rods, cones, or other natural elements
Extraocular motion	Difficulty in gazing upward and maintaining convergence
Intraocular pressure	Increased pressure
Refractive power	Increased hyperopia and myopia Presbyopia Increased lens size Nuclear sclerosis (lens) Ciliary muscle atrophy
Tear secretion	Decreased tearing Decreased lacrimal gland function Decreased goblet cell secretion
Corneal function	Loss of endothelial integrity Posterior surface pigmentation

From Kane RL, Ouslander JG, Abrass JB: *Essentials of clinical geriatrics,* New York, 1988, McGraw-Hill.

saying. These changes certainly have some impact on how the elder's cognition is perceived. While elderly persons may be able to process questions and answer them correctly if they could hear them or deduce them from the speaker's facial expression, they can be labeled confused or demented if they give an incorrect answers because they cannot hear the questions.

Taste changes with aging, in that there is a loss of taste bud receptors.[69] The flavors of sweet, sour, salt, and bitter are known to become blurred with this bud loss.[15] The sensations brought about by touch may also diminish with sensory nerve losses, especially in the presence of debilitating diseases such as diabetes, stroke, or Parkinson's disease. Finally, the ability to smell and the acuity of the olfactory nerve decrease with age as decreases the number of fibers. Cognitive reactions to such common danger signals as smoke or rotten food are impaired, not because of impaired cognition of the event, but because the appropriate sensory input to process the situation has not been received.

A careful nursing assessment is important in order to determine the possible causes of cognitive change. Psychologic changes in aging can also be brought about by changes in family structure and cultural norms, by ageism, and by changing coping patterns. Mental disorders that affect at least 10% of all elders over the age of 65 years may take the form of emotional problems or cognitive disorders.[2,4,38] Specific mental disorders in the elderly, such as depression, have been the subject of detailed study. Estimates of the prevalence of depression vary widely depending upon the sample characteristics, ranging from 15% to 60% of elders over 65 years old.[69] While it seems that the illness affects elders in much the same way it affects younger individuals, certain patterns of symptoms, as well as the elders' overall susceptibility, may be different from those of younger counterparts. Further, certain disorders that can cause depression must be ruled out before treatment ensues (see Table 24-6).

Reed noted that the incidence of depression was high in the elderly, yet little research has been done on the oldest old (those 80-100 years of age).[59] She examined a sample of 55 (36 females and 19 males) who ranged in age from 80 to 97. The researcher used a variety of qualitative and quantitative methods to examine whether self-transcendence was related to mental health in the oldest old. Reed defined self-transcendence as the management of boundaries between self, others, and the environment as evidenced by introspective examination; concern for others, and the integration of past, present, and future time. She found that elders who integrated time, were at ease with the physical changes of aging, and continued activities that provided inner satisfaction were the least depressed.

Alzheimer's disease (AD) is probably one of the most devastating diseases of older people, affecting 2 to 3

Table 24-6. **Disorders that cause depression**

Disorder	Examples
Neoplasm	Carcinomatosis, cancer of the pancreas, primary cerebral tumor, cerebral metastasis
Infection	Tuberculosis, subacute bacterial endocarditis, neurosyphilis, hepatitis, encephalitis, postencephalitic states
Cardiovascular disease	Post-myocardial infarction, congestive heart failure
Metabolic disorders	Hyperthyroidism, hypothyroidism, hyperparathyroidism, Cushing's disease, Addison's disease, hyponatremia, hypokalemia, pernicious anemia, severe anemia (any cause), protein deficiency, avitaminosis (especially vitamin B deficiencies), diabetes, uremia, hepatic disease, Wilson's disease
Degenerative disease	Parkinson's disease, Huntington's disease, primary degenerative dementia
Miscellaneous conditions	Pancreatitis, collagen vascular disorders, chronic subdural hematoma
Drug effects	Neuroleptics, barbiturates, meprobamate, benzodiazepines, alcohol, steroids, L-dopa, digitalis, methyldopa, reserpine, propranolol, hydralazine, guanethidine, clonidine

From Lehmann HE: Affective disorders in the aged, *Psych Clin North Am* 5:33, 1982.

million people. This number is expected to triple in the next 15 years, and it is estimated that $38 billion a year are spent annually in direct costs.[51] Previously, it was commonly believed that senility symptoms were a part of normal aging. Alzheimer's disease research has demonstrated clearly that this is not the case. The incidence of Alzheimer's disease increases with age. The criteria for a probable diagnosis of AD include (1) typical dementia, ascertained by objective mental status examination; (2) deficits in at least two cognitive functions; (3) progression without altered consciousness; and (4) exclusion of other diseases, by adequate evaluation, that could cause the dementia. At this time definite Alzheimer's disease can be determined only by examination of the brain (at autopsy), observing for the customary neurofibrillary tangles that are paired helical protein filaments. However, progress is being made in the development of a laboratory test for the diagnosis of Alzheimers by examining spinal fluid for the presence of an amyloid beta-protein precursor.[42] To date there is no known prevention or cure for this disease.

Management of AD centers around the management of symptoms with concomitant caregiver support. The heartbreaking behavioral changes, often including the

Table 24-7. **The four phases of Alzheimer's disease**

Phase	Observable changes
I	Onset is insidious. Spontaneity, energy, and initiative are decreased; slowness is increased. Word-finding is difficult. Learning times and reacting are slower. Anger is easier. Familiarity is sought and prefered.
II	Supervision with detailed activities such as banking is needed. Speech and understanding are much slower. Train of though is lost.
III	Personality change is marked (can be depressed). Directions must be specific and repeated for safety. Recent memory is poor. Disorientation is easy. People are incorrectly identified. Behavior is lethargic.
IV	Apathy is noticeable. Memory is poor or absent. Person can't be alone. Urinary incontinence is present. Individuals aren't recognized.

loss of recognition of loved ones, requires very thoughtful care planning, which must be individualized. Families need to know that AD is a progressive disorder of the brain affecting memory, thought, and language. The stages of AD are shown in Table 24-7.

The progression of the phases is individual, and changes may be rapid or occur over the course of several years. The major nursing role in caring for individuals and families with AD varies according to the stage of the disease, the families' responses and the support system in place. Helping families plan for the appropriate supervision of the older person, as well as making plans to ensure the safety of the AD victim, are key issues. AD victims may be unaware of such dangers as fire, traffic, or the ingestion of poisonous substances. At the same time, care-givers need to be cognizant of their own safety. AD victims can become extremely combative and violent, with mood swings. The nurse can help the family by explaining that this behavior is a part of the disease and not a personal attack. There may be tremendous guilt on the part of a family who decide they can no longer provide care for the AD victim. When nursing home placement is discussed, it is important to be sensitive to the emotional-laden impact such a discussion evokes. Sometimes, with adequate respite care services and appropriate home health aides, the elder can be maintained at home; but that is often prohibitively expensive and nonreimbursable by insurance. Appropriate financial counseling is needed, and the nurse needs to know to whom AD families can be referred for this specific information.

Support groups, usually listed in telephone directors, can provide important peer understanding for families and victims. The Alzheimer's Disease and Related Disorders Association is a national association with a network of chapters across the country. The nurse can direct families to the nearest local chapter.

Self-Perception and Self-Concept

The variability of elderly individuals is never so apparent as in the observation of self-concept.[39] Most people know of an elderly person with numerous physical disabilities who says things are going well and generally perceives life in a positive light. Conversely, other elders come to mind who seem healthy and monetarily well off but complain bitterly about their lot in life. According to Gordon, self-perception of self-concept includes "the individual's attitudes about himself or herself, perception of abilities (cognitive, affective, or physical), body image, identity, general sense of worth, and general emotional pattern."[24] Generally personality traits in individuals tend to remain constant throughout life. Individuals who have had a positive attitude in their younger years generally keep a positive outlook as they age.[2-5,22]

Coping and Stress

The depletion of reserves in elderly individuals makes them vulnerable to stress. The various ways they cope have been organized into three major groupings by Moos and Billings.[46] These are (1) appraisal-focused coping, which concerns defining the meaning of the situation; (2) problem-focused coping, which focuses on dealing with the reality of the situation by modifying the source of the threat, handling the consequences of the problem, or changing the individual self impacted upon; and (3) emotion-focused coping, which is aimed at the management of the emotions aroused by an event. The box on this page lists the components of each coping process. It seems likely that an individual utilizes parts of each grouping at the same time, depending on his or her personality and the given situation.[41]

Physiologically, elderly individuals have a more difficult time maintaining homeostasis because age reduces the function of the numerous organs. This places the elderly at risk for increased morbidity from pathologic changes. Most age-related changes are not severe enough to result in any major impairments in function. However, under stress, physiologic reserves are pushed beyond their capacity, and disorders, as well as functional decline become apparent. For example, there can be declines in the immune system, renal and pulmonary function, glucose tolerance, and cardiac function. Clinical examples provided by Rowe and Wang[61] include the following:

1. Aging is associated with significant progressive reductions in the dopamine content of the substantia nigra. These decreases may interact with pathophysiologic changes to account for the increasing prevalence of Parkinson's disease in late life, as well as increased susceptibility to extraprya-midal side effects.
2. Age-related reductions in pulmonary function are dramatic, lending to increased susceptibility to certain pneumonia.
3. Normal renal functions can be reduced by as much as 40% from that found in young adults.

These age-related changes clearly show that an elderly person is unable to ward off stressors with the same strength as a younger individual.

❑ ❑ THREE MAJOR GROUPINGS FOR THE APPRAISAL AND COPING PROCESSES

Appraisal-focused coping
- Logical analysis
- Cognitive redefinition
- Cognitive avoidance

Problem-focused coping
- Seeking information or advice
- Taking problem-solving action
- Developing alternate rewards

Emotion-focused coping
- Affective regulation
- Resigned acceptance
- Emotional discharge

Source: Moos R, Billings A: *Conceptualizing and measuring coping resources and processes.* In Goldberger L, Breynitz S, editors: *Handbook of stress: theoretical and clinical aspects,* New York, 1986, Free Press.

Value and Belief Pattern

The values and beliefs of elderly individuals are influenced by a lifetime of contact with various norms, cultures, and experiences, McCullough describes the "value history" as one way of ascertaining the basic beliefs held by an older individual, its main function being to provide a record of what a person would choose for himself or herself if competency became impaired.[43] Henderson and McConnell point out that value histories have two major limitations.[28]

First, the majority of clinicians are not trained in eliciting such information; and second, such information may not be valid under different conditions. For example, a healthy older adult may make one set of choices but change them after the onset of some acute illness. However, the basic idea that values and beliefs are important and play a crucial role in the decision-making patterns of aging persons is important. Clearly, their viewpoints will vary considerably. Variables such as sex, religion, ethnic background, birth order, and socioeconomic status all play roles in the values and beliefs of people whether they are young or old.

Spiritual well-being is one dimension with important meaning to many elderly. Guidelines have been developed that can help nurses gain insight into their elderly patients. The six considered can be found in the box below.

Self-esteem and life satisfaction have long been studied in relation to aging.[27,37,62] In one study, life satisfaction, defined as a cognitive measure of aspirations relative to one's achievements and progress toward goals, was studied in elderly black females.[68] Twenty-one urban, noninstitutionalized black women over 60 years old were randomly assigned to 2 treatment groups to study the effect of meditation and relaxation training versus didactic stress management. After a 10-week session, statistical significance was identified for life satisfaction and self-esteem for the meditation and relaxation group. This study has important implications because it suggests not only that life satisfaction and self-esteem can be improved in old age but also that the two interventions have different results. More research needs to be conducted in order to understand the variations in life satisfaction scores and self-esteem measures as they vary with race, religion, ethnicity, and socioeconomic status.

❑ ❑ SPIRITUAL ASSESSMENT

- What is the person's concept of God or spirit?
- What is the person's source of strength and hope?
- What is the significance to the person of religious rituals and practices?
- What is the perceived relationship between the person's spiritual beliefs and level of function?
- What unusual events (paranormal or normal) has the person experienced?
- Under what circumstances did these occur?

Source: Ebersole P, Hess P: *Aging as a peak experience.* In *Toward healthy aging: human needs nursing responses,* ed 3, St Louis, 1990, Mosby.

Health Perception and Management

After age 65 there is a progressive increase in the use of health services. The average hospital stay for persons age 65 to 74 was 8.2 days, compared with 9.5 days for the 86-year-and-over group. Older people account for 44% of all days in hospital.[75] Use of physician services also increases with age. It is known that the chance of needing professional help increases with age. Among the 65-to-74-year-old group, 82% reported seeing a physician in the previous year, while in the over-75-year age group, 87% had been treated by a physician in the past year. In 1988, older people had more contacts with doctors per year (9 versus 5) than those under 65.[75]

Although health declines and utilization of health care resources increases, it is important that some clinical variables do not change at all with aging. For example, the mythical disorder known as "anemia in old age" was once used to explain low hematocrit in the elderly. Today it is widely understood that hematocrit values remain constant over time and that a low value indicates the need for medical intervention.

Distinct from the aging process are the diseases associated with aging as a function of the passage of time. For example, exposure to certain environmental agents or dietary toxins over time may finally manifest in symptoms in late life. Skin cancer resulting from prolonged sun exposure is an example.[69]

There is evidence that some age-related changes may alter the common presentation of a given disease. The classic example is hyperthryoidism, which is characterized by agitation, anxiety, and a palpable thyroid gland. The heart rate increases, blood pressure rises, and there are hyperactive deep-tendon reflexes. With aging, the clinical presentation is very different. The thyroid may not be palpable, and there may be no hyperactivity or irritability. The elderly person may seem almost lethargic.

Another example is related to physiologic changes that mimic certain diseases. The changes in glucose tolerance with age imitate diabetes and can cause a false-positive oral glucose-tolerance test. This last example has profound implications on the way elders are diagnosed and greated if inappropriate laboratory values are used to evaluate certain body systems. Nurses educated about the physiologic changes and unusual disease presentations in old age are in an excellent position to give care to the elderly. They are also an invaluable resource to peers who may be aware of these changes.

The elderly themselves need to learn this information

❑ ❑ RECOMMENDED HEALTH SCREENINGS FOR THOSE 65 AND OLDER

History (screening)

Prior symptoms of transient ischemic attacks
- Dietary intake
- Physical activity
- Tobacco, alcohol, and drug use
- Functional status at home

Physical exam (screening)

Height and weight
- Blood pressure
- Visual acuity
- Hearing and hearing aids
- Clinical breast exam

Laboratory or diagnostic procedures (screening)

Nonfasting total blood cholesterol
- Dipstick urinalysis
- Mammogram
- Thyroid function tests

Diet and exercise (counseling)

Fat, cholesterol, complex carbohydrates, fiber, sodium, and calcium
- Caloric balance
- Exercise program

Substance use (counseling)

Tobacco cessation
- Alcohol and other drugs
- Limiting alcohol consumption
- Driving or other dangerous activities under the influence
- Treatment for abuse

Injury prevention (counseling)

Prevention of falls
- Safety belts
- Smoke detectors
- Smoking near bedding or upholstery
- Water heater temperature
- Safety helmets

Dental health
- Regular dental visits
- Tooth brushing and flossing

Other preventive measures
- Glaucoma testing by eye specialist

Immunizations
- Tetanus-diphtheria booster
- Influenza vaccine
- Pneumococcal vaccine

Problems to remain alert for
- Depression symptoms
- Suicide risk factors
- Abnormal bereavement
- Changes in cognitive function
- Medications that increase risk of falls
- Signs of physical abuse or neglect
- Malignant skin lesions
- Peripheral arterial disease
- Tooth decay, gingivitis, loose teeth

Adapted from Fisher M, editor: *Guide to clinical preventive services,* Baltimore, 1989, Williams & Wilkins.

as well. Both the elderly and the health care provider may believe that certain symptoms are attributable to the aging process while in fact there is a disease state present.[69] Such treatable conditions as iron deficiency anemia, foot disease that interferes with mobility, or oral pathology that interferes with food ingestion may go undetected because the elderly person sees the problem as inevitable or trivial. Nursing care that includes effective health teaching can do much to prevent the needless suffering of elderly who need medical treatment.[60]

Health maintenance practices, such as regular medical checkups and appointments made if new symptoms occur, can make a dramatic impact on the well-being of older individuals (see the box above).

ENVIRONMENTAL PROCESSES

Natural Processes

PHYSICAL AGENTS

Older adults are exposed to the same physical pollutants as their younger counterparts. Water pollution, air pollution, and noise-pollution are all potential health risks. Sensorineural hearing losses can result from environmental influences, such as noise trauma over years of exposure to loud noise.

Chronic obstructive pulmonary diseases in the elderly

includes bronchitis, asthma, emphysema, and bronchiectasis. Aged men today were perhaps the first generation to smoke all their adult lives. Results of the smoking occurred slowly over time and problems were may times not seen until lung damage had already occurred. Research has shown that because smoking can initiate and promote disease processes it is one of the most important negative predictors of longevity. For example, smokers have a 70% greater risk of coronary heart disease than do nonsmokers.[72]

Exposure to various air pollutants, such as coal or asbestos dust, also puts today's aged men at increased risk for pulmonary conditions. For older adults with pulmonary conditions, smog and other air pollutants cause increased discomfort and difficulty in breathing. During periods when the air pollution is above normal levels, older adults need to stay inside so they can continue to breathe easily.

BIOLOGIC AND BACTERIAL AGENTS

Structural changes, diminished immune response, and environmental factors predispose older adults to respiratory problems. Conditions that affect the respiratory system, particularly in older men, are among the most common life-threatening disorders–the fifth leading cause of death in this group.[49]

Respiratory disease, particularly pneumonia, is responsible for 25% of mortality in the aged.[69] Signs and symptoms manifested in the young are not commonly seen in the aged. The tendency toward atypical responses can easily lead to an incorrect diagnosis. In persons with normal immune function, vaccination against pneumococcus is approximately 60% to 75% effective.[21] Vaccine should be given once during the life-span to all individuals with chronic cardiac or pulmonary disease and conditions predisposing to pneumococcal infection and to all persons more than 65 years of age.

INFLUENZA

The older adult is susceptible to influenza viruses, and most influenza-related deaths occur in the elderly.[10] Nurses who work in various settings can help the older adult with simple suggestions, such as avoiding crowded placed–movies, restaurants, and shopping malls–when it is known that the influenza virus is prevalent. The threat of an immediate attack of influenza prompts some older adults, particularly the frail and ill, to receive an inoculation to prevent its onset (see box on p. 634). Influenza vaccine can markedly reduce the incidence of complications, hospitalizations, and death from the disease. Unfortunately, only 20% of elders routinely receive the vaccine.[10] The influenza vaccine, composed of inactivated whole virus or virus subunits grown in chick embryo cells, should be given annually to all older adults with chronic conditions, such as pulmonary or cardiac problems; those in long-term care facilities; and all persons more than 65 years of age. Vaccination is contraindicated in persons with an allergy to eggs.

One research study done on 160 adults aged 65 to 94 examined self-initiated health promotion activities related to the influenza virus.[10] The results of the interviews revealed that the sample's preventive measures were taking the vaccine, avoiding people with influenza, dressing warmly, and trying to eat balanced meals. The elders used the symptoms of elevated temperature and body aches to self-diagnose the virus. To manage the illness, they reported that they took a variety of over-the-counter medications. The second most common activity was to increase fluid consumption, especially fruit juices. Most of the subjects also reduced their intake of solid food and their activities and increased their rest periods. In this study the subjects did not identify any hazards associated with the virus and reported that they did not usually seek professional care.

TUBERCULOSIS

Tuberculosis (TB) is on the increase in the Western world and is still a threat to the older age group. This disease is prevalent in long-term care facilities and thought to be a repeat of infection acquired very early in life or a repeat primary infection. Several researchers have suggested that the increased incidence of active TB in the older adult represents a drop in immune system function.[21] This is troublesome given the advent of the drug-resistant TB.

Diagnosis of this disease in the older adult requires a high degree of clinical expertise.Signs and symptoms of tuberculosis include fatigue, anorexia, nausea, fever, night sweats, and weight loss; but atypical disease presentations often occur in the elderly. For example, they may show only weight loss and anorexia. Current therapy for tuberculosis includes Isoniazid 300 mg/day and Rifampin 600 mg/day orally for 9 months.[21]

CHEMICAL AGENTS

Although the elderly are only 12% of the U.S. population, they utilize 25% of prescription and over-the-counter medications.[11] Medication use and misuse create a health problem for older adults that is not exclusively their fault. It is evident that as a person ages the chance of experiencing a drug reaction is increased; and each additional prescribed or over-the-counter preparation taken multiplies the possibility of an adverse reaction.

Physiologic changes that are a natural result of aging profoundly influence drug therapy in the older adult. Medications must be absorbed, distributed, metabolized,

Table 24-8. **Normal age-related changes capable of altering pharmacokinetics**

Functions	Physiologic change	Comments
Absorption	1. Reduced splanchnic blood flow	Reduced ability to absorb medication taken by oral route. In many elderly this is balanced by a decrease in bowel motility, allowing increased time for absorption to occur.
	2. Reduced parietal cell functioning	Less HCl acid production with age can alter "form" of medication to that less or more absorbable; i.e., dietary iron, ferric, must be converted at acid pH to absorbable form, ferrous; ernteric coated aspirin may be broken down earlier than desired.
	3. Reduced cell number	Changes in cell number may result in more drug per unit cell. This is a particular problem with neuroleptic medications, often leading to exaggerated and even paradoxical responses.
Distribution	1. Changes in body composition	Increases in body fat with age may lead to excessive storage of fat-soluble medications (i.e., vitamin D); reduced ICF and ECF may lead to a reduced volume of distribution of water-soluble medications (i.e., alcohol), leaving more available for toxic effects.
	2. Thickening of basement membranes	May impair permeability of medication into cells.
	3. Reduced blood flow	May reduce ability of medication to reach desired site of action: suboptimal effect may occur despite a therapeutic blood level.
Metabolism and clearance	1. Decline in renal function	Renal function declines 0.6% per year after maturity. Potential for drug overdosing is ever present.
	2. Decreased cell numbers	May reduce metabolism of medication at cellular level.
	3. Subtle changes in liver function	Although rarely of clinical significance in persons with normal liver function tests, changes may result as a function of age, i.e., reduced first-pass clearance in the liver of propranolol.

From Gambert S: *Handbook of geriatrics,* New York, 1987, Plenum.

and cleared from the body (Table 24-8). Even when medications are taken as prescribed by the physical, the age-related changes discussed previously may increase the risk of unwanted or untoward side effects (see the box on p. 650).

The nurse needs to educate older adults with both written and oral instructions. Use of calendars, color-coded charts, and clocks may serve as reminders. The better informed this population is about their medications, the better they will be able to respond to the regimens prescribed by their primary physicians.

Medication compliance is problematic. Graveley and Oseasohn[25] examined medication compliance in 249 veterans ranging in age from 65 to 87. The subjects were prescribed from 1 to 19 medications, with a mean number of 3.9 medications per man. They found that only 27% of the sample was compliant. Surprisingly, there was no significant relationship between the use of memory aids and compliance. Compliance significantly decreased as the number of medications increased. Compliance was also significantly related to age, marital status, and ethnicity. The old old, unmarried Anglos (white) were the most compliant. Given the subjects, explanations for their noncompliance, the researchers suggested that clients be included in the planning and scheduling of medication routines.

ALCOHOL

Although current data indicate that alcohol problems among older adults have been underestimated and hidden, elders drink less than other age groups.[1] Alcoholism rates for the elderly are estimated at 2.2% of those aged 65 to 74 and 1.2% of those over 75.[1,6,65] Alcohol abuse in elders often goes unnoticed because the symptoms may be similar to those of other common problems of aging, and the affected individuals are no longer in the work force where they can be observed. The elderly are more vulnerable to the effects of alcohol because their systems do not detoxify and excrete as efficiently as those of younger persons.[69]

When nurses are conducting their assessment, it is

❑ ❑ MEDICATIONS FREQUENTLY IMPLICATED IN ORGANIC AFFECTIVE DISORDERS

CNS drugs

- Benzodiazepines
- Alcohol
- Tricyclic antidepressants
- Levodopa
- Amantadine
- Major tranquilizers
- Stimulants (rebound)

Antihypertensives

- Beta-blockers
- Clonidine
- Reserpine
- Methyldopa
- Prazosin

Chemotherapeutic drugs

- Vincristine
- L-asparaginase
- Interferon

Steroids

- Prendisone
- Estrogen preparations

Anticonvulsants

- Procarbazine

Others

- Cimetidine
- Digitalis

From Cassel CK, Riesenberg DE, Sorenson LB, Walsh JR, editors: *Geriatric medicine,* New York, 1990, Springer-Verlag.

important for them to ask about drug use and alcohol consumption. They must remember to discuss alcohol consumption with family, because older people often deny they have drinking problems. In cases of alcohol abuse, nurses must not convey a judgmental attitude but look at the cause of the behavior rather than the behavior itself. When older adults seek active treatment for their alcoholism, their prognosis is many times better than it is for their younger counterparts.

NUTRITION

Coronary artery disease increases with age and represents the major cause of heart disease and death in older Americans. Factors responsible for the narrowing of the blood vessels in this disease are not definitely known. However, it is thought that the narrowing can be caused by plaques that contain fat and cholesterol crystals in combination with calcium salts, connective tissue, scar tissue, and carbohydrates.

A diet high in animal products, and hence cholesterol, has been one of the factors most frequently included in the search for the cause of coronary artery disease. Each 1% decrease in serum cholesterol is thought to reduce the risk of heart disease by 2%.[71] More recently, dietary consumption of refined sugars has also been implicated. Although aging represents an important risk factor, the effect of aging itself on the development of coronary artery disease is not known.

CARCINOGENS

Dodd notes that "Cancer is largely a disease of older persons, with 67 years of age being the median age of occurrence."[12] Sixty percent of all cancer occurs after age 60, with an incidence reaching almost 1 to 10 by age 70. The cancers that commonly occur at age 65 and older are non-Hodgkin's lymphoma, lung, prostate, colon and rectum, pancreas, bladder, stomach, skin, breast, and uterus.[12,77]

Bladder cancers in older men occur frequently in chemical, rubber, and cable workers and in individuals who are exposed to antioxidants, solvents, or other carcinogens. The high-risk occupations that potentiate bladder cancer include asphalt, coal tar, and pitch workers; gas stokers; still cleaners; dyestuff users; rubber workers; textile dyers; paint manufacturers; and leather and shoe workers.[29]

A great deal of controversy surrounds the association of bladder cancer in the older adult with drinking coffee and beverages with artificial sweeteners and with smoking cigarettes. However, there has been no evidence to date to conclusively support or refute the claim that smoking, the use of large quantities of sodium or saccharin, or drinking coffee causes bladder cancer.[29] It is important for the nurse obtaining a health history from a client with urinary complaints to elicit a detailed occupational history. Exposure to specifically known carcinogenic agents, as well as involvement in high-risk occupations and concomitant urinary symptoms, should raise the suspicion of bladder cancer.

Of all the known risk factors for skin cancer, most experts believe that ultraviolet radiation from the sun is the leading cause[12] (Table 24-9). Fortunately, the most carcinogenic of the ultraviolet wavelengths can be blocked by sun-screening agents. Older adults should be cautioned about sitting in the sun for long periods of time without first applying para-aminobenzoic acid (PABA) and should be urged to avoid the times when sunlight is most intense (10 A.M. to 3 P.M.).[45]

In an examination of an elderly client, it is important

Table 24-9. **Risk factors for skin cancer**

Agent: Exogenous	Ultraviolet radiation from the sunlight Ionizing radiation x-rays, radium, medical exposure to radiation Petroleum, including coal tar and creosote preparations Long-term exposure to wind, sun, and sea Increases markedly in latitudes where the sun shines longer and exposure is greater
Host: Endogenous	Caucasions Fair complexions, such as fair-haired people of Irish, Scottish, Scandinavian lineage Xeroderma pigmentosum, which is a rare recessively inherited deficiency in one of the enzymes that repairs DNA after ultraviolet injury. Premalignant lesions: Senile keratosis Leukoplakia–a white patch that adheres to the skin Arsenical keratosis–caused by exposure to aresenic

From American Cancer Society: *Sense in the sun,* Pub No 2611-LE, New York, 1976, The Society.

to remember that the vast majority of both basal cell and squamous cell cancers occur on sun-exposed areas. The typical client with carcinoma of the skin is an elderly man showing signs of chronic exposure to solar rays (farmer, laborer, rancher).

The most important nursing interventions for older adults are first, recognition of the effects of years of maladaptive habits or hazards of occupational exposure manifesting themselves during this stage of development; second, periodic monitoring and screening of clients; and finally, alertness to the early signs and symptoms of cancers that occur during this stage, which should be taught during a screening programs' educational phase.

ACCIDENTS

The major causes of accidental death in the elderly are car accidents, falls, suffocation, fires, and poisoning.[52] Older adults are predisposed to age-related factors, such as a decrease in muscle strength and reaction time, that increase vulnerability to environmental hazards. Decreased sensory acuity and impaired balance further diminish their ability to interpret the environment (see Fig. 24-5). Because of this, falls are the greatest cause of accidents in persons over 70 years of age. Fifty percent of accidents are caused by environmental factors, such as broken stairs, icy sidewalks, inadequate lighting, frayed rugs, or exposed electrical cords.[52] A simple accident can cause not only weeks of immobilization for older adults but psychologic trauma as well. This is evidenced by their loss of confidence and self-esteem. They suddenly feel old and may become confused (see box on p. 634).

❑ ❑ **RISK FACTORS FOR FALLS**

- Use of medications or alcohol
- Poor physical condition
- Changes in visual acuity
- Inner ear disturbance
- Foot problems
- Gait and balance disorders
- Hazards in home and community

Of the 200,000 hip fractures that occur in the United States each year, 74% occur in individuals over 65 years of age. One third of women and one sixth of men who live to be 90 will have factrured a hip.[1] Those living alone are more likely to fall than those living with a spouse or family. It is estimated that two thirds of the falls by older adults may be preventable. For other risk factors for falls see the box above. The nurse is in a good position to help clients modify their environment and prevent all types of accidents, not only falls. See Table 24-10 for frequent causes of accidents and specific preventive nursing interventions.

As nurses evaluate client's homes they should teach about some of the dangers: frayed wires on electrical appliances can produce sparks that start fires, and loose scatter rugs can calls falls. Health teaching should incorporate the concept of accident prevention.

THERMAL CHANGES

The older adult's ability to feel changes in heat and cold is impaired.[69] Because of this, there are documented cases of older adults who died from the effects of heat waves or cold spells. During periods of heat and humidity, older persons usually need increased fluids and salt intake. They should stay in cool quarters, remain quiet, have more rest periods, and refrain from going out of doors when the temperature goes above 90° F. Sweating, which tends to be delayed and reduced in the old, can be facilitated by wearing light-colored, lightweight cotton clothing.[15] If sweating ceases, the older person may be at risk for heat stroke. Heat may

Table 24-10. **Frequent in-home accidents of older adults and nursing interventions**

Area of attention	Intervention
Stairways	• Secure handrails • Stairways illuminated with light switches at both top and bottom of stairways. • Nonskid treads for steps.
Bedroom	• Nightlights • Tacked down carpet • Discourage use of throw rugs • Furniture securely placed that will not obstruct clear pathways • Extension cords and telephone wires not loose and in walking areas
Bathroom	• Handrails used near tub and toilet • Nonskid mats in tub area • Bath thermometer for tub hot water
Kitchen	• Nonflammable, lightweight loose clothing when cooking • Needed dishes and cooking devices at reasonable heights • Stepstools according to specifications and only if not alone • Keep off wet floor and refrain from using slippery wax • Never climb on chairs • Keep emergency numbers handy • Locks are to be easy to open in times of emergency • Cook at front of the stove rather than at the back
Living Room	• Furniture that is easy to get in and out of • Fire detectors installed at appropriate places
Outdoors	• Stairs free of breaks and cracks, clear of snow and ice • Safe handrails • Good lighting for stairs and walkways

Table 24-11. **Factors that predispose the older adult to hypothermia**

Cause	Type
Environment	Wet, winter, sub-freezing temperatures
Medications	Major tranquilizers, alcohol
CNS Disease	Stroke, dementia, Parkinson's disease
Habits	Wear more clothing in cold temperatures rather than seeking warm shelter
Illness	Pneumonia and CHF may coincide with hypothermia
Autonomic nervous dysfunction	Age-prevalent illness or medication use may lower sympathetic response to stress

Table 24-12. **Nursing interventions for hypothermia**

Symptom	Interventions
Cold to touch	Warm hands and feet
Slow respirations	Cover with blanket
Bradycardia	Temperature to 70° F in room
Low blood pressure	Wear hat to bed at night
Slurred speech	Wear several layers of clothing
Drowsiness	Increase activity
Temperature 95° F rectally	Decrease alcohol intake

contribute to sepsis, mycodarial infarction, and cerebral vascular accidents, especially in diabetic patients. Factors that predispose the older adult to hyperthermia are listed in Table 24-11.

The clinical picture of hypothermia is often nonspecific, and the condition may remain unrecognized unless a core temperature is obtained. Often a mild alteration in mental status or a sinus bradycardia may be the only presenting sign.[21] Risk of hypothermia results when indoor temperatures are between 50° and 65° F. When this happens, the person may exhibit a dulling of the mind and fail to call for relief.[21] Several nursing interventions for hypothermia are listed in Table 24-12.

Social Processes

FAMILY ROLES AND RELATIONSHIPS

It has already been noted that role changes in late life have a significant impact on the older adult. Widowhood, retirement, and relocation can result in profound feelings of loss. The death of a spouse or significant other is a trauma of extreme complexity. For some, it may be a time of tremendous sadness and yet a time of resolution. For example, an older person who has lived through a spouse's terminal illness may be very sad and yet believe his or her partner is better off and at some peace in death. Conversely, a sudden death with no warning, as in the case of a myocardial infarction, can devastate beyond imagination. Kübler-Ross describes the grief stages of death and dying that nurses must understand fully as they counsel others.[36] These stages are denial, anger, bargaining, depression, and acceptance. Nursing care needs to respond to the individual experience of bereavement.

There is little agreement why certain life events trigger ineffectual behavioral responses. One explanation is the disengagement theory that states with aging "there is an inevitable mutual withdrawal or disengagement resulting in decreased interaction between the aging person and others in the Social System he belongs to."[11] The researchers who wrote this believe that disengagement is a universal process intrinsic to the species. Palmore

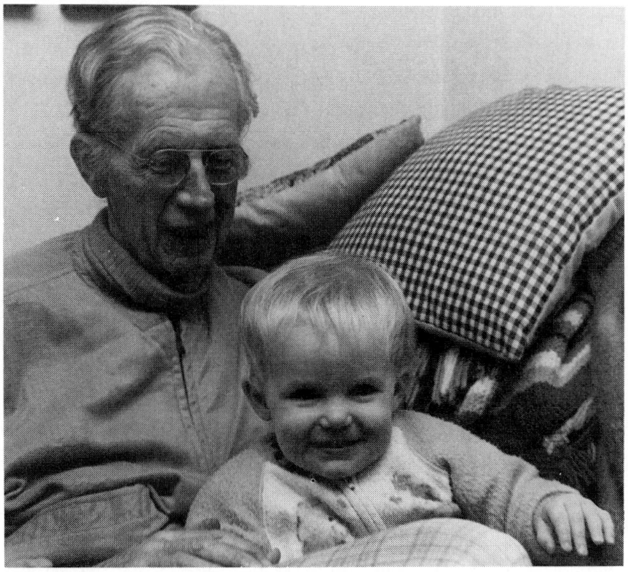

Fig. 24-6. Older persons who remain engaged are happier and healthier. (Photograph by Douglas Bloomquist.)

refuted this idea in a 10-year study of volunteers that examined their activity and degree of social engagement.[54] The generalizability of the findings of this study are limited partly because of the upper-class socioeconomic background of the subjects. Other researchers also question the notion of disengagement. Activity theorists state that involvement in a variety of activities and roles is ideal and that those older persons who remain engaged are happier and healthier (Fig. 24-6). Personality and its expression over time is considered a major determinant in how engaged or active one is in late life. Other variables, such as health, bereavement, and habit affect engagements as well. Health promotion activities related to this area center around an understanding of an individual's usual behavior and any unexpected or unexplained deviation in that behavior.

It is important to recognize that new roles come with aging while other roles are lost. Whereas grandparenting and mentorship are two roles that may be added to life with age, roles such as daughter, sister, wife, secretary, volunteer, and so forth may be lost. Nursing care should be directed toward helping the older adult identify the meaning of the role and its subsequent loss so as to work through any reactions to the loss. Most people adapt to the continuum of life and can easily understand death as a part of life. In cases where this is more traumatic, support groups, such as bereavement groups, may be very helpful. Along with role losses and gains come role changes and reversals. A retired couple may find that it is now the husband who is doing chores that were once the domain of the wife–cooking, cleaning, ironing, and so forth. Similarly, the older female may find herself in the new role of "family accountant." Role changes may be necessary, helpful, and welcomed but also very threatening. The nurse can be a support to older adults going through role changes by eliciting reactions and facilitating communication about those reactions. Significant others, such as adult children, neighbors, and friends, can provide important support in an ongoing way.

RETIREMENT

Retirement is tied in as closely with aging as is the loss of a spouse or close friends and the changes in personal vigor related to declining health. An older individuals may also decide to sell his or her house either for financial gain or to reduce the work of home maintenance. In some, such changes are welcomed; and for others, these changes are quite devastating.

Retirement is currently viewed as a normal transition in our society, although such thinking has gone back and forth over the decades. Before Social Security began in 1935, there was no specific age at which a person stopped working. In fact, at that time, our society was primarily an agricultural one. It would be a laughable notion to the farmers of that time to simply stop working on a sixty-fifth birthday. Today, with a highly industrialized and technologically sophisticated society, choices are available. Although mandatory retirement is no longer the rule, many look forward to retiring at 65 to relax and enjoy and "golden years." With average lifespans increasing, that can mean 20 years of retirement.

For those who view retirement in a positive light, it is seen as a time that is peaceful and less stressful than the work years. Retirement is presented as desirable, a time to reflect on life and enjoy the remaining time with loved ones and friends. For healthy older individuals who have an adequate amount of money, this can be a time for travel, golf, painting lessons, and other activities, such as volunteering, which require time that was unavailable during the work years. For those who view retirement negatively, it is simply a long void at the end of life that is full of ill health and financial difficulty. Loneliness is a real fear.[40]

Retirement need not be thought of as an all-or-nothing proposition. Part-time work or volunteer activities can both add to the structure of retired years and supplement a fixed income. In 1988 the American Association of Retired Persons reported that 12% of those over 65 work full time and 52% work part time.[75]

Nursing interventions surrounding the subject of retirement need to recognize the views, health, and resources of the older person. There are no standard nursing care plans that take into account the variability among older adults, and it would be a mistake to address the topic without a clear psychosocial history beforehand.

ELDER MISTREATMENT

It is tragic that the same society that can produce the genius to extend the average lifespan is also responsible for a phenomenon called elder mistreatment, a term that encompasses a variety of events that harm elderly individuals. Abuse and neglect cross all socioeconomic state and have been identified in all races and religious denominations.

Estimates suggest that approximately 700,000 to 1,200,000 of the nation's elderly are victims of "elder mistreatment," the umbrella term that includes trauma, unattended medical problems, poor hygiene or dehydration, substandard housing, battering, verbal abuse, forced confinement, or other types of harm that can occur at the hands of family, neighbors, strangers, or professional caregivers.[56]

A major impediment to the study of elder mistreatment is the lack of a common definition among researchers. Since there is no national clearinghouse for the study of elder abuse, many definitions have been proposed and are currently used (Table 24-13).

Many of these definitions have commonalities, but it is not possible to compare data from current studies, given the diverse meanings and possibilities of interpretation inherent in such definitions. It is true, however, that all these definitions reflect a relationship between an elderly person and a person acting as a caregiver with a focus upon whether a particular act was intentional or unintentional.[19] The five major theories generally proposed to account for elder mistreatment are given in the left box on p. 655.

These theories must be considered in light of one another to get a feeling for the full range of events that can cause elder mistreatment. They are limited, and to date they are useful only as guidelines to critical thinking about mistreatment. Certain signs of abuse, neglect, and

***Table 24-13.* Definitions of elder abuse**

Source	Definition
O'Malley, Segal, and Perez (1979), adapted from Connecticut Department of Aging	Abuse: The willful infliction of physical pain, injury, or debilitating mental anguish; unreasonable confinement; or deprivation by a caretaker of services that are necessary to maintain mental and physical health.
Block and Sinnott (1979)	1. Physical abuse: malnutrition; injuries, e.g., bruises, welts, sprains, dislocations, abrasions, or lacerations. 2. Psychologic abuse: verbal assault, threat, fear, isolation. 3. Material abuse: theft, misuse of money or property. 4. Medical abuse: withholding of medications or aids required.
Douglass, Hickey, and Noele (1980)	1. Passive neglect: being ignored, left alone, isolated, forgotten. 2. Active neglect: withholding of companionship, medicine, food, exercise, assistance to bathroom. 3. Verbal or emotional abuse: name-calling, insults, treating as a child, frightening, humiliation, intimidation, threats. 4. Physical abuse: being hit, slapped, bruised, sexually molested, cut, burned, physically restrained.
Lau and Kosberg (1979)	1. Physical abuse: direct beatings; withholding personal care, food, medical care; lack of supervision. 2. Psychologic abuse: verbal assaults, threats, provoking fear, isolation. 3. Material abuse: monetary or material theft or misuse. 4. Violation of rights: being forced out of one's dwelling or forced into another setting.
Wolf and Pillemer (1984)	1. Physical abuse: infliction of physical pain or injury, physical coercion (confinement against one's will), e.g., slapped, bruised, sexually molested, cut, burned, physically restrained. 2. Psychologic abuse: the infliction of mental anguish, e.g., called names, treated as child, frightened, humiliated, intimidated, threatened, isolated. 3. Material abuse: the illegal or improper exploitation and/or use of funds or other resources. 4. Active neglect: refusal or failure to fulfill a caretaking obligation, including a conscious and intentional attempt to inflict physical or emotional stress on the elder, e.g., deliberate abandonment or deliberate denial of food or health-related services. 5. Passive neglect: refusal or failure to fulfill a caretaking obligation, excluding a conscious and intentional attempt to inflict physical or emotional distress on the elder, e.g., abandonment, nonprovision of services.

From Fulmer T, O'Malley FA: *Inadequate care of the elderly: a health care perspective on abuse and neglect,* New York, 1987, Springer Publishing.

❑ ❑ FIVE MAJOR THEORIES OF ELDER MISTREATMENT

1. Impairment of the elderly person

This theory proposes that dependency brought about by age and disease-related impairment may put an elder at high risk for mistreatment. However, we know that the majority of elders with dependency needs are not mistreated, so by itself, this theory provides only a part of the picture.

2. Nonnormal care providers

This theory holds that abusive behavior as a result of alcoholism, psychiatric disease, mental retardation, or drug abuse in the elder is exhibited because the abuser is unable to control his or her impulses and abuse ensues.

3. Transgenerational violence

Theories from this set propose that mistreatment occurs because the abuser has learned violence as a normative behavior. An offshoot of this theory contends that there may also be an element of retribution in this behavior. That is, if a child grows up as a victim of abuse and later becomes responsible for the care of an aging parent, he or she may abuse that elder as revenge for past abuse.

4. Stressed caregiver

Theories related to stressed caregivers focus on the relationships between the amount of stress in the life of the caregiver and mistreatment of the elderly. Life crises, such as the loss of a job, legal problems, or death of a loved one could provide the pivotal stress that triggers abuse. Here too, we know that while stressful life events occur in families every day, abuse of old people is not the outcome. Stress is a common element in abusive situations, however, and cannot be overlooked. Rigorous research studies need to be conducted to understand the role of stress more clearly as it is related to mistreatment.

5. Exchange theory

This theory examines the interrelationship between the elder and the abuser and contends that the abusive behavior will continue to occur as long as the abuser feels some sense of "gain" from the act. This theory would fit with the belief that social isolation is dangerous for elders; and only with increased visibility by outsiders will the abusive behavior decrease.

inadequate care should be carefully evaluated (see the right box on this page). These signs, which may provide the only signal that things are not going well for the elder, should be carefully reviewed. The decision to report abuse is complex. Elders, unlike children, are adults and may not want the abuse reported. It is also difficult to assess abuse, and an incorrect assessment of abuse can be devastating to the elder and family. When the situation is clear, the nurse should follow the guidelines of her institution or state reporting laws. Adult protective service agencies are generally available to assist the abused elder. Summaries of reporting laws are available in the literature.[71]

❑ ❑ SIGNS OF ELDER MISTREATMENT

Contusions	Decubiti
Lacerations	Untreated but previously treated conditions
Abrasions	Dehydration
Fractures	Misuse of medications
Sprains	Malnutrition
Dislocations	Freezing
Burns	Poor hygiene
Oversedation	Depression
Anxiety	
Over- or under-medication	

Adapted from O'Malley TA, et al: Identifying and preventing family mediated abuse and neglect of elderly persons, *Ann Intern Med* 98:998, 1983; Fulmer T, O'Malley TA: *Inadequate care of the elderly: a health care perspective on abuse and neglect,* New York, 1987, Springer Publishing.

CULTURE AND ETHNICITY

In 1989, 13% of Whites, 8% of Blacks, and 5% of Hispanics were age 65 or over.[75] These dramatic discrepancies show the higher mortality among nonwhites at all age levels. It is expected that these proportions will remain relatively stable over the next two decades and then shift toward the mortality curve for whites.[76]

Each successive cohort of the population includes a blend of immigrants to this country. Ebersole and Hess provide a comprehensive discussion on the topic of culture and ethnicity. They emphasize that ethnicity and culture are not to be used interchangeably–ethnicity reflects social status and support subsystems, as well as culture.[15] Culture and ethnicity must be studied individually with each group.

However, nursing care must be delivered with an appreciation for the differences inherent in different cultures. For a detailed discussion of this topic, the reader should see Chapter 2.

POLICY AND LEGISLATION

Nowhere is there more political activity than in the groups responsible for social policy and aging.[18] The political impact of the "graying of America" has been enormous, and there are now more than 100 separate federal authorizations for programs benefiting older persons. This large number creates problems of consistency, equity, and authority. Further, several large programs, including the Social Security Administration, the

Health Care Financing Administration, and the Department of Veterans Affairs have difficulty with coordination because of their size and the great number of cases they handle.

Federal expenditures for older adults (either directly or indirectly) constitute over 25% of the current federal budget. The majority goes to old age and retirement programs, disability, Medicare, and Medicaid.[67,75]

Persons over 65 have a very difficult time paying for goods and services once they retire and must live on fixed incomes (Table 24-14). As a group, older people have lower socioeconomic status than other adults, but there has been an overall reduction in the poverty rate for elders; in 1965 it was 28.5%, in 1991 it was 12%.[34] In 1992 the median income of families headed by someone 65 or older was $23,179, about 62% of the median income of families with heads of household aged 25 to 65.[34] Persons 85 or older are likely to have even greater financial difficulty and are most likely to have incomes below or just above the poverty level (Table 24-15). A 1987 U.S. Bureau of the Census report documented that the poverty rate for persons over 85 was 17.6%, nearly twice the rate for those 65 to 74.[70] Older women are more likely to have financial problems than older men, with a median income of only half that of the men ($6425 versus $11,544). This trend is serious and likely to continue for the foreseeable future. Finally, Blacks and Hispanics have tremendous financial problems that become devastating in old age. Thirty-two percent of older black adults and 22% of older Hispanics have incomes below 125% of the poverty level.[70]

The financial picture presented in the preceding paragraph is of great concern because the United States is contributing enormous financial resources to programs for old people yet hundreds of thousands of the elderly population are not making ends meet.

Table 24-14. **Major sources of income for older couples in 1988**

Source	Percentage
Social Security	39
Asset Income	25
Earnings	17
Public and private pensions	17
Other sources	3

Source: Fowles CM: *A profile of older Americans: 1990,* Washington, DC, 1990, AARP Fulfillment.

Table 24-15. **Persons below poverty level by race and age**

Age	All races	White	Black	Hispanic
22-44	10.7%	8.5%	25.1%	21.2%
45-64	9.1%	7.4%	23.5%	20.4%
65+	12.2%	10.1%	33.9%	27.4%

Source: US Department of Health and Human Services: *Health status of minorities and low income groups,* ed 3, Washington, DC, 1991, The Department.

Financing Health Care for Elders

Public hospitals have historically served as the major care provider for the indigent, including older adults. The first comprehensive program began in 1966 when Medicare and Medicaid come into existence (Titles XVIII and XIX of the Social Security Act). These programs were developed as a way of improving access to health care for the elderly and indigent (see Fig. 24-7). Government health benefits today cover 63% of the elderly's

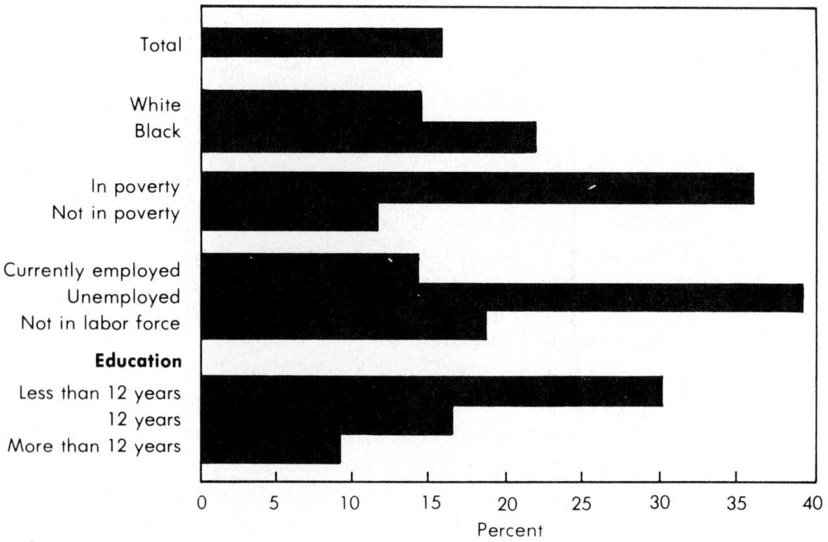

Fig. 24-7. Persons without health care coverage. (From US Department of Health and Human Services: Health United States 1991 and Prevention Profile, May 1992.)

health expenses, compared to 26% of the expenses of those under age 65.[26]

Handbooks available to the public describe benefits and eligibility requirements under Social Security, Medicare, and Medicaid.[44,73] The complexity of the system can easily overwhelm the average individual who is trying to learn the benefits coverage. Most states have information numbers listed in telephone directories. These information services can be extremely helpful. See Chapter 3 for a more comprehensive discussion of these topics.

THE HEALTH CARE DELIVERY SYSTEM FOR OLDER ADULTS

The elderly require a wide range of services that ideally exist on a continuum and are responsive to variations in the health of individuals.[17,55,58,74] During a serious acute illness, it is obvious that hospitalization may be required; but it is less obvious how much health care support will be needed after hospitalization. Fig. 24-8 identifies the array of services available with an indication of the degree of restriction each places on the elderly. It should be noted that not all services listed are available in all geographic areas, nor are they all within a price range that could be afforded by every older person. For example, retirement villages require a substantial down payment in order to enter them. Likewise, dental service coverage ranges in price depending upon whether there is an emergency need or routine prophylactic care (see box on p. 634). Encouraging to note in the current health care delivery system are the increasing number of new services available to the over-65 age group.

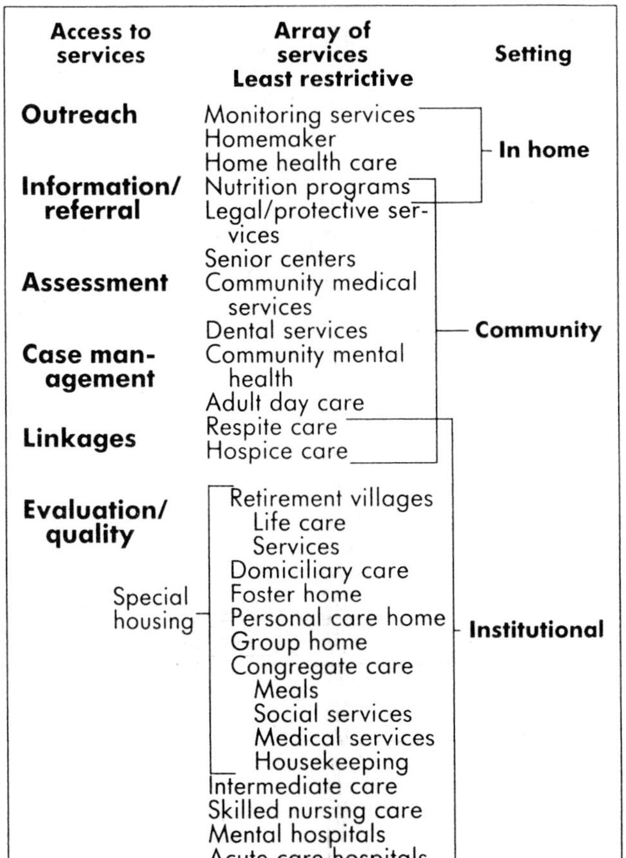

Fig. 24-8. Continuum of care for the elderly. (From Wetle T: *Handbook of geriatric care,* East Hanover, NJ, 1982, Sandoz.)

RESOURCES ON TEACHING FOR HEALTH MAINTENANCE, PROMOTION, AND PREVENTION OF ILLNESS

Today's elderly enjoy a quality of living unknown to their ancestors. However, with increased longevity, the difficulties of chronic health problems have virtually replaced the acute diseases of the past. Therefore, nursing interventions for health promotion are targeted more toward maintaining the older person's current level of function than to introducing curative activities. The nurse who specializes in the care of older adults can do much to promote the health and well-being of this group through education, research, and practice.[35]

In the educational realm, curriculums should be continually evaluated to ensure that appropriate and accurate content related to aging is evident. This is very important for nursing assistant and home health aide curriculums as well. The quality of care depends on the clinician's knowledge base in gerontologic nursing. Education for the older person is equally important and begins with an assessment of the level of understanding he or she has about health promotional activities.

The American Association of Retired Persons (AARP) provides many services to those over 55. One of these services is the distribution of booklets that outline the association's many publications.[57] Many other groups also provide lists of publications, such as the Center for the Study of Aging.[8] The topics in all the publication lists reflect a broad range of concerns common in older adults and are generally presented in a self-help manner. Among the topics covered are smoking, exercise, nutrition, and wellness. Each serves as a guide for the older person as he or she tries to negotiate a system or learn more about a health problem. They are written in layperson's terms and are easily understandable. They are also printed in large letters to accommodate vision changes in the elderly. This self-help method is especially important for older adults who may feel uncomfortable addressing questions related to finances or sexuality to nurses and physicians.

Educational seminars for older adults are an important way to teach health promotion activities. Teaching can be conducted formally in classrooms or informally while other activities are ongoing.

Previous chapters in this book have discussed various self-help groups, such as Alcoholics Anonymous and Smoking Cessation groups. These groups are certainly important to older adults as well. However, the elderly person may not be able to attend meetings of these groups because of monetary problems or physical restrictions. Such meetings can be held on-site in nursing homes or after church in order to make them more accessible.

Research needs in the area of health promotion in older adults include substantiation that commonly held beliefs apply equally to older adults. Nurse researchers involved with sleep disorders clinics, for example, provide the science necessary to understand how many hours of sleep an older adult needs in order to feel well. Clinically, this information has important applications when it comes to planning nighttime activities in rest homes and scheduling breakfast hours.

Many examples of research-based practice questions come to mind. Do older people cope differently with the stressors of life? As people age, exactly how do their caloric needs change? Do men and women change in the same manner? Do they change gradually or suddenly? The same questions could be posed for activity, exercise, rest, and sleep. Nurse researchers provide the data to make informed decisions about health promotional activity.

Older adults derive the same benefits from health promotional activity as their younger counterparts. They should not be viewed as "too old" to stop smoking, exercise, diet, or change bad health habits. Nurses can do much to change common stereotypes about the elderly. Stereotypes impede the ability of nurses to provide the best possible care for older adults. The potential for improvement is apparent, and nurses have an obligation to advance new ways of thinking about health promotion and older adults.

SUMMARY

- The average American life expectancy is over 70 years of age for both males and females.
- The fastest growing age group is those over the age of 85.
- Aging causes physiologic changes in body function.
- Many problems of old age are related to lifestyle problems.
- Some of the dysfunctional aspects of aging have extrinsic causes, such as environmental pollution.
- Nursing care can improve the quality of life in the older person.
- The elderly are as susceptible as any age group to society's problems, such as homelessness, mistreatment, and drug and alcohol abuse.

References

1. Beck JC, editor: *Geriatrics review syllabus: a core curriculum in geriatric medicine,* New York, 1989, American Geriatrics Society.
2. Belsky JK: *The psychology of aging, theory, research, practice,* Monterey, Calif, 1990, Brooks/Cole Publishing.
3. Bengston VL, Reedy M, Gordon C: *Summary of research on age changes or age differences in cognitive components of self-concepts. Study using self-conception scale.* In Birren JE, Schaie KW, editors: *Handbook of the psychology of aging,* ed 3, San Diego, 1990, Academic Press.
4. Birren JE, Schaie KW: *Handbook of the psychology of aging,* ed 3, San Diego, 1990, Academic Press.
5. Brigan OG, Kagan J, editors: *Constancy and change: a view of the issues.* In *Constancy and change in human development,* Cambridge, Mass, 1980, Harvard University Press.
6. Buchsbaum DG, et al: Screening for drinking disorders in the elderly using the CAGE questionnaire, *J Am Geriatr Soc* 40(7):662-665, 1992.
7. Carlson E: Redrawing America, *AARP Bulletin* 33(6):1, 1992.
8. Center for the Study of Aging: *Books for the professional and the public on aging health and fitness,* Washington, DC, 1991, Serif Press.
9. Chronic and other disabling conditions impair the quality of life of many Americans, Washington, DC, 1991, US Public Health Service, Office of Disease Prevention and Health Promotion.
10. Conn V: Self-care actions taken by older adults for influenza and colds, *Nurs Res* 40(3):176-181, 1991.
11. Cumming E, Henry WE: *Growing old,* New York, 1961, Basic Books.
12. Dodd GD: Cancer control and the older person: an overview, *Cancer* (suppl) 68(11):2493-2495, 1991.
13. Dowd TT: Discovering older women's experience of urinary incontinence, *Res Nurs Health* 14:179-186, 1991.
14. Duaran R, London E, Rapoport S: *Changes in the structure and energy metabolism of the aging brain.* In Schneider EL, Rowe JW, editors: *Handbook of the biology of aging,* ed 3, San Diego, 1990, Academic Press.
15. Ebersole P, Hess P: *Toward healthy aging: human needs and nursing responses,* ed 3, St Louis, 1990, Mosby.
16. Exercise improves elder's health, MD tells Congress, *Nurse RX* 2(4):1, 1992.
17. Fisher M, editor: *Guide to clinical preventive services,* Baltimore, 1989, Williams & Wilkins.
18. Fowles CM: *A profile of older Americans: 1990,* Washington, DC, 1990, AARP Fulfillment.
19. Fulmer T, O'Malley FA: *Inadequate care of the elderly. A health care perspective on abuse and neglect,* New York, 1987, Springer.
20. Gallagher-Thompson D, et al: The relations among caregiver stress, "sundowning" symptoms, and cognitive decline in Alzheimer's disease, *J Am Geriatr Soc* 40(8):807-810, 1992.
21. Gambert S: *Handbook of geriatrics,* New York, 1987, Plenum.
22. George L: The happiness syndrome: neurological and substantive issues in the study of social-psychological well-being in adulthood, *Gerontologist* 19:210, 1979.
23. Goldman J: *Decline in organic function with age.* In Rossman I, editor: *Clinical geriatrics,* ed 3, Philadelphia, 1986, JB Lippincott.
24. Gordon M: *Manual of nursing diagnosis,* New York, 1985, McGraw-Hill.
25. Graveley EA, Oseasohn CS: Multiple drug regimens: medication compliance among veterans 65 years and older, *Res*

Nurs Health 14:51-58, 1991.
26. Grimaldi PL: Congress slices medicare physician fees, *Nurs Manag* 22(1):22-24, 1991.
27. Havighurst RJ: Successful aging, *Gerontologist* 1:88, 1961.
28. Henderson JL, McConnell ES: *Ethical considerations.* In Matteson MA, McConnell ES, editors: *Gerontological nursing concepts and practice,* Philadelphia, 1987, WB Saunders.
29. Higginson J: *Human cancer: epidemiology and environmental causes,* Cambridge, UK, 1992, Cambridge Press.
30. Horwath CC, Worsley A: Dietary supplement use in a randomly selected group of elderly Australians: results from a large nutrition and health survey, *J Am Geriatr Soc* 37(8):689-696, 1989.
31. Jarvik L: *Genetic aspects of aging.* In Rossman I, editor: *Clinical geriatrics,* ed 3, Philadelphia, 1986, JB Lippincott.
32. Kane RL, Ouslander JG, Abrass IB: *Essentials of clinical geriatrics,* New York, 1984, McGraw-Hill.
33. Kolanowski AM: Restlessness in the elderly: the effect of artificial lighting, *Nurs Res* 39(3):181-183, 1990.
34. Krause N, Wray LA: Psychosocial correlates of health and illness among minority elders, *Generations* 15(4):25-30, 1991.
35. Kubok PA, Baldwin JH: From preventive health behavior to health prmotion: advancing a positive construct of health, *Adv Nurs Sci* 14(4):50-63, 1992.
36. Kübler-Ross E: *On death and dying,* New York, 1978, Macmillan.
37. Kurtz JG, Wolk S: Continued growth and life satisfaction, *Gerontologist* 15:80-83, 1975.
38. Larue A, Dessorville C, Jarvik LF: *Aging and mental disorders.* In Birren JE, Schaie KW, editors: *Handbook of the psychology of aging,* New York, 1990, Van Nostrand Reinhold.
39. Lehmann HE: Affective disorders of the aged, *Psych Clin North Am* 5:33, 1982.
40. Lemon BW, Bengston VL and Peterson JA: An exploration of the activity theory of aging: activity types and life satisfaction among in-movers to a retirement community, *J Gerontol* 27:511-523, 1987.
41. Liberman MA: *Adaptive processes in later life.* In Datan N, Ginsberg L, editors: *Lifespan developmental psychology: normative life crises,* New York, 1975, Academic Press.
42. Maugh TH: Scientists detail new early test for Alzheimers, *Los Angeles Times,* August 22, 1992.
43. McCullough LB: Medical care in elderly patients with diminished competence: an ethical analysis, *J Am Geriatr Soc* 32:151-153, 1984.
44. *Medicare and Medigap update,* Washington, DC, 1992, United Seniors Health Cooperative.
45. Mettlin C, et al: Prevention and detection in older persons, *Cancer* (suppl) 68(11): 2530-2533, 1991.
46. Moos R, Billings A: *Conceptualizing and measuring coping resources and processes.* In Goldberger L, Breynitz S, editors: *Handbook of stress: theoretical and clinical aspects,* New York, 1986, Free Press.
47. Nagler W: The case for exercise, *Update on Aging* 8(1):1, Milltown, NJ, 1992, Gerontology Institute of New Jersey.
48. National Academy of Sciences: *Recommended dietary allowances,* ed 10, Washington, DC, 1989, US Government Printing Office.
49. National Center for Health Statistics: *Health: United States,* DHHS Pub No 90-1232, Public Health Service, Washington, DC, 1990, US Government Printing Office.
50. National Center for Health Statistics: *Current estimates from the nation, NIA.* Biennial report to the Congress, US Department of Health and Human Services, Public Health Service, Bethesda, Md, 1986, US Government Printing Office.
51. National Center for Health Statistics, Bloom B: *Use of selective preventive care procedures, US 1982.* Vital health statistics series 10, No 157, DHHS Pub No PHS 86-1585, Public Health Service, Washington, DC, September 1986, US Government Printing Office.
52. National Committee for Injury Prevention and Control: *Injury prevention: meeting the challenge,* New York, 1989, Oxford University Press.
53. Ouslander J, et al: Prospective evaluation of an assessment strategy for geriatric urinary incontinence *J Amer Geriatr Soc* 37(8):715-724, 1989.
54. Palmore E: The effects of aging on activities and attitudes, *Gerontologist* 8:259-263, 1968.
55. Perspectives in health promotion and aging, *The National Resource Center on Health Promotion and Aging* 6(3):1-3 1991.
56. Pillemer K, Finkelhor D: Causes of elder abuse: caregiver stress versus problem relatives, *Am J Orthopsych* 59(2):179-187, 1989.
57. Publications List of AARP: The National Center on Health Promotion and Aging, Washington, DC, American Association of Retired Persons.
58. Rabins PV: Prevention of mental disorder in the elderly: current perspectives and future prospects, *J Am Geriatr Soc* 40:727-733, 1992.
59. Reed PG: Self-transcendence and mental health in the oldest-old adults, *Nurs Res* 40(1):5-11, 1991.
60. Rowe JW, Minaker KL: *Geriatric medicine.* In Finch E, Schneider EL, editors: *Handbook of the biology of aging,* New York, 1987, Von Nostrand Reinhold.
61. Rowe JW, Wang S: *The biology and physiology of aging.* In Rowe JW, Besdine RW, editors: *Geriatric medicine,* ed 2, Boston, 1987, Little, Brown.
62. Ryff CD: Successful aging: a developmental approach, *Gerontologist* 22(2):209-213, 1982.
63. Salzman C: *Clinical geriatric psychopharmacology,* New York, 1984, McGraw-Hill.
64. Schaie KW: *Age changes in intelligence.* In Sprott RL, editor: *Age, learning, ability and intelligence,* New York, 1980, Von Nostrand Reinhold.
65. Scherr PA, et al: Light to moderate alcohol consumption and mortality in the elderly, *J Am Geriatr Soc* 40(7):651-657, 1992.
66. Sprott RL, editor: *Age, learning, ability and intelligence,* New York, 1980, Von Nostrand Reinhold.
67. Strain RM: *Medigap reform, special interest highlights,* White Plains, NY, 1992, Office for the Aging.
68. Thomas BL: Self esteem and life satisfaction, *J Geron Nurs* 14(12):25-29, 1988.
69. Timiras PS, editor: *Physiological basis of geriatrics,* New York, 1988, Macmillan.
70. US Bureau of the Census: *Money income and poverty status of families and persons in the US: 1986,* Current Population Reports Series P-60 No 1SZ, Washington, DC, July 1987, The Bureau.
71. US Department of Health and Human Services: *Healthy people 2000: national health promotion and disease prevention objectives,* Boston, 1992, Jones & Bartlett.
72. US Department of Health and Human Services: *Medicare,* Pub No 05-10043, Baltimore, 1992, Social Security Administration.
73. US Department of Health and Human Services: *The Medicare 1992 handbook,* Pub No HCFA 10050, Baltimore, 1992, Health Care Financing Administration.
74. US Department of Health and Human Services: *Promoting health, preventing disease: objectives for the nation,* Public Health Service, Washington, DC, 1988, US Government Printing Office.
75. US Senate Special Committee on Aging in Conjunction with the AARP, FCOA, and the US AA: *Aging America: trends and projections,* Washington, DC, 1991, US Government Printing Office.
76. Williams S: *Nutrition and diet therapy,* ed 6, St Louis, 1989, Mosby.
77. Yanik R, Reis LG: Cancer in the aged, *Cancer* (suppl) 68(11):2502-2510, 1991.

UNIT FIVE

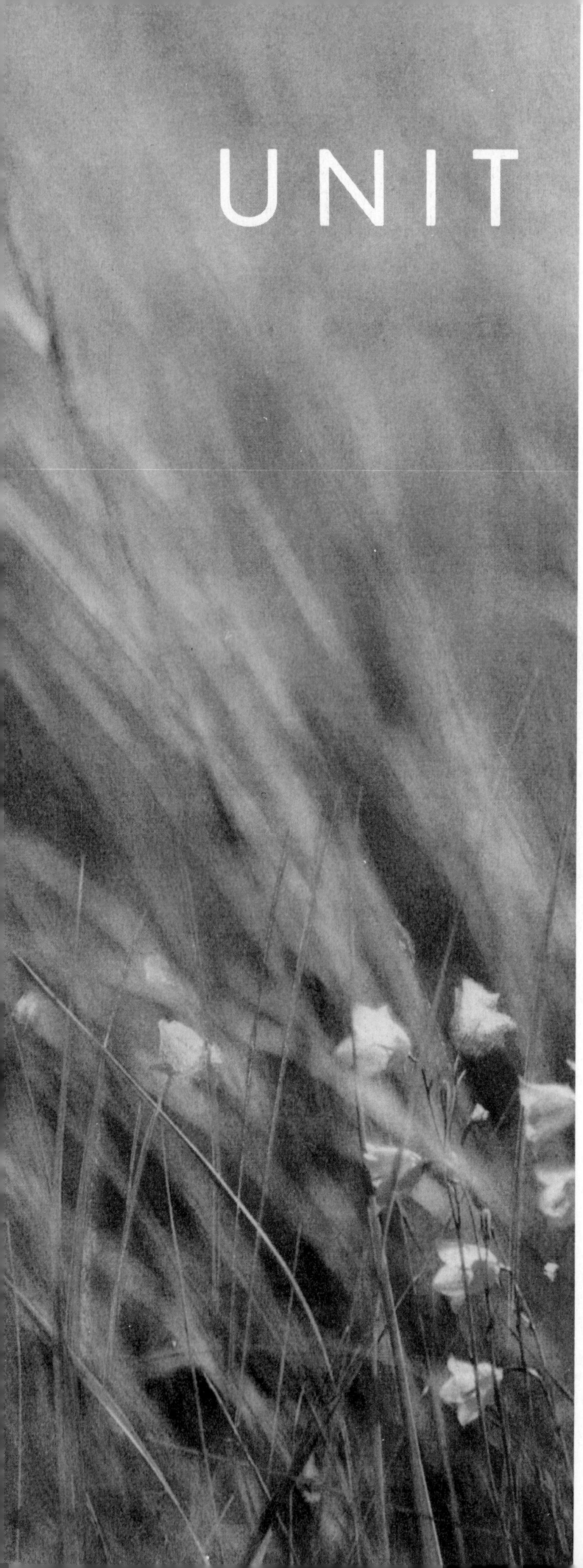

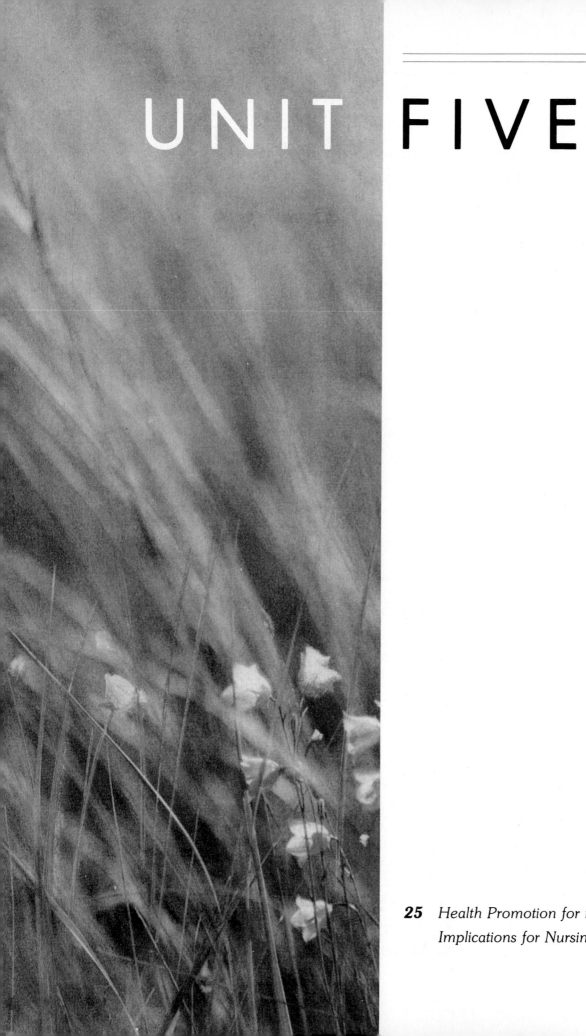

Trends

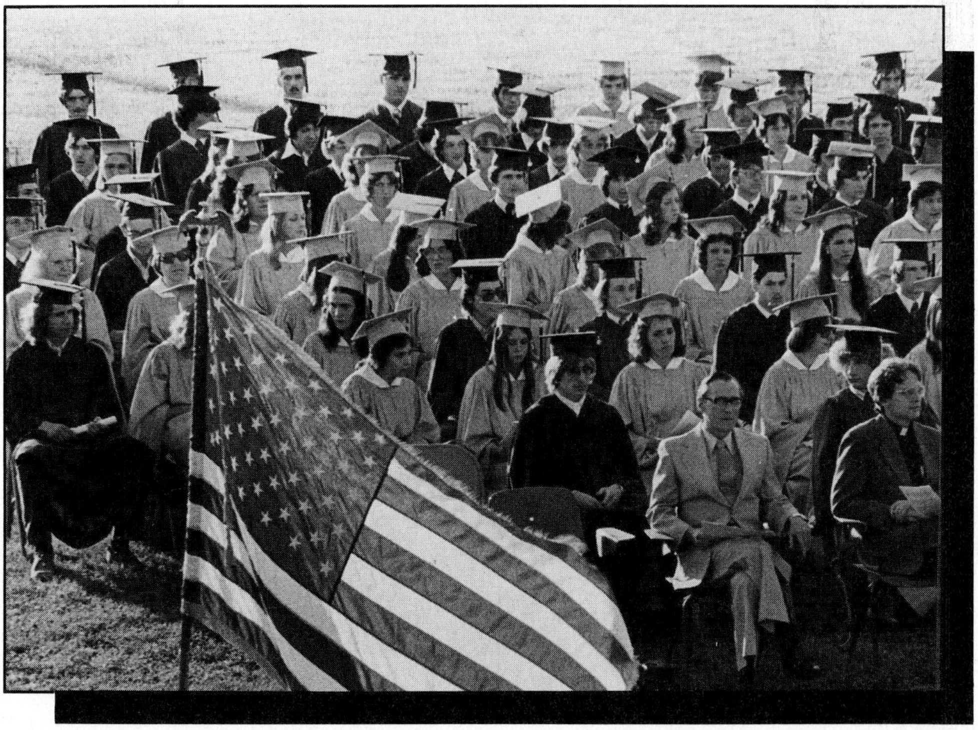

CHAPTER

25

Susan Simmons

Health Promotion for the Year 2000: Implications for Nursing

Objectives

After completing this chapter, the nurse will be able to

- *Identify nursing's contribution to the achievement of the Healthy People 2000 objectives.*
- *Summarize significant activities across public and private sectors to achieve the Healthy People 2000 objectives.*
- *Describe three health promotion priorities of the 1990s which influence nursing practice, research, and education.*
- *Discuss nursing's future role in health promotion policy development, practice, research, and education.*

Nursing's long-standing focus on health-related experiences across the lifespan is now reflected across a broad spectrum of endeavors in health promotion practice, research, and education. Such a focus, along with similar efforts from other disciplines, has inspired the development of public policy guidelines, such as *Healthy People 2000: National Health Promotion and Disease Prevention Objectives.*[27] The preceding chapters have illustrated the importance of this document in directing national attention toward improved health and well-being for all Americans by the year 2000.

Nurses are uniquely positioned among health professionals to act on the opportunities for promoting health. With an enduring emphasis on health promotion and disease prevention, nurses–as primary care providers, educators, and researchers–are critical links between the philosophy of *Healthy People 2000* and activities that promote its implementation. Opportunities for action involve defining and implementing relevant professional activities that support achievement of the year 2000 goals and objectives.

This chapter identifies the role of nursing in health promotion and disease prevention throughout the 1990s. Future directions for nursing–in terms of policy development, practice, research, and education–are provided within the context of three prevailing health promotion priorities: (1) achievement of the *Healthy People 2000* objectives, (2) the role of prevention in health care reform, and (3) health promotion for underserved populations. The chief premise for this discussion is that nurses have the vision, expertise, and experience required to provide leadership and support for a national health care system that emphasizes health promotion and disease prevention.

HEALTH PROMOTION PRIORITIES OF THE 1990s

Achievement of the *Healthy People 2000* Objectives

BACKGROUND

As a comprehensive blueprint for health promotion and disease prevention, *Healthy People 2000* represents the commitment of over 10,000 interested parties–citizens, community groups, professional organizations, and government agencies, among others–to the attainment of three overarching goals:

- Increasing the span of healthy life
- Reducing health disparities
- Achieving access to preventive services for all Americans

To assist in reaching these goals, 300 measurable objectives have been established in 22 priority areas, organized under the categories of health promotion, health protection, and preventive services. Health promotion objectives pertain to lifestyle choices about physical activity and fitness, nutrition, tobacco, alcohol and other drugs, family planning, mental health, and violent behavior. Health protection objectives address environmental or regulatory measures for occupational safety and health, food and drug safety, unintentional injuries and oral health. Preventive services objectives consist of screening, immunization, and counseling interventions provided by primary care providers, including nurses, nurse practitioners, physicians, and physician assistants.

The nursing literature is replete with philosophies of practice, research, and education that mirror the goals of objectives of *Healthy People 2000*. The first broad goal–increasing the span of healthy life for all Americans–reflects nursing's focus on clinical and research endeavors to prevent premature death and disease and improve quality of life. The second broad goal–reducing health disparities–corresponds with nursing's rich legacy of caring for those who bear a disproportionate share of preventable illness due to age, gender, race, ethnicity, or socioeconomic status. The third broad goal–achieving access to preventive services–parallels nursing's priority of establishing and reinforcing provider-patient partnerships in the interest of health promotion.

IMPLEMENTATION EFFORTS

The *Healthy People 2000* process began with intensive planning and continues with implementation, including the adoption and adaptation of objectives by numerous public and private organizations. Given the breadth of the objectives and the challenges they pose, sustained support is critical from federal, state, and local governments; professional and community organizations; schools; worksites; and voluntary agencies.

Public Health Service. Agencies within the Public Health service (PHS) have been assigned lead responsibility for each of the 22 priority areas. These agencies coordinate federal action toward achievement of the *Healthy People 2000* objectives, and involve key nongovernmental organizations in developing strategies to achieve the objectives. One such responsibility is to monitor progress through the collection of data. For example, PHS grant announcements now indicate the priority areas supported by the available funds. *Healthy People 2000: Public Health Service Action*[28] lays out the major PHS initiatives across the 22 priority areas of *Health People 2000*.

State Health Departments. By 1992, 21 states had set state health objectives for the year 2000, modeled on the national effort. Another 26 states now have health objectives under development for the year 2000. In support of both state and national health objectives, the states are implementing and evaluating their own prevention programs and policies and improving their surveillance and data capabilities. *Healthy People 2000: State Action*[29] provides an overview of the states' objective-setting process, with particular attention to the use of coalitions and partnerships with nongovernmental groups, and serves as a directory of state program resources.

Healthy People 2000 Consortium. The consortium consists of more than 300 membership organizations–representing professional, voluntary, and private sectors as well as 54 state and territorial health departments–all committed to advancing the year 2000 objectives. More than 20 general and specialty nursing organizations are members of the *Healthy People 2000* consortium. Periodic meetings are being held throughout the 1990s to assess progress and stimulate further action by these organizations. *Healthy People 2000: Consortium Action*[26] describes a broad range of activities initiated by consortium members to help achieve the year 2000 objectives.

HEALTHY PEOPLE 2000 PROGRESS REVIEWS

The first round of *Healthy People 2000* progress reviews for all 22 priority areas was completed in 1992. While many of these progress reviews identified significant improvements, gains were not universal across priority areas or population groups. There is growing evidence that the health status of Americans is characterized by unacceptable disparities linked to age, racial and ethnic identity, economic status, and gender. Consequently, a series of crosscutting *Healthy People 2000* progress reviews is currently underway for special population groups, including adolescents, older adults, women, persons with low income, persons with disabilities, and minority populations.

Trends in selected *Healthy People 2000* objectives for women are identified in Table 25-1. As the data indicate, both positive and negative trends can be seen across priority areas for women. Priority areas showing a positive trend for women include (1) a slight decrease in the prevalence of cigarette smoking, (2) a significant increase in the percentage of women who receive clinical breast examinations and mammograms, and (3) a decrease in the incidence of gonorrhea and pelvic

Table 25-1. Trends in *Healthy People 2000* objectives for women

Objective		1987 Baseline	1990	1991	Year 2000 target
1.2	*Overweight prevalence*				
	Persons 20 years+	26%	27%	28%	20%
	Women 20 years+	27%	27%	28%	20%
	Low income women 20 years+	37%	37%	39%	25%
	Black women 20 years+	44%	42%	44%	30%
2.7	*Weight loss practices among people 12 years+*				
	Overweight women 18 years+	30%	29%	22%	50%
3.4	*Cigarette smoking prevalence*				
	Persons 20 years+	29%	26%	26%	15%
	Women 20 years+	27%	23%	24%	15%
	Pregnant women	25%	19%	20%	10%
3.7	*Smoking cessation/abstinence during pregnancy*	39%		31%	60%
5.1	*Adolescents who have ever had sexual intercourse*				
	Women 15 years	27%	43%	45%	15%
	Women 17 years	50%	67%	65%	50%
7.1	*Homicides* (per 100,000)				
	Total population	8.5	10.1		7.2
	Black women aged 15-34	20.2	22.1		16.0
9.7	*Hip fractures* (per 100,000)				
	Persons 65 years+	714	776	814	607
	White women 65 years+	2721	3075	3791	2177
14.11	*Prenatal care* (% live births)	76.0%	75.8%		90%
	Black women	60.8%	60.6%		90%
	Hispanic women	61.0%	60.2%		90%
	Native American women	57.6%	57.9%		90%
16.3	*Breast cancer deaths* (age adjusted per 100,000 women)	23.0	23.1		20.6
16.4	*Cervical cancer deaths* (age adjusted per 100,000 women)	2.8	2.8		1.3
16.11	*Breast examinations/mammograms*				
	Women 40 years+ (ever received)	36%	60%		80%
	Women 50 years+ (received in preceding 1-2 years)	25%	47%	54%	60%
16.12	*Pap tests*				
	Received in preceding 3 years	75%		59%	85%
	Low-income women 18 years+	64%		50%	80%
19.1	*Gonorrhea incidence* (per 100,000)	300	278	249	225
	Women 15-44 years	501	493	419	290
19.6	*Pelvic inflammatory disease* (per 100,000)				
	Women 15-44 years	311	261		250

From statistics compiled by the *Healthy People 2000* Data Unit, National Center for Health Statistics, Centers for Disease Control and Prevention, US Public Health Service, 1993.

inflammatory disease. Priority areas showing neither a positive nor a negative trend include (1) women who receive prenatal care in the first trimester of pregnancy and (2) numbers of breast and cervical cancer deaths. Priority areas showing a negative trend for women include (1) overweight prevalence, (2) weight loss practices among overweight women, (3) smoking cessation and abstinence during pregnancy, (4) homicides in black women, (5) hip fractures in older white women, and (6) women who undergo cervical cancer screening.

The Role of Prevention in Health Care Reform

BACKGROUND

The current high-cost health care delivery system, which emphasizes acute hospital care as opposed to primary and preventive care, has served as a fundamental catalyst for recent health care reform efforts. Both policy makers and the American public have come to realize that the ultimate solution to the current health care crisis is comprehensive reform in the financing, organization, and provision of health care services within an integrated and coordinated system.

The concept of equitable access to preventive care for all Americans has been nourished in recent years by the demonstrated effectiveness of clinical preventive services in reducing premature morbidity and mortality.[25] Yet an equal opportunity for health promotion through preventive care remains unrealized for a growing percentage of citizens. According to the National Association of Community Health Centers,[7] approximately 50 million Americans were underserved in 1990. Given that an estimated 37 million citizens are without health insurance[6] and that 20 million more have insufficient coverage in the event of a serious illness,[20] equitable access to primary and preventive care has become one of the pivotal health priorities of the 1990s. Nursing's long-standing support of health promotion for underserved groups can serve as a touchstone for achieving equitable access to preventive health services for all Americans.

CLINICAL EFFECTIVENESS OF PREVENTIVE HEALTH CARE

The clinical effectiveness of preventive health care was identified in the U.S. Preventive Services Task Force report, *Guide to Clinical Preventive Services.*[25] This report provides age-, gender-, and risk factor-specific recommendations for the prevention of over 60 major causes of morbidity and mortality. The methodology of the report involved a thorough examination of the quality of scientific evidence for the effectiveness of screening tests, immunizations, and counseling interventions. A relevant finding for nursing was the recommendation that counseling to change personal health behaviors long before the onset of clinical disease is the most promising role for health promotion in current health are practice (see box to the right on this page). The task force report advises that both practitioners and clients assume responsibility for health promotion, with the client being empowered for behavioral change.

COST-EFFECTIVENESS OF PREVENTIVE HEALTH CARE

The belief that prevention be judged on the criterion of whether the gains in health are a reasonable return for the costs occurs at a time when the nation continues to endure the economic burden of preventable illness and death (Table 25-2). The portion of the Gross National Product going to health care rose from 5.3% in 1960 to 12.2% ($666 billion) in 1990.[17] The diagnosis and treatment of diseases, including heart disease, cancer, injuries and HIV/AIDS, have outstripped society's ability to pay for what are essentially preventable conditions.

The reality of skyrocketing health care expenditures has ushered in cost-effectiveness analysis as a method for determining how financial resources are, and should be, used in health care. The specific purpose of cost-effectiveness analysis is to help clinicians and policy makers focus on investments that bring the most health for the required expenditure, with outcomes reported either as a single measure (e.g., years of life saved) or as several measures combined on a single scale (e.g., quality-adjusted life years.)[5] Cost-effectiveness analyses of preventive services have included (as of 1993) screenings for lead, cholesterol, breast cancer, and cervical cancer. The fact that most counseling interventions have not been analyzed for cost-effectiveness is consistent with the finding that primary care physicians spend less than 15% of their time counseling clients on weight reduction, cholesterol reduction, smoking cessation, and breast self-examination.[31] A primary care provider survey, which is currently being sponsored by the PHS to track provider-related *Healthy People 2000* objectives, should help to determine the nature and amount of preventive health care delivered by primary care provid-

❑ ❑ RECOMMENDATIONS FOR CLIENT EDUCATION AND COUNSELING

1. Develop a therapeutic alliance through provider-client partnerships.
2. Counsel all clients in an age-, gender-, and culturally appropriate manner.
3. Ensure that clients understand the relationship between behavior and health. (Keep in mind that knowledge is a necessary, but not a sufficient, stimulus for change.)
4. Work with clients to assess barriers to behavior change.
5. Gain commitment from clients to change.
6. Involve clients in selecting risk factors to change.
7. Use a combination of strategies (e.g., individual counseling, group classes, audiovisual aids, written materials, community resources).
8. Design a behavior-modification plan.
9. Monitor progress through follow-up contact.
10. Share responsibility for client education with other health professionals.

From US Preventive Services Task Force: *Guide to clinical preventive services: an assessment of the effectiveness of 169 interventions,* Baltimore, 1989, Williams & Wilkins.

***Table 25-2.* Costs of treatment for selected preventable conditions**

Condition	Overall magnitude	Avoidable intervention*	Cost per patient†
Heart disease	500,000 deaths/yr 284,000 bypass surgeries/yr	Coronary bypass surgery	$30,000
Cancer	510,000 deaths/yr 1 million new cases/yr	Lung cancer Rx Cervical cancer Rx	$30,000 $29,000
Injuries	142,500 deaths/yr 2.3 million hospitalizations/yr 177,000 spinal cord injuries	Quadriplegia Rx/rehabilitation Severe head injury Rx/rehabilitation	$570,000 (lifetime) $310,000
Alcoholism	105,000 alcohol related deaths/yr 18.5 million alcohol abusers	Liver transplant	$250,000
Low birth weight baby (LBWB)	23,000 deaths/yr 260,000 LBWB/yr	Neonatal intensive care for LBWB Care for very LBWB	$10,000 $31,000
Inadequate	Lacking basic immunization series: 20% to 30% aged 2 yr or younger	Congenital rubella	$422,000 (lifetime)

From data compiled and updated to June 1991 dollars by the Office of Disease Prevention and Health Promotion, US Public Health Service.
*Examples (other interventions may apply).
†Representative first-year costs, except as noted. Not indicated are non-health care costs, such as lost economic productivity.

ers, including nurse practitioners and nurses.

A number of fundamental questions remain concerning the cost-effectiveness of preventive health care. It has been estimated that providing coverage for preventive services is likely to increase costs in the short term.[24] Furthermore, preventive services vary in clinical and cost-effectiveness when performed by health care providers using different guidelines and methods. A third consideration involves the differential costs per year for services that have undergone cost-effectiveness analysis, suggesting that personal and social values may influence whether a preventive intervention is judged to be cost-effective.

Because the U.S. health care delivery system has evolved with a bias toward coverage for acute illness, it has been difficult to include coverage for preventive services in most public and private insurance plans. At a time of heightened attention to health care reform, it is critical that preventive services of known effectiveness be incorporated into a comprehensive benefits package for all Americans. A core set of clinical preventive services–immunizations, screening, and counseling–was recently prepared for inclusion in an overall benefits package.[30] These services are specified according to age- and gender-specific periodic health examinations in order to assure their economic efficience in primary care settings.

Health Promotion for Underserved Populations

BACKGROUND

Between 1980 and 1989, the percentage of individuals under age 65 without health insurance increased from 13% to 16%. Among those persons most likely to be uninsured were Blacks (22%), persons with incomes below the poverty line (36%), the unemployed (39%), and persons with less than 12 years of education (30%). Between 1984 and 1989, persons with higher incomes were more likely to receive their care through ambulatory visits, whereas persons with lower incomes were more likely to use acute care hospitals for their primary source of care. In 1990, less than 1% of Medicaid funds were directed to early and periodic screening, rural health clinics, and family planning services.[17]

According to a report on the 1987 *National Medical Expenditure Survey* (NMES),[1] persons who are uninsured or who have inadequate coverage usually forego primary and preventive health care. Additional evidence of this primary care underservice is found in the Robert Wood Johnson Foundation's National Access to Care Surveys,[21-23] which identify factors associated with utilization of health care services. The most recent survey indicated that 43 million Americans (18% of the population) did not have a health care provider, clinic, or hospital as a regular source of health care, representing a 7% increase over an earlier survey. At the same time, the percentage of persons who reported having no ambulatory visit in the prior 12 months rose significantly, from 19% to 33%. Underserved populations were affected disproportionately, with a significantly higher percentage of poor, uninsured, and ethnic minority individuals reporting no regular source of care, no ambulatory visits within the preceding 12 months, and fair or poor health status.

HEALTH PROFILES OF UNDERSERVED POPULATIONS

Infants. Perhaps no other indicator of health is as dramatic for underserved populations as the infant mortality rate. Although the mortality rate for American infants dropped from 29.2 per 1000 live births in 1950 to 9.1 per 1000 births in 1990,[17] the U.S. infant mortality rate continues to rank among the lowest of industrialized nations. And despite an overall downward trend, the infant mortality rates for racial and ethnic minority groups have remained consistently higher than the national average. For example, black infants are twice as likely as white infants to die before their first birthday and are twice as likely to be born weighing less than 2500 g.[17]

Poor pregnancy outcomes are influenced by late or no prenatal care, racial/ethnic minority status, low income, low educational level, unemployment, being unmarried, and teen pregnancy.[10] Women living in poverty are three times more likely that nonpoor women to obtain late prenatal care or none at all. In 1989, early prenatal care was used by only 57% of Mexican American and American Indian women and 62% of black, Central and South American, and Puerto Rican women, compared with 79% of white women.[17]

Children and Adolescents. As in the case of underserved mothers and infants, the adverse health status of disadvantaged children is associated with a variety of social disadvantages, including poverty, limited parental education, extramarital births, adolescent parenthood, and racial/ethnic minority status. Underserved children are more likely to die during early childhood; more likely to experience acute illnesses, injuries, lead poisoning, or child abuse; and more likely to suffer from nutrition-related problems, chronic illnesses, and developmental disabilities.[13]

The 1986 National Access to Care Survey[21] showed that 15% of all poor children lack a regular source of health care–twice the percentage of nonpoor children. An analysis of preventive care use by school-aged children demonstrated that those in families living in poverty were 52% less likely to receive routine medical and dental examinations.[18] Poor families are more likely to seek their care in acute care settings, such as hospital emergency rooms, which are not designed to provide primary or preventive care services. Yet because they engage in fewer health-promoting behaviors than the nonpoor, families living in poverty are in greater need of preventive health care. Inadequate knowledge of the importance of preventive behaviors and services, insufficient funds, preoccupation with immediate survival issues, and feelings of powerlessness are all cited as reasons why families living in poverty do not have preventive care patterns that are favorable to the health of infants and children.[14]

For the leading causes of death among adolescents–unintentional injuries, homicide, and suicide–racial/ethnic minority groups experience disproportionately higher rates. Between 1985 and 1989, the homicide rate for black males aged 15 to 24 years increased by 74%. The suicide rate for Native American youth is nearly twice the rate for white youth.[17] Low-income adolescents have significantly higher rates of sexually transmitted diseases, unintended pregnancy, depression, and substance abuse.[27] Adolescents without health insurance, often from poor working families, are more likely to delay seeking health care.[11]

Adults. The health and preventive care patterns of adults, like those of infants and children, are shaped by a mosaic of economic, ethnic, and other social characteristics. For example, health disparities between black and white adults are seen by a shorter life expectancy for Blacks as well as a higher incidence of preventable conditions, including cardiovascular disease, cancer, diabetes, homicide, and obesity.[17] As in the case of other underserved groups, low-income adults are more likely to use hospital emergency room as their routine source of health care and are more likely to delay seeking needed care.[19]

The tendency for adult populations at greater risk for disease to be less likely to receive preventive services has been observed for specific screening procedures. This "reverse targeting" tendency was predicted primarily by inadequate insurance coverage in a sample of middle-aged women who received four screening tests: blood pressure checkup, clinical breast examination, Papanicolaou test, and glaucoma examination. Lack of insurance was more prevalent among Blacks (20%), the poor (35%), those without a high school education (19%), and those in fair or poor health (18%).[32] The impact of insurance status has also been demonstrated in studies of screening mammography, which showed that having no insurance and being non-White, poor, and older were all associated with less likelihood of receiving a screening mammogram in the past year.[3,33]

Among all age groups, older adults represent those who are most in need of clinical preventive services to offset disabling and life-threatening conditions. Especially important for this age group are screening tests for breast, cervical, and colorectal cancers; cardiovascular disease; and immunizations against pneumococcal disease and influenza.[27] Yet public and private insurers have not traditionally covered the cost of primary and secondary preventive services.As a result, the delivery of health care to older adults is often fragmented, with individuals having no primary care provider as case manager.

The current Medicare structure leaves older women especially vulnerable due to the inadequate coverage of chronic conditions typically experienced by more women than men. Older women who have only Medicare coverage are more likely than men to have illnesses with moderate to high out-of-pocket expenses.[8] Given the predominance of poverty among older women, out-of-pocket expenses become more of a hardship in this population, who have limited or no coverage for primary and secondary preventive services.

The Homeless. For some underserved populations, unstable or dangerous physical environments, isolation, and the lack of adequate and available health services exacerbate the already high rates of preventable illness and death. Perhaps for no other group is the convergence of economic hardship, social isolation, and physical and mental disability more apparent than for homeless individuals and families. The Institute of Medicine's report, *Homelessness, Health and Human Needs,*[9] revealed that families with children are the fastest-growing group among the homeless.Data show that homeless children experience higher numbers of upper respiratory infections, malnutrition, skin diseases, and traumas. In addition, these children have immunization delays, elevated blood lead levels, and increased rates of child abuse and hospital admissions.[12] A study of homeless adults in South Carolina found that the majority of respondents had no insurance coverage, knew little about the availability of health services, and had no regular source of primary health care.[15] A survey of shelters serving women in Chicago revealed that most of the women did not view prenatal care as a high priority, in large part because they were fearful of losing their infants if they listed the shelter as their place of residence.[4]

Nursing Leadership in Health Promotion: Implications for Policy Development

The health promotion priorities discussed in this chapter pose a dramatic challenge for nurse clinicians, educators and researchers. Now is the time for nurses, as individuals and as a group, to play a key role in a health care system that underscores health promotion and disease prevention. Because nurses believe in and practice the principles of primary and preventive health care, their leadership and participation in health promotion policy development is critical during the current era of health care reform. Through a perspective on the development of community-based, health-promotion programs, nurses can bring a balance to decisions made about the appropriate use of health care resources. Likewise, as members of clinical and academic institutions, nurses can influence policy by communicating the principles of health promotion.

The preventive services delivered by nurses–health assessment, screening, and counseling–are necessary toois to empower clients to promote and maintain optimum health and well-being. Achieving the year 2000 objectives is possible only by a comprehensive implementation of preventive health care at the community level, including worksites, schools, homes, and neighborhood settings. In collaboration with other professional and business groups, nurses can empower clients to become active participants in defining their health needs, in making informed decisions to meets such needs, and ultimately, in adopting healthy lifestyles.

The current and future demand for primary care providers will continue to spur the need for training nurse practitioners and other advanced practice nurses. Meeting such a demand can be met if nursing students at the undergraduate level are introduced early to the concepts and practical application of health promotion and disease prevention. Curricula which provide clinical experiences directed toward maximizing health will enable nurses to fulfill innovative roles in a reformed health care system. Given the increasing focus on self-care in disease prevention and health promotion, nurses can respond directly to clients' needs by focusing on health promotion and by supporting clients as they learn new ways to work and live.

In the area of research, there is a heightened need for nurses to test individual, family, and community-level interventions which optimize health and well-being. Due to the evidence that maximum effectiveness in lifestyle modification occurs through a combination of educational and environmental interventions, future research should identify the ideal combination of these interventions under different conditions. In addition, nurse researchers need to examine the relationship between the delivery of preventive health care and cost, access, utilization, and health outcomes associated with such care.

Given the acknowledged importance of health promotion and preventive care in health care reform deliberations, it is critical to articulate an agenda that will assure nursing's role of leadership and active participation. The beginnings of such an agenda is evident in the report, *Nursing's Agenda for Health Care Reform,*[2] a broad-based strategy that calls for a nationally defined standard package of primary and preventive health services. A central theme in this report is the development of provider-client relationships targeted to activities that will improve health outcomes in a cost-effective manner. By acting on this agenda, nursing can assume a position of leadership in promoting the health of all Americans. Three principal goals for nurses to consider include the following:

1. *Participate in health promotion policy development.* Cultivating nursing leadership in health policy development involves time, funds, expertise, authority, and education.[16] While nurses continue to focus on the care of individuals in acute settings, there should be equal support for altering the contexts which result in preventable illness and disability. Professional attention to health-promoting environments and behaviors provides an entry point to the development of community-based models of primary care that emphasize health promotion and disease prevention.

   Manuscripts, monographs, and other formal viewpoints should be developed by nursing groups concerned with economic, practice, education, or research issues in health promotion. In an effort to build strong linkages, nurses should present position papers before a variety of professional and government policy makers. One approach would be to evaluate the *Healthy People 2000* report[27] and identify how nursing initiatives support achievement of the year 2000 objectives. By directly linking disciplinary policies and programs to the national prevention agenda, nurses can more fully participate in health promotion policy development.

2. *Influence public expectations about health promotion.* Presentations and other forms of public dialogue and education will help to raise awareness of the value of individual and community health promotion. Nurses have the collective capacity to change the philosophy of the system from selling health care in the marketplace to creating a milieu for health behavior change. Encouraging meaningful community participation in addressing health issues provides a significant opportunity to narrow the gap between what is possible in terms of health promotion in this country and what is the reality.

   Increasing consumer demand for preventive health care as well as provider willingness to offer such care is largely influence by the coverage of preventive services in health insurance plans. Nurses should participate in a broad range of activities that evaluate options for expanding coverage of preventive health care. In addition, nurses should lobby for equitable reimbursement of preventive services delivery. One approach might be to advocate a periodic preventive health visit fee, which would specify a science-based package of preventive services for different population groups.

3. *Promote equitable access to preventive health care.* Given the higher rates of preventable conditions among underserved populations, there is a justified need to promote the distribution and utilization of preventive health services. Community-based efforts that combine public and private resources should be targeted to those most in need of preventive health care. Delivery models that focus on the integration of preventive and primary care should be expanded into more areas.

   Preventive health care delivery should be based on a broad research agenda that encompasses multiple health and social science perspectives. Nurses should participate in areas of research that will influence both personal and community health in a cost-effective manner. Service delivery can also benefit from an expanded health services research agenda that fosters collaboration with other disciplines, such as nutrition and education. Most importantly, preventive health care should be adapted to the health and social problems of specific groups and supplemented as needed by the services of social workers, nutritionists, translaters, and outreach workers. Alternative forms of preventive service delivery should also be examined, including mobile vans, schools and worksite clinics, and other community-based sites.

SUMMARY

In this chapter, priority issues and future directions for nursing in the area of health promotion have been examined. Current health care reform efforts pose significant opportunities and challenges for nurse clinicians, educators, and researchers. with an enduring emphasis on health promotion and disease prevention, nurses are critical links for promoting the nation's health. As the 21st century approaches, nurses have the vision, expertise, and experience to truly make a difference in the health of American women, men, and children. This chapter has demonstrated that nursing is committed to realizing an equal opportunity for improved health through preventive health care. Through a combination of leadership, creativity and determination, nurses can and will establish a healthier future for all Americans.

References

1. Agency for Health Care Policy and Research: *National medical expenditure survey: health insurance, use of health services and health care expenditures,* Rockville, Md, 1991, US Public Health Service.
2. American Nurses' Association: *Nursing's agenda for health care reform,* Kansas City, Mo, 1991, The Association.
3. Anda RF, et al: Screening mammography for women 50 years of age and older: practices and trends, *Am J Prev Med* 6(3)123-129.
4. Barge FC, Norr KF: Homeless shelter policies for women in an urban environment, *Image: J Nurs Scholarship* 23(3):145-149, 1991.
5. Eisenberg JM: *Discussion of economic barriers to preventive services: clinical obstacle or fiscal defense?* In Battista RN, Lawrence RS, editors: *Implementing preventive services,* New York, 1988, Oxford.
6. Friedman E: the uninsured: from dilemma to crisis, *JAMA* 265:2491-2495, 1991.
7. Hawkins DR, Rosenbaum S: *Lives in the balance: a national, state and county profile of America's medically underserved,* Washington, DC, 1992, National Association of Community Health Centers.
8. Horton JA, editor: *The women's health data book: a profile of women's health in the United States,* Washington, DC, 1992, Jacobs Institute of Women's Health.
9. Institute of Medicine: *Homelessness, health and human needs,* Washington, DC, 1988, National Academy Press.
10. Institute of Medicine: *Preventing low birth weight,* Washington, DC, 1985, National Academy Press.
11. Jenkins RR: Social dynamics and health care in adolescence, *J Health Care Poor Underserved* 2(1):106-112, 1992.
12. Klerman LV: *Children with special problems that affect their health. In Alive and well? A research and policy review of health programs for poor young children,* New York, 1991, National Center for Children in Poverty, Columbia University School of Public Health.
13. Klerman LV: *The health problems of chidlren in poverty. In Alive and well? A research and policy review of health programs for poor young children,* New York, 1991, National Center for Children in Poverty, Columbia University School of Public Health.
14. Klerman LV: *The impact of poverty on health. In Alive and well? A research and policy review of health programs for poor young children,* New York, 1991, National Center for Children in Poverty, Columbia University School of Public Health.
15. Malloy C, Christ MA, Hohlock FJ: The homeless: social isolates, *J Comm Health Nurs* 7(1):25-36, 1992.
16. Milio N: Developing nursing leadership in health policy, *J Prof Nurs* 5(6):315-321, 1989.
17. National Center for Health Statistics, Centers for Disease Control and Prevention: *Health United States 1991,* Hyattsville, Md, 1992, US Public Health Service.
18. Newacheck PW, Halfon N: Preventive care use by school-aged children: differences by socioeconomic status, *Pediatrics* 82(3):462-468, 1988.
19. Pane GA: Health care access problems of medically indigent emergency walk-in patients, *Ann Emer Med* 20(7):730-733, 1991.
20. Pepper Commission, Bipartisan Commission on Comprehensive Health Care: *A call for action,* Washington, DC, 1990, US Government Printing Office.
21. Robert Wood Johnson Foundation: *Access to health care in the United States: results of a 1986 survey, special report,* Princeton, NJ, 1987, The Foundation.
22. Robert Wood Johnson Foundation: *A new survey on access to medical care, special report,* Princeton, NJ, 1978, The Foundation.
23. Robert Wood Johnson Foundation: *Updated report on access to health care for the American people, special report,* Princeton, NJ, 1983, The Foundation.
24. Russell L: *Is prevention better than cure?,* Washington, DC, 1986, Brookings Institution.
25. US Preventive Services Task Force: *Guide to clinical preventive services: an assessment of the effectiveness of 169 interventions,* Baltimore, 1989, Williams & Wilkins.
26. US Public Health Service: *Healthy people 2000: consortium action,* Washington, DC, 1993, US Public Health Service.
27. US Public Health Service: *Healthy people 2000: national health promotion and disease prevention objectives,* Washington, DC, 1990, US Public Health Service.
28. US Public Health Service: *Healthy people 2000: public health service action,* Washington, DC, 1993, US Public Health Service.
29. US Public Health Service: *Healthy people 2000: state action,* Washington, DC, 1993, US Public Health Service.
30. US Public Health Service: Preventive services in the clinical setting: what works and what it costs, Washington, DC, 1993, US Public Health Service (unpublished).
31. Woodwell DA: *Office visits to internists,* Advance Data, Vital and Health Statistics 209, National Center for Health Statistics Pub No 216, Washington, DC, 1989.
32. Woolhandler S, Himmelstein DU: Reverse targeting of preventive care due to lack of health insurance, *JAMA* 259(19):2872-2874, 1988.
33. Zapka JG, Stoddard AM, Costanza ME, Greene HL: Breast cancer screening by mammography: utilization and associated factors, *Am J Public Health* 79(11):1499-1502.

Index

Page numbers in *italics* indicate illustrations. Page numbers followed by a *t* indicate tables.

D